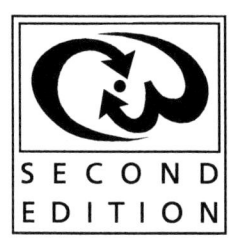

The CenterWatch Directory of
Drugs in Clinical Trials

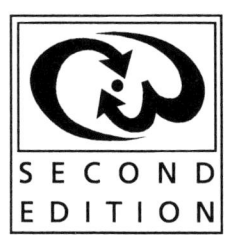

The CenterWatch Directory of
Drugs in Clinical Trials

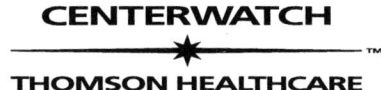

Project Manager
Kristen Eschmann

Medical Advisor
Alan Sugar, M.D.

Research
Sarah Dineen
Nicole Pettit
Jamien Richardson

Publisher
Ken Getz

Design and Production
Paul Gualdoni

Contact Information
For further information about *The CenterWatch Directory of Drugs in Clinical Trials* or any other CenterWatch publication or service, call (617) 856-5900.

© Copyright 2001 CenterWatch, Boston, MA.

All rights reserved. Printed in the United States of America. No part of this work may be reproduced, stored in a retrieval system or transmitted in any form or by any means—electronic, mechanical, photocopying, recording or otherwise—without prior written permission from CenterWatch.

ISBN: 1-930624-18-2

Preface to the Second Edition

The drug development pipeline continues to produce a great variety of new drugs for the treatment of existing and new indications. These represent only a fraction of those compounds that have been studied in the laboratory. The success of CenterWatch's first edition of *The Directory of Drugs in Clinical Trials* supported the belief that a compendium of drugs in clinical development would be a useful reference source. As the number of agents being actively studied continues to increase, it is important that this reference source be updated and we have done just that. The first edition contained references to approximately 1,100 drugs. This edition presents information on approximately 1,900 drugs and more than 400 indications.

This second edition is written for the health care professional and the sophisticated lay person. Scientific language is used throughout and as much information as could be accumulated from press releases, presentations at meetings, company contacts and medical literature has been included. We have aspired to provide information on as many new therapies as possible—still, this is not an exhaustive resource as information on some drugs has not been made available.

We have expanded the second edition of *The Directory of Drugs in Clinical Trials* to cover all active clinical trials. This edition focuses on drugs in development from phase I, II and III and includes information on some NDAs that have been submitted or withdrawn. Additionally, we have expanded our coverage of active clinical trails to include trials conducted worldwide. It is important to note that this directory does not include the relatively small number of drugs being developed independently by the NIH.

We have also added another index to make the directory an easier searchable resource. Now, there are three indexes: The first is an alphabetical listing of the drugs described in the text. It should be noted that trade names for the same drug compound may vary in different countries. Registration, trademark symbols and designations are not shown to make the presentation of the drug descriptions consistent. The second lists the indications for treatment. Thus, the reader will be able to find new drugs by name or a series of drugs used for treatment of a particular disease. The third lists the company and their drugs alphabetically. It is important to remember, however, that since these compounds are still experimental and in development, there is no guarantee of benefit and these agents can only be obtained through participation in a clinical research study.

A profiled drug may be listed more than once if it has more than one formulation, such as oral pill versus intravenous solution. Multiple indications, if available, are listed in the same record for the same formulation of the clinical test medication. Also, some drug delivery devices have been included since they may represent a significant clinical improvement. In some instances, the descriptions are presented separately for those clinical trials using combination therapies.

Although most of the drugs listed in this edition are still experimental, the FDA may have approved some for use in the United States by the time this book is published. Other drugs have been approved for use in countries outside of the United States and may or may not ever be approved by the FDA. Some of the drugs mentioned in the first edition, and even in this second edition, may no longer be available because of unfavorable results in clinical studies. Also, companies developing these drugs often merge or move and change their phone numbers and addresses. Thus, all information concerning phase of development, continued availability of the drug, trade and generic name, and contact information needs to be continuously verified.

To keep you abreast of the latest developments in the clinical pipeline, we have incorporated the content of *The Directory of Drugs in Clinical Trials* into an online database located at the company web site www.centerwatch.com. By providing your email address when you purchase the second edition of this book, you will be emailed a protected username and password to freely search the database and view weekly updates on the drugs in the clinical pipeline.

This book can, and should be used in conjunction with the Clinical Trials Listing service provided by CenterWatch. At this web site, the most up-to-date information on clinical studies can be obtained. Many, if not most, of the drugs listed on that web site will be described in this book. Furthermore, both the Trial Result database and FDA Approval database located on the CenterWatch web site will inform you of the latest advances in drug development.

This book contains information on the next wave of medical advances. However, no one knows which of these drugs will be approved, which will make a critical difference in the treatment of specific diseases, and which will fall by the wayside. For patients reading this book and in search of new possible therapies for their condition, we recommend taking this information to their health care providers so that the information can be incorporated into a suitable treatment plan. Participation in clinical studies is often best accomplished when the patient's primary physician helps with explanations and support of the study subject.

We encourage reader feedback on this new second edition and hope that the book meets your needs with respect to providing useful information on new drugs in the developmental pipeline.

Kristen Eschman, Managing Editor
Alan Sugar, M.D., Medical Advisor

Contents

Foreword 9

1. **Cardiovascular Disease** 11
2. **Hematology** 47
3. **Neurology** 71
4. **Psychology** 121
5. **Oncology** 149
6. **Infectious Disease and Immunology** 285
7. **Pulmonary and Respiratory** 353
8. **Endocrine and Metabolism** 379
9. **Gastroenterology** 401
10. **Urology** 445
11. **Musculoskeletal** 485
12. **Dermatology** 513
13. **Ophthalmology** 537
14. **Otolaryngology** 547
15. **Women's Disorders** 557
16. **Men's Disorders** 573
17. **Pediatric Illnesses** 595

Indexes 635

  Manufacturers Index 637

  Therapeutic Indications Index 673

  Scientific and Trade Name Index 697

  Pediatric Manufacturers Index 710

  Pediatric Therapeutic Indications Index 718

  Pediatric Scientific and Trade Name Index 723

Appendixes 727

  Useful Websites 729

  About CenterWatch 733

Foreword

Today every clinician, health professional, and patient is extremely interested to know about "coming attractions" with regard to medical therapies in their area(s) of interest. Until now it has only been possible to do this for new drugs through a great deal of research in hard-to-find sources, often very expensive ones that are beyond the budget of someone who wants to consult the resource only occasionally.

CenterWatch, a highly respected publisher in the clinical trials industry, has provided just this type of resource. The current book is both inexpensive and easy to use. The most frequently sought information on drugs under development includes:

- Indication(s) for use
- Study phase status
- Clinical trial results
- Mechanism of action
- Formulation
- Manufacturer and contact information

The data for these entries have been verified or have come directly from many research scientists, physicians, and other healthcare professionals in academia, private practice, and industry. The data is then organized by indication, drug name ,and phase, which is very useful and facilitates the book's use as a reference tool.

The number of physicians involved in clinical trials has never been larger. A great deal of this growth has occurred among independent physicians in private practice clinics as well as in various types of managed care clinics outside the traditional academic environment. This rapid growth, in part at the expense of academic medical centers, has led to a reassessment—and confirmation—of interest within the academic centers in sponsored clinical trials being conducted in their setting. Some forward-looking academic centers now have a more "customer-oriented" attitude toward the pharmaceutical industry. Specifically, the process of research contract approvals, protocol, and informed consent reviewed by institutional IRBs (Institutional Review Boards), and the internal administrative procedures of the institution have now been more efficiently organized and operated.

These activities already have helped increase the number of clinical trials conducted by those academic institutions and have helped to re-adjust the balance between trials conducted by academicians and by independent physicians. It is hoped that the remaining academic centers will address this issue for the advantage of faculty and patients—both beneficiaries when new drugs are introduced more rapidly.

Clinical trials have reached a golden age where contemporary views of good science and good medicine are widely understood in regulatory agencies, academic centers, and the pharmaceutical industry.

This coming of age, from the start of modern clinical trials in the late 1940s until the present, is a remarkable achievement for an entire field to reach a mature stage in such a short time. There is still a great deal of research to do in testing new clinical designs, exploring how clinical data can best be analyzed with statistics, and studying many other issues and questions. Nonetheless, the questions of determining how much data to collect on a new drug, and what type of clinical data to collect prior to marketing is generally understood by regulatory agencies, pharmaceutical companies, and practicing physicians.

This book also serves to educate those less familiar with the process of drug development and clinical trials. At the same time, it is a valuable reference for those more skilled, or at least knowledgeable, in this art and science.

Readers will find periodic updates of this material useful, not only for providing current data, but for telling the story of the many turns and unexpected twists that drugs often take during their development and product lifetime. This varies from those that are never marketed and are "stillborn," to those such as morphine and opium whose lifetime is measured in tens, if not hundreds of generations.

Bert Spilker, PhD, MD
Senior Vice President
Scientific & Regulatory Affairs
PhRMA

1 | Cardiovascular Disease

Population with illnesses in this category	158 million[1]
Drugs in the development pipeline	630[2]
Number of drugs in preclinical testing	254
Number of drugs in clinical testing	188

Source: 1. World Health Organization, worldwide figures 2. Parexel

The Pharmaceutical Research Manufacturers of America (PhRMA) has estimated the annual cost of cardiovascular disease in the United States as $298.2 billion. This amount includes all health expenditures and estimates of loss of productivity resulting from morbidity and mortality. According to the American Heart Association, almost 61 million Americans suffer from one or more forms of cardiovascular disease, including hypertension, coronary heart disease, myocardial infarction, chest pain, stroke, and rheumatic fever/rheumatic heart disease. These diseases cause close to one million deaths each year.

CenterWatch has identified approximately 150 drugs in clinical development for cardiovascular treatment. Indications with the largest number of drugs being tested include congestive heart failure, myocardial infarction, and hypertension. According to PhRMA, these new medicines represent a 20% increase in drug development efforts for cardiovascular disease since 1999. Many of these new therapies in the pipeline use cutting-edge technologies and new scientific approaches to these diseases. These include a vaccine that may be able to increase levels of "good" cholesterol, or HDL, by blocking its transition into "bad" cholesterol, or LDL; a medicine now used to treat rheumatoid arthritis that may be able to block a substance that damages the heart and causes congestive heart failure; and a gene therapy that prompts the growth of new blood vessels to bypass clogged arteries.

Coronary heart disease is the most common cause of death in both men and women in the United States. Of the one million cardiac fatalities seen each year, about half are caused by coronary heart disease. Coronary heart disease occurs when the coronary arteries become thickened or clogged by deposits of cholesterol, and cannot supply enough blood to the heart. A heart attack results when a blood clot obstructs a coronary artery supplying blood to the heart. This causes an inadequate flow of oxygenated and nutrient-enriched blood and results in the death of a portion of the heart muscle.

As many as 1.1 million Americans suffer heart attacks each year. Every 29 seconds, someone in the U.S. will suffer a heart attack, and every minute, someone will die from one. It is estimated that 7.3 million Americans over the age of 20 have a history of myocardial infarction. There are currently an estimated 15 drugs in the clinical pipeline for the prevention and/or treatment of myocardial infarction. Annual costs for such development are estimated by CenterWatch to be between $70 million and $90 million.

The FDA has approved five new drugs indicated for the treatment of cardiovascular disease. One of these products, TNKase, may help to reduce the growing number of heart attack victims. TNKase (tenecteplase), a thrombolytic, has been FDA approved for the reduction of mortality associated with acute myocardial infarction. It is the first thrombolytic to date that can be administered over five seconds and in one dose, which is selected based on the weight of the patient. TNKase works by stimulating the innate clot-dissolving mechanism by activating plasminogen, a naturally occurring substance secreted by endothelial cells in response to injury to the artery walls that contributes to clot formation. When TNKase activates plasminogen, it converts into plasmin, which breaks down the fibrin mesh that binds the clot together. The clot is then dissolved, restoring blood flow to the heart.

Despite the advances put forth from such efforts, cardiovascular illness and death can be prevented most effectively by controlling the risk factors associated with heart disease. The list of controllable factors is led by high blood pressure, also known as hypertension. Over 50 million Americans ages six years and older, and one in four adults, suffer from high blood pressure. Along with high blood cholesterol and smoking, hypertension doubles a patient's chance of developing heart disease. Hypertension seldom causes symptoms but it can cause severe damage to major organs over time—leading to heart attack, stroke, or kidney failure. Exercising regularly, maintaining a healthy weight, and not smoking can help control one's blood pressure. Others need assistance from blood pressure medications.

In September 2000, the FDA approved Atacand HCT for the treatment of hypertension. Atacand HCT consists of an angiotensin II receptor antagonist and the diuretic, hydrochlorothiazide. This combination medication has a dual mechanism of action: inhibition of the effects of angiotenisin II, an agent that causes vasoconstriction and hypertension, and increased sodium and water elimination through the effects of the diuretic.

CenterWatch has identified an estimated 20 drugs currently involved in clinical trials for the treatment of hypertension. Expenditure for this indication will range from $80 million to $100 million this year. These drugs are categorized as diuretics, beta blockers, calcium channel blockers, angiotensin-converting enzyme (ACE) inhibitors, alpha blockers, and centrally acting drugs that act on the brain to reduce neural impulses that may cause blood vessels to constrict. Many of these products treat other types of heart conditions in addition to lowering blood pressure.

Angina

abciximab, c7E3
ReoPro

MANUFACTURER
Centocor

DESCRIPTION
ReoPro is an antiplatelet drug being tested for acute ischemic stroke, acute myocardial infarction, and angina. This biological drug is a fragment (Fab) of a monoclonal antibody that binds to the glycoprotein (IIb/IIIa) receptor of human platelets and inhibits their clumping together.

ReoPro has recently completed a phase II trial for acute ischemic stroke and the overall results have shown that it improves the subject's clinical condition. ReoPro is unique because it can work when given up to 24 hours after a stroke, unlike other drugs that must be given within the first three hours. Also, none of the subjects suffered from symptomatic intracranial bleeding (ICH), a potential fatal side effect of current therapy.

A preliminary analysis showed that after three months of treatment, 35 percent of the subjects treated with any dose of abciximab had minimal or no remaining disability, compared with the 20 percent of subjects who received the placebo. In addition, half of the subjects treated with abciximab showed improved function in carrying out daily activities compared with 40 percent that were given the placebo. There was also a trend toward improved neurological functioning.

ReoPro is also being tested in a phase III trial for acute myocardial infarction and for angina. It is approved by the FDA as an add-on therapy to heart procedures (percutaneous coronary interventions, such as balloon angioplasty and stent placement) for the prevention of heart blood flow problems.

INDICATION(S) AND RESEARCH PHASE
Angina – Phase III
Heart Disease – Phase III
Strokes – Phase II completed
Myocardial Infarction – Phase III
Cardiac Surgery – FDA approved

amlodipine besylate
Norvasc

MANUFACTURER
Pfizer

DESCRIPTION
Norvasc is the besylate salt of amlodipine, a long acting calcium channel blocker. The drug blocks the flow of calcium ions across the cell membrane into vascular smooth muscle and cardiac muscle. Additionally, Norvasc is a peripheral arterial vasodilator that acts directly on vascular smooth muscle to reduce peripheral vascular resistance and blood pressure.

Norvasc has been approved by the FDA for the treatment of hypertension, chronic stable angina, and vasospastic angina in adults.

It is currently in phase III trials for hypertension in children between the ages of six and 17 years.

INDICATION(S) AND RESEARCH PHASE
Pediatric, hypertension – Phase III
Hypertension – FDA approved
Angina – FDA approved

AR69931
unknown

MANUFACTURER
AstraZeneca

DESCRIPTION
AR69931 is an enzyme inhibitor of thrombin that may help block this protein's ability to form blood clots. This drug is currently in a phase II study to prevent angina and thrombosis.

INDICATION(S) AND RESEARCH PHASE
Angina – Phase II
Thrombosis – Phase II

bivalirudin
Angiomax

MANUFACTURER
The Medicines Company

DESCRIPTION
Angiomax, formerly called Hirulog, is a synthetic derivate of hirudin, an anticoagulant from the leech medicinals that inhibits the formulation of blood clots. Angiomax is in a phase II trial at the Duke University Medical Center testing 50–100 subjects with heparin-induced thrombocytopenia (HIT) or heparin-induced thrombocytopenia and thrombosis syndrome (HITTS).

The FDA approved Angiomax on May 17, 2000 for use as an anticoagulant in subjects with unstable angina undergoing percutaneous transluminal coronary angioplasty (PTCA). Angiomax is intended for use with aspirin and has been studied only in subjects receiving concomitant aspirin. The FDA approval was based on data from double-blinded clinical trials of 4,312 subjects.

INDICATION(S) AND RESEARCH PHASE
Thrombosis – Phase II
Angina – FDA approved

diltiazem HCl/hydrochlorothiazide
Cardizide SR

MANUFACTURER
Elan Pharmaceutical Research

DESCRIPTION
Cardizide SR is a sustained release (SR) oral drug made to slowly deliver the combination therapy of a calcium blocker (diltiazem hydrochloride) and a diuretic (hydrochlorothiazide) to treat angina. The diltiazem is thought to work by inhibiting the movement (influx) of calcium ions during membrane depolarization of heart muscle and vascular smooth muscle in blood vessels. In effect, this calcium antagonism decreases cardiac muscle contraction and lowers vascular resistance. In turn, oxygen demand decreases on the heart giving relief from angina. Cardizide SR also combines the water reducing effect of a traditional diuretic, which may help relieve heart pain. Clinical trials testing for relief from angina are in phase III.

INDICATION(S) AND RESEARCH PHASE
Angina – Phase III

esprolol
unknown

MANUFACTURER
Selectus Pharmaceuticals

DESCRIPTION
Esprolol is a potent, rapidly acting drug to be taken sublingually. It is classified as a β-adrenergic blocker that may lessen heart rate and increase blood pressure during physical exertion.

This compound completed a phase IIb clinical trial to evaluate the effects of esprolol on exercise tolerance in angina pectoris subjects. During the trial all exercise parameters and negative exercise induced angina symptoms were significantly improved.

Esprolol is currently in a phase II trial for panic disorders and cardiovascular effects of acute anxiety and migraine. A phase I trial of esprolol was conducted in healthy subjects, showing the drug to be well tolerated with only mildly adverse effects.

In addition, a follow-up phase II trial was conducted to evaluate esprolol's ability to lessen the effects of β-receptor stimulation in healthy subjects better than standard challenge doses of isoproterenol, and to assess the drug's rate of onset of action and duration of effect. Esprolol's therapeutic effect was seen within ten minutes and lasted for two to four hours.

INDICATION(S) AND RESEARCH PHASE
Angina – Phase IIb completed
Migraine and Cluster Headaches – Phase II
Panic Disorders – Phase II
Anxiety – Phase II

fibrinogen-receptor antagonist
unknown

MANUFACTURER
Aventis

DESCRIPTION
This drug is in a phase II trial for both prevention and treatment of unstable angina and myocardial infarction. It works by blocking a receptor for the protein precursor, fibrinogen, that is involved in blood clot structure formation.

INDICATION(S) AND RESEARCH PHASE
Angina – Phase II
Myocardial Infarction – Phase II

GP II b/II a
Cromafiban

MANUFACTURER
COR Therapeutics

DESCRIPTION
Cromafiban is a small molecule that blocks platelets from clumping (an aggregation inhibitor) together. This drug is being tested in phase II trials for treatment of acute coronary disease, unstable angina, and stroke.

INDICATION(S) AND RESEARCH PHASE
Angina – Phase II
Coronary Artery Disease – Phase II
Strokes – Phase II

human albumin microspheres
Optison

MANUFACTURER
Molecular Biosystems

DESCRIPTION
Optison is an ultrasound contrast agent. It is made up of human albumin microspheres in an injectable suspension octafluoropropane formulation. Indicated for use in subjects with myocardial perfusion problems, Optison aids doctors in heart imaging.

The completed phase II clinical trials consisted of six studies in 376 subjects with a wide range of known or suspected coronary artery diseases. In all studies, Optison Myocardial Contrast Echocardiography (MCE) was found to compare favorably with standard clinical tests, whether Single Photon Emission Computed Tomography (SPECT) or coronary angiography. Of the six, three studies have been performed in subjects with known or suspected coronary artery disease including those with recent heart attacks undergoing pharmacologic stress echo test, two evaluated Optison with exercise stress echo, and another involved subjects presenting to the Emergency Room with unexplained chest pain.

INDICATION(S) AND RESEARCH PHASE
Angina – Phase II completed
Coronary Artery Disease – Phase II completed
Heart Disease – Phase II completed

PEG-hirudin
unknown

MANUFACTURER
Knoll Pharmaceutical

DESCRIPTION
PEG-hirudin is a modified drug that originally was discovered and derived from the active secretion product of leeches. It has the ability to stop coagulation of blood and acts as an antithrombin agent to dissolve blood clots. Trials are currently in phase II for use in unstable angina and peripheral bypass surgery.

INDICATION(S) AND RESEARCH PHASE
Angina – Phase II
Cardiac Surgery – Phase II

ranolazine, CVT-303
unknown

MANUFACTURER
CV Therapeutics

DESCRIPTION
Ranolazine belongs to a class of therapies called pFOX (partial fatty acid oxidation) inhibitors, and is administered in an oral sustained release formulation. It is currently in development for the treatment of chronic stable angina, the chest pain associated with coronary artery disease. Ranolazine may work by causing a partial shift in the heart's energy source from fatty acids to glucose, a more oxygen efficient source of energy.

CV Therapeutics has started a second pivotal phase III for ranolazine. This study is known as the CARISA (Combination Assessment of Ranolazine in Stable Angina) trial and will enroll about 450 subjects. It is a double-blind, placebo-controlled trial of ranolazine used in combination with other anti-anginal drugs. The primary endpoint for evaluation is the duration of time a subject spends exercising on a treadmill before experiencing chest pain.

In addition, a phase II trial for congestive heart failure was initiated in December 2000, testing ranolazine in an oral formulation.

INDICATION(S) AND RESEARCH PHASE
Angina – Phase III
Congestive Heart Failure – Phase II

RSR13
unknown

MANUFACTURER
Allos Therapeutics

DESCRIPTION
RSR13 is a synthetic small molecule that increases the release of oxygen from hemoglobin, the oxygen carrying protein contained within red blood cells. The presence of oxygen in tumors is an essential part of the effectiveness of radiation therapy in cancer treatment. By increasing tumor oxygenation, RSR13 has the potential to enhance the effectiveness of standard radiation therapy.

In November 2000, positive preliminary phase II results of induction chemotherapy, followed by radiation therapy plus RSR13, for Stage IIIA and IIIB non-small cell lung cancer were announced. Data from the first 30 of 47 subjects demonstrated that 87% had a complete or partial response of their tumors within the radiation therapy portal in the chest.

Additionally, Allos Therapeutics is conducting a 408 subject, randomized, multi-center, international phase III trial to confirm that RSR13, when used in combination with radiation therapy, significantly improves the survival of subjects with brain metastases.

INDICATION(S) AND RESEARCH PHASE
Angina – Phase I completed
Myocardial Infarction – Phase II
Brain Cancer – Phase III
Lung Cancer – Phase II
Glomerulonephritis (GBM) – Phase II completed

tedisamil
Tedangin

MANUFACTURER
Solvay Pharmaceuticals

DESCRIPTION
Tedangin (tedisamil) is a drug that exerts anti-ischemic and anti-arrhythmic effects by blocking the flux of potassium to and from cells. It is being evaluated in a phase II trial for atrial fibrillation and a phase III trial for angina pectoris (chronic stable type).

INDICATION(S) AND RESEARCH PHASE
Angina – Phase III
Arrhythmia – Phase II

TP-9201
unknown

MANUFACTURER
Integra LifeSciences

DESCRIPTION
TP-9201 inhibits a platelet membrane receptor (glycoprotein IIb/IIIa) and a cyclic peptide (RGD) for treatment of several cardiovascular diseases. Blood clots can be prevented from growing and propagating by stopping platelets from aggregating together. Potential treatments being tested for this therapy include myocardial infarction, angioplasty, unstable angina, and stroke.

Integra Life Sciences has acquired Telios Pharmaceuticals and they have suspended clinical research between phases I and II until a development partner is found.

INDICATION(S) AND RESEARCH PHASE
Angina – Phase I/II
Heart Disease – Phase I/II
Strokes – Phase I/II
Myocardial Infarction – Phase I/II

Arrhythmia

amindarone-best, SR-33589
unknown

MANUFACTURER
Sanofi-Synthelabo Pharmaceuticals

DESCRIPTION
SR-33589 is a new medication similar in action to amiodarone, a drug currently usd to treat cardiac arrythmias. SR-33589, however, may have a better side effect profile than the older drug. Currently, it is being studied in Phase II clinical trials and will be administered as an oral medication.

Amiodarone is an antiarrythmic drug currently used primarily to treat abnormal heartbeats in the upper (atrial) and lower (ventricular) chambers of the heart. It can be used for potentially deadly ventricular arrythmias called ventricular tachyarrythmias. When it is used to treat atrial fibrillation, a less serious form of arrythmia, it can help reduce the subject's risk of stroke. Amiodarone works by selectively blocking certain electrolyte channels in cardiac tissue, thus reducing the contractility of the heart muscle. The main problem with amiodarone is that over 75% of subjects experience serious side effects and toxicities from its use.

SR-33589 is from the same class of compounds as amiodarone, but has slightly different action within the body, and thus may possibly result in fewer side effects. In preliminary studies, it showed a similar efficacy in the treatment of arrythmias as amiodarone. Further study is necessary to confirm these early results.

INDICATION(S) AND RESEARCH PHASE
Arrhythmia – Phase II

amiodarone HCl
Amio-Aqueous IV

MANUFACTURER
Academic Pharmaceuticals

DESCRIPTION

Amio-Aqueous IV is an intravenously formulated drug being evaluated for different types of heart arrhythmias, such as treatment of incessant ventricular tachycardia and supraventricular arrhythmia. Amiodarone is considered a class III antiarrhythmic because it lengthens the electrical activity of the heart. The clinical trials are in phase III.

INDICATION(S) AND RESEARCH PHASE
Arrhythmia – Phase III

azimilide
Stedicor

MANUFACTURER
Procter & Gamble Pharmaceuticals

DESCRIPTION
Stedicor is an anti-arrhythmic oral drug initially indicated for atrial fibrillation, a common upper chamber heart arrhythmia. It's an active, chemically unique, class III antiarrhythmic agent that prolongs the heart's electrical recovery time (cardiac refractoriness) long enough to interrupt the abnormal cycle. Stedicor works by blocking potassium movement through both fast and slow channels in the heart's pacemaker-like cells.

Stedicor also significantly reduces the risk of recurrence in subjects with symptomatic paroxysmal supraventricular tachycardia (PSVT). Stedicor is currently in phase III trials for treatment of arrhythmia.

INDICATION(S) AND RESEARCH PHASE
Arrhythmia – Phase III

CVT-510
unknown

MANUFACTURER
CV Therapeutics

DESCRIPTION
CVT-510 is a selective adenosine A1 receptor stimulator for the treatment of atrial arrhythmias. Atrial arrhythmias are abnormal electrical impulses that are created within the atria at a high rate. These impulses travel through the atrioventricular (AV) node and cause the ventricles to beat too quickly to allow efficient pumping of blood. CVT-510 works by slowing electrical impulses through the AV node, an important regulator of heart rate.

By selectively stimulating the adenosine A1 receptor, which slows rapid heart rate, and without stimulating the adenosine A2 receptor, which lowers blood pressure, CVT-510 may be able to intervene immediately in the arrhythmia process, without the undesirable effects of lowering blood pressure. If phase II testing goes well, the types of atrial arrhythmias that may be treated are atrial flutter, atrial fibrillation, and paroxysmal atrial tachycardia.

INDICATION(S) AND RESEARCH PHASE
Arrhythmia – Phase II

DTI-0009
unknown

MANUFACTURER
Fujisawa Healthcare

DESCRIPTION
DTI-0009 is a novel A-1 adenosine facilitator for treatment of fast heart rate arrhythmia called tachyarrythmia. In such cases the heart beats faster than one hundred times per minute. DTI-0009 is being tested for braking this abnormal cardiac cycle. DTI-0009 is in partnership with Discovery Therapeutics.

DTI-0009, in an intravenous formulation, is being tested in a phase II multicenter trial to determine the dosage necessary to normalize the heart rate and to convert the atrial fibrilliation to normal cardiac rhythm.

Results from Phase I trials demonstrated DTI-0009 to be safe, well tolerated, and to be highly bioavailable after oral administration, as well as lasting long enough in the blood stream enabling it for chronic use.

Fujisawa Healthcare has acquired U.S. rights to DTI-0009 in an intravenous formulation. Discovery Therapeutics has retained rights to DTI-0009 as an oral product and an intravenous product in markets outside the United States.

INDICATION(S) AND RESEARCH PHASE
Arrhythmia – Phase II

GW 473178
unknown

MANUFACTURER
GlaxoSmithKline

DESCRIPTION
GW 473178 is a thrombin inhibitor being developed for use in subjects with atrial fibrillation and venous thrombosis. It is currently in phase I trials.

INDICATION(S) AND RESEARCH PHASE
Arrhythmia – Phase I
Thrombosis – Phase I

SB 207266
unknown

MANUFACTURER
GlaxoSmithKline

DESCRIPTION
SB 207266 is a 5HT4 receptor antagonist. It is currently in phase II trials for the treatment of atrial fibrillation.

INDICATION(S) AND RESEARCH PHASE
Arrhythmia – Phase II

SB-237376
unknown

MANUFACTURER
GlaxoSmithKline

DESCRIPTION
SB-237376 is a potassium/calcium channel blocker. It is being tested in phase II trials for the treatment of cardiac arrhythmia.

INDICATION(S) AND RESEARCH PHASE
Arrhythmia – Phase II

SB 424323
unknown

MANUFACTURER

GlaxoSmithKline

DESCRIPTION
SB 424323 is an indirect thrombin inhibitor currently in phase I trials for prevention of embolization in atrial fibrillation and stroke prevention.

INDICATION(S) AND RESEARCH PHASE
Arrhythmia – Phase I
Strokes – Phase I

tedisamil
Tedangin

MANUFACTURER
Solvay Pharmaceuticals

DESCRIPTION
Tedangin (tedisamil) is a drug that exerts anti-ischemic and anti-arrhythmic effects by blocking the flux of potassium to and from cells. It is being evaluated in a phase II trial for atrial fibrillation and a phase III trial for angina pectoris (chronic stable type).

INDICATION(S) AND RESEARCH PHASE
Angina – Phase III
Arrhythmia – Phase II

Blood Cancer

LGD-1550
unknown

MANUFACTURER
Ligand Pharmaceuticals

DESCRIPTION
LGD-1550 is being formulated to limit the proliferation and spread of head, neck, and cervical cancers; it is to be given orally and is currently in phase II trials. Retinoids are a group of substances, one being vitamin A, thought to be responsible for growth, bone development, vision, and skin integrity. It is thought that retinoids act against cancer by regulating the process by which cells reproduce themselves (gene transcription regulation). Studies have shown that subjects with metastatic cancer have lower levels of retinoid activity in their bodies. LGD-1550 works by binding to retinoid receptors in cells, thereby stimulating retinoid activity.

Preliminary studies have shown that retinoids may inhibit cell proliferation and promote cell differentiation. Cancer arises when there is uncontrolled growth of immature cells. Retinoids act to slow cell division and stimulates cell maturation, making it less likely that these mature cells will be transformed into cancerous cells. Retinoids have also been shown in early studies to boost the effects of other anticancer medications.

Trials of LGD-1550 for head and neck cancer, cervical cancer, and solid and hematological tumors are in phase II testing.

INDICATION(S) AND RESEARCH PHASE
Blood Cancer – Phase II
Cancer/Tumors (Unspecified) – Phase II
Cervical Dysplasia/Cancer – Phase II
Head and Neck Cancer – Phase II

Cardiac Ischemia

enoxaparin sodium
Lovenox/Clexane

MANUFACTURER
Aventis

DESCRIPTION
Lovenox/Clexane is in phase III trials for the prevention of deep-vein thrombosis (DVT) in trauma adult subjects and pediatric subjects.

Lovenox/Clexane is also being tested in a phase III trial for the prevention of acute cardiac ischemia following stent placement. A stent is placed inside the coronary artery to keep it open to help the blood flow. Lovenox/Clexane may prevent blood clots from forming around the stent area.

INDICATION(S) AND RESEARCH PHASE
Thrombosis – Phase III
Pediatric, Thrombosis – Phase III
Cardiac Ischemia – Phase III

RSR13
unknown

MANUFACTURER
Allos Therapeutics

DESCRIPTION
RSR13 is a synthetic small molecule that increases the release of oxygen from hemoglobin, the oxygen carrying protein contained within red blood cells. The presence of oxygen in tumors is an essential part of the effectiveness of radiation therapy in cancer treatment. By increasing tumor oxygenation, RSR13 has the potential to enhance the effectiveness of standard radiation therapy.

In November 2000, positive preliminary phase II results of induction chemotherapy, followed by radiation therapy plus RSR13, for Stage IIIA and IIIB non-small cell lung cancer were announced. Data from the first 30 of 47 subjects demonstrated that 87% had a complete or partial response of their tumors within the radiation therapy portal in the chest.

Additionally, Allos Therapeutics is conducting a 408 subject, randomized, multi-center, international phase III trial to confirm that RSR13, when used in combination with radiation therapy, significantly improves the survival of subjects with brain metastases.

INDICATION(S) AND RESEARCH PHASE
Angina – Phase I completed
Myocardial Infarction – Phase II
Brain Cancer – Phase III
Lung Cancer – Phase II
Glomerulonephritis (GBM) – Phase II completed

TP10
unknown

MANUFACTURER
AVANT Immunotherapeutics

DESCRIPTION
TP10 is a genetically engineered (recombinant) soluble complement receptor-1 (sCR1). Complement-1 is a naturally occurring substance that binds to antibodies as part of the immune response to infection or foreign bodies. Clinical trials are testing

TP10 in an intravenous formulation for a variety of disorders including the treatment of acute respiratory distress syndrome (ARDS), reperfusion injury, heart attack, cardiac surgery, organ reperfusion, xenotransplantation, allotransplantation, and post-surgical complications in infants.

A phase IIb trial was initiated in January 2001 in approximately 30 infants undergoing high risk cardiac surgery utilizing cardiopulmonary bypass. The trial will be conducted at seven sites in the United States.

INDICATION(S) AND RESEARCH PHASE
Acute Respiratory Distress Syndrome (ARDS) – Phase II/III
Cardiac Ischemia – Phase I/II
Cardiac Surgery – Phase IIb
Myocardial Infarction – Phase I/II
Pediatric, Post-surgical Complications – Phase I/II
Pediatric, Cardiac Surgery – Phase IIb

vascular endothelial growth factor-2 gene therapy (gtVEGF-2)
unknown

MANUFACTURER
Human Genome Sciences

DESCRIPTION
Vascular endothelial growth factor-2 gene therapy (gtVEGF-2) is used to treat subjects suffering from coronary artery disease. The active ingredient in this drug product is a novel gene that encodes the protein VEGF-2, which scientists believe is the body's signal to grow new blood and lymph vessels. Laboratory studies show that the gene is active in the formation of new blood vessels, a process known as angiogenesis. The laboratory studies demonstrate that this gene also is active in the regeneration of lymphatic vessels, which resulted in reduced swelling and edema. This swelling is caused by lymph fluid seepage which occurs normally.

Vascular endothelial growth factor-2 gene therapy is currently in two phase I/II trials treating subjects that suffer from refractory myocardial ischemia. One trial is using a catheter inserted through a small incision in the subject's groin and directed to the heart using X-ray imaging. A needle is then advanced out of the catheter and used to inject DNA into the inner wall of the heart. The second trial is using direct injection of DNA into the inner wall of the heart, through an incision in the chest wall.

In the future, Vascular Genetics plans to submit additional INDs for other indications for this gene therapy product, including lymphedema and other coronary artery diseases.

INDICATION(S) AND RESEARCH PHASE
Myocardial Ischemia – Phase I/II
Coronary Artery Disease – Phase I/II

Cardiac Surgery

ancrod
Viprinex

MANUFACTURER
Knoll Pharmaceutical

DESCRIPTION
Viprinex is a venom derived from snakes (viper *Agkistrodon rhodostoma*). It is a defibrinogenator being tested in phase III trials for treatment of ischemic stroke, as well as for establishing and maintaining anticoagulation in heparin-intolerant subjects undergoing cardiopulmonary bypass surgery.

INDICATION(S) AND RESEARCH PHASE
Cardiac Surgery – Phase III
Strokes – Phase III
Thrombosis – Phase III

antithrombin III, rhATIII
unknown

MANUFACTURER
Genzyme Genetics Division

DESCRIPTION
Antithrombin-III (AT-III) is a genetically altered form of a naturally occurring plasma protein that helps control blood clotting. This drug has just finished phase III testing for prevention of thrombosis, specializing in subjects undergoing cardiac surgery requiring cardiopulmonary bypass. This therapy may be helpful in subjects who have either acquired or hereditary AT-III deficiencies, by restoring heparin sensitivity to heparin-resistant subjects experiencing cardiopulmonary bypass.

INDICATION(S) AND RESEARCH PHASE
Thrombosis – Phase III completed
Cardiac Surgery – Phase III completed

BCX-1470
unknown

MANUFACTURER
BioCryst Pharmaceuticals

DESCRIPTION
BCX-1470 inhibits complement activation during cardiopulmonary bypass surgery. The complement cascade is part of the body's normal defense system against invasive bacteria, viruses, and foreign substances. When one of these foreign bodies is detected, the complement cascade activates a series of enzymes that attack these harmful substances.

During cardiopulmonary bypass surgery, a person's blood is pumped through a heart-lung machine, which can accidentally activate the complement cascade, thereby damaging healthy tissue when the blood is returned back into the subject. BCX-1470 may inhibit the complement cascade by blocking the activation of its initial enzymes (factor D and C1s). BCX-1470 may help subjects during bypass surgery. Clinical trials in phase II will evaluate this drug's ability to prevent excessive bleeding, inflammation, and heart muscle damage. This drug is manufactured in an intravenous formulation.

INDICATION(S) AND RESEARCH PHASE
Cardiac Surgery – Phase II

blood substitute
Hemolink

MANUFACTURER
Hemosol

DESCRIPTION

Hemolink is a type of artificial blood or blood substitute. It is a human hemoglobin-based oxygen carrier for use in coronary artery bypass grafting surgery (CABG), commonly known as a bypass.

Hemolink is currently being tested in a phase III trial on some 300 subjects undergoing CABG in Canada and the United Kingdom. According to the company, Hemolink is being evaluated in conjunction with a blood conservation strategy called intraoperative autologous donation (IAD) through a technique known as acute normovolemic hemodilution (ANH). One to four units of a subject's blood are removed just prior to undergoing cardiopulmonary bypass surgery. The subject's blood is then replaced with Hemolink to maintain an adequate amount of circulating hemoglobin throughout surgery. At the end of surgery, the subjects' own blood is returned as required, along with blood recovered by cell salvage techniques.

This study is part of a broader phase III program, which is planned to include two additional clinical trials during 2001. One trial involves 600 subjects in the United States and uses a very similar cardiac protocol. The goal of the clinical trials is to see if there is evidence that Hemolink reduces or avoids subject exposure to human donated (allogeneic) blood. The benefit of avoiding donated blood is to decrease the potential risk of unknown contamination.

In addition, a phase I/II trial was initiated in December 2000 in 18 subjects with non-small cell lung cancer who are experiencing chemotherapy associated anemia. The trial is expected to be complete in the fourth quarter of 2001.

INDICATION(S) AND RESEARCH PHASE
Cardiac Surgery – Phase III
Lung Cancer – Phase I/II

---

heparinase I
Neutralase

MANUFACTURER
IBEX Technologies

DESCRIPTION
Neutralase is being evaluated as a heparin neutralization agent for use after coronary bypass surgery. This enzyme-based drug is a purified natural heparinase that breaks up heparin. IBEX Technologies states that heparin neutralization is required in over 400,000 coronary bypass procedures annually in the United States and a further 250,000 in other countries.

Neutralase is currently in a phase III trial in the United States for use in cardiac surgery. The first objective of this trial is to demonstrate that Neutralase reverses the anticoagulant effects of heparin to prevent blood clots. The second criteria is to compare Neutralase's effect against protamine, the currently used anticoagulant drug. One advantage of Neutralase may be its ability to preserve the antithrombotic properties of heparin. There is also a phase II trial under way for use in angioplasty.

INDICATION(S) AND RESEARCH PHASE
Cardiac Surgery – Phase III
Angioplasty – Phase II

PEG-hirudin
unknown

MANUFACTURER
Knoll Pharmaceutical

DESCRIPTION
PEG-hirudin is a modified drug that originally was discovered and derived from the active secretion product of leeches. It has the ability to stop coagulation of blood and act as an antithrombin agent to dissolve blood clots. Trials are currently in phase II testing for use in unstable angina and peripheral bypass surgery.

INDICATION(S) AND RESEARCH PHASE
Angina – Phase II
Cardiac Surgery – Phase II

---

perfluorohexane emulsion
Imagent

MANUFACTURER
Alliance Pharmaceutical

DESCRIPTION
Imagent is a perfluorochemical-based microbubble intravenous contrast agent. It is used along with an ultrasound for the evaluation of cardiac function and myocardial perfusion, and detection of organ lesions and blood flow abnormalities, for which the drug is currently in phase III trials. Imagent is being tested in phase II trials for the organ perfusion evaluation of tumors in the breast, kidney, liver, and prostate gland.

INDICATION(S) AND RESEARCH PHASE
Cardiac Function – Phase III
Cancer/Tumors (Unspecified) – Phase III

---

pexelizumab
unknown

MANUFACTURER
Alexion

DESCRIPTION
Pexelizumab is an anti-inflammatory C5 Inhibitor monoclonal antibody fragment. In January 2001, preliminary results of a double-blind, placebo-controlled phase IIb trial indicated that pexelizumab significantly reduced a composite endpoint of death or myocardial infarction at 30 days in subjects undergoing coronary artery bypass graft surgery (CABG) with cardiopulmonary bypass (CPB). Subjects were separated into two groups, those undergoing only CABG with CPB (approximately 90%) or subjects undergoing CABG with concomitant valve surgery during CPB. Results showed that pexelizumab suppressed complement in CPB subjects, with bolus (pexelizumab 2.0 mg/kg) and bolus plus infusion (pexelizumab 2.0 mg/kg bolus, pexelizumab infusion at 0.05 mg/kg/hr) regimens showing complete suppression for four and 24 hours, respectively. Alexion is developing pexelizumab in collaboration with Procter & Gamble Pharmaceuticals.

INDICATION(S) AND RESEARCH PHASE
Cardiac Surgery – Phase IIb completed
Myocardial Infarction – Phase IIb completed

rNAPc2
unknown

MANUFACTURER
Corvas International

DESCRIPTION
Recombinant Nematode Anticoagulant Protein c2 (rNAPc2) is a recombinant protein that was originally discovered by Corvas scientists in blood-feeding hookworms. It is a potent inhibitor of the factor VIIa/tissue factor protease complex, which is required for the initiation of blood clot formation.

Results of a phase II trial of rNAPc2 demonstrated that, in the largest subject cohort, rNAPc2 reduced the risk of developing deep vein thrombosis (DVT) by greater than 50% compared to a contemporary historical control of low molecular weight heparin (LMWH). The open-label dose-ranging trial was conducted in 293 subjects undergoing unilateral knee replacement at sites in the United States, Canada, the Netherlands, and Italy. The incidence of total DVT in the largest cohort was 12.2% in 74 evaluated subjects treated with rNAPc2 versus an incidence of 25–27% treated with a historical control for LMWH. The incidence of major bleeding following rNAPc2 prophylaxis was 2.3% versus a historical control value of 3% for LMWH.

rNAPc2 is also being evaluated in a phase IIa trial in subjects undergoing elective percutaneous transluminal coronary angioplasty (PTCA). The purpose of the PTCA trial is to establish safety prior to conducting additional trials in subjects with unstable angina.

INDICATION(S) AND RESEARCH PHASE
Thrombosis – Phase II
Cardiac Surgery – Phase IIa

TP10
unknown

MANUFACTURER
AVANT Immunotherapeutics

DESCRIPTION
TP10 is a genetically engineered (recombinant) soluble complement receptor-1 (sCR1). Complement-1 is a naturally occurring substance that binds to antibodies as part of the immune response to infection or foreign bodies. Clinical trials are testing TP10 in an intravenous formulation for a variety of disorders including the treatment of acute respiratory distress syndrome (ARDS), reperfusion injury, heart attack, cardiac surgery, organ reperfusion, xeno-transplantation, allotransplantation, and post-surgical complications in infants.

A phase IIb trial was initiated in January 2001 in approximately 30 infants undergoing high risk cardiac surgery utilizing cardiopulmonary bypass. The trial will be conducted at seven sites in the United States.

INDICATION(S) AND RESEARCH PHASE
Acute Respiratory Distress Syndrome (ARDS) – Phase II/III
Cardiac Ischemia – Phase I/II
Cardiac Surgery – Phase IIb
Myocardial Infarction – Phase I/II
Pediatric, Post-surgical Complications – Phase I/II
Pediatric, Cardiac Surgery – Phase IIb

unknown
Vascugel

MANUFACTURER
Curis

DESCRIPTION
Vascugel is currently in phase I trials for the reduction of intimal hyperplasia after coronary artery bypass graft (CABG) surgery.

INDICATION(S) AND RESEARCH PHASE
Cardiac Surgery – Phase I

Cholesterol, High Levels

AGI-1067
unknown

MANUFACTURER
AtheroGenics

DESCRIPTION
AGI-1067 is an oral compound being evaluated in phase II trials for reducing cholesterol and treating atherosclerosis, as well as for treatment of post-angioplasty restenosis, in which the diseased blood vessel has become clogged up again after stent placement. A stent is a metallic scaffold that is placed inside the blood vessel to keep the wall from collapsing and allowing blood flow to remain normal. Occasionally, the stent needs replacement when atherosclerotic plaques build up to block the passageway. AGI-1067 works by using a composite vascular protectant technology that may reduce the need for restenosis. AGI-1067 is being developed under an agreement between AtheroGenics and Schering-Plough Corporation.

INDICATION(S) AND RESEARCH PHASE
Peripheral Vascular Disease – Phase II
Cholesterol - high levels – Phase II
In-stent Restenosis – Phase II

BAY 13-9952
unknown

MANUFACTURER
Bayer Corporation

DESCRIPTION
BAY 13-9952 is a novel inhibitor of a specific class of proteins called apolipoprotein-B. Normally, the B-apolipoproteins are recognized by specific cell-surface receptors that help capture and store them, especially in the liver. BAY 13-9952 is being tested in a phase II trial to reduce the body storage of cholesterol and triglycerides. If this therapy works, it may help prevent atherosclerosis.

INDICATION(S) AND RESEARCH PHASE
Cholesterol, High Levels – Phase II

cerivastatin sodium
Certa

MANUFACTURER
Takeda Chemical Industries

DESCRIPTION

Certa is an HMG CoA reductase inhibitor. Takeda is conducting phase III trials in Japan to investigate the use of high dose Certa for the treatment of hypercholesterolemia.

INDICATION(S) AND RESEARCH PHASE
Cholesterol, High Levels – Phase III

CETP vaccine, CETi-1
unknown

MANUFACTURER
AVANT Immunotherapeutics

DESCRIPTION
CETi-1 is an antigen derived from cholesteryl ester transfer protein (CETP), a protein that transfers cholesterol from HDL to LDL. Immunization with this protein results in the production of antibodies which can inhibit the function of CETP. Inhibition of this transfer by interfering with the protein would result in an increase in HDL levels, and therefore, might decrease the risk of cardiovascular disease. In January 2001, positive results were obtained from a phase I trial of CETi-1 in 48 healthy adult subjects. The vaccine was well tolerated, and the only adverse reaction reported during the trial was not related to study medication. Additionally, limited evidence of an immune response was reported in one subject treated with the highest dose of the vaccine. CETi-1 is being developed for the treatment of subjects with low levels of HDL cholesterol.

INDICATION(S) AND RESEARCH PHASE
Cholesterol, High Levels – Phase I completed

colsevelam/simvastatin
Cholestagel/Zocor

MANUFACTURER
GelTex Pharmaceuticals

DESCRIPTION
This drug trial combines Cholestagel (colsevelam) and Zocor (simvastatin) together for the treatment of high cholesterol levels in the blood (hypercholesterolemia). This lipid-lowering regime uses a second generation of Cholestagel. Clinical studies have completed phase II and development is ready for the next stage of phase III.

INDICATION(S) AND RESEARCH PHASE
Cholesterol, High Levels – Phase II/III

estrogen/pravastatin
Premarin/Pravachol

MANUFACTURER
Bristol-Myers Squibb

DESCRIPTION
This combination study is testing the effects of both Premarin and Pravachol together to lower cholesterol levels in postmenopausal women. Premarin works with conjugated estrogen hormones to decrease cholesterol. Pravachol stops cholesterol from being stored by inhibiting a liver enzyme known as HMG-CoA reductase. Pravachol may also reduce the risk of cardiac events in subjects both with and without congestive heart disease; it was approved by the FDA for the prevention of stroke and second heart attacks in subjects with normal cholesterol levels. Clinical trials are in phase III development using both these oral drugs together for treating hypercholesterolemia.

INDICATION(S) AND RESEARCH PHASE
Cholesterol, High Levels – Phase III

ezetimibe
unknown

MANUFACTURER
Schering-Plough Corporation

DESCRIPTION
Ezetimibe is an orally administered lipid-lowering agent that belongs to a class of novel intestinal absorption inhibitors. The drug is being developed both as a monotherapy and for co-administration with statins for the treatment of high cholesterol. Both methods of administration are in phase III trials. Ezetimibe is being developed under an agreement between Schering-Plough and Merck.

INDICATION(S) AND RESEARCH PHASE
Cholesterol, High Levels – Phase III

unknown
Lovastatin XL

MANUFACTURER
Andrx

DESCRIPTION
Lovastatin XL is a cholesterol-lowering compound designed to provide extended delivery of lovastatin, especially to the liver. The compound works by inhibiting the liver enzyme HMG-CoA reductase, which is used in the manufacture of cholesterol.

In November 2000, phase III trial results of Lovastatin XL for the treatment of dyslipidemia indicated that the drug's effectiveness is similar to that of other potent HMG-CoA reductase inhibitors. A majority of subjects achieved therapeutic goals on the starting dose, and Lovastatin XL was generally well tolerated with no unexpected safety concerns identified. Andrx anticipates filing an NDA in 2001.

INDICATION(S) AND RESEARCH PHASE
Cholesterol, High Levels – Phase III completed

ursodiol
Urso

MANUFACTURER
Axcan Pharma

DESCRIPTION
Urso is an oral tablet composed of a bile acid (ursodeoxycholic acid) found in small amounts in normal human bile and in larger quantities in the bile of certain bears. This drug has been marketed in the United States for the treatment of primary biliary cirrhosis (PBC) since 1998. It is also approved in Canada for the treatment of cholestatic liver diseases, such as PBC, and the dissolution of gallstones. Additionally, Urso is being tested in phase II trials for at least 5 other indications: the treatment of high cholesterol blood levels (hypercholesterolemia), treatment with chemo-preven-

tion of colorectal polyps, treatment of colorectal cancer, treatment of non-alcoholic steatohepatitis, and treatment of viral hepatitis. The drug is licensed by Sanofi-Synthelabo to Axcan Pharma in a joint venture with Schwarz Pharma.

INDICATION(S) AND RESEARCH PHASE
Cholesterol, High Levels – Phase II
Colon Polyps – Phase II
Colorectal Cancer – Phase II
Hepatitis – Phase II

ZD-4522, S-4522
Crestor

MANUFACTURER
AstraZeneca

DESCRIPTION
Crestor is a cholesterol-lowering superstatin that works by inhibiting the enzyme HMG-CoA reductase. It currently is being tested in phase III trials for treating high cholesterol levels in the blood. The company plans to file for regulatory approval in the United States, Europe, and Japan.

According to phase II data, ZD-4522 reduced low-density lipoprotein cholesterol levels up to 65% and increased high-density lipoprotein cholesterol levels up to 14%. The trial evaluated ZD-4522 over six weeks in subjects ranging in ages 18–70, with mild-to-moderate hypercholesterolemia. The first stage of the program involved 142 subjects in a double-blind trial. In the second stage, 64 subjects were randomized to treatment. Direct comparisons between ZD-4522 and currently available statins will occur during the planned phase III program.

INDICATION(S) AND RESEARCH PHASE
Cholesterol, High Levels – Phase III

Congestive Heart Failure

BMS-186295, SR-47436 (irbesartan)
Avapro

MANUFACTURER
Bristol-Myers Squibb

DESCRIPTION
Avapro (irbesartan) is an approved drug (September 1997) in the United States for the treatment of hypertension. Avapro is a very selective, long-acting angiotensin-II receptor antagonist. By inhibiting the potent vasoconstrictor, angiotensin-II, Avapro works to lower blood pressure.

The company is trying to extend the product line by conducting a phase III trial for the indication of diabetic neuropathy. Avapro alters the renin-angiotensin-aldosterone system, which includes hormones involved with kidney function. The drug has also completed a phase III trial for the treatment of heart failure, with a phase IV trial planned for 2001.

INDICATION(S) AND RESEARCH PHASE
Neuropathy, Diabetic – Phase III
Congestive Heart Failure – Phase III completed
Hypertension – FDA approved

BMS-186716, omapatrilat
Vanlev

MANUFACTURER
Bristol-Myers Squibb

DESCRIPTION
Vanlev is a combination medicine made of two enzyme inhibitors for angiotensin converting enzyme (ACE) and neural endopeptidase (NEP). This dual drug mixture is being evaluated in phase II trials for the treatment of heart failure and phase III trials for hypertension.

In April 2000 Bristol-Myers Squibb voluntarily withdrew its current NDA for Vanlev as a treatment for hypertension because of questions regarding the side effect angioedema. Angioedema is a localized swelling that generally affects the face, throat, lips, or tongue which can be triggered by food and commonly used drugs such as ACE-inhibitors, nonsteroidal anti-inflammatory agents, and some antibiotics. The company plans to continue with further controlled trials and identify additional data to answer the FDA's questions.

INDICATION(S) AND RESEARCH PHASE
Congestive Heart Failure – Phase II
Hypertension – NDA withdrawn

BMS-193884
unknown

MANUFACTURER
Bristol-Myers Squibb

DESCRIPTION
BMS-193884 is an endothelin-A receptor stimulator for both congestive heart failure and male erectile dysfunction. It is made in an oral formulation. Clinical testing is in phase II.

INDICATION(S) AND RESEARCH PHASE
Congestive Heart Failure – Phase II
Erectile Dysfunction – Phase II

candesartan cilexetil
Atacand

MANUFACTURER
AstraZeneca

DESCRIPTION
Atacand (candesartan cilexetil) is an angiotensin II receptor blocker (ARB) being tested for the treatment of hypertension. Results of two multicenter, double-blind, randomized studies in more than 1,200 hypertensive subjects demonstrated Atacand to be significantly more effective in lowering both diastolic and systolic blood pressure than the most prescribed ARB Cozaar (losartan). During the double-blind treatment period, subjects were randomized to receive either 16 mg of Atacand or 50 mg of losartan. At week two, all subjects were titrated to double their current dose to 32 mg of Atacand or 100 mg of losartan. Duration of treatment was eight weeks unless a subject was discontinued due to an adverse event, had an insufficient therapeutic response, or withdrew consent. The incidence of discontinuation was only 2.7% for Atacand and 1.8% for losartan. The most commonly reported adverse events for both

medications were headache, dizziness, sinusitis, and respiratory infection.

The drug is currently being tested in phase III trials for hypertension outcomes (SCOPE study), congestive heart failure outcomes (CHARM study), and diabetic retinopathy. Pediatric phase III trials for hypertension are ongoing. Atacand Plus (a diuretic formula) is FDA approved for hypertension in adults.

INDICATION(S) AND RESEARCH PHASE
Hypertension – Phase III
Pediatric, Hypertension – Phase III
Congestive Heart Failure – Phase III
Diabetic Retinopathy – Phase III

candesartan cilexetil
Blopress

MANUFACTURER
Takeda Chemical Industries

DESCRIPTION
Blopress is an angiotensin II receptor antagonist being developed in phase III trials in Japan for the treatment of congestive heart failure. Additionally, the drug is in phase II trials in Japan for diabetic nephropathy.

INDICATION(S) AND RESEARCH PHASE
Congestive Heart Failure – Phase III
Diabetes Mellitus Types I and II – Phase II

captopril
Captelan

MANUFACTURER
Elan Pharmaceutical Research

DESCRIPTION
Captelan is a once-daily oral product made available by a technology that improves oral drug delivery. Captelan is a specific competitive inhibitor of the angiotensin I converting enzyme (ACE), the enzyme responsible for converting angiotensin I to angiotensin II. As an ACE inhibitor, Captelan has the potential to lower blood pressure and to indirectly reduce the workload on the heart. Clinical testing is in phase II for hypertension and congestive heart failure.

INDICATION(S) AND RESEARCH PHASE
Congestive Heart Failure – Phase II
Hypertension – Phase II

carvedilol
Coreg

MANUFACTURER
GlaxoSmithKline

DESCRIPTION
Coreg is a nonselective β-adrenergic blocking agent with α1-blocking activity. It is administered in tablet formulation and is rapidly and extensively absorbed by the body. An international study of Coreg in subjects with advanced chronic heart failure, called COPERNICUS (Carvedilol Prospective Randomized Cumulative Survival Trial), was stopped early by its steering committee due to a significant survival benefit seen with the drug. The study, which was conducted in over 300 medical centers in 21 countries, enrolled more than 2,200 subjects with advanced heart failure who had symptoms at rest or on minimal exertion but who did not require hospitalization in the intensive care unit or intravenous pharmacologic support. The mortality rate in the Coreg group was significantly lower than in the placebo group, and there were fewer serious adverse effects with Coreg treatment.

The drug was approved in May 1997 for the treatment of mild or moderate heart failure. It is currently in phase III trials for severe heart failure, and pediatric phase III trials are under way for congestive heart failure in children ages one to 18 years old.

INDICATION(S) AND RESEARCH PHASE
Congestive Heart Failure – Phase III
Pediatric, Congestive Heart Failure – Phase III

CVT-124
Adentri

MANUFACTURER
Biogen

DESCRIPTION
Adentri is believed to act by blocking the selective adenosine A-1 receptor that is present in several locations within the kidney. The selectivity of this compound offers the potential to promote excretion of excess fluid without causing side effects such as renal failure, diuretic resistance, or potassium loss.

This drug was shown to be active in a placebo-controlled, phase II trial evaluating various doses of Adentri in comparison to and in combination with furosemide for congestive heart failure. Biogen plans to move ahead with phase III studies. Adentri has also been evaluated in 70 subjects and it was shown that the glomerular filtration rate (GFR), a measure of kidney function, is preserved, while causing useful increases in sodium and urine excretion. Other useful indications may include acute renal failure following kidney transplantation, and high risk surgical procedures.

INDICATION(S) AND RESEARCH PHASE
Kidney Disease – Phase II
Congestive Heart Failure – Phase II

endothelin A receptor antagonist
unknown

MANUFACTURER
Aventis

DESCRIPTION
This drug is a novel endothelin-A receptor antagonist currently being tested in a phase II trial for chronic heart failure. Hoechst Marion Roussel is collaborating development of this program with Knoll Pharmaceuticals.

INDICATION(S) AND RESEARCH PHASE
Congestive Heart Failure – Phase II

etanercept
Enbrel

MANUFACTURER
Wyeth-Ayerst

DESCRIPTION
Enbrel binds to tumor necrosis factor

(TNF), which is one of the dominant cytokines or proteins associated with normal immune function and the series of reactions that cause the inflammatory process of rheumatoid arthritis. Enbrel inhibits the binding of TNF molecules to the TNF receptor (TNFR) sites. The binding of these sites inactivates TNF, resulting in significant reduction in inflammatory cascade. Enbrel has been FDA approved for treatment of rheumatoid arthritis in adults and children.

Results from postmarketing studies demonstrated that Enbrel can have serious adverse effects such as infection, sepsis, and death. According to the company, subjects who are predisposed to infection, such as those with advanced or poorly controlled diabetes, are at greater risk of experiencing side effects. In addition, use of Enbrel should be terminated in subjects with current infections or sepsis. Allergic reactions to Enbrel or its components are also a possibility.

Trial results showed that nearly 75% of children with severe, long-standing juvenile rheumatoid arthritis (JRA) respond to Enbrel. In the first segment of the study, 74% of children (51 of 69) between the ages of four and 17 showed an improvement in disease response when treated with Enbrel for three months. In the second segment, half of these 51 subjects received Enbrel and half received a placebo. Seventy-two percent of those who received Enbrel completed the second segment without worsening of JRA symptoms, compared to 19% who took a placebo.

Enbrel is currently in phase III trials for the treatment of psoriasis and congestive heart failure.

Enbrel is co-marketed by Immunex and Wyeth-Ayerst.

INDICATION(S) AND RESEARCH PHASE
Rheumatoid Arthritis – FDA approved
Pediatric, Juvenile Rheumatoid Arthritis – FDA approved
Psoriasis and Psoriatic Disorders – Phase III
Congestive Heart Failure – Phase III

---

fenoldopam mesylate, SK&F-82526
Corlopam

MANUFACTURER
Elan Pharmaceutical Research

DESCRIPTION
Corlopam is a dopamine-1 receptor facilitator that opens up blood vessels throughout the body (a systemic vasodilator). This drug is being tested in phase II trials for the treatment of congestive heart failure and acute renal failure.

INDICATION(S) AND RESEARCH PHASE
Congestive Heart Failure – Phase II
Kidney Disease – Phase II

HMR-1883/1098
unknown

MANUFACTURER
Aventis

DESCRIPTION
HMR-1883/1098 is a K-ATP channel blocker in a phase II study for treatment of sudden cardiac death. Although it is unknown why the heart stops within 24 hours of the onset of an acute illness, in greater than 90% of the cases the coronary arteries seem to be involved.

INDICATION(S) AND RESEARCH PHASE
Congestive Heart Failure – Phase II

---

nesiritide
Natrecor

MANUFACTURER
Scios

DESCRIPTION
Human B-type natriuretic peptide (BNP) is a naturally occurring hormone produced predominantly in the ventricles of the heart. A number of published studies indicate that endogenous levels of BNP are elevated in fluid-overload states such as congestive heart failure, which suggests that production of BNP may be a natural regulatory response to a failing heart.

Two pivotal trial results demonstrated Natrecor, a recombinant form of human BNP, significantly improves hemodynamic function and may represent a new treatment for congestive heart failure. The first trial enrolled 127 subjects at 23 sites and the second enrolled 305 subjects at 46 sites. Both trials tested Nesiritide at two different doses.

Scios first submitted an NDA for Natrecor in April 1998. In April 1999, Scios received a non-approval letter from the FDA for Natrecor, but was encouraged to study the drug in more subjects. After obtaining additional data, Scios submitted an amendment to the NDA for Natrecor in January of 2001. The company expects FDA review of the application by July of 2001.

INDICATION(S) AND RESEARCH PHASE
Congestive Heart Failure – NDA submitted

---

ranolazine, CVT-303
unknown

MANUFACTURER
CV Therapeutics

DESCRIPTION
CVT-303 belongs to a class of therapies called pFOX (partial fatty acid oxidation) inhibitors, and is administered in an oral sustained release formulation. It is currently in development for the treatment of chronic stable angina, the chest pain associated with coronary artery disease. Ranolazine may work by causing a partial shift in the heart's energy source from fatty acids to glucose, which is a more oxygen efficient source of energy.

CV Therapeutics has started a second pivotal phase III for CVT-303. This study is known as the CARISA (Combination Assessment of Ranolazine in Stable Angina) trial and will enroll about 450 subjects. It is a double-blind, placebo-controlled trial of CVT-303 used in combination with other anti-anginal drugs. The primary endpoint for evaluation is the duration of exercise on a treadmill.

In addition, a phase II trial for congestive heart failure was initiated in December 2000 testing ranolazine in an oral formulation.

INDICATION(S) AND RESEARCH PHASE
Angina – Phase III
Congestive Heart Failure – Phase II

SB 217242
unknown

MANUFACTURER
GlaxoSmithKline

DESCRIPTION
SB 217242 is an oral, broad-spectrum antagonist targeted to endothelin receptors. It is currently being tested in a phase II trial for the treatment of congestive heart failure. Previous clinical trials were discontinued for the indications of chronic obstructive pulmonary disease (COPD) and benign prostatic hypertrophy (BPH).

INDICATION(S) AND RESEARCH PHASE
Congestive Heart Failure – Phase II
Lung Disease – Trial discontinued
Prostate Disorders – Trial discontinued

SLV 306
unknown

MANUFACTURER
Solvay Pharmaceuticals

DESCRIPTION
SLV 306 is an anti-hypertensive drug being tested in phase II trials for the treatment of both hypertension and congestive heart failure.

INDICATION(S) AND RESEARCH PHASE
Congestive Heart Failure – Phase II
Hypertension – Phase II

somatropin, r-hGH
Serostim

MANUFACTURER
Serono Laboratories

DESCRIPTION
Serostim is a recombinant human growth hormone in trials for several indications. The drug is currently marketed for the treatment of cachexia, or AIDS wasting. Serostim is in phase III trials for treatment of growth hormone deficiency in adults and for short bowel syndrome, and phase II trials for lipodystrophy and congestive heart failure.

INDICATION(S) AND RESEARCH PHASE
Acquired Immune Deficiency (AIDS) and AIDS-Related Infections – FDA approved
Hormone Deficiencies – Phase III
Gastrointestinal Diseases and Disorders, miscellaneous – Phase III
Lipodystrophy – Phase II
Congestive Heart Failure – Phase II

TBC-11251
unknown

MANUFACTURER
Texas Biotechnology

DESCRIPTION
TBC-11251 is a small molecule that blocks the endothelin-A receptor. This drug is being evaluated in a phase II trial for the treatment of congestive heart failure and pulmonary hypertension associated with chronic obstructive pulmonary disease (COPD) or primary pulmonary hypertension. It is an oral formulation.

INDICATION(S) AND RESEARCH PHASE
Congestive Heart Failure – Phase II
Chronic Obstructive Pulmonary Disease (COPD) – Phase II
Lung Disease – Phase II

TBC-3711
unknown

MANUFACTURER
Texas Biotechnology

DESCRIPTION
TBC-3711 is an oral endothelin A receptor antagonist (ETA). Endothelin is a potent vasoconstrictor that exerts its effects through the activation of endothelin A and B receptors. The endothelin A receptor is believed to contribute to increase pulmonary and systemic artery pressures. Thus in blocking the endothelin A receptor, vasoconstriction may be prevented or reserved. TBC-3711 is being co-developed with ICOS Corporation and is currently in phase I development for congestive heart failure and essential hypertension.

The company plans to initiate a phase II trial for either congestive heart failure or essential hypertension by the second half of 2001.

INDICATION(S) AND RESEARCH PHASE
Congestive Heart Failure – Phase I
Hypertension – Phase I

TCV-116, candesartan cilexetil
unknown

MANUFACTURER
Takeda Chemical Industries

DESCRIPTION
TCV-116 is an angiotensin II receptor antagonist being developed for the treatment of congestive heart failure. It is currently in phase III trials in both the United States and Europe.

INDICATION(S) AND RESEARCH PHASE
Congestive Heart Failure – Phase III

toborinone
unknown

MANUFACTURER
Otsuka America Pharmaceutical

DESCRIPTION
Toborinone is an injectable cardiovascular drug that is in phase III testing for preventing acute heart failure. It works by inhibiting a muscle enzyme, phosphodiesterase III, thereby increasing the ability of the heart to contract more effectively. Toborinone acts as a vasodilator, dilating veins and arteries in a balanced manner, as was observed in experimental models of acute heart failure. Toborinone may prove to be another alternative to commercially available vasodilators to treat heart failure.

INDICATION(S) AND RESEARCH PHASE

Congestive Heart Failure – Phase III

unknown
Etomoxir

MANUFACTURER
MediGene AG

DESCRIPTION
Etomoxir is a highly active and specific inhibitor of carnitine-palmitoyl-transferase-1 (CPT1), a key enzyme of mitochondrial fatty acid oxidation. The inhibition of this enzyme leads to a shift from fatty acid oxidation to glucose oxidation, a more efficient supplier of energy in the diseased heart. Results from MediGene's unique Integrated Target Definition (ITD) technology platform, a program applied to identify, characterize, and validate genes causing heart disease, had indicated that the oxidation of fatty acids is pathologically increased in congestive heart failure (CHF) subjects. Etomoxir is believed to tackle this deregulation of heart metabolism and bring real therapeutic benefits in CHF. Clinical phase II trials for Etomoxir to treat CHF subjects are currently ongoing.

INDICATION(S) AND RESEARCH PHASE
Congestive Heart Failure – Phase II

valsartan
Diovan

MANUFACTURER
Novartis

DESCRIPTION
Diovan is an oral angiotensin II receptor antagonist in phase III development for the treatment of post- and pre-myocardial infarction and congestive heart failure. Diovan blocks the action of angiotensin II (AT-II), a hormone formed when a precursor (angiotensin I) is cleaved by an enzyme in the lungs and blood vessels. In this manner, Diovan blocks the vasoconstriction of blood vessels and the aldosterone-secreting effects of AT-II.

Diovan has been FDA approved for the treatment of hypertension in elderly subjects. It is currently being marketed by Novartis with this indication.

INDICATION(S) AND RESEARCH PHASE
Congestive Heart Failure – Phase III
Myocardial Infarction – Phase III
Hypertension – FDA approved

VAS 991
unknown

MANUFACTURER
Vasogen

DESCRIPTION
VAS 991 is an immuno modulator being developed by Vasogen for the treatment of congestive heart failure. A two-center phase II clinical trial of VAS 991 in subjects with congestive heart failure (CHF) is under way.

INDICATION(S) AND RESEARCH PHASE
Congestive Heart Failure – Phase II

YM-087, conivaptan
unknown

MANUFACTURER
Yamanouchi Pharmaceutical

DESCRIPTION
YM-087 is a receptor antagonist to the peptide hormone vasopressin, which is released by the hypothalamus to regulate water balance in the body. The drug is currently in phase III trials for the treatment of hyponatremia, and phase II trials for the treatment of heart failure. It is being developed in both Europe and the United States. The drug is also part of Yamanouchi's domestic pipeline; YM-087 is in phase II trials for both hyponatremia and heart failure. YM-087 is manufactured in oral and injectable formulations.

INDICATION(S) AND RESEARCH PHASE
Congestive Heart Failure (United States and Japan) – Phase II
Hyponatremia (United States) – Phase III
Hyponatremia (Japan) – Phase II

Coronary Artery Disease

Ad5FGF4
Generx

MANUFACTURER
Berlex Laboratories

DESCRIPTION
Generx is a novel growth factor gene FGF-4 therapy being developed in phase II/III trials for the treatment of subjects with stable exertional angina due to coronary artery disease. Berlex Laboratories has a collaborative agreement with Collateral Therapeutics for development of this drug.

INDICATION(S) AND RESEARCH PHASE
Coronary Artery Disease – Phase II/III

AI-700
unknown

MANUFACTURER
Acusphere

DESCRIPTION
AI-700 is a third-generation ultrasound contrast agent being tested in a phase II trial for assessing myocardial perfusion. A1-700 is a patented porous microparticle made of synthetic polymer that acts as an intravenous delivery system for gas. These synthetic polymer microspheres have high mechanical strength and produce minimal shadowing which prolong the duration of imaging. Earlier ultrasound agents are made from natural materials such as albumin, liposomes, and sugars that are not as strong as this new contrast agent.

Results from previous studies showed AI-700 to be long-lasting and uniform after one intravenous bolus injection without resorting to the complex administration procedures of other agents.

INDICATION(S) AND RESEARCH PHASE
Coronary Artery Disease – Phase II

cariporide mesylate, HOE-642

unknown

MANUFACTURER
Aventis

DESCRIPTION
HOE-642 (cariporide mesylate) is a sodium/hydrogen ion exchange inhibitor that is being tested for the treatment of coronary artery disease and acute myocardial infarction in phase II/III trials. Both intravenous and oral formulations of HOE-642 were made for clinical evaluation.

INDICATION(S) AND RESEARCH PHASE
Coronary Artery Disease – Phase II/III
Myocardial Infarction – Phase II/III

enoxaparin sodium/tirofiban
Lovenox/Aggrastat

MANUFACTURER
Aventis

DESCRIPTION
Lovenox (enoxaparin sodium) and Aggrastat (tirofiban) are in development as a combination therapy for acute coronary syndromes. Tirofiban, a small-molecule, non-peptide drug in a class of intravenous medicines known as glycoprotein (GP) IIb/IIIa receptor antagonists, works by blocking platelet aggregation, a key step in the formation of blood clots. Enoxaparin, a low-molecular-weight heparin, is a blood-thinning agent that inhibits thrombin, an enzyme present throughout the circulatory system that, when activated by injury to a blood vessel, facilitates the formation of a blood clot.

Currently, acute coronary syndrome subjects may receive tirofiban in combination with unfractionated heparin. However, unlike unfractionated heparin, low-molecular-weight heparins such as enoxaparin are easier to administer and do not require laboratory monitoring and frequent dose adjustments.

Results of the international ACUTE II trial demonstrated that treatment with Lovenox injection in combination with Aggrastat is well tolerated in subjects with acute coronary syndromes. ACUTE II was a multicenter, double-blind phase II trial that enrolled 525 subjects with unstable angina or non-Q-wave myocardial infarction. Tirofiban/enoxaparin and tirofiban/heparin treatment produced similar rates of major and minor bleeding up to 24 hours after drug cessation, using criteria from the trials of Thrombolysis In Myocardial Infarction (TIMI).

INDICATION(S) AND RESEARCH PHASE
Coronary Artery Disease – Phase IIb

eptifibatide
Integrilin

MANUFACTURER
COR Therapeutics

DESCRIPTION
Integrilin (eptifibatide) is a GP IIb-IIIa inhibitor that helps prevent platelet clumping and possible complete blockage of coronary arteries. Integrilin works by blocking the GPIIb-IIIa receptor, which is located on platelets and is responsible for their clumping. The drug is FDA approved for the treatment of subjects with acute coronary syndrome, including subjects who are to be managed medically and those undergoing percutaneous coronary intervention.

Traditional heart attack therapies, known as fibrinolytics, break up the fibrin strands that hold together the blood clot. These therapies, however, do not prevent continued platelet clumping and can indirectly stimulate clot reformation. As a result, Integrilin is being tested in combination with the fibrinolytic alteplase in heart attack subjects.

In November 2000, results of a phase II trial showed that Integrilin combined with half-dose alteplase significantly improved blood flow through clogged arteries supplying oxygen-starved heart muscle when compared with full-dose alteplase alone. Integrilin is also in phase II trials in combination with reduced-dose TNKase (tenecteplase), a fibrinolytic developed by Genentech.

Integrilin is being co-developed by COR Therapeutics and Schering-Plough Corporation.

INDICATION(S) AND RESEARCH PHASE
Coronary Artery Disease – FDA approved
Myocardial Infarction – Phase II

GP IIb/II a
Cromafiban

MANUFACTURER
COR Therapeutics

DESCRIPTION
Cromafiban is a small molecule that acts as an aggregation inhibitor, blocking platelets from clumping together. This drug is being tested in phase II trials for treatment of acute coronary disease, unstable angina, and strokes.

INDICATION(S) AND RESEARCH PHASE
Angina – Phase II
Coronary Artery Disease – Phase II
Strokes – Phase II

human albumin microspheres
Optison

MANUFACTURER
Molecular Biosystems

DESCRIPTION
Optison is an ultrasound contrast agent. It is made up of human albumin microspheres in an injectable suspension octafluoropropane formulation. Indicated for use in subjects with myocardial perfusion problems, Optison helps doctors in heart imaging.

The completed phase II clinical trials consisted of six studies in 376 subjects with a wide range of known or suspected coronary artery diseases. In all studies, Optison Myocardial Contrast Echocardiography (MCE) was found to compare favorably with the standard clinical tests, whether Single Photon Emission Computed Tomography (SPECT) or coronary angiography. Of the six, three studies were performed in subjects with known or suspected coronary artery disease including those with recent heart attacks undergoing pharmacologic stress echo test, two evaluated Optison with exercise stress echo, and another involved subjects presenting to the Emergency Room with unexplained chest pain.

INDICATION(S) AND RESEARCH PHASE
Angina – Phase II completed
Coronary Artery Disease – Phase II completed
Heart Disease – Phase II completed

monoclonal antibody (Mab), anti-VEGF
unknown

MANUFACTURER
Genentech

DESCRIPTION
The anti-VEGF antibody is a novel inhibitor of angiogenesis that may hinder the growth of cancer tumors by starving their blood supply. This humanized monoclonal antibody is a protein directed against vascular endothelial growth factor (VEGF) to block blood vessel growth in the treatment of solid tumors, for which this drug is involved in a phase II trial. Coronary artery disease is another indication being tested in phase II clinical trials.

INDICATION(S) AND RESEARCH PHASE
Cancer/Tumors (Unspecified) – Phase II
Coronary Artery Disease – Phase II

MRE0470
unknown

MANUFACTURER
King Pharmaceuticals

DESCRIPTION
MRE0470 is a second generation derivative of adenosine which the body uses for high energy chemical transactions by bonding to specific recognition sites or receptors on the surface of cells. When this adenosine analog binds selectively to the A2a receptor, it is thought to open up the blood vessels of the heart (coronary vasodilatation). In the second half of 1999, MRE0470 began a phase II trial for the diagnosis and treatment of coronary artery disease.

INDICATION(S) AND RESEARCH PHASE
Coronary Artery Disease – Phase II

raloxifene, LY-139481
Evista

MANUFACTURER
Eli Lilly

DESCRIPTION
Evista is a selective estrogen receptor modulator for prevention of coronary events (heart attack or cardiac death) in postmenopausal women. A phase III trial is assessing Evista's effect on secondary prevention of coronary events. Evista is also being tested in a phase III study for the prevention of breast cancer.

INDICATION(S) AND RESEARCH PHASE
Coronary Artery Disease – Phase III
Breast Cancer – Phase III

trafermin
Fiblast

MANUFACTURER
Chiron Corporation

DESCRIPTION
Fibroblast growth factor (FGF) is normally synthesized in response to insufficient blood supply caused by diseased arteries. Fiblast is a recombinant form of basic fibroblast growth factor (bFGF) developed to stimulate new blood vessel growth in the hearts of subjects with severe coronary artery disease. The drug is currently in phase II trials for coronary artery disease and has completed a phase II trial for treatment of peripheral vascular disease.

Scios has licensed rights to develop Fiblast to several companies, including Chiron. In November 1999, Scios and Chiron entered into a patent and license agreement under which Scios has licensed to Chiron its rights in human bFGF. Additionally, Scios has licensed FGF to Kaken Pharmaceutical of Japan for development in Japan, China, Taiwan and South Korea. Kaken has initially investigated the use of FGF as a wound healing treatment and is seeking approval to market FGF in Japan.

INDICATION(S) AND RESEARCH PHASE
Coronary Artery Disease – Phase II
Peripheral Vascular Disease – Phase II completed

vascular endothelial growth factor-121 (VEGF)
BioByPass

MANUFACTURER
GenVec

DESCRIPTION
Vascular endothelial growth factor-121 (VEGF) incorporates the VEGF gene into a replication-deficient adenovirus vector. VEGF is the body's potent natural growth factor that stimulates endothelial cells in blood vessels to migrate, replicate, and form new blood vessels.

BioByPass is being tested in phase II trials for coronary artery disease (CAD) and peripheral vascular disease (PVD).

INDICATION(S) AND RESEARCH PHASE
Coronary Artery Disease – Phase II
Peripheral Vascular Disease – Phase II

vascular endothelial growth factor-2 gene therapy (gtVEGF-2)
unknown

MANUFACTURER
Human Genome Sciences

DESCRIPTION
Vascular endothelial growth factor-2 gene therapy (gtVEGF-2) is in development in phase I/II trials for the treatment of coronary artery disease. The active ingredient in this drug product is a novel gene that encodes the protein VEGF-2, which scientists believe is the body's signal to grow new blood and lymph vessels. Laboratory studies show that this gene is active in the formation of new blood vessels, a process known as angiogenesis. The laboratory studies demonstrate that the gene is also active in the regeneration of lymphatic vessels, which results in reduced swelling and edema. This

swelling is caused by lymph fluid seepage which occurs normally.

Vascular Endothelial Growth Factor-2 gene therapy is currently in two phase I/II trials treating subjects that suffer from refractory myocardial ischemia. One trial uses a catheter inserted through a small incision in the subject's groin and directed to the heart using X-ray imaging. A needle is then advanced out of the catheter and used to inject DNA into the inner wall of the heart. The second trial uses direct injection of DNA into the inner wall of the heart, through an incision in the chest wall.

In the future, Vascular Genetics plans to submit additional INDs for other indications for this gene therapy product, including lymphedema and other coronary artery diseases.

INDICATION(S) AND RESEARCH PHASE
Cardiac Ischemia – Phase I/II
Coronary Artery Disease – Phase I/II

VEGF121
unknown

MANUFACTURER
Scios

DESCRIPTION
Vascular endothelial growth factor (VEGF) is one of a number of cytokines associated with angiogenesis. A 121 residue isoform of DNA encoding VEGF has been cloned and is called BioByPass angiogen. When expressed, this gene encodes biologically active VEGF. Phase II trials for VEGF121 are under way for the treatment of coronary artery disease and peripheral vascular disease.

INDICATION(S) AND RESEARCH PHASE
Coronary Artery Disease – Phase II
Peripheral Vascular Disease – Phase II

YM-337
unknown

MANUFACTURER
Yamanouchi Pharmaceutical

DESCRIPTION
YM-337 is an antibody, made in an injectable formulation, that blocks the platelet cell surface receptor glycoprotein (IIb/IIIa). The drug is being developed for high-risk Percutaneous Transluminal Coronary Angioplasy (PTCA), an established therapy for subjects with coronary artery disease. It is being evaluated in Europe and the United States in phase II trials.

INDICATION(S) AND RESEARCH PHASE
Coronary Artery Disease – Phase II

Heart Disease

abciximab, c7E3
ReoPro

MANUFACTURER
Centocor

DESCRIPTION
ReoPro is an antiplatelet drug being tested for acute ischemic stroke, acute myocardial infarction, and angina. This biological drug is a fragment (Fab) of a monoclonal antibody that binds to the glycoprotein (IIb/IIIa) receptor of human platelets and inhibits their clumping together.

ReoPro has recently completed a phase II trial for acute ischemic stroke and the overall results have shown that it improves the subject's clinical condition. ReoPro is unique because it can work when given up to 24 hours after a stroke, unlike other drugs that must be given within the first three hours. Also, none of the subjects suffered from symptomatic intracranial bleeding (ICH), a potential fatal side effect of current therapy.

A preliminary analysis showed that after three months of treatment, 35 percent of the subjects treated with any dose of abciximab had minimal or no remaining disability, compared with the 20 percent of subjects who received the placebo. In addition, half of the subjects treated with abciximab showed improved function in carrying out daily activities compared with 40 percent that were given the placebo. There was also a trend toward improved neurological functioning.

ReoPro is also being tested in a phase III trial for acute myocardial infarction and for angina. It is approved by the FDA as an add-on therapy to heart procedures (percutaneous coronary interventions, such as balloon angioplasty and stent placement) for the prevention of heart blood flow problems.

INDICATION(S) AND RESEARCH PHASE
Angina – Phase III
Heart Disease – Phase III
Strokes – Phase II completed
Myocardial Infarction – Phase III
Cardiac Surgery – FDA approved

BB-10153
unknown

MANUFACTURER
British Biotech plc

DESCRIPTION
BB-10153 is a genetically engineered protein, which has shown thrombolytic and anti-thrombotic properties in preclinical models. It may have potential use in the treatment of cardiovascular diseases, including heart attacks and strokes. This drug has successfully completed a phase I trial. Plans are under consideration for both the design of the phase II program as well as partnering with another company for development and marketing.

INDICATION(S) AND RESEARCH PHASE
Heart Disease – Phase I/II
Strokes – Phase I/II

daptomycin
Cidecin

MANUFACTURER
Cubist Pharmaceuticals

DESCRIPTION
Cidecin is a novel antibiotic lipopeptide for the treatment of skin and soft tissue infections, urinary tract infections in hospitalized subjects, and bacteremia. The drug is made

in an intravenous formulation. Cidecin is in phase III trials for skin infections and urinary tract infections, as well as a phase II trial for bacterial infections and a phase II/III trial for heart disease.

INDICATION(S) AND RESEARCH PHASE
Skin Infections/Disorders – Phase III
Bacterial Infection – Phase II
Urinary Tract Infections – Phase II/III
Heart Disease – Phase II/III

human albumin microspheres
Optison

MANUFACTURER
Molecular Biosystems

DESCRIPTION
Optison is an ultrasound contrast agent. It is made up of human albumin microspheres in an injectable suspension octafluoropropane formulation. Indicated for use in subjects with myocardial perfusion problems, Optison aids doctors in heart imaging.

The completed phase II clinical trials consisted of six studies in 376 subjects with a wide range of known or suspected coronary artery diseases. In all studies, Optison Myocardial Contrast Echocardiography (MCE) was found to compare favorably with standard clinical tests, whether Single Photon Emission Computed Tomography (SPECT) or coronary angiography. Of the six, three studies have been performed in subjects with known or suspected coronary artery disease including those with recent heart attacks undergoing pharmacologic (drug) stress echo test, two evaluated Optison with exercise stress echo, and another involved subjects presenting to the Emergency Room with unexplained chest pain.

INDICATION(S) AND RESEARCH PHASE
Angina – Phase II completed
Coronary Artery Disease – Phase II completed
Heart Disease – Phase II completed

human muscle cells, cardiac disease
unknown

MANUFACTURER
Diacrin

DESCRIPTION
Diacrin is developing a therapy involving isolated and expanded muscle cells from human tissue. According to the company, these cells may be transplanted into damaged heart muscle to potentially repair injury due to a heart attack. The cells would be isolated from a muscle biopsy of a heart attack subject, allowing transplantation of the subject's own cells into the heart, in order to avoid any rejection. A phase I trial is currently being held at the Temple University Hospital for the treatment of myocardial infarction and heart failure.

INDICATION(S) AND RESEARCH PHASE
Myocardial Infarction – Phase I
Heart Disease – Phase I

LDP-01
unknown

MANUFACTURER
LeukoSite

DESCRIPTION
LDP-01 is a genetically engineered, humanized monoclonal antibody directed to attach to β-2 integrin, the cell marker on white blood cells. LDP-01 is being tested in phase II trials for the prevention of post-ischemic reperfusion injury such as that resulting from organ transplantation, stroke, or heart attack. This drug may enhance organ survival and reduce the time required for the transplanted organ to function in kidney transplant subjects.

INDICATION(S) AND RESEARCH PHASE
Heart Disease – Phase II
Kidney Transplant Surgery – Phase II
Strokes – Phase II

liposomal prostaglandin E1, PGE-1
Liprostin

MANUFACTURER
Endovasc

DESCRIPTION
Liprostin is a liposomal encapsulation of prostaglandin E-1 (PGE-1), a potent vasodilator, platelet inhibitor, and antithrombotic compound. The effect of PGE-1 on cytokine production by antigen presenting cells is being studied using Liprostin. Liprostin is being evaluated in phase III trials for the treatment of cardiovascular diseases such as restenosis angioplasty.

Positive results were reported from a phase I trial of Liprostin in healthy volunteers. Liprostin was well tolerated and caused few side effects, all of which were minimal and short term, when administered to the maximum tolerated dose. The company plans to initiate phase II trials in subjects with critical limb ischemia.

INDICATION(S) AND RESEARCH PHASE
Heart Disease – Phase III
In-stent Restenosis – Phase III
Critical Limb Ischemia – Phase I completed

OPC-18790
unknown

MANUFACTURER
Otsuka America Pharmaceutical

DESCRIPTION
OPC-18790 is an inotropic agent that works by increasing the contractility of the heart so that the cardiac muscle beats stronger. Both injectable and tablet formulations were tested in phase II trials for general heart disease indications. However, clinical trial activity in phase III has been suspended as Otsuka America Pharmaceutical searches for a development partner.

INDICATION(S) AND RESEARCH PHASE
Heart Disease – Trial halted

TP-9201
unknown

MANUFACTURER
Integra LifeSciences

DESCRIPTION

TP-9201 inhibits a platelet membrane receptor (glycoprotein IIb/IIIa) and a cyclic peptide (RGD) for treatment of several cardiovascular diseases. Blood clots can be prevented from growing and propagating by stopping platelets from aggregating together. Potential treatments being tested for this therapy may include myocardial infarction, angioplasty, unstable angina, and stroke.

Integra Life Sciences have acquired Telios Pharmaceuticals and they has suspended clinical research between phases I and II until a development partner is found.

INDICATION(S) AND RESEARCH PHASE

Angina – Phase I/II on hold
Heart Disease – Phase I/II on hold
Strokes – Phase I/II on hold

unknown
Resten-NG

MANUFACTURER
AVI BioPharma

DESCRIPTION

Resten-NG is the first compound from the company's third-generation NeuGene antisense technology platform being tested for the treatments of cardiovascular restenosis and cancer in phase I and II trials. Resten-NG is designed to treat cardiovascular restenosis by inhibiting the production of a cellular transcription factor, the oncogene c-myc.

Results from preclinical trials show Resten-NG preserves vessel passageways and prevents arterial wall thickening. Delivering the compound to the site of angioplasty blocks growth and proliferation events in the vessel walls.

A phase II trial will test Resten-NG in 100 subjects undergoing angioplasty procedures. A new drug delivery phase I trial will study this compound's level of bioavailability via the oral route of administration. Trials will take place at Lenox Hill Hospital in New York under the direction of Dr. Martin Leon and Dr. Jeffrey Moses, Chief of Interventional Cardiology at the hospital.

Additionally, a phase I/II trial is under way testing Resten-NG with Oncomyc-NG for treatment of cancer.

INDICATION(S) AND RESEARCH PHASE

Heart Disease – Phase I/II
Cancer/Tumors (Unspecified) – Phase I completed

unknown
Tranilast

MANUFACTURER
GlaxoSmithKline

DESCRIPTION

Tranilast is an endothelial cell proliferation/migration inhibitor. It is currently in phase III trials for restenosis, a recurrent narrowing of the coronary arteries that can occur following percutaneous transluminal coronary angioplasty (PTCA).

INDICATION(S) AND RESEARCH PHASE

Heart Disease – Phase III

unknown
Levovist

MANUFACTURER
Berlex Laboratories

DESCRIPTION

Levovist is a diagnostic contrast agent for ultrasound imaging of the left ventricle. It may be used to help enhance ultrasound pictures of the large left ventricular heart muscle. This agent is in a phase III trial.

INDICATION(S) AND RESEARCH PHASE

Heart Disease – Phase III

Hemophilia

antihemophilic factor
Alphanate

MANUFACTURER
Alpha Therapeutic

DESCRIPTION

Alphanate is a heat-treated human blood factor approved by the FDA to treat hemophilia A. It is a highly purified Factor VIII, which is normally responsible for clotting blood to prevent hemorrhage. A phase IV trial is being conducted to further expand the safety and pharmacology characteristics.

A phase III study was completed in children seven years and older for the treatment of von Willebrand's disease, a bleeding disorder.

INDICATION(S) AND RESEARCH PHASE

Hemophilia – Phase IV/FDA approved
Pediatric, von Willebrand's disease – Phase III completed

factor VIII gene therapy
unknown

MANUFACTURER
Transkaryotic Therapies

DESCRIPTION

Factor VIII gene therapy, utilizing Transkaryotic Therapy, is being developed for the treatment of hemophilia A. Transkaryotic Therapy is the company's non-viral gene therapy system. A sample of a subject's cells are removed and genetically engineered to produce a desired protein for extended periods of time. The genetically engineered cells are then injected back into the subjects. The blood clotting protein factor VIII is deficient in subjects with hemophilia A, and in this manner, therapeutic delivery of the protein can be established.

Data from six subjects in a phase I trial for hemophilia A demonstrated that Transkaryotic Therapies' factor VIII gene therapy was safe and well tolerated. Following implantation of 100–400 million genetically modified cells, four of six subjects demonstrated decreased bleeding frequency and/or factor VIII usage. Additionally, two subjects did not experience spontaneous bleeds for approximately one year following treatment.

INDICATION(S) AND RESEARCH PHASE

Hemophilia – Phase I completed

factor VIII gene therapy

unknown

MANUFACTURER
Chiron Corporation

DESCRIPTION
Factor VIII gene therapy is designed to insert the gene coding for factor VIII into a person's cells. Factor VIII is an important protein in the blood clotting system. Subjects with hemophilia A lack adequate circulating factor VIII. Once factor VIII is reintroduced into the body and sufficiently expressed, bleeding episodes should be drastically reduced.

This therapy is currently in phase I trials.

INDICATION(S) AND RESEARCH PHASE
Hemophilia – Phase I

r-FVIIa
NovoSeven

MANUFACTURER
Novo Nordisk

DESCRIPTION
The coagulant NovoSeven is a recombinant factor VIIa developed for the treatment of hemophilia in subjects with inhibitors to factor VIIa. This recombinant protein induces hemostasis, stopping bleeding at the site of injury independent of the presence of factor VIII or factor IX, by forming complexes with exposed tissue factor (TF). In the United States, NovoSeven has been approved for the treatment of bleeding episodes in hemophilia A or B subjects with inhibitors to factor VIII or factor IX.

NovoSeven began phase III trials for the prevention and treatment of bleeding episodes in subjects with coagulopathy, the inability of the blood to clot normally, associated with liver disease.

INDICATION(S) AND RESEARCH PHASE
Hemophilia – FDA approved
Liver Disease – Phase III

unknown
Coagulin-B

MANUFACTURER
Avigen

DESCRIPTION
Coagulin-B is an AAV vector, which carries the gene for factor IX, the missing or deficient protein that causes hemophilia B. Coagulin-B is designed to deliver the factor IX gene into the subjects' muscle or liver cells where it will continuously produce factor IX. Results show Coagulin-B to be safe and well tolerated in all subjects, with no side effects observed. Coagulin-B is currently in phase III trials.

INDICATION(S) AND RESEARCH PHASE
Hemophilia – Phase III

Hyperlipidemia

BMS-201038
unknown

MANUFACTURER
Bristol-Myers Squibb

DESCRIPTION
BMS-201038 is an oral inhibitor of the microsomal transport protein (MTP) for lowering fat (lipid) levels in the blood. BMS-201038 is being evaluated in a phase II trial with special attention to the two important criteria of morbidity and mortality.

INDICATION(S) AND RESEARCH PHASE
Hyperlipidemia – Phase II

Hypertension

BMS-186716, omapatrilat
Vanlev

MANUFACTURER
Bristol-Myers Squibb

DESCRIPTION
BMS-186716 is a combination medicine made of two enzyme inhibitors for angiotensin converting enzyme (ACE) and neural endopeptidase (NEP). This dual drug mixture is being evaluated in phase II trials for the treatment of heart failure and phase III trials for hypertension.

In April 2000 Bristol-Myers Squibb voluntarily withdrew its NDA for Vanlev as a treatment for hypertension due to questions regarding the side effect angioedema. Angioedema is a localized swelling that generally affects the face, throat, lips, or tongue which can be triggered by food and commonly used drugs such as ACE-inhibitors, nonsteroidal anti-inflammatory agents, and some antibiotics. The company plans to continue with further controlled trials and identify additional data to answer the FDA's questions.

INDICATION(S) AND RESEARCH PHASE
Congestive Heart Failure – Phase II
Hypertension – NDA withdrawn

bosentan
Tracleer

MANUFACTURER
Actelion Pharmaceuticals

DESCRIPTION
Tracleer is an orally active dual endothelin receptor agonist, blocking the action of endothelin at two different receptors (ETA and ETB). Endothelin is a potent vasoconstrictor, narrowing blood vessels, and appears to play a fundamental mechanistic role in the development of pulmonary hypertension (PHT). Results of a double-blind, placebo-controlled phase III trial of Tracleer showed that subjects receiving the drug experienced significant improvements in exercise ability and hemodynamics, including blood flow and circulation. At 12 weeks, subjects in the Tracleer group demonstrated a 20% increase in exercise ability compared to placebo in the standardized six-minute walk test. Actelion plans to soon complete NDA filing.

INDICATION(S) AND RESEARCH PHASE
Hypertension – Phase III completed

candesartan cilexetil

Hypertension/33

Atacand

MANUFACTURER
AstraZeneca

DESCRIPTION
Atacand (candesartan cilexetil) is an angiotensin II receptor blocker (ARB) being tested for the treatment of hypertension. Results of two multicenter, double-blind, randomized studies in more than 1,200 hypertensive subjects demonstrated Atacand to be significantly more effective in lowering both diastolic and systolic blood pressure than the most prescribed ARB Cozaar (losartan). During the double-blind treatment period, subjects were randomized to receive either 16 mg of Atacand or 50 mg of losartan. At week two, all subjects were titrated to double their current dose to 32 mg of Atacand or 100 mg of losartan. Duration of treatment was eight weeks unless a subject discontinued due to an adverse event, had an insufficient therapeutic response, or withdrew consent. The incidence of discontinuation was only 2.7% for Atacand and 1.8% for losartan. The most commonly reported adverse events for both medications were headache, dizziness, sinusitis, and respiratory infection.

The drug is currently being tested in phase III trials for hypertension outcomes (SCOPE study), congestive heart failure outcomes (CHARM study), and diabetic retinopathy. Pediatric phase III trials for hypertension are ongoing. Atacand Plus (a diuretic formula) is FDA approved for hypertension in adults.

INDICATION(S) AND RESEARCH PHASE
Hypertension – Phase III
Pediatric, Hypertension – Phase III
Congestive Heart Failure – Phase III
Diabetic Retinopathy – Phase III

captopril
Captelan

MANUFACTURER
Elan Pharmaceutical Research

DESCRIPTION
Captelan is a once-daily oral product made available by a technology that improves oral drug delivery. Captelan is a specific competitive inhibitor of the angiotensin I converting enzyme (ACE), the enzyme responsible for converting angiotensin I to angiotensin II. As an ACE inhibitor, Captelan has the potential to lower blood pressure and to indirectly reduce the workload on the heart. Clinical testing is in phase II for hypertension and congestive heart failure.

INDICATION(S) AND RESEARCH PHASE
Congestive Heart Failure – Phase II
Hypertension – Phase II

CS-866
unknown

MANUFACTURER
Sankyo

DESCRIPTION
CS-866 is an antihypertensive drug that works by blocking the receptor on angiotensin II, a very potent, natural agent that raises blood pressure. CS-866, as a treatment for hypertension, is in an oral formulation and is currently in a phase III trial. Sankyo is collaborating development of this product with Recordati Industria Chimica e Farmaceutica S.p.A.

INDICATION(S) AND RESEARCH PHASE
Hypertension – Phase III

diltiazem HCl
Verzem

MANUFACTURER
Verex Laboratories

DESCRIPTION
Verzem is an oral tablet formulation of a calcium channel blocker (diltiazem hydrochloride). This drug works by inhibiting the influx of calcium ions during the normal electrical discharge, or membrane depolarization, of cardiac and vascular smooth muscle. For the treatment of hypertension, Verzem is thought to relax blood vessel muscles, which decreases peripheral vascular resistance; for angina, it may reduce oxygen demand in heart muscle. Verzem is currently in a phase II trial for hypertension.

INDICATION(S) AND RESEARCH PHASE
Hypertension – Phase II

GW 660511
unknown

MANUFACTURER
GlaxoSmithKline

DESCRIPTION
GW 660511 is an angiotensin-converting enzyme (ACE)/neutral-endopeptidase enzyme (NEP) inhibitor being developed for the treatment of hypertension. It is currently in phase I trials.

INDICATION(S) AND RESEARCH PHASE
Hypertension – Phase I

isradipine
unknown

MANUFACTURER
Elan Pharmaceutical Research

DESCRIPTION
Isradipine is a calcium channel blocker being evaluated in a once-daily formulation, using the Insoluble Drug Absorption System (INDAS) manufactured by Elan Pharmaceutical Research. Clinical testing is in a phase II trial for treating hypertension.

INDICATION(S) AND RESEARCH PHASE
Hypertension – Phase II

lercanidipine
unknown

MANUFACTURER
Forest Laboratories

DESCRIPTION
Lercanidipine belongs to the dihydropyridine calcium channel blocker class of antihypertensives. The drug is currently marketed in 19 countries, and clinical testing has

shown it to have comparable efficacy to other drugs in its class. Forest Laboratories has entered into an agreement with Recordati of Milan, Italy, for the marketing of lercanidipine in the United States. The drug is currently in phase III trials for hypertension in the United States, and it is expected that an NDA will be filed for approval in the United States mid-2001.

INDICATION(S) AND RESEARCH PHASE
Hypertension – Phase III

Sitaxsentan
unknown

MANUFACTURER
ICOS Corporation

DESCRIPTION
Sitaxsentan is an endothelin receptor antagonist with a long duration of action and high specificity for Type A endothelin (ETA) receptors. Blocking ETA may reverse the vasoconstrictive effects of endothelin-1 (ET-1) on the pulmonary vasculature, while maintaining the vasodilator functions of the Type B (ETB) receptor.

Sitaxsentan is being developed by ICOS and Texas Biotechnology for the treatment of pulmonary hypertension. They expect to enroll subjects in a phase IIb/III trial in the first quarter of 2001.

INDICATION(S) AND RESEARCH PHASE
Hypertension – Phase II/III

SLV 306
unknown

MANUFACTURER
Solvay Pharmaceuticals

DESCRIPTION
SLV 306 is an anti-hypertensive drug being tested in phase II trials for treatment of hypertension and congestive heart failure.

INDICATION(S) AND RESEARCH PHASE
Congestive Heart Failure – Phase II
Hypertension – Phase II

SPP 100
unknown

MANUFACTURER
Speedel Pharma

DESCRIPTION
SPP 100 is an oral renin inhibitor being developed in a phase II fast-track program. The ongoing multicenter trial for the treatment of hypertension, involving 300 subjects, will establish the dose-response of the blood pressure lowering effect. SPP 100 was licensed to Speedel from Novartis.

INDICATION(S) AND RESEARCH PHASE
Hypertension – Phase II

TBC-3711
unknown

MANUFACTURER
Texas Biotechnology

DESCRIPTION
TBC-3711 is an oral endothelin A receptor antagonist (ETA). Endothelin is a potent vasoconstrictor that exerts its effects through the activation of endothelin A and B receptors. The endothelin A receptor is believed to contribute to increased pulmonary and systemic artery pressures. Thus in blocking the endothelin A receptor, vasoconstriction may be prevented or reserved. The company plans to initiate a phase II trial for either congestive heart failure or essential hypertension by the second half of 2001. TBC-3711 is being co-developed with ICOS Corporation and is currently in phase I development for congestive heart failure and essential hypertension.

INDICATION(S) AND RESEARCH PHASE
Congestive Heart Failure – Phase I
Hypertension – Phase I

TCV-116C
unknown

MANUFACTURER
Takeda Chemical Industries

DESCRIPTION
TCV-116C is a combination of TCV-116, an angiotensin II receptor antagonist, and a diuretic. The drug is in phase II trials in Japan for the treatment of hypertension.

INDICATION(S) AND RESEARCH PHASE
Hypertension – Phase II

telmisartan
unknown

MANUFACTURER
GlaxoSmithKline

DESCRIPTION
Telmisartan is an angiotensin II receptor antagonist. Binding sites for angiotensin II are found in many tissues, including vascular smooth muscle and adrenal gland. Blockade of these binding sites inhibits vasoconstriction and facilitates blood flow, thereby reducing blood pressure.

Telmisartan is currently in phase III trials, in combination with hydrochlorothiazide (HCTZ), for the treatment of hypertension. HCTZ is a diuretic commonly prescribed in combination with other antihypertensives. HCTZ flushes excess water and sodium from the body by increasing urine formation. This decreases the amount of fluid in the blood vessels, thereby increasing blood flow and reducing blood pressure.

INDICATION(S) AND RESEARCH PHASE
Hypertension – Phase III

unknown
Beraprost

MANUFACTURER
United Therapeutics

DESCRIPTION
Beraprost is a chemically-stable oral form of prostacyclin that dilates blood vessels, prevents platelet aggregation and prevents proliferation of smooth muscle cells surrounding blood vessels. It is in phase III trials for both early-stage peripheral vascular disease and early-stage pulmonary hypertension, in an immediate-release oral formulation.

UT-15
unknown

MANUFACTURER
United Therapeutics

DESCRIPTION
UT-15 is a formulation of prostacyclin that is delivered continuously through the MiniMed subcutaneous system. UT-15 is a particularly long-lived and stable version of prostacyclin, and because the MiniMed system operates by subcutaneous infusion rather than intravenous injection, there is less risk of infection. The product is in phase II development for the treatment of late-stage peripheral vascular disease and has also been developed for treatment of pulmonary hypertension.

In November 2000, United Therapeutics announced that the NDA submitted for UT-15 for the treatment of pulmonary hypertension was accepted by the FDA. The company anticipates a six-month priority review status.

INDICATION(S) AND RESEARCH PHASE
Hypertension – NDA submitted
Peripheral Vascular Disease – Phase II

valsartan
Diovan

MANUFACTURER
Novartis

DESCRIPTION
Diovan is an oral angiotensin II receptor antagonist in phase III development for the treatment of post- and pre-myocardial infarction and congestive heart failure. Diovan blocks the action of angiotensin II (AT-II), a hormone formed when a precursor (angiotensin I) is cleaved by an enzyme in the lungs and blood vessels. In this manner, Diovan blocks the vasoconstriction of blood vessels and the aldosterone-secreting effects of AT-II.

Diovan has been FDA approved for the treatment of hypertension in elderly subjects. It is currently being marketed by Novartis with this indication.

INDICATION(S) AND RESEARCH PHASE
Congestive Heart Failure – Phase III
Myocardial Infarction – Phase III
Hypertension – FDA approved

In-stent Restenosis

unknown
Antrin/Photoangioplasty

MANUFACTURER
Pharmacyclics

DESCRIPTION
Antrin is in a phase II trial for peripheral arterial disease (PAD). Photoangioplasty uses a laser light to activate an injected drug, which dissolves plaque in blood vessels. Upon exposure to light, the compound manufactures oxygen free radicals that cause mild damage to the plaque but leave healthy tissue alone.

The phase II trial is evaluating the therapy as both a primary treatment of PAD and for preventing restenosis following balloon angioplasty. The trial consists of 375 subjects using two active treatment arms and one control arm. The company hopes the conclusions of the phase II trial will be measurable improvement at 180 days in angiography, ankle-brachial index (ABI), treadmill tests, intravascular ultrasonography (IVUS), and Ruetherford-Becker classification scores.

INDICATION(S) AND RESEARCH PHASE
In-stent Restenosis – Phase II
Peripheral Arterial Occlusive Disease – Phase II

AGI-1067
unknown

MANUFACTURER
AtheroGenics

DESCRIPTION
AGI-1067 is an oral compound being evaluated for reducing cholesterol and treating atherosclerosis. The specific indication being tested in phase II clinical trials is post-angioplasty restenosis, in which the diseased blood vessel has become clogged up again after stent placement. A stent is a metallic scaffold that is placed inside the blood vessel to keep the wall from collapsing and allowing blood flow to remain normal. Occasionally, the stent needs replacement when atherosclerotic plaques build up to block the passageway. AGI-1067 works by using a composite vascular protectant technology that may reduce the need for restenosis. AGI-1067 is being developed under an agreement between AtheroGenics and Schering-Plough Corporation.

INDICATION(S) AND RESEARCH PHASE
Peripheral Vascular Disease – Phase II
Cholesterol, High Levels – Phase II
In-stent Restenosis – Phase II

liposomal prostaglandin E1, PGE-1
Liprostin

MANUFACTURER
Endovasc

DESCRIPTION
Liprostin is a liposomal encapsulation of prostaglandin E-1 (PGE-1), a potent vasodilator, platelet inhibitor, and antithrombotic compound. The effect of PGE-1 on cytokine production by antigen presenting cells is being studied using Liprostin. Liprostin is being evaluated in phase III trials for the treatment of cardiovascular diseases such as restenosis angioplasty.

Positive results were reported from a phase I trial of Liprostin in healthy volunteers. Liprostin was well tolerated and caused few side effects, all of which were minimal and short term, when administered to the maximum tolerated dose. The company plans to initiate phase II trials in subjects with critical limb ischemia.

INDICATION(S) AND RESEARCH PHASE
Heart Disease – Phase III

In-stent Restenosis – Phase III
Critical Limb Ischemia – Phase I completed

Limb Preservation and Amputation

AS-013
Circulase

MANUFACTURER
Alpha Therapeutic

DESCRIPTION
Circulase is being tested in a phase II/III study for the prevention of limb amputation in subjects with severe ischemia. Circulase may help blood flow in the arms and legs.

INDICATION(S) AND RESEARCH PHASE
Limb Preservation and Amputation – Phase II/III

Memory Loss

SIB-1508Y
unknown

MANUFACTURER
Sibia Neurosciences

DESCRIPTION
SIB-1508Y is a nicotinic acetylcholine receptor (nAChR)-selective drug being developed for the treatment of Parkinson's disease, memory loss, and attention deficit hyperactivity disorder (ADHD). SIB-1508Y is being tested in phase II trials as both a single therapeutic agent and combined with L-dopa for treatment of Parkinson's disease.

INDICATION(S) AND RESEARCH PHASE
Attention Deficit Hyperactivity Disorder (ADHD) – Phase II
Memory Loss – Phase II
Parkinson's Disease – Phase II

Myocardial Infarction

abciximab, c7E3
ReoPro

MANUFACTURER
Centocor

DESCRIPTION
ReoPro is an antiplatelet drug being tested for acute ischemic stroke, acute myocardial infarction, and angina. This biological drug is a fragment (Fab) of a monoclonal antibody that binds to the glycoprotein (IIb/IIIa) receptor of human platelets and inhibits their clumping together.

ReoPro has recently completed a phase II trial for acute ischemic stroke and the overall results have shown that it improves the subject's clinical condition. ReoPro is unique because it can work when given up to 24 hours after a stroke, unlike other drugs that must be given within the first three hours. Also, none of the subjects suffered from symptomatic intracranial bleeding (ICH), a potential fatal side effect of current therapy.

A preliminary analysis showed that after three months of treatment, 35 percent of the subjects treated with any dose of abciximab had minimal or no remaining disability, compared with the 20 percent of subjects who received the placebo. In addition, half of the subjects treated with abciximab showed improved function in carrying out daily activities compared with 40 percent that were given the placebo. There was also a trend toward improved neurological functioning.

ReoPro is also being tested in a phase III trial for acute myocardial infarction and for heart pain angina. It is approved by the FDA as an add-on therapy to heart procedures (percutaneous coronary interventions, such as balloon angioplasty and stent placement) for the prevention of heart blood flow problems.

INDICATION(S) AND RESEARCH PHASE
Angina – Phase III
Heart Disease – Phase III
Strokes – Phase II completed
Myocardial Infarction – Phase III
Cardiac Surgery – FDA approved

AMISTAD-II
Pallacor

MANUFACTURER
King Pharmaceuticals

DESCRIPTION
Pallacor is an adenosine allosteric modulator that works by making the heart beat more regularly. Studies are under way for the treatment of acute myocardial infarction in combination with blood clot therapy (thrombolysis) and angioplasty.

INDICATION(S) AND RESEARCH PHASE
Myocardial Infarction – Phase III

AMP-579
unknown

MANUFACTURER
Aventis

DESCRIPTION
AMP-579 is an adenosine A-1/A-2 receptor stimulator (agonist) for myocardial protection. The study is in phase II for reperfusion injury and cardioprotection in acute myocardial infarction (AMI). AMP-579 is made in an intravenous formulation.

INDICATION(S) AND RESEARCH PHASE
Myocardial Infarction – Phase II

cariporide mesylate, HOE-642
unknown

MANUFACTURER
Aventis

DESCRIPTION
HOE-642 (cariporide mesylate) is a sodium/hydrogen ion exchange inhibitor that is being tested for the treatment of coronary artery disease and acute myocardial infarction in phase II/III trials. Both intravenous and oral formulations of HOE-642 were made for clinical evaluation.

INDICATION(S) AND RESEARCH PHASE
Coronary Artery Disease – Phase II/III

Myocardial Infarction – Phase II/III

eptifibatide
Integrilin

MANUFACTURER
COR Therapeutics

DESCRIPTION
Integrilin (eptifibatide) is a GP IIb-IIIa inhibitor that helps prevent platelet clumping and possible complete blockage of coronary arteries. Integrilin works by blocking the GPIIb-IIIa receptor, which is located on platelets and is responsible for their clumping. The drug is FDA approved for the treatment of subjects with acute coronary syndrome, including subjects who are to be managed medically and those undergoing percutaneous coronary intervention.

Traditional heart attack therapies, known as fibrinolytics, break up the fibrin strands that hold together the blood clot. These therapies, however, do not prevent continued platelet clumping and can indirectly stimulate clot reformation. As a result, Integrilin is being tested in combination with the fibrinolytic alteplase in heart attack subjects.

In November 2000, results of a phase II trial showed that Integrilin combined with half-dose alteplase significantly improved blood flow through clogged arteries supplying oxygen-starved heart muscle when compared with full-dose alteplase alone. Integrilin is also in phase II trials in combination with reduced-dose TNKase (tenecteplase), a fibrinolytic developed by Genentech.

Integrilin is being co-developed by COR Therapeutics and Schering-Plough Corporation.

INDICATION(S) AND RESEARCH PHASE
Coronary Artery Disease – FDA approved
Myocardial Infarction – Phase II

fibrinogen-receptor antagonist
unknown

MANUFACTURER
Aventis

DESCRIPTION
This drug is in a phase II trial for both prevention and treatment of unstable angina and myocardial infarction. It works by blocking a receptor for the protein precursor, fibrinogen, that is involved in blood clot structure formation.

INDICATION(S) AND RESEARCH PHASE
Angina – Phase II
Myocardial Infarction – Phase II

H376/95
unknown

MANUFACTURER
AstraZeneca

DESCRIPTION
H376/95 belongs to a new class of oral anticoagulants. This drug prevents clot formation in a different manner than low-molecular-weight heparin and the anticoagulant warfarin. It exerts its effect in the final stage of clot formation by inhibiting the activity of thrombin, a clot-forming substance.

Positive phase II results for the prevention of leg vein blood clots in subjects undergoing elective total knee replacement surgery were announced in December 2000. In the dose-determining trial, a 24-mg dose of H376/95 resulted in a 15.8% incidence of venous thromboembolism (VTE) compared to a 22.7% incidence with injections of enoxaparin. In subjects receiving H376/95, the lowest incidence of VTE was seen with the 24-mg dose.

Phase III trials are now being conducted for both the prevention and treatment of VTE and the prevention of stroke in subjects with atrial fibrillation. A phase I/II study is ongoing for post myocardial infarction.

INDICATION(S) AND RESEARCH PHASE
Venous Thromboembolism (VTE) – Phase III
Strokes – Phase III
Myocardial Infarction – Phase I/II

human muscle cells, cardiac disease
unknown

MANUFACTURER
Diacrin

DESCRIPTION
Diacrin is developing a therapy involving isolated and expanded muscle cells from human tissue. According to the company, these cells may be transplanted into damaged heart muscle to potentially repair injury due to a heart attack. The cells would be isolated from a muscle biopsy of a heart attack subject, allowing transplantation of the subject's own cells into the heart, in order to avoid any rejection. A phase I trial is currently being held at the Temple University Hospital for the treatment of myocardial infarction and heart failure.

INDICATION(S) AND RESEARCH PHASE
Myocardial Infarction – Phase I
Heart Disease – Phase I

lanoteplase, BMS-200980
unknown

MANUFACTURER
Genetics Institute

DESCRIPTION
Lanoteplase is a novel "clot buster." It is a longer acting, genetically recombined form of an activator for plasminogen, which is the inactive precursor for plasmin, the main enzyme responsible for chopping up fibrin blood clots. This plasminogen activator is administered in a single injection.

Lanoteplase is being tested in a phase III trial for its ability to quickly dissolve blood clots associated with recent acute myocardial infarctions.

INDICATION(S) AND RESEARCH PHASE
Myocardial Infarction – Phase III

pexelizumab
unknown

MANUFACTURER
Alexion

DESCRIPTION

Pexelizumab is an anti-inflammatory C5 inhibitor monoclonal antibody fragment. In January 2001, preliminary results of a double-blind, placebo-controlled phase IIb trial indicated that pexelizumab significantly reduced a composite endpoint of death or myocardial infarction at 30 days in subjects undergoing coronary artery bypass graft surgery (CABG) with cardiopulmonary bypass (CPB). Subjects were separated into two groups, those undergoing only CABG with CPB (approximately 90%) or subjects undergoing CABG with concomitant valve surgery during CPB. Results showed that pexelizumab suppressed complement in CPB subjects, with bolus (pexelizumab 2.0 mg/kg) and bolus plus infusion (pexelizumab 2.0 mg/kg bolus, pexelizumab infusion at 0.05 mg/kg/hr) regimens showing complete suppression for four and 24 hours, respectively. Alexion is developing pexelizumab in collaboration with Procter & Gamble Pharmaceuticals.

INDICATION(S) AND RESEARCH PHASE
Cardiac Surgery – Phase IIb completed
Myocardial Infarction – Phase IIb completed

rPSGL-Ig
unknown

MANUFACTURER
Wyeth-Ayerst

DESCRIPTION
rPSGL-Ig is a p-selectin antagonist being evaluated as a potential treatment to prevent the reformation of blood clots. It is currently being developed in phase II trials in subjects being treated for acute myocardial infarction.

INDICATION(S) AND RESEARCH PHASE
Myocardial Infarction – Phase II

SB 214857
Lotrafiban

MANUFACTURER
GlaxoSmithKline

DESCRIPTION
Lotrafiban is an orally active glycoprotein (IIb/IIIa) blocker of the fibrinogen receptor. The company decided to terminate clinical investigation of lotrafiban, which was in a phase III trial to evaluate its utility in preventing recurrent strokes and heart attacks. This decision was based on the recommendation of an independent data and safety monitoring board, which found a lack of efficacy and raised safety concerns.

INDICATION(S) AND RESEARCH PHASE
Myocardial Infarction – Trial discontinued
Strokes – Trial discontinued

TP10
unknown

MANUFACTURER
AVANT Immunotherapeutics

DESCRIPTION
TP10 is a genetically engineered (recombinant) soluble complement receptor-1 (sCR1). Complement-1 is a naturally occurring substance that binds to antibodies as part of the immune response to infection or foreign bodies. Clinical trials are testing TP10 in an intravenous formulation for a variety of disorders including the treatment of acute respiratory distress syndrome (ARDS), reperfusion injury, heart attack, cardiac surgery, organ reperfusion, xenotransplantation, allotransplantation, and post-surgical complications in infants.

A phase IIb trial was initiated in January 2001 in approximately 30 infants undergoing high risk cardiac surgery utilizing cardiopulmonary bypass. The trial will be conducted at seven sites in the United States.

INDICATION(S) AND RESEARCH PHASE
Acute Respiratory Distress Syndrome (ARDS) – Phase II/III
Cardiac Ischemia – Phase I/II
Cardiac Surgery – Phase IIb
Myocardial Infarction – Phase I/II
Pediatric, Post-surgical Complications – Phase I/II
Pediatric, Cardiac Surgery – Phase IIb

unknown
Amiscan

MANUFACTURER
Draximage

DESCRIPTION
Amiscan is a technetium-99m labelled derivative of D-glucaric acid used for the imaging of acute myocardial infarction (AMI) or heart attack. Amiscan was developed in conjunction with Molecular Targeting Technology and is in phase I clinical trials. The first trial will enroll 10 subjects and will be conducted at the Centre Hospitalier de l'Université de Montréal, Canada.

INDICATION(S) AND RESEARCH PHASE
Myocardial Infarction – Phase I

valsartan
Diovan

MANUFACTURER
Novartis

DESCRIPTION
Diovan is an oral angiotensin II receptor antagonist in phase III development for the treatment of post- and pre-myocardial infarction and congestive heart failure. Diovan blocks the action of angiotensin II (AT-II), a hormone formed when a precursor (angiotensin I) is cleaved by an enzyme in the lungs and blood vessels. In this manner, Diovan blocks the vasoconstriction of blood vessels and the aldosterone-secreting effects of AT-II.

Diovan has been FDA approved for the treatment of hypertension in elderly subjects. It is currently being marketed by Novartis with this indication.

INDICATION(S) AND RESEARCH PHASE
Congestive Heart Failure – Phase III
Myocardial Infarction – Phase III
Hypertension – FDA approved

Peripheral Arterial Occlusive Disease

Peripheral Vascular Disease

unknown
Antrin/Photoangioplasty

MANUFACTURER
Pharmacyclics

DESCRIPTION
Antrin is in a phase II trial for peripheral arterial disease (PAD). Photoangioplasty uses a laser light to activate an injected drug, which dissolves plaque in blood vessels. Upon exposure to light, the compound manufactures oxygen free radicals that cause mild damage to the plaque but leaves healthy tissue alone.

The phase II trial is evaluating the therapy as both a primary treatment of PAD and for preventing restenosis following balloon angioplasty. The trial consists of 375 subjects using two active treatment arms and one control arm. The company hopes the conclusions of the phase II trial will be measurable improvement at 180 days in angiography, ankle-brachial index (ABI), treadmill tests, intravascular ultrasonography (IVUS), and Ruetherford-Becker classification scores.

INDICATION(S) AND RESEARCH PHASE
In-stent Restenosis – Phase II
Peripheral Arterial Occlusive Disease – Phase II

ifetroban sodium, BMS-180291
unknown

MANUFACTURER
Bristol-Myers Squibb

DESCRIPTION
BMS-180291 is ifetroban sodium, an oral drug that may prevent the formation of blood clots. It works much like aspirin, by inhibiting the clumping, or aggregation, of platelets which are elements in the blood that promote coagulation. Ifetroban was designed to be given once a day to prevent thrombosis and ischemia.

According to the company, in animal studies ifetroban has been shown to reduce the tissue injury caused by inadequate blood flow related to coronary artery obstruction. If successful, BMS-180291 could replace current treatments for acute and chronic ischemic heart disease, such as calcium channel blockers and β blockers.

BMS-180291-02 is currently in a phase II trial for treatment of venous ulcers, with studies run jointly by PRI and ConvaTec. Phase II trials are also ongoing in the United States and Europe for cardiovascular indications. In addition, an exploratory phase II trial is taking place to evaluate ifetroban as a treatment for subjects with intermittent claudication, or leg pain, from peripheral arterial disease.

INDICATION(S) AND RESEARCH PHASE
Peripheral Vascular Disease – Phase II
Venous Leg Ulcers – Phase II
Peripheral Arterial Occlusive Disease – Phase II

MS-325
AngioMARK

MANUFACTURER
Mallinckrodt

DESCRIPTION
AngioMARK is a radiology contrast agent that makes pictures clearer for Magnetic Resonance Imaging (MRI) of large arteries. The agent is injected into the blood vessels and is especially useful to diagnose diseases of the aorta and its branches to the abdomen and legs, such as aortoiliac occlusive disease in subjects with known or suspected peripheral vascular disease or abdominal aortic aneurysm.

AngioMARK is in phase III trials, one of which compares the diagnostic accuracy of AngioMARK-enhanced MRI with that of X-ray angiography, the current standard procedure for diagnosing vascular disease. This study is designed to enroll 600 subjects at over 50 sites in the United States, Canada, and Europe.

INDICATION(S) AND RESEARCH PHASE
Vascular Diseases – Phase III
Peripheral Arterial Occlusive Disease – Phase III
Peripheral Vascular Disease – Phase III

prourokinase
Abbokinase

MANUFACTURER
Abbott Laboratories

DESCRIPTION
Abbokinase is a tissue plasminogen activator (TPA), which is a type of clot buster. It is being tested in phase III trials for the treatment of stroke and peripheral arterial occlusion. For strokes, the drug is given by intra-arterial administration to the brain.

INDICATION(S) AND RESEARCH PHASE
Peripheral Arterial Occlusive Disease – Phase III
Strokes – Phase III

unknown
Genvascor

MANUFACTURER
Collateral Therapeutics

DESCRIPTION
Genvascor is a non-surgical angiogenic gene therapy product for the treatment of subjects with peripheral vascular disease. Genvascor uses an adenovirus, a deactivated cold virus, vector to deliver FGF-4, a growth factor gene that triggers the production of a protein that causes new blood vessels to grow in ischemic regions of the leg. Collateral Therapeutics believes these vessels could provide an alternate route for blood flow around clogged or blocked arteries in the legs. A phase I/II trial is being conducted on 130 subjects at 10 major European medical centers.

INDICATION(S) AND RESEARCH PHASE
Peripheral Arterial Occlusive Disease – Phase I/II

Peripheral Vascular Disease

AC3056
unknown

Peripheral Vascular Disease

MANUFACTURER
Amylin Pharmaceuticals

DESCRIPTION
AC3056 is an antioxidant that inhibits vascular cell adhesion molecule expression. AC3056 has been tested in phase I trials for the prevention of restenosis following angioplasty and other procedures to open clogged arteries, as well as for the treatment of atherosclerosis. In a single-dose, double-blind, placebo-controlled study, 26 healthy subjects received an oral formulation of AC3056. Peak plasma levels of AC3056 observed in the study were comparable to levels necessary to exhibit vascular protective properties in preclinical studies. No safety concerns were noted.

INDICATION(S) AND RESEARCH PHASE
Peripheral Vascular Disease – Phase I completed

AGI-1067
unknown

MANUFACTURER
AtheroGenics

DESCRIPTION
AGI-1067 is an oral compound being evaluated for reducing cholesterol and treating atherosclerosis. The specific indication being tested in phase II clinical trials is post-angioplasty restenosis, in which the diseased blood vessel has become clogged up again after stent placement. A stent is a metallic scaffold that is placed inside the blood vessel to keep the wall from collapsing and allowing blood flow to remain normal.

Occasionally, the stent needs replacement when atherosclerotic plaques build up to block the passageway. AGI-1067 works by using a composite vascular protectant technology that may reduce the need for restenosis. AGI-1067 is being developed under an agreement between AtheroGenics and Schering-Plough Corporation.

INDICATION(S) AND RESEARCH PHASE
Peripheral Vascular Disease – Phase II
Cholesterol, High Levels – Phase II
In-stent Restenosis – Phase II

avasimibe
unknown

MANUFACTURER
Pfizer

DESCRIPTION
Avasimibe is a lipid-regulating ACAT inhibitor developed to prevent the accumulation of atherosclerotic plaque occurring in peripheral vascular disease. ACAT inhibitors function based on the theory that a drug stopping the production of an enzyme known as ACAT should reduce the accumulation of plaque that clogs and hardens arteries. In addition, ACAT inhibitors may also reduce total cholesterol levels. In early studies, avasimibe did not show the adrenal toxicity that has been seen with competitor compounds in this class. The drug is currently in phase III trials.

INDICATION(S) AND RESEARCH PHASE
Peripheral Vascular Disease – Phase III

CP-529,414
unknown

MANUFACTURER
Pfizer

DESCRIPTION
The administering of CP-529,414 results in dramatic increases in HDL levels. Pfizer is currently completing phase II trials for the treatment of peripheral vascular disease, and is exploring combinations with cholesterol-lowering agents such as Lipitor.

INDICATION(S) AND RESEARCH PHASE
Peripheral Vascular Disease – Phase II

ifetroban sodium, BMS-180291
unknown

MANUFACTURER
Bristol-Myers Squibb

DESCRIPTION
BMS-180291 is ifetroban sodium, an oral drug that may prevent the formation of blood clots. It works much like aspirin, by inhibiting the clumping, or aggregation, of platelets which are elements in the blood that promote coagulation. Ifetroban was designed to be given once a day to prevent thrombosis and interruption of ischemia.

According to the company, in animal studies ifetroban has been shown to reduce the tissue injury caused by inadequate blood flow related to coronary artery obstruction. If successful, BMS-180291 could replace current treatments for acute and chronic ischemic heart disease, such as calcium channel blockers and β blockers.

BMS-180291-02 is currently in a phase II trial for treatment of venous ulcers, with studies run jointly by PRI and ConvaTec. Phase II trials are also ongoing in the United States and Europe for cardiovascular indications. In addition, an exploratory phase II trial is taking place to evaluate ifetroban as a treatment for subjects with intermittent claudication, or leg pain, from peripheral arterial disease.

INDICATION(S) AND RESEARCH PHASE
Peripheral Vascular Disease – Phase II
Venous Leg Ulcers – Phase II
Peripheral Arterial Occlusive Disease – Phase II

iloprost
unknown

MANUFACTURER
Berlex Laboratories

DESCRIPTION
Iloprost is a novel prostacyclin derivative for peripheral vascular diseases, which are disorders of the arms and legs involving arteries and veins. Prostacyclins protect blood vessels, and are normally made and broken down by the body. Berlex Laboratories is conducting a phase III trial with iloprost.

INDICATION(S) AND RESEARCH PHASE
Peripheral Vascular Disease – Phase III

MS-325
AngioMARK

MANUFACTURER
Mallinckrodt

DESCRIPTION
AngioMARK is a radiology contrast agent that makes pictures clearer for Magnetic Resonance Imaging (MRI) of large arteries. The agent is injected into the blood vessels and is especially useful to diagnose diseases of the aorta and its branches to the abdomen and legs, such as aortoiliac occlusive disease in subjects with known or suspected peripheral vascular disease or abdominal aortic aneurysm.

AngioMARK is in phase III trials, one of which compares the diagnostic accuracy of AngioMARK-enhanced MRI with that of X-ray angiography, the current standard procedure for diagnosing vascular disease. This study is designed to enroll 600 subjects at over 50 sites in the United States, Canada, and Europe.

INDICATION(S) AND RESEARCH PHASE
Vascular Diseases – Phase III
Peripheral Arterial Occlusive Disease – Phase III
Peripheral Vascular Disease – Phase III

propionyl-L-carnitine
Dromos

MANUFACTURER
Sigma-Tau Pharmaceuticals

DESCRIPTION
Dromos (propionyl-L-carnitine) is an oral derivative of levocarnitine, a naturally occurring substance needed in energy metabolism. Levocarnitine is a carrier molecule in the transport of long-chain fatty acids across the inner mitochondrial membrane where the body makes energy. Fatty acids are used as an energy substrate or fuel for the cells to burn.

Dromos has demonstrated unique cardiovascular effects in clinical studies. This drug is being tested in an oral formulation for treatment of peripheral vascular disease. A narrowing or obstruction of a large or medium artery supplying the limbs causes peripheral arterial disease. The primary symptom is pain during leg movement or intermittent claudication. Peripheral arterial disease of the lower extremities affects about 2% of the overall population, becoming more prevalent with age. It is a major cause of disability in the United States. Sigma-Tau S.p.A. has completed phase III clinical trials in 6,000 subjects with peripheral arterial disease and chronic heart failure in clinical trials conducted in both Europe and the United States.

INDICATION(S) AND RESEARCH PHASE
Peripheral Vascular Disease – Phase III

SB 435495
unknown

MANUFACTURER
GlaxoSmithKline

DESCRIPTION
SB 435495 is an Lp-PLA2 inhibitor being developed for the treatment of atherosclerosis. It is currently in phase I development.

INDICATION(S) AND RESEARCH PHASE
Peripheral Vascular Disease – Phase I

trafermin
Fiblast

MANUFACTURER
Chiron Corporation

DESCRIPTION
Fibroblast growth factor (FGF) is normally synthesized in response to insufficient blood supply caused by diseased arteries. Fiblast is a recombinant form of basic fibroblast growth factor (bFGF) developed to stimulate new blood vessel growth in the hearts of subjects with severe coronary artery disease. The drug is currently in phase II trials for coronary artery disease and has completed a phase II trial for treatment of peripheral vascular disease.

Scios has licensed rights to develop Fiblast to several companies, including Chiron. In November 1999, Scios and Chiron entered into a patent and license agreement under which Scios has licensed to Chiron its rights in human bFGF. Additionally, Scios has licensed FGF to Kaken Pharmaceutical of Japan for development in Japan, China, Taiwan, and South Korea. Kaken has initially investigated the use of FGF as a wound healing treatment and is seeking approval to market FGF in Japan.

INDICATION(S) AND RESEARCH PHASE
Coronary Artery Disease – Phase II
Peripheral Vascular Disease – Phase II completed

unknown
Beraprost

MANUFACTURER
United Therapeutics

DESCRIPTION
Beraprost is a chemically stable oral form of prostacyclin that dilates blood vessels, prevents platelet aggregation, and prevents proliferation of smooth muscle cells surrounding blood vessels. It is in phase III trials for both early-stage peripheral vascular disease and early-stage pulmonary hypertension, in an immediate-release oral formulation.

INDICATION(S) AND RESEARCH PHASE
Peripheral Vascular Disease – Phase III
Hypertension – Phase III

unknown
VasoCare

MANUFACTURER
Vasogen

DESCRIPTION
Vasogen's proprietary VasoCare therapy has been developed to target immune processes that lead to inflammatory damage to the vascular endothelium. In November 2000, Vasogen announced positive clinical trial results of VasoCare therapy in subjects with peripheral vascular disease (PVD). The randomized, double-blind, placebo-controlled trial, completed in 81 subjects at two centers in the United Kingdom, achieved its primary endpoint. The trial showed that significantly more subjects receiving VasoCare therapy had a greater than 50% increase in

their walking distances compared to placebo. In addition to enabling subjects to walk farther before the onset of pain, VasoCare therapy was shown to be long lasting, well tolerated, and free of significant adverse side effects. Phase II trials are currently under way.

INDICATION(S) AND RESEARCH PHASE
Peripheral Vascular Disease – Phase II

UT-15
unknown

MANUFACTURER
United Therapeutics

DESCRIPTION
UT-15 is a formulation of prostacyclin that is delivered continuously through the MiniMed subcutaneous system. UT-15 is a particularly long-lived and stable version of prostacyclin, and because the MiniMed system operates by subcutaneous infusion rather than intravenous injection, there is less risk of infection. The product is in phase II development for the treatment of late-stage peripheral vascular disease and has also been developed for treatment of pulmonary hypertension.

In November 2000, United Therapeutics announced that the NDA submitted for UT-15 for the treatment of pulmonary hypertension was accepted by the FDA. The company anticipates a six-month priority review status.

INDICATION(S) AND RESEARCH PHASE
Hypertension – NDA submitted
Peripheral Vascular Disease – Phase II

vascular endothelial growth factor-121 (VEGF)
BioByPass

MANUFACTURER
GenVec

DESCRIPTION
Vascular endothelial growth factor-121 (VEGF) incorporates the VEGF gene into a replication-deficient adenovirus vector. VEGF is the body's potent natural growth factor that stimulates endothelial cells in blood vessels to migrate, replicate, and form new blood vessels.

BioByPass is being tested in phase II trials for coronary artery disease (CAD) and peripheral vascular disease (PVD).

INDICATION(S) AND RESEARCH PHASE
Coronary Artery Disease – Phase II
Peripheral Vascular Disease – Phase II

VEGF121
unknown

MANUFACTURER
Scios

DESCRIPTION
Vascular endothelial growth factor (VEGF) is one of a number of cytokines associated with angiogenesis. A 121 residue isoform of DNA encoding VEGF has been cloned and is called BioByPass angiogen. When expressed, this gene encodes biologically active VEGF. Phase II trials for VEGF121 are under way for the treatment of coronary artery disease and peripheral vascular disease.

INDICATION(S) AND RESEARCH PHASE
Coronary Artery Disease – Phase II
Peripheral Vascular Disease – Phase II

Thrombosis

ancrod
Viprinex

MANUFACTURER
Knoll Pharmaceutical

DESCRIPTION
Viprinex is a venom derived from snakes (viper *Agkistrodon rhodostoma*). It is a defibrinogenator being tested in phase III trials for treatment of ischemic (cerebral) stroke, as well as for establishing and maintaining anticoagulation in heparin-intolerant subjects undergoing cardiopulmonary bypass surgery.

INDICATION(S) AND RESEARCH PHASE
Cardiac Surgery – Phase III
Strokes – Phase III
Thrombosis – Phase III

antithrombin III, rhATIII
unknown

MANUFACTURER
Genzyme Genetics Division

DESCRIPTION
Antithrombin-III (AT-III) is a genetically altered form of a naturally occurring plasma protein that helps control blood clotting. This drug has just finished phase III testing for prevention of thrombosis, specializing in subjects undergoing cardiac surgery requiring cardiopulmonary bypass. This therapy may be helpful in subjects who have either acquired or hereditary AT-III deficiencies, by restoring heparin sensitivity to heparin-resistant subjects experiencing cardiopulmonary bypass.

INDICATION(S) AND RESEARCH PHASE
Thrombosis – Phase III completed
Cardiac Surgery – Phase III completed

AR69931
unknown

MANUFACTURER
AstraZeneca

DESCRIPTION
AR69931 is an enzyme inhibitor of thrombin that may help block this protein's ability to form blood clots. This drug is currently in a phase II study to prevent angina and thrombosis.

INDICATION(S) AND RESEARCH PHASE
Angina – Phase II
Thrombosis – Phase II

AZD 6140 (AR-C126532)
unknown

MANUFACTURER
AstraZeneca

DESCRIPTION
AZD 6140 is a P2T antagonist in an oral formulation, indicated for the treatment of arterial thrombosis. It is currently in phase I trials.

INDICATION(S) AND RESEARCH PHASE
Thrombosis – Phase I

bivalirudin
Angiomax

MANUFACTURER
The Medicines Company

DESCRIPTION
Angiomax, formerly called Hirulog, is a synthetic derivate of hirudin, an anticoagulant from the leech medicinals, that inhibits the formulation of blood clots. Angiomax is in a phase II trial at the Duke University Medical Center testing 50–100 subjects with heparin-induced thrombocytopenia (HIT) or heparin-induced thrombocytopenia and thrombosis syndrome (HITTS).

The FDA approved Angiomax on May 17, 2000 for the use as an anticoagulant in subjects with unstable angina undergoing percutaneous transluminal coronary angioplasty (PTCA). Angiomax is intended for use with aspirin and has been studied only in subjects receiving concomitant aspirin. The FDA approval was based on data from double-blind clinical trials of 4,312 subjects.

INDICATION(S) AND RESEARCH PHASE
Thrombosis – Phase II
Angina – FDA approved

CCI-1004
unknown

MANUFACTURER
Conjuchem

DESCRIPTION
CCI-1004, a new generation thrombin inhibitor that prevents local blood clot formation, is in phase I/II trials for the treatment of thrombosis. The trial is taking place at five sites and involves 12 hemodialysis subjects.

CCI-1004 can be delivered locally to a defined site in the body. It bonds to locally fixed proteins, and as a result, high levels of sustained drug activity in a specific area are obtained. This limits the systemic exposure of CCI-1004 and reduces the side effects, such as systemic bleeding, as seen with classic anticoagulants.

INDICATION(S) AND RESEARCH PHASE
Thrombosis – Phase I/II

desirudin/recombinant hirudin
Revasc

MANUFACTURER
Aventis

DESCRIPTION
Desirudin is a recombined form of hirudin, the active oral secretion product of leeches, known for its ability to prevent blood coagulation. Desirudin is being tested in a phase II trial for the prevention of deep vein thrombosis (DVT) after orthopedic (hip) surgery.

INDICATION(S) AND RESEARCH PHASE
Orthopedic (hip) Surgery – Phase III
Thrombosis – Phase III

DPC-444
unknown

MANUFACTURER
Du Pont

DESCRIPTION
DPC-444 is a pharmaceutical agent that is radioactively labeled with Tc-99m. This radiopharmaceutical is currently being tested for blood clot, or thrombosis, imaging in a phase III trial. A phase III trial for the detection of silent ischemia in type II diabetes has been completed.

INDICATION(S) AND RESEARCH PHASE
Thrombosis – Phase III
Diabetes Mellitus Types I and II – Phase III completed

enoxaparin sodium
Lovenox/Clexane

MANUFACTURER
Aventis

DESCRIPTION
Lovenox/Clexane is in trials for the prevention of deep-vein thrombosis (DVT) in adult trauma subjects and in pediatric subjects.

Lovenox/Clexane is also being tested in a phase III trial for the prevention of acute cardiac ischemia (not enough oxygen being delivered to the heart muscle) following stent placement. A stent, a medical device, is placed inside the coronary artery (an important oxygen rich blood vessel supplying the heart) to keep it open to help the blood flow. Lovenox/Clexane may prevent blood clots from forming around the stent area.

INDICATION(S) AND RESEARCH PHASE
Thrombosis – Phase III
Pediatric, Thrombosis – Phase III
Cardiac Ischemia – Phase III

GW 473178
unknown

MANUFACTURER
GlaxoSmithKline

DESCRIPTION
GW 473178 is a thrombin inhibitor being developed for use in subjects with atrial fibrillation and venous thrombosis. It is currently in phase I trials.

INDICATION(S) AND RESEARCH PHASE
Arrhythmia – Phase I
Thrombosis – Phase I

melagatran
unknown

MANUFACTURER
AstraZeneca

DESCRIPTION

Melagatran is an inhibitor of thrombin, the enzyme responsible for blood clot formation. This drug is being evaluated in a phase III clinical trial for the treatment of venous thrombosis, in a subcutaneous formulation.

INDICATION(S) AND RESEARCH PHASE
Thrombosis – Phase III

NCX 4016
unknown

MANUFACTURER
NicOx SA

DESCRIPTION
NCX 4016 is a nitric oxide-releasing derivative of acetylsalicylic acid, the active ingredient in aspirin. NCX 4016 may be able to provide the antithrombotic effects of aspirin with less gastric damage or toxicity. Also, studies suggest that nitric oxide itself may provide antithrombotic activity, and NCX 4016, unlike other treatments, may inhibit almost all phases of the blood clotting process. The compound is in phase I development for pain, inflammation, and prevention of cardiovascular diseases including thrombosis.

INDICATION(S) AND RESEARCH PHASE
Pain, Acute or Chronic – Phase I
Thrombosis – Phase I

ORG-31540/SR-90107A
unknown

MANUFACTURER
Organon

DESCRIPTION
ORG-31540/SR-90107A is a synthetic 5-unit multi-sugar (pentasaccharide) that may be used in the prevention and treatment of blood clots, or thrombi, that form in the veins and arteries. It is a synthetic antithrombotic with its molecular shape modeled after antithrombin III, a protein molecule involved in blood clotting.

Results of an international phase III program demonstrated that ORG31540/SR90107A provided a superior benefit over enoxaparin in major orthopedic surgery subjects, with an overall relative risk reduction of 50% and a similar safety profile. Four multicenter phase III trials compared the two drugs in the prevention of venous thromboembolism (VTE): EPHESUS (hip replacement surgery), PENTATHLON (hip replacement surgery), PENTHIFRA (hip fracture surgery), and PENTAMAKS (major knee surgery).

Future indications may include prevention and/or treatment of deep vein thrombosis, pulmonary embolism, and coronary and peripheral arterial disease. ORG-31540/SR-90107A is being co-developed by Sanofi-Synthelabo and Organon.

INDICATION(S) AND RESEARCH PHASE
Orthopedic Surgery – Phase III completed
Thrombosis – Phase III completed

poloxamer 188 N.F., CRL-5861
Flocor

MANUFACTURER
CytRx Corporation

DESCRIPTION
Flocor is an injectable drug that may improve blood flow. It is a type of surfactant, a purified form of poloxamer 188, non-ionic copolymer, which is a surface-active agent, like soap, that helps reduce surface tension on blood cells to keep fluids flowing.

Flocor is in a phase I/II study in subjects with acute lung injury. This clinical trial is being conducted at Vanderbilt University Medical Center in Nashville, Tennessee. In acute lung injury, arterial and venous microvascular obstructions contribute to the severity of pulmonary dysfunction. Flocor is being evaluated for the prevention of secondary platelet aggregation and stasis-related capillary obstruction, and the development and propagation of dynamic blood clots, or thrombi.

Flocor is also being evaluated in a pivotal phase III study for the treatment of the acute painful crisis in sickle cell subjects ages ten and over, and a phase I study in sickle cell subjects with acute chest syndrome.

INDICATION(S) AND RESEARCH PHASE
Anemia, Sickle Cell – Phase III
Anemia, Sickle Cell – Phase I
Lung Injury – Phase I/II
Thrombosis – Phase I/II
Pediatric, Sickle Cell Disease – Phase III

rNAPc2
unknown

MANUFACTURER
Corvas International

DESCRIPTION
Recombinant Nematode Anticoagulant Protein c2 (rNAPc2) is a recombinant protein that was originally discovered by Corvas scientists in blood-feeding hookworms. It is a potent inhibitor of the factor VIIa/tissue factor protease complex, which is required for the initiation of blood clot formation.

Results of a phase II trial of rNAPc2 demonstrated that, in the largest subject cohort, rNAPc2 reduced the risk of developing deep vein thrombosis (DVT) by greater than 50% compared to a contemporary historical control of low molecular weight heparin (LMWH). The open-label dose-ranging trial was conducted in 293 subjects undergoing unilateral knee replacement at sites in the United States, Canada, the Netherlands, and Italy. The incidence of total DVT in the largest cohort was 12.2% in 74 evaluated subjects treated with rNAPc2 versus an incidence of 25–27% treated with a historical control for LMWH. The incidence of major bleeding following rNAPc2 prophylaxis was 2.3% versus a historical control value of 3% for LMWH.

rNAPc2 is also being evaluated in a phase IIa trial in subjects undergoing elective percutaneous transluminal coronary angioplasty (PTCA). The purpose of the PTCA trial is to establish safety prior to conducting additional trials in subjects with unstable angina.

INDICATION(S) AND RESEARCH PHASE
Thrombosis – Phase II
Cardiac Surgery – Phase IIa

SR-34006
unknown

MANUFACTURER
Sanofi-Synthelabo Pharmaceuticals

DESCRIPTION
SR-34006 is a new drug that may be a safer, more controllable anticoagulant than the ones currently in clinical use. Thrombosis occurs when some injury to the blood vessel lining or some medical predisposition causes platelets to aggregate within the blood vessel. This inappropriate clot formation attracts other structural proteins such as fibrin, which further enlarges the blood clot, or thrombus. The thrombus either remains lodged within the vessel, blocking blood flow and causing venous obstruction, or may dislodge from its site of origin, travel to the lungs, and cause a life-threatening blood clot in the lungs, a pulmonary embolus.

Subjects with blood disorders, limited mobility, recent surgery, or heart arrythmias are at greater risk for thrombus formation and therefore, should be on anticoagulant therapy, most often being coumadin therapy. The challenge with coumadin is that blood levels do not correlate well with the doses given, and therefore, subjects need to be monitored closely to guard against inadequate or excessive anticoagulation.

SR-34006 is a synthetic molecule with anticoagulant action. In preliminary studies, it was well tolerated with a better side effect profile than that of established anti-coagulants. The doses given may produce therapeutic blood levels more controllably and precisely than with coumadin. This linear dose-blood level relationship may further reduce potentially serious side effects and toxicities. It is designed to be given in a once-weekly regimen and is currently in phase II trials.

INDICATION(S) AND RESEARCH PHASE
Thrombosis – Phase II

technetium-99m-labeled FBD
Fibrimage

MANUFACTURER
Draximage

DESCRIPTION
Fibrimage is a radioactively labeled (technetium-99m) peptide for imaging an active thrombus, or blood clot formation in deep vein thrombosis. It is an intravenously administered product based on fibrin-binding domain (FBD), a genetically engineered (recombinant) polypeptide that binds fibrin. Fibrimage is currently in a phase III multicenter trial in Canada, during which subjects are given the drug and have images taken at two time points.

INDICATION(S) AND RESEARCH PHASE
Thrombosis – Phase III

unknown
Argatroban

MANUFACTURER
Texas Biotechnology

DESCRIPTION
A phase II multi-center, placebo-controlled trial (ARGIS-1) is evaluating the use of Argatroban in patients with acute ischemic stroke. Aragtroban is a direct thrombin inhibitor which may influence the primary clot causing a stroke, as well as the collateral and microcirculation of the brain in and around the original infarction. Through this mechanism, it is possible that additional clots may be prevented from forming. It is approved in Japan for this indication and is FDA approved as an anticoagulant for the prophylaxis or treatment of thrombosis in patients with heparin-induced thrombocytopenia.

INDICATION(S) AND RESEARCH PHASE
Strokes – Phase II
Thrombosis – FDA approved

ZD4927
unknown

MANUFACTURER
AstraZeneca

DESCRIPTION
ZD4927 is a factor Xa inhibitor indicated for the treatment of thrombosis. It is currently in phase I trials.

INDICATION(S) AND RESEARCH PHASE
Thrombosis – Phase I

Vascular Diseases

ApoA-I Milano
unknown

MANUFACTURER
Esperion Therapeutics

DESCRIPTION
ApoA-I Milano is a high density lipoprotein that is believed to protect against vascular disease by extracting cholesterol from the artery wall and transporting it to the liver for removal. ApoA-I Milano is currently in phase I trials for cardiovascular and metabolic diseases.

INDICATION(S) AND RESEARCH PHASE
Vascular Diseases – Phase I
Metabolic Disease – Phase I

MS-325
AngioMARK

MANUFACTURER
Mallinckrodt

DESCRIPTION
AngioMARK is a radiology contrast agent that makes pictures clearer for Magnetic Resonance Imaging (MRI) of large arteries. The agent is injected into the blood vessels and is especially useful to diagnose diseases of the aorta and its branches to the abdomen and legs, such as aortoiliac occlusive disease in subjects with known or suspected peripheral vascular disease or abdominal aortic aneurysm.

AngioMARK is in phase III trials, one of which compares the diagnostic accuracy of AngioMARK-enhanced MRI with that of X-ray angiography, the current standard procedure for diagnosing vascular disease. This study is designed to enroll 600 subjects at over 50 sites in the United States, Canada, and Europe.

INDICATION(S) AND RESEARCH PHASE
Vascular Diseases – Phase III
Peripheral Arterial Occlusive Disease –
  Phase III
Peripheral Vascular Disease – Phase III

2 | Hematology

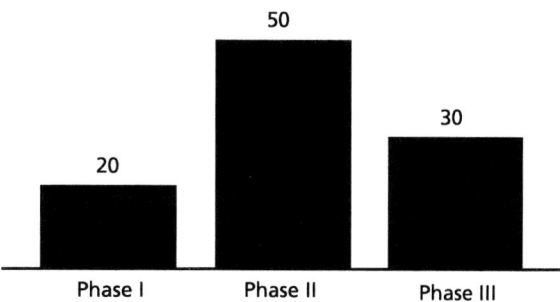

Drugs in the development pipeline

Phase I: 20
Phase II: 50
Phase III: 30

Source: CenterWatch, 2001

CenterWatch has identified over 100 drugs currently involved in clinical trials for the treatment of hematological diseases. The three hematological disorders most widely studied include leukemia, lymphoma, and myeloma. Each of these conditions is a malignancy of the bone marrow and lymph nodes.

According to the American Cancer Society, each year 28,000 adults and more than 2,500 children in the United States develop new cases of leukemia, and approximately 22,000 will die from the disease. Leukemia is the leading cause of death in children under age 15. Leukemia is a malignant disease of the bone marrow and blood. It is characterized by the uncontrolled growth of blood cells. The common types of leukemia are myelogenous or lymphocytic, each of which can be acute or chronic. Acute leukemia is a rapidly progressing disease that results in the accumulation of immature, functionless cells in the marrow and blood. The marrow often can no longer produce enough normal red and white blood cells and platelets. Anemia develops in virtually all patients with leukemia. The lack of normal white cells impairs the body's defense against infections. Thrombocytopenia results in bruising and easy bleeding. Chronic leukemia progresses more slowly and permits greater numbers of more mature, functional cells to be made.

Though still high, death rates for leukemia have dropped 21% in adults under the age of 65 in the past 20 years and 57% in children over the last three decades. This decline in mortality reflects the strides being made in research and treatment of the disease. CenterWatch estimates that between $160 million and $190 million will be spent this year in clinical research on the 35 drugs in the pipeline for treatment of leukemia. The aim of treatment is complete remission, meaning that there is no evidence of the disease and the patient returns to good health, with normal blood and marrow cells. For leukemia, a complete remission that lasts five years after treatment often indicates cure.

Lymphoma is a general term for a group of cancers that originate in the lymphatic system, which includes the lymph nodes, the spleen, the gastrointestinal tract, and the thymus in children. Lymphoma results when a lymphocyte undergoes a malignant change Approximately 454,000 members of the U.S. population are living with lymphoma and over 62,000 new cases are expected to be diagnosed this year. Similar to that in leukemia, the rate of recovery from lymphoma has seen a significant turnaround in the past 30 years. Less than 20 years ago the majority of children with lymphoma did not live five years after diagnosis. Today the five year survival rate is almost 80 percent. These advances are largely due to the development of effective combination therapy regimens for the treatment of these diseases. CenterWatch estimates that between $50 million and $70 million will be spent this year developing the 14 drugs in the pipeline for the treatment of lymphomas.

Myeloma is a malignancy of plasma cells. Patients with myeloma develop bone pain, and may be susceptible to many different infections. Malignant plasma cells produce an abnormal protein called monoclonal immunoglobulin. The onset of myeloma interferes with normal production of antibodies. Each year approximately 14,000 new cases of myeloma will be diagnosed and 11,500 people will die from the disease. CenterWatch reports that 14 drugs are currently being developed for treatment of myeloma, with an estimated cost of $65 million to $80 million this year.

The use of chemotherapy, usually in combinations of two or more drugs, is largely responsible for the dramatic improvement in managing leukemia, lymphoma, and myeloma. Approximately 40 different drugs are now being used in the treatment of these diseases. Lymphoma patients, and some patients with acute lymphocytic leukemia, also can be treated with radiation therapy. Chemotherapy plus radiation may also be useful for select patients with lymphoma. Bone marrow transplantation was introduced about 30 years and is now standard therapy for selected patients with leukemia, lymphoma, and myeloma.

Clinical development for the treatment of leukemia, lymphoma, and myeloma can be placed in one of four areas. New drug developments are currently evaluating the use of thalidomide to stop the progression of myeloma, and interferon-alpha for the treatment of chronic myelogenous leukemia. Antibody treatment, immune cell administration, and vaccine development are three types of immunotherapy currently being explored. Immunotherapy is designed to enhance the immune system's ability to suppress leukemia, lymphoma, or myeloma progression and to minimize toxic effects on normal tissues.

The malignant cells of patients have mechanisms that may allow them to escape the damaging effects of chemotherapy agents. These cells are, or become, less responsive to therapy. Approaches to reversing multi-drug resistance are being evaluated. Lastly, through gene therapy, scientists are studying two approaches directed at attacking leukemic cells by turning off the oncogene or its product, the oncoprotein, therefore preventing the tranformation of a normal cell into a malignant cell.

Anemia

CPC-111
Cordox

MANUFACTURER
Questcor

DESCRIPTION
Cordox is a fructose-1,6-diphosphate, a naturally occurring small molecule that has a protective effect on cells, especially red blood cells. This drug is being evaluated in a phase III trial for its ability to improve the biochemical and physical characteristics of stored human red blood cells. According to Questcor, Cordox is expected to increase the shelf-life of blood from the current maximum level of 42 days to eight to ten weeks.

In 2000, a trial evaluating Cordox as an analgesic agent for the treatment of sickle cell disease painful crises was terminated. As of January 2001, the data from enrolled subjects is under review. A pediatric phase II trial for treatment of sickle cell disease has been completed.

INDICATION(S) AND RESEARCH PHASE
Anemia, Sickle cell – Phase Discontinued
Blood Preservative – Phase III
Pediatric, Sickle Cell Disease – Phase II completed

decitabine
unknown

MANUFACTURER
SuperGen

DESCRIPTION
Decitabine is an investigational chemotherapeutic agent in development for the treatment of sickle cell anemia and a variety of solid tumors and hematological malignancies, including myelodysplastic syndrome, non-small cell lung cancer, and chronic myelogenous leukemia. Decitabine inhibits DNA methyltransferase activity, and in this manner, presumably reactivates tumor suppressor genes.

In October 2000, results of a phase I/II trial of decitabine for sickle cell anemia demonstrated that it produced a response in 100% of subjects tested. The trial enrolled a total of eight subjects. Five had shown no response to hydroxyurea (HU) after one year of treatment, two had a moderate but unsustained response to HU, and one subject was not treated with HU. After administration of decitabine, the five subjects previously treated with HU experienced an average 35-fold increase of fetal hemoglobin levels compared to levels during HU treatment. The two subjects who responded briefly to HU experienced an average fetal hemoglobin level increase of 52% with decitabine, and the one subject who had not received HU treatment experienced a greater than 50% increase in fetal hemoglobin levels.

INDICATION(S) AND RESEARCH PHASE
Myelodysplastic Syndrome – Phase III
Lung Cancer – Phase II
Anemia – Phase I/II completed
Leukemia – Phase II

erythropoietin
Procrit

MANUFACTURER
R.W. Johnson Pharmaceutical Research Institute

DESCRIPTION
Procit (erythropoietin) is currently in phase III trials for anemia.

INDICATION(S) AND RESEARCH PHASE
Anemia – Phase III

gene-activated erythropoietin
Dynepo

MANUFACTURER
Transkaryotic Therapies

DESCRIPTION
Dynepo is a human erythropoietin produced through the use of gene activation technology. Sequences of DNA are inserted into human cells, activating a portion of the endogenous human gene and stimulating production of the gene-activated erythropoietin, Dynepo. Erythropoietin is a hormone that stimulates red blood cell production and is used as a treatment for anemia. Phase III trials have been completed for Dynepo as a treatment for anemia associated with renal disease and a NDA has been filed. Phase III trials are under way for anemia associated with chemotherapy. Dynepo is being co-developed by Aventis and Transkaryotic Therapies.

INDICATION(S) AND RESEARCH PHASE
Anemia – NDA submitted
Anemia – Phase III

hemoglobin glutamer-250 (bovine)
Hemopure

MANUFACTURER
Biopure Corporation

DESCRIPTION
Hemopure is a hemoglobin-based oxygen therapy solution originally derived from cows. Hemoglobin is a naturally produced protein containing iron that red blood cells use to transport oxygen from the lungs to the rest of the body. This blood substitute product is being tested for cases of anemia where more red blood cells and oxygen exchange would be needed. Hemopure is given intravenously and phase III trials are ongoing in the United States and recently have been expanded in Canada. Therapeutic uses may include sickle cell anemia, cardiopulmonary bypass surgery, and trauma. Biopure has completed a phase III trial evaluating Hemopure as an alternative to red blood cell transfusion in orthopedic surgery subjects.

INDICATION(S) AND RESEARCH PHASE
Anemia – Phase III
Orthopedic Surgery – Phase III completed

MDX-33
unknown

MANUFACTURER
Medarex

DESCRIPTION

MDX-33 is a humanized monoclonal antibody being evaluated for its ability to decrease the activity of monocytes, macrophages, or other white blood cells that can destroy healthy platelets or red blood cells. MDX-33 is in development for the treatment of autoimmune blood disorders such as idiopathic thrombocytopenia purpura (ITP) and autoimmune hemolytic anemia. Phase II trials for anemia are currently under way.

Results of a phase II trial of MDX-33 suggested the drug was well tolerated in adult subjects with chronic ITP. Additionally, a single dose of MDX-33 appeared to substantially elevate platelet counts in all subjects treated with the optimal dose. The dose-escalating, double-blind, placebo-controlled trial consisted of 30 adults with chronic ITP. MDX-33 is being developed through a corporate alliance between Medarex and Aventis Behring.

INDICATION(S) AND RESEARCH PHASE

Anemia – Phase II
Thrombocytopenia – Phase II completed

novel erythropoiesis stimulating protein (NESP)
unknown

MANUFACTURER
Amgen

DESCRIPTION

Novel erythropoiesis stimulating protein (NESP) is a compound that stimulates bone marrow to produce more red blood cells. NESP is currently in phase III trials to treat anemia associated with chronic renal failure, especially for pre-dialysis subjects.

INDICATION(S) AND RESEARCH PHASE

Anemia – Phase III
Kidney Disease – Phase III

poloxamer 188 N.F., CRL-5861
Flocor

MANUFACTURER
CytRx Corporation

DESCRIPTION

Flocor is an injectable drug that may improve blood flow. It is a type of surfactant, a purified form of poloxamer 188, non-ionic copolymer, which is a surface-active agent, like soap, that helps reduce surface tension on blood cells to keep fluids flowing.

Flocor is in a phase I/II study in subjects with acute lung injury. This clinical trial is being conducted at Vanderbilt University Medical Center in Nashville, Tennessee. In acute lung injury, arterial and venous microvascular obstructions contribute to the severity of pulmonary dysfunction. Flocor is being evaluated for the prevention of secondary platelet aggregation and stasis-related capillary obstruction, and the development and propagation of dynamic blood clots, or thrombi.

Flocor is also being evaluated in a pivotal phase III study for the treatment of the acute painful crisis in sickle cell subjects ages ten and over, and a phase I study in sickle cell subjects with acute chest syndrome.

INDICATION(S) AND RESEARCH PHASE

Anemia, Sickle Cell – Phase III
Anemia, Sickle Cell – Phase I
Lung Injury – Phase I/II
Thrombosis – Phase I/II
Pediatric, Sickle Cell Disease – Phase III

pyridoxalated hemoglobin polyoxyethylene (PHP)
unknown

MANUFACTURER
Apex Bioscience

DESCRIPTION

Apex Bioscience has manufactured a human red blood cell substitute called pyridoxalated hemoglobin polyoxethylene (PHP). The primary indication is for nitric oxide-induced shock, which may lead to therapy in the treatment of surgical septic shock. Other indications may include anemia and as a helpful aid to cancer chemotherapy. Phase III trials are expected to begin in 2001.

INDICATION(S) AND RESEARCH PHASE

Anemia – Phase II/III completed
Effects of Chemotherapy – Phase II/III completed
Sepsis and Septicemia – Phase II/III

RF-1010
unknown

MANUFACTURER
SuperGen

DESCRIPTION

RF-1010 is a hormone-like drug resembling a naturally occurring human product. This non-masculine, non-androgenic hormone is being tested for the treatment of blood cell disorders. It is currently in a phase II trial for treatment of aplastic anemia.

INDICATION(S) AND RESEARCH PHASE

Anemia – Phase II

RF-1012
unknown

MANUFACTURER
SuperGen

DESCRIPTION

SuperGen is developing RF-1012 to counteract the anemia, or red cell depletion, and leukopenia, or white cell depletion, often associated with chemotherapy and radiotherapy treatments. This drug is currently being evaluated in phase II trials, and is to be given in an intravenous formulation. Cancer treatments usually work by targeting steps in the process of cell replication, since cells usually become cancerous due to uncontrolled cell division. However, by giving systemic drugs that block cell division, cells undergoing normal division and growth may be unharmed, especially in the bone marrow where new red and white blood cells are born. This total body exposure to the drug may result in very low levels of red blood cells and white blood cells. This situation leads to fatigue, pallor, susceptibility to infections, and organ failure.

RF-1012 is a protective agent that may potentially limit the effect of chemotherapy and radiotherapy on normal, growing blood cells. This protective ability is crucial since cancer treatment regimens are frequently stopped because of severe anemia or leukopenia. This agent may also prevent life-threatening infections secondary to white blood cell depletion, congestive heart failure, and other organ damage resulting from a decline in red blood cells.

INDICATION(S) AND RESEARCH PHASE
Anemia – Phase II
Effects of Chemotherapy – Phase II
White Blood Cell Disorders – Phase II

unknown
MARstem

MANUFACTURER
Maret Pharmaceuticals

DESCRIPTION
MARstem is a peptide that resembles the human hormone angiotensin. The compound has shown promise as a therapy to stimulate the formation of red blood cells, white blood cells, and platelets when they are below normal levels. In preclinical studies, the drug was shown to minimize neutropenia following chemotherapy or radiation. It is a common effect of chemotherapy to lower the blood levels of neutrophils, which are a specialized type of granular white blood cells. Since neutrophils serve as the first line of defense for the immune system, decreased numbers may predispose to certain infections.

MARstem is in phase I development as a multilineage hematopoietic therapy to treat or prevent pancytopenia following chemotherapy in breast cancer subjects. It is also in phase I/II trials for the treatment of anemia in chronic renal failure subjects.

INDICATION(S) AND RESEARCH PHASE
Breast Cancer – Phase I
Anemia – Phase I/II

Bone Marrow Transplant

anti B-7 humanized antibodies
unknown

MANUFACTURER
Wyeth-Ayerst

DESCRIPTION
Anti B-7 humanized antibodies are being developed for the prevention of graft versus host disease (GvHD) following haploidentical bone marrow transplant and for preventing kidney rejection. Clinical trials are currently in phase I/II development.

INDICATION(S) AND RESEARCH PHASE
Immunosuppressive – Phase I/II
Kidney Transplant Surgery – Phase I/II
Bone Marrow Transplant – Phase I/II

immune globulin intravenous
Venoglobulin-S

MANUFACTURER
Alpha Therapeutic

DESCRIPTION
Venoglobulin-S is a solution of antibodies being tested in two phase III trials. The first is trial for prevention of infection, or prophylaxis, from the hepatitis A virus. The second is for prevention of acute graft versus host disease (GVHD) in bone marrow transplant subjects. Drug therapy can be helpful in preventing the body from rejecting a transplanted organ, or in the opposite case of the organ rejecting its new host.

This immune globulin product may replace missing antibodies, especially in subjects that have a compromised immune system or primary immunodeficiencies, which may be present at birth. It is given to a subject by intramuscular injection.

INDICATION(S) AND RESEARCH PHASE
Bone Marrow Transplant – Phase III
Hepatitis – Phase III

keratinocyte growth factor-2 (KGF-2)
Repifermin

MANUFACTURER
Human Genome Sciences

DESCRIPTION
Repifermin is a genomics-derived therapeutic protein drug, known as keratinocyte growth factor-2 (KGF-2). It is in a phase II study for the treatment of mucositis associated with bone marrow transplantation for the treatment of cancer. This trial is a randomized, double-blind, placebo-controlled, dose-escalation study that is being conducted at several sites in the United States. In addition, Repifermin is in a phase IIb trial for topical wound healing treatment of venous ulcers and a phase II trial for inflammatory bowel disease (IBD).

Results from phase I clinical trials showed that systemically administered Repifermin is safe and well tolerated in healthy human subjects at doses proposed for subsequent clinical studies. None of the subjects withdrew from the study or required dose modification because of adverse effects.

KGF-2 stimulates the growth of keratinocyte cells, which make up 95% of the epidermal cells. Together, keratinocyte and melanocyte cells form the epidermis of the body. The company claims that KGF-2 has demonstrated beneficial effects on both the dermal and epidermal tissues of the skin, healing full-thickness wounds in a short period of time. In mucositis, Repifermin may stimulate the creation of new mucosal tissue.

INDICATION(S) AND RESEARCH PHASE
Bone Marrow Transplant – Phase II
Skin Wounds – Phase IIb
Inflammatory Bowel Disease – Phase II

lisofylline, CT-1501R
ProTec

MANUFACTURER
Cell Therapeutics

DESCRIPTION
ProTec is a supportive care agent being tested for prevention or reduction of the occurrence of serious or fatal infection, mucositis, and mortality among cancer subjects receiving high-dose radiation and/or chemothera-

py. Most cancer therapies have toxic effects that cause serious problems for subjects, including low white blood cell counts and inflammation of the intestinal mucous membranes. Serious infection is a very common adverse effect of high dose cancer treatment, especially when the epithelial cells that line the gastrointestinal tract are damaged and no longer form a protective barrier from infectious bacteria. According to Cell Therapeutics, ProTec may protect this barrier and decrease the number of life-threatening infections in cancer subjects following bone marrow transplant. Enrollment has been completed in a phase III bone marrow transplant trial among unrelated donors, and results are pending.

Lisofylline was investigated in a phase III trial for newly diagnosed acute myeloid leukemia (AML), in subjects undergoing high dose induction chemotherapy. Results demonstrated ProTec did not reduce the number of new neutropenia associated infections. Though a lower number of fungal infections were observed, Cell Therapeutics indicated that they will terminate all ProTec research activity.

Some of the ProTec research trials with Cell Therapeutics were under collaboration and license agreement for joint development with Ortho Biotech, R.W. Johnson, and BioChem Pharma.

INDICATION(S) AND RESEARCH PHASE
Bone Marrow Transplant – Trial discontinued
Leukemia – Trial discontinued
Effects of Chemotherapy – Trial discontinued
Head and Neck Cancer – Trial discontinued

MDX-22
unknown

MANUFACTURER
Medarex

DESCRIPTION
MDX-22 is used to purge leukemia cells from the bone marrow of acute myeloid leukemia (AML) subjects who are undergoing a transplant of their own bone marrow. This therapy uses a monoclonal antibody to attack the abnormal leukemia cells. MDX-22 is currently in a phase II trial.

INDICATION(S) AND RESEARCH PHASE
Leukemia – Phase II
Bone Marrow Transplant – Phase II

recombinant human GM-CSF
Leucotropin

MANUFACTURER
Cangene Corporation

DESCRIPTION
Leucotropin was being tested in phase III trials in Canada to evaluate the drug's role in reversing hematologic toxicity induced by chemotherapy and bone marrow transplantation. Leucotropin is a protein that stimulates white blood cell growth. The trials included approximately 100 subjects and were expected to take 12 months to complete. Due to slow enrollment, the trials were discontinued in early 2001.

The trials were monitoring the impact of treatment on white blood cell counts, which affect rates of infection following high-dose cancer chemotherapy. Leucotropin is produced recombinantly in *Streptomyces* bacteria, using Cangene's Cangenus manufacturing system.

INDICATION(S) AND RESEARCH PHASE
Bone Marrow Transplant – Trial Discontinued
Effects of Chemotherapy – Trial Discontinued

tresperimus
unknown

MANUFACTURER
Fournier Research

DESCRIPTION
Tresperimus is a new immunosuppressive drug being formulated to protect bone marrow transplant subjects from graft versus host disease. It is currently in a phase III trial. Graft versus host disease is a potentially lethal condition that arises when the immunologically active, transplanted bone marrow cells attack the subject's immunocompromised body. This complication can cause anorexia, diarrhea, low white cell and platelet counts, growth retardation, and death.

Tresperimus may prevent graft versus host disease by stimulating the production of CD4 suppressor cells, immune cells that act to suppress the immunogenic activity of the donated bone marrow cells. This drug may also result in decreased amounts of another type of immune cell (CD8 cells), which acts to destroy tissue that the immune cells see as foreign. In other words, tresperimus may act to reduce the amount of destructive, attacker immune cells, while increasing the immune cells which act to suppress the potentially damaging immune reactions that lead to graft versus host disease. Further studies are needed to determine the precise clinical efficacy of this new immunosuppressive medication.

INDICATION(S) AND RESEARCH PHASE
Bone Marrow Transplant – Phase III

Hemochromatosis

ICL 670
unknown

MANUFACTURER
Novartis

DESCRIPTION
ICL 670 is an iron chelator being developed for oral administration. It is in phase II trials for the treatment of chronic iron overload.

INDICATION(S) AND RESEARCH PHASE
Hemochromatosis – Phase II

Hemophilia

antihemophilic factor
Alphanate

MANUFACTURER
Alpha Therapeutic

DESCRIPTION

Alphanate is a heat-treated human blood factor approved by the FDA to treat hemophilia A. It is a highly purified factor VIII, which is normally responsible for clotting blood to prevent hemorrhage. A phase IV trial is being conducted to further expand the safety and pharmacology characteristics.

A phase III study was completed for the treatment of von Willebrand's disease, another type of bleeding disorder, in children 7 years and older.

INDICATION(S) AND RESEARCH PHASE
Hemophilia – FDA approved/Phase IV
Pediatric, von Willebrand's disease – Phase III completed

factor VIII gene therapy
unknown

MANUFACTURER
Transkaryotic Therapies

DESCRIPTION
Factor VIII gene therapy, utilizing Transkaryotic Therapies, is being developed for the treatment of hemophilia A. Transkaryotic Therapies is the company's non-viral gene therapy system. A sample of a subject's cells are removed and genetically engineered to produce a desired protein for extended periods of time. The genetically engineered cells are then injected back into the subjects. The blood clotting protein factor VIII is deficient in subjects with hemophilia A, and in this manner therapeutic delivery of the protein can be established.

In December 2000, data from six subjects in a phase I trial for hemophilia A demonstrated that Transkaryotic Therapies' factor VIII gene therapy was safe and well tolerated. Following implantation of 100–400 million genetically modified cells, four of six subjects demonstrated decreased bleeding frequency and/or factor VIII usage. Additionally, two subjects did not experience spontaneous bleeds for approximately one year following treatment.

INDICATION(S) AND RESEARCH PHASE
Hemophilia – Phase I completed

factor VIII gene therapy
unknown

MANUFACTURER
Chiron Corporation

DESCRIPTION
Factor VIII gene therapy is designed to insert the gene coding for factor VIII into a person's cells. Factor VIII is an important protein in the blood clotting system. Subjects with hemophilia A lack adequate circulating factor VIII. Once factor VIII is reintroduced into the body and sufficiently expressed, bleeding episodes should be drastically reduced.

This therapy is currently in phase I trials.

INDICATION(S) AND RESEARCH PHASE
Hemophilia – Phase I

r-FVIIa
NovoSeven

MANUFACTURER
Novo Nordisk

DESCRIPTION
The coagulant NovoSeven is a recombinant factor VIIa developed for the treatment of hemophilia in subjects with inhibitors to factor VIIa. This recombinant protein induces hemostasis, stopping bleeding at the site of injury, independent of the presence of factor VIII or factor IX, by forming complexes with exposed tissue factor (TF). In the United States, NovoSeven has been approved for the treatment of bleeding episodes in hemophilia A or B subjects with inhibitors to factor VIII or factor IX.

NovoSeven is also in phase III trials for the prevention and treatment of bleeding episodes in subjects with coagulopathy, the inability of the blood to clot normally, associated with liver disease as well as phase II trials for coagulopathy associated with bone marrow transplantation and stroke.

INDICATION(S) AND RESEARCH PHASE
Bone Marrow Transplant – Phase II
Hemophilia – FDA approved
Liver Disease – Phase III
Stroke – Phase II

unknown
Coagulin-B

MANUFACTURER
Avigen

DESCRIPTION
Coagulin-B is an adeno-associated virus (AAV) vector, which carries the gene for factor IX, the missing or deficient protein that causes hemophilia B. Coagulin-B is designed to deliver the factor IX gene into the subject's muscle or liver cells where it will continuously produce factor IX. Results show Coagulin-B to be safe and well tolerated in all subjects treated with no untoward side effects of any kind being observed.

INDICATION(S) AND RESEARCH PHASE
Hemophilia – Phase III

Hemorrhage

Corleukin NIF
unknown

MANUFACTURER
Pfizer

DESCRIPTION
Corleukin NIF is an intravenous biosynthetic neutrophil inhibitory factor (NIF) being developed as an anti-inflammatory agent for treatment of ischemic stroke and hemorrhagic shock. Corleukin NIF prevents neutrophils from adhering to endothelial cells lining the blood vessels. Clinical trials are in phase II.

Future indications may include the treatment of adult respiratory distress syndrome. Pfizer has licensed Corleukin NIF from Corvas International and is responsible for the development of the compound.

INDICATION(S) AND RESEARCH PHASE
Hemorrhage – Phase II
Strokes – Phase II

fibrin sealant
unknown

MANUFACTURER
V.I. Technologies

DESCRIPTION
Fibrin sealant is being evaluated in a phase III trial for the prevention of hemorrhaging following surgery or accidental trauma. This drug is derived from human blood plasma and made of a combination of two proteins, fibrinogen and thrombin, both of which facilitate blood clotting.

INDICATION(S) AND RESEARCH PHASE
Hemorrhage – Phase III

hemoglobin
PolyHeme

MANUFACTURER
Northfield Laboratories

DESCRIPTION
PolyHeme is a solution of chemically modified hemoglobin derived from human blood. Hemoglobin is the oxygen-carrying component of the human red blood cell. First, hemoglobin is extracted from red blood cells and filtered to remove impurities. The purified hemoglobin is then chemically modified using a multi-step process to create a polymerized form of hemoglobin designed to avoid the undesirable effects historically associated with hemoglobin-based blood substitutes, including vasoconstriction, kidney dysfunction, liver dysfunction and gastrointestinal distress. Then the modified hemoglobin is incorporated into a solution which can be administered as an alternative to transfused blood. The result of this process is the product PolyHeme.

One unit of PolyHeme contains 50 grams of modified hemoglobin, approximately the same amount of hemoglobin delivered by one unit of transfused blood. PolyHeme is used for the treatment of subjects with acute blood loss resulting from trauma, surgery, and emergencies. PolyHeme is currently in phase III trials.

INDICATION(S) AND RESEARCH PHASE
Hemorrhage – Phase III

Hypercalcemia

zoledronate
Zometa

MANUFACTURER
Novartis

DESCRIPTION
Zometa is an intravenous bisphosphonate osteoclast inhibitor. In September 2000, Novartis announced it had received an approvable letter from the FDA for Zometa for the treatment of hypercalcemia of malignancy (HCM), the most common life-threatening metabolic complication associated with cancer. Zometa is also in phase II development for the treatment of post-menopausal osteoporosis and phase III development for bone metastasis treatment and prevention.

INDICATION(S) AND RESEARCH PHASE
Osteoporosis – Phase II
Hypercalcemia – FDA approvable letter
Bone Metastases – Phase III

Leukemia

aldesleukin, interleukin-2 (IL-2)
Proleukin

MANUFACTURER
Chiron Corporation

DESCRIPTION
Proleukin is a genetically engineered, recombinant form of interleukin-2, a naturally occurring immune modulator. Proleukin is being evaluated in a phase III trial for leukemia and non-Hodgkin's lymphoma and a phase II study for HIV infection. Proleukin was approved in July 2000 for advanced-stage kidney cancer and melanoma.

INDICATION(S) AND RESEARCH PHASE
HIV Infection – Phase III
Leukemia – Phase III
Lymphoma, Non-Hodgkin's – Phase III
Renal Cell Carcinoma – FDA approved
Melanoma – FDA approved

aminopterin
unknown

MANUFACTURER
ILEX Oncology

DESCRIPTION
Aminopterin is an anti-folate in the same family as methotrexate, a widely used anti-cancer drug. Although aminopterin has been around for many years, it went out of common use because it was difficult to synthesize and there were some concerns about its toxicity. Aminopterin kills tumor cells by interfering with their ability to synthesize DNA. It is currently being tested in phase II studies for the treatment of metastatic endometrial cancer resistant to methotrexate and other drugs, and acute lymphocytic leukemia. Aminopterin has received an orphan drug status for acute lymphocytic leukemia.

INDICATION(S) AND RESEARCH PHASE
Endometrial Cancer – Phase II
Leukemia – Phase II

AR-522
Annamycin

MANUFACTURER
Aronex Pharmaceuticals

DESCRIPTION
Annamycin is an anthracycline analogue intended to overcome multi-drug resistance and irreversible cardiotoxicity associated with anthracycline agents. The compound is being tested in a phase II trial for treatment of refractory breast cancer. Other indications being evaluated include acute myelogenous leukemia (AML), acute lymphocytic leukemia (ALL), and chronic myelogenous leukemia (CML), all of which are currently in phase I/II trials. Annamycin is made in a liposomal formulation.

Leukemia/55

INDICATION(S) AND RESEARCH PHASE
Breast Cancer – Phase II
Leukemia – Phase I/II

---

arsenic trioxide (ATO)
Trisenox

MANUFACTURER
Cell Therapeutics

DESCRIPTION
Trisenox is believed to act by killing cancer cells through apoptosis, or programmed cell death. Though the mechanism of action for Trisenox is not fully understood, it is thought that the drug induces apoptosis in ways different from other anti-cancer agents, such as retinoids.

Trisenox is currently FDA approved to treat acute promyelocytic leukemia (APL) and is currently in fourteen different trials in the United States for other types of leukemia, prostate cancer, multiple myeloma, renal cell cancer, cervical cancer, and bladder cancer.

INDICATION(S) AND RESEARCH PHASE
Leukemia – Phase I
Lymphoma, Non-Hodgkin's – Phase II
Leukemia – Phase II
Leukemia – Phase III
Multiple Myeloma – Phase II
Prostate Cancer – Phase II
Renal Cell Carcinoma – Phase II
Cervical Dysplasia/Cancer – Phase II
Bladder Cancer – Phase II
Leukemia – FDA approved

BCX-34
unknown

MANUFACTURER
BioCryst Pharmaceuticals

DESCRIPTION
BCX-34 is an inhibitor of the enzyme purine nucleoside phosphorylase (PNP), which may be essential for T-cells to replicate. T-cells are part of the body's immune system that normally attacks invading bacteria and viruses. When T-cells multiply abnormally or attack healthy body tissue, then the resulting disorders are considered proliferative diseases, such as cutaneous T-cell lymphoma (CTCL) and T-cell leukemia. All trials for BCX-34 were discontinued.

INDICATION(S) AND RESEARCH PHASE
HIV Infection – Phase II discontinued
Psoriasis – Phase I/II discontinued
Lymphomas – Phase II discontinued
Leukemia – Trial discontinued

---

clofarabine
unknown

MANUFACTURER
Bioenvision

DESCRIPTION
Clofarabine, a 2-fluoro-2-chloro sustituted purine nucleoside analog, is currently undergoing phase II trials at the M.D. Anderson Cancer Center in Houston. The drug is being given to fludarabine-resistant patients with acute lymphocytic leukemia and patients with acute myelogenous leukemia. Trials are being conducted in both adult and pediatric patients.

Clofarabine's unique mechanism of action stems from its nulcleoside structural features, where both the purine and ribose rings are halogenated. This purine analog inhibits DNA synthesis in two critical junctures, DNA polymerse I and RNA reductase, and is one of the most potent nucleoside analogs developed to date.

INDICATION(S) AND RESEARCH PHASE
Leukemia – Phase II
Pediatric, Leukemia – Phase II

CTLA4-Ig
unknown

MANUFACTURER
Repligen Corporation

DESCRIPTION
CTLA4-Ig is a key regulator that signals the immune system to "turn off." CTLA4-Ig, an injectable form of CTLA4, is a T-cell regulatory protein that may prevent graft versus host disease (GVHD) by down regulating the immune response. According to Repligen, CTLA4-Ig has the potential to inactivate only those cells that are initiating an unwanted immune response, without compromising the body's ability to fight infections.

Results of a phase I trial demonstrated that CTLA4-Ig prevented the development of GVHD in eight of 11 evaluable subjects receiving a stem cell transplantation for leukemia.

Additionally, in October 2000, Repligen received approval from the FDA to initiate a phase II clinical trial to determine if CTLA4-Ig, in combination with T-cell depletion, can reduce the incidence or severity of GVHD in subjects receiving a stem cell transplant from a genetically mismatched donor.

INDICATION(S) AND RESEARCH PHASE
Leukemia – Phase II
Immunosuppressant – Phase I completed

---

daunorubicin citrate
DaunoXome

MANUFACTURER
Gilead Sciences

DESCRIPTION
DaunoXome is the anticancer agent daunorubicin, formulated in tiny, closed lipid spheres called liposomes. This liposomal form has demonstrated improved drug delivery throughout the body and extends the time the drug remains in the body. In some cases, liposomal drugs may gather near the site of a tumor, thereby increasing its treatment effect. It is unknown how DaunoXome works to deliver daunorubicin to solid tumors, but it is thought to make the blood vessels of the tumor more leaky. When the drug gets inside the tumor, daunorubicin exerts its anticancer effect.

DaunoXome has received FDA approval as a first-line chemotherapy agent for advanced AIDS-related Kaposi's sarcoma. Additionally, this anticancer drug is being tested in phase II trials for leukemias and the treatment of non-Hodgkin's lymphoma.

Adverse effects of DaunoXome may include a triad of back pain, flushing, and chest tightness, which was reported in 13.8% of the subjects, treated with DaunoXome. This triad is reported to generally occur during the first five minutes of the infusion.

INDICATION(S) AND RESEARCH PHASE
Leukemia – Phase II
Lymphoma, Non-Hodgkin's – Phase II
Kaposi's Sarcoma – FDA approved

decitabine
unknown

MANUFACTURER
SuperGen

DESCRIPTION
Decitabine is an investigational chemotherapeutic agent in development for the treatment of sickle cell anemia and a variety of solid tumors and hematological malignancies, including myelodysplastic syndrome, non-small cell lung cancer, and chronic myelogenous leukemia. Decitabine inhibits DNA methyltransferase activity, and in this manner, presumably reactivates tumor suppressor genes.

In October 2000, results of a phase I/II trial of decitabine for sickle cell anemia demonstrated that it produced a response in 100% of subjects tested. The trial enrolled a total of eight subjects. Five had shown no response to hydroxyurea (HU) after one year of treatment, two had a moderate but unsustained response to HU, and one subject was not treated with HU. After administration of decitabine, the five subjects previously treated with HU experienced an average 35-fold increase of fetal hemoglobin levels compared to levels during HU treatment. The two subjects who responded briefly to HU experienced an average fetal hemoglobin level increase of 52% with decitabine, and the one subject who had not received HU treatment experienced a greater than 50% increase in fetal hemoglobin levels.

INDICATION(S) AND RESEARCH PHASE
Myelodysplastic Syndrome – Phase III
Lung Cancer – Phase II
Anemia – Phase I/II completed

Leukemia – Phase II

denileukin diftitox
Ontak

MANUFACTURER
Ligand Pharmaceuticals

DESCRIPTION
Ontak, previously known as DAB389IL-2, is a novel, targeted, cytotoxic biologic. The cytotoxic diphtheria toxin is fused to a subunit of IL-2 and therefore is delivered only to cells that express the IL-2 receptor (IL-2R). IL-2R may be expressed in a variety of malignant cells, including chronic lymphocytic leukemia cells.

A phase II trial for treatment of leukemia was initiated in January 2001 at the Comprehensive Cancer Center of the Wake Forest University School of Medicine in Winston-Salem, NC, in subjects diagnosed with fludarabine-refractory, CD25-positive, B-cell chronic lymphocytic leukemia.

Additionally, results of a phase III trial showed that Ontak induced substantial and durable partial and complete responses, 30% response overall, in subjects with persistent or refractory cutaneous T-cell lymphoma (CTCL). Overall, 21 of 71 CTCL subjects treated with Ontak had an objective response. There was a trend suggesting a dose effect for those subjects with more advanced disease, as an objective response was seen in two of 21 and nine of 24 subjects with at least stage IIb disease, treated with nine or 18 U/kg/d, respectively. Fifty-three of the 71 subjects entered had significant pruritus at baseline and 36 of these experienced clinically significant improvements.

Based on these results, in February 1999, the FDA granted Seragen, a subsidiary of Ligand, marketing approval for Ontak for the treatment of subjects with persistent or recurrent CTCL whose malignant cells express the CD25 component of the IL-2 receptor.

INDICATION(S) AND RESEARCH PHASE
Leukemia – Phase II
Lymphomas – FDA approved

flavopiridol, HMR-1275
unknown

MANUFACTURER
Aventis

DESCRIPTION
Flavopiridol is a cyclin-dependent kinase (CDK) inhibitor, included in a new class of drugs for cancer therapy. It is being tested in phase II trials as a treatment for chronic lymphatic leukemia, esophageal cancer, and non-small cell lung cancer.

INDICATION(S) AND RESEARCH PHASE
Esophageal Cancer – Phase II
Leukemia – Phase II
Lung Cancer – Phase II

G3139
Genasense/Mylotarg

MANUFACTURER
Genta

DESCRIPTION
Genasense is an antisense fragment of DNA, which when incorporated into the human genome will inhibit the synthesis of messenger RNA coded for by the bcl-2 gene. This results in the reduction of bcl-2 protein expression in certain malignancies. In many human cancers the bcl-2 protein is believed to be a major factor in inhibiting apoptosis, and in contributing to resistance of those cancers to treatment with anticancer drugs. Preclinical studies using the bcl-2 protein showed enhanced cancer effects when Genasense was combined with various types of chemotherapeutic agents.

A phase II trial was initiated in January 2001 using Genasense in combination with Mylotarg (gemtuzumab ozogamicin), from Wyeth/Genetics Institute, for the treatment of acute myeloid leukemia.

INDICATION(S) AND RESEARCH PHASE
Leukemia – Phase II

G3139
Genasense

MANUFACTURER
Genta

DESCRIPTION
Genasense is an antisense fragment of DNA, which when incorporated into the human genome will inhibit the synthesis of messenger RNA coded for by the bcl-2 gene. This results in the reduction of bcl-2 protein expression in certain malignancies. In many human cancers the bcl-2 protein is believed to be a major factor in inhibiting apoptosis, and in contributing to resistance to treatment with anticancer drugs. Preclinical studies using bcl-2 protein showed enhanced cancer effects when Genasense was combined with various types of chemotherapeutic agents.

A phase III trial was initiated in March 2001 testing Genasense as a single agent in subjects suffering from chronic lymphocytic leukemia.

INDICATION(S) AND RESEARCH PHASE
Leukemia – Phase III

gene therapy, leukemia
unknown

MANUFACTURER
Bioenvision

DESCRIPTION
Bioenvision's gene therapy product, for the treatment of leukemia, is currently in phase I and II trials.

INDICATION(S) AND RESEARCH PHASE
Leukemia – Phase I/II

GL-331
unknown

MANUFACTURER
Genelabs Technologies

DESCRIPTION
GL-331 is a enzyme inhibitor of topoisomerase II. It is a semi-synthetic derivative of podophyllotoxin, a chemotherapeutic agent designed to overcome multi-drug resistant (MDR) cancers. Indications for phase II clinical testing included leukemia, non-small cell lung cancer, colon malignancies, and renal cell carcinoma. Trials for the drug were discontinued during phase IIa testing.

INDICATION(S) AND RESEARCH PHASE
Colon Malignancies – Phase II Discontinued
Leukemia – Phase II discontinued
Lung Cancer – Phase II discontinued
Renal Cell Carcinoma – Phase II Discontinued

GPX-100
Adriamycin

MANUFACTURER
Gem Pharmaceuticals

DESCRIPTION
Adriamycin is a noncardiotoxic version of the anticancer drug Adriamycin. Adriamycin, an anthracycline, is a commonly used drug in the treatment of cancers, including metastatic breast cancer. The cytotoxic effect of Adriamycin on malignant cells and its toxic effects on various organs are thought to be related to genetic insertion and cell membrane lipid binding activities. Intercalation inhibits both nucleotide replication and enzyme activity of DNA and RNA polymerases. The interaction of Adriamycin with topoisomerase II to form DNA-cleavable complexes appears to be an important mechanism of Adriamycin cell-killing activity. The drug's cellular membrane binding may affect a variety of cellular functions.

Unfortunately, Adriamycin and related drugs may produce irreversible damage to the heart if the subject receives too many doses. Thus, although Adriamycin may eliminate the tumor, if the cancer returns the drug often cannot be administered again because of the significant risk of heart failure and possible death. The company claims to have developed a platform technology that allows the chemical conversion of any standard anthracycline to a closely related analog that cannot be converted to the cardiotoxic metabolite by the body. Adriamycin is presently in clinical trials for treatment of metastatic breast cancer, pediatric trials for leukemia, and solid tumor cancers.

INDICATION(S) AND RESEARCH PHASE
Cancer/Tumors (Unspecified) – Phase II
Breast Cancer – Phase II
Leukemia – Phase II
Pediatric, Leukemia – Phase II

imatinib, STI 571
Glivec

MANUFACTURER
Novartis

DESCRIPTION
Glivec is a Bcr-Abl tyrokinase inhibitor, an oral signal transduction inhibitor. Glivec works by blocking signals within cancer cells that express the Bcr-Abl protein, thus preventing a series of chemical reactions that elicit cell proliferation. Glivec is currently in phase III trials for acute lymphocytic leukemia and an NDA has been submitted for chronic myeloid leukemia. It is also in a phase I trial for Philadelphia-positive leukemia for ages newborn to 16 years.

INDICATION(S) AND RESEARCH PHASE
Leukemia – NDA submitted
Pediatric, Leukemia – Phase I

immunotherapeutic AML
Ceplene

MANUFACTURER
Maxim Pharmaceuticals

DESCRIPTION
Ceplene, previously Maxamine, is a histamine-2 (H-2) receptor agonist that is being co-administered with immunotherapies, including cytokines and interleukin-2 (IL-2). Clinical testing includes treatment of acute myelogenous leukemia (AML), chronic hepatitis C, malignant melanoma, multiple myeloma, and renal cell carcinoma.

Results from a phase III 300 subject trial evaluating Maxamine (histamine dihydrochloride) as a treatment for stage IV malignant melanoma, indicated that Maxamine used in combination with a lower dose of IL-2 improved survival rates compared to the same doses of IL-2 alone. Treatment with Maxamine and IL-2 improved overall survival, increased survival rates at 12, 18, and 24 months, and improved time-to-disease progression over treatment with IL-2 alone. Twenty-five percent of subjects treated with Maxamine and lower-dose IL-2 survived for a 24-month period. Overall response was achieved in 38% of the subjects treated with Maxamine and lower-dose IL-2. The company received an NDA non-approvable letter in January 2001 because the FDA stated that the phase III trial forming the basis of the NDA was not adequate, as a single study, to support approval.

INDICATION(S) AND RESEARCH PHASE
Hepatitis – Phase II
Leukemia – Phase III completed
Malignant Melanoma – NDA denied
Multiple Myeloma – Phase II
Renal Cell Carcinoma – Phase II

interferon alfa-2b
PEG-Intron

MANUFACTURER
Schering-Plough Corporation

DESCRIPTION
PEG-Intron is a long-acting antiviral/biological response modifier. Phase III trials are in progress for treatment of chronic myelogenous leukemia and malignant melanoma, in addition to a phase II trial for treatment of solid tumors.

PEG-Intron was developed by Enzon for Schering-Plough, who own the exclusive rights. The drug was approved by the FDA for the treatment of hepatitis C in January 2001.

INDICATION(S) AND RESEARCH PHASE
Cancer/Tumors (Unspecified) – Phase II
Hepatitis – FDA approved
Leukemia – Phase III
Malignant Melanoma – Phase III

LDI-200
unknown

MANUFACTURER
Milkhaus Laboratory

DESCRIPTION
LDI-200, in a subcutaneous formulation, is in phase II/III trials for treatment of prostate cancer, and has completed a phase II trial for treatment of leukemia and a phase II/III trial for myelodysplastic syndrome.

LDI-200 demonstrated positive results in a small phase II/III open label crossover trial in subjects with myelodysplastic syndrome. The control consisted of subjects given supportive therapy of transfusions and antibiotics, who became eligible for treatment if their disease progressed more rapidly than anticipated. A total of 23 subjects were treated using LDI-200, and seven showed significant clinical response.

INDICATION(S) AND RESEARCH PHASE
Leukemia – Phase II completed
Prostate Cancer – Phase II/III
Myelodysplastic Syndrome – Phase II/III completed

LDP-03
Campath

MANUFACTURER
BTG International

DESCRIPTION
Campath is a genetically engineered monoclonal antibody targeted to the CD52 antigen that is a surface marker on abnormal human lymphocytes. This biological drug therapy is being tested for the treatment of chronic lymphocytic leukemia (CLL) that has not responded to conventional chemotherapy. It works by attacking these cancerous white blood cells and tagging them for immune system disposal.

BTG International reported that phase II and III trials have been completed. In the phase II study, subjects enrolled at the 20 clinical sites in the United States and Europe received 30 mg of Campath on an outpatient basis, as an infusion, three times a week, for four to 12 weeks. The dose was gradually raised over the first week to 30 mg, in order to reduce the incidence and severity of infusion-related adverse events. Subjects also received anti-infective treatment as a precaution to reduce the risk of opportunistic infections. The primary evaluation factor for this trial was the overall response rate, and the study objective was to show a major response rate of at least 20%. Response rate was assessed by an independent review panel in accordance with the National Cancer Institute's guidelines for the diagnosis and treatment of CLL.

The company combined the phase III results with those from phase II studies, and submitted a Biologics License Application seeking Food and Drug Administration (FDA) approval under the FDA's fast track accelerated approval procedure. BTG International is developing Campath in a joint venture with LeukoSite.

INDICATION(S) AND RESEARCH PHASE
Leukemia – NDA submitted

liposomal ether lipid
TLC ELL-12

MANUFACTURER
The Liposome Company

DESCRIPTION
TLC ELL-12 is a liposomal ether lipid that may have efficacy in the treatment of several cancers. This drug has exhibited significant anti-tumor activity, but did not have the hemolytic side effects common in this type of ether lipid when therapeutic doses were used in experimental models. It does not appear to be myelosuppressive.

TLC ELL-12 is currently being developed in phase I trials for the treatment of lung cancer, multiple myeloma, leukemia, and prostate cancer.

INDICATION(S) AND RESEARCH PHASE
Lung Cancer – Phase I
Multiple Myeloma – Phase I
Leukemia – Phase I
Prostate Cancer – Phase I

lisofylline, CT-1501R
ProTec

MANUFACTURER
Cell Therapeutics

DESCRIPTION
ProTec is a supportive care agent being tested for prevention or reduction of the occurrence of serious or fatal infection, mucositis, and mortality among cancer subjects receiving high-dose radiation and/or chemotherapy. Most cancer therapies have toxic effects that cause serious problems for subjects, including low white blood cell counts and inflammation of the intestinal mucous membranes. Serious infection is a very common adverse effect of high dose cancer treatment, especially when the epithelial cells that line the gastrointestinal tract are damaged and no longer form a protective barrier from infectious bacteria. According to Cell Therapeutics, ProTec may protect this barrier and decrease the number of life-threatening infections in cancer subjects following bone marrow transplant. Enrollment has been completed in a phase III bone marrow transplant trial among unrelated donors, and results are pending.

Additionally, a phase II study began in late 1998 that enrolled 12–20 subjects in a single-center trial for treatment of head and neck cancer.

Lisofylline was investigated in a phase III trial for newly diagnosed acute myeloid leukemia (AML), in subjects undergoing high dose induction chemotherapy. In Results demonstrated ProTec did not reduce the number of new neutropenia associated infections. Though a lower number of fungal infections were observed, Cell Therapeutics indicated that they will terminate all ProTec research activity.

Some of the ProTec research trials with Cell Therapeutics were under collaboration and license agreement for joint development with Ortho Biotech, R.W. Johnson, and BioChem Pharma.

INDICATION(S) AND RESEARCH PHASE
Bone Marrow Transplant – Trial discontinued
Leukemia – Trial discontinued
Effects of Chemotherapy – Trial discontinued
Head and Neck Cancer – Trial discontinued

MDX-22
unknown

MANUFACTURER
Medarex

DESCRIPTION
MDX-22 is used to purge leukemia cells from the bone marrow of acute myeloid leukemia (AML) subjects who are undergoing a transplant of their own bone marrow. This therapy uses a monoclonal antibody to attack the abnormal leukemia cells. MDX-22 is currently in a phase II trial.

INDICATION(S) AND RESEARCH PHASE
Leukemia – Phase II
Bone Marrow Transplant – Phase II

peginterferon alfa-2a
Pegasys

MANUFACTURER
Hoffmann-La Roche

DESCRIPTION
Pegasys is a longer-lasting form of interferon, which is a naturally produced immune boosting substance. This drug is given in an injectable formulation that is being tested in phase III trials for treatments of complications of hepatitis C, malignant melanoma, renal cell carcinoma, and chronic myelogenous leukemia.

INDICATION(S) AND RESEARCH PHASE
Hepatitis – Phase III
Malignant Melanoma – Phase II
Renal Cell Carcinoma – Phase II
Leukemia – Phase III

pentostatin
Nipent

MANUFACTURER
SuperGen

DESCRIPTION
Nipent (pentostatin) belongs to a group of drugs called antimetabolites. Nipent inhibits the enzyme adenosine deaminase, leading to cytotoxicity and cell death. This drug is in trials for rheumatoid arthritis, non-Hodgkin's lymphoma, and chronic lymphocytic leukemia.

In December 2000, results of a phase II trial of Nipent indicated the drug has significant 75% overall response rate in the treatment of graft versus host disease (GVHD). Twelve subjects with steroid refractory GVHD received Nipent as salvage therapy after each had previously failed all other treatments. A phase III trial is now under way.

INDICATION(S) AND RESEARCH PHASE
Leukemia – Phase III
Lymphoma, Non-Hodgkin's – Phase II
Rheumatoid Arthritis – Phase II
Immunosuppressive – Phase III

RFS-2000
Rubitecan

MANUFACTURER
SuperGen

DESCRIPTION
Rubitecan is a novel drug in the late stages of phase III development for treating advanced pancreatic cancer. It works by inhibiting the enzyme topoisomerase-I. Rubitecan is made in an oral formulation, which is advantageous for outpatient treatment compared to intravenous type cancer drugs that may require a visit to a hospital setting.

In addition to treating pancreatic cancer, Rubitecan is being evaluated in phase II trials for treatment of a variety of solid tumors, such as in breast, colorectal, lung, ovarian, and prostate cancers, as well as metastatic melanoma and advanced gastric carcinoma. Additional phase II trials in the United States and Europe are testing Rubitecan in blood cancers such as chronic myelomonocytic leukemia.

Results demonstrated Rubitecan was given to a group of end-stage pancreatic cancer subjects who failed all previous conventional therapies. Of the 60 subjects who completed Rubitecan treatment, 31.7% responded favorably with half of the subjects staying alive (the median survival) at 18.6 months. Additionally, 31.7% were stabilized with a 9.7 month median survival rate, and 36.6% were non-responders with a 6.8 month median survival rate.

SuperGen announced that the company has also started a phase III trial of Rubitecan in combination with gemcitabine for the treatment of subjects with pancreatic cancer. This combination therapy trial is being conducted at a cancer center in Philadelphia.

Some expected side effects reported are blood toxicities, bladder irritation (cystitis), and some gastrointestinal disorders.

INDICATION(S) AND RESEARCH PHASE
Pancreatic Cancer – Phase III
Breast Cancer – Phase II
Colorectal Cancer – Phase II
Gastric Cancer – Phase II
Leukemia – Phase II
Malignant Melanoma – Phase II
Ovarian Cancer – Phase II
Lung Cancer – Phase II
Prostate Cancer – Phase II
Myelodysplastic Syndrome – Phase III

SMART M195
unknown

MANUFACTURER
Protein Design Labs

DESCRIPTION
SMART M195 is a radioactive compound that is linked to a humanized monoclonal antibody. Radiotherapy using alpha particle emitting isotopes, bismuth-213, has been used for some years to treat different forms of cancer. This combination therapy is a specialized targeting method that allows the monoclonal antibody to hunt down and attach itself to the cancer cell, which gives the adjoining radioactive isotope a greater chance, by proximity, to kill the cancer.

SMART M195 is currently in a phase III trial for treatment of acute myeloid leukemia using radiotherapy. This biologic product is also being tested in two other phase II studies for the indications of acute promyelocytic leukemia and myelodysplastic syndrome.

INDICATION(S) AND RESEARCH PHASE
Leukemia – Phase III
Leukemia – Phase II
White Blood Cell Disorders,
  Myelodysplastic Syndrome – Phase II

tiazofurin
Tiazole

MANUFACTURER
ICN Pharmaceuticals

DESCRIPTION
Tiazole is a nucleoside analogue that resembles part of the energy rich substrates used for building genetic coded materials. This drug is being assessed in a phase II/III trial for acute and chronic myelogenous Leukemia. ICN Pharmaceuticals and the National Cancer Institute sponsor this clinical study.

INDICATION(S) AND RESEARCH PHASE
Leukemia – Phase II/III

TNP-470
unknown

MANUFACTURER
Takeda Chemical Industries

DESCRIPTION
TNP-470 is a synthetically modified form of the antibiotic fumagillin. This drug inhibits new blood vessel growth and is being tested in phase II trials for treatment of adults with malignant solid tumors. It is also being evaluated in a phase I trial in children with solid tumors, lymphomas, and acute leukemias.

INDICATION(S) AND RESEARCH PHASE
Cancer/Tumors (Unspecified) – Phase II
Pediatric, Solid Tumors – Phase I
Pediatric, Leukemia – Phase I
Pediatric, Lymphomas – Phase I

tretinoin
Atragen

MANUFACTURER
Aronex Pharmaceuticals

DESCRIPTION
Atragen is a liposomal, intravenous formulation of tretinoin, or all-trans retinoic acid. Tretinoin induces cell differentiation in rapidly proliferating cells, such as those observed in malignant diseases. Additionally, Atragen appears to affect the cellular signaling mechanisms that become unbalanced in cancer cells.

Results of a phase II trial of Atragen monotherapy for acute promyelocytic leukemia (APL) indicated its potential to induce complete remission. The trial was conducted in Peru, and included 16 subjects with newly diagnosed or previously untreated APL who were treated with Atragen every other day as a single agent for a maximum of 28 doses. Fourteen subjects (87.5%) achieved morphologic remission, and 28.6% of these subjects also attained molecular remission. The safety profile observed in the subject population is similar to that reported with the currently approved oral formulation of Atra.

Aronex is also conducting phase II trials to evaluate the compound for the treatment of non-Hodgkin's lymphoma, hormone-resistant prostate cancer, acute myelogenous leukemia (AML), and renal cell carcinoma in combination with interferon-alpha.

In January 2001, Aronex announced that the FDA has denied approval of the company's NDA for Atragen as a treatment for subjects with APL, for whom therapy with tretinoin (all-trans retinoic acid or Atra) is necessary, but for whom an intravenous administration is required.

INDICATION(S) AND RESEARCH PHASE
Lymphoma, Non-Hodgkin's – Phase II
Prostate Cancer – Phase II
Renal Cell Carcinoma – Phase I/II
Leukemia, APL – NDA denied
Leukemia, AML – Phase II

Trisenox/dexamethasone
unknown

MANUFACTURER
Cell Therapeutics

DESCRIPTION

Trisenox was FDA approved in injection formulation for treatment of acute promyelocytic leukemia in September 2000. Trisenox is believed to act by killing cancer cells through apoptosis, or programmed cell death. The mechanism of action for Trisenox is not fully understood, but it is believed that the drug induces apoptosis differently than other anti-cancer agents, such as retinoids.

Phase II trials are testing Trisenox in combination with dexamethasone, a high dose steroid, for treatment of multiple myeloma.

INDICATION(S) AND RESEARCH PHASE

Leukemia – FDA approved
Multiple Myeloma – Phase II

troxacitabine, BCH-4556
Troxatyl

MANUFACTURER
BioChem Pharma

DESCRIPTION

Troxatyl is a dioxolane nucleoside analog being investigated as an anti-cancer agent. The drug is a complete DNA chain terminator and DNA polymerase inhibitor. It acts by incorporating itself into the growing DNA chain of cancer cells, interfering with their ability to replicate further. Currently, Troxatyl is being evaluated as a single agent or in combination therapy in a number of ongoing single and multicenter trials for hematologic malignancies including acute myeloid leukemia, chronic myeloid leukemia in blastic phase, and lymphoproliferative disorders such as lymphoma, chronic lymphocytic leukemia, and myeloma. It is also being evaluated as a single agent for treatment of pancreatic cancer and in combination therapy in a number of solid tumors. Troxatyl is currently in phase II development.

INDICATION(S) AND RESEARCH PHASE

Cancer/Tumors (Unspecified) – Phase II
Colorectal Cancer – Phase II
Head and Neck Cancer – Phase II
Leukemia – Phase II
Lung Cancer – Phase II
Malignant Melanoma – Phase II
Ovarian Cancer – Phase II
Pancreatic Cancer – Phase II
Prostate Cancer – Phase II
Renal Cell Carcinoma – Phase II
Lymphomas – Phase II

unknown
L-Vax

MANUFACTURER
AVAX Technologies

DESCRIPTION

L-Vax is a cancer vaccine against leukemia in subjects with acute myelogenous leukemia (AML) being tested on 40 subjects in a phase I/II trial at the University of Texas M.D. Anderson Cancer Center. L-Vax will be prepared from blood samples from the subjects, obtained after their first relapse. AVAX uses a process known as haptenization for the L-Vax vaccine, which alters the tumor cells and makes them appear foreign to the subject's immune system. According to the company, when the hapten-modified cells are injected into subjects, they stimulate the immune system to recognize the cancer cells and destroy them. In addition, subjects in second remission will receive seven weekly L-Vax vaccinations. AVAX will evaluate whether L-Vax induces an immune response against subjects, leukemia cells and if it prevents or delays another response.

INDICATION(S) AND RESEARCH PHASE
Leukemia – Phase I/II

unknown
Vasogen IMT

MANUFACTURER
Vasogen

DESCRIPTION

Vasogen immune modulation therapy (IMT) is being developed for the treatment of chronic lymphocytic leukemia (CLL). The company's immune modulation therapies target the destructive inflammatory processes that lead to disease. This inhibition of inflammatory responses is thought to be mediated by anti-inflammatory cytokines, including interleukin-10, produced by the activation of regulatory immune cells. Vasogen IMT is currently in phase II development.

INDICATION(S) AND RESEARCH PHASE
Leukemia – Phase II

unknown
Clofarabine

MANUFACTURER
Bioenvision

DESCRIPTION

Clofarabine is currently undergoing a phase II trial at the M. D. Anderson Cancer Center in Houston for treatment of leukemia and lymphomas. The drug is being given to fludarabine-resistant subjects with chronic lymphocytic leukemia and to subjects with acute leukemia. A phase I trial is also under way, testing Clofarabine as a treatment for solid tumors. Early results have been positive, and Bioenvision is currently looking for a development partner to help fund further trials with Clofarabine.

INDICATION(S) AND RESEARCH PHASE

Lymphomas – Phase II
Leukemia – Phase II
Cancer/Tumors (Unspecified) – Phase I

vaccine, cancer
Gvax

MANUFACTURER
Cell Genesys

DESCRIPTION

Gvax is an allogenic compound involving genetic modification of prostate cancer cell lines. These cancer cells have been irradiated and modified to secrete granulocyte-macrophage colony stimulating factor (GM-CSF), a hormone that plays a key role in stimulating the body's immune response to vaccines. The compound is in phase II trials for prostate and pancreatic cancer, and phase I/II trials for lung cancer, leukemia, and malignant melanoma.

The Gvax prostate cancer vaccine demonstrated anti-tumor activity in an initial phase II trial in subjects with advanced metastatic prostate cancer who have not responded to hormone therapy. Prior to initiating a phase III trial, Cell Genesys plans to run further trials of Gvax prostate cancer vaccine in 2001, employing a higher potency version of the same product. Future phase III trials in hormone refractory prostate cancer subjects may compare the Gvax vaccine in combination with chemotherapy to chemotherapy alone.

INDICATION(S) AND RESEARCH PHASE
Prostate Cancer – Phase II
Lung Cancer – Phase I/II completed
Malignant Melanoma – Phase I/II
Vaccines – Phase I/II
Pancreatic Cancer – Phase II
Leukemia – Phase I/II

Lymphomas

APL400-020 V-B
Genevax-TCR

MANUFACTURER
Wyeth-Lederle Vaccines

DESCRIPTION
Genevax-TCR is a novel DNA-based vaccine in early clinical testing for T-cell lymphomas and other autoimmune diseases. Treatment of cutaneous T-cell lymphoma is an orphan indication currently being evaluated in a phase I/II trial.

INDICATION(S) AND RESEARCH PHASE
Autoimmune Diseases – Phase I/II
Lymphomas – Phase I/II

arsenic trioxide (ATO)
Trisenox

MANUFACTURER
Cell Therapeutics

DESCRIPTION
Trisenox is believed to act by killing cancer cells through apoptosis, or programmed cell death. Though the mechanism of action for Trisenox is not fully understood, it is thought that the drug induces apoptosis in ways different from other anti-cancer agents, such as retinoids.

Trisenox is currently FDA approved to treat acute promyelocytic leukemia (APL) and is currently in fourteen different trials in the United States for other types of leukemia, prostate cancer, multiple myeloma, renal cell cancer, cervical cancer, and bladder cancer.

INDICATION(S) AND RESEARCH PHASE
Leukemia – Phase I
Lymphoma, Non-Hodgkin's – Phase II
Leukemia – Phase II
Leukemia – Phase III
Multiple Myeloma – Phase II
Prostate Cancer – Phase II
Renal Cell Carcinoma – Phase II
Cervical Dysplasia/Cancer – Phase II
Bladder Cancer – Phase II
Leukemia – FDA approved

BCX-34
unknown

MANUFACTURER
BioCryst Pharmaceuticals

DESCRIPTION
BCX-34 is an inhibitor of the enzyme purine nucleoside phosphorylase (PNP), which may be essential for T-cells to replicate. T-cells are part of the body's immune system that normally attacks invading bacteria and viruses. When T-cells multiply abnormally or attack healthy body tissue, then the resulting disorders are considered proliferative diseases, such as cutaneous T-cell lymphoma (CTCL) and T-cell leukemia. All trials for BCX-34 were discontinued.

INDICATION(S) AND RESEARCH PHASE
HIV Infection – Phase II discontinued
Psoriasis – Phase I/II discontinued
Lymphomas – Phase II discontinued
Leukemia – Trial discontinued

daunorubicin citrate
DaunoXome

MANUFACTURER
Gilead Sciences

DESCRIPTION
DaunoXome is the anticancer agent daunorubicin, formulated in tiny, closed lipid spheres called liposomes. This liposomal form has demonstrated improved drug delivery throughout the body and extends the time the drug remains in the body. In some cases, liposomal drugs may gather near the site of a tumor, thereby increasing its treatment effect. It is unknown how DaunoXome works to deliver daunorubicin to solid tumors, but it is thought to make the blood vessels of the tumor more leaky. When the drug gets inside the tumor, daunorubicin exerts its anticancer effect.

DaunoXome has received FDA approval as a first-line chemotherapy agent for advanced AIDS-related Kaposi's sarcoma. Additionally, this anticancer drug is being tested in phase II trials for leukemias and the treatment of non-Hodgkin's lymphoma.

Adverse effects of DaunoXome may include a triad of back pain, flushing, and chest tightness, which was reported in 13.8% of the subjects treated with DaunoXome. This triad is reported to generally occur during the first five minutes of the infusion.

INDICATION(S) AND RESEARCH PHASE
Leukemia – Phase II
Lymphoma, Non-Hodgkin's – Phase II
Kaposi's sarcoma – FDA approved

denileukin diftitox
Ontak

MANUFACTURER
Ligand Pharmaceuticals

DESCRIPTION
Ontak, previously known as DAB389IL-2, is a novel, targeted, cytotoxic biologic. The cytotoxic diphtheria toxin is fused to a subunit of IL-2 and therefore is delivered only to cells that express the IL-2 receptor (IL-2R). IL-2R may be expressed in a variety of malignant cells, including chronic lymphocytic leukemia cells. A phase II trial for treatment of leukemia was initiated in

January 2001 at the Comprehensive Cancer Center of the Wake Forest University School of Medicine in Winston-Salem, NC, in subjects diagnosed with fludarabine-refractory, CD25-positive, B-cell chronic lymphocytic leukemia.

Additionally, results of a phase III trial showed that Ontak induced substantial and durable partial and complete responses, 30% response overall, in subjects with persistent or refractory cutaneous T-cell lymphoma (CTCL). Overall, 21 of 71 CTCL subjects treated with Ontak had an objective response. There was a trend suggesting a dose-effect for those subjects with more advance disease, as an objective response was seen in two of 21 and nine of 24 subjects with at least stage IIb disease, treated with nine or 18(u)kg/d, respectively. Fifty-three of the 71 subjects entered had significant pruritus at baseline and 36 of these experienced clinically significant improvements.

Based on the results, in February 1999, the FDA granted Seragen, a subsidiary of Ligand, marketing approval for Ontak for the treatment of subjects with persistent or recurrent CTCL whose malignant cells express the CD25 component of the IL-2 receptor.

INDICATION(S) AND RESEARCH PHASE
Leukemia – Phase II
Lymphomas – FDA approved

FLT3 ligand
Mobist

MANUFACTURER
ImClone Systems

DESCRIPTION
Mobist is a hematopoietic growth factor being tested outside the body. It is a stem cell mobilizer and potential anti-tumor agent. Mobist is being evaluated in phase II trials for treatment of breast cancer, solid tumors, non-Hodgkin's lymphoma, and ovarian cancer.

INDICATION(S) AND RESEARCH PHASE
Cancer/Tumors (Unspecified) – Phase II
Breast Cancer – Phase II
Lymphomas, Non-Hodgkin's – Phase II
Ovarian Cancer – Phase II

gullium maltolate
unknown

MANUFACTURER
Titan Pharmaceuticals

DESCRIPTION
Gullium is a semi-metallic element that has shown some therapeutic activity in metabolic bone disease, hypercalcemia of malignancy, and cancer. Gullium maltolate can displace divalent iron from the iron transporting protein, transferrin; thus gullium maltolate causes interference with iron metabolism through the inhibition of enzymes requiring divalent iron. In addition, gullium appears to form salts with calcium and phosphate and get incorporated into bone. The bone that is incorporated with gullium appears to be at least as strong as normal bone however, appears to be more resistant to degradation by osteoclasts and tumor cells. This drug is currently in phase I/II trials for treatment of prostate and bladder cancer, lymphomas, myeloma, and HIV infection.

INDICATION(S) AND RESEARCH PHASE
Prostate Cancer – Phase I/II
Lymphomas – Phase I/II
Myeloma – Phase I/II
Bladder Cancer – Phase I/II
HIV Infection – Phase I/II

hypericin
VIMRxyn

MANUFACTURER
Nexell Therapeutics

DESCRIPTION
VIMRxyn (hypericin) is a light-activated, topically applied formulation of aromatic polycyclic dione (APD-1), a synthetic agent directed against retroviruses. This drug is being tested in phase I/II trials for treatment of skin diseases including psoriasis, cutaneous T-cell lymphoma, and warts.

Nexell has also manufactured an oral, once-daily formulation of APD-1. This drug form is being evaluated for the treatment of malignant gliomas. Subject enrollment has been completed for this trial.

INDICATION(S) AND RESEARCH PHASE
Cancer/Tumors (Unspecified) – Phase I/II
Lymphomas – Phase I/II
Psoriasis and Psoriatic Disorders – Phase I/II
Skin Infections/Disorders – Phase I/II

organ transplantation system
AlloMune

MANUFACTURER
BioTransplant

DESCRIPTION
AlloMune is an organ transplantation system for the creation of specific immune tolerance in solid organ transplants from human donor organs, using a novel anti-CD2 antibody/immunosuppressive monoclonal antibody (MAb). The drug is designed to re-educate the recipient's immune system to recognize the foreign tissue as "self." The AlloMune system for cancer applications is designed to attack tumor cells more aggressively than the subject's own immune defenses. Phase I/II trials are being conducted for therapy refractory lymphoma, kidney transplant surgery, and for use as an immunosuppressant.

INDICATION(S) AND RESEARCH PHASE
Immunosuppressive – Phase I/II
Kidney Transplant Surgery – Phase I/II
Lymphomas – Phase I/II

TNP-470
unknown

MANUFACTURER
Takeda Chemical Industries

DESCRIPTION
TNP-470 is a synthetically modified form of the antibiotic fumagillin. This drug inhibits new blood vessel growth and is being tested in phase II trials for treatment of adults with malignant solid tumors. It is also being

evaluated in a phase I trial in children with solid tumors, lymphomas, and acute leukemias.

INDICATION(S) AND RESEARCH PHASE
Cancer/Tumors (Unspecified) – Phase II
Pediatric, Solid Tumors – Phase I
Pediatric, Leukemia – Phase I
Pediatric, Lymphomas – Phase I

unknown
Clofarabine

MANUFACTURER
Bioenvision

DESCRIPTION
Clofarabine is currently undergoing a phase II trial at the M.D. Anderson Cancer Center in Houston for treatment of leukemia and lymphomas. The drug is being given to fludarabine-resistant subjects with chronic lymphocytic leukemia and to subjects with acute leukemia. A phase I trial is also under way, testing Clofarabine as a treatment for solid tumors. Early results have been positive, and Bioenvision is currently looking for a development partner to help fund further trials with Clofarabine.

INDICATION(S) AND RESEARCH PHASE
Lymphomas – Phase II
Leukemia – Phase II
Cancer/Tumors (Unspecified) – Phase I

unknown
Beta LT

MANUFACTURER
LifeTime Pharmaceuticals

DESCRIPTION
Beta LT is a new anti-cancer agent designed to stimulate the immune system, therefore having an anti-cancer effect. Positive results were noted in two-phase I/II trials testing Beta LT as a treatment for progressing pre-malignant myeloma-related disease (MGUS) and for cancer treatment in subjects having the advanced disease. The 14 subjects treated received the target dose for up to one year with no serious side effects except for mild bowel habit changes in one subject. The trial took place at McGill University Jewish General Hospital in Montreal, Canada.

INDICATION(S) AND RESEARCH PHASE
Lymphomas – Phase I/II completed
Multiple Myeloma – Phase I/II completed

vaccine, cancer
unknown

MANUFACTURER
Genzyme Genetics Division

DESCRIPTION
This cancer vaccine is made from proteins associated with tumors taken from the individual subject. Phase I/II clinical trials are testing the vaccine in subjects suffering from B-cell lymphoma and multiple myeloma.

INDICATION(S) AND RESEARCH PHASE
Lymphomas – Phase I/II
Multiple Myeloma – Phase I/II

vaccine, lymphoma
Vaxid

MANUFACTURER
Vical

DESCRIPTION
Vaxid is a DNA protective vaccine being developed in phase III trials for the treatment of B-cell lymphoma. According to Vical, immunization of post-chemotherapy subjects with Vaxid could result in the elimination of residual disease and the prevention of relapse. The vaccine was developed using Vical's proprietary naked DNA delivery technology. It is manufactured in an intramuscular injection formulation.

INDICATION(S) AND RESEARCH PHASE
Lymphomas – Phase III

Multiple Myeloma

AE-941
Neovastat

MANUFACTURER
AEterna Laboratories

DESCRIPTION
Neovastat is an angiogenesis inhibitor being tested in a phase III trial for treatment of non-small cell lung cancer and a phase II trial for moderate to severe psoriasis. A phase I trial for treatment of macular degeneration has been completed.

A phase II trial for multiple myeloma was initiated in October 2000 and will treat 120 subjects and include approximately 20 sites across North America and Europe. Trial results are expected by summer 2002.

Additionally, a phase III trial was initiated in May 2000 for kidney cancer that will include 270 subjects at sites in North America and Europe.

INDICATION(S) AND RESEARCH PHASE
Lung Cancer – Phase III
Psoriasis and Psoriatic Disorders – Phase II
Multiple Myeloma – Phase II
Renal Cell Carcinoma – Phase III
Macular Degeneration – Phase I completed

APC8020
Mylovenge

MANUFACTURER
Dendreon Corporation

DESCRIPTION
Mylovenge is a therapeutic vaccine designed to trigger the immune system to recognize and destroy cancer cells. It involves isolating dendritic cells from a subject's blood and activating them with a protein, called an M component or idiotype, that is specific to each subject. The activated dendritic cells are infused back into the subject's body to stimulate an immune response.

Long-term follow-up data from phase II trials involving multiple myeloma and amyloidosis subjects were presented in December 2000. The trials indicated that Mylovenge caused disease regression or stabilization in more than 30% of subjects. In some subjects, these benefits were found to extend more than 18 months following treatment.

INDICATION(S) AND RESEARCH PHASE
Amyloidosis – Phase II completed
Multiple Myeloma – Phase II completed

arsenic trioxide (ATO)
Trisenox

MANUFACTURER
Cell Therapeutics

DESCRIPTION
Trisenox is believed to act by killing cancer cells through apoptosis, or programmed cell death. Though the mechanism of action for Trisenox is not fully understood, it is thought that the drug induces apoptosis in ways different from other anti-cancer agents, such as retinoids.

Trisenox is currently FDA approved to treat acute promyelocytic leukemia (APL) and is currently in fourteen different trials in the United States for other types of leukemia, prostate cancer, multiple myeloma, renal cell cancer, cervical cancer, and bladder cancer.

INDICATION(S) AND RESEARCH PHASE
Leukemia – Phase I
Lymphoma, Non-Hodgkin's – Phase II
Leukemia – Phase II
Leukemia – Phase III
Multiple Myeloma – Phase II
Prostate Cancer – Phase II
Renal Cell Carcinoma – Phase II
Cervical Dysplasia/Cancer – Phase II
Bladder Cancer – Phase II
Leukemia – FDA approved

CDC 801
SelCIDs

MANUFACTURER
Celgene Corporation

DESCRIPTION
SelCIDs, selective cytokine inhibitory drugs, are oral immunotherapeutic agents that treat various inflammatory diseases by inhibiting phosphodiesterase type-4 enzyme (PDE-4). The inhibition of PDE-4 decreases production of tumor necrosis factor-alpha (TNF-α), a protein manufactured by cells of the immune system. This inhibition reduces the level of circulating TNF-α and, therefore, its ability to cause inflammation in cells. At normal levels, the protein is essential for effective immune function. However, overproduction of TNF as a result of age, genetics, and other influences contributes to the pathology of numerous diseases.

SelCIDs are in phase II trials for the following indications: inflammatory bowel disease, rheumatoid arthritis, multiple sclerosis, tuberculosis, autoimmune diseases, multiple myeloma, and mycobacteriosis such as leprosy.

INDICATION(S) AND RESEARCH PHASE
Inflammatory Bowel Disease – Phase II
Rheumatoid Arthritis – Phase II
Multiple Sclerosis – Phase II
Asthma – Phase Discontinued
Tuberculosis – Phase II
Autoimmune Diseases – Phase II
Bacterial Infection – Phase II
Multiple Myeloma – Phase II

immunotherapeutic, AML
Ceplene

MANUFACTURER
Maxim Pharmaceuticals

DESCRIPTION
Ceplene, previously Maxamine, is a histamine-2 (H-2) receptor agonist that is being co-administered with immunotherapies, including cytokines and interleukin-2 (IL-2). Clinical testing includes treatment of acute myelogenous leukemia (AML), chronic hepatitis C, malignant melanoma, multiple myeloma, and renal cell carcinoma.

Results from a phase III 300 subject trial evaluating Ceplene (histamine dihydrochloride) as a treatment for stage IV malignant melanoma, indicated that Ceplene used in combination with a lower dose of IL-2 improved survival rates compared to the same doses of IL-2 alone. Treatment with Ceplene and IL-2 improved overall survival, increased survival rates at 12, 18, and 24 months, and improved time-to-disease progression over treatment with IL-2 alone. Twenty-five percent of subjects treated with Ceplene and lower-dose IL-2 survived for a 24-month period. Overall response was achieved in 38% of the subjects treated with Ceplene and lower-dose IL-2. The company received an NDA non-approvable letter in January 2001 because the FDA stated that the phase III trial forming the basis of the NDA was not adequate, as a single study, to support approval.

INDICATION(S) AND RESEARCH PHASE
Hepatitis – Phase II
Leukemia – Phase III completed
Malignant Melanoma – NDA denied
Multiple Myeloma – Phase II
Renal Cell Carcinoma – Phase II

LDP-341, PS-341
unknown

MANUFACTURER
Millennium Pharmaceuticals

DESCRIPTION
LDP-341 is a proteasome inhibitor being developed for the treatment of cancer. In tumor cells, proteasome inhibition produces cellular stress by stabilizing cell cycle regulatory proteins and disrupting cell proliferation, ultimately leading to apoptosis, or cell death. In preclinical studies, LDP-341 has shown activity against multiple myeloma cells, resulting in the inducement of apoptosis. The anti-tumor action of LDP-341 on multiple myeloma cells appears to involve both direct and indirect inhibition of factors which promote tumor growth. LDP-341 also appears to increase the effectiveness of other anti-cancer drugs by overcoming cellular resistance, a major cause of chemotherapy failure.

LDP-341 is currently in a phase I trial in subjects with advanced hematological malignancies. Preliminary results presented in December 2000 showed that LDP-341 reduced serum myeloma protein levels and myeloma cell numbers in bone marrow in two of three subjects with advanced multiple myeloma. The drug was well tolerated by these subjects and appeared to have induced a complete response in one subject and a reduction in bone marrow plasma cells in another.

INDICATION(S) AND RESEARCH PHASE
Blood Cancer – Phase I
Multiple Myeloma – Phase I

liposomal ether lipid
TLC ELL-12

MANUFACTURER
The Liposome Company

DESCRIPTION
TLC ELL-12 is a liposomal ether lipid that may have efficacy in the treatment of several cancers. This drug has exhibited significant anti-tumor activity, but did not have the hemolytic side effects common in this type of ether lipid when therapeutic doses were used in experimental models. It does not appear to be myelosuppressive.

TLC ELL-12 is currently being developed in phase I trials for the treatment of lung cancer, multiple myeloma, leukemia, and prostate cancer.

INDICATION(S) AND RESEARCH PHASE
Lung Cancer – Phase I
Multiple Myeloma – Phase I
Leukemia – Phase I
Prostate Cancer – Phase I

monoclonal antibody
BrevaRex MAb

MANUFACTURER
AltaRex

DESCRIPTION
BrevaRex MAb is a cancer immunotherapeutic being developed for the treatment of MUC1 expressing cancers. Multiple myeloma cells express tumor associated antigens that are ideal targets for immunotherapy. One such antigen is the core protein of MUC1. The ability of an antibody to bind to MUC1 is largely dependent on the extent of mutation of the antigen. In contrast to breast and other common cancers, MUC1 in multiple myeloma subjects is highly mutated in virtually every subject, thereby making antibody therapy targeting the core peptide appear more promising.

Results of a phase I trial in late-stage cancer subjects with substantial tumor burden indicated that BrevaRex MAb was well tolerated and without significant adverse effects. Immune responses were induced to both the antibody and the tumor associated antigen, MUC1, to which BrevaRex MAb is targeted.

Due to the limited therapy options for multiple myeloma, the BrevaRex clinical development program could possibly be accelerated under U.S. regulations. AltaRex expects to conduct the next trial in the second half of 2001, and if favorable results are obtained, phase II/IIb trials may be initiated.

INDICATION(S) AND RESEARCH PHASE
Multiple Myeloma – Phase I/II

skeletal targeted radiotherapy (STR)
unknown

MANUFACTURER
NeoRx Corporation

DESCRIPTION
Skeletal targeted radiotherapy (STR) uses a molecule that targets the bone as a means of administering radiation to the bone and bone marrow for the treatment of multiple myeloma. The molecule tightly binds Holmium-166, a beta emitting radionuclide.

NeoRx reported that a completed phase II trial of STR resulted in nine of 17 subjects having achieved completed regression of their tumors. Trials for multiple myeloma are currently in phase III.

INDICATION(S) AND RESEARCH PHASE
Multiple Myeloma – Phase III

thalidomide
Thalomid

MANUFACTURER
Celgene Corporation

DESCRIPTION
Thalomid is an oral formulation of the immunomodulatory agent thalidomide. Thalidomide has a notorious history of having caused birth defects when the medical profession unsuspectingly prescribed it for pregnant women as a treatment for nausea and insomnia. Celgene is investigating new applications for the drug, while being particularly mindful of the potential risks of thalidomide treatment. Thalomid is currently being tested for numerous indications in the areas of oncology and immunology.

INDICATION(S) AND RESEARCH PHASE
Multiple Myeloma – Phase II
Myelodysplastic Syndrome – Phase II
Leukemia – Phase II
Brain Cancer – Phase II
Liver Cancer – Phase II
Kidney Cancer – Phase II
Prostate Cancer – Phase II
Kaposi's Sarcoma – Phase II
Cachexia – Phase II
Recurrent Aphthous Stomatitis – Phase III
Crohn's Disease – Phase II
Inflammatory Bowel Disease – Phase II
Sarcoidosis – Phase II
Scleroderma – Phase II

Trisenox/dexamethasone
unknown

MANUFACTURER
Cell Therapeutics

DESCRIPTION
Trisenox was FDA approved in injection formulation for treatment of acute promyelocytic leukemia in September 2000. Trisenox is believed to act by killing cancer cells through apoptosis, or programmed cell death. The mechanism of action for Trisenox is not fully understood, but it is believed that the drug induces apoptosis differently than other anti-cancer agents, such as retinoids.

Phase II trials are testing Trisenox in combination with dexamethasone, a high dose steroid, for treatment of multiple myeloma.

INDICATION(S) AND RESEARCH PHASE
Leukemia – FDA approved
Multiple Myeloma – Phase II

unknown
Beta LT

MANUFACTURER
LifeTime Pharmaceuticals

DESCRIPTION
Beta LT is a new anti-cancer agent designed to stimulate the immune system, therefore having an anti-cancer effect. Positive results were noted in two-phase I/II trials testing Beta LT as a treatment for progressing pre-malignant myeloma-related disease (MGUS) and for cancer treatment in subjects having the advanced disease. The 14 subjects treated received the target dose for up to one year with no serious side effects except for mild bowel habit changes in one subject. The trial took place at McGill University Jewish General Hospital in Montreal, Canada.

INDICATION(S) AND RESEARCH PHASE
Lymphomas – Phase I/II completed
Multiple Myeloma – Phase I/II completed

vaccine, cancer
unknown

MANUFACTURER
Genzyme Genetics Division

DESCRIPTION
This cancer vaccine is made from proteins associated with tumors taken from the individual subject. Phase I/II clinical trials are testing the vaccine in subjects suffering from B-cell lymphoma and multiple myeloma.

INDICATION(S) AND RESEARCH PHASE
Lymphomas – Phase I/II
Multiple Myeloma – Phase I/II

Wobe-Mugos-E
unknown

MANUFACTURER
Mucos Pharma GmbH

DESCRIPTION
Wobe-Mugos-E is an enzyme combination of papain, trypsin, and chymotrypsin in an oral formulation being tested for improving the general health of cancer subjects. It may reduce the need for additional medications, such as pain relievers and antiemetics, during or after chemotherapy.

Wobe-Mugos-E is an alpha-macroglobulin that binds interleukins, TGF-β, TNF receptor I and II, hyperactive T-cells, and CRP. Results showed Wobe-Mugos-E, given palliatively, increased the subject's appetite and there was a reduction in fatigue and depression. Leukopenia and thrombopenia induced by cancer cytostatic agents and radiation were reduced.

Clinical trials in phase II/III are evaluating this enzyme combination for multiple myeloma and effects of chemotherapy. Wobe-Mugos-E is given as a dose of three tablets, three times daily for one-half hour before meals.

INDICATION(S) AND RESEARCH PHASE
Multiple Myeloma – Phase II/III
Effects of Chemotherapy – Phase II/III

YM-529, minodronate
unknown

MANUFACTURER
Yamanouchi Pharmaceutical

DESCRIPTION
YM-529 is a bisphosphonate being evaluated for the treatment of multiple myeloma and bone metastasis with breast cancer. The drug is manufactured in both oral and injectable formulations. It is in phase III trials and is part of Yamanouchi's domestic pipeline.

INDICATION(S) AND RESEARCH PHASE
Multiple Myeloma – Phase III
Breast Cancer – Phase III

Red Blood Cell Disorders

flumecinol
Zixoryn

MANUFACTURER
Farmacon

DESCRIPTION
Zixoryn is being tested as an oral treatment and prevention of hyperbilirubinemia. Bilirubin is a red bile pigment that is formed from hemoglobin, an essential oxygen-carrying component of red blood cells. Zixoryn is in a phase II trial for subjects with hyperbilirubinemia.

INDICATION(S) AND RESEARCH PHASE
Red Blood Cell Disorders – Phase II

psoralen, S-59
unknown

MANUFACTURER
Cerus Corporation

DESCRIPTION
Psoralen uses ultraviolet-A light to initiate a platelet pathogen inactivation system. This invitro process works on blood temporarily drawn outside of the body for sterilization of viruses, bacteria, and other pathogens that may be present. Psoralen is being tested in phase III trials with blood components used in transfusions, including platelets, fresh frozen plasma (FFP), and red blood cells. The purpose is to enhance the safety of blood transfusions by inactivating pathogens in the blood components.

Psoralen may also help inactivate white blood cells, which are responsible for a variety of adverse transfusion reactions. This therapy may be useful for treatment of thrombocytopenia, and red and white blood cell disorders.

A phase III thrombocytopenia trial in the United States is under way with ten to 12 sites enrolling approximately 600 thrombocytopenic subjects. The European phase III trial will involve four sites and 100 subjects.

A pathogen inactivation system for FFP also is in phase III trials in the United States, with a target goal of 175 subjects with congenital or acquired coagulation factor deficiencies and those with thrombocytopenic purpura who need large volume FFP transfusions, enrolled at multiple sites. Cerus Corporation is developing psoralen in collaboration with Baxter Healthcare.

68/Red Blood Cell Disorders

INDICATION(S) AND RESEARCH PHASE
Bacterial Infection – Phase III
Red Blood Cell Disorders – Phase III
Thrombocytopenia – Phase III
Viral Infection – Phase III
White Blood Cell Disorders – Phase III

Thrombocytopenia

5c8 (anti CD-40 ligand antibody)
Antova

MANUFACTURER
Biogen

DESCRIPTION
Biogen has engineered 5c8 (anti CD-40 ligand antibody), a humanized monoclonal antibody for the potential treatment of a number of autoimmune disorders. These include idiopathic thrombocytopenic purpura (ITP), systemic lupus erythematosus, kidney transplantation, and factor VIII antibody inhibition.

In the aforementioned autoimmune diseases, it is thought that activated white blood cells, called T-cell lymphocytes, bind to other tissue cells through a cell surface receptor, the CD-40 ligand. Abnormal antibodies are produced that will then recognize healthy body tissues as foreign, and thereby cause an inflammatory response. The 5c8 antibody may stop this abnormal immune cycle by binding to the CD-40 ligand and inhibiting its ability to bind with its receptor on a variety of other normal cells.

Biogen is considering future trials testing 5c8 for other autoimmune diseases, including multiple sclerosis and other types of transplant surgeries.

INDICATION(S) AND RESEARCH PHASE
Thrombocytopenia – Phase II
Systemic Lupus Erythematosus – Phase II
Kidney Transplant Surgery – Phase II
Factor VIII Antibody Inhibition – Phase II

argatroban
unknown

MANUFACTURER
Sanofi-Synthelabo Pharmaceuticals

DESCRIPTION
Argatroban is being tested in phase II trials to prevent thrombocytopenia, characterized by low platelet levels that can occur as a result of inappropriate immune reactions. Low platelet counts often occur after taking heparin, a commonly used blood thinner. Heparin may instigate an immune reaction in which the body attacks its own platelets. One to two percent of subjects treated with heparin for more than four days develop this complication. This condition can cause limb loss, life-threatening blood clots throughout the body, heart attacks, or strokes.

INDICATION(S) AND RESEARCH PHASE
Thrombocytopenia – Phase II

CBP-1011
Colirest

MANUFACTURER
Inkine Pharmaceutical Company

DESCRIPTION
Colirest is an oral steroid-like drug in phase III development for the treatment of idiopathic thrombocytopenic purpura (ITP). ITP is a disorder in which the immune system attacks its own platelets, targeting them with antibodies, then destroying the resulting immune complexed platelets. Preliminary studies indicate that Colirest may help increase platelet counts.

Additionally, phase II trials for the treatment of Crohn's disease have been completed, and the drug is also in development for ulcerative colitis. In December 2000, positive results were announced for a multicenter open-label phase II trial of Colirest in subjects with mild or moderate active ulcerative colitis. Nine of 11 evaluable subjects completed eight weeks of Colirest treatment. Seven of the nine responded to Colirest treatment in the Disease Activity Index (DAI) and Investigator Global Assessment (IGA) evaluations. Inkine plans to move Colirest into later stage pivotal trials.

INDICATION(S) AND RESEARCH PHASE
Thrombocytopenia – Phase III
Crohn's Disease – Phase II completed
Irritable Bowel Syndrome – Phase II completed

MDX-33
unknown

MANUFACTURER
Medarex

DESCRIPTION
MDX-33 is a humanized monoclonal antibody being evaluated for its ability to decrease the activity of monocytes, macrophages, or other white blood cells that can destroy healthy platelets or red blood cells. It is in trials for the treatment of autoimmune blood disorders such as idiopathic thrombocytopenia purpura (ITP) and autoimmune hemolytic anemia.

Results of a phase II trial of MDX-33 suggested the drug was well tolerated in adult subjects with chronic ITP. A single dose of MDX-33 appeared to substantially elevate platelet counts in all subjects treated with the optimal dose. The dose-escalating, double-blind, placebo-controlled trial consisted of 30 adults with chronic ITP. MDX-33 is being developed through a corporate alliance between Medarex and Aventis Behring.

INDICATION(S) AND RESEARCH PHASE
Anemia – Phase II
Thrombocytopenia – Phase II completed

PI-88
unknown

MANUFACTURER
Progen Industries

DESCRIPTION
PI-88 will be evaluated in phase II trials for the prevention of blood clots in thromboembolic diseases and angioplasty induced restenosis in 2001. Results from previous trials have shown PI-88 to be a potent antithrombotic and anticoagulant with a unique mode of action. According to Progen Industries, PI-88 inhibits growth of

vascular smooth muscle cells, restenosis, in animal models that are analogues to balloon angioplasty. Balloon angioplasty is a surgical procedure in which a balloon-tipped catheter is used to widen blocked arteries. Local vascular irritation occurs in 30% of cases of people who have received the angioplasty procedure. Local vascular irritation induces rapid growth of smooth muscle cells surrounding the artery, which causes re-blockage of the artery.

PI-88 will also be entering phase II trials for treatment of cancer in early 2001.

INDICATION(S) AND RESEARCH PHASE
Thrombocytopenia – Phase II
Cancer/Tumors (Unspecified) – Phase II
Angioplasty – Phase II

psoralen, S-59
unknown

MANUFACTURER
Cerus Corporation

DESCRIPTION
Psoralen uses ultraviolet-A light to initiate a platelet pathogen inactivation system. This invitro process works on blood temporarily drawn outside of the body for sterilization of viruses, bacteria, and other pathogens that may be present. Psoralen is being tested in phase III trials with blood components used in transfusions, including platelets, fresh frozen plasma (FFP), and red blood cells. The purpose is to enhance the safety of blood transfusions by inactivating pathogens in the blood components.

Psoralen may also help inactivate white blood cells, which are responsible for a variety of adverse transfusion reactions. This therapy may be useful for treatment of thrombocytopenia, and red and white blood cell disorders.

A phase III thrombocytopenia trial in the United States is under way with ten to 12 sites enrolling approximately 600 thrombocytopenic subjects. The European phase III trial will involve four sites and 100 subjects.

A pathogen inactivation system for FFP also is in phase III trials in the United States, with a target goal of 175 subjects with congenital or acquired coagulation factor deficiencies and those with thrombocytopenic purpura who need large volume FFP transfusions, enrolled at multiple sites. Cerus Corporation is developing psoralen in collaboration with Baxter Healthcare.

INDICATION(S) AND RESEARCH PHASE
Bacterial Infection – Phase III
Red Blood Cell Disorders – Phase III
Thrombocytopenia – Phase III
Viral Infection – Phase III
White Blood Cell Disorders – Phase III

YM-294, oprelvekin
unknown

MANUFACTURER
Yamanouchi Pharmaceutical

DESCRIPTION
YM-294 is an injectable thrombocytopoietic factor (rhIL-11) being evaluated for its effectiveness in preventing chemotherapy-induced thrombocytopenia. The drug is in phase III trials and is part of Yamanouchi's domestic pipeline. The company is developing the drug with Genetics Institute.

INDICATION(S) AND RESEARCH PHASE
Thrombocytopenia – Phase III

White Blood Cell Disorders

alitretinoin, ALRT-1057
Panretin

MANUFACTURER
Ligand Pharmaceuticals

DESCRIPTION
Panretin is 9-cis retinoic acid, and is chemically related to vitamin A. It activates all known retinoid receptors. Activation of retinoid receptors regulates the expression of genes controlling processes related to cell differentiation and proliferation. A topical gel formulation of Panretin has been on the market since February 1999 for the treatment of lesions associated with Kaposi's sarcoma.

Currently, Panretin in oral capsule formulation is being evaluated for the treatment of breast and pediatric cancers in phase II trials, and for treatment of myelodysplastic syndrome, bronchial metaplasia, and psoriasis in phase II/III trials.

INDICATION(S) AND RESEARCH PHASE
Breast Cancer – Phase II
Lung Cancer – Phase II/III
Pediatric, Cancer – Phase II
Psoriasis and Psoriatic Disorders – Phase II/III
White Blood Cell Disorders, Myelodysplastic Syndrome – Phase II/III
Kaposi's Sarcoma – FDA approved

LDI-200
unknown

MANUFACTURER
Milkhaus Laboratory

DESCRIPTION
LDI-200, in a subcutaneous formulation, is in phase II/III trials for treatment of prostate cancer, and has completed a phase II trial for treatment of leukemia and a phase II/III trial for myelodysplastic syndrome.

LDI-200 demonstrated positive results in a small phase II/III open label crossover trial in subjects with myelodysplastic syndrome. The control consisted of subjects given supportive therapy of transfusions and antibiotics, who became eligible for treatment if their disease progressed more rapidly than anticipated. A total of 23 subjects were treated using LDI-200, and seven showed significant clinical response.

INDICATION(S) AND RESEARCH PHASE
Leukemia – Phase II completed
Prostate Cancer – Phase II/III
White Blood Cell Disorders, Myelodysplastic Syndrome – Phase III completed

psoralen, S-59
unknown

MANUFACTURER

Cerus Corporation

DESCRIPTION

Psoralen uses ultraviolet-A light to initiate a platelet pathogen inactivation system. This invitro process works on blood temporarily drawn outside of the body for sterilization of viruses, bacteria, and other pathogens that may be present. Psoralen is being tested in phase III trials with blood components used in transfusions, including platelets, fresh frozen plasma (FFP), and red blood cells. The purpose is to enhance the safety of blood transfusions by inactivating pathogens in the blood components.

Psoralen may also help inactivate white blood cells, which are responsible for a variety of adverse transfusion reactions. This therapy may be useful for treatment of thrombocytopenia, and red and white blood cell disorders.

A phase III thrombocytopenia trial in the United States is under way at ten to 12 sites enrolling approximately 600 thrombocytopenic subjects. The European phase III trial will involve four sites and 100 subjects.

A pathogen inactivation system for FFP also began phase III trials in July 1999 in the United States, with a target goal of 175 subjects with congenital or acquired coagulation factor deficiencies and those with thrombocytopenic purpura who need large volume FFP transfusions, enrolled at multiple sites. Cerus Corporation is developing psoralen in collaboration with Baxter Healthcare.

INDICATION(S) AND RESEARCH PHASE
Bacterial Infection – Phase III
Red Blood Cell Disorders – Phase III
Thrombocytopenia – Phase III
Viral Infection – Phase III
White Blood Cell Disorders – Phase III

RF-1012
unknown

MANUFACTURER
SuperGen

DESCRIPTION
SuperGen is developing RF-1012 to counteract the anemia, or red cell depletion, and leukopenia, or white cell depletion, often associated with chemotherapy and radiotherapy treatments. This drug is currently being evaluated in phase II trials, and is to be given in an intravenous formulation. Cancer treatments usually work by targeting steps in the process of cell replication, since cells usually become cancerous due to uncontrolled cell division. However, by giving systemic drugs that block cell division, cells undergoing normal division and growth may be unharmed, especially in the bone marrow where new red and white blood cells are born. This total body exposure to the drug may result in very low levels of red blood cells and white blood cells. This situation leads to fatigue, pallor, susceptibility to infections, and organ failure.

RF-1012 is a protective agent that may potentially limit the effect of chemotherapy and radiotherapy on normal, growing blood cells. This protective ability is crucial since cancer treatment regimens are frequently stopped because of severe anemia or leukopenia. This agent may also prevent life-threatening infections secondary to white blood cell depletion, congestive heart failure, and other organ damage resulting from a decline in red blood cells.

INDICATION(S) AND RESEARCH PHASE
Anemia – Phase II
Effects of Chemotherapy – Phase II
White Blood Cell Disorders – Phase II

SD/01
unknown

MANUFACTURER
Amgen

DESCRIPTION
SD/01 is a sustained duration granulocyte colony stimulating factor (G-CSF) molecule being tested in phase III trials for treatment of chemotherapy induced neutropenia. Granulocytes and neutrophils are types of white blood cells that help the immune system protect the body from foreign substances. SD/01 consists of the protein G-CSF, to which poly(ethylene) glycol (PEG) has been bound. PEGylated proteins stay circulating longer in the body; therefore it is thought that subjects may require fewer injections.

SD/01 is also currently in a phase III trial in breast cancer subjects.

INDICATION(S) AND RESEARCH PHASE
Breast Cancer – Phase III
Effects of Chemotherapy – Phase III
White Blood Cell Disorders – Phase III

SMART M195
unknown

MANUFACTURER
Protein Design Labs

DESCRIPTION
SMART M195 is a radioactive compound that is linked to a humanized monoclonal antibody. Radiotherapy using alpha particle emitting isotopes, bismuth-213, has been used for some years to treat different forms of cancer. This combination therapy is a specialized targeting method that allows the monoclonal antibody to hunt down and attach itself to the cancer cell, which gives the adjoining radioactive isotope a greater chance, by proximity, to kill the cancer.

SMART M195 is currently in a phase III trial for treatment of acute myeloid leukemia using radiotherapy. This biologic product is also being tested in two other phase II studies for the indications of acute promyelocytic leukemia and myelodysplastic syndrome.

INDICATION(S) AND RESEARCH PHASE
Leukemia – Phase III
Leukemia – Phase II
White Blood Cell Disorders,
    Myelodysplastic Syndrome – Phase II

3 | Neurology

Population with illnesses in this category	160 million[1]
Drugs in the development pipeline	329[2]
Number of drugs in preclinical testing	188
Number of drugs in clinical testing	130

Source: 1. World Health Organization, worldwide figures 2. Parexel

Little is known about the causes of the diseases related to the brain and nervous system. Due to this lack of information, scientists have had great difficulty in finding cures for such diseases as Alzheimer's, Parkinson's, and epilepsy. CenterWatch has identified approximately 250 drugs currently in clinical development for the treatment of neurological diseases. These efforts have led to the approval of many effective medications. However, those that do exist often cause severe side effects that may limit patient use.

Alzheimer's disease is a progressive, neurodegenerative disease affecting more than ten million people worldwide and four million in the United States. It is the fourth leading cause of death in the United States. Alzheimer's causes impaired memory, thinking and behavior, leading to eventual functional decline and loss of independence for the patient. Early diagnosis and treatment can delay a decline in the patient's ability to perform activities of daily living, reduce behavioral disturbances, and improve cognitive performance.

Hallmarks of the disease seem to be the presence of amyloid plaques and neurofibrillary tangles in the brain tissue. There is also a decrease in the neurotransmitter acetylcholine, which is thought to play a major role in memory and cognition. Current treatment includes three different acetylcholinesterase inhibitors, which block the breakdown of acetylcholine. These drugs cannot halt or reverse the progression of Alzheimer's, but only alleviate some symptoms in some patients. Aricept (donepezil hydrochloride) dominates the market over the older treatment Cognex (tacrine). In 2000, Exelon (rivastigmine tartrate) was approved by the FDA for treatment of mild to moderate Alzheimer's. During trials, subjects treated with the drug showed significant benefit on daily living activities and behavioral symptoms, and showed some cognitive improvement.

There have been other drugs in late stage development, but many trials have been halted due to failure to produce statistically significant results. CenterWatch has identified 27 drugs in the clinical pipeline for treatment of Alzheimer's. The industry will spend an estimated $120 million to $140 million this year researching these medicines. Acetylcholinesterase inhibitors continue to dominate the pipeline. There is a potentially promising vaccine in development that may be able to clear amyloid plaques from the brains of Alzheimer's patients and prevent new plaques from forming. These actions would both relieve the symptoms and improve brain function. The vaccine is a synthetic form of the naturally occurring beta amyloid protein and is designed to prompt the body to produce small proteins that tag the amyloid for removal by scavenger cells in the brain.

Parkinson's disease affects over one and a half million people in the United States. Symptoms include muscle stiffness, tremors, slowness of movement, poor balance, and walking problems. The disease occurs when neurons in the brain that release dopamine are destroyed. Dopamine is a neurotransmitter that enables people to move normally and smoothly. Though the cause is unknown, it is thought that Parkinson's results from a combination of genetic predisposition and a presently unidentified environmental factor.

CenterWatch estimates that between $120 million and $135 million will be spent on the clinical development of 22 drugs for the treatment of Parkinson's disease this year. Selegiline is a monamine oxidase inhibitor (MAOI) that works against the enzyme that breaks down dopamine. Elan Pharmaceuticals is developing Zelapar, a new oral disintegrating formulation of selegiline that may provide rapid action with a smaller daily dose. Another MAOI currently in clinical trials is TVP-1012, from Teva Pharmaceuticals. This medication is said to have five times the potency of selegiline and may produce fewer side effects. Levodopa/carbidopa treatments combine levodopa, a dopamine precursor molecule that is converted to dopamine upon entering the brain, with carbidopa, which optimizes the amount of levodopa received by the brain while reducing its side effects. Additionally, there are many dopamine agonists in development and in use. Unfortunately though, many of the most successful drugs for treatment of Parkinson's disease come with undesirable side effects and often lose their effectiveness in advanced stages of the disease. Recent studies of the transplantation of porcine cells into the brains of people with Parkinson's disease showed that too much dopamine was being produced, which resulted in additional movement problems in the study subjects. Moreover, there appears to be no satisfactory way to treat this dopamine overproduction with medication. The result is that further critical analysis of transplantation of cells for the treatment of Parkinson's and other diseases is being conducted.

Epilepsy is a neurological dysfunction in which sudden and excessive bursts of electrical energy are emitted in the brain. These seizures can result from a number of events, including congenital malformations, head injuries, brain tumors, aneurysms, metabolic problems, infections, or for no apparent reason at all. Over two million Americans are affected by this disease and CenterWatch estimates that $55 million to $70 million is spent each year on the development of anti-convulsants used to control seizure activity.

The type of seizure determines what medication will be an effective treatment. Partial seizures, during which a person may or may not maintain consciousness, affect only one hemisphere of the brain. During general seizures, consciousness is partially or completely lost and contraction and relaxation of muscles occurs, producing the classic picture of a "seizure." Symptoms vary widely depending on seizure type. Approximately 30% to 50% of epileptics may continue to experience seizures despite treatment with medications currently available.

Depending on the type of seizure, an anticonvulsant is prescribed and dosage is increased until therapeutic blood levels are reached. Since most of these drugs have side effects, it is optimal to use only one medication. Anticonvulsants increase the threshold at which neurons fire. These drugs affect the neuron by interfering with the passage of ions, e.g., sodium, calcium, or potassium through channels in the neural cell membrane, thus reducing the chance of ion-dependent seizure activity. They may also work to increase levels of GABA (gamma amino butyric acid), a seizure-inhibiting molecule, and to decrease levels of glutamate, a seizure-promoting molecule.

In 2000, the FDA approved two new drugs for the treatment of epilepsy. Trileptal (oxcarbazepine) is for use as a monotherapy or adjunctive therapy in the treatment of partial seizures in adults and as adjunctive therapy in children ages four to 16. Zonegran (zonisamide) capsules were approved for adjunctive therapy for treatment of partial epileptic seizures in adults.

There are currently 15 drugs in the pipeline being developed for treatment of epilepsy. Pregabalin, in phase III trials being conducted by Pfizer, is a gabapentin analogue intended to increase GABA and decrease glutamate. Novartis is testing Rufinamide in pediatric trials. This drug induces anticonvulsant activity by blocking sodium channels in neurons. A unique phase I study is being conducted using porcine fetal neural cells to control epilepsy. Diacrin Laboratories is transplanting these cells into epileptic foci in the brain to study whether they will have an inhibitory effect on hyperexicitable regions of the human brain.

For the many adults and children suffering from these and other neurological diseases not adequately controlled by available medications, the drugs currently in the pipeline may hold the promise of effective treatment with fewer side effects and toxicities.

Alzheimer's Disease

acetyl-L-carnitine
Alcar

MANUFACTURER
Sigma-Tau Pharmaceuticals

DESCRIPTION
Alcar, an orally formulated drug, is being evaluated in phase III studies for early onset Alzheimer's disease and diabetic peripheral neuropathy. Alcar causes the growth and repair of neurons through the stimulation of nerve growth factor, which should lessen the cognitive deterioration resulting from Alzheimer's disease.

INDICATION(S) AND RESEARCH PHASE
Alzheimer's Disease – Phase III
Diabetes Prevention – Phase III

AIP-001
unknown

MANUFACTURER
Wyeth-Ayerst

DESCRIPTION
Wyeth-Ayerst and Elan are collaborating to develop an Alzheimer's disease immunotherapeutic aimed at modulating fl-amyloid plaque deposition. AIP-001 is currently in phase I development.

INDICATION(S) AND RESEARCH PHASE
Alzheimer's Disease – Phase I

AN-1792
unknown

MANUFACTURER
Elan Pharmaceutical Research

DESCRIPTION
AN-1792 is in a phase I trial for the treatment of Alzheimer's disease.

INDICATION(S) AND RESEARCH PHASE
Alzheimer's Disease – Phase I

aripiprazole, OPC-14597, OPC-31
expected to be Abilitat

MANUFACTURER
Bristol-Myers Squibb

DESCRIPTION
Aripiprazole is an oral drug that is a mixed dopamine receptor agonist/antagonist that is being developed to improve positive and negative symptoms due to schizophrenia and treat dementia/psychosis in Alzheimer's subjects. Currently, clinical testing is at the phase III level, with NDA filing planned for late 2001 for schizophrenia treatment.

The company reported that early studies with aripiprazole, a blocker at postsynaptic D_{2A} receptors, and a stimulator at presynaptic dopamine autoreceptors, show reduction in psychotic symptoms with a favorable extrapyramidal side effect profile. Animal models indicate the drug has less potential to cause side effects because of the relative lack of upregulation of D_2 receptors in the striatum of the brain.

INDICATION(S) AND RESEARCH PHASE
Schizophrenia and Schizoaffective Disorders – Phase III
Alzheimer's Disease – Phase III

CEP-1347
unknown

MANUFACTURER
Cephalon

DESCRIPTION
CEP-1347 is a selective inhibitor of the stress-activated protein kinase pathway, an intracellular signaling pathway, which is an essential component of the stress response leading to neuronal death. Working through a novel mechanism of action, CEP-1347 is the first orally active molecule in a new class of compounds to enter clinical testing in Parkinson's disease and is currently in a phase I/II trial. In animal models CEP-1347 has greatly reduced degeneration of dopamine neurons in the brain, indicating that it may delay or completely stop the progress of Parkinson's disease. The company H. Lundback A/S has the licensing rights in Europe.

INDICATION(S) AND RESEARCH PHASE
Parkinson's Disease – Phase I/II
Alzheimer's Disease – Phase I/II

CX-516, BDP-12
Ampalex

MANUFACTURER
Cortex Pharmaceuticals

DESCRIPTION
Ampalex is an ampakine (AMPA) receptor enhancer being developed for the treatment of Alzheimer's disease and cognitive dysfunction associated with schizophrenia. The drug has completed a phase I/II trial.

INDICATION(S) AND RESEARCH PHASE
Alzheimer's Disease – Phase I/II
Schizophrenia and Schizoaffective Disorders – Phase I/II completed

donepezil hydrochloride, E2020
Aricept

MANUFACTURER
Eisai

DESCRIPTION
Aricept is an acetylcholinesterase inhibitor. The enzyme acetylcholinesterase breaks down acetylcholine. By inhibiting this process, Aricept causes a greater concentration of acetylcholine. Acetylcholine is a neurotransmitter associated with memory, which means that greater concentrations of it could significantly improve the conditions of Alzheimer's disease. In addition, Aricept is in phase II trials in children seven to 16 years old who are suffering from attention deficit/hyperactivity disorder.

Aricept is currently in development in Japan, Europe and the United States. Aricept is being co-promoted by Pfizer.

INDICATION(S) AND RESEARCH PHASE
Alzheimer's Disease – NDA submitted in Japan
Dementia – Phase III

76/Alzheimer's Disease

Attention Deficit/Hyperactivity Disorder (ADHD) – Phase II
Pediatric, Attention Deficit Disorder – Phase II

DPC-543, DMP-543
unknown

MANUFACTURER
Du Pont

DESCRIPTION
DPC-543, formerly named DMP-543, enhances neurotransmitter release in the brain. It is being tested in phase II clinical trials for the treatment of Alzheimer's disease.

INDICATION(S) AND RESEARCH PHASE
Alzheimer's Disease – Phase II

dronabinol
Marinol

MANUFACTURER
Unimed Pharmaceuticals

DESCRIPTION
Marinol is an oral pill formulation of dronabinol, which is a synthetic marijuana derivative that is being tested in phase IIIb clinical trials for the treatment of dementia, including dementia in Alzheimer's disease. This naturally occurring cannabinoid has complex effects on the central nervous system. Marinol is approved by the FDA for anorexia associated with weight loss in AIDS subjects, and nausea and vomiting associated with cancer chemotherapy.

The company reported that this drug is only legally available in a synthetic form of the psychoactive component of marijuana, and a recent study found it has a very low potential for drug abuse. Marinol is available in round, soft gelatin capsules of 2.5 mg, 5 mg, and 10 mg.

INDICATION(S) AND RESEARCH PHASE
Alzheimer's Disease – Phase II
Dementia – Phase II

FK960
unknown

MANUFACTURER
Fujisawa Healthcare

DESCRIPTION
FK960 is a novel antidementia drug being tested in a phase II clinical study for the treatment of mild to moderate Alzheimer's disease.

INDICATION(S) AND RESEARCH PHASE
Alzheimer's Disease – Phase II

galantamine hydrobromide
Reminyl

MANUFACTURER
Janssen Research Foundation

DESCRIPTION
Reminyl (galantamine) is a nicotinic modulator that is being developed for the treatment of chronic fatigue syndrome (CFS), Alzheimer's disease, and dementia. This drug works by slowing down or reversibly inhibiting acetylcholinesterase, which is the enzyme responsible for degrading the neurotransmitter acetylcholine. It is produced in an oral tablet formulation.

Study results show that volunteers with Alzheimer's treated with Reminyl exhibited improved memory, behavior, and ability to perform activities of daily living. In addition, a second study suggested that the cognitive and functional benefits of galantamine may be sustained for at least 12 months. Reminyl is being developed by the Janssen Research Foundation under a co-development agreement with Shire Pharmaceuticals. An NDA was filed with the FDA in September 1999 and the company received an approvable letter in August 2000.

INDICATION(S) AND RESEARCH PHASE
Alzheimer's Disease – FDA approved
Chronic Fatigue Syndrome – Phase II
Dementia – Phase III

GT-2331
Perceptin

MANUFACTURER
Gliatech

DESCRIPTION
Perceptin is a selective histamine H3 receptor antagonist which is being developed for potential use in central nervous system diseases involving attention/learning or sleep disorders. Perceptin is being evaluated in a phase II trial for treatment of attention deficit/hyperactivity disorder (ADHD) and in a phase I/II for Alzheimer's disease and sleep disorders.

According to the company, histamine is a chemical messenger released from certain neurons in the brain, which regulates sleep/wake states and modulates levels of arousal and alertness in the conscious state. The histamine H3 receptor is predominantly found in the brain where it regulates the release of histamine.

Phase I clinical studies have demonstrated that Perceptin is safe, well tolerated, and amenable to once daily dosing.

The phase II trial for ADHD is a multi-dose, double-blind, randomized placebo-controlled clinical trial to evaluate the safety and preliminary efficacy of Perceptin at varying doses. The company expects to enroll up to 120 adult subjects.

INDICATION(S) AND RESEARCH PHASE
Alzheimer's Disease – Phase I/II
Attention Deficit/Hyperactivity Disorder (ADHD) – Phase II
Sleep Disorders – Phase I/II

leteprinim potassium, AIT-082
Neotrofin

MANUFACTURER
NeoTherapeutics

DESCRIPTION
Neotrofin is composed of the purine compound hypoxanthine, which is linked with the antiarrhythmic drug procainamide. Results of a double-blind, dose-escalating phase II trial of Neotrofin indicated that the

compound facilitated brain activity in Alzheimer's disease subjects, leading to improvements in memory, attention and judgement. The improvements were dose-related, with 500 mg and 1,000 mg doses producing more benefit than the 150 mg dose. The trial supported NeoTherapeutics' decision to initiate a one-year trial in early 2001 at doses of 500 mg and 1,000 mg in subjects with moderate Alzheimer's disease.

Neotrofin is also in development for indications other than Alzheimer's disease, including peripheral neuropathy (preclinical) and other neurodegenerative diseases (research). In March 2001, NeoTherapeutics announced that it has begun a 12-week, double-blind, placebo-controlled phase II trial of Neotrofin in Parkinson's disease. Also in March, the company announced the initiation of a phase II trial in subacute spinal cord injured patients.

INDICATION(S) AND RESEARCH PHASE
Alzheimer's Disease – Phase III
Parkinson's Disease – Phase II
Spinal Cord Injuries – Phase II
Neuropathy – Preclinical
Neurodegenerative Disease – Research

memantine
unknown

MANUFACTURER
Neurobiological Technologies

DESCRIPTION
Memantine is an orally available compound that appears to restore the function of damaged nerve cells and reduce abnormal excitatory signals. This is accomplished by the modulation of *N*-methyl-D-aspartate (NMDA) receptor activity.

Memantine is in trials for diabetic neuropathy (phase II completed), AIDS-related dementia and neurological function (phase II), and moderate to severe dementia and Alzheimer's disease (phase III). Forest Laboratories intends to prepare an NDA for submission around the end of 2001 for the treatment of Alzheimer's disease, but will also begin additional phase III trials in both mild to moderate and moderately severe to severe Alzheimer's disease.

Forest Laboratories has entered into an agreement with Merz & Co. (collaborator of Neurobiological Technologies), for the development and marketing of memantine in the United States.

INDICATION(S) AND RESEARCH PHASE
Alzheimer's Disease – Phase III
Acquired Immune Deficiency Syndrome (AIDS) and AIDS-Related Infections – Phase II
Neuropathy, Diabetic – Phase II completed

modafinil
Provigil

MANUFACTURER
Cephalon

DESCRIPTION
Provigil (modafinil) is a dopamine-releasing agent that increases excitatory glutamatergic transmission. It is being developed in phase III trials for the prevention of daytime sleepiness associated with obstructive sleep apnea, hypersomnia, and shiftwork. Phase II trials are being conducted for the prevention of excessive daytime sleepiness associated with Alzeimer's disease and Parkinson's disease.

A phase II trial has been completed using Provigil as a treatment for sleep apnea and fatigue associated with multiple sclerosis. This drug is also currently in a phase III trial for the treatment of sleepiness regardless of cause, with an NDA filing planned for late 2001.

Additionally, Provigil is currently in phase I/II trials for ADHD in pediatric subjects.

INDICATION(S) AND RESEARCH PHASE
Multiple Sclerosis – Phase II completed
Sleep Disorders – Phase III
Pediatric, Attention Deficit/Hyperactivity Disorder (ADHD) – Phase I/II
Parkinson's Disease – Phase II
Alzheimer's Disease – Phase II

NGD 97-1
unknown

MANUFACTURER
Neurogen Corporation

DESCRIPTION
NGD 97-1 is a selective GABA inverse agonist being developed for the treatment of Alzheimer's disease and other dementias. In preclinical models, this type of drug reduced the activity of the GABA system in a manner that produced memory enhancing effects. NGD 97-1 is in phase II development; to date, results indicate the drug is well tolerated.

INDICATION(S) AND RESEARCH PHASE
Alzheimer's Disease – Phase II
Dementia – Phase I

nicotinamide adenine dinucleotide (NAD)
Memex

MANUFACTURER
Telluride Pharmaceutical

DESCRIPTION
Memex is an oral tablet that contains reduced fl-nicotinamide adenine dinucleotide (NAD), a disodium salt with no starch. NAD is obtained from yeast and it is an essential co-factor of numerous enzymes such as NAD-dehydrogenase. Since cellular ATP production, which provides needed energy to the body, is coupled to the NAD content in the cell, the company believes that a medication that would help subjects with Alzheimer's disease regain their normal cellular energy production capacity would be effective. This reasoning includes the relative observation that the more NAD present in a cell, the more ATP is produced, and therefore the more energy a cell has available.

The company reported that in an open label trial, 470 subjects who received NAD orally were compared to 415 subjects who received NAD intravenously. The oral form of NAD produced a beneficial clinical effect comparable to that of the intravenously administered NAD. Motor skills improved considerably in these subjects, in particular, walking, posture, speech, and mimicry.

This observation provides indirect evidence that the oral form of NAD was absorbed and transported in the blood to the target organs, where it was taken up by the cells. The mechanism of action appears to be an increase in energy production produced by the oral administration of NAD. The coenzyme triggers increased NAD ubiquinone reductase activity due to increased production of ATP.

In addition, results from an invivo study showed that Memex stimulates the production of dopamine and epinephrine in the striatum of the rat brain. Dopamine and epinephrine are responsible for physiological functions such as walking, upright position, alertness, vigilance, and mental concentration. Since these functions are impaired in subjects with Alzheimer's Disease, Memex could have an additional beneficial effect.

Memex is currently being tested in a phase II/III clinical trial for Alzheimer's disease.

INDICATION(S) AND RESEARCH PHASE
Alzheimer's Disease – Phase II/III

NS-2330
unknown

MANUFACTURER
NeuroSearch A/S

DESCRIPTION
NS-2330 is a monoamine reuptake inhibitor in development for the treatment of Alzheimer's disease. NS-2330 increases the activity of dopamine and norepinephrine by inhibiting their uptake or degradation, and its mechanism of action also increases the release of acetylcholine in the brain. Since the function of all three neurotransmitters is affected in Alzheimer's disease, NS2330 may prove more beneficial than compounds that solely increase the amount of acetylcholine. NS2330 is currently in phase II development.

INDICATION(S) AND RESEARCH PHASE
Alzheimer's Disease – Phase II

NXY-059
unknown

MANUFACTURER
AstraZeneca

DESCRIPTION
NXY-059 is a neuroprotective agent in a phase IIb/III trial for the treatment of stroke in the United States. A phase I trial was initiated in Japan for acute stroke in December 2000. Furthermore, an NDA filing with the FDA is expected in late 2002. NXY-059 is being developed in partnership with Centaur Pharmaceuticals.

INDICATION(S) AND RESEARCH PHASE
Alzheimer's Disease – Phase II
Strokes – Phase IIb/III
Strokes – Phase I in Japan

phenserine
unknown

MANUFACTURER
Axonyx

DESCRIPTION
Phenserine is a highly selective, reversible acetylcholinesterase inhibitor, a mechanism known to improve memory and cognition in Alzheimer's subjects. Since phase I trials found phenserine to be safe and well tolerated, phase II trials were initiated in April 2000. Phenserine may prove to target the brain while disappearing rapidly from the blood, which would reduce toxicities and side effects.

INDICATION(S) AND RESEARCH PHASE
Alzheimer's Disease – Phase II

propentofylline, HWA-285
unknown

MANUFACTURER
Aventis

DESCRIPTION
Propentofylline is a novel compound that is being developed for the treatment of Alzheimer's disease and vascular dementia. This drug may work through glial cell modulation in the central nervous system. Clinical trials were formerly in phase III for both neuronal disorders. Currently development of the drug has been discontinued.

INDICATION(S) AND RESEARCH PHASE
Alzheimer's Disease – Phase III
  Discontinued
Dementia – Phase III Discontinued

quetiapine fumarate
Seroquel

MANUFACTURER
AstraZeneca

DESCRIPTION
Seroquel is an atypical antipsychotic medication, which belongs to a new chemical class, the dibenzothiazepine derivatives. Although the exact mechanism of action is unknown, scientists believe that Seroquel is a receptor antagonist for a combination of neurotransmitters, including dopamine type 2 (D_2) and serotonin type 2 ($5HT_2$).

Seroquel is approved for the management of the manifestations of psychotic disorders. The antipsychotic effectiveness has been proven in schizophrenic subjects for a six-week short-term usage.

Additionally, Seroquel is being tested in trials for the management of psychosis in Alzheimer's disease, line extension studies for the treatment of mania, bipolar disorder and schizophrenia are also under way for the granule formulation of the drug as well as for schizophrenia in a sustained-release formulation.

INDICATION(S) AND RESEARCH PHASE
Alzheimer's Disease – Phase III
Bipolar Disorders – Phase III
Manic Disorders – Phase III
Schizophrenia and Schizoaffective Disorders
  – Phase III

SIB-1553A
unknown

MANUFACTURER
Sibia Neurosciences

DESCRIPTION
SIB-1553A is a nicotinic acetylcholine

receptor (nAChR)-selective drug that is being developed for the treatment of Alzheimer's disease. Drugs that raise brain chemical levels of the neurotransmitter acetylcholine have demonstrated improvement in the symptoms of Alzheimer's disease. Currently, SIB-1553A is being tested in a phase II trial for this indication.

INDICATION(S) AND RESEARCH PHASE
Alzheimer's Disease – Phase II

SR-57746
unknown

MANUFACTURER
Sanofi-Synthelabo Pharmaceuticals

DESCRIPTION
SR-57746 is treating both Alzheimer's disease and amyotrophic lateral sclerosis (ALS, or Lou Gehrig's disease), both diseases that are caused by the death of nerve cells. A substance known as nerve growth factor (NGF) can potentially counteract this destructive process. NGF is responsible for synapse formation between neurons and also protects against neuronal death. In particular, NGF stimulates the growth of a type of nerve cell called cholinergic neurons that are the first cells to degenerate in Alzheimer's disease.

Unfortunately, it is very difficult to administer NGF since it cannot cross the blood-brain barrier and gain direct access to brain tissue. Therefore, scientists are developing compounds such as SR-57746, which enhance the effect of existing NGF on cell survival and neuron growth and development. SR-57746 may also lead to increased production of NGF itself. The result may be improvement in several aspects of Alzheimer's disease, including mood disorders, psychosis, aggressiveness, and restlessness. The same NGF-enhancing properties may make SR-57746 an effective therapy for ALS subjects as well, the only difference being the affected cells in ALS are the motor neurons in the spinal cord, not the brain neurons as in Alzheimer's. Further study will investigate whether this new medication can stabilize these two debilitating conditions.

INDICATION(S) AND RESEARCH PHASE
Amyotrophic Lateral Sclerosis (ALS) – Phase III
Alzheimer's Disease – Phase II

TAK-147
unknown

MANUFACTURER
Takeda Chemical Industries

DESCRIPTION
TAK-147 is an acetylcholinesterase inhibitor being developed for the treatment of senile dementia of the Alzheimer's disease type. It is currently in phase III trials in Japan.

INDICATION(S) AND RESEARCH PHASE
Dementia – Phase III
Alzheimer's Disease – Phase III

TVP-1012, rasagiline mesylate
unknown

MANUFACTURER
Teva Pharmaceutical Industries

DESCRIPTION
TVP-1012 is an inhibitor of monoamine oxidase B (MAO-B). MAO inhibitors have been used for many years to treat depression; however, they have the potential to cause a hypertensive crisis when taken concurrently with sympathomimetic drugs (such as amphetamines, dopamine, L-dopa, and epinephrine) or certain foods (such as cheeses or fava beans containing tyramine). TVP-1012 may present a better safety profile than previously approved MAO inhibitors. The drug is currently in phase III trials for the treatment of Parkinson's disease and phase II trials for Alzheimer's disease.

INDICATION(S) AND RESEARCH PHASE
Parkinson's Disease – Phase III
Alzheimer's Disease – Phase II

unknown
Memantine

MANUFACTURER
Forest Laboratories

DESCRIPTION
Memantine is an orally active, non-competitive N-methyl-D-aspartate (NMDA) antagonist. Memantine is the first NMDA receptor antagonist that has shown activity treating Alzheimer's disease and vascular dementia.

Forest Laboratories holds the rights to the United States market for Memantine. On August 11, 2000, Lundbeck acquired the exclusive rights from the Merz & Co to a series of European markets and the markets in Canada, Australia, and South Africa. For Japan memantine is under development by Merz' collaborating partner Suntory Ltd.

INDICATION(S) AND RESEARCH PHASE
Alzheimer's Disease – Phase III

unknown
Arecoline

MANUFACTURER
Cogent Pharmaceuticals

DESCRIPTION
Arecoline, a muscarinic receptor agonist for subjects suffering from Alzheimer's disease completed phase I trials in February 2000 that include 22 subjects. The once-a-day proprietary transdermal patch delivery demonstrated it was able to deliver arecoline at levels equal to intravenous doses that in prior published studies showed improvement in cognitive ability. The company is now actively looking for a partner to initiate phase II trials.

INDICATION(S) AND RESEARCH PHASE
Alzheimer's Disease – Phase I completed

Amyotrophic Lateral Sclerosis (ALS)

AVP-923
unknown

MANUFACTURER
AVANIR Pharmaceuticals

Amyotrophic Lateral Sclerosis

DESCRIPTION
AVP-923 is in a phase II/III trial for the treatment of emotional liability in neurodegenerative disease. Approximately 100 subjects with Lou Gehrig's disease (amyotrophic lateral sclerosis or ALS) will be tested at 11 sites in the United States. The trial is being monitored by INC Research and is expected to continue through July 2001. The company plans to initiate a second clinical trial in 2001 that will be conducted in multiple sclerosis.

INDICATION(S) AND RESEARCH PHASE
Amyotrophic Lateral Sclerosis (ALS) – Phase I
Neuropathy – Phase II/III
Neuropathic pain – Phase II/III
Emotional lability – Phase II

---

brain-derived neurotrophic factor, BDNF
unknown

MANUFACTURER
Regeneron Pharmaceuticals

DESCRIPTION
Brain-derived neurotrophic factor (BDNF) is a naturally occurring human protein that promotes the survival of spinal neurons. It is being developed for the treatment of amyotrophic lateral sclerosis (ALS), commonly known as Lou Gehrig's disease.

BDNF is currently in phase II/III trials for ALS. Partnerships for development of the protein include Amgen and Sumitomo Pharmaceuticals.

INDICATION(S) AND RESEARCH PHASE
Amyotrophic Lateral Sclerosis (ALS) – Phase II/III

SR-57746
unknown

MANUFACTURER
Sanofi-Synthelabo Pharmaceuticals

DESCRIPTION
SR-57746 is treating both Alzheimer's and amyotrophic lateral sclerosis (ALS, or Lou Gehrig's Disease), both diseases that are caused by the death of nerve cells. A substance known as nerve growth factor (NGF) can potentially counteract this destructive process. NGF is responsible for synapse formation between neurons and also protects against neuronal death. In particular, NGF stimulates the growth of a type of nerve cell called cholinergic neurons that are the first cells to degenerate in Alzheimer's disease.

Unfortunately, it is very difficult to administer NGF since it cannot cross the blood-brain barrier and gain direct access to brain tissue. Therefore, scientists are developing compounds such as SR-57746, which enhance the effect of existing NGF on cell survival and neuron growth and development. SR-57746 may also lead to increased production of NGF itself. The result may be improvement in several aspects of Alzheimer's disease, including mood disorders, psychosis, aggressiveness, and restlessness. The same NGF-enhancing properties may make SR-57746 an effective therapy for ALS subjects as well, the only difference being the affected cells in ALS are the motor neurons in the spinal cord, not the brain neurons as in Alzheimer's. Further study will investigate whether this new medication can stabilize these two debilitating conditions.

INDICATION(S) AND RESEARCH PHASE
Amyotrophic Lateral Sclerosis (ALS) – Phase III
Alzheimer's Disease – Phase II

Attention Deficit/Hyperactivity Disorder (ADHD)

altropane
unknown

MANUFACTURER
Boston Life Sciences

DESCRIPTION
Altropane is a radioactive molecule that binds specifically to the dopamine transporter (DAT) in the brain. The actual number of DATs in the midbrain can be measured using Altropane along with SPECT imaging. A measurement of DATs may be useful because data suggest there is an abnormally high amount in the midbrain of individuals with ADHD. A phase II/III trial involving 40 subjects is under way. The company plans to initiate two parallel phase III studies in adults between the ages of 20 and 40 years. Upon completion of these trials, the company will file for marketing approval using altropane to aid in the diagnosis of ADHD in adults. Afterwards, the company plans to initiate a phase III trial testing altropane in the diagnosis of ADHD in children.

Additionally, phase III results showed that altropane is able to differentiate Parkinson's movement disorders (including Parkinson's disease) from other movement disorders. The phase III trial included 95 subjects having the clinical diagnosis of Parkinsonian syndrome (PS) and 70 subjects having non-movement disorders with clinical features similar to PS but whose symptoms are caused by something other than a destruction of dopamine producing cells.

INDICATION(S) AND RESEARCH PHASE
Parkinson's Disease – Phase III completed
Attention Deficit/Hyperactivity Disorder (ADHD) – Phase II/III

CNS stimulant
unknown

MANUFACTURER
Elan Pharmaceutical Research

DESCRIPTION
This central nervous system (CNS) stimulant is being developed for the treatment of attention deficit/hyperactivity disorder (ADHD). This drug is being tested in a phase II trial using the CODAS delivery technology.

INDICATION(S) AND RESEARCH PHASE
Attention Deficit/Hyperactivity Disorder (ADHD) – Phase II

+DDMS

unknown

MANUFACTURER
Sepracor

DESCRIPTION
+DDMS is a serotonin, norepinephrine, and dopamine reuptake inhibitor. It is the single isomer version of Meridia, developed and marketed by Knoll Pharmaceuticals. The drug is currently in phase I studies for the treatment of different central nervous system disorders, including depression and attention deficit/hyperactivity disorder (ADHD).

INDICATION(S) AND RESEARCH PHASE
Attention Deficit/Hyperactivity Disorder (ADHD) – Phase I
Depression – Phase I
Neurologic Disorders – Phase I

d-methylphenidate HCl
unknown

MANUFACTURER
Celgene Corporation

DESCRIPTION
D-methylphenidate hydrochloride (d-MPH) is a chirally pure, single isomer version of Ritalin in an oral formulation. It is being tested in a phase III study for the treatment of attention deficit/hyperactivity disorder (ADHD) in children.

INDICATION(S) AND RESEARCH PHASE
Pediatric, Attention Deficit/Hyperactivity Disorder (ADHD) – Phase III

donepezil hydrochloride, E2020
Aricept

MANUFACTURER
Eisai

DESCRIPTION
Aricept is an acetylcholinesterase inhibitor. The enzyme acetylcholinesterase breaks down acetylcholine. By inhibiting this process, Aricept causes a greater concentration of acetylcholine. Acetylcholine is a neurotransmitter associated with memory, which means that greater concentrations of it could significantly improve the conditions of Alzheimer's disease. In addition, Aricept is in phase II trials in children seven to 16 years old who are suffering from attention deficit/hyperactivity disorder.

Aricept is currently in development in Japan, Europe, and the United States. Aricept is being co-promoted by Pfizer.

INDICATION(S) AND RESEARCH PHASE
Alzheimer's Disease – NDA submitted in Japan
Dementia – Phase III
Attention Deficit/Hyperactivity Disorder (ADHD) – Phase II
Pediatric, Attention Deficit Disorder – Phase II

GT-2331
Perceptin

MANUFACTURER
Gliatech

DESCRIPTION
Perceptin is a selective histamine H3 receptor antagonist which is being developed for potential use in central nervous system diseases involving attention/learning or sleep disorders. Perceptin is being evaluated in a phase II trial for treatment of attention deficit/hyperactivity disorder (ADHD) and in a phase I/II for Alzheimer's disease and sleep disorders.

According to the company, histamine is a chemical messenger released from certain neurons in the brain, which regulates sleep/wake states and modulates levels of arousal and alertness in the conscious state. The histamine H3 receptor is predominantly found in the brain where it regulates the release of histamine.

Phase I clinical studies have demonstrated that Perceptin is safe, well tolerated, and amenable to once daily dosing.

The phase II trial for ADHD is a multi-dose, double-blind, randomized placebo-controlled clinical trial to evaluate the safety and preliminary efficacy of Perceptin at varying doses. The company expects to enroll up to 120 adult subjects.

INDICATION(S) AND RESEARCH PHASE
Alzheimer's Disease – Phase I/II
Attention Deficit/Hyperactivity Disorder (ADHD) – Phase II
Sleep Disorders – Phase I/II

GW 320659, 1555U88
unknown

MANUFACTURER
GlaxoSmithKline

DESCRIPTION
GW 320659 is a noradrenaline reuptake inhibitor being tested in phase II trials for the treatment of attention deficit/hyperactivity disorder (ADHD).

INDICATION(S) AND RESEARCH PHASE
Attention Deficit/Hyperactivity Disorder (ADHD) – Phase II

mecamylamine HCl
Inversine

MANUFACTURER
Layton Bioscience

DESCRIPTION
Inversine is being evaluated in a phase III trial for the treatment of Tourette's syndrome in young adult subjects and a phase III trials for attention deficit/hyperactivity disorder (ADHD) in pediatric subjects.

INDICATION(S) AND RESEARCH PHASE
Pediatric, Tourette's Syndrome – Phase III
Pediatric, Attention Deficit/Hyperactivity Disorder – Phase III

methylphenidate
MethyPatch

MANUFACTURER
Noven Pharmaceuticals

DESCRIPTION
Noven Pharmaceutical's MethyPatch, a transdermal methylphenidate patch, is in phase III development. Methylphenidate is the active ingredient found in Ritalin,

82/Attention Deficit/Hyperactivity Disorder (AD/HD)

Novartis Pharmaceuticals' approved drug for attention deficit/hyperactivity disorder (ADHD). The patch is being developed to address the social concerns of children needing to take an oral pill each day. The company hopes that a discreet patch will eliminate the stigma children suffer from taking an oral medication during the school day, as well as eliminating drug diversion and abuse issues that affect the pill formulation. The company expects to file an NDA in the first half of 2001.

INDICATION(S) AND RESEARCH PHASE
Pediatric, Attention Deficit/Hyperactivity Disorder (ADHD) – Phase III

methylphenidate
MR Racemate

MANUFACTURER
Celltech Chiroscience plc

DESCRIPTION
A modified release (MR) formulation of methylphenidate is currently being developed for the treatment of attention deficit\hyperactivity disorder (ADHD). The problem with approved methylphenidate treatment is the drug's short duration of action. The MR formulation should eliminate the need for mid-day dosing and should increase compliance with drug use instructions by children.

A UK Marketing Authority Application was granted at the end of 1999 for the existing racemic IR formulation. The drug is in phase III trials in the United States.

INDICATION(S) AND RESEARCH PHASE
Attention Deficit\Hyperactivity Disorder (ADHD) – Phase III

methylphenidate
Ritalin LA

MANUFACTURER
Novartis

DESCRIPTION
Ritalin LA, a time-release product, is an NK-1 substance P antagonist. Ritalin is an established treatment for attention deficit/hyperactivity disorder (ADHD) that works by increasing attention and decreasing restlessness in children and adults who are overactive, cannot concentrate for very long or are easily distracted, and are impulsive. An application has been submitted overseas for Ritalin LA for the treatment of attention deficit disorders.

INDICATION(S) AND RESEARCH PHASE
Attention Deficit/Hyperactivity Disorder (ADHD) – MAA submitted
Pediatric, Attention Deficit/Hyperactivity Disorder (ADHD) – MAA submitted

methylphenidate HCl
unknown

MANUFACTURER
Medeva plc

DESCRIPTION
Methylphenidate is a stimulant used for the treatment of attention deficit/hyperactivity disorder (ADHD). Methylphenidate HCl modified release capsules utilize Eurand's novel Diffucaps technology, a multi-particulate bead delivery system with each bead acting as a drug reservoir. Each bead is coated with a chosen polymer to provide a unique release profile. Customized release profiles can then be achieved by incorporating different types of beads into each capsule.

Phase III trial results of the formulation demonstrated that the capsules control the symptoms of ADHD throughout the school day without the need for a second midday dose. Three hundred fourteen children with ADHD between the ages of six and 15 were evaluated in the randomized, double-blind, placebo-controlled trial. The primary efficacy measure was the difference from baseline on the teacher's version of the Conners' Global Index (CGI). The estimated mean improvement from baseline was 7.9 for methylphenidate modified release capsules compared to 1.2 for placebo.

INDICATION(S) AND RESEARCH PHASE
Pediatric, Attention Deficit/Hyperactivity Disorder (ADHD) – Phase III

modafinil
Provigil

MANUFACTURER
Cephalon

DESCRIPTION
Provigil (modafinil) is a dopamine-releasing agent that increases excitatory glutamatergic transmission. It is being developed in phase III trials for the prevention of daytime sleepiness associated with obstructive sleep apnea, hypersomnia, and shiftwork. Phase II trials are being conducted for the prevention of excessive daytime sleepiness associated with Alzheimer's disease and Parkinson's disease.

A phase II trial has been completed using Provigil as a treatment for sleep apnea and fatigue associated with multiple sclerosis. This drug is also currently in a phase III trial for the treatment of sleepiness regardless of cause, with an NDA filing planned for late 2001.

Provigil is currently in phase I/II trials for ADHD in pediatric subjects.

INDICATION(S) AND RESEARCH PHASE
Multiple Sclerosis – Phase II completed
Sleep Disorders – Phase III
Pediatric, Attention Deficit/Hyperactivity Disorder – Phase I/II
Parkinson's Disease – Phase II
Alzheimer's Disease – Phase II

SIB-1508Y
unknown

MANUFACTURER
Sibia Neurosciences

DESCRIPTION
SIB-1508Y is a nicotinic acetylcholine receptor (nAChR)-selective drug that is being developed for the treatment of Parkinson's disease, other cognitive disorders, and attention deficit/hyperactivity disorder (ADHD). SIB-1508Y is being tested in phase II trials as both a single therapeutic agent and combined with L-dopa for treatment of Parkinson's disease.

INDICATION(S) AND RESEARCH PHASE
Attention Deficit/Hyperactivity Disorder (ADHD) – Phase II
Memory Loss – Phase II
Parkinson's Disease – Phase II

SLI 381
Adderall

MANUFACTURER
Shire Pharmaceuticals

DESCRIPTION
SLI 381 is a once-a-day formulation of Adderall in development for the treatment of attention deficit/hyperactivity disorder (ADHD). Adderall is an amphetamine compound that produces central nervous system stimulant activity. Trial results indicated the drug may control symptoms of ADHD throughout the day and into the evening. Compared with placebo, subjects given SLI 381 demonstrated significant improvement on both the SKAMP Rating Scale and the PERMP Derived Measures throughout the day and into evening time points. The effects of SLI 381 on these scales also lasted until later in the day and longer than those of Adderall 10 mg. An NDA that includes this trial was submitted to the FDA in October 2000.

INDICATION(S) AND RESEARCH PHASE
Attention Deficit/Hyperactivity Disorder (ADHD) – NDA submitted

SPD 420
unknown

MANUFACTURER
Shire Pharmaceuticals

DESCRIPTION
Ampakine CX516 (designated as SPD 420) is being evaluated for the treatment of attention deficit/hyperactivity disorder (ADHD). The drug is being developed for worldwide use in both adult and pediatric subjects.

INDICATION(S) AND RESEARCH PHASE
Attention Deficit/Hyperactivity Disorder (ADHD) – Phase I completed
Pediatric, Attention Deficit/Hyperactivity Disorder (ADHD) – Phase I completed

SPD 503
unknown

MANUFACTURER
Shire Pharmaceuticals

DESCRIPTION
SPD 503 is being evaluated for the treatment of both adult and pediatric attention deficit/hyperactivity disorder (ADHD). SPD 503 is in phase I trials, and a proof of concept study is expected to begin in the first half of 2001.

INDICATION(S) AND RESEARCH PHASE
Attention Deficit/Hyperactivity Disorder (ADHD) – Phase I
Pediatric, Attention Deficit/Hyperactivity Disorder (ADHD) – Phase I

tomoxetine
unknown

MANUFACTURER
Eli Lilly

DESCRIPTION
Tomoxetine, a noradrenergic compound, is in development for the treatment of attention deficit/hyperactivity disorder (ADHD). It is being tested in phase II trials in children ages six and older.

INDICATION(S) AND RESEARCH PHASE
Pediatric, Attention Deficit/Hyperactivity Disorder (ADHD) – Phase III

Brain Cancer

CI-1042, ONYX-015
unknown

MANUFACTURER
Onyx Pharmaceuticals

DESCRIPTION
CI-1042 (ONYX-015) is a tumor-selective, modified adenovirus that has been genetically engineered to replicate in and kill cancer cells that possess a mutated oncogene called p53, while sparing normal cells with functioning p53. p53 is a tumor suppressor gene that is mutated in approximately 50% of all human cancers. CI-1042 is in development for several indications, including pancreatic cancer, liver metastases of colorectal cancer, and lung cancer.

In November 2000, results of a phase II trial demonstrated that CI-1042 administered as a single-agent replicates and causes tumor regression in refractory head and neck cancer. CI-1042 was shown to selectively target cancer cells containing a mutant p53 gene, while sparing normal cells with a functioning p53 gene. Of the 19 subjects who received the standard dosing regimen, four (21%) had an objective response, including two complete responses and two partial responses. CI-1042 is being co-developed with Pfizer.

INDICATION(S) AND RESEARCH PHASE
Colorectal Cancer – Phase II
Pancreatic Cancer – Phase II
Head and Neck Cancer – Phase III
Cervical Dysplasia/Cancer – Phase I completed
Lung Cancer – Phase II
Bladder Cancer – Phase I completed
Brain Cancer – Phase I completed

cidofovir
Vistide

MANUFACTURER
Gilead Sciences

DESCRIPTION
Vistide is being tested as an injectable formulation for treatment of central nervous system infections and hepatitis B virus respiratory tumors, and tumors or disorders of the larynx. The drug is in phase I/II trials for HBV respiratory tumors, laryngeal papillomatosis, and progressive multifocal leukoencephalopathy.

INDICATION(S) AND RESEARCH PHASE
Hepatitis – Phase I/II

Laryngeal Tumors/Disorders – Phase I/II
Viral Infection – Phase I/II
Brain Cancer – Phase I/II

docetaxel hydrate
Taxotere

MANUFACTURER
Aventis

DESCRIPTION
Many drugs for the treatment of cancer and other diseases originate in plants, many of them highly poisonous. Taxotere (docetaxel hydrate), an agent that inhibits the formation of new protoplasm, is derived from the renewable evergreen needles of the genus *Taxus* (Yew). Taxotere acts by disrupting the microtubular network in cells that is essential for cell division and many other cellular functions. The drug is approved for use in the United States for treatment of refractory breast, refractory non-small cell lung cancer (NSCLC), and treatment of locally advanced or metastatic breast cancer.

New phase II/III clinical trials under way in head and neck, gastric, and ovarian cancers, as well as either alone or in combination with other chemotherapy agents in the earlier stages of breast cancer, NSCLC and others tumors.

Phase I extension studies are under way for brain metastases and lung cancer.

INDICATION(S) AND RESEARCH PHASE
Gastric Cancer – Phase II/III
Head and Neck Cancer – Phase II/III
Lung Cancer – Phase II/III
Ovarian Cancer – Phase II/III
Breast Cancer – Phase III/IV
Brain Cancer – Phase I
Lung Cancer – Phase I

hypericin
VIMRxyn

MANUFACTURER
Nexell Therapeutics

DESCRIPTION
VIMRxyn (hypericin) is a light-activated and topically applied formulation of aromatic polyclinic dione (APD-1), which is a synthetic agent directed against retroviruses. This drug is being tested for treatment of specific skin diseases including psoriasis, cutaneous T-cell lymphoma, and warts.

VIMRx Pharmaceuticals has also manufactured an oral, once-daily formulation of aromatic polyclinic dione (APD-1). This drug form is being evaluated for the treatment of malignant gliomas. Subject enrollment has now completed for this trial.

INDICATION(S) AND RESEARCH PHASE
Brain Cancer – Phase I/II
Lymphomas – Phase I/II
Psoriasis and Psoriatic Disorders – Phase I/II
Skin Infections/Disorders – Phase I/II

INGN-201
Adenoviral p53

MANUFACTURER
Introgen Therapeutics

DESCRIPTION
The p53 tumor suppressor gene (INGN-201) has been tested for a variety of solid tumor cancers. In those trials, the drug was administered by intratumoral injection. The drug was well tolerated according to the company, and additional trials are under way using an intravenous infusion in order to reach more types of cancers. The tumor-suppressing p53 gene encodes a protein that responds to damage involving cellular DNA by terminating cell division. An adenoviral vector delivers normal p53 genes into cancer cells of the subject to attempt to restore normal cellular control.

The developers of INGN-201 have signed a Cooperative Research and Development Agreement (CRADA) with the National Cancer Institute to evaluate the potential effectiveness and superiority of the drug over other treatments against breast, ovarian, bladder, prostate, and brain cancers in phase I/II and phase II trials. A phase III trial in head and neck cancer was initiated in March 2000.

INDICATION(S) AND RESEARCH PHASE
Head and Neck Cancer – Phase III
Bladder Cancer – Phase I
Brain Cancer – Phase I
Breast Cancer – Phase I
Ovarian Cancer – Phase I
Prostate Cancer – Phase I
Lung Cancer – Phase II
Cancer/Tumors (Unspecified) – Phase I

interferon beta-1a
Avonex

MANUFACTURER
Biogen

DESCRIPTION
Interferons are proteins naturally produced by the body to help fight viral infections and regulate the immune system. Avonex is a biosynthetic compound that contains the same arrangement of amino acids as the interferon-beta produced by the body. It is believed that Avonex regulates the body's immune response to decrease an attack against myelin, a possible mechanism for the nervous system destructive in multiple sclerosis.

Approved by the FDA for the treatment of relapsing forms of multiple sclerosis, Avonex is currently in phase II trials for the treatment of brain cancer and idiopathic pulmonary fibrosis (IPF). For IPF, treatment is aimed at minimizing the disease progression from inflammation to fibrosis.

In January 2001, results of a phase III trial of Avonex (interferon beta-1a) for the treatment of secondary progressive multiple sclerosis (MS) demonstrated that the drug reduced the progression of disability by 27% versus treatment with placebo. IMPACT (International Multiple Sclerosis Secondary Progressive Avonex Controlled Trial) was a randomized, double-blind, placebo-controlled trial involving 436 subjects at 42 sites in the United States, Canada and Europe.

INDICATION(S) AND RESEARCH PHASE
Pulmonary Fibrosis – Phase II
Brain Cancer – Phase II
Multiple Sclerosis – Phase III

interleukin-4 fusion toxin,

NBI-3001
unknown

MANUFACTURER
Neurocrine Biosciences

DESCRIPTION
IL-4 fusion toxin is being tested in a phase II trial for the treatment of glioblastoma multiforme (GBM), malignant brain tumors. According to the company, preclinical data suggest that when infused directly into a glioblastoma, IL-4 fusion toxin kills tumor cells but not healthy brain cells.

IL-4 fusion toxin is a protein in which a blood cell derived growth factor (IL-4) has been joined with a *Pseudomonas* exotoxin, a potent toxin that can destroy cancer cells. IL-4 has a very high affinity for binding to its receptors, which are highly expressed on malignant brain tumors, but not on normal brain cells. IL-4 binds tightly to the IL-4 receptors on the surface of the glioblastoma cells and delivers the exotoxin directly into the cell, resulting in cell death. IL-4 fusion toxin is administered via a special catheter that permits delivery directly into the brain tumor.

Results from a phase I/II testing NBI-3001 demonstrated 56% of the 31 subjects tested exhibited a reduction in tumor size. The phase I/II trial took place at nine leading neurosurgery centers in the United States and Germany. The 31 subjects being treated had end-stage (grade 4) recurrent glioblastoma, unresponsive to surgery and radiotherapy and were treated with intratumoral infusions of IL-4 for up to four days.

The company claims that these findings show the drug to be safe and that it demonstrates anti-tumor effects in the majority of subjects receiving it. Phase III pivotal trials of IL-4 fusion toxin, which was granted fast track designation by the FDA in 1999, are estimated to begin in 2001.

INDICATION(S) AND RESEARCH PHASE
Brain Cancer – Phase II completed

marimastat, BB-2516
unknown

MANUFACTURER
British Biotech plc

DESCRIPTION
Marimastat is an inhibitor of matrix metalloproteinase (MMP), a family of naturally occurring enzymes that are over-produced in a number of disease states, especially in cancer, where MMPs are involved in the spread and local growth of tumors. Both angiogenesis and metastasis require MMPs during tumor invasion. Anti-angiogenic strategies, unlike other therapeutic approaches, do not aim to directly destroy or "kill" the tumor or cause tumor regression. Rather, they are designed to prevent the further growth of tumors by limiting their blood supply. Because peripheral tumor cells could theoretically survive on a diffusion-dependent basis, anti-angiogenic drugs may prove most effective when given in combination with other standard cytotoxic regimens. Marimastat is in phase III development for the treatment of cancer.

In 1999, British Biotech and Schering-Plough Corporation signed an agreement to develop and commercialize British Biotech's metalloproteinase inhibitors, including marimastat.

INDICATION(S) AND RESEARCH PHASE
Pancreatic Cancer – Phase III
Lung Cancer – Phase III
Breast Cancer – Phase III
Brain Cancer – Phase III completed
Ovarian Cancer – Phase III

matrix metalloprotease inhibitor (MMP)
Prinomastat

MANUFACTURER
Agouron Pharmaceuticals

DESCRIPTION
Prinomastat is an orally active, synthetic molecule designed to potently and selectively inhibit certain members of a family of enzymes known as a matrix metalloproteases that are believed to be involved in tumor angiogenesis, invasion, and metastasis. According to the company, based on their mechanism of action, MMP inhibitors may prove to have potential in reducing the invasiveness of malignant brain tumor cells.

The most common side effects of Prinomastat have been observed in the joints, and include stiffness, joint swelling, and in a few subjects, some limits on the mobility of certain joints, most often in the shoulders and hands. All these effects were reported reversible and were effectively managed by treatment rests and dose reductions.

Matrix metalloprotease inhibitors are in trials for the treatment of hormone-refractory prostate cancer combined with mitoxantrone and prednisone and a phase II for treatment of osteoarthritis.

Additionally, Prinomastat in combination with chemotherapy for subjects with newly diagnosed glioblastoma multiforme following surgery with radiation therapy is in a phase II trial.

Two phase III trials for advanced non-small cell lung cancer and prostate cancer were halted in August 2000 due to the drug's lack of effectiveness in subjects with late-stage disease.

Subjects who are interested in finding more information on the drug Prinomastat can call the toll free number (888) 849-6482.

INDICATION(S) AND RESEARCH PHASE
Lung Cancer – Halted
Prostate Cancer – Halted
Osteoarthritis – Phase II
Brain Cancer – Phase II
Macular Degeneration – Phase II

MDX-447, H-447
unknown

MANUFACTURER
Medarex

DESCRIPTION
MDX-477 is a novel biological drug designed to stimulate an immune response against cancer cells. Certain cancer cells contain and express large amounts of unique proteins (such as epidermal growth factor receptors), which MDX-477 is directed to recognize. MDX-477 attaches itself both to these cancer proteins and to macrophages that specialize in killing foreign material.

The binding together of the cancer and the immune cells by MDX-477 signals the body to destroy the tumor. MDX-477 may offer a new therapeutic alternative to cancer subjects who may have been unresponsive to conventional therapies. This agent is unique since it has two receptors on its surface, one that can attract the cancer cell, and the other that can attract a killer immune cell. This dual nature of the drug is why it is known as a "bispecific antibody."

This type of drug is designed to be more efficient than current anti-cancer therapies, and may have effects that last longer. This technology may also be useful in the development of an "anti-cancer vaccine" in the future. MDX-477 is currently being tested as an intravenous solution in phase II trials for multiple tumor indications, which include brain, bladder, breast, head and neck, and lung cancer.

INDICATION(S) AND RESEARCH PHASE
Brain Cancer – Phase II
Bladder Cancer – Phase II
Breast Cancer – Phase II
Head and Neck Cancer – Phase II
Lung Cancer – Phase II

motexafing adolinium
Xcytrin

MANUFACTURER
Pharmacyclics

DESCRIPTION
Xcytrin (motexafing adolinium) Injection is a novel drug that augments the activity of radiation. Preclinical and clinical data indicate that after repeated injections Xcytrin accumulates selectively in tumors and increases the vulnerability of cancer cells to the effects of radiation or chemotherapy without increasing damage to surrounding healthy cells.

Positive results from the lead-in phase of an ongoing phase III trial of Xcytrin for brain metastases were announced in October 2000. Tumor response was observed in 68% of subjects evaluable by MRI scans, with a median reduction in tumor volume of 83%. Seventy-seven percent of the 25 subjects were free from neurologic progression.

INDICATION(S) AND RESEARCH PHASE
Brain Cancer – Phase III

prolifeprosan 20/carmustine
Gliadel

MANUFACTURER
Aventis

DESCRIPTION
One of the most common intravenous chemotherapy agents used to treat primary brain tumors is carmustine, which is also known as BCNU. BCNU can be useful in treating brain tumors like glioblastoma malignancies (GBM). However, when BCNU is given intravenously, it can cause some serious side effects such as bone marrow damage, which interferes with new blood cell formation.

The Gliadel wafer was developed to deliver BCNU directly to the site of the recurrent brain tumor. After neurosurgical removal of GBM tissue, eight dime-sized Gliadel wafers are implanted in the space the tumor once occupied. Each wafer contains a precise amount of BCNU. Over the next two to three weeks, the wafers slowly dissolve, bathing the surrounding cells with BCNU. The goal of Gliadel wafer therapy is to kill the remaining small tumor cells that were previously undetectable during surgical removal, thereby extending subject survival.

Circumventing intravenous delivery by direct placement may decrease drug related adverse effects. The Gliadel wafers were being tested in phase III clinical trials as adjunctive therapy for the treatment of recurrent GBM. Currently development of this drug therapy has been discontinued.

INDICATION(S) AND RESEARCH PHASE
Brain Cancer – Phase III Discontinued

RSR13
unknown

MANUFACTURER
Allos Therapeutics

DESCRIPTION
RSR13 is a synthetic small molecule that increases the release of oxygen from hemoglobin, the oxygen carrying protein contained within red blood cells. The presence of oxygen in tumors is an essential part of the effectiveness of radiation therapy in cancer treatment. By increasing tumor oxygenation, RSR13 has the potential to enhance the effectiveness of standard radiation therapy.

Positive preliminary phase II results of induction chemotherapy, followed by radiation therapy plus RSR13, for stage IIIA and IIIB non-small cell lung cancer were announced. Data from the first 30 of 47 subjects demonstrated that 87% had a complete or partial response of their tumors within the radiation therapy portal in the chest. Additionally, Allos Therapeutics is conducting a randomized, multicenter, international phase III trial in 408 subjects to confirm that RSR13, when used in combination with radiation therapy, significantly improves the survival of subjects with brain metastases.

INDICATION(S) AND RESEARCH PHASE
Angina – Phase I completed
Cardiac Ischemia – Phase II
Brain Cancer – Phase III
Lung Cancer – Phase II
Myocardial Infarction – Phase II completed

SU101
unknown

MANUFACTURER
Sugen

DESCRIPTION
SU-101 is a synthetic, platelet-derived growth factor receptor, which blocks the essential enzyme, tyrosine kinase. This drug may be helpful for the treatment of end-stage malignant glioma, a tumor of nerve tissue. The drug is being tested in phase III trials for refractory brain and prostate cancers, and phase II studies for non-small cell lung and ovarian cancers.

INDICATION(S) AND RESEARCH PHASE
Brain Cancer – Phase III
Prostate Cancer – Phase III

Lung Cancer – Phase II
Ovarian Cancer – Phase II

SU101/BCNU
unknown

MANUFACTURER
Sugen

DESCRIPTION
SU-101 is a synthetic, platelet-derived growth factor receptor, which blocks the essential enzyme, tyrosine kinase. This drug may be useful for the treatment of end-stage malignant glioma, a tumor of nerve tissue. The drug is being tested in phase II trials for refractory brain cancers.

SU101 in combination with BCNU is being tested in phase II trials for treating brain cancer.

INDICATION(S) AND RESEARCH PHASE
Brain Cancer – Phase II

T67
unknown

MANUFACTURER
Tularik

DESCRIPTION
T67 is an anti-cancer compound that binds irreversibly to tubulin and inhibits the growth of multi-drug resistant tumors. Tubulin is a protein that polymerizes into chains to form microtubules. Microtubules are essential for cell division, and by disrupting their function, T67 produces cell death and potentially causes tumor shrinkage.

The drug is currently in phase II trials in subjects with non-small cell lung cancer, glioma, colorectal cancer, and breast cancer. It is also in a phase I/II trial for the treatment of hepatocellular carcinoma. These trials are being conducted in the United States, the United Kingdom, Hong Kong, and Taiwan.

INDICATION(S) AND RESEARCH PHASE
Lung Cancer – Phase II
Brain Cancer – Phase II
Colorectal Cancer – Phase II
Breast Cancer – Phase II
Hepatocellular Carcinoma – Phase I/II

temozolomide
Temodar

MANUFACTURER
Schering-Plough Corporation

DESCRIPTION
Temodar is an oral cytotoxic chemotherapeutic agent belonging to a class of compounds known as imidazotetrazines. Temodar has been approved by the FDA for the treatment of adult subjects with anaplastic astrocytoma at the first relapse with disease progression on a nitrosourea- and procarbazine-containing drug regimen. It is currently in phase II trials for the treatment of a variety of solid tumors.

INDICATION(S) AND RESEARCH PHASE
Brain Cancer – FDA approved
Cancer/Tumors (Unspecified) – Phase II

thalidomide
Thalomid

MANUFACTURER
Celgene Corporation

DESCRIPTION
Thalomid is an oral formulation of the immunomodulatory agent thalidomide. Thalidomide has a notorious history of having caused birth defects when the medical profession unsuspectingly prescribed it for pregnant women as a treatment for nausea and insomnia. Celgene is investigating new applications for the drug, while being particularly mindful of the potential risks of thalidomide treatment. Thalomid is currently being tested for numerous indications in the areas of oncology and immunology.

INDICATION(S) AND RESEARCH PHASE
Multiple Myeloma – Phase II
Myelodysplastic Syndrome – Phase II
Leukemia – Phase II
Brain Cancer – Phase II
Liver Cancer – Phase II
Kidney Cancer – Phase II
Prostate Cancer – Phase II
Kaposi's Sarcoma – Phase II
Cachexia – Phase II
Recurrent Aphthous Stomatitis – Phase III
Crohn's Disease – Phase II
Inflammatory Bowel Disease – Phase II
Sarcoidosis – Phase II
Scleroderma – Phase II

XR5000
unknown

MANUFACTURER
Xenova

DESCRIPTION
XR5000 is a topoisomerase I and II inhibitor being developed for the treatment of common solid tumors. Three phase II trials are under way at a number of European centers for XR5000. The trials are being conducted on an "open-label" basis and target three cancer types: ovarian, non-small cell lung, and glioblastoma. The results of a fourth phase II trial, in which the efficacy of XR5000 was investigated in subjects with colorectal cancer, were announced in June 2000. No complete or partial responses to treatment were observed after two courses of treatment with XR5000. Two subjects showed stable disease and 13 subjects experienced disease progression. The company is not planning any further recruitment for this indication.

INDICATION(S) AND RESEARCH PHASE
Lung Cancer – Phase II
Ovarian Cancer – Phase II
Brain Cancer – Phase II

Chronic Fatigue Syndrome

2CVV
unknown

MANUFACTURER
Milkhaus Laboratory

DESCRIPTION

Chronic Fatigue Syndrome

2CVV is an orally formulated therapy that was being tested for chronic fatigue syndrome. Trials have completed phase II and are suspended indefinitely from further development.

INDICATION(S) AND RESEARCH PHASE
Chronic Fatigue Syndrome – Phase II discontinued

galantamine hydrobromide
Reminyl

MANUFACTURER
Janssen Research Foundation

DESCRIPTION
Reminyl (galantamine) is a nicotinic modulator that is being developed for the treatment of both chronic fatigue syndrome (CFS) and Alzheimer's disease. This drug works by slowing down or reversibly inhibiting acetylcholinesterase, which is the enzyme responsible for degrading the neurotransmitter acetylcholine. It is produced in an oral tablet formulation.

Study results show that volunteers with Alzheimer's treated with Reminyl exhibited improved memory, behavior, and ability to perform activities of daily living. In addition, a second study suggested that the cognitive and functional benefits of galantamine may be sustained for at least 12 months.

Reminyl is being developed by the Janssen Research Foundation under a co-development agreement with Shire Pharmaceuticals. An NDA was filed with the FDA in September 1999 and the company received an approvable letter in August 2000. Reminyl is FDA approved for the treatment of Alzheimer's disease.

INDICATION(S) AND RESEARCH PHASE
Alzheimer's Disease – FDA approved
Chronic Fatigue Syndrome – Phase II
Dementia – Phase III

poly I:poly C-12-U
Ampligen

MANUFACTURER
Hemispherx Biopharma

DESCRIPTION
Ampligen is a novel therapeutic treatment composed of polyribonucleotide and synthetic nucleic acid for the treatment of metastatic renal carcinoma, as an orphan indication. This intravenous drug is being evaluated in phase II/III trials for renal carcinoma, phase I/II for malignant melanoma, and phase III for chronic fatigue syndrome and HIV.

INDICATION(S) AND RESEARCH PHASE
Renal Cell Carcinoma – Phase II/III
Malignant Melanoma – Phase I/II
Chronic Fatigue Syndrome – Phase III
HIV Infection – Phase III

Chronic Pain

oxycodone
unknown

MANUFACTURER
Alza (Sequus Pharmaceuticals)

DESCRIPTION
Oxycodone is in a phase I trial for the treatment of chronic pain.

INDICATION(S) AND RESEARCH PHASE
Chronic Pain – Phase I

ziconotide, SNX-111
unknown

MANUFACTURER
Elan Pharmaceutical Research

DESCRIPTION
Ziconotide is an omega-conotoxin that blocks the entry of calcium ions into nerve cells. An NDA has been accepted for ziconotide as a treatment for chronic pain in conjunction with Medtronic using their SynchroMed implantable pump for direct administration into the cerebrospinal fluid. Ziconotide binds in the human spinal cord at the site where pain signals originate. The SynchroMed pump is the size of a hockey puck, and it is implanted in the chest and refilled by syringe.

INDICATION(S) AND RESEARCH PHASE
Chronic Pain – NDA submitted

Dementia

donepezil hydrochloride, E2020
Aricept

MANUFACTURER
Eisai

DESCRIPTION
Aricept is an acetylcholinesterase inhibitor. The enzyme acetylcholinesterase breaks down acetylcholine. By inhibiting this process, Aricept causes a greater concentration of acetylcholine. Acetylcholine is a neurotransmitter associated with memory, which means that greater concentrations of it could significantly improve the conditions of Alzheimer's disease. In addition, Aricept is in phase II trials in children seven to 16 years old who are suffering from attention deficit/hyperactivity disorder.

Aricept is currently in development in Japan, Europe, and the United States. Aricept is being co-promoted by Pfizer.

INDICATION(S) AND RESEARCH PHASE
Alzheimer's Disease – NDA submitted in Japan
Dementia – Phase III
Pediatric, Attention Deficit/Hyperactivity Disorder (ADHD) – Phase II

dronabinol
Marinol

MANUFACTURER
Unimed Pharmaceuticals

DESCRIPTION
Marinol is an oral pill formulation of dronabinol, which is a synthetic marijuana derivative that is being tested in phase IIIb clinical trials for the treatment of dementia, including dementia in Alzheimer's disease. This naturally occurring cannabinoid has

complex effects on the central nervous system. Marinol is approved by the FDA for anorexia associated with weight loss in AIDS subjects, and nausea and vomiting associated with cancer chemotherapy.

The company reported that this drug is the only legally available synthetic form of the psychoactive component of marijuana, and a recent study found it has a very low potential for drug abuse. Marinol is available in round, soft gelatin capsules of 2.5 mg, 5 mg, and 10 mg.

INDICATION(S) AND RESEARCH PHASE
Alzheimer's Disease – Phase II
Dementia – Phase II

galantamine hydrobromide
Reminyl

MANUFACTURER
Janssen Research Foundation

DESCRIPTION
Reminyl (galantamine) is a nicotinic modulator that is being developed for the treatment of both chronic fatigue syndrome (CFS) and Alzheimer's disease. This drug works by slowing down or reversibly inhibiting acetylcholinesterase, which is the enzyme responsible for degrading the neurotransmitter acetylcholine. It is produced in an oral tablet formulation.

Study results show that volunteers with Alzheimer's treated with Reminyl exhibited improved memory, behavior, and ability to perform activities of daily living. In addition, a second study suggested that the cognitive and functional benefits of galantamine may be sustained for at least 12 months. Reminyl is being developed by the Janssen Research Foundation under a co-development agreement with Shire Pharmaceuticals. Reminyl is approved for the treatment of Alzheimer's disease.

INDICATION(S) AND RESEARCH PHASE
Alzheimer's Disease – FDA approved
Chronic Fatigue Syndrome – Phase II
Dementia – Phase III

NGD 97-1
unknown

MANUFACTURER
Neurogen Corporation

DESCRIPTION
NGD 97-1 is a selective GABA inverse agonist being developed for the treatment of Alzheimer's disease and other dementias. In preclinical models, this type of drug reduced the activity of the GABA system in a manner that produced memory enhancing effects. NGD 97-1 is in phase I development; to date, results indicate the drug is well tolerated.

INDICATION(S) AND RESEARCH PHASE
Alzheimer's Disease – Phase I
Dementia – Phase I

olanzapine
Zyprexa

MANUFACTURER
Eli Lilly

DESCRIPTION
Zyprexa is an approved antipsychotic agent that may work by inhibiting receptors for several CNS neurotransmitters, including dopamine and serotonin type 2 ($5HT_2$).

There was an NDA filed in June 2000 for Zyprexa in a short-acting intramuscular (SAIM) injectable formulation for the treatment of agitation in schizophrenia, bipolar I disorder, and dementia.

This drug is in phase II trials for treatment of depressive episodes associated with bipolar disorder and for the long-term relapse prevention in bipolar affective disorder, with NDA filing planned for late 2002.

Zyprexa is also in a phase II trial in a four-week depot formulation.

INDICATION(S) AND RESEARCH PHASE
Bipolar Disorders – Phase II
Bipolar Disorders – NDA submitted
Schizophrenia and Schizoaffective Disorders – NDA submitted
Dementia – NDA submitted

propentofylline, HWA-285
unknown

MANUFACTURER
Aventis

DESCRIPTION
Propentofylline is a novel compound that is being developed for the treatment of Alzheimer's disease and vascular dementia. This drug may work through glial cell modulation in the central nervous system. Clinical trials were formerly in phase III for both neuronal disorders. Currently development of the drug has been discontinued.

INDICATION(S) AND RESEARCH PHASE
Alzheimer's Disease – Phase III Discontinued
Dementia – Phase III Discontinued

TAK-147
unknown

MANUFACTURER
Takeda Chemical Industries

DESCRIPTION
TAK-147 is an acetylcholinesterase inhibitor being developed for the treatment of senile dementia of the Alzheimer's disease type. It is currently in phase III trials in Japan.

INDICATION(S) AND RESEARCH PHASE
Dementia – Phase III
Alzheimer's Disease – Phase III

Epilepsy

NPS 1776, alifatic amide
unknown

MANUFACTURER
Abbott Laboratories

DESCRIPTION
NPS 1776 is an orally active small molecule in development for the treatment of epilepsy, bipolar disorders, and other neurological disorders. In March 2000, NPS licensed NPS 1776 to Abbott Laboratories for further development.

Data were presented on two double-blind, placebo-controlled phase I trials of healthy volunteers, conducted in the United Kingdom last year to evaluate single-dose and multiple-dose regimens. In the first phase I trial, a total of 18 volunteers were given an ascending dose of NPS 1776 ranging from 100mg to 1,600 mg three times daily. In the multiple-dose phase I study, a total of 36 volunteers were given NPS 1776 for 10 days at three doses three times daily ranging from 1,200 mg to 2,400 mg. In both studies, NPS 1776 was well tolerated and there were no clinically important changes in vital signs, clinical lab evaluations, or standard neurological exams.

INDICATION(S) AND RESEARCH PHASE
Epilepsy – Phase I completed
Bipolar Disorders – Phase I completed

fosphenytoin sodium injection
unknown

MANUFACTURER
Pfizer

DESCRIPTION
Fosphenytoin is a phosphate ester of phenytoin that has been classified "1S" (new molecular entity) by the FDA. It is freely soluble in aqueous solutions, including standard intravenous solutions. After administration, fosphenytoin is rapidly converted (within eight to 15 minutes) to phenytoin by phosphatases found in a number of tissues. Unlike phenytoin, fosphenytoin can be given rapidly intravenously and promptly achieves therapeutic levels. It is rapidly absorbed when given IM, and is well tolerated. The drug is 100% bioavailable, and it is bioequivalent to phenytoin (10 mL fosphenytoin is equivalent to 5 mg intravenous phenytoin). Side effects are minor and transient. Unlike benzodiazepines and barbiturates, fosphenytoin does not cause respiratory or CNS depression; thus subjects can breathe well enough to compensate for metabolic acidosis, and think well enough after recovery to cooperate with diagnostic evaluation. Fosphenytoin sodium injection has been approved for the treatment of seizures in adults and currently an NDA has been submitted to treat pediatric subjects.

INDICATION(S) AND RESEARCH PHASE
Epilepsy – FDA approved
Pediatric, Epilepsy – NDA submitted

GABA agonist, anxiolytic
unknown

MANUFACTURER
DOV Pharmaceutical

DESCRIPTION
This unspecified gamma-amino butyric acid (GABA) analogue-anti-epileptic is used for the treatment of panic disorder and for sleep induction. Both trials are currently in phase I.

INDICATION(S) AND RESEARCH PHASE
Sleep Disorders – Phase I
Epilepsy – Phase I

gabapentin
Neurontin

MANUFACTURER
Pfizer

DESCRIPTION
Neurontin is an anticonvulsant used with other medications to treat certain types of seizures, including elementary partial and complex partial seizures, with and without secondary generalization. This drug has been approved by the FDA for the treatment of epilepsy in adults. An NDA has been submitted for Neurontin as a treatment for epilepsy in pediatric subjects. In addition, Neurontin may be used in the future for the treatment of generalized and social anxiety disorders, panic disorder, and bipolar disorder.

INDICATION(S) AND RESEARCH PHASE
Epilepsy – FDA approved
Pediatric, Epilepsy – NDA submitted

ganaxolone, CCD-1042
unknown

MANUFACTURER
CoCensys

DESCRIPTION
Ganaxolone is being developed to prevent migraine headaches. This drug is a synthetic epalon-based compound that works as an allosteric receptor modulator of the neurotransmitter, gamma-amino butyric acid (GABA). Epalons are naturally occurring neuroactive compounds.

Ganaxolone is being tested for both an oral suspension and tablet formulation. The company reported that phase II trials are completed for migraine prophylaxis.

In addition, ganaxolone is being evaluated in a phase II trial for the treatment of catamenial (related to menstruation) epilepsy. Seizure research includes the orphan indication of infantile spasms and the treatment of adult subjects experiencing complex partial seizures. Furthermore, a phase II trial is being conducted in pediatric subjects from two months to 15 years of age suffering from epilepsy.

INDICATION(S) AND RESEARCH PHASE
Epilepsy – Phase II
Migraine and Cluster Headaches – Phase II
Pediatric, Epilepsy – Phase II

GW 273293
unknown

MANUFACTURER
GlaxoSmithKline

DESCRIPTION
GW 273293 is a sodium channel inhibitor in phase II trials for the treatment of epilepsy and bipolar disorders.

INDICATION(S) AND RESEARCH PHASE
Bipolar Disorders – Phase II
Epilepsy – Phase II

porcine neural cells, focal epilepsy
unknown

MANUFACTURER
Diacrin

DESCRIPTION

Porcine neural cells, when transplanted into the brain of a subject that suffers from focal epilepsy may have an inhibitory effect on the hyperexcitable brain region. Currently, development is focused on subjects who experience loss of consciousness or have complex partial seizures. A six person, phase I study is being held at the Beth Israel Deaconess Medical Center and Brigham and Women's Hospital in Boston.

INDICATION(S) AND RESEARCH PHASE
Epilepsy – Phase I

pregabalin
unknown

MANUFACTURER
Pfizer

DESCRIPTION

Pregabalin is being developed for the treatment of neuropathic pain, epilepsy, a variety of anxiety disorders, and chronic pain syndromes. In February 2001, Pfizer announced it has restricted the use of pregabalin for certain subjects in clinical trials. The restriction follows an analysis by the FDA of previously submitted results from a chronic administration mouse study that showed increased evidence of a tumor type in the mice. A similar dosing study in rats did not show increases in any tumor type, nor were these results seen in any other toxicological screen or study. The planned submission of the NDA for neuropathic pain and epilepsy is expected to proceed as previously announced.

INDICATION(S) AND RESEARCH PHASE
Pain, Acute or Chronic – Phase III
Epilepsy – Phase III

remacemide
unknown

MANUFACTURER
AstraZeneca

DESCRIPTION

Remacemide blocks a cell receptor for the amino acid neurotransmitter N-methyl-D-aspartate (NMDA). This NMDA receptor antagonist produces a neuroprotective effect. The drug has completed a phase II trial for the treatment of Parkinson's disease, and is in studies for Huntington's chorea and epilepsy. According to the company, remacemide may help alleviate neuropathic pain associated with these neurologic diseases.

INDICATION(S) AND RESEARCH PHASE
Epilepsy – Phase II/III
Huntington's Disease – Phase III
Parkinson's Disease – Phase II completed

retigabine
unknown

MANUFACTURER
ASTA Medica AG

DESCRIPTION

Retigabine is a potassium channel agent with GABAergic activity being developed for the treatment of partial onset epilepsy. Gamma-amino butyric acid (GABA) is an inhibitory neurotransmitter that may help suppress seizure activity. Clinical testing of retigabine is in phase II studies. ASTA Medica AG has a collaborative development agreement for this product with Wyeth-Ayerst Division, American Home Products.

INDICATION(S) AND RESEARCH PHASE
Epilepsy – Phase II

SB 204269
unknown

MANUFACTURER
GlaxoSmithKline

DESCRIPTION

SB 204269 is an anticonvulsant drug designed for the treatment of epilepsy. It is currently in phase II development.

INDICATION(S) AND RESEARCH PHASE
Epilepsy – Phase II

SPD 418
unknown

MANUFACTURER
Shire Pharmaceuticals

DESCRIPTION

SPD 418 is being developed for the treatment of epilepsy. The compound is in phase I trials in the United States.

INDICATION(S) AND RESEARCH PHASE
Epilepsy – Phase I

SPD 421
unknown

MANUFACTURER
Shire Pharmaceuticals

DESCRIPTION

SPD 421 is a prodrug of valproic acid initially being evaluated for the treatment of epilepsy. Valproic acid enhances brain gamma-aminobutyric acid (GABA) levels, which activates GABA receptors and inhibits nerve impulse propagation. SPD 421 was in-licensed from D-Pharm in March 2000, where it was known as DP-VPA. A phase I trial has been completed.

INDICATION(S) AND RESEARCH PHASE
Epilepsy – Phase I completed

topiramate tablet
Topamax

MANUFACTURER
R.W. Johnson Pharmaceutical Research Institute

DESCRIPTION

Topamax is being tested in phase III trials for monotherapy in neuropathic pain in a tablet formulation. It is in phase II trials for bipolar mania and was approved in May 2000 for epilepsy.

INDICATION(S) AND RESEARCH PHASE
Epilepsy – FDA approved

Pain, Acute or Chronic – Phase III
Bipolar Disorders – Phase II

TVP-1901
unknown

MANUFACTURER
Teva Pharmaceutical Industries

DESCRIPTION
TVP-1901 is a broad-spectrum, anti-epileptic agent. The compound has proven active in a wide range of relevant animal models. Additionally, TVP-1901 may prove useful as a treatment for additional indications, such as bipolar disease and neuropathic pain. An early phase II European trial has been completed in subjects with refractory epilepsy with TVP-1901 as an add-on therapy for a period of up to 13 weeks.

INDICATION(S) AND RESEARCH PHASE
Epilepsy – Phase II

Huntington's Disease

porcine fetal cells
NeuroCell-HD

MANUFACTURER
Diacrin

DESCRIPTION
NeuroCell-HD is a preparation of fetal porcine (pig) neural cells and/or precursors, which is coated with anti-MHC-1 antibodies. This preparation is being studied in a phase I/II clinical trial as a replacement therapy for human brain cells (neurons) lost to Huntington's disease. This indication has an orphan drug status. NeuroCell-HD is made for surgical transplantation directly into the brain.
According to the company, preliminary data suggest the product is safe, and efficacy data are currently being evaluated. Diacrin has a joint agreement with Genzyme Tissue Repair for development of the NeuroCell-HD program.

INDICATION(S) AND RESEARCH PHASE
Huntington's Disease – Phase I/II

remacemide
unknown

MANUFACTURER
AstraZeneca

DESCRIPTION
Remacemide blocks a cell receptor for the amino acid neurotransmitter N-methyl-D-aspartate (NMDA). This NMDA receptor antagonist produces a neuroprotective effect. The drug has completed a phase II trial for the treatment of Parkinson's disease, and is studies for Huntington's chorea and epilepsy. According to the company, remacemide may help alleviate neuropathic pain associated with these neurologic diseases.

INDICATION(S) AND RESEARCH PHASE
Epilepsy – Phase II/III
Huntington's Disease – Phase III
Parkinson's Disease – Phase II completed

Insomnia

epalon, CCD-3693
unknown

MANUFACTURER
CoCensys

DESCRIPTION
CCD-3693 is a GABA receptor antagonist/synthetic version of epalons, used as a hypnotic for the treatment of insomnia and sleep disorders. The drug is in a phase I trial.

INDICATION(S) AND RESEARCH PHASE
Insomnia – Phase I
Sleep Disorders – Phase I

NBI-34060
unknown

MANUFACTURER
Neurocrine Biosciences

DESCRIPTION
NBI-34060 is a gamma-amino butyric acid (GABA) receptor stimulator that binds to specific sites on the GABA receptor—the same sites that are targeted by benzodiazepines. It is expected to offer an improved side effect profile because it is a non-benzodiazepine.
Preclinical studies have shown that NBI-34060 may produce a more rapid onset of sleep and fewer next-day hangover effects compared to currently marketed products. Also, NBI-34060 has been shown to have minimal interaction with alcohol and may not produce rapid tolerance or amnesia at effective sleep promoting doses.
As of January 2001, NBI-34060 is in multiple phase II trials for insomnia. The company plans on initiating phase III trials later in 2001.

INDICATION(S) AND RESEARCH PHASE
Insomnia – Phase II
Sleep Disorders – Phase II

NGD 96-1
unknown

MANUFACTURER
Neurogen Corporation

DESCRIPTION
NGD 96-1 belongs to a group of drugs that modulate specific GABA receptor subtypes. GABA is a principal inhibitory neurotransmitter in the central nervous system, affecting neuronal membranes via GABA receptors throughout the brain. In collaboration with Pfizer, Neurogen is attempting to develop drugs that modulate GABA receptor subtypes differently than currently marketed products. NGD 96-1 is currently in phase I trials for the treatment of insomnia, focusing on the onset of the drug, duration of action, and pharmacology.

INDICATION(S) AND RESEARCH PHASE
Insomnia – Phase I

racemic zoplicone
Zopiclone

MANUFACTURER
Sepracor

DESCRIPTION
Zopiclone is a new agent developed by Sepracor that is to be taken orally in the treatment of insomnia. It is currently in phase III clinical trials. Benzodiazepine medications such as Valium or Ativan are commonly used to relieve insomnia; however, the danger of these drugs is that they can lead to tolerance, addiction, and severe, sometimes life-threatening withdrawal symptoms. Scientists have been attempting to find a way to develop a medication that relieves insomnia as well as benzodiazepine drugs do, while not leading to tolerance and addiction.

Zopiclone is a non-benzodiazepine hypnotic drug that has been shown in preliminary clinical trials to be as effective at relieving insomnia as the benzodiazepines. It also appears from early studies that in short-term use (less than four weeks), Zopiclone may not have a high potential to cause tolerance, dependence, or addiction. Its use also might result in fewer residual clinical effects, such as difficulty waking and reduced morning concentration, than seen with the benzodiazepines. In addition, after a subject stops taking zopiclone, the subject may experience less of a problem re-establishing normal sleep patterns (rebound insomnia) than with other insomnia agents. Since drugs used to treat insomnia are frequently used for longer time periods in clinical practice, further studies may be necessary to evaluate the long-term safety and efficacy of Zopiclone.

INDICATION(S) AND RESEARCH PHASE
Insomnia – Phase III

Memory Loss

SIB-1508Y
unknown

MANUFACTURER
Sibia Neurosciences

DESCRIPTION
SIB-1508Y is a nicotinic acetylcholine receptor (nAChR)-selective drug that is being developed for the treatment of Parkinson's disease, other cognitive disorders, and attention deficit/hyperactivity disorder (ADHD). SIB-1508Y is being tested in phase II trials as both a single therapeutic agent and combined with L-dopa for treatment of Parkinson's disease.

INDICATION(S) AND RESEARCH PHASE
Attention Deficit/Hyperactivity Disorder (ADHD) – Phase II
Memory Loss – Phase II
Parkinson's Disease – Phase II

Meningitis

nystatin, AR-121
Nyotran

MANUFACTURER
Aronex Pharmaceuticals

DESCRIPTION
Nyotran is an intravenous liposomal formulation of nystatin being developed for the treatment of serious systemic, opportunistic fungal infections. Phase III trials have been completed for systemic fungal infections and confirmed cryptococcal meningitis. Additionally, phase II trials have been completed for candidiasis and aspergillosis.

Nyotran is under agreement with Abbott Laboratories for worldwide commercialization. Abbott will fund clinical development and will submit marketing registration outside the United States.

INDICATION(S) AND RESEARCH PHASE
Aspergillosis – Phase II completed
Candidiasis – Phase II completed
Systemic Fungal Infections – Phase III completed
Meningitis – Phase III completed

opebecan, rBPI-21, recombinant human bactericidal/permeability-increasing protein
Neuprex

MANUFACTURER
XOMA Corporation

DESCRIPTION
Neuprex is a systemic formulation of recombinant bactericidal/permeability-increasing protein; rBPI-21, for the treatment of severe meningococcemia, a rare systemic gram-negative bacterial infection that primarily affects children. The active molecule in Neuprex, rBPI-21, binds to endotoxin molecules (LOS and LPS, lipopolysaccharide) in living bacteria, disrupting their cell walls, killing the bacteria or making them more susceptible to antibiotics. Phase III data were released in September 2000 for both pediatric and adult trials.

XOMA is pursuing at least four indications for Neuprex: One indication is severe meningococcemia in children who become infected with these harmful bacteria that attack their brain and spinal cord's protective sheathing after entering the bloodstream. The gram-negative bacteria, called *Neisseria meningitidis*, cause meningococcemia and produce spiking high fever and a classic rigid stiff neck. Shock and death may occur in just a few hours after infection.

Also, there is a 1,650-subject phase III trauma trial evaluating whether Neuprex can prevent serious lung complications (pneumonia and Acute Respiratory Distress Syndrome (ARDS)). Subjects are enrolled after experiencing a severe accident in which they have lost at least two units of blood. More than 800 subjects have enrolled. Supporting this study was a previous 401-subject phase II trial that ended, with the results published in the Journal of Trauma on April 28, 1999.

Acute intra-abdominal infection is the third potential use for Neuprex in combination with other antibiotics. The drug is currently in phase I/II trials for this indication.

Finally, a phase II trial is currently enrolling subjects who have had part of their liver removed during surgery. Neuprex may prevent infection and complications after this major surgery.

INDICATION(S) AND RESEARCH PHASE
Bacterial Infection – Phase III
Pediatric, Meningococcemia – Phase III

completed
Meningitis – Phase III
Acute Respiratory Distress Syndrome (ARDS) – Phase III
Pneumonia – Phase III
Liver Disease – Phase II
Intra-abdominal Infection – Phase I/II

vaccine, meningococcal C conjugate
Meningitec

MANUFACTURER
Wyeth-Ayerst

DESCRIPTION
Meningitec is a conjugate vaccine for the prevention of meningococcal Group C disease. In October 1999, the vaccine was approved for use in the United Kingdom. Meningitec is being evaluated in clinics in combination with the pneumococcal conjugate vaccine.

INDICATION(S) AND RESEARCH PHASE
Meningitis – Phase III
Pediatric, Meningococcal Group C Meningitis – Phase III
Vaccines – Phase III

vaccine, meningococcus C
unknown

MANUFACTURER
Chiron Corporation

DESCRIPTION
Chiron Corporation is working on a new vaccine for meningococcal bacterial infections. The bacteria known as *Neisseria meningitidis* produce these infections. This organism can cause a variety of diseases ranging from benign upper respiratory infections to serious blood infections, which can lead to rashes, muscle and joint aches, and meningitis. Meningococcal meningitis begins when the organism crosses the meninges, which are the membranes surrounding the brain and spinal cord. This bacterial invasion into the central nervous system can result in fever, neck stiffness, headache and coma. In a third of affected subjects, overwhelming infection causes the body to go into shock with associated blood clotting problems, lung and heart infections, and death. If subjects survive, they could experience residual problems such as deafness, paralysis, and mental retardation. Approximately half of all cases of meningococcal meningitis occur in children under the age of 15 years, with most cases of meningitis occurring among infants three to eight months of age.

INDICATION(S) AND RESEARCH PHASE
Pediatric, meningitis – Phase III
Pediatric, vaccines – Phase III

Migraine and Cluster Headaches

ALX-0646
unknown

MANUFACTURER
NPS Allelix Corp

DESCRIPTION
ALX-0646 is one of a new generation of triptans that affect serotonin [5-hydroxytryptamine (5HT)] receptors. The drug is designed to selectively act on specific 5HT receptors in the brain to relieve migraine symptoms and may be less likely to cause cardiovascular side effects commonly associated with other migraine drugs. ALX-0646 has completed phase I trials in the UK; additional toxicology studies are ongoing and will be completed prior to beginning clinical trials in the United States. Forest Laboratories has entered into an agreement with NPS Allelix for the development and worldwide marketing of ALX-0646.

INDICATION(S) AND RESEARCH PHASE
Migraine and Cluster Headaches – Phase I completed

botulinum toxin type A, AGN-191622
Botox

MANUFACTURER
Allergan

DESCRIPTION
Botulinum toxin type A, a purified neurotoxin complex, has been used as a therapeutic agent since the 1960s. At a normal neuromuscular junction, a nerve impulse triggers the release of acetylcholine, which causes the muscle to contract. Botox reduces excessive muscle activity by blocking the release of acetylcholine at the neuromuscular junction. It is currently being tested in an injectable formulation for pediatric cerebral palsy, muscle spasticity, and brow furrow.

In addition, Botox is being tested in a phase II trial for the prevention of migraine headaches and a phase III study for lower back pain.

Botox was FDA approved in December 2000 for the treatment of adults with cervical dystonia. When injected into the affected muscles, Botox decreases the severity of abnormal head position and neck pain associated with this condition by blocking the release of the neurotransmitter acetylcoline from the peripheral nerve terminal to the muscle.

INDICATION(S) AND RESEARCH PHASE
Migraine and Cluster Headaches – Phase II
Musculoskeletal Diseases – FDA approved
Pain, Acute or Chronic – Phase III
Pediatric, Juvenile Cerebral Palsy – Phase III

CNS-5161
unknown

MANUFACTURER
Cambridge NeuroScience

DESCRIPTION
CNS-5161, a non-competitive blocker of the *N*-methyl-D-aspartate (NMDA) ion-channel complex, is a small molecule with various biological mechanisms that is being developed for the treatment of neuropathic pain and migraine. Ions travel across nerve cell membranes through protein conduits known as ion channels. Ion channels play a critical role in injury and disease. When the brain is subjected to severe insult such as stroke or traumatic brain injury, blood flow to the brain cells is reduced, a condition

known as ischemia. Nerve cells respond to ischemia by releasing excess quantities of a neurotransmitter called glutamate. In turn, this agent binds to specific receptor sites activating key ion channels on nerve cells. Through these open channels, calcium ions flood into the cells at toxic levels, causing a cascade reaction that can lead to cell death.

Ion-channel blockers may act on specific nerve cells in a variety of ways including the inhibition of glutamate function. Inhibiting glutamate function may minimize the damage that occurs in some disorders of the central nervous system. Rather than competing with glutamate for receptor sites on the nerve cell, ion-channel inhibitors actually block the ion channel itself.

INDICATION(S) AND RESEARCH PHASE
Migraine and Cluster Headaches – Phase II

dotarizine
unknown

MANUFACTURER
Mylan

DESCRIPTION
Dotarizine was being tested in clinical trials for the prophylaxis of migraine headaches. A phase II study was completed and a cardiac safety problem of QTc prolongation was identified. This ECG electrophysiologic prolongation has the potential to cause heart arrythmias.

The phase III program was designed to include two double-blind clinical trials, enrolling 800 subjects. Once initiated, the company estimates that the trials would be completed in 12 to 18 months. Dosing was supposed to have begun in mid-1999, but the design of phase III development was delayed. The company is reassessing the development project.

INDICATION(S) AND RESEARCH PHASE
Migraine and Cluster Headaches – Phase III

eletriptan
Relpax

MANUFACTURER
Pfizer

DESCRIPTION
Relpax is an oral drug that targets serotonin $5HT_{1d}$ receptors, which is found in intracranial blood vessels and sensory nerves. It is being studied for treatment of pain from migraine headaches. The efficacy of Relpax was demonstrated in Pfizer's NDA in seven randomized, double-blind clinical studies. The drug has a rapid onset of action, superior efficacy, and a lower headache recurrence rate than those reported for other triptans. Pfizer has received an approvable letter from the FDA.

INDICATION(S) AND RESEARCH PHASE
Migraine and Cluster Headaches – FDA recommend approval letter

esprolol
unknown

MANUFACTURER
Selectus Pharmaceuticals

DESCRIPTION
Esprolol is a potent, rapidly acting drug to be taken under the tongue. It is classified as a beta-adrenergic blocker that may lessen heart rate and blood pressure increases during physical exertion.

This compound completed a phase IIb clinical trial to evaluate the effects of esprolol on exercise tolerance in angina pectoris subjects. During the trial all exercise parameters and negative exercise induced angina symptoms were significantly improved.

In addition, esprolol is in a phase II study for panic disorders and cardiovascular effects of acute anxiety and migraine. Results from a Phase I trial of esprolol demonstrated the drug was well tolerated with only mild adverse effects. In addition, a follow-up phase II trial was conducted to evaluate the ability of esprolol to lessen the effects of beta receptor stimulation by standard challenge doses of isoproterenol in healthy volunteers, and to assess the drug's rate of onset of action and the duration of effect. Esprolol's therapeutic effect was seen within ten minutes and lasted for two to four hours.

INDICATION(S) AND RESEARCH PHASE
Angina – Phase IIb completed
Migraine and Cluster Headaches – Phase II
Panic Disorders – Phase II

frovatriptan
unknown

MANUFACTURER
Elan Pharmaceutical Research

DESCRIPTION
Frovatriptan is a serotonin ($5HT_1$) antagonist that is being developed for the treatment of migraine headaches. This triptan blocker received an approvable letter in May 2000 for their NDA that was submitted.

INDICATION(S) AND RESEARCH PHASE
Migraine and Cluster Headaches – FDA approvable letter

ganaxolone, CCD-1042
unknown

MANUFACTURER
CoCensys

DESCRIPTION
Ganaxolone is being developed to prevent migraine headaches. This drug is a synthetic epalon-based compound that works as an allosteric receptor modulator of the neurotransmitter, gamma-amino butyric acid (GABA). Epalons are naturally occurring neuroactive compounds.

Ganaxolone is being tested for both an oral suspension and tablet formulation. The company reported that phase II trials are completed for migraine prophylaxis.

In addition, ganaxolone is being evaluated in a phase II trial for the treatment of catamenial (related to menstruation) epilepsy. Seizure research includes the orphan indication of infantile spasms and the treatment of adult subjects experiencing complex partial seizures. Furthermore, a phase II trial is being conducted in pediatric subjects from two months to 15 years of age suffering from epilepsy.

INDICATION(S) AND RESEARCH PHASE

Epilepsy – Phase II
Migraine and Cluster Headaches – Phase II
Pediatric, Epilepsy – Phase II

GW 468816
unknown

MANUFACTURER
GlaxoSmithKline

DESCRIPTION
GW 468816 is a glycine receptor antagonist in phase I development for the treatment of migraine prophylaxis and smoking cessation.

INDICATION(S) AND RESEARCH PHASE
Migraine and Cluster Headaches – Phase I
Smoking Cessation – Phase I

MT 100
unknown

MANUFACTURER
Pozen

DESCRIPTION
MT 100 is an oral treatment for migraine headache and associated symptoms. Trial results indicate MT 100 provides rapid and sustained migraine relief with minimal side effects. Phase III trials for MT 100 were completed in late November 2000, and the company expects to file an NDA in late 2001.

INDICATION(S) AND RESEARCH PHASE
Migraine and Cluster Headaches – Phase III completed

MT 400
unknown

MANUFACTURER
Pozen

DESCRIPTION
MT 400 is a proprietary product concept combining a triptan drug with a long-acting, non-steroidal anti-inflammatory agent, which is designed to provide faster and more sustained release for the treatment of migraine headaches. A phase II trial was initiated in November 2000 and the trial is expected to include 800 subjects from 35 sites.

INDICATION(S) AND RESEARCH PHASE
Migraine and Cluster Headaches – Phase II

MT 500
unknown

MANUFACTURER
Pozen

DESCRIPTION
MT 500 is a selective serotonin $5HT_{2B}$ receptor antagonist for migraines. A large phase II trial will be initiated in the first half of 2000. The company reported that results from phase I trials showed MT 500 to have a favorable safety profile.

INDICATION(S) AND RESEARCH PHASE
Migraine and Cluster Headaches – Phase II

naratriptan
Naramig, Amerge

MANUFACTURER
GlaxoSmithKline

DESCRIPTION
Naramig (naratriptan) is a selective 5-hydroxytryptamine1 ($5HT_1$) receptor subtype agonist. It is currently in phase III trials for menstrual migraine prophylaxis. Naramig is also marketed as Amerge.

INDICATION(S) AND RESEARCH PHASE
Migraine and Cluster Headaches – Phase III

propranolol
Migrastat

MANUFACTURER
Questcor

DESCRIPTION
Migrastat (propranolol) is a nasal spray in development for the treatment of migraine headaches. Propranolol is an antagonist that competes with beta-adrenergic receptor stimulating agents for available beta receptor sites. The drug is currently in phase II development. Propranolol is approved by the FDA for oral and parenteral use for a variety of other indications.

INDICATION(S) AND RESEARCH PHASE
Migraine and Cluster Headaches – Phase II

s-fluoxetine
unknown

MANUFACTURER
Sepracor

DESCRIPTION
S-Fluoxetine is a single-isomer derivative of Prozac that is being tested for prophylaxis of migraine headaches in phase II clinical trials.

INDICATION(S) AND RESEARCH PHASE
Migraine and Cluster Headaches – Phase II

selective serotonergic agent
unknown

MANUFACTURER
Nastech

DESCRIPTION
Nastech is developing a selective serotonergic agent, or "triptan", with nasal administration for the treatment of migraine pain. Migraine symptoms may be due to local cranial vasodilation and/or the release of vasoactive and pro-inflammatory peptides from sensory nerve endings, which can lead to nausea and vomiting in severe migraine pain sufferers. These changes may be caused by alterations in the neurotransmitter serotonin. Triptans mimic certain actions of serotonin by activating 5-HT receptors, which constrict blood vessels that may be dilated and distended during a migraine attack.

The company has commenced enrollment in a phase I trial in the United States. The objective of the multidose trial is to determine nasal absorption, tolerance and safety of the agent in healthy volunteers.

INDICATION(S) AND RESEARCH PHASE
Migraine and Cluster Headaches – Phase I

sumatriptan
Imigran, Imitrex

MANUFACTURER
GlaxoSmithKline

DESCRIPTION
Imigran (sumatriptan) is a 5-hydroxytryptamine ($5HT_1$) agonist for the treatment of migraine headaches. $5HT_1$ receptors are found on the cells of cranial artery endothelia. When the receptors are activated by sumatriptan, the resulting vasoconstriction provides relief of migraine symptoms. A needle-free injection formulation of the drug is in phase II trials. Additionally, a Marketing Authorization Application (MAA) and an NDA have been submitted for a nasal formulation for the treatment of adolescent migraine. Imigran is also marketed under the trade name Imitrex.

INDICATION(S) AND RESEARCH PHASE
Pediatric – NDA submitted
Pediatric, Adolescent Migraine – NDA submitted, MAA submitted
Migraine and Cluster Headaches – Phase II

zolmitriptan
Zomig IN

MANUFACTURER
AstraZeneca

DESCRIPTION
Zomig IN is an intranasal formulation of a second generation selective serotonin ($5HT_1$ agonist) receptor stimulator being evaluated in a phase III trial for the treatment of migraines.

Zomig IN is an agent belonging to a new class of drugs treating migraines known as "triptans," which target specific subtype receptors of the neurotransmitter, serotonin. Triptans are considered "abortive" drugs, since they stop the pain before it has started by constricting blood vessels in the brain associated with serotonergic nerve projections. It is thought that migraine headaches may occur due to dilation of these blood vessels. These triptans may also reduce inflammation in the nerves that signal the pain of a migraine headache.

INDICATION(S) AND RESEARCH PHASE
Migraine and Cluster Headaches – Phase III

zolmitriptan
Zomig FM

MANUFACTURER
AstraZeneca

DESCRIPTION
Zomig FM is a second generation selective serotonin ($5HT_1$ agonist) receptor stimulator being tested in a phase III trial for the treatment of acute migraine attacks and associated symptoms in adults.

Zomig FM is an agent belonging to a new class of drugs treating migraines known as "triptans," which target specific subtype receptors of the neurotransmitter, serotonin. Tripans are considered "abortive" drugs, since they stop the pain before it has started by constricting blood vessels in the brain associated with serotonergic nerve projections. It is thought that migraine headaches may occur due to dilation of these blood vessels. These triptans may also reduce inflammation in the nerves that signal the pain of a migraine headache.

INDICATION(S) AND RESEARCH PHASE
Migraine and Cluster Headaches – Phase III

zolmitriptan
Zomig Cluster

MANUFACTURER
AstraZeneca

DESCRIPTION
Zomig Cluster is an oral formulation of a second generation selective serotonin ($5HT_1$ agonist) receptor stimulator being tested in a phase III trial for the treatment of cluster headaches due to migraines.

Zomig Cluster targets a "cluster" headache, which is a one-sided headache usually occurring in or around the eye and typically for a short duration. A cluster headache usually lasts several minutes to several hours in a group or series and thus is called a cluster because it occurs in a group or series.

Zomig Cluster is an agent belonging to a new class of drugs treating migraines known as "triptans," which target specific subtype receptors of the neurotransmitter, serotonin. Tripans are considered "abortive" drugs, since they stop the pain before it has started by constricting blood vessels in the brain associated with serotonergic nerve projections. It is thought that migraine headaches may occur due to dilation of these blood vessels. These triptans may also reduce inflammation in the nerves that signal the pain of a migraine headache.

INDICATION(S) AND RESEARCH PHASE
Migraine and Cluster Headaches – Phase III

zolmitriptan
Zomig

MANUFACTURER
AstraZeneca

DESCRIPTION
Zomig is an agent belonging to a new class of drugs treating migraines known as "triptans," which target specific subtype receptors of the neurotransmitter, serotonin. Tripans are considered "abortive" drugs, since they stop the pain before it has started by constricting blood vessels in the brain associated with serotonergic nerve projections. It is thought that migraine headaches may occur due to dilation of these blood vessels. These triptans may also reduce inflammation in the nerves that signal the pain of a migraine headache.

Zomig capsules are currently FDA approved for treating adult migraines, and the company is conducting clinical trials to expand the drug label to include pediatric subjects who experience migraine headaches.

INDICATION(S) AND RESEARCH PHASE
Migraine and Cluster Headaches – NDA submitted

Pediatric, Migraine – NDA submitted

zolmitriptan
Zomig Aura

MANUFACTURER
AstraZeneca

DESCRIPTION
Zomig Aura is an oral formulation of a second generation selective serotonin ($5HT_1$ agonist) receptor stimulator in a phase III trial for the treatment of aura headaches due to migraines.

Zomig Aura treats the special migraines called "aura," which are headaches that usually occur just a few minutes before the initial migraine attack. Symptoms may take the form of a feeling of elation, a clearer awareness of color, variations in mood, an increase in energy, or a feeling of hunger or thirst. Some subjects might even experience depression. Aura migraines can be positive, such as seeing bright lights or stars or negative, such as seeing blind spots or only part of a visual field. The warnings may also distort figures or shapes. Some people may get a tingling sensation in their arms or legs, or even smell a strange odor.

Zomig Aura is an agent belonging to a new class of drugs treating migraines known as "triptans," which target specific subtype receptors of the neurotransmitter, serotonin. Tripans are considered "abortive" drugs, since they stop the pain before it has started by constricting blood vessels in the brain associated with serotonergic nerve projections. It is thought that migraine headaches may occur due to dilation of these blood vessels. These triptans may also reduce inflammation in the nerves that signal the pain of a migraine headache.

INDICATION(S) AND RESEARCH PHASE
Migraine and Cluster Headaches – Phase III

Multiple Sclerosis

CDC 801
SelCID

MANUFACTURER
Celgene Corporation

DESCRIPTION
SelCIDs (selective cytokine inhibitory drugs) are oral immunotherapeutic agents that treat various inflammatory diseases by inhibiting phosphodiesterase type 4 enzyme (PDE-4). The inhibition of PDE-4 decreases production of tumor necrosis factor-alpha (TNF-α), a protein manufactured by cells of the immune system. This inhibition reduces the level of circulating TNF-α and, therefore, its ability to cause inflammation in cells. At normal levels, the protein is essential for effective immune function. However, overproduction of TNF as a result of age, genetics, and other influences contributes to the pathology of numerous diseases.

SelCIDs are in phase II trials for the following indications: inflammatory bowel disease, rheumatoid arthritis, multiple sclerosis, asthma, tuberculosis, autoimmune diseases, and mycobacterial infections such as leprosy.

INDICATION(S) AND RESEARCH PHASE
Inflammatory Bowel Disease – Phase II
Rheumatoid Arthritis – Phase II
Multiple Sclerosis – Phase II
Asthma – Phase Discontinued
Tuberculosis – Phase II
Autoimmune Diseases – Phase II
Bacterial Infection – Phase II
Multiple Myeloma – Phase II

fampridine
Neurelan

MANUFACTURER
Acorda Therapeutics

DESCRIPTION
Neurelan is a (4-aminopyridine) potassium channel blocker that is being tested in trials for the treatment of multiple sclerosis (MS) and spinal cord injuries. In this study, Neurelan is delivered using the Intestinal Protective Drug Absorption System (IPDAS) in a sustained-release formulation. Neurelan has an orphan indication status for the symptomatic relief of MS.

INDICATION(S) AND RESEARCH PHASE
Multiple Sclerosis – Phase II/III
Spinal Cord Injuries – Phase II

glatiramer acetate
Copaxone (oral)

MANUFACTURER
Teva Pharmaceutical Industries

DESCRIPTION
Copaxone is currently approved in an injectable formulation for the treatment of relapsing-remitting multiple sclerosis (RR-MS). A new oral formulation of the drug is being tested in more than 1,500 RR-MS subjects in a multinational phase III trial (CORAL). The trial is planned to involve 178 study sites around the world, including 57 in the United States.

INDICATION(S) AND RESEARCH PHASE
Multiple Sclerosis – Phase III

glatiramer acetate
Copaxone

MANUFACTURER
Teva Pharmaceutical Industries

DESCRIPTION
Copaxone (glatiramer acetate for injection) has been approved by the FDA for the treatment of relapsing-remitting multiple sclerosis. Currently, a phase III trial (PROMISE) is being conducted at 54 clinical sites in over 900 subjects with primary-progressive multiple sclerosis. Two-thirds of the recruited subjects receive Copaxone and one-third receive placebo.

INDICATION(S) AND RESEARCH PHASE
Multiple Sclerosis – Phase III

interferon beta-1b
Betaseron

MANUFACTURER
Chiron Corporation

DESCRIPTION

Betaseron (interferon beta-1b) alters the expression of surface antigens on myelin cells, controlling the body's destructive immune response to them. Study results show that it reduces the frequency of hypointense T1 lesions in subjects with secondary progressive multiple sclerosis.

Chiron/Berlex have currently filed an NDA for the indication of secondary progressive multiple sclerosis and are awaiting approval for this indication.

Betaseron is currently being marketed in the United States for the treatment of early stage, relapsing-remitting MS. It is manufactured by Chiron and marketed in the United States and Canada by Berlex. It is also being marketed by Schering AG in Europe as Betaferon for the treatment of secondary progressive MS, as well as for early stage, relapsing-remitting MS.

INDICATION(S) AND RESEARCH PHASE
Multiple Sclerosis – NDA submitted

interferon beta-1a
Avonex

MANUFACTURER
Biogen

DESCRIPTION
Interferons are proteins naturally produced by the body to help fight viral infections and regulate the immune system. Avonex is a biosynthetic compound that contains the same arrangement of amino acids as the interferon-beta produced by the body. It is believed that Avonex regulates the body's immune response to decrease an attack against myelin, a possible mechanism for the nervous system destructive in multiple sclerosis.

Approved by the FDA for the treatment of relapsing forms of multiple sclerosis, Avonex is currently in phase II trials for the treatment of brain cancer and idiopathic pulmonary fibrosis (IPF). For IPF, treatment is aimed at minimizing the disease progression from inflammation to fibrosis.

In January 2001, results of a phase III trial of Avonex (interferon beta-1a) for the treatment of secondary progressive multiple sclerosis (MS) demonstrated that the drug reduced the progression of disability by 27% versus treatment with placebo. IMPACT (International Multiple Sclerosis Secondary Progressive Avonex Controlled Trial) was a randomized, double-blind, placebo-controlled trial involving 436 subjects at 42 sites in the United States, Canada, and Europe.

INDICATION(S) AND RESEARCH PHASE
Pulmonary Fibrosis – Phase II
Brain Cancer – Phase II
Multiple Sclerosis – Phase III completed

IR208
NeuroVax

MANUFACTURER
Immune Response Corporation

DESCRIPTION
IR208 is a synthetic T-cell receptor (TCR) vaccine being developed for the treatment of multiple sclerosis. Clinical testing for the IR208 vaccine is in phase I/II.

INDICATION(S) AND RESEARCH PHASE
Multiple Sclerosis – Phase I/II
Vaccines – Phase I/II

micellar paclitaxel
unknown

MANUFACTURER
Angiotech Pharmaceuticals

DESCRIPTION
Micellar paclitaxel is being developed for the treatment of secondary progressive multiple sclerosis, rheumatoid arthritis, and severe psoriasis. A double-blind, placebo-controlled, phase I trial produced positive results in the treatment of rheumatoid arthritis (RA). Enrolled patients were between 21 and 75 years of age, presented Class I to III of RA severity, and had failed treatment with at least one disease-modifying anti-rheumatic drug, such as methotrexate. The drug was determined to be safe and well-tolerated in all 15 patients enrolled in the study. Of those patients treated with micellar paclitaxel that completed the study, 25% had a clinical response defined by a series of measures consistent with the American College of Rheumatology (ACR) 20% improvement criteria. A larger phase II study may be initiated in 2001. Trials for multiple sclerosis and psoriasis are currently in phase II.

INDICATION(S) AND RESEARCH PHASE
Multiple Sclerosis – Phase II
Rheumatoid Arthritis – Phase I completed
Psoriasis and Psoriatic Disorders – Phase II

modafinil
Provigil

MANUFACTURER
Cephalon

DESCRIPTION
Provigil (modafinil) is a dopamine-releasing agent that increases excitatory glutamatergic transmission. It is being developed in phase III trials for the prevention of daytime sleepiness associated with obstructive sleep apnea, hypersomnia, and shift work. Phase II trials are being conducted for the prevention of excessive daytime sleepiness associated with Alzheimer's disease and Parkinson's disease.

A phase II trial has been completed using Provigil as a treatment for sleep apnea and fatigue associated with multiple sclerosis. This drug is also currently in a phase III trial for the treatment of sleepiness regardless of cause, with an NDA filing planned for late 2001.

Additionally, Provigil is in phase I/II trials for ADHD in pediatric subjects.

INDICATION(S) AND RESEARCH PHASE
Multiple Sclerosis – Phase II completed
Sleep Disorders – Phase III
Pediatric, Attention Deficit/Hyperactivity Disorder (ADHD) – Phase I/II
Parkinson's Disease – Phase II
Alzheimer's Disease – Phase II

natalizumab
Antegren

MANUFACTURER

Elan Pharmaceutical Research

DESCRIPTION
Antegren is a humanized monoclonal antibody that belongs to a new class of potential therapeutics known as alpha4-integrin inhibitors. It is designed to block immune cell adhesion to blood vessel walls and subsequent migration of lymphocytes into tissue. Antegren binds to the cell surface receptors known as alpha4beta1 (VLA-4) and alpha4beta7.

Positive results were announced from preliminary analyses of two large phase II trials of Antegren in subjects with multiple sclerosis (MS) and Crohn's disease. The first double-blind, placebo-controlled trial included 213 MS subjects and was conducted at 26 sites in the United States, Canada, and the United Kingdom. The primary endpoint of a reduction in new gadolinium enhancing lesions compared to placebo over the six-month treatment period was achieved with a high degree of statistical significance. The second trial included 240 subjects with moderate to severe Crohn's disease and was conducted at 38 sites in eight European countries. Statistically significant positive results were obtained for multiple endpoints, including induction of remission as measured by the Crohn's Disease Activity Index.

Elan Corporation and Biogen plan to initiate phase III trials in 2001 for both MS and Crohn's disease. Additionally, Antegren is being studied in a phase II trial for inflammatory bowel disease. In August 2000, Biogen and Elan announced a worldwide, exclusive collaboration to develop, manufacture, and commercialize Antegren.

INDICATION(S) AND RESEARCH PHASE
Multiple Sclerosis – Phase II completed
Inflammatory Bowel Disease – Phase II
Crohn's Disease – Phase II completed

NBI-5788, MSP-771
unknown

MANUFACTURER
Neurocrine Biosciences

DESCRIPTION
NBI-5788 is a vaccine that is being developed for the treatment of relapsing-remitting and progressive multiple sclerosis. It is composed of an altered peptide ligand product. NBI-5788 is being tested in phase II trials. Neurocrine Biosciences has a collaborative development agreement with Novartis Pharmaceuticals for this vaccine.

INDICATION(S) AND RESEARCH PHASE
Multiple Sclerosis – Phase II

pirfenidone
Deskar

MANUFACTURER
Marnac

DESCRIPTION
Deskar is a broad-spectrum antifibrotic drug being tested in clinical trials for treatment of fibrotic conditions. These diseases include pulmonary fibrosis, uterine fibroids, peritoneal sclerosis, and scleroderma. The drug is also a tumor necrosis factor (TNF)-alpha agent, which is effective in multiple sclerosis. The phase II trials for pulmonary fibrosis and multiple sclerosis use a capsule formulation of Deskar.

INDICATION(S) AND RESEARCH PHASE
Pulmonary Fibrosis – Phase II
Multiple Sclerosis – Phase II

recombinant human interferon beta-1a
Rebif

MANUFACTURER
Serono Laboratories

DESCRIPTION
Rebif is an interferon beta-1a product being developed for a variety of indications. These include non-small cell lung cancer, chronic hepatitis C, Crohn's disease, ulcerative colitis, Guillain-Barre syndrome, secondary progressive multiple sclerosis, and rheumatoid arthritis. Rebif has been approved in several countries for the treatment of relapsing-remitting multiple sclerosis.

INDICATION(S) AND RESEARCH PHASE
Multiple Sclerosis – Phase III
Lung Cancer – Phase II
Hepatitis – Phase II
Crohn's Disease – Phase II
Inflammatory Bowel Disease – Phase II
Neurologic Disorders, Guillain-Barré Syndrome – Phase II
Rheumatoid Arthritis – Phase II

T-cell peptide vaccines
unknown

MANUFACTURER
Immune Response Corporation

DESCRIPTION
T-cell receptor (TCR) peptide vaccines are composed of TCR peptides (BV5S2, BV6S5 and BV13S1) in incomplete Freud's adjuvant (IFA). The rationale for the vaccines is to elicit an antibody response to the T-cell receptor and thereby decrease T-cell activity. This would have anti-inflammatory effects. The IFA should enhance the immunogenicity of peptides. A phase I/II trial will evaluate T-cell receptor (TCR) peptide vaccines for safety, the ability to increase anti-inflammatory immune responses, and changes in neurologic evaluations including MRI (magnetic resonance imaging) in multiple sclerosis.

INDICATION(S) AND RESEARCH PHASE
Multiple Sclerosis – Phase I/II
Vaccines – Phase I/II

T-cell receptor vaccine
unknown

MANUFACTURER
Immune Response Corporation

DESCRIPTION
Immune Response has developed a vaccine of T-cell receptor (TCR) peptides which may induce the immune system to suppress the aberrant T cells that are active in rheumatoid arthritis, psoriasis, and multiple sclerosis. While these cells are suppressed, the other normal cells should not be affected. The vaccine is designed to treat the pre-

sumed cause of the disease, not just the symptoms. Three trials have recently been completed with the TCR vaccine for treatment of multiple sclerosis (phase I), rheumatoid arthritis (phase IIb), and psoriasis (phase II).

INDICATION(S) AND RESEARCH PHASE
Multiple Sclerosis – Phase I completed
Psoriasis and Psoriatic Disorders – Phase II completed
Rheumatoid Arthritis – Phase IIb completed

thalidomide
Thalomid

MANUFACTURER
Celgene Corporation

DESCRIPTION
Thalomid is an oral formulation of the immunomodulatory agent thalidomide. Thalidomide has a notorious history of having caused birth defects when the medical profession unsuspectingly prescribed it for pregnant women as a treatment for nausea and insomnia. Celgene is investigating new applications for the drug, while being particularly mindful of the potential risks of thalidomide treatment. Thalomid is currently being tested for numerous indications in the areas of oncology and immunology.

INDICATION(S) AND RESEARCH PHASE
Multiple Myeloma – Phase II
Myelodysplastic Syndrome – Phase II
Leukemia – Phase II
Brain Cancer – Phase II
Liver Cancer – Phase II
Kidney Cancer – Phase II
Prostate Cancer – Phase II
Kaposi's Sarcoma – Phase II
Cachexia – Phase II
Recurrent Aphthous Stomatitis – Phase III
Crohn's Disease – Phase II
Inflammatory Bowel Disease – Phase II
Sarcoidosis – Phase II
Scleroderma – Phase II

TM27, ATM027, TCAR
unknown

MANUFACTURER
AVANT Immunotherapeutics

DESCRIPTION
TM27 is a genetically engineered, humanized monoclonal antibody (MAb) being developed for the treatment of multiple sclerosis. It is composed of a T-cell antigen receptor (TCAR). TM27 is being evaluated in phase II clinical trials in subjects with multiple sclerosis. AVANT Immunotherapeutics has a joint development agreement with AB Astra, Sweden.

INDICATION(S) AND RESEARCH PHASE
Multiple Sclerosis – Phase II

unknown
AnergiX.MS

MANUFACTURER
Corixa Corporation

DESCRIPTION
AnergiX.MS is an MHC-class II molecule loaded with a multiple sclerosis-associated peptide, in development for the treatment of multiple sclerosis. A phase I/II trial has been completed. A phase I trial using AnergiX.MS for the treatment of chronic progressive multiple sclerosis (MS) was completed. The company is seeking a development partner prior to initiating a phase II trial.

INDICATION(S) AND RESEARCH PHASE
Multiple Sclerosis – Phase I/II completed

Neuroblastoma

vaccine, allogenic and autologous neuroblastoma cells
unknown

MANUFACTURER
St. Jude Children's Research Hospital

DESCRIPTION
Currently, phase II/III clinical trials are evaluating gene-modified cancer vaccines using autologous and allogenic tumor cells from interleukin-2 (IL-2) secreting neuroblastomas after autologous bone marrow transplant in first remission. According to the researchers, they are conducting parallel clinical trials in children with recurrent neuroblastoma who are receiving either allogenic or autologous tumor cells that are gene modified to secrete small amounts of IL-2.

In the autologous trial, one subject had a complete tumor response, one had a partial response, and three had stable disease following the tumor immunogen alone. Four of the five subjects with tumor responses had coexisting neuroblastoma-specific cytotoxic T-lymphocyte activity, as opposed to only one of the subjects with non-responsive disease. These results show a promising correlation between immune response and clinical outcome with autologous vaccines.

In the allogenic group, one child had a very good partial response, five had stable disease, and four had progressive disease. Although immunization with autologous vaccine produces superior immune responses, these results offer encouragement for the continued pursuit of allogenic vaccine strategies in human cancer.

INDICATION(S) AND RESEARCH PHASE
Pediatric, Neuroblastoma – Phase II/III
Pediatric, Vaccines – Phase II/III

Neurodegenerative Disease

leteprinim potassium, AIT-082
Neotrofin

MANUFACTURER
NeoTherapeutics

DESCRIPTION
Neotrofin is composed of the purine compound hypoxanthine, which is linked with the antiarrhythmic drug procainamide. Results of a double-blind, dose-escalating phase II trial of Neotrofin indicated that the compound facilitated brain activity in Alzheimer's disease subjects, leading to improvements in memory, attention and judgement. The improvements were dose-

related, with 500 mg and 1,000 mg doses producing more benefit than the 150 mg dose. The trial supported NeoTherapeutics' decision to initiate a one-year trial in early 2001 at doses of 500 mg and 1,000 mg in subjects with moderate Alzheimer's disease.

Neotrofin is also in development for indications other than Alzheimer's disease, including peripheral neuropathy (preclinical) and other neurodegenerative diseases (research). In March 2001, NeoTherapeutics announced that it has begun a 12-week, double-blind, placebo-controlled phase II trial of Neotrofin in Parkinson's disease. Also in March, the company announced the initiation of a phase II trial in subacute spinal cord injured patients.

INDICATION(S) AND RESEARCH PHASE
Alzheimer's Disease – Phase III
Parkinson's Disease – Phase II
Spinal Cord Injuries – Phase II
Neuropathy – Preclinical
Neurodegenerative Disease – Research

Neurologic Disorders

+DDMS
unknown

MANUFACTURER
Sepracor

DESCRIPTION
+DDMS is a serotonin, norepinephrine, and dopamine reuptake inhibitor. It is the single isomer version of Meridia, developed and marketed by Knoll Pharmaceuticals. The drug is currently in phase I studies for the treatment of different central nervous system disorders, including depression and attention deficit/hyperactivity disorder (ADHD).

INDICATION(S) AND RESEARCH PHASE
Attention Deficit/Hyperactivity Disorder (ADHD) – Phase I
Depression – Phase I
Neurologic Disorders – Phase I

dimethyl sulfoxide, DMSO
unknown

MANUFACTURER
Topical Technologies

DESCRIPTION
Dimethyl sulfoxide (DMSO) is a topical medication being developed for the treatment of two indications: palmar-plantar dystensia syndrome caused by anti-cancer drugs and soft-tissue injury following extravasation of cytotoxic drugs. An orphan drug status has been granted for both of these indications.

According to the company, dimethyl sulfoxide has a history of use in the wood industry as a commercial solvent since 1953. Since it penetrates the skin deeply and quickly without apparent damage, DMSO can carry other drugs with it across membranes. It is more successful ferrying some drugs, such as morphine sulfate, penicillin, steroids, and cortisone, than others, such as insulin. What DMSO can carry depends on the molecular weight, shape, and electrochemistry of the molecules. This property may enable DMSO to act as a new drug delivery system that may lower the risk of infection occurring when the skin is penetrated.

DMSO, while approved for topical use over much of the world, has had a long and controversial history with the FDA due to concerns about eye problems and other issues.

INDICATION(S) AND RESEARCH PHASE
Connective Tissue Diseases – Phase II
Effects of Chemotherapy – Phase III
Neurologic Disorders – Phase III

recombinant human interferon beta-1a
Rebif

MANUFACTURER
Serono Laboratories

DESCRIPTION
Rebif is an interferon beta-1a product being developed for a variety of indications. These include non-small cell lung cancer, chronic hepatitis C, Crohn's disease, ulcerative colitis, Guillain-Barré syndrome, secondary progressive multiple sclerosis, and rheumatoid arthritis. Rebif has been approved in several countries for the treatment of relapsing-remitting multiple sclerosis.

INDICATION(S) AND RESEARCH PHASE
Multiple Sclerosis – Phase III
Lung Cancer – Phase II
Hepatitis – Phase II
Crohn's Disease – Phase II
Inflammatory Bowel Disease – Phase II
Neurologic Disorders, Guillain-Barré Syndrome – Phase II
Rheumatoid Arthritis – Phase II

Neuropathy

AVP-923
unknown

MANUFACTURER
AVANIR Pharmaceuticals

DESCRIPTION
AVP-923 is in a phase II/III trial for the treatment of emotional lability in neurodegenerative disease. Approximately 100 subjects with Lou Gehrig's disease (amyotrophic lateral sclerosis or ALS) will be tested at 11 sites in the United States. The trial is being monitored by INC Research and is expected to continue through July 2001. The company plans to initiate a second clinical trial in 2001 that will be conducted in multiple sclerosis.

INDICATION(S) AND RESEARCH PHASE
Amyotrophic Lateral Sclerosis (ALS) – Phase I
Neuropathy – Phase II/III
Neuropathic pain – Phase II/III
Emotional lability – Phase II

leteprinim potassium, AIT-082
Neotrofin

MANUFACTURER
NeoTherapeutics

DESCRIPTION

Neotrofin is composed of the purine compound hypoxanthine, which is linked with the antiarrhythmic drug procainamide. Results of a double-blind, dose-escalating phase II trial of Neotrofin indicated that the compound facilitated brain activity in Alzheimer's disease subjects, leading to improvements in memory, attention and judgement. The improvements were dose-related, with 500 mg and 1,000 mg doses producing more benefit than the 150 mg dose. The trial supported NeoTherapeutics' decision to initiate a one-year trial in early 2001 at doses of 500 mg and 1,000 mg in subjects with moderate Alzheimer's disease.

Neotrofin is also in development for indications other than Alzheimer's disease, including peripheral neuropathy (preclinical) and other neurodegenerative diseases (research). In March 2001, NeoTherapeutics announced that it has begun a 12-week, double-blind, placebo-controlled phase II trial of Neotrofin in Parkinson's disease. Also in March, the company announced the initiation of a phase II trial in subacute spinal cord injured patients.

INDICATION(S) AND RESEARCH PHASE
Alzheimer's Disease – Phase III
Parkinson's Disease – Phase II
Spinal Cord Injuries – Phase II
Neuropathy – Preclinical
Neurodegenerative Disease – Research

Neuropathy, Diabetic

BMS-186295, SR-47436 (irbesartan)
Avapro

MANUFACTURER
Bristol-Myers Squibb

DESCRIPTION
Avapro (irbesartan) is an approved drug (September 1997) in the United States and indicated for the treatment of hypertension. Avapro is a very selective, long-acting angiotensin-II receptor antagonist. By inhibiting the potent vasoconstrictor, angiotensin-II, Avapro works to lower blood pressure.

The company is trying to extend the product line by conducting a phase III trial for the indication of diabetic neuropathy and a phase IV for heart failure is planned for 2001.

INDICATION(S) AND RESEARCH PHASE
Neuropathy, Diabetic – Phase III
Congestive Heart Failure – Phase III completed

LY-333531
unknown

MANUFACTURER
Eli Lilly

DESCRIPTION
LY-333531 is an enzyme inhibitor (of PKC). It is being tested in diabetes subjects in a phase II trial for the treatment of neuropathy and eye disease (macular edema), which are pathological diabetic complications.

INDICATION(S) AND RESEARCH PHASE
Neuropathy, Diabetic – Phase II
Eye Disorders/Infections – Phase II

memantine
unknown

MANUFACTURER
Neurobiological Technologies

DESCRIPTION
Memantine is an orally available compound that appears to restore the function of damaged nerve cells and reduce abnormal excitatory signals. This is accomplished by the modulation of N-methyl-D-aspartate (NMDA) receptor activity.

Memantine is in trials for diabetic neuropathy (phase II completed), AIDS-related dementia and neurological function (phase II), and moderate to severe dementia and Alzheimer's disease (phase III). Forest Laboratories intends to prepare an NDA for submission around the end of 2001 for the treatment of Alzheimer's disease, but will also begin additional phase III trials in both mild to moderate and moderately severe to severe Alzheimer's disease.

Forest Laboratories has entered into an agreement with Merz & Co. (collaborator of Neurobiological Technologies), for the development and marketing of memantine in the United States.

INDICATION(S) AND RESEARCH PHASE
Alzheimer's Disease – Phase III
Acquired Immune Deficiency Syndrome (AIDS) and AIDS-Related Infections – Phase II
Neuropathy, Diabetic – Phase II completed

timcodar dimesylate
Timcodar

MANUFACTURER
Vertex Pharmaceuticals

DESCRIPTION
Timcodar dimesylate is an orally bioavailable neuroprotective agent being evaluated in a phase II trial for reversal of neural dysfunction in subjects with diabetic neuropathy. This neurophilin compound is made up of small molecules that may promote nerve growth and recovery of nerve function.

In 1998, Vertex began collaborating with Schering AG on the discovery, development, and commercialization of neurophilin ligands for the treatment of neurological disease. Vertex and Schering AG are working to clarify the development track for Timcodar.

INDICATION(S) AND RESEARCH PHASE
Neuropathy, Diabetic – Phase II

zenarestat
unknown

MANUFACTURER
Pfizer

DESCRIPTION
Pfizer announced in October 2000 that it is suspending development of its aldose reductase inhibitor research candidate, zenarestat, for the treatment of diabetic neuropathy. The company based its decision on an evaluation of safety data from two large phase III trials. In a small number of subjects, zenarestat was noted to have

potential renal toxicity, which appears to be dose dependent with the majority of cases at the highest dose (1,200 mg/day). However, with regard to efficacy, zenarestat was shown in phase II development to have a beneficial effect on nerve conduction velocity, which was confirmed in an interim efficacy analysis of one of the phase III trials.

INDICATION(S) AND RESEARCH PHASE
Neuropathy, Diabetic – Phase II discontinued

Pain, Acute or Chronic

ABT-594, epibatidine
unknown

MANUFACTURER
Abbott Laboratories

DESCRIPTION
In 1976, scientists with the National Institutes of Health (NIH) isolated a compound from the skin of *Epipedobates tricolor*, an Ecuadorian frog. Named epibatidine, this alkaloid (a nitrogen containing compound) was found to block pain 200 times more effectively than morphine, without morphine's addictive and harmful side effects. A potent antinociceptive agent for acute and persistent pain, this compound works predominately by an action at central neuronal acetylcholine receptors (nAChRs).

After successfully eliminating the paralyzing effects of the poison, epibatidine is now being tested for hepatic encephalopathy in subjects with advanced liver disease. Most analgesics modulate the feeling of pain by binding to opiate receptors. Epibatidine has a very low affinity for the nicotine receptors in the neuromuscular junction that cause the paralysis effect, but it has a high affinity for the nicotine receptors in the central nervous system that regulate pain perception.

INDICATION(S) AND RESEARCH PHASE
Hepatic Encephalopathy – Phase II
Pain, Acute or Chronic – Phase II

acetaminophen/ dextromethorphan
HydrocoDex

MANUFACTURER
Algos Pharmaceutical

DESCRIPTION
HydrocoDex is a novel *N*-methyl-D-aspartate (NMDA) enhanced narcotic combination of acetaminophen and dextromethorphan. This NMDA combination with antagonist drugs has been approved for human use in other applications. HydrocoDex is currently being tested in phase II/III trials in an oral formulation for acute and/or chronic pain.

INDICATION(S) AND RESEARCH PHASE
Pain, Acute or Chronic – Phase II/III

ADX-153
unknown

MANUFACTURER
Andrx

DESCRIPTION
ADX-153 is being engineered to deliver pain relieving (analgesic) medications to affected areas in a more efficient, targeted manner. Currently, one of the most active areas of drug development is the formulation of new drug delivery systems, including new methods of controlled-release and targeted action. The goal is to ensure that drugs are delivered to their particular target sites without being inactivated or destroyed, leaving their potency intact.

ADX-153 is a chemical union of the active analgesic medication and a protein container. When this container comes into contact with fluids in the digestive tract, it changes shape and begins to allow the slow release of the pain medication. Because of this slower, more controlled release, this drug can be given in a once daily dose that may result in fewer side effects.

Drugs already in clinical use could potentially become much more effective if their transport system to affected sites in the body were improved. More precise delivery of pain medications could result in better pain relief and the ability to use smaller dosages of the drug to achieve equivalent effects, thus minimizing the drug's potential side effects and toxicities.

INDICATION(S) AND RESEARCH PHASE
Pain, Acute or Chronic – Phase II

asimadoline
unknown

MANUFACTURER
Merck KgaA

DESCRIPTION
Asimadoline is a pain reliever that is being evaluated in a phase II trial for osteoarthritis. It works by stimulating specific kappa receptors on nerve cells in the peripheral nervous system. As a peripherally effective opioid or synthetic narcotic, asimadoline may inhibit the pain associated with the inflammatory changes of osteoarthritis.

An additional benefit may be that asimadoline lacks the potential for addiction or substance abuse, since this agent exerts its effect only in the periphery, and has not shown any significant adverse events associated with the central nervous system. According to the company, asimadoline has thus far proved to be well tolerated in clinical investigations.

INDICATION(S) AND RESEARCH PHASE
Osteoarthritis – Phase II
Pain, Acute or Chronic – Phase II

BCH-3963, LEF576
unknown

MANUFACTURER
BioChem Pharma

DESCRIPTION
BCH-3963 is an injectable delivery form of a new class of pain relievers that work by binding selectively to peripherally located pain (mu opioid) receptors. This drug does not enter the central nervous system (CNS) to treat pain. Therefore, BCH-3963 has the potential to cause fewer neurological

adverse effects, such as the physical dependence associated with morphine, making it potentially suitable for treatment of chronic as well as acute pain. Although BioChem and Astra have a collaborative research agreement, Astra is primarily responsible for the global clinical development of BCH-3963.

INDICATION(S) AND RESEARCH PHASE
Pain, Acute or Chronic – Phase II

benzestrom
Esterom

MANUFACTURER
Entropin

DESCRIPTION
Esterom is a topical treatment for impaired range of motion associated with acute lower back sprain and acute painful shoulders. The product name is derived from its chemical identity and medical purpose since it is an ester that improves the range of motion (ROM) of subjects suffering from a painful shoulder sprain/strain. Esterom solution is a mixture of components in a propylene, glycol water solution. It contains benzolyecgonine and ecgonine, their hydroxypropyl esters, and other hydrolytic by-products. Esterom's mechanism of action is currently unknown.

The company reported that results from a previous phase II trial testing Esterom demonstrated effectiveness in the improvement of range of motion associated with impaired shoulder function and acute lower back sprain. Currently, this drug is being tested in a phase III trial that will enroll 600 subjects experiencing only shoulder pain. The trial will consist of two segments, a phase IIIa and a phase IIIb.

INDICATION(S) AND RESEARCH PHASE
Pain, Acute or Chronic – Phase III
Musculoskeletal Diseases – Phase III

bupivacaine
DepoBupivacaine

MANUFACTURER
Skye Pharma

DESCRIPTION
Bupivacaine is a drug classified as a local anesthetic. It is an amino-amide compound that causes reversible blockade of nerve impulses to control pain. DepoBupivacaine is administered via injection and provides sustained release using the DepoFoam slow release, lipid-based delivery system. It is thought that the local anesthetic receptors are protein bound receptors located near the sodium channel. Bupivacaine is highly protein bound, which results in a slower dissociation from the receptor and a subsequent prolonged effect. Reported side effects include tremors, cardiovascular abnormalities, and drug hypersensitivity. Bupivacaine is being tested in phase II trials for the relief of pain.

INDICATION(S) AND RESEARCH PHASE
Pain, Acute or Chronic – Phase II

clondine gel
unknown

MANUFACTURER
Curatek

DESCRIPTION
Clondine gel is in phase III trials testing 600 subjects for the treatment of peripheral neuropathic pain and painful diabetic neuropathy at 20 sites in the United States.

Although clondine is widely prescribed in both a transdermal path and oral formulation, it has also been shown to act as a potent local analgesic. According to Curateck, the gel formulation is being designed to provide concentrated, site-specific therapy over the complete painful area without blocking motor or sensory nerve function. Results from early trials using clondine gel showed it to be effective with minimal side effects.

INDICATION(S) AND RESEARCH PHASE
Pain, Acute or Chronic – Phase III

COX 189
unknown

MANUFACTURER
Novartis

DESCRIPTION
COX 189 is an oral, non-steroidal anti-inflammatory/analgesic belonging to the COX-2 inhibitor class. COX 189 has yielded promising results in dental pain relief, in addition to demonstrating relief of pain due to osteoarthritis and rheumatoid arthritis comparable to Voltaren (diclofenac). It is currently in phase III development.

INDICATION(S) AND RESEARCH PHASE
Rheumatoid Arthritis – Phase III
Osteoarthritis – Phase III
Pain, Acute or Chronic – Phase III

CT-3
unknown

MANUFACTURER
Atlantic Pharmaceuticals

DESCRIPTION
CT-3 is an analgesic and anti-inflammatory drug that is a synthetic derivative of tetrahydrocannabinol (THC), the active ingredient in marijuana. CT-3 is in phase I trials in Paris, France.

Results from animal studies demonstrated CT-3 has analgesic and anti-inflammatory properties at microgram doses without neurological or gastrointestinal side effects, which are the common side effects of current anti-inflammatory drugs.

INDICATION(S) AND RESEARCH PHASE
Inflammation – Phase I
Pain, Acute or Chronic – Phase I/II

dexamethasone
IontoDex

MANUFACTURER
Iomed

DESCRIPTION
IontoDex is being developed for the treatment of acute local inflammation, for the treatment of ocular disease, and for systemic (whole body) pain control. IontoDex is

comprised of the drug dexamethasone, an anti-inflammatory steroid, delivered by the proprietary iontophoretic drug delivery device Phoresor. Iontophoresis is a needle-free method of delivering certain types of medication directly into and through the skin using a mild, low-level electric current. Programming the system's electric current levels to achieve the desired dose, delivery rate or pattern of delivery can control the amount of drug delivered. This drug is in phase III trials.

INDICATION(S) AND RESEARCH PHASE
Eye Disorders/Infections – Phase III
Pain, Acute or Chronic – Phase III
Skin Wounds – Phase III

diclofenac
unknown

MANUFACTURER
Pharmos Corporation

DESCRIPTION
Diclofenac is a non-steroidal anti-inflammatory drug (NSAID) for the treatment of local pain and inflammation. This topically formulated drug is in phase I/II trials.

INDICATION(S) AND RESEARCH PHASE
Pain, Acute or Chronic – Phase I/II

DPI-3290
unknown

MANUFACTURER
Delta Pharmaceutical Group

DESCRIPTION
DPI-3290 is pain reliever or analgesic agent that works by stimulating both delta and mu receptors. This intravenous drug is being developed for the treatment of severe post-operative pain. Current strong analgesics, such as morphine, act on mu receptors to suppress pain. These opioids also produce many unwanted side effects, such as nausea, vomiting, constipation, and respiratory depression.

The Delta Pharmaceutical Group has developed DPI-3290 based on a novel class of delta opioid receptors, which have the promise to provide strong analgesia without the serious side effects caused by currently approved drugs, such as respiratory depression, nausea, and vomiting.

The company reported that in early clinical trials DPI-3290 showed that it could potentially deliver potent analgesia exceeding that of morphine. Currently, this mixed delta/mu agonist is being tested in a phase II trial for the relief of severe pain, immediately after surgery.

INDICATION(S) AND RESEARCH PHASE
Pain, Acute or Chronic – Phase II

etodolac
Lodine

MANUFACTURER
Elan Pharmaceutical Research

DESCRIPTION
Lodine is a non-steroidal anti-inflammatory (NSAID) pain reliever (analgesic) that has been on the market in an oral tablet formulation since 1991 for acute and long-term treatment of osteoarthritis and rheumatoid arthritis. Lodine is currently being tested in a new formulation, a once daily Intestinal Protective Drug Absorption System (IPDAS) for controlled release delivery. Elan Pharmaceutical Research has a development and marketing agreement with Wyeth-Ayerst for this agent.

INDICATION(S) AND RESEARCH PHASE
Osteoarthritis – Phase III
Rheumatoid Arthritis – Phase III
Pain, Acute or Chronic – Phase III

fentanyl
unknown

MANUFACTURER
Elan Pharmaceutical Research

DESCRIPTION
Fentanyl is a well-regarded opioid (synthetic narcotic) that has 75-100 times more analgesic potency than morphine, as well as a more rapid onset of action and shorter duration of effect. Unlike morphine, it does not provoke histamine release and is therefore not as commonly associated with vascular dilatation and systemic hypotension. These phase I/II trials are currently testing the administration of fentanyl through the Medipad Continuous System. A unique "pump in a patch" system, Medipad provides controlled parenteral (injectable) delivery in a simple, subject-friendly format. It is a low-cost, disposable, single-use system that combines microinfusion technology with an integral subcutaneous probe. An adhesive backing fixes the system against the user's chest or abdomen where it continuously dispenses a drug for up to 48 hours.

INDICATION(S) AND RESEARCH PHASE
Pain, Acute or Chronic – Phase I/II

fentanyl transdermal system
Duragesic

MANUFACTURER
Alza (Sequus Pharmaceuticals)

DESCRIPTION
Duragesic is a 72-hour transdermal (across the skin) system for management of chronic pain in subjects who require continuous opioid (synthetic narcotic) pain relief that cannot be managed by lesser means such as acetaminophen-opioid combinations or non-steroidal analgesics.

Duragesic is marketed by Janssen Pharmaceutica. It is currently in phase III trials for the treatment of chronic pain in pediatric subjects two to 16 years of age.

INDICATION(S) AND RESEARCH PHASE
Pain, Acute or Chronic – Phase III
Pediatric, Pain Management – Phase III

GW 406381
unknown

MANUFACTURER
GlaxoSmithKline

DESCRIPTION
GW 406381 is a second generation cyclooxygenase-2 inhibitor being developed

for the treatment of pain, including inflammatory pain. It is currently in phase I trials.

INDICATION(S) AND RESEARCH PHASE
Pain, Acute or Chronic – Phase I

HCT 3012
unknown

MANUFACTURER
NicOx SA

DESCRIPTION
HCT 3012 is a nitric-oxide derivative of the non-steroidal anti-inflammatory drug (NSAID) naproxen. In animal models of rheumatoid inflammatory disorders, pain, and arthritis, HCT 3012 exhibited significantly lower gastric toxicity than naproxen. AstraZeneca, NicOx S.A.'s development partner has initiated a phase II trial in Europe for pain and inflammation.

INDICATION(S) AND RESEARCH PHASE
Pain, Acute or Chronic – Phase II

hydromorphone
unknown

MANUFACTURER
Alza (Sequus Pharmaceuticals)

DESCRIPTION
This trial is testing a new 24-hour OROS controlled-release delivery system for pain relief caused by severe chronic conditions. The benefit may be around-the-clock relief of pain using this delivery system and a synthetic narcotic.

INDICATION(S) AND RESEARCH PHASE
Pain, Acute or Chronic – Phase III

ketoprofen patch
unknown

MANUFACTURER
Noven Pharmaceuticals

DESCRIPTION
Noven Pharmaceuticals is developing a ketoprofen transdermal patch for the treatment of joint pain. Ketoprofen is a non-steroidal anti-inflammatory drug (NSAID), which works by reducing hormones that cause inflammation and pain in the body. The transdermal patch technology allows ketoprofen to be delivered directly to the site of pain, instead of initially passing through the gastrointestinal tract. According to the company, this is expected to reduce gastrointestinal toxicity. The ketoprofen patch is in phase II trials.

INDICATION(S) AND RESEARCH PHASE
Pain, Acute or Chronic – Phase II

LEF
unknown

MANUFACTURER
AstraZeneca

DESCRIPTION
LEF is a peripheral mu-agonist in an intravenous formulation. It is currently in phase II trials for the treatment of acute or chronic pain.

INDICATION(S) AND RESEARCH PHASE
Pain, Acute or Chronic – Phase II

MH-200, morphine hydrochloride
unknown

MANUFACTURER
Takeda Chemical Industries

DESCRIPTION
MH-200 is being evaluated as an analgesic for severe pain due to cancer (high content/concentration preparation). The drug is currently under application in Japan.

INDICATION(S) AND RESEARCH PHASE
Pain, Acute or Chronic – Under application in Japan

MK-663
unknown

MANUFACTURER
Merck & Co.

DESCRIPTION
MK-663 belongs to a relatively new class of non-steroidal anti-inflammatory drugs (NSAIDs) called Cox-2 inhibitors. MK-663 is designed to specifically inhibit cyclooxygenase-2 (Cox-2), which is one of several enzymes that lead to the production of substances that cause acute or chronic discomfort in joints with the associated pain and inflammation of arthritis.

Clinical studies have shown that Cox-2 inhibitors work with the body to help it strengthen the system and prevent activation of several enzymes of the arachidonic acid metabolism. Consequently, the inhibitors prevent the formulation of eicosanoids, which are short-lived chemical agents that control a large number of physiological functions. Cox-2 inhibitors counteract the formation of at least two undesired biochemicals: prostaglandins that are responsible for short-term joint discomfort, and also leukotrienes that are responsible for long-term joint discomfort. By inhibiting prostaglandin synthesis and counteracting the destructive changes in healthy joints caused by leukotrienes, the extract Cox-2 is the first dual inhibitor available.

The company reported favorable results from a phase II trial that showed MK-663 relieved pain better than the placebo in 617 subjects with osteoarthritis of the knee. Currently, MK-663 is being tested in phase III trials for the treatment and relief of pain associated with rheumatoid arthritis.

INDICATION(S) AND RESEARCH PHASE
Pain, Acute or Chronic – Phase III
Rheumatoid Arthritis – Phase III
Chemotherapy – Phase III

morphine
unknown

MANUFACTURER
Nastech Pharmaceutical

DESCRIPTION
Nastech's intranasal morphine formulation is being evaluated for the treatment of breakthrough pain. The intranasal formula-

tion allows the opioid to be absorbed directly into systemic circulation for a faster therapeutic effect. Results of a phase II trial showed the product to be safe and efficacious in the treatment of eight episodes of breakthrough pain. The treatment group consisted of thirteen subjects suffering from moderate-to-severe chronic pain with daily episodes of breakthrough pain. Sixty-six percent of breakthrough pain episodes were treated successfully within 20 minutes with the nasal formulation. Significantly, five treatments resulted in a total pain score that was below the baseline level of medication used for chronic therapy, meaning that subjects experienced less pain than they feel on a chronic basis. Pain relief typically began within five minutes, and six subjects sustained their total pain score below baseline up to the period of discharge from the study.

INDICATION(S) AND RESEARCH PHASE
Pain, Acute or Chronic – Phase II completed

morphine sulfate
Morphelan

MANUFACTURER
Ligand Pharmaceuticals

DESCRIPTION
Morphelan is a once-daily oral morphine presentation that utilizes Elan's SODAS release technology. The controlled-release beads produced by the SODAS technology range from 1 to 2 mm in diameter. Each bead begins as an inert core onto which the drug is applied followed by a number of layers of soluble and insoluble polymers combined with other excipients to produce the rate controlling layer. Within the gastrointestinal tract the soluble polymers dissolve leaving pores within the outer membrane. Fluid then enters the core of the beads and dissolves the drug. The resultant solution then diffuses out in a controlled, predetermined manner allowing for prolonged invivo dissolution and absorption phases. Morphelan is being tested in phase III trials for pain relief.

Morphelan is also being tested in a transdermal delivery system called MediPad.

A "pump in a patch" system, MediPad provides controlled parenteral (injectable) delivery in a low-cost, disposable, single-use system that combines microinfusion technology with an integral subcutaneous probe. An adhesive backing fixes the system against the user's chest or abdomen where it continuously dispenses drug for up to 48 hours.

INDICATION(S) AND RESEARCH PHASE
Pain, Acute or Chronic – Phase III

nabumetone Q
unknown

MANUFACTURER
GlaxoSmithKline

DESCRIPTION
Nabumetone Q is a non-steroidal anti-inflammatory drug (NSAID). It is currently in phase III trials for the treatment of osteoarthritis and pain.

INDICATION(S) AND RESEARCH PHASE
Osteoarthritis – Phase III
Pain, Acute or Chronic – Phase III

NCX 4016
unknown

MANUFACTURER
NicOx SA

DESCRIPTION
NCX 4016 is a nitric oxide-releasing derivative of acetylsalicylic acid, the active ingredient in aspirin. According to the company, NCX 4016 may be able to provide the antithrombotic effects of aspirin with less gastric damage or toxicity. Also, studies suggest that nitric oxide itself may provide antithrombotic activity, and NCX 4016, unlike other treatments, may inhibit almost all phases of the blood clotting process. The compound is in phase I development for pain, inflammation, and prevention of cardiovascular diseases including thrombosis.

INDICATION(S) AND RESEARCH PHASE
Pain, Acute or Chronic – Phase I
Thrombosis – Phase I

NCX 701
unknown

MANUFACTURER
NicOx SA

DESCRIPTION
NCX 701 is a derivative of paracetamol (acetaminophen) which results in the release of nitric oxide (NO). It is being evaluated for the treatment of pain in a phase I trial in France. This study was initiated in December 2000 and will include 40 subjects.

Preclinical trials demonstrated NCX 701 to have significantly better analgesic activity than paracetamol and to be a potent anti-inflammatory compound with absence of the liver toxicity characteristic of paracetamol. The anti-inflammatory effect of the NO compound is a paradoxical finding and one that prompts further investigation. In the meantime, the drug seems effective and may be the first in a line of NO-NSAID derivatives.

INDICATION(S) AND RESEARCH PHASE
Pain, Acute or Chronic – Phase I

neurotrophin-3, NT-3
unknown

MANUFACTURER
Regeneron Pharmaceuticals

DESCRIPTION
This drug is an injectable formulation of neurotrophin-3, a naturally occurring human protein. It acts on the neurons of the intestinal tract and is being tested for severe constipation and various constipating conditions caused by spinal cord injuries, narcotic analgesics, and Parkinson's disease. NT-3 is currently in phase II development.

INDICATION(S) AND RESEARCH PHASE
Constipation – Phase II
Spinal Cord Injuries – Phase II
Parkinson's Disease – Phase II
Pain, Acute or Chronic – Phase II

NO-naproxen
unknown

MANUFACTURER
AstraZeneca

DESCRIPTION
NO-naproxen is a nitric oxide non-steroidal anti-inflammatory drug (NSAID) derivative. It is currently in phase I trials for the treatment of acute or chronic pain.

INDICATION(S) AND RESEARCH PHASE
Pain, Acute or Chronic – Phase I

oxycodone hydrochloride/ dextromethorphan hydrobromide
OxyCoDex

MANUFACTURER
Algos Pharmaceutical

DESCRIPTION
OxycoDex is a novel NMDA (*N*-methyl-D-aspartate) enhanced narcotic being developed for the management of moderate to severe pain. In the nervous system, chemical messengers called neurotransmitters bind to receptors embedded in the cell membranes of neurons. One of the neurotransmitters, glutamate, binds to the NMDA receptor. When activated by glutamate, the NMDA receptor opens a channel in the cell membrane setting off a series of reactions necessary for normal function of the brain.

When impaired, nerve cells are unable to control the normal release of neurotransmitters and "dump" excess glutamate into the extracellular environment. Excess glutamate results in overexcitation of the NMDA receptor allowing excess calcium to enter the affected neurons. These neurons may then swell and rupture, releasing more glutamate into the surrounding area, which in turn overexcites NMDA receptors on adjacent neurons. This cascade of neuronal injury, referred to as "excitotoxicity," follows acute conditions such as stroke and traumatic brain injury. As an NMDA antagonist combined with an analgesic, OxycoDex may significantly improve pain relief over currently available analgesics.

INDICATION(S) AND RESEARCH PHASE
Pain, Acute or Chronic – Phase I/II

pancrelipase
Viokase

MANUFACTURER
Axcan Pharma

DESCRIPTION
Viokase is a pancreatic enzyme preparation containing standardized lipase, protease, and amylase in fixed proportions. It is indicated for the treatment of subjects with exocrine pancreatic enzyme deficiency as is often associated with cystic fibrosis, chronic pancreatitis, and post-pancreatectomy. It has been prescribed for years to assist in the digestion and absorption of food. Axcan is currently conducting phase II trials of Viokase at elevated dosages (8,000 units/day) to alleviate pain often associated with pancreatic disorders.

INDICATION(S) AND RESEARCH PHASE
Pain, Acute or Chronic – Phase II
Pancreatic Disorders – Phase II

pregabalin
unknown

MANUFACTURER
Pfizer

DESCRIPTION
Pregabalin is being developed for the treatment of neuropathic pain, epilepsy, a variety of anxiety disorders, and chronic pain syndromes. In February 2001, Pfizer announced it has restricted the use of pregabalin for certain subjects in clinical trials. The restriction follows an analysis by the FDA of previously submitted results from a chronic administration mouse study that showed an increased evidence of a tumor type in the mice. A similar dosing study in rats did not show increases in any tumor type, nor were these results seen in any other toxicological screen or study. The planned submission of the NDA for neuropathic pain and epilepsy is expected to proceed as previously announced.

INDICATION(S) AND RESEARCH PHASE
Pain, Acute or Chronic – Phase III
Epilepsy – Phase III

propiram
Dirame

MANUFACTURER
Roberts Pharmaceutical

DESCRIPTION
Dirame is an orally administered analgesic that works through the central nervous system to reduce pain. This agent binds (as a mixed agonist/antagonist) to opioid (morphine-like) receptors and blocks painful stimuli. Dirame is being tested in phase III trials for the treatment of moderate to severe pain, especially in osteoarthritis.

INDICATION(S) AND RESEARCH PHASE
Pain, Acute or Chronic – Phase III
Osteoarthritis – Phase III

ropivacaine HCl
Naropin

MANUFACTURER
AstraZeneca

DESCRIPTION
Naropin is a sodium channel blocker that is currently in phase III as a spinal anesthesia and for intra-articular administration. An NDA was submitted in December 2000 for approval for a single-dose administration of Naropin injection for regional anesthesia in pediatric subjects to fulfill the company's pediatric phase IV commitment to the FDA and seeks approval for acute pain management in children one to 12 years old. Naropin has been FDA approved as an obstetric anesthesia and regional anesthesia for surgery, as well as for the management of post-operative pain.

INDICATION(S) AND RESEARCH PHASE
Pain, Acute or Chronic – Phase III
Pediatric, Spinal Anesthesia and for Intra-Articular Administration – FDA approved

RSD 921
unknown

MANUFACTURER
Nortran Pharmaceuticals

DESCRIPTION
RSD 921 is a novel sodium channel blocker designed to function as a local anesthetic. An ion channel is a membrane protein that controls the flow of ions such as sodium, potassium, and calcium in and out of cells. The regulation of these ion concentrations can affect many processes, including nerve signal transmission and muscle contraction.

INDICATION(S) AND RESEARCH PHASE
Pain, Acute or Chronic – Phase II completed

topiramate tablet
Topamax

MANUFACTURER
R.W. Johnson Pharmaceutical Research Institute

DESCRIPTION
Topamax is being tested in phase III trials for monotherapy in neuropathic pain in a tablet formulation. It is also in phase II trials for bipolar mania, and was approved in May 2000 for epilepsy.

INDICATION(S) AND RESEARCH PHASE
Epilepsy – FDA approved
Pain, Acute or Chronic – Phase III
Bipolar Disorders – Phase II

unknown
Lidocaine

MANUFACTURER
Celltech Chiroscience plc

DESCRIPTION
Lidocaine (needleless anesthetic injection) is in phase II development for the treatment of pain. Celltech Chiroscience has established a collaborative venture with PowderJect Pharmaceuticals for the development of local anesthetic products delivered via PowderJect's proprietary needle-free drug injector technology.

INDICATION(S) AND RESEARCH PHASE
Pain, Acute or Chronic – Phase II

ZD-4953
unknown

MANUFACTURER
AstraZeneca

DESCRIPTION
ZD-4953 is being developed in phase II clinical trials for the treatment of moderate pain. This analgesic drug works through the central nervous system to block painful stimuli.

INDICATION(S) AND RESEARCH PHASE
Pain, Acute or Chronic – Phase II

Parkinson's Disease

altropane
unknown

MANUFACTURER
Boston Life Sciences

DESCRIPTION
Altropane is a radioactive molecule that binds specifically to the dopamine transporter (DAT) in the brain. The actual number of DATs in the midbrain can be measured using Altropane along with SPECT imaging. A measurement of DATs may be useful because data suggest there is an abnormally high amount in the midbrain of individuals with ADHD.

A phase II/III trial involving 40 subjects began in early 2000. The company plans to initiate two parallel phase III studies in adults between the ages of 20 and 40 years. Upon completion of these trials, the company will file for marketing approval using altropane to aid in the diagnosis of ADHD in adults. Afterwards, the company plans to initiate a phase III trial testing altropane in the diagnosis of ADHD in children.

Additionally, phase III results showed that altropane is able to differentiate Parkinson's movement disorders (including Parkinson's disease) from other movement disorders. The phase III trial included 95 subjects having the clinical diagnosis of Parkinsonian syndrome (PS) and 70 subjects having non-movement disorders with clinical features similar to PS but whose symptoms are caused by something other than a destruction of dopamine producing cells.

INDICATION(S) AND RESEARCH PHASE
Parkinson's Disease – Phase III completed
Attention Deficit/Hyperactivity Disorder (ADHD) – Phase II/III

apomorphine
unknown

MANUFACTURER
Pentech Pharmaceuticals

DESCRIPTION
Pentech Pharmaceuticals is developing apomorphine for the treatment of on/off fluctuations associated with drugs used to treat late-stage Parkinson's disease. This dopamine receptor agonist is being tested in a phase III trials for the treatment of Parkinson's disease. It has been formulated by Pentech in a sublingual tablet with a high dosage regimen.

INDICATION(S) AND RESEARCH PHASE
Parkinson's Disease – Phase III

apomorphine
unknown

MANUFACTURER
Britannia Pharmaceuticals Limited

DESCRIPTION
Apomorphine stimulates dopamine receptors as a drug agonist. It is being tested in a phase II trial in the United States for the treatment of on/off fluctuations associated with late-stage Parkinson's disease. The FDA has granted this indication as having an orphan drug status. Apomorphine has been previously approved in the United Kingdom.

INDICATION(S) AND RESEARCH PHASE
Parkinson's Disease – Phase II

brasofensine, NS-2214, BMS-204756
unknown

MANUFACTURER
NeuroSearch A/S

DESCRIPTION
Brasofensine is an orally administered dopamine reuptake inhibitor. When the neurotransmitter dopamine is released into the synaptic cleft, brasofensine prevents it from entering back into the nerve cell, thereby allowing a longer period of neural stimulation. Brasofensine is being tested in phase II trials for the treatment of Parkinson's disease.

INDICATION(S) AND RESEARCH PHASE
Parkinson's Disease – Phase II

CEP-1347
unknown

MANUFACTURER
Cephalon

DESCRIPTION
CEP-1347 is a selective inhibitor of the stress-activated protein kinase pathway, an intracellular signaling pathway, which is an essential component of the stress response leading to neuronal death. Working through a novel mechanism of action, CEP-1347 is the first orally active molecule in a new class of compounds to enter clinical testing in Parkinson's disease and is currently in a phase I/II trial.

In animal models CEP-1347 has greatly reduced degeneration of dopamine neurons in the brain, indicating that it may delay or completely stop the progress of Parkinson's disease.

The company H. Lundback A/S has the licensing rights in Europe.

INDICATION(S) AND RESEARCH PHASE
Parkinson's Disease – Phase I/II
Alzheimer's Disease – Phase I/II

CPI-1189
unknown

MANUFACTURER
Centaur Pharmaceuticals

DESCRIPTION
CPI-1189 completed a phase IIa trial for AIDS dementia complex (ADC) in May 2000. The trial was conducted in conjunction with the Neuro AIDS Research Consortium. It included 64 HIV subjects with cognitive and motor impairment. Subjects either received 100 mg a day or 50 mg a day of CPI-1189 or the placebo over ten weeks, with a 12-week open-label follow-on for those who volunteered. CPI-1189 is also in phase IIa trials for Parkinson's disease.

INDICATION(S) AND RESEARCH PHASE
Acquired Immune Deficiency Syndrome (AIDS) and AIDS-Related Infections – Phase IIa completed
Parkinson's Disease – Phase IIa

entacapone
Comtan

MANUFACTURER
Novartis

DESCRIPTION
Comtan is a catechol-O-methyltransferase (COMT) inhibitor approved by the FDA for the treatment of Parkinson's disease. The drug is used together with carbidopa/levodopa to treat people with Parkinson's disease who experience the signs and symptoms of end-of-dose "wearing-off." The recommended dose of Comtan is 200 mg with each levodopa dose, up to eight times daily.

INDICATION(S) AND RESEARCH PHASE
Parkinson's Disease – Phase IV

etilevodopa, TV-1203
unknown

MANUFACTURER
Teva Pharmaceutical Industries

DESCRIPTION
TV-1203, the ethyl ester of levodopa, is being developed as a replacement for levodopa in the treatment of Parkinson's disease. TV-1203 may provide superior clinical benefits to levodopa due to its solubility in aqueous solution. This solubility allows for rapid and predictable absorption with increased bioavailability. According to the company, TV-1203 may be particularly useful for advanced Parkinsonian subjects suffering from fluctuations in response to levodopa therapy. Phase III trials are currently under way.

INDICATION(S) AND RESEARCH PHASE
Parkinson's Disease – Phase III

FKBP-neuroimmunophilin ligands
unknown

MANUFACTURER
Guilford Pharmaceuticals

DESCRIPTION
Neuroimmunophilin ligands are orally active drugs that stimulate nerve growth. They are thought to cross the blood-brain barrier and may be useful in the treatment of neurological diseases and neurodegenerative disorders. These compounds are currently undergoing phase II trials for the treatment of Parkinson's disease. Other indications may include Alzheimer's disease, traumatic brain and spinal cord injuries, and ALS.

INDICATION(S) AND RESEARCH PHASE
Parkinson's Disease – Phase II

leteprinim potassium, AIT-082
Neotrofin

MANUFACTURER
NeoTherapeutics

DESCRIPTION
Neotrofin is composed of the purine compound hypoxanthine, which is linked with the antiarrhythmic drug procainamide. Results of a double-blind, dose-escalating phase II trial of Neotrofin indicated that the

compound facilitated brain activity in Alzheimer's disease subjects, leading to improvements in memory, attention and judgement. The improvements were dose-related, with 500 mg and 1,000 mg doses producing more benefit than the 150 mg dose. The trial supported NeoTherapeutics' decision to initiate a one-year trial in early 2001 at doses of 500 mg and 1,000 mg in subjects with moderate Alzheimer's disease.

Neotrofin is also in development for indications other than Alzheimer's disease, including peripheral neuropathy (preclinical) and other neurodegenerative diseases (research). In March 2001, NeoTherapeutics announced that it has begun a 12-week, double-blind, placebo-controlled phase II trial of Neotrofin in Parkinson's disease. Also in March, the company announced the initiation of a phase II trial in subacute spinal cord injured patients.

INDICATION(S) AND RESEARCH PHASE
Alzheimer's Disease – Phase III
Parkinson's Disease – Phase II
Spinal Cord Injuries – Phase II
Neuropathy – Preclinical
Neurodegenerative Disease – Research

levodopa/carbidopa
Duodopa

MANUFACTURER
NeoPharma

DESCRIPTION
Duodopa is a levodopa/carbidopa formulation delivered directly to the small intestine (duodenum). A possible advantage of this formulation may be the avoidance of irregular gastric emptying, providing subjects with continuous exposure to the drug. A phase III trial for the treatment of Parkinson's disease is planned for early 2001.

INDICATION(S) AND RESEARCH PHASE
Parkinson's Disease – Phase III

modafinil
Provigil

MANUFACTURER
Cephalon

DESCRIPTION
Provigil (modafinil) is a dopamine-releasing agent that increases excitatory glutamatergic transmission. It is being developed in phase III trials for the prevention of daytime sleepiness associated with obstructive sleep apnea, hypersomnia, and shift work. Phase II trials are being conducted for the prevention of excessive daytime sleepiness associated with Alzheimer's disease and Parkinson's disease.

INDICATION(S) AND RESEARCH PHASE
Multiple Sclerosis – Phase II completed
Sleep Disorders – Phase III
Pediatric, Attention Deficit/Hyperactivity Disorder – Phase I/II
Parkinson's Disease – Phase II
Alzheimer's Disease – Phase II

N-0923
unknown

MANUFACTURER
Schwarz Pharma

DESCRIPTION
Subjects with Parkinson's disease are currently treated with drugs that have to be taken several times a day and have significant side effects. However, N-0923 is a dopamine D-2 receptor agonist delivered in a transdermal patch to be applied once a day. This product may provide an improved therapeutic effect by eliminating fluctuations in the level of active ingredients. Currently, N-0923 is being tested in a phase IIb trial for adjunctive treatment to levidopa/carbidopa for Parkinson's disease.

INDICATION(S) AND RESEARCH PHASE
Parkinson's Disease – Phase IIb

neurotrophin-3, NT-3
unknown

MANUFACTURER
Regeneron Pharmaceuticals

DESCRIPTION
This drug is an injectable formulation of neurotrophin-3, a naturally occurring human protein. It acts on the neurons of the intestinal tract and is being tested for severe constipation and various constipating conditions caused by spinal cord injuries, narcotic analgesics, and Parkinson's disease. NT-3 is currently in phase II development.

INDICATION(S) AND RESEARCH PHASE
Constipation – Phase II
Spinal Cord Injuries – Phase II
Parkinson's Disease – Phase II
Pain, Acute or Chronic – Phase II

nitrone radical trap (NRT)
unknown

MANUFACTURER
Centaur Pharmaceuticals

DESCRIPTION
Nitrone Radical Trap (NRT) is an oxidative stress reducing neuroprotective compound for the treatment of Parkinson's disease, AIDS, and stroke. NRTs are designed to combine with free radicals to create a less reactive molecule.

A phase IIb/III trial for stroke will include about 150 subjects who will first receive a bolus and be evaluated for safety and tolerability. If this trial is successful, the subjects will then receive a continuous infusion for 72 hours. The company states that data from a phase IIa study have demonstrated favorable results.

INDICATION(S) AND RESEARCH PHASE
Acquired Immune Deficiency Syndrome (AIDS) and AIDS-Related Infections – Phase IIa
Parkinson's Disease – Phase IIa
Strokes – Phase II/III

porcine fetal cells
NeuroCell-PD

MANUFACTURER
Diacrin

DESCRIPTION

NeuroCell-PD is a preparation of fetal porcine (pig) neural cells that is being tested in a phase II/III clinical trial as a replacement therapy for some of the human brain cells (neurons) lost to Parkinson's disease. NeuroCell-PD is for surgical transplantation directly into the brain. Diacrin has an equally shared joint agreement with Genzyme Tissue Repair for development of the NeuroCell-PD program.

INDICATION(S) AND RESEARCH PHASE
Parkinson's Disease – Phase II/III

remacemide
unknown

MANUFACTURER
AstraZeneca

DESCRIPTION
Remacemide blocks a cell receptor for the amino acid neurotransmitter *N*-methyl-D-aspartate (NMDA). This NMDA receptor antagonist produces a neuroprotective effect. The drug has completed a phase II trial for the treatment of Parkinson's disease, and is in phase III studies for Huntington's chorea and epilepsy. According to the company, remacemide may help alleviate neuropathic pain associated with these neurologic diseases.

INDICATION(S) AND RESEARCH PHASE
Epilepsy – Phase II/III
Huntington's Disease – Phase III
Parkinson's Disease – Phase II completed

riluzole
Rilutek

MANUFACTURER
Aventis

DESCRIPTION
Rilutek is an approved drug for the treatment of amyotrophic lateral sclerosis (ALS), also known as Lou Gehrig's disease. It belongs to the chemical class of benzothiazoles. The mechanism of action of Rilutek is unknown, but it is thought to be mediated through several modes, including inhibited release of glutamate and the inactivation of sodium channels. Currently, Rilutek is being tested in phase III trials for the treatment of Parkinson's disease.

INDICATION(S) AND RESEARCH PHASE
Parkinson's Disease – Phase III

ropinirole
ReQuip

MANUFACTURER
GlaxoSmithKline

DESCRIPTION
ReQuip, an orally administered anti-Parkinsonian drug, is a non-ergoline dopamine agonist. ReQuip's exact mechanism of action is unknown; however, it may produce its effects through the stimulation of post-synaptic dopamine D_2-type receptors within the caudate-putamen in the brain. A controlled-release formulation of the drug is currently in phase II development.

INDICATION(S) AND RESEARCH PHASE
Parkinson's Disease – Phase II

selegiline
Zelapar

MANUFACTURER
Elan Pharmaceutical Research

DESCRIPTION
Selegiline is a monoamine oxidase B (MAO-B) inhibitor that prevents the breakdown of dopamine in the brain. Zelapar is a new formulation of selegiline that dissolves instantly in the mouth without water. The tablet contains only 1.25 mg of selegiline, which is a sufficient dose for efficacy, but low enough to hopefully decrease side effects. Zelapar is in phase III development for the treatment of Parkinson's disease in the United States. Zelapar is already approved in the United Kingdom.

INDICATION(S) AND RESEARCH PHASE
Parkinson's Disease – Phase III

selgiline
Eldepryl

MANUFACTURER
Somerset Pharmaceuticals

DESCRIPTION
Eldepryl is FDA approved for the treatment of Parkinson's disease when given orally. This new formulation is a transdermal patch, which will allow for improved adherence and more optimal pharmacokinetics. It is in a phase III trial for the treatment of depression and Parkinson's disease.

INDICATION(S) AND RESEARCH PHASE
Depression – Phase III
Parkinson's Disease – Phase III

SIB-1508Y
unknown

MANUFACTURER
Sibia Neurosciences

DESCRIPTION
SIB-1508Y is a nicotinic acetylcholine receptor (nAChR)-selective drug that is being developed for the treatment of Parkinson's disease, other cognitive disorders, and attention deficit/hyperactivity disorder (ADHD). SIB-1508Y is being tested in phase II trials as both a single therapeutic agent and combined with L-dopa for treatment of Parkinson's disease.

INDICATION(S) AND RESEARCH PHASE
Attention Deficit/Hyperactivity Disorder (ADHD) – Phase II
Memory Loss – Phase II
Parkinson's Disease – Phase II

SLV 308
unknown

MANUFACTURER
Solvay Pharmaceuticals

DESCRIPTION
SLV 308 is currently in phase II development for the treatment of depression and

Parkinson's disease.

INDICATION(S) AND RESEARCH PHASE
Depression – Phase II
Parkinson's Disease – Phase II

spheramine
unknown

MANUFACTURER
Titan Pharmaceuticals

DESCRIPTION
Spheramine is a novel cell therapy product. It utilizes normal human cells called retinal pigmented epithelial (RPE) cells, which secrete dopamine and can be propagated in cell culture to produce large amounts of cells. Since Parkinson's disease involves a depletion of dopaminergic nerve cells, it is thought that the replacement of the neurotransmitter dopamine may help lessen the symptoms of this disorder. Spheramine is being tested in a phase I/II trial at Emory University that will assess the safety and preliminary efficacy of the drug in subjects with later stage Parkinson's disease.

INDICATION(S) AND RESEARCH PHASE
Parkinson's Disease – Phase I/II

TVP-1012, rasagiline mesylate
unknown

MANUFACTURER
Teva Pharmaceutical Industries

DESCRIPTION
TVP-1012 is an inhibitor of monoamine oxidase B (MAO-B). MAO inhibitors have been used for many years to treat depression; however, they have the potential to cause a hypertensive crisis when taken concurrently with sympathomimetic drugs (such as amphetamines, dopamine, L-dopa, and epinephrine) or certain foods (such as cheeses or fava beans containing tyramine). TVP-1012 may present a better safety profile than previously approved MAO inhibitors. The drug is currently in phase III trials for the treatment of Parkinson's disease and phase II trials for Alzheimer's disease.

INDICATION(S) AND RESEARCH PHASE
Parkinson's Disease – Phase III
Alzheimer's Disease – Phase II

Sleep Disorders

BMS-214778
unknown

MANUFACTURER
Bristol-Myers Squibb

DESCRIPTION
BMS-214778 is a melatonin agonist used in the treatment of sleep disorders. Phase II trials of this drug were suspended mid-2000 pending an internal R&D review.

INDICATION(S) AND RESEARCH PHASE
Sleep Disorders – Phase II halted

doxylamine
unknown

MANUFACTURER
Nastech Pharmaceutical

DESCRIPTION
Doxylamine is being tested in phase II/III trials as a night-time sleep aid. This therapy may be helpful as a short-term treatment of insomnia. It is made in a nasal spray formulation. Nastech Pharmaceutical has a development agreement with Pfizer for this drug.

INDICATION(S) AND RESEARCH PHASE
Sleep Disorders – Phase II/III

epalon, CCD-3693
unknown

MANUFACTURER
CoCensys

DESCRIPTION
CCD-3693 is a GABA receptor antagonist/synthetic version of epalons, used as a hypnotic for the treatment of insomnia and sleep disorders. The drug is in a phase I trial.

INDICATION(S) AND RESEARCH PHASE
Insomnia – Phase I
Sleep Disorders – Phase I

GABA agonist, anxiolytic
unknown

MANUFACTURER
DOV Pharmaceutical

DESCRIPTION
This unspecified gamma-amino butyric acid (GABA) analogue-anti-epileptic is used for the treatment of panic disorder and for sleep induction. Both trials are currently in phase I.

INDICATION(S) AND RESEARCH PHASE
Sleep Disorders – Phase I
Epilepsy – Phase I

GT-2331
Perceptin

MANUFACTURER
Gliatech

DESCRIPTION
Perceptin is a selective histamine H3 receptor antagonist which is being developed for potential use in central nervous system diseases involving attention/learning or sleep disorders. Perceptin is being evaluated in a phase II trial for treatment of attention deficit/hyperactivity hisorder (ADHD) in a multi-dose, double-blind, randomized, placebo-controlled clinical trial that is evaluating the safety and preliminary efficacy of Perceptin at varying doses. The company expects to enroll up to 120 adult subjects. In addition, it is being tested in phase I/II trials for Alzheimer's disease and sleep disorders.

According to the company, histamine is a chemical messenger released from certain neurons in the brain, which regulates sleep/wake states and modulates levels of arousal and alertness in the conscious state. The histamine H3 receptor is predominantly found in the brain where it regulates the release of histamine.

Phase I clinical studies have demonstrated

that Perceptin is safe, well tolerated, and amenable to once-daily dosing.

INDICATION(S) AND RESEARCH PHASE
Alzheimer's Disease – Phase I/II
Attention Deficit/Hyperactivity Disorder (ADHD) – Phase II
Sleep Disorders – Phase I/II

modafinil
Provigil

MANUFACTURER
Cephalon

DESCRIPTION
Provigil (modafinil) is a dopamine-releasing agent that increases excitatory glutamatergic transmission. It is being developed in phase III trials for the prevention of daytime sleepiness associated with obstructive sleep apnea, hypersomnia, and shift work. Phase II trials are being conducted for the prevention of excessive daytime sleepiness associated with Alzheimer's disease and Parkinson's disease.

INDICATION(S) AND RESEARCH PHASE
Multiple Sclerosis – Phase II completed
Sleep Disorders – Phase III
Pediatric, Attention Deficit/Hyperactivity Disorder – Phase I/II
Parkinson's Disease – Phase II
Alzheimer's Disease – Phase II

NBI-34060
unknown

MANUFACTURER
Neurocrine Biosciences

DESCRIPTION
NBI-34060 is a gamma-amino butyric acid (GABA) receptor stimulator that binds to specific sites on the GABA receptor—the same sites that are targeted by benzodiazepines. It is expected to offer an improved side effect profile because it is a non-benzodiazepine.

Preclinical studies have shown that NBI-34060 may produce a more rapid onset of sleep and fewer next-day hangover effects compared to currently marketed products. Also, NBI-34060 has been shown to have minimal interaction with alcohol and may not produce rapid tolerance or amnesia at effective sleep promoting doses.

NBI-34060 is in multiple phase II trials for insomnia and plans on initiating phase III trials later in 2001.

INDICATION(S) AND RESEARCH PHASE
Insomnia – Phase II
Sleep Disorders – Phase II

sodium oxybate (GHB)
Xyrem

MANUFACTURER
Orphan Medical

DESCRIPTION
Sodium oxybate (GHB) is a naturally occurring neurotransmitter in the brain, which is involved in sleep regulation. Xyrem is administered as an oral solution for the treatment of narcolepsy and cataplexy. Cataplexy is a form of narcolepsy, characterized by loss of muscle control in response to strong emotion. Other treatments for narcolepsy do not address this syndrome and their effectiveness can be diminished over time due to drug tolerance. They may also have unpleasant side effects such as weight gain, palpitations, dry mouth, and loss of sense of self. Xyrem offers an alternative to these treatments. A phase IIIb trial is under way to assess the drug's efficacy in controlling excessive daytime sleepiness (EDS). The company submitted an NDA in October 2000. In addition, phase III trials for children 12 years and older have been completed.

INDICATION(S) AND RESEARCH PHASE
Sleep Disorders – NDA submitted
Pediatric, Cataplexy – Phase III completed

SR-46349
unknown

MANUFACTURER
Sanofi-Synthelabo Pharmaceuticals

DESCRIPTION
SR-46349 blocks the action of $5HT_2$ receptors in the body. Normally, these receptors are responsible for absorbing 5HT, a precursor of serotonin, back into neurons. Inadequate levels of serotonin outside nerve cells can lead to depressive states. The action of SR-46349 allows serotonin to circulate longer in the body and in greater amounts. Because this drug acts on a specific receptor, there may be fewer side effects associated with its use. Common anti-depressant side effects include nausea, anorexia, and sexual dysfunction. Further study will determine whether these side effects are fewer with the use of SR-46349.

INDICATION(S) AND RESEARCH PHASE
Sleep Disorders – Phase IIb
Schizophrenia and Schizoaffective Disorders – Phase IIb
Depression – Phase IIb

thGRF 1-44
unknown

MANUFACTURER
Theratechnologies

DESCRIPTION
ThGRF 1-44 is a growth hormone releasing factor analogue indicated for the treatment of chronic obstructive pulmonary disease (COPD) and sleep impairment. An IND has been filed in Canada for a phase II trial for sleep impairment.

INDICATION(S) AND RESEARCH PHASE
Chronic Obstructive Pulmonary Disease (COPD) – Phase II
Sleep Disorders – Phase II

unknown
Gaboxadol

MANUFACTURER
H. Lundbeck A/S

DESCRIPTION
Gaboxadol is a gamma-amino butyric acid A (GABAA) agonist which, in preclinical studies has demonstrated an improvement

in the sleep pattern. The company H. Lundbeck has entered into a license agreement with Garching Innovation GmbH (acting on behalf of the Max Planck Institutes) for Gaboxadol.

INDICATION(S) AND RESEARCH PHASE
Sleep Disorders – Phase II

Spinal Cord Injuries

fampridine
Neurelan

MANUFACTURER
Acorda Therapeutics

DESCRIPTION
Neurelan is a 4-aminopyridine potassium channel blocker that is being tested in a phase II/III trial for the treatment of multiple sclerosis (MS). In this study, Neurelan is delivered using the Intestinal Protective Drug Absorption System (IPDAS) in a sustained-release formulation. Neurelan has an orphan indication status for the symptomatic relief of MS.

INDICATION(S) AND RESEARCH PHASE
Multiple Sclerosis – Phase II/III
Spinal Cord Injuries – Phase II

neurotrophin-3, NT-3
unknown

MANUFACTURER
Regeneron Pharmaceuticals

DESCRIPTION
This drug is an injectable formulation of neurotrophin-3, a naturally occurring human protein. It acts on the neurons of the intestinal tract and is being tested for severe constipation and various constipating conditions caused by spinal cord injuries, narcotic analgesics, and Parkinson's disease. NT-3 is currently in phase II development.

INDICATION(S) AND RESEARCH PHASE
Constipation – Phase II
Spinal Cord Injuries – Phase II

Parkinson's Disease – Phase II
Pain, Acute or Chronic – Phase II

recombinant human bone morphogenic protein-2 (rhBMP-2)
unknown

MANUFACTURER
Genetics Institute

DESCRIPTION
Recombinant human bone morphogenic protein-2 (rhBMP-2) has shown positive results in accelerating bone and cartilage repair in a variety of situations, including severe orthopedic trauma, oral and maxillofacial surgery, and spinal fusion. This genetically engineered drug works as a growth factor that stimulates new bone development. Genetics Institute, which is a subsidiary of American Home Products, is researching rhBMP-2 in a development partnership with Yamanouchi.

INDICATION(S) AND RESEARCH PHASE
Orthopedics – Phase III
Oral Medicine – Phase III
Musculoskeletal Diseases – Phase III
Spinal Cord Injuries – Phase III

Strokes

ancrod
Viprinex

MANUFACTURER
Knoll Pharmaceutical

DESCRIPTION
Viprinex is a venom derived from a snake (viper *Agkistrodon rhodostoma*). It is a defibrinogenator being tested for treatment of ischemic (cerebral) stroke. Viprinex is also being evaluated for establishing and maintaining anticoagulation in heparin-intolerant subjects undergoing cardiopulmonary bypass surgery.

INDICATION(S) AND RESEARCH PHASE
Cardiac Surgery – Phase III
Strokes – Phase III

Thrombosis – Phase III

BB-10153
unknown

MANUFACTURER
British Biotech plc

DESCRIPTION
British Biotech plc stated that BB-10153 is a genetically engineered protein, which has shown thrombolytic and anti-thrombotic properties in preclinical models. It may have potential use in the treatment of cardiovascular diseases including heart attack and stroke. This drug has completed a phase I trial showing that it is well tolerated in healthy volunteers. Plans are under consideration for both the design of the phase II program as well as partnering with another company for development and marketing.

INDICATION(S) AND RESEARCH PHASE
Heart Disease – Phase I/II
Strokes – Phase I/II

citicoline sodium
CerAxon

MANUFACTURER
Interneuron Pharmaceuticals

DESCRIPTION
CerAxon is believed to have multiple mechanisms of action, which may limit stroke-induced brain damage by the following three methods: First, limiting the extent of the infarct, or tissue caused by interrupted blood flow, by preventing the accumulation of toxic free fatty acids. Second, promoting recovery of brain function by providing two components, cytidine and choline, required in the formation of nerve cell membranes. Lastly, promoting the synthesis of acetylcholine, a neurotransmitter associated with memory or cognitive function.

CerAxon is currently in a phase III study to treat ischemic stroke. The trial consists of 900 subjects in 170 hospitals throughout the United States and Canada. The subjects are being treated with 2,000 milligrams of the CerAxon tablets daily or with matching placebo tablets for six weeks, with an additional six-week follow-up period. Treatment was initiated within 24 hours following the stroke. The goal of the trial is the change in neurological function of subjects between the time of enrollment and the end of the 12-week follow-up period, as measured by the National Institutes of Health (NIH) stroke scale scores.

Preliminary results indicated that CerAxon failed to meet its primary endpoint, which was improvement of neurological function among subjects with moderate to severe ischemic stroke. The company is currently analyzing the data and given the unfavorable results will need to seriously evaluate further development of this drug.

INDICATION(S) AND RESEARCH PHASE
Strokes – Phase III

clomethiazole
Zendra

MANUFACTURER
AstraZeneca

DESCRIPTION
Zendra was developed as a neuroprotective agent. It was being tested in a phase III clinical trial for the treatment of ischemic stroke. As of December 2000, development of this drug had been discontinued.

INDICATION(S) AND RESEARCH PHASE
Strokes – Phase III discontinued

corleukin NIF
unknown

MANUFACTURER
Pfizer

DESCRIPTION
Corleukin NIF is an intravenous biosynthetic neutrophil inhibitory factor (NIF) being developed as an anti-inflammatory agent for treatment of ischemic stroke and hemorrhagic shock. Corleukin NIF prevents neutrophils from adhering to endothelial cells lining the blood vessels. Clinical trials are in phase II.

Future indications may include the treatment of adult respiratory distress syndrome. Pfizer has licensed corleukin NIF from Corvas International and is responsible for the development of the compound.

INDICATION(S) AND RESEARCH PHASE
Hemorrhage – Phase II
Strokes – Phase II

GP IIb/IIa
Cromafiban

MANUFACTURER
COR Therapeutics

DESCRIPTION
Cromafiban is a small molecule that blocks platelets from clumping (an aggregation inhibitor) together. This drug is being tested in phase II trials for treatment of acute coronary disease, unstable angina, and stroke.

INDICATION(S) AND RESEARCH PHASE
Angina – Phase II
Coronary Artery Disease – Phase II
Strokes – Phase II

H376/95
unknown

MANUFACTURER
AstraZeneca

DESCRIPTION
H376/95 belongs to a new class of oral anticoagulants. The drug prevents clot formation in a different manner than low-molecular-weight heparin and the anticoagulant warfarin. It exerts its effect in the final stage of clot formation by inhibiting the activity of a clot-forming substance called thrombin.

Positive phase II results for the prevention of leg vein blood clots in subjects undergoing elective total knee replacement surgery were announced in December 2000. In the dose-determining trial, a 24-mg dose of H376/95 resulted in a 15.8% incidence of venous thromboembolism (VTE) (blood clot) compared to a 22.7% incidence with injections of enoxaparin. In the subjects receiving H376/95, the lowest incidence of VTE was seen with the 24-mg dose.

Phase III trials are now being conducted for both the prevention and treatment of VTE and the prevention of stroke in subjects with atrial fibrillation. A phase I/II study is ongoing for post myocardial infarction.

INDICATION(S) AND RESEARCH PHASE
Venous Thromboembolism – Phase III
Strokes – Phase III
Myocardial Infarction – Phase I/II

ion-channel blocker
Aptiganel

MANUFACTURER
Cambridge NeuroScience

DESCRIPTION
Aptiganel, formerly called Cerestat, is an ion-channel blocker that was being studied for the treatment of stroke and traumatic brain injury. Phase III trials were halted in 1997. The company is currently seeking further development opportunities.

INDICATION(S) AND RESEARCH PHASE
Strokes – Phase III halted
Traumatic Brain Injuries – Phase III halted

LBS-neurons
unknown

MANUFACTURER
Layton Bioscience

DESCRIPTION
LBS-neurons are human neuronal cells being tested for the treatment of fixed neurological deficits resulting from stroke. This therapy is made in an injectable formulation.

INDICATION(S) AND RESEARCH PHASE
Strokes – Phase IIb

LDP-01
unknown

MANUFACTURER
LeukoSite

DESCRIPTION
LDP-01 is a genetically engineered, humanized monoclonal antibody directed to attach to the cell surface marker, beta2 integrin, on white blood cells. LDP-01 is being tested in phase II trials for the prevention of post-ischemic reperfusion injury such as that resulting from organ transplantation, stroke, and heart attack. This drug may enhance organ survival and reduce the time required for the transplanted organ to function in kidney transplant subjects.

INDICATION(S) AND RESEARCH PHASE
Heart Disease – Phase II
Kidney Transplant Surgery – Phase II
Strokes – Phase II

---

leteprinim potassium, AIT-082
Neotrofin

MANUFACTURER
NeoTherapeutics

DESCRIPTION
Neotrofin is composed of the purine compound hypoxanthine, which is linked with the antiarrhythmic drug procainamide. Results of a double-blind, dose-escalating phase II trial of Neotrofin indicated that the compound facilitated brain activity in Alzheimer's disease subjects, leading to improvements in memory, attention and judgement. The improvements were dose-related, with 500 mg and 1,000 mg doses producing more benefit than the 150 mg dose. The trial supported NeoTherapeutics' decision to initiate a one-year trial in early 2001 at doses of 500 mg and 1,000 mg in subjects with moderate Alzheimer's disease.

Neotrofin is also in development for indications other than Alzheimer's disease, including peripheral neuropathy (preclinical) and other neurodegenerative diseases (research). In March 2001, NeoTherapeutics announced that it has begun a 12-week, double-blind, placebo-controlled phase II trial of Neotrofin in Parkinson's disease. Also in March, the company announced the initiation of a phase II trial in subacute spinal cord injured patients.

INDICATION(S) AND RESEARCH PHASE
Alzheimer's Disease – Phase III
Parkinson's Disease – Phase II
Spinal Cord Injuries – Phase II
Neuropathy – Preclinical
Neurodegenerative Disease – Research

---

licostinel, ACEA-1021
unknown

MANUFACTURER
CoCensys

DESCRIPTION
Licostinel is a blocker of glycine receptors (glystasins) that is being tested in a phase II trial for the treatment of cerebral ischemic events, including stroke and head trauma. Licostinel is available in an intravenous formulation. Future indications may include tinnitus and possibly treatment of eye disorders and substance abuse.

INDICATION(S) AND RESEARCH PHASE
Strokes – Phase II

---

nitrone radical trap (NRT)
unknown

MANUFACTURER
Centaur Pharmaceuticals

DESCRIPTION
Nitrone radical trap (NRT) is an oxidative stress reducing neuroprotective compound for the treatment of Parkinson's disease and for stroke. NRT is also being tested in a phase IIa trial for AIDS dementia complex. NRTs are designed to combine with free radicals to create a less reactive molecule.

INDICATION(S) AND RESEARCH PHASE
Acquired Immune Deficiency Syndrome (AIDS) and AIDS-Related Infections – Phase IIa
Parkinson's Disease – Phase IIa
Strokes – Phase II/III

NPS 1506
unknown

MANUFACTURER
NPS Allelix Corp

DESCRIPTION
NPS 1506 is a novel neuroprotectant designed as a treatment for stroke. The drug works by blocking calcium channels controlled by *N*-methyl-D-aspartate (NMDA) receptors, which are located on neurons. During a stroke or other brain injury, oxygen deprivation triggers an accumulation of glutamate, an excitatory chemical neurotransmitter that opens NMDA receptors. This results in an influx of calcium, which can lead to disruption of normal cellular processes. NPS 1506 prevents this excessive calcium influx, and therefore may stabilize cell chemistry and minimize cell death. Phase I trials of NPS 1506 have been completed; however, trials of the drug have been put on financial hold until a corporate partner is obtained to assist with further development.

INDICATION(S) AND RESEARCH PHASE
Strokes – Phase I completed
Depression – Phase Ib

NS-1209, SPD-502
unknown

MANUFACTURER
NeuroSearch A/S

DESCRIPTION
NS-1209 is a glutamate antagonist that may prove effective as a neuroprotective agent. It is thought that high concentrations of glutamate in the brain might play a role in neuronal death following a stroke or heart attack. After a stroke, dying neurons release high concentrations of various neurotransmitters including glutamate. These neurotransmitters diffuse out of the primary area of damage into surrounding areas of the brain causing excessive stimulation leading to further brain cell death. NS-1209 is in development for the treatment of neuronal damage following stroke and other acute neurodegenerative conditions.

Shire Pharmaceuticals has in-licensed

this project (designated SPD-502) from NeuroSearch A/S and has marketing rights outside of certain Nordic countries.

INDICATION(S) AND RESEARCH PHASE
Strokes – Phase I

NXY-059
unknown

MANUFACTURER
AstraZeneca

DESCRIPTION
NXY-059 is a neuroprotective agent that completed a phase IIa trial for Alzheimer's disease, is in a phase IIb/III trial for the treatment of stroke in the United States and a phase I trial was initiated in Japan for acute stroke in December 2000. Furthermore, an NDA filing with the FDA is expected in late 2002. NXY-059 is being developed in partnership with Centaur Pharmaceuticals.

INDICATION(S) AND RESEARCH PHASE
Alzheimer's Disease – Phase II
Strokes – Phase IIb/III
Strokes – Phase I in Japan

porcine neural cells, stroke
unknown

MANUFACTURER
Diacrin

DESCRIPTION
Transplanted porcine neural cells have been found to improve the condition of a subject who has suffered a stroke by repairing neural connections and damaged tissue.

Transplanted porcine fetal neural cells form solid grafts that integrate with normal brain tissue. Extensive neural outgrowth from the graft to the surrounding brain has been observed in clinical studies. Transplanted cells have the capacity to form new synaptic connections and release chemicals that promote neural cell growth.

Currently this therapy is in a six-subject phase I study in Boston at the Beth Israel Deaconess Medical Center and Brigham and Women's Hospital. However, the study has been temporarily discontinued due to adverse events.

INDICATION(S) AND RESEARCH PHASE
Strokes – Phase I halted

prourokinase
Abbokinase

MANUFACTURER
Abbott Laboratories

DESCRIPTION
Prourokinase is a tissue plasminogen activator (TPA), which is a type of clot buster. It is being tested in phase III trials for the treatment of stroke and peripheral arterial occlusion. For strokes prourokinase is given by intra-arterial administration to the brain.

INDICATION(S) AND RESEARCH PHASE
Peripheral Arterial Occlusive Disease – Phase III
Strokes – Phase III

SB 249417
unknown

MANUFACTURER
GlaxoSmithKline

DESCRIPTION
SB 249417 is an anti-factor IX monoclonal antibody being developed for the treatment of severe sepsis, septic shock, and stroke. It is currently in phase I development.

INDICATION(S) AND RESEARCH PHASE
Sepsis and Septicemia – Phase I
Strokes – Phase I

TP-9201
unknown

MANUFACTURER
Integra LifeSciences

DESCRIPTION
TP-9201 inhibits a platelet membrane receptor (glycoprotein IIb/IIIa) and a cyclic peptide (RGD) for treatment of several cardiovascular diseases. Blood clots can be prevented from growing and propagating by stopping platelets from aggregating together. Potential treatments being tested for this therapy may include myocardial infarction, angioplasty, unstable angina, and stroke.

Integra Life Sciences has acquired Telios Pharmaceuticals and they have suspended clinical research between phases I and II until a development partner is found.

INDICATION(S) AND RESEARCH PHASE
Angina – Phase I/II
Heart Disease – Phase I/II
Strokes – Phase I/II

unknown
Argatroban

MANUFACTURER
Texas Biotechnology

DESCRIPTION
A phase II multi-center, placebo-controlled trial (ARGIS-1) is evaluating the use of Argatroban in patients with acute ischemic stroke. Aragtroban is a direct thrombin inhibitor which may influence the primary clot causing a stroke, as well as the collateral and microcirculation of the brain in and around the original infarction. Through this mechanism, it is possible that additional clots may be prevented from forming. It is approved in Japan for this indication and is FDA approved as an anticoagulant for the prophylaxis or treatment of thrombosis in patients with heparin-induced thrombocytopenia.

INDICATION(S) AND RESEARCH PHASE
Strokes – Phase II
Thrombosis – FDA approved

YM-872
unknown

MANUFACTURER
Yamanouchi Pharmaceutical

DESCRIPTION

DESCRIPTION
YM-872 is an injectable AMPA antagonist in trials for the treatment of acute ischemic stroke. Clinical trials have reached phase II testing. The drug is being developed in the United States and Europe.

INDICATION(S) AND RESEARCH PHASE
Strokes – Phase II

Tourette's Syndrome

mecamylamine HCl
Inversine

MANUFACTURER
Layton Bioscience

DESCRIPTION
Inversine is being evaluated in a phase III trials for the treatment of Tourette's syndrome and attention deficit/hyperactivity disorder (ADHD) in pediatric subjects.

INDICATION(S) AND RESEARCH PHASE
Pediatric, Tourette's Syndrome – Phase III
Pediatric, Attention Deficit/Hyperactivity Disorder (ADHD) – Phase III

Traumatic Brain Injuries

dexanabinol, HU-211
unknown

MANUFACTURER
Pharmos Corporation

DESCRIPTION
Dexanabinol is a novel synthetic compound developed to protect against damage associated with severe traumatic brain injury (TBI) and stroke. Dexanabinol may inhibit the synthesis, release, and activity of certain neuro-toxic chemicals when administered within hours after the traumatic event. This inhibition, in turn, would block a cascade of events leading to cell death, and help prevent a damaging increase in intracranial pressure (ICP). An analysis of results from a phase II trial focusing on TBI demonstrated that the drug significantly improved orientation and memory among conscious subjects and prevented the elevation of ICP.

A phase III trial was initiated in January 2001 at 40 centers in Europe and 30 centers in the United States will be initiated later in 2001, testing dexanabinal in 860 subjects suffering from severe traumatic brain injury.

INDICATION(S) AND RESEARCH PHASE
Traumatic Brain Injuries – Phase III

ion-channel blocker
Aptiganel

MANUFACTURER
Cambridge NeuroScience

DESCRIPTION
Aptiganel, formerly called Cerestat, is an ion-channel blocker that was being studied for the treatment of stroke and traumatic brain injury. Phase III trials were halted in 1997. The company is currently seeking further development opportunities.

INDICATION(S) AND RESEARCH PHASE
Strokes – Phase III halted
Traumatic Brain Injuries – Phase III halted

Vestibular Hypofunction

scopolamine
unknown

MANUFACTURER
Elan Transdermal Technologies

DESCRIPTION
Scopolamine acts as a central nervous system depressant. It is an alkaloid derived from plants of the Solanaceae family (deadly nightshade), particularly *Datura metel* and *Scopolia carniolica*. The drug is in phase II trials for the prevention of motion sickness and for treatment of gastrointestinal disorders, central and peripheral nervous system disorders, and vertigo. It is administered in a transdermal patch formulation.

INDICATION(S) AND RESEARCH PHASE
Gastrointestinal Diseases and Disorders, Miscellaneous – Phase II
Vestibular Hypofunction – Phase II

4 | Psychiatry

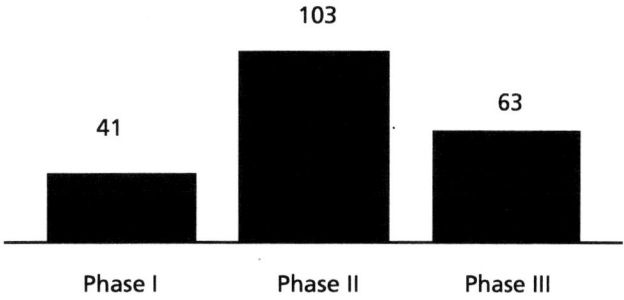

Drugs in the development pipeline

Phase I: 41
Phase II: 103
Phase III: 63

Source: CenterWatch, 2001

The National Institute for Mental Health estimates that the annual cost to the United States for treatment, social service and disability payments, lost productivity, and premature mortality due to mental illness is more than $150 billion. Approximately 10% of total national health care expenditures are spent on treating mental illness. In the United States today, over 50 million people suffer from some form of mental illness. It is the second leading cause of disability and premature mortality. Mental disorders collectively account for more than 15% of the overall burden of all diseases, which is slightly more than that associated with all forms of cancer. About one in five Americans experiences a mental disorder in the course of a year.

CenterWatch has identified close to 200 drugs involved in clinical development for the treatment of various psychiatric disorders. The psychiatric/neurological diseases currently dominating the pipeline include depression, anxiety disorders, Alzheimer's disease, and schizophrenia. Despite being extensively researched, the cause of most diseases of the brain and nervous system remain a mystery to scientists.

According to the Pharmaceutical Research Manufacturers of America (PhRMA) depression occurs in almost 19 million Americans and costs the economy an estimated $44 billion a year, including $12 billion in lost work days. As high as this cost is, the cost in human suffering is greater. Depressive illnesses interfere with normal functioning and cause pain and suffering to those with the disorder and those around them. Depression affects nearly twice as many women as men. It is estimated that more than six percent of nine to 17 year olds are depressed. Unfortunately, nearly two-thirds of those suffering from depression do not seek treatment.

A depressive disorder is an illness involving the body, mood, and thoughts. Symptoms often include persistent sadness, feelings of hopelessness and guilt, loss of interest, fatigue, insomnia, and irritability. In some cases, classified as bipolar disorder, manic symptoms also occur. Though the cause of depression is unknown, it is suggested that a combination of genetic, psychological, and environmental factors are responsible. A variety of antidepressant medications and psychotherapies are used to treat depressive disorders. A growing amount of evidence supports the view that people with depression have an imbalance of the brain's neurotransmitters, the chemicals that allow nerve cells in the brain to communicate with each other. Many scientists believe that an imbalance in serotonin, one of these neurotransmitters, may be an important factor in the development and severity of depression.

The most often prescribed medications are classified as selective serotonin reuptake inhibitors (SSRIs) and monamine oxidase inhibitors (MAOIs). Both work to increase serotonin levels in the brain. Brain imaging research is revealing that in depression, neural circuits responsible for moods, thinking, sleep, appetite, and behavior fail to function properly, and that the regulation of critical neurotransmitters is impaired. CenterWatch has identified over 50 drugs in the pipeline for treatment of depression. The research and development of these treatments will cost the industry an estimated $215 million to $260 million this year.

There is a new medicine in the pipeline, being developed by Merck, that may produce fewer side effects than currently used treatments. This drug blocks the action of the neuropeptide substance P, which is thought to be involved in regulating emotion.

PhRMA estimates that the United States economy spends nearly $50 million each year on costs due to the more than 19 million Americans suffering from anxiety disorders, the country's most common mental illness. Anxiety disorders include such diagnoses as generalized anxiety disorder, panic disorder, obsessive-compulsive disorder, post-traumatic stress disorder, social phobia, and other numerous other phobias. They are chronic and relentless, and fill people's lives with overwhelming anxiety and fear.

Like depression, anxiety disorders are complex and probably result from a combination of genetic, behavioral, developmental, and other factors. It is thought that anxiety disorders may result from an imbalance of the chemical serotonin, which transports signals between nerve cells in the brain. Other neurotransmitters that may be perturbed in anxiety include norepinephrine, gamma-aminobutyric acid, corticotropin-releasing hormone, and cholecystokinin. Using brain imaging technologies and neurochemical techniques, scientists are finding that a network of interacting structures are responsible for the emotions of fear and anxiety. Exciting new research focuses on the amygdala, which is believed to serve as a communications hub between the parts of the brain that process incoming sensory signals and those that interpret them. It will signal that a threat is present and trigger a response of fear or anxiety.

Although medications cannot cure an anxiety disorder, they may be able to control symptoms and allow one to lead a normal life. Many SSRIs and MAOIs originally indicated for treatment of depression have also been found to be effective in treating anxiety disorders. Other commonly prescribed anti-anxiety medications come from the class of high-potency benzodiazepines, which relieve symptoms quickly with few side effects, but can only be taken for short periods of time due to the development of tolerance and their addictive potential. Buspirone, from the azipirone class, is a newer anti-anxiety medication, used to treat generalized anxiety disorder. Biovail Corporation International plans a NDA filing in 2001 for a once-daily formulation of buspirone, currently in a phase III trial. In addition to this drug, CenterWatch has identified 25 treatments presently in clinical development to treat anxiety disorders, which will cost the industry an estimated $90 million to $110 million in 2001.

According to PhRMA, schizophrenia costs the United States economy over $32 million annually. There are approximately 2.5 million adults in the United States living with schizophrenia, a devastating brain disorder that is the most chronic and disabling of the severe mental illnesses. Psychosis, marked by hallucinations and delusions, is a common symptom of schizophrenia. People with schizophrenia often experience visual and/or auditory hallucinations and paranoid ideation. These symptoms may leave them fearful and withdrawn. Their speech and behavior can be so disorganized that they may be incomprehensible or frightening to others. Available treatments can relieve many symptoms, but most people with schizophrenia continue to suffer some symptoms throughout their lives and it is estimated that no more than one in five recovers completely. Some people cannot be helped by available treatments because of the unpleasant side effects of many drugs.

Antipsychotic drugs, which block dopamine receptors, provide the best treatment currently available to treat schizophrenia, but they cannot cure the disease or ensure that there will be no further psychotic episodes. A reduction in psychotic symptoms and improvement in daily functioning is seen in the majority of people treated with such drugs. Today, the atypical antidepressants are primarily perscribed. They have a different mechanism of action than the original antidepressants and display fewer side effects. In February 2001 the FDA approved Pfizer's Geodon (ziprasidone) in both oral and injectable formulations for the control of agitated behavior associated with schizophrenia. The injectable formulation may be especially helpful in treating this violent, uncooperative behavior due to its rapid onset of action.

CenterWatch reports that there are currently 24 drugs in the pipeline being evaluated for the treatment of schizophrenia. The annual cost for this clinical development is estimated at $100 million to $130 million. One treatment showing positive phase III results is aripiprazole. Bristol-Meyers Squibb reports that its partnering company, Otsuka, has discovered a potentially best-in-class agent for treatment of schizophrenia. In trials, aripiprazole was favorable compared to haloperidol, an atypical antipsychotic currently used for schizophrenia treatment.

Addictions

amino-cyclopropane carboxylic acid
unknown

MANUFACTURER
Annovis

DESCRIPTION
Amino-cyclopropane carboxylic acid is an ion channel regulator/neuroprotectant being evaluated for use in the treatment of depression, addiction, and anxiety.

INDICATION(S) AND RESEARCH PHASE
Depression – Phase I
Anxiety Disorders – Phase I
Addictions – Phase I

DOV 216303
unknown

MANUFACTURER
DOV Pharmaceutical

DESCRIPTION
DOV 216303 is an unspecified antidepressant for alcohol addiction in phase I trials.

INDICATION(S) AND RESEARCH PHASE
Addictions – Phase I
Alcohol Dependence – Phase I

NS-2359
unknown

MANUFACTURER
NeuroSearch A/S

DESCRIPTION
NS-2359 is a monoamine (MAO) reuptake inhibitor in development for the treatment of cocaine addiction. The drug prevents dopamine from being reabsorbed in the brain, thereby allowing a longer period of neural stimulation. Because prolonged cocaine use leads to decreased dopamine activity (and increased withdrawal symptoms), this mechanism of action may prove to be an effective therapy. As of November 2000, NS-2359 has completed phase I development.

INDICATION(S) AND RESEARCH PHASE
Addictions – Phase I completed

Affective Disorders

CE-1050
unknown

MANUFACTURER
Core Group plc

DESCRIPTION
CE-1050 is in a phase II trial for the treatment of behavioral disorders.

INDICATION(S) AND RESEARCH PHASE
Affective Disorders – Phase II

Alcohol Dependence

acamprosate
unknown

MANUFACTURER
Lipha Pharmaceuticals

DESCRIPTION
Acamprosate is being tested in phase III trials as an anti-alcohol dependence drug. It may be useful in integrated relapse-prevention treatment and to help with behavioral modification programs.

INDICATION(S) AND RESEARCH PHASE
Alcohol Dependence – Phase III

DOV 216303
unknown

MANUFACTURER
DOV Pharmaceutical

DESCRIPTION
DOV 216303 is an unspecified antidepressant for alcohol addiction in phase I trials.

INDICATION(S) AND RESEARCH PHASE
Addictions – Phase I
Alcohol Dependence – Phase I

IP501
unknown

MANUFACTURER
Interneuron Pharmaceuticals

DESCRIPTION
IP501 is a purified phospholipid, which helps to repair damaged cells. It is indicated for the treatment and prevention of alcohol-induced cirrhosis of the liver and hepatitis-C. IP501 is currently in phase III trials. The drug is in tablet form.

INDICATION(S) AND RESEARCH PHASE
Alcohol Dependence – Phase III
Hepatitis – Phase III
Liver Disease – Phase III

Anorexia

SR-27897B
unknown

MANUFACTURER
Sanofi-Synthelabo Pharmaceuticals

DESCRIPTION
CCK_A (cholecystokinin-A) is a molecule that is secreted from the lining of the small intestine, and is also present in the central nervous system. It is a substance that causes many different actions throughout the body, including gallbladder contraction, release of pancreatic digestive enzymes, and promotion of the feeling of digestive fullness, or satiety. CCK promotes cell growth and division, especially in the pancreas. It also has a regulating effect on the amount of the neurotransmitters dopamine and serotonin present in the body.
SR-27897 is a potent substance that blocks the receptors to which CCK would ordinarily bind, thus blocking CCK's effects on the body. By negating the action of CCK, people may lose their sense of satiety, potentially making SR-27897 a good therapy for

anorexia. In addition, CCK's probable role in the pathogenesis of pancreatic cancer (since it can cause abnormal pancreatic cell division) may also be reduced with the use of SR-27897. Potential applications for this drug may also include treatment for autism, although no clinical trials for this indication are under way as of yet.

INDICATION(S) AND RESEARCH PHASE
Pancreatic Cancer – Phase II
Anorexia – Phase II

Anxiety Disorders

amino-cyclopropane carboxylic acid
unknown

MANUFACTURER
Annovis

DESCRIPTION
Amino-cyclopropane carboxylic acid is an ion channel regulator/neuroprotectant being evaluated for use in the treatment of depression, addiction, and anxiety.

INDICATION(S) AND RESEARCH PHASE
Depression – Phase I
Anxiety Disorders – Phase I
Addictions – Phase I

buspirone
unknown

MANUFACTURER
Biovail Corporation International

DESCRIPTION
This new formulation, which allows for once daily administration of Buspirone, is in a phase III trial for the treatment of generalized anxiety disorders. An NDA filing is planned for early 2001.

INDICATION(S) AND RESEARCH PHASE
Anxiety Disorders – Phase III

buspirone HCl

BuSpar

MANUFACTURER
Bristol-Myers Squibb

DESCRIPTION
BuSpar is a serotonin/dopamine antagonist in a phase III trial for the treatment of generalized anxiety disorders (GAD) in a once daily transdermal patch delivery formulation. An NDA was filed, but development was discontinued in September 2000 as a result of insufficient efficacy of the transdermal formulation.

INDICATION(S) AND RESEARCH PHASE
Anxiety Disorders – Trial discontinued

CRF receptor antagonist (partnered), NBI-37582
unknown

MANUFACTURER
Neurocrine Biosciences

DESCRIPTION
Neurocrine Biosciences is developing both a proprietary corticotropin releasing factor-1 (CRF) receptor antagonist and a compound in partnership with Janssen Pharmaceutica. CRF functions as a neurotransmitter in the brain and plays a critical role in coordinating the body's response to stress. The CRF_1 receptor subtype largely mediates these effects. In preclinical models, selective CRF_1 receptor antagonists block stress-related responses providing evidence that this novel mechanism may result in improved anti-anxiety and antidepressant properties. In addition, some data suggest that CRF_1 antagonists may have a more rapid onset of action and a reduced side effect profile compared to currently marketed antidepressants.

INDICATION(S) AND RESEARCH PHASE
Depression – Phase I
Anxiety Disorders – Phase I

CRF receptor antagonist (proprietary)
unknown

MANUFACTURER
Neurocrine Biosciences

DESCRIPTION
Neurocrine Biosciences is developing both a proprietary corticotropin releasing factor-1 (CRF) receptor antagonist and a compound in partnership with Janssen Pharmaceutica. CRF functions as a neurotransmitter in the brain and plays a critical role in coordinating the body's response to stress. The CRF_1 receptor subtype largely mediates these effects. In preclinical models, selective CRF_1 receptor antagonists block stress-related responses providing evidence that this novel mechanism may result in improved anti-anxiety and antidepressant properties. In addition, some data suggests that CRF_1 antagonists may have a more rapid onset of action and a reduced side effect profile compared to currently marketed antidepressants.

In December 2000, Neurocrine Biosciences announced the initiation of a phase I trial with its proprietary CRF_1 receptor antagonist compound for the treatment of anxiety and depression. The trial is being conducted in 48 normal, healthy subjects and is designed to evaluate safety, tolerability, pharmacokinetics, and pharmacodynamics over a range of escalating doses.

INDICATION(S) AND RESEARCH PHASE
Anxiety Disorders – Phase I
Depression – Phase I

DU125530
unknown

MANUFACTURER
Solvay Pharmaceuticals

DESCRIPTION
DU125530 is a 5-hydroxy-tryptamine 1A ($5\text{-}HT_{1A}$) antagonist being developed for the treatment of anxiety and major depression. $5\text{-}HT_{1A}$ antagonists increase serotonin levels in the brain, and may provide beneficial effects as antidepressants. DU125530 is currently in phase II trials.

INDICATION(S) AND RESEARCH PHASE
Depression – Phase II

Anxiety Disorders – Phase II

flesinoxan
unknown

MANUFACTURER
Solvay Pharmaceuticals

DESCRIPTION
Flesinoxan is a serotonin agonist used for the treatment of generalized anxiety disorder and major depressive disorder. The phase III trial was discontinued in 2000.

INDICATION(S) AND RESEARCH PHASE
Anxiety Disorders – Phase III discontinued
Depression – Phase III discontinued

fluvoxamine maleate
Fluvoxamine-CR

MANUFACTURER
Solvay Pharmaceuticals

DESCRIPTION
Fluvoxamine-CR is a controlled-release version of Luvox—a selective serotonin reuptake inhibitor approved in the United States for the treatment of obsessive compulsive disorder (OCD). The drug is being developed under an agreement with Elan Pharmaceuticals. An NDA has been submitted for the treatment of OCD and social anxiety.

INDICATION(S) AND RESEARCH PHASE
Obsessive-Compulsive Disorders – NDA submitted
Anxiety Disorders – NDA submitted

GW 150013
unknown

MANUFACTURER
GlaxoSmithKline

DESCRIPTION
GW 150013 is a cholecystokinin-B (CCK$_B$) receptor antagonist. It is currently in phase II trials for the treatment of anxiety disorders.

INDICATION(S) AND RESEARCH PHASE
Anxiety Disorders – Phase II

LY-354740
unknown

MANUFACTURER
Eli Lilly

DESCRIPTION
LY-354740 is a glutamate receptor agonist used as a smoking cessation aid and in the treatment of anxiety. This drug is currently in a phase II trial.

INDICATION(S) AND RESEARCH PHASE
Smoking Cessation – Phase II
Anxiety Disorders – Phase II

MK-869
unknown

MANUFACTURER
Merck & Co.

DESCRIPTION
MK-869 is a substance P receptor antagonist for the treatment of chemotherapy induced emesis. Substance P acts on neurokinin-1 (NK$_1$) receptors in areas of the brain stem associated with vomiting.

Results from the phase II trial showed that MK-869 prevented nausea and vomiting induced by cisplatin. The phase II trial included 150 subjects who received granisetron and dexamethasone followed by therapy with cisplatin. Acute emesis (within 24 hours) and delayed emesis (days 2-5) were evaluated. In the acute-emesis evaluation 93% of the subjects in the first two groups had no vomiting compared to 67% given placebo. Then, in the delayed-emesis evaluation 82% of the subjects in group one, 78% in group two, and 33% in group three had no vomiting. There were no serious adverse events reported.

INDICATION(S) AND RESEARCH PHASE
Anxiety Disorders – Phase III
Bipolar Disorders – Phase III
Depression – Phase III
Effects of Chemotherapy – Phase III

NAD299
unknown

MANUFACTURER
AstraZeneca

DESCRIPTION
NAD299 is a 5-HT$_{1A}$ antagonist indicated for the treatment of anxiety and depression. It is currently in phase II trials.

INDICATION(S) AND RESEARCH PHASE
Anxiety Disorders – Phase II
Depression – Phase II

NGD 91-1
unknown

MANUFACTURER
Neurogen Corporation

DESCRIPTION
NGD 91-1 is a gamma-amino butyric acid (GABA) receptor partial agonist used in the treatment of anxiety without sedation. After a phase Ib trial was completed, the compound did not advance to phase II because of concerns regarding absorption following oral administration.

INDICATION(S) AND RESEARCH PHASE
Anxiety Disorders – Phase Ib discontinued

NGD 91-2
unknown

MANUFACTURER
Pfizer

DESCRIPTION
NGD 91-2 is gamma-amino butyric acid (GABA) receptor subtype modulator (GABA partial agonist) used to treat generalized anxiety disorder. NGD 91-2 completed a phase I trial, but the follow-on compound NGD 91-3 has advanced to phase II as the lead candidate in this program.

INDICATION(S) AND RESEARCH PHASE
Anxiety Disorders – Phase I completed

NGD 91-3
unknown

MANUFACTURER
Neurogen Corporation

DESCRIPTION
NGD 91-3 belongs to a group of drugs that modulate specific GABA receptor subtypes. GABA (gamma-amino butyric acid) is a principal inhibitory neurotransmitter in the central nervous system, affecting neuronal membranes via GABA receptors throughout the brain. The purpose of the drugs is to treat anxiety and depression without side effects such as sedation, memory impairment, or delayed onset of action. NGD 91-3 is being tested in a phase II trial.

INDICATION(S) AND RESEARCH PHASE
Anxiety Disorders – Phase II

NGD 98-1
unknown

MANUFACTURER
Pfizer

DESCRIPTION
NGD 98-1 is an orally administered corticotropin releasing antagonist. It is being studied for the treatment of stress-related disorders, including depression and anxiety. It is currently in a phase II trial.

INDICATION(S) AND RESEARCH PHASE
Depression – Phase II
Anxiety Disorders – Phase II

NKP 608
unknown

MANUFACTURER
Novartis

DESCRIPTION
NKP 608 is an oral neurokinin-1 (NK$_1$) substance P antagonist being tested for the treatment of anxiety disorders. Early phase II trials have shown promising results.

INDICATION(S) AND RESEARCH PHASE
Anxiety Disorders – Phase II

NS-2710
unknown

MANUFACTURER
NeuroSearch A/S

DESCRIPTION
NS-2710 is a gamma-amino butyric acid (GABA) receptor modulator that is being developed for the treatment of anxiety disorders. GABA is a major inhibitory neurotransmitter in the brain that interacts with many specific receptors, one of which is the GABA receptor. It is believed that modulation of this GABA receptor complex can play a role in the reduction of anxiety. NS-2710 is in phase II development.

INDICATION(S) AND RESEARCH PHASE
Anxiety Disorders – Phase II

pagoclone
unknown

MANUFACTURER
Pfizer

DESCRIPTION
Pagoclone is partial agonist of gamma-amino butyric acid (GABA) receptors. GABA is an inhibitory neurotransmitter that may help suppress anxious activity. A phase II trial was initiated in January 2001 evaluating pagoclone for the treatment of generalized anxiety disorder. In addition, a phase III for panic disorders was initiated in August 2000. Interneuron licensed worldwide rights to develop and commercialize pagoclone to Warner-Lambert Company, which is now part of Pfizer.

INDICATION(S) AND RESEARCH PHASE
Anxiety Disorders – Phase II
Panic Disorders – Phase III

paroxetine
Paxil, Seroxat

MANUFACTURER
GlaxoSmithKline

DESCRIPTION
Paxil (paroxetine) is an orally administered selective serotonin reuptake inhibitor (SSRI) currently approved to treat a variety of mood and anxiety disorders. FDA approval has been received for the treatment of depression, obsessive compulsive disorder (OCD), panic disorder, and social anxiety disorder or social phobia. This drug is sold under the brand name Paxil in the United States and Seroxat in Europe.

Paxil is currently in phase III trials for the treatment of depression in a dispersible tablet formulation. NDAs have also been submitted for the treatment of generalized anxiety disorders and post-traumatic stress disorder.

INDICATION(S) AND RESEARCH PHASE
Post-traumatic Stress Disorders – NDA submitted
Anxiety Disorders – NDA submitted
Depression – Phase III

PH94B
unknown

MANUFACTURER
Pherin Pharmaceuticals

DESCRIPTION
PH94B is a vomeropherin being developed for the treatment of acute anxiety disorders. Vomeropherins act by triggering local chemosensory receptors in the human vomeronasal organ, which elicits a nerve impulse to the hypothalamus region of the brain. The drug is being developed under a partnership between Pherin Pharmaceuticals and Janssen Pharmaceutica.

INDICATION(S) AND RESEARCH PHASE
Anxiety Disorders – Phase I

SR-142801, osanetant
unknown

MANUFACTURER
Sanofi-Synthelabo Pharmaceuticals

DESCRIPTION

Sanofi Laboratories is developing a new medication, SR-142801, that could become a new treatment for schizophrenia and major depression. It is currently in phase IIa clinical trials for the treatment of anxiety, psychosis, and schizophrenia and a phase II trial for major depressive disorder. It will be formulated as an oral medication. It is thought that both schizophrenia and depression are related to low serotonin levels in the brain. The molecule from which serotonin is made, 5-HT, is manufactured by certain cells (enterochromaffin cells) located in the gut. When these cells are stimulated, they release 5-HT into the circulation, spurring greater production of serotonin.

There are certain cell receptors (NK_3 receptors) found in the body that when activated, can prevent the release of 5-HT by the enterochromaffin cells, resulting in lower serotonin production. If the action of NK_3 receptors is blocked, then the levels of 5-HT and serotonin might increase. SR-142801, in preliminary studies, was shown to block the serotonin-lowering action of NK_3 receptors and thus may lead to increased 5-HT and serotonin levels in the body. Further study is necessary to determine the precise efficacy of this new compound.

INDICATION(S) AND RESEARCH PHASE

Schizophrenia and Schizoaffective Disorders – Phase IIa
Depression – Phase II
Anxiety Disorders – Phase IIa
Psychosis – Phase IIa

substance P antagonist candidates
unknown

MANUFACTURER
Merck & Co.

DESCRIPTION

Substance P antagonist candidates are in a phase IIa trial for the treatment of neuropsychiatric diseases, including depression and anxiety disorders.

INDICATION(S) AND RESEARCH PHASE
Depression – Phase IIa
Anxiety Disorders – Phase IIa

sunepitron, CP-93,393
unknown

MANUFACTURER
Pfizer

DESCRIPTION

Sunepitron is a 5-hydroxytryptamine-1A (5-HT$_{1A}$) agonist for the treatment of anxiety. This drug is currently in a phase III trial.

INDICATION(S) AND RESEARCH PHASE
Anxiety Disorders – Phase III

unknown
Siramesine

MANUFACTURER
Forest Laboratories

DESCRIPTION

Siramesine is a selective sigma-2 ligand in developing for treatment of anxiety disorders. Use of sigma ligands for this type of treatment is a completely new principle. Siramesine is a potent compound that has been shown to be effective against both anxiety and depression in a number of models. H. Lundbeck A/S is in partnership with Forest Laboratories.

INDICATION(S) AND RESEARCH PHASE
Anxiety Disorders – Phase II

vomeropherin, PH-80
unknown

MANUFACTURER
Pherin Pharmaceuticals

DESCRIPTION

Vomeropherin, in a nasal spray formulation, is in a phase I trial for the treatment of premenstrual syndrome and of anxiety disorders.

INDICATION(S) AND RESEARCH PHASE
Premenstrual Syndrome – Phase I
Anxiety Disorders – Phase I

Attention Deficit/Hyperactivity Disorder (ADHD)

altropane
unknown

MANUFACTURER
Boston Life Sciences

DESCRIPTION

Altropane is a radioactive molecule that binds specifically to the dopamine transporter (DAT) in the brain. The actual number of DATs in the midbrain can be measured using altropane along with SPECT imaging. A measurement of DATs may be useful because data suggest there is an abnormally high amount in the midbrain of individuals with ADHD. A phase II/III trial involving 40 subjects is under way. The company plans to initiate two parallel phase III studies in adults between the ages of 20 and 40 years. Upon completion of these trials, the company will file for marketing approval using altropane to aid in the diagnosis of ADHD in adults. Afterwards, the company plans to initiate a phase III trial testing altropane in the diagnosis of ADHD in children.

Additionally, phase III results showed that altropane is able to differentiate Parkinson's movement disorders (including Parkinson's disease) from other movement disorders. The phase III trial included 95 subjects having the clinical diagnosis of Parkinsonian syndrome (PS) and 70 subjects having non-movement disorders with clinical features similar to PS but whose symptoms are caused by something other than a destruction of dopamine producing cells.

INDICATION(S) AND RESEARCH PHASE
Parkinson's Disease – Phase III completed
Pediatric, Attention Deficit/Hyperactivity Disorder (ADHD) – Phase III

CNS stimulant
unknown

MANUFACTURER
Elan Pharmaceutical Research

DESCRIPTION
This central nervous system (CNS) stimulant is being developed for the treatment of attention deficit/hyperactivity disorder (ADHD). This drug is being tested in a phase II trial using the CODAS delivery technology.

INDICATION(S) AND RESEARCH PHASE
Pediatric, Attention Deficit/Hyperactivity Disorder (ADHD) – Phase II

dl-methylphenidate HCl
unknown

MANUFACTURER
Celgene Corporation

DESCRIPTION
Dl-methylphenidate hydrochloride (dl-MPH) is a chirally pure, single isomer version of Ritalin in an oral formulation. It is being tested in a phase III study for the treatment of attention deficit/hyperactivity disorder (ADHD) in children.

INDICATION(S) AND RESEARCH PHASE
Pediatric, Attention Deficit/Hyperactivity Disorder (ADHD) – Phase III

donepezil hydrochloride, E2020
Aricept

MANUFACTURER
Eisai

DESCRIPTION
Aricept is an acetylcholinesterase inhibitor. The enzyme acetylcholinesterase breaks down acetylcholine. By inhibiting this process, Aricept causes a greater concentration of acetylcholine. Acetylcholine is a neurotransmitter associated with memory, which means that greater concentrations of it could significantly improve the conditions of Alzheimer's disease. In addition, Aricept is in phase II trials in children seven to 16 years old who are suffering from attention deficit/hyperactivity disorder.

Aricept is currently in development in Japan, Europe, and the United States. Aricept is being co-promoted by Pfizer.

INDICATION(S) AND RESEARCH PHASE
Alzheimer's Disease – NDA submitted, (Japan)
Dementia – Phase III
Attention Deficit/Hyperactivity Disorder (ADHD) – Phase II
Pediatric, Attention Deficit/Hyperactivity Disorder – Phase II

GT-2331
Perceptin

MANUFACTURER
Gliatech

DESCRIPTION
Perceptin is a selective histamine H_3 receptor antagonist, which is being developed for potential use in central nervous system diseases involving attention/learning or sleep disorders. Perceptin is being evaluated in a phase II trial for treatment of attention deficit/hyperactivity disorder (ADHD), Alzheimer's disease, and sleep disorders.

Histamine is a chemical messenger released from certain neurons in the brain, which regulates sleep/wake states and modulates levels of arousal and alertness in the conscious state. The histamine H_3 receptor is predominantly found in the brain where it regulates the release of histamine.

Phase I clinical studies have demonstrated that Perceptin is safe, well tolerated, and amenable to once daily dosing.

The phase II trial for ADHD is a multi-dose, double-blind, randomized, placebo-controlled clinical trial to evaluate the safety and preliminary efficacy of Perceptin at varying doses. The company expects to enroll up to 120 adult subjects.

INDICATION(S) AND RESEARCH PHASE
Alzheimer's Disease – Phase I complete
Attention Deficit/Hyperactivity Disorder (ADHD) – Phase II
Sleep Disorders – Phase I complete

GW 320659, 1555U88
unknown

MANUFACTURER
GlaxoSmithKline

DESCRIPTION
GW 320659 is a noradrenaline reuptake inhibitor being tested in phase II trials for the treatment of attention deficit/hyperactivity disorder (ADHD).

INDICATION(S) AND RESEARCH PHASE
Attention Deficit/Hyperactivity Disorder (ADHD) – Phase II

mecamylamine HCl
Inversine

MANUFACTURER
Layton Bioscience

DESCRIPTION
Inversine is being evaluated in phase III trials for the treatment of Tourette's syndrome in young adult subjects and attention deficit/hyperactivity disorder (ADHD) in pediatric subjects.

INDICATION(S) AND RESEARCH PHASE
Pediatric, Tourette's Syndrome – Phase III
Pediatric, Attention Deficit/Hyperactivity Disorder (ADHD) – Phase III

methylphenidate
MethyPatch

MANUFACTURER
Noven Pharmaceuticals

DESCRIPTION
MethyPatch, a transdermal methylphenidate patch, is in phase III development. Methylphenidate is the active ingredient found in Ritalin, Novartis Pharmaceuticals' approved drug for attention deficit/hyperactivity disorder (ADHD). The patch is being developed to address the social concerns of children needing to take an oral pill each

day. The company hopes that a discreet patch will eliminate the stigma children suffer from taking an oral medication during the school day, as well as eliminating drug diversion and abuse issues that affect the pill formulation. The company expects to file an NDA in the first half of 2001.

INDICATION(S) AND RESEARCH PHASE
Pediatric, Attention Deficit/Hyperactivity Disorder (ADHD) – Phase III

methylphenidate
Ritalin LA

MANUFACTURER
Novartis

DESCRIPTION
Ritalin LA, a timed-release product, is an NK_1 substance P antagonist. Ritalin is an established treatment for attention deficit/hyperactivity disorder (ADHD) that works by increasing attention and decreasing restlessness in children and adults who are overactive, cannot concentrate for very long or are easily distracted, and are impulsive. An application has been submitted overseas for Ritalin LA for the treatment of attention deficit disorders.

INDICATION(S) AND RESEARCH PHASE
Attention Deficit/Hyperactivity Disorder (ADHD) – MAA submitted

methylphenidate
MR Racemate

MANUFACTURER
Celltech Chiroscience plc

DESCRIPTION
A modified release (MR) formulation of methylphenidate is currently being developed for the treatment of attention deficit/hyperactivity disorder (ADHD). The problem with approved methylphenidate treatment is the drug's short duration of action. The MR formulation should eliminate the need for mid-day dosing and should increase compliance with drug use instructions by children.

A UK Marketing Authority Application was granted at the end of 1999 for the existing racemic IR formulation. The drug is in phase III trials in the United States.

INDICATION(S) AND RESEARCH PHASE
Attention Deficit/Hyperactivity Disorder (ADHD) – Phase III

methylphenidate HCl
unknown

MANUFACTURER
Medeva plc

DESCRIPTION
Methylphenidate is a stimulant used for the treatment of attention deficit/hyperactivity disorder (ADHD). Methylphenidate HCl modified-release capsules utilize Eurand's novel Diffucaps technology, a multi-particulate bead delivery system with each bead acting as a drug reservoir. Each bead is coated with a chosen polymer to provide a unique release profile. Customized release profiles can then be achieved by incorporating different types of beads into each capsule.

Phase III trial results of the formulation demonstrated that the capsules control the symptoms of ADHD throughout the school day without the need for a second midday dose. Three hundred fourteen children with ADHD between the ages of six and 15 were evaluated in the randomized, double-blind, placebo-controlled trial. The primary efficacy measure was the difference from baseline on the teacher's version of the Conners' Global Index (CGI). The estimated mean improvement from baseline was 7.9 for methylphenidate modified-release capsules compared to 1.2 for placebo.

INDICATION(S) AND RESEARCH PHASE
Pediatric, Attention Deficit/Hyperactivity Disorder (ADHD) – Phase III completed

modafinil
Provigil

MANUFACTURER
Cephalon

DESCRIPTION
Provigil (modafinil) is a dopamine-releasing agent that increases excitatory glutamatergic transmission. It is being developed in phase III trials for the prevention of daytime sleepiness associated with obstructive sleep apnea, hypersomnia, and shift work. Phase II trials are being conducted for the prevention of excessive daytime sleepiness associated with Alzheimer's disease and Parkinson's disease.

A phase II trial has been completed using Provigil as a treatment for sleep apnea and fatigue associated with multiple sclerosis. This drug is also in a phase III trial for the treatment of sleepiness regardless of cause, with an NDA filing planned for late 2001.

Additionally, Provigil is currently in phase I/II trials for ADHD in pediatric subjects.

INDICATION(S) AND RESEARCH PHASE
Multiple Sclerosis – Phase II completed
Sleep Disorders – Phase III
Pediatric, Attention Deficit/Hyperactivity Disorder – Phase I/II
Attention Deficit/Hyperactivity Disorder (ADHD) – Phase I/II
Parkinson's Disease – Phase II
Alzheimer's Disease – Phase II

SIB-1508Y
unknown

MANUFACTURER
Sibia Neurosciences

DESCRIPTION
SIB-1508Y is a nicotinic acetylcholine receptor (nAChR)-selective drug that is being developed for the treatment of Parkinson's disease, other cognitive disorders, and attention deficit/hyperactivity disorder (ADHD). SIB-1508Y is being tested in phase II trials as both a single therapeutic agent and combined with L-dopa for treatment of Parkinson's disease.

INDICATION(S) AND RESEARCH PHASE
Attention Deficit/Hyperactivity Disorder (ADHD) – Phase II
Memory Loss – Phase II

SLI 381
Adderall

MANUFACTURER
Shire Pharmaceuticals

DESCRIPTION
SLI 381 is a once-a-day formulation of Adderall in development for the treatment of attention deficit/hyperactivity disorder (ADHD). Adderall is an amphetamine compound that produces central nervous system stimulant activity. Trial results indicated the drug may control symptoms of ADHD throughout the day and into the evening. Compared with placebo, subjects given SLI 381 demonstrated significant improvement on both the SKAMP Rating Scale and the PERMP Derived Measures throughout the day and into evening time points. The effects of SLI 381 on these scales also lasted until later in the day and longer than those of Adderall 10 mg. An NDA that includes this trial was submitted to the FDA in October 2000.

INDICATION(S) AND RESEARCH PHASE
Attention Deficit/Hyperactivity Disorder (ADHD) – NDA submitted

SPD 420
unknown

MANUFACTURER
Shire Pharmaceuticals

DESCRIPTION
Ampakine CX516 (designated as SPD 420) is being evaluated for the treatment of attention deficit/hyperactivity disorder (ADHD). The drug is being developed for worldwide use in both adult and pediatric subjects.

INDICATION(S) AND RESEARCH PHASE
Attention Deficit/Hyperactivity Disorder (ADHD) – Phase I completed
Pediatric, Attention Deficit/Hyperactivity Disorder (ADHD) – Phase I completed

SPD 503
unknown

MANUFACTURER
Shire Pharmaceuticals

DESCRIPTION
SPD 503 is being evaluated for the treatment of both adult and pediatric attention deficit/hyperactivity disorder (ADHD). SPD 503 is in phase I trials, and a proof of concept study is expected to begin in the first half of 2001.

INDICATION(S) AND RESEARCH PHASE
Attention Deficit/Hyperactivity Disorder (ADHD) – Phase I
Pediatric, Attention Deficit/Hyperactivity Disorder (ADHD) – Phase I

tomoxetine
unknown

MANUFACTURER
Eli Lilly

DESCRIPTION
Tomoxetine, a noradrenergic compound, is in development for the treatment of attention deficit/hyperactivity disorder (ADHD). It is being tested in phase III trials in children ages six and older.

INDICATION(S) AND RESEARCH PHASE
Pediatric, Attention Deficit/Hyperactivity Disorder (ADHD) – Phase III

Autism

secretin
unknown

MANUFACTURER
Repligen Corporation

DESCRIPTION
Secretin is a hormone that stimulates the pancreas as part of normal digestion. It is currently approved by the FDA for the diagnosis of gastrinoma and the assessment of pancreatic function. Anecdotal off-label use of secretin in pediatric autism has led to interest in its potential as a treatment.

In March 2000, Repligen initiated a phase II trial that will evaluate three doses of secretin over nine weeks in more than 100 children. In November 2000, the company announced it has completed subject recruitment for the phase II trial of secretin for pediatric autism. Data should be available during the first quarter of 2001.

INDICATION(S) AND RESEARCH PHASE
Pediatric, Autism – Phase II
Gastrointestinal Diseases and Disorders, Miscellaneous – FDA approved

Bipolar Disorders

NPS 1776, alifatic amide
unknown

MANUFACTURER
Abbott Laboratories

DESCRIPTION
NPS 1776 is an orally active small molecule in development for the treatment of epilepsy, bipolar disorders, and other neurological disorders. In March 2000, NPS licensed NPS 1776 to Abbott Laboratories for further development.

Results were presented on two double-blind, placebo-controlled phase I trials of healthy volunteers, conducted in the United Kingdom last year to evaluate single-dose and multiple-dose regimens. In the first phase I trial, a total of 18 volunteers were given an ascending dose of NPS 1776 ranging from 100 mg to 1,600 mg three times daily. In the multiple-dose phase I study, a total of 36 volunteers were given NPS 1776 for ten days at three doses three times daily ranging from 1,200 mg to 2,400 mg. In both studies, NPS 1776 was well tolerated and there were no clinically important changes in vital signs, clinical lab evaluations, or standard neurological exams.

INDICATION(S) AND RESEARCH PHASE
Epilepsy – Phase I completed
Bipolar Disorders – Phase I completed

GW 273293
unknown

MANUFACTURER
GlaxoSmithKline

DESCRIPTION
GW 273293 is a sodium channel inhibitor in phase II trials for the treatment of epilepsy and bipolar disorders.

INDICATION(S) AND RESEARCH PHASE
Bipolar Disorders – Phase II
Epilepsy – Phase II

MK-869
unknown

MANUFACTURER
Merck & Co.

DESCRIPTION
MK-869 is a substance P receptor antagonist for the treatment of chemotherapy induced emesis. Substance P acts on neurokinin-1 (NK_1) receptors in areas of the brain stem associated with vomiting.

Results from the phase II trial showed that MK-869 prevented nausea and vomiting induced by cisplatin. The phase II trial included 150 subjects who received granisetron and dexamethasone followed by therapy with cisplatin. Acute emesis (within 24 hours) and delayed emesis (days 2–5) were evaluated. In the acute-emesis evaluation 93% of the subjects in the first two groups had no vomiting compared to 67% given placebo. Then, in the delayed-emesis evaluation 82% of the subjects in group one, 78% in group two, and 33% in group three had no vomiting. There were no serious adverse events reported.

INDICATION(S) AND RESEARCH PHASE
Anxiety Disorders – Phase III
Bipolar Disorders – Phase III
Depression – Phase III
Effects of Chemotherapy – Phase III

olanzapine
Zyprexa

MANUFACTURER
Eli Lilly

DESCRIPTION
Zyprexa is an approved antipsychotic agent that may work by inhibiting receptors for several CNS neurotransmitters, including dopamine and serotonin type 2 ($5-HT_2$).

There was an NDA filed in June 2000 for Zyprexa in a short-acting intramuscular (SAIM) injectable formulation for the treatment of agitation in schizophrenia, bipolar I disorder, and dementia.

This drug is in phase II trials for treatment of depressive episodes associated with bipolar disorder and for the long-term relapse prevention in bipolar affective disorder, with NDA filing planned for late 2002. Zyprexa is also in a phase II trial in a four-week depot formulation.

INDICATION(S) AND RESEARCH PHASE
Bipolar Disorders – Phase II
Bipolar Disorders – NDA submitted
Schizophrenia and Schizoaffective Disorders – NDA submitted
Dementia – NDA submitted

quetiapine fumarate
Seroquel

MANUFACTURER
AstraZeneca

DESCRIPTION
Seroquel is an atypical antipsychotic medication, which belongs to a new chemical class, the dibenzothiazepine derivatives. Although the exact mechanism of action is unknown, scientists believe that Seroquel is a receptor antagonist for a combination of neurotransmitters, including dopamine type 2 (D_2) and serotonin type 2 ($5-HT_2$).

Seroquel is approved for the management of the manifestations of psychotic disorders. The antipsychotic effectiveness has been proven in schizophrenic subjects for a 6-week short-term usage.

Seroquel is being tested in phase III trials for the management of psychosis in Alzheimer's disease and line extension studies for the treatment of mania. Phase III trials for bipolar disorder and schizophrenia are also under way for the granule formulation of the drug as well as for schizophrenia in a sustained-release formulation.

INDICATION(S) AND RESEARCH PHASE
Alzheimer's Disease – Phase III
Bipolar Disorders – Phase III
Manic Disorders – Phase III
Schizophrenia and Schizoaffective Disorders – Phase III

risperidone
Risperdal

MANUFACTURER
Janssen Pharmaceutica

DESCRIPTION
Risperdal is an antipsychotic medication that belongs to a new chemical class, the benzisoxazole derivatives. As with other antipsychotic drugs, the exact mechanism of action is unknown, but researchers believe that Risperdal works as a receptor antagonist for a combination of neurotransmitters, including dopamine type 2 (D_2) and serotonin type 2 ($5-HT_2$).

Risperdal has already been FDA approved in tablet and oral solutions to treat schizophrenia and schizoaffective disorder, though the company is conducting further studies for first-break treatment and relapse prevention for these indications.

Risperdal is currently in phase III trials for the treatment of conduct disorder in pediatric subjects ages 5-16 years old in both an oral and tablet formulation and for treatment of schizophrenia in I.M. depot formulation.

Janssen Pharmaceutica terminated their collaborative agreement for development and marketing with SmithKline Beecham in 1999.

INDICATION(S) AND RESEARCH PHASE
Bipolar Disorders – Phase III
Conduct Disorder – Phase III
Pediatric, Schizophrenia, and Schizoaffective Disorders – Phase III

SPD 417, carbamazepine
Carbatrol

MANUFACTURER
Shire Pharmaceuticals

DESCRIPTION
Carbatrol (carbamazepine) is being evaluated for the treatment of bipolar disorder. Carbatrol has previously been approved by the FDA as a treatment for seizures and trigeminal neuralgia.

INDICATION(S) AND RESEARCH PHASE
Bipolar Disorders – Phase III

topiramate tablet
Topamax

MANUFACTURER
R.W. Johnson Pharmaceutical Research Institute

DESCRIPTION
Topamax is being tested in trials for monotherapy in neuropathic pain and bipolar disorders in a tablet formulation. It was approved in May 2000 for epilepsy.

INDICATION(S) AND RESEARCH PHASE
Epilepsy – FDA approved
Pain, Acute or Chronic – Phase III
Bipolar Disorders – Phase II

Conduct Disorder

risperidone
Risperdal

MANUFACTURER
Janssen Pharmaceutica

DESCRIPTION
Risperdal is an antipsychotic medication that belongs to a new chemical class, the benzisoxazole derivatives. As with other antipsychotic drugs, the exact mechanism of action is unknown, but researchers believe that Risperdal works as a receptor antagonist for a combination of neurotransmitters, including dopamine type 2 (D_2) and serotonin type 2 (5-HT_2).

Risperdal has already been FDA approved in tablet and oral solutions to treat schizophrenia and schizoaffective disorder, though the company is conducting further studies for first-break treatment and relapse prevention for these indications.

Risperdal is currently in phase III trials for the treatment of conduct disorder in pediatric subjects ages 5-16 years old in both an oral and tablet formulation and for treatment of schizophrenia in I.M. depot formulation.

Janssen Pharmaceutica terminated their collaborative agreement for development and marketing with SmithKline Beecham in 1999.

INDICATION(S) AND RESEARCH PHASE
Bipolar Disorders – Phase III
Pediatric, Conduct Disorder – Phase III
Schizophrenia and Schizoaffective Disorders – Phase III

Depression

5-HT1A partial agonist
Ariza

MANUFACTURER
Organon

DESCRIPTION
Ariza, a 5 hydroxytryptamine-1A (5-HT_{1A}) partial agonist, is in a phase III trial for the treatment of depression. An NDA filing is planned for summer 2001.

INDICATION(S) AND RESEARCH PHASE
Depression – Phase III

amino-cyclopropane carboxylic acid
unknown

MANUFACTURER
Annovis

DESCRIPTION
Amino-cyclopropane carboxylic acid is an ion channel regulator/neuroprotectant being evaluated for use in the treatment of depression, addiction, and anxiety.

INDICATION(S) AND RESEARCH PHASE
Depression – Phase I
Anxiety Disorders – Phase I
Addictions – Phase I

antidepressant
unknown

MANUFACTURER
Merck KgaA

DESCRIPTION
The company is developing this drug for the treatment of depression. Clinical trials are in phase II.

INDICATION(S) AND RESEARCH PHASE
Depression – Phase II

befloxatone
Osanetant

MANUFACTURER
Sanofi-Synthelabo Pharmaceuticals

DESCRIPTION
Osanetant is a selective and reversible monoamine oxidase (MAO) type A inhibitor, primarily being studied for the treatment of depression. Future indications may include atypical depression, social phobias, and panic disorder. The phase III trial conducted in 2000 was discontinued due to insufficient results.

INDICATION(S) AND RESEARCH PHASE
Depression – Phase III discontinued

citalopram HBr
Escitalopram

MANUFACTURER
Forest Laboratories

DESCRIPTION
Escitalopram, the active isomer of Celexa (citalopram HBr), is in development for the treatment of depression. In its current formulation, citalopram is a racemic mixture. The S-isomer of citalopram is the active isomer with respect to antidepressant effects,

while the R-isomer does not contribute to antidepressant activity. Escitalopram contains only the S-isomer.

In December 2000, results of a phase III trial indicated that escitalopram produced significant improvement relative to placebo at 10 mg/day and 20 mg/day doses.

INDICATION(S) AND RESEARCH PHASE
Depression – NDA submitted

CP-122,721
unknown

MANUFACTURER
Pfizer

DESCRIPTION
CP-122,721 is a neurokinin 1 (NK$_1$) antagonist being developed as a treatment for depression. The drug is in a phase II trial, with phase III planned for early 2001.

INDICATION(S) AND RESEARCH PHASE
Depression – Phase II

CRF receptor antagonist (partnered), NBI-37582
unknown

MANUFACTURER
Neurocrine Biosciences

DESCRIPTION
Neurocrine Biosciences is developing both a proprietary corticotropin releasing factor-1 (CRF) receptor antagonist and a compound in partnership with Janssen Pharmaceutica. CRF functions as a neurotransmitter in the brain and plays a critical role in coordinating the body's response to stress. The CRF$_1$ receptor subtype largely mediates these effects.

In preclinical models, selective CRF$_1$ receptor antagonists block stress-related responses providing evidence that this novel mechanism may result in improved anti-anxiety and antidepressant properties. In addition, some data suggest that CRF$_1$ antagonists may have a more rapid onset of action and a reduced side effect profile compared to currently marketed anti-depressants.

INDICATION(S) AND RESEARCH PHASE
Depression – Phase I
Anxiety Disorders – Phase I

CRF receptor antagonist (proprietary)
unknown

MANUFACTURER
Neurocrine Biosciences

DESCRIPTION
Neurocrine Biosciences is developing both a proprietary corticotropin releasing factor-1 (CRF) receptor antagonist and a compound in partnership with Janssen Pharmaceutica. CRF functions as a neurotransmitter in the brain and plays a critical role in coordinating the body's response to stress. The CRF$_1$ receptor subtype largely mediates these effects.

In pre-clinical models, selective CRF$_1$ receptor antagonists block stress-related responses providing evidence that this novel mechanism may result in improved anti-anxiety and antidepressant properties. In addition, some data suggest that CRF$_1$ antagonists may have a more rapid onset of action and a reduced side effect profile compared to currently marketed anti-depressants.

In December 2000, Neurocrine Biosciences announced the initiation of a phase I trial with its proprietary CRF$_1$ receptor antagonist compound for the treatment of anxiety and depression. The trial is being conducted in 48 normal, healthy subjects and is designed to evaluate safety, tolerability, pharmacokinetics, and pharmacodynamics over a range of escalating doses.

INDICATION(S) AND RESEARCH PHASE
Anxiety Disorders – Phase I
Depression – Phase I

CX-619, ORG-24448
unknown

MANUFACTURER
Cortex Pharmaceuticals

DESCRIPTION
CX-619, ORG-24448 is in a phase I trial for the treatment of depression.

INDICATION(S) AND RESEARCH PHASE
Depression – Phase I

DU125530
unknown

MANUFACTURER
Solvay Pharmaceuticals

DESCRIPTION
DU125530 is a 5-hydroxy-tryptamine 1A (5-HT$_{1A}$) antagonist being developed for the treatment of anxiety and major depression. 5-HT$_{1A}$ antagonists increase serotonin levels in the brain, and may provide beneficial effects as antidepressants. DU125530 is currently in phase II trials.

INDICATION(S) AND RESEARCH PHASE
Depression – Phase II
Anxiety Disorders – Phase II

duloxetine HCl, LY-248686
unknown

MANUFACTURER
Eli Lilly

DESCRIPTION
Duloxetine hydrochloride is an antidepressant that works by inhibiting the reuptake of norepinephrine and serotonin. This reuptake inhibitor blocks the neurotransmitters from re-entering the nerve cells, and thereby allows a longer period of synaptic stimulation in the brain. Duloxetine is being tested in phase III studies for the treatment of depression. An NDA filing is planned for late 2001 or early 2002.

INDICATION(S) AND RESEARCH PHASE
Depression – Phase III
Urinary Incontinence – Phase III

flesinoxan
unknown

MANUFACTURER
Solvay Pharmaceuticals

DESCRIPTION
Flesinoxan is a serotonin agonist used for the treatment of generalized anxiety disorder and major depressive disorder. The phase III trial was discontinued in 2000.

INDICATION(S) AND RESEARCH PHASE
Anxiety Disorders – Phase III discontinued
Depression – Phase III discontinued

fluoxetine HCl
Prozac

MANUFACTURER
Eli Lilly

DESCRIPTION
Prozac is a serotonin reuptake inhibitor used for the treatment of panic disorder, post-traumatic stress disorder, depression and obsessive-compulsive disorder in children and adolescents, pre-menstrual dysphoric disorder in adolescents, and dysthymia. Prozac is currently in phase III trials, with the patent expiring 8/2/01 following the end of a pediatric extension. An NDA filing is planned for 2001 for the treatment of panic disorder.

INDICATION(S) AND RESEARCH PHASE
Panic Disorders – Phase III
Post-Traumatic Stress Disorders – Phase III
Depression – Phase III
Pediatric, Obsessive-Compulsive Disorder – Phase III
Pediatric, Pre-menstrual Dysphoric Disorder – Phase III
Pediatric, Dysthemia – Phase III

fluoxetine HCl
unknown

MANUFACTURER
Eli Lilly

DESCRIPTION
Fluoxetine HCl (formerly known as DuraPac) is a serotonin reuptake inhibitor antidepressant, administered in once-weekly doses. An NDA has been filed.

INDICATION(S) AND RESEARCH PHASE
Depression – NDA submitted

fluoxetine/olanzapine
Zyp/Zac

MANUFACTURER
Eli Lilly

DESCRIPTION
Fluoxetine/olanzapine is a Prozac/Zyprexa combination for the treatment and resistance of depression and psychotic depression. It is in a phase II trial, with NDA filing planned for 2002.

INDICATION(S) AND RESEARCH PHASE
Depression – Phase II

gepirone
Geppar (proposed to PTO)

MANUFACTURER
Fabre-Kramer Pharmaceuticals

DESCRIPTION
Gepirone is a once-daily formulation used in the treatment of major depression and major depression with anxiety. Gepirone has completed a phase III trial and the company is in preparation to submit an NDA.

INDICATION(S) AND RESEARCH PHASE
Depression – Phase III completed

GW 597599
unknown

MANUFACTURER
GlaxoSmithKline

DESCRIPTION
GW 597599 is a neurokinin-1 (NK_1) receptor antagonist. It is currently in phase I trials for the treatment of depression.

INDICATION(S) AND RESEARCH PHASE
Depression – Phase I

GW 650250
unknown

MANUFACTURER
GlaxoSmithKline

DESCRIPTION
GW 650250 is a mixed monoamine reuptake inhibitor. It is currently in phase II trials for the treatment of depression.

INDICATION(S) AND RESEARCH PHASE
Depression – Phase II

GW-650250A, NS-2389
unknown

MANUFACTURER
GlaxoSmithKline

DESCRIPTION
GW-650250A, NS-2389 is a mixed monoamine reuptake inhibitor used in the treatment of depression. Phase II trials for this drug were suspended in August 2000 due to safety concerns. Development will be delayed six months while further preclinical toxicology studies are carried out.

INDICATION(S) AND RESEARCH PHASE
Depression – Phase II on hold

INN-00835
unknown

MANUFACTURER
Innapharma

DESCRIPTION
INN-00835 is a novel antidepressant that is being studied in two formulations; subcutaneous and sublingual forms. This drug is a synthetic peptide with a potential for rapid onset of action.

INDICATION(S) AND RESEARCH PHASE
Depression – Phase II completed

JO-1784, CI-1019
unknown

MANUFACTURER
Pfizer

DESCRIPTION
JO-1784, CI-1019 is an igmesine sigma agonist used as a treatment for depression. The phase III trial of this drug was discontinued in 2000.

INDICATION(S) AND RESEARCH PHASE
Depression – Phase III discontinued

LU 26-054, SSRI
unknown

MANUFACTURER
Forest Laboratories

DESCRIPTION
LU 26-054, SSRI is an escitalo selective serotonin reuptake inhibitor. The drug is an s-enantiomer of citalopram (Celexa) used for the treatment of depression. It is currently in a phase III trial, with an NDA filing planned for mid 2001.

INDICATION(S) AND RESEARCH PHASE
Depression – Phase III

MK-869
unknown

MANUFACTURER
Merck & Co.

DESCRIPTION
MK-869 is a substance P receptor antagonist for the treatment of chemotherapy induced emesis. Substance P acts on neurokinin-1 (NK_1) receptors in areas of the brain stem associated with vomiting.

Results from the phase II trial showed that MK-869 prevented nausea and vomiting induced by cisplatin. The phase II trial included 150 subjects who received granisetron and dexamethasone followed by therapy with cisplatin. Acute emesis (within 24 hours) and delayed emesis (days 2-5) were evaluated. In the acute-emesis evaluation 93% of the subjects in the first two groups had no vomiting compared to 67% given placebo. Then, in the delayed-emesis evaluation 82% of the subjects in group one, 78% in group two, and 33% in group three had no vomiting. There were no serious adverse events reported.

INDICATION(S) AND RESEARCH PHASE
Anxiety Disorders – Phase III
Bipolar Disorders – Phase III
Depression – Phase III
Effects of Chemotherapy – Phase III

moclobemide
unknown

MANUFACTURER
Dainippon Pharmaceutical

DESCRIPTION
Moclobemide is currently in a phase II trial for the treatment of depression.

INDICATION(S) AND RESEARCH PHASE
Depression – Phase II

NAD299
unknown

MANUFACTURER
AstraZeneca

DESCRIPTION
NAD299 is a $5\text{-}HT_{1A}$ antagonist indicated for the treatment of anxiety and depression. It is currently in phase II trials.

INDICATION(S) AND RESEARCH PHASE
Anxiety Disorders – Phase II
Depression – Phase II

nefazodone metabolite
Serzone-ER

MANUFACTURER
Sepracor

DESCRIPTION
Serzone-ER is a nefazodone metabolite in an extended-release capsule formulation. This drug is currently in a phase III trial for the treatment of depression.

INDICATION(S) AND RESEARCH PHASE
Depression – Phase III

neurokinin antagonist
unknown

MANUFACTURER
AstraZeneca

DESCRIPTION
This drug, a neurokinin antagonist, is in a phase II trial for the treatment of depression.

INDICATION(S) AND RESEARCH PHASE
Depression – Phase II

NGD 98-1
unknown

MANUFACTURER
Pfizer

DESCRIPTION
NGD 98-1 is an orally administered corticotropin releasing antagonist. It is being studied for the treatment of stress-related disorders, including depression and anxiety. It is currently in a phase II trial.

INDICATION(S) AND RESEARCH PHASE
Depression – Phase II
Anxiety Disorders – Phase II

NK-1
unknown

MANUFACTURER
Hoffmann-La Roche

DESCRIPTION
NK-1 is currently in a phase I trial for the treatment of depression and deficits associated with schizophrenia.

INDICATION(S) AND RESEARCH PHASE
Schizophrenia and Schizoaffective Disorders – Phase I
Depression – Phase I

NPS 1506
unknown

MANUFACTURER
NPS Allelix Corp

DESCRIPTION
NPS 1506 is a novel neuroprotectant designed as a treatment for stroke. The drug works by blocking calcium channels controlled by *N*-methyl-D-asparate (NMDA) receptors, which are located on neurons. During a stroke or other brain injury, oxygen deprivation triggers an accumulation of glutamate, an excitatory chemical neurotransmitter that opens NMDA receptors. This results in an influx of calcium, which can lead to disruption of normal cellular processes. NPS 1506 prevents this excessive calcium influx, and therefore may stabilize cell chemistry and minimize cell death. Phase I trials of NPS 1506 have been completed; however, trials of the drug have been put on financial hold until a corporate partner is obtained to assist with further development.

NPS-1506 has completed trials for the treatment of depression (phase Ib) and stroke (phase I).

INDICATION(S) AND RESEARCH PHASE
Strokes – Phase I completed
Depression – Phase Ib completed

NS-2389
unknown

MANUFACTURER
NeuroSearch A/S

DESCRIPTION
NS-2389 is a monoamine reuptake inhibitor in development for the treatment of depression. Monoamine reuptake inhibitors block the reabsorption of specific neurotransmitters, which therefore accumulate in the brain and can provide a longer period of neural stimulation. The increase of three particular neurotransmitters—serotonin, norepinephrine, and dopamine—is the basis for NS-2389 treatment. NS-2389 is in phase II development.

INDICATION(S) AND RESEARCH PHASE
Depression – Phase II

OPC-14523
unknown

MANUFACTURER
Otsuka America Pharmaceutical

DESCRIPTION
OPC-14523 is in a phase II trial for the treatment of major depressive disorder.

INDICATION(S) AND RESEARCH PHASE
Depression – Phase II

ORG-12962
unknown

MANUFACTURER
Organon

DESCRIPTION
ORG-12962, a selective, 5-HT$_{2C}$ receptor agonist, is in a phase II trial for the treatment of depression.

INDICATION(S) AND RESEARCH PHASE
Depression – Phase II

ORG-34167
unknown

MANUFACTURER
Organon

DESCRIPTION
ORG-34167 is in a phase I trial for the treatment of depression.

INDICATION(S) AND RESEARCH PHASE
Depression – Phase I

ORG-34517
unknown

MANUFACTURER
Organon

DESCRIPTION
ORG-34517 is in a phase II trial for the treatment of depression.

INDICATION(S) AND RESEARCH PHASE
Depression – Phase II

paroxetine
Paxil, Seroxat

MANUFACTURER
GlaxoSmithKline

DESCRIPTION
Paxil (paroxetine) is an orally administered selective serotonin reuptake inhibitor (SSRI) currently approved to treat a variety of mood and anxiety disorders. FDA approval has been received for the treatment of depression, obsessive-complusive disorder (OCD), panic disorder, and social anxiety disorder or social phobia. This drug is sold under the brand name Paxil in United States and Seroxat in Europe.

Paxil is currently in phase III trials for the treatment of depression in a dispersible tablet formulation. NDAs have also been submitted for the treatment of generalized anxiety disorders and post-traumatic stress disorder.

INDICATION(S) AND RESEARCH PHASE
Post-Traumatic Stress Disorders – NDA submitted
Anxiety Disorders – NDA submitted
Depression – Phase III

R 107474
unknown

MANUFACTURER
Janssen Pharmaceutica

DESCRIPTION
R107474, an alpha-2 antagonist, was in a phase II trial that was discontinued in 2000. R107474 was being evaluated for the treatment of depression.

INDICATION(S) AND RESEARCH PHASE
Depression – Phase II discontinued

R-fluoxetine
unknown

MANUFACTURER
Sepracor

DESCRIPTION
R-fluoxetine is the R-isomer of Prozac, a selective serotonin reuptake inhibitor for the treatment of depression, developed and marketed by Eli Lilly. Prozac contains both R- and S-isomers of fluoxetine. The Company believes that R-fluoxetine will allow for faster relief, better efficacy, and fewer side effects in subjects being treated for depression. Additional indications may also be a possibility, such as anxiety. All further development and marketing of drugs containing R-fluoxetine have been taken over by Eli Lilly who has chosen to discontinue trials.

INDICATION(S) AND RESEARCH PHASE
Depression – Trial discontinued

SB 243213
unknown

MANUFACTURER
GlaxoSmithKline

DESCRIPTION
SB 243213 is a 5-hydroxytryptamine 2c (5-HT_{2c}) receptor antagonist. It is currently in phase I development for the treatment of depression.

INDICATION(S) AND RESEARCH PHASE
Depression – Phase I

SB 659746A, EMD 68843
unknown

MANUFACTURER
GlaxoSmithKline

DESCRIPTION
SB 659746A is a selective serotonin reuptake inhibitor (SSRI) and 5-hydroxytryptamine 1A (5-HT_{1A}) receptor partial agonist. It is currently in phase II trials for the treatment of depression.

INDICATION(S) AND RESEARCH PHASE
Depression – Phase II

selgiline
Eldepryl

MANUFACTURER
Somerset Pharmaceuticals

DESCRIPTION
Eldepryl is FDA approved for the treatment of Parkinson's disease when given orally. This new formulation is a transdermal patch, which will allow for improved adherence and more optimal pharmacokinetics. It is in a phase III trial for the treatment of depression and Parkinson's disease.

INDICATION(S) AND RESEARCH PHASE
Depression – Phase III
Parkinson's Disease – Phase III

SLV 308
unknown

MANUFACTURER
Solvay Pharmaceuticals

DESCRIPTION
SLV 308 is currently in phase II development for the treatment of depression and Parkinson's disease.

INDICATION(S) AND RESEARCH PHASE
Depression – Phase II
Parkinson's Disease – Phase II

SR-142801, osanetant
unknown

MANUFACTURER
Sanofi-Synthelabo Pharmaceuticals

DESCRIPTION
Sanofi Laboratories is developing a new medication, SR-142801 that could become a new treatment for schizophrenia and major depression. It is currently in phase IIa clinical trials for the treatment of anxiety, psychosis, and schizophrenia and a phase II trial for major depressive disorder. It will be formulated as an oral medication. It is thought that both schizophrenia and depression are related to low serotonin levels in the brain. The molecule from which serotonin is made, 5-HT, is manufactured by enterochromaffin cells located in the gut. When these cells are stimulated, they release 5-HT into the circulation, spurring greater production of serotonin.

There are certain cell receptors (NK_3 receptors) found in the body that when activated, can prevent the release of 5-HT by the enterochromaffin cells, resulting in lower serotonin production. If the action of NK_3 receptors is blocked, then the levels of 5-HT and serotonin might increase. SR-142801, in preliminary studies, was shown to block the serotonin-lowering action of NK_3 receptors and thus may lead to increased 5-HT and serotonin levels in the body. Further study is necessary to determine the precise efficacy of this new compound.

INDICATION(S) AND RESEARCH PHASE
Schizophrenia and Schizoaffective Disorders – Phase IIa
Depression – Phase II
Anxiety Disorders – Phase IIa
Psychosis – Phase IIa

SR-46349
unknown

MANUFACTURER
Sanofi-Synthelabo Pharmaceuticals

DESCRIPTION
SR-46349 blocks the action of 5-HT_2 receptors in the body. Normally, these receptors are responsible for absorbing 5-HT, a precursor of serotonin, back into neurons. Inadequate levels of serotonin outside nerve cells can lead to depressive states. The action of SR-46349 allows serotonin to circulate longer in the body and in greater amounts. Because this drug acts on a specific receptor, there may be fewer side effects associated with its use. Common antidepressant side effects include nausea,

anorexia, and sexual dysfunction. Further study will determine whether these side effects are fewer with the use of SR-46349.

SR-46349 is in trials for the treatment of sleep apnea, depression and schizophrenia.

INDICATION(S) AND RESEARCH PHASE
Sleep Disorders – Phase IIb
Schizophrenia and Schizoaffective Disorders – Phase IIb
Depression – Phase IIb

SR-48692
unknown

MANUFACTURER
Sanofi-Synthelabo Pharmaceuticals

DESCRIPTION
SR-48692 is a neurotensin antagonist for the treatment of colon cancer, prostate cancer, depression, psychosis, and schizophrenia. It is an oral formulation.

INDICATION(S) AND RESEARCH PHASE
Colon Malignancies – Phase II
Prostate Cancer – Phase II
Schizophrenia and Schizoaffective Disorders – Phase IIa
Psychosis – Phase IIa
Depression – Phase II

SR-58611
unknown

MANUFACTURER
Sanofi-Synthelabo Pharmaceuticals

DESCRIPTION
SR-58611 is a new compound that may be an effective treatment for depression. There are many receptors and neurotransmitters that play a part in the pathology of depression. One of these, the beta receptor, has a strong effect on mood. In fact, a common side effect of beta blockers, anti-hypertensive drugs that block this receptor, is depression. It is thought that the action of the beta receptors stimulates the production and release of important neurotransmitters such as norepinephrine and serotonin, two substances that can alleviate the symptoms of depression.

SR-58611 is a medication that increases the activity of these beta receptors. Beta receptors are found throughout the body and have many different actions on many different organs. By focusing on one specific kind of beta receptor, the beta$_3$ receptor, scientists hope this compound will have an antidepressant effect, but will not produce any other cardiac or respiratory side effects. The increased activity of the beta$_3$ receptor may lead to increased levels of norepinephrine and serotonin, and thereby, improve depressive symptoms. Scientists are also interested in SR-58611 as a possible weight loss aid.

The drug is currently in a phase IIa trial.

INDICATION(S) AND RESEARCH PHASE
Depression – Phase IIa

substance P antagonist candidates
unknown

MANUFACTURER
Merck & Co.

DESCRIPTION
Substance P antagonist candidates are in a phase IIa trial for the treatment of neuropsychiatric diseases, including depression and anxiety disorders.

INDICATION(S) AND RESEARCH PHASE
Depression – Phase IIa
Anxiety Disorders – Phase IIa

TAK-637
unknown

MANUFACTURER
Takeda Chemical Industries

DESCRIPTION
TAK-637 is an NK$_1$ receptor antagonist being developed for the treatment of various indications. It is currently in phase I trials in Japan for urinary incontinence. Additionally, TAK-637 is in phase II trials in Europe and the United States for urinary incontinence, depression, and irritable bowel syndrome.

INDICATION(S) AND RESEARCH PHASE
Urinary Incontinence – Phase I (Japan)
Urinary Incontinence – Phase II
Depression – Phase II
Irritable Bowel Syndrome (IBS) – Phase II

Unknown
TritAb

MANUFACTURER
Protherics

DESCRIPTION
TritAb is an antibody product made to offset the toxic effects of overdoses of tricyclic antidepressants (TCAs). This antidote is made from specialized monoclonal antibodies that target TCAs. TritAb is being tested in both pediatric and adult subjects. Phase III development is scheduled to be initiated. The TritAb program for reversal of antidepressant toxicity has an orphan drug status.

INDICATION(S) AND RESEARCH PHASE
Depression – Phase II/III
Overdose/Drug Toxicity – Phase II/III
Pediatric, Depression – Phase II

YKP-10A
unknown

MANUFACTURER
Janssen Pharmaceutica

DESCRIPTION
YKP-10A is a fourth-generation antidepressant. Although the final formulation is not yet determined, this compound is being tested in phase II trials for the treatment of depression. YKP-10A was licensed from SK Corporation Bio-Pharmaceutical R&D Center.

INDICATION(S) AND RESEARCH PHASE
Depression – Phase II

YKP-10A
unknown

MANUFACTURER
SK Corporation Bio-Pharmaceutical R&D Center

DESCRIPTION
YKP-10A is a fourth-generation antidepressant. Although the final formulation is not yet determined, this compound is being tested in phase II trials for the treatment of depression.

INDICATION(S) AND RESEARCH PHASE
Depression – Phase II

YM-992
unknown

MANUFACTURER
Yamanouchi Pharmaceutical

DESCRIPTION
YM-992 is an oral selective 5-HT reuptake inhibitor and noradrenaline augmenting 5-HT$_{2A}$ antagonist. The drug is in phase II trials for depression. It is being developed in Europe and the United States.

INDICATION(S) AND RESEARCH PHASE
Depression – Phase II

Manic Disorders

quetiapine fumarate
Seroquel

MANUFACTURER
AstraZeneca

DESCRIPTION
Seroquel is an atypical antipsychotic medication, which belongs to a new chemical class, the dibenzothiazepine derivatives. Although the exact mechanism of action is unknown, scientists believe that Seroquel is a receptor antagonist for a combination of neurotransmitters, including dopamine type 2 (D$_2$) and serotonin type 2 (5-HT$_2$).

Seroquel is approved for the management of the manifestations of psychotic disorders. The antipsychotic effectiveness has been proven in schizophrenic subjects for a 6-week short-term usage.

It is being tested in phase III trials for the management of psychosis in Alzheimer's disease and line extension studies for the treatment of mania. Phase III trials for bipolar disorder and schizophrenia are also under way for the granule formulation of the drug as well as for schizophrenia in a sustained release formulation.

INDICATION(S) AND RESEARCH PHASE
Alzheimer's Disease – Phase III
Bipolar Disorders – Phase III
Manic Disorders – Phase III
Schizophrenia and Schizoaffective Disorders – Phase III

Obsessive-Compulsive Disorders

fluvoxamine maleate
Fluvoxamine-CR

MANUFACTURER
Solvay Pharmaceuticals

DESCRIPTION
Fluvoxamine-CR is a controlled-release version of Luvox—a selective serotonin reuptake inhibitor approved in the United States for the treatment of obsessive-compulsive disorder (OCD). The drug is being developed under an agreement with Elan Pharmaceuticals. An NDA has been submitted for the treatment of OCD and social anxiety.

INDICATION(S) AND RESEARCH PHASE
Obsessive-Compulsive Disorders – NDA submitted
Anxiety Disorders – NDA submitted

Panic Disorders

esprolol
unknown

MANUFACTURER
Selectus Pharmaceuticals

DESCRIPTION
Esprolol is a potent, rapidly acting, drug to be taken under the tongue. It is classified as a beta-adrenergic blocker that may lessen heart rate and blood pressure increases during physical exertion.

This compound completed a Phase IIb clinical trial to evaluate the effects of esprolol on exercise tolerance in angina pectoris subjects. During the trial all exercise parameters and negative exercise induced angina symptoms were significantly improved.

In addition, esprolol is in a Phase II study for panic disorders and cardiovascular effects of acute anxiety and migraine. A Phase I trial of esprolol was conducted in healthy volunteers and the drug was well tolerated with only mild adverse effects. In addition, a follow up Phase II trial was conducted to evaluate the ability of esprolol to lessen the effects of beta receptor stimulation by standard challenge doses of isoproterenol in healthy volunteers, and to assess the drug's rate of onset of action and the duration of effect. Esprolol's therapeutic effect was seen within ten minutes and lasted for two to four hours.

INDICATION(S) AND RESEARCH PHASE
Angina – Phase IIb completed
Migraine and Cluster Headaches – Phase II
Panic Disorders – Phase II

fluoxetine HCl
Prozac

MANUFACTURER
Eli Lilly

DESCRIPTION
Prozac is a serotonin reuptake inhibitor used for the treatment of panic disorder, post-traumatic stress disorder, depression and obsessive-compulsive disorder in children and adolescents, pre-menstrual dysphoric disorder in adolescents, and dysthymia. Prozac is currently in phase III trials, with the patent expiring August 2, 2001, following the end of a pediatric extension. An NDA filing is planned for 2001 for the treatment of panic disorder.

INDICATION(S) AND RESEARCH PHASE

Panic Disorders – Phase III
Post-Traumatic Stress Disorders – Phase III
Depression – Phase III
Pediatric, Obsessive-Compulsive Disorder – Phase III
Pediatric, Pre-Menstrual Dysphoric Disorder – Phase III
Pediatric, Dysthymia – Phase III

pagoclone
unknown

MANUFACTURER
Pfizer

DESCRIPTION
Pagoclone is a partial agonist of gamma-amino butyric acid (GABA) receptors. GABA is an inhibitory neurotransmitter that may help suppress anxious activity. A phase II trial was initiated in January 2001 evaluating pagoclone for the treatment of generalized anxiety disorder. In addition, a phase III for panic disorders was initiated in August 2000. Interneuron licensed worldwide rights to develop and commercialize pagoclone to Warner-Lambert Company, which is now part of Pfizer.

INDICATION(S) AND RESEARCH PHASE
Anxiety Disorders – Phase II
Panic Disorders – Phase III

Post-Traumatic Stress Disorders

fluoxetine HCl
Prozac

MANUFACTURER
Eli Lilly

DESCRIPTION
Prozac is a serotonin reuptake inhibitor used for the treatment of panic disorder, post-traumatic stress disorder, depression and obsessive-compulsive disorder in children and adolescents, pre-menstrual dysphoric disorder in adolescents, and dysthymia. Prozac is currently in phase III trials, with the patent expiring August 2, 2001, following the end of a pediatric extension. An NDA filing is planned for 2001 for the treatment of panic disorder.

INDICATION(S) AND RESEARCH PHASE
Panic Disorders – Phase III
Post-Traumatic Stress Disorders – Phase III
Depression – Phase III
Pediatric, Obsessive-Compulsive Disorder – Phase III
Pediatric, Pre-Menstrual Dysphoric Disorder – Phase III
Pediatric, Dysthymia – Phase III

paroxetine
Paxil, Seroxat

MANUFACTURER
GlaxoSmithKline

DESCRIPTION
Paxil (paroxetine) is an orally administered selective serotonin reuptake inhibitor (SSRI) currently approved to treat a variety of mood and anxiety disorders. FDA approval has been received for the treatment of depression, obsessive complusive disorder (OCD), panic disorder, and social anxiety disorder or social phobia. This drug is sold under the brand name Paxil in the United States and Seroxat in Europe.

Paxil is currently in phase III trials for the treatment of depression in a dispersible tablet formulation. NDAs have also been submitted for the treatment of generalized anxiety disorders and post-traumatic stress disorder.

INDICATION(S) AND RESEARCH PHASE
Post-Traumatic Stress Disorders – NDA submitted
Anxiety Disorders – NDA submitted
Depression – Phase III

Premenstrual Syndrome

vomeropherin, PH-80
unknown

MANUFACTURER
Pherin Pharmaceuticals

DESCRIPTION
Vomeropherin, in a nasal spray formulation, is in a phase I trial for the treatment of premenstrual syndrome. This drug is also in a phase I trial for the treatment of anxiety disorders.

INDICATION(S) AND RESEARCH PHASE
Premenstrual Syndrome – Phase I
Anxiety Disorders – Phase I

Psychosis

DTA 201
unknown

MANUFACTURER
Novartis

DESCRIPTION
DTA 201 is a dopamine D_3 receptor antagonist being developed in an oral formulation. It is currently in phase II trials for the treatment of psychosis.

INDICATION(S) AND RESEARCH PHASE
Psychosis – Phase II

DU127090
unknown

MANUFACTURER
Solvay Pharmaceuticals

DESCRIPTION
DU127090 is an atypical antipsychotic drug that has mixed (agonist/antagonist) receptor activity with the neurotransmitters dopamine ($D_{2/3/4}$) and serotonin. The drug is being evaluated in phase II trials for the treatment of psychosis.

Solvay is the originator of the compound and retains the marketing rights in the United States, Canada, Mexico, and Japan, while Lundbeck gains the marketing rights for Europe and the rest of the World. Lundbeck and Solvay will jointly market the product in Brazil and Argentina.

INDICATION(S) AND RESEARCH PHASE
Psychosis – Phase II

Lu 35-139
unknown

MANUFACTURER
H. Lundbeck A/S

DESCRIPTION
Lu 35-139 is being evaluated as a rapidly acting therapy for both the positive and the negative symptoms of schizophrenia. It may have fewer extrapyramidal or cardiovascular side effects than existing therapies. Lu 35-139 is in a phase I trial for psychosis.

INDICATION(S) AND RESEARCH PHASE
Psychosis – Phase I

SR-142801, osanetant
unknown

MANUFACTURER
Sanofi-Synthelabo Pharmaceuticals

DESCRIPTION
Sanofi Laboratories is developing a new medication, SR-142801, that could become a new treatment for schizophrenia and major depression. It is currently in phase IIa clinical trials for the treatment of anxiety, psychosis, and schizophrenia and a phase II trial for major depressive disorder. It will be formulated as an oral medication. It is thought that both schizophrenia and depression are related to low serotonin levels in the brain. The molecule from which serotonin is made, 5-HT, is manufactured by certain cells (enterochromaffin cells) located in the gut. When these cells are stimulated, they release 5-HT into the circulation, spurring greater production of serotonin.

There are certain cell receptors (NK_3 receptors) found in the body that, when activated, can prevent the release of 5-HT by the enterochromaffin cells, resulting in lower serotonin production. If the action of NK_3 receptors is blocked, then the levels of 5-HT and serotonin might increase. SR-142801, in preliminary studies, was shown to block the serotonin-lowering action of NK_3 receptors and thus may lead to increased 5-HT and serotonin levels in the body. Further study is necessary to determine the precise efficacy of this new compound.

INDICATION(S) AND RESEARCH PHASE
Schizophrenia and Schizoaffective Disorders – Phase IIa
Depression – Phase II
Anxiety Disorders – Phase IIa
Psychosis – Phase IIa

SR-48692
unknown

MANUFACTURER
Sanofi-Synthelabo Pharmaceuticals

DESCRIPTION
SR-48692 is a neurotensin antagonist for treatment of colon cancer, prostate cancer, depression, psychosis, and schizophrenia. It is in an oral formulation.

INDICATION(S) AND RESEARCH PHASE
Colon Malignancies – Phase II
Prostate Cancer – Phase II
Schizophrenia and Schizoaffective Disorders – Phase IIa
Psychosis – Phase IIa
Depression – Phase II

Schizophrenia and Schizoaffective Disorders

amisulpride, SL 91.1076
Solian

MANUFACTURER
Sanofi-Synthelabo Pharmaceuticals

DESCRIPTION
Solian is an anti-psychotic drug for the treatment of schizophrenia. Phase III trials were discontinued in the United States because the company doesn't consider it will be worthwhile to file an NDA due to the FDA's supplemental information request and Solian's patent expiration date of 2002/2003. Solian is currently marketed on the European market.

INDICATION(S) AND RESEARCH PHASE
Schizophrenia and Schizoaffective Disorders – Phase III discontinued

amisulpride, SL 91.1077
Solian

MANUFACTURER
Sanofi-Synthelabo Pharmaceuticals

DESCRIPTION
The drug amisulpride is an anti-psychotic for the treatment of schizophrenia. Its phase III trial was discontinued in 2000 and the company does not consider NDA filing worthwhile due to the FDA's supplemental information request and Solian's patent expiration date of 2002/2003. The drug is marketed in Europe.

INDICATION(S) AND RESEARCH PHASE
Schizophrenia and Schizoaffective Disorders – Phase III discontinued

aripiprazole, OPC-14597, OPC-31
expected to be Abilitat

MANUFACTURER
Bristol-Myers Squibb

DESCRIPTION
Aripiprazole is an oral drug that is a mixed dopamine receptor agonist/antagonist that is being developed to improve positive and negative symptoms due to schizophrenia, and treat dementia/psychosis in Alzheimer's subjects. Currently, clinical testing is at the phase III level, with NDA filing planned for late 2001 for schizophrenia treatment.

The company reported that early studies with aripiprazole, an antagonist at postsynaptic D_{2A} receptors, and an agonist at presynaptic dopamine autoreceptors, show reduction in psychotic symptoms with a favorable extrapyramidal side effect profile. Animal models indicate the drug has less potential to cause side effects because of the relative lack of upregulation of D_2 receptors in the striatum of the brain.

INDICATION(S) AND RESEARCH PHASE
Schizophrenia and Schizoaffective Disorders

blonanserin, AD-5423
unknown

MANUFACTURER
Dainippon Pharmaceutical

DESCRIPTION
Blonanserin, a dopamine D_2 receptor with serotonin 5-HT_2 receptor antagonist, is an antipsychotic agent developed to improve both the negative and positive symptoms of schizophrenia. This drug is currently in a phase III trial and is seeking license to market outside of Japan.

INDICATION(S) AND RESEARCH PHASE
Schizophrenia and Schizoaffective Disorders – Phase III

CX-516, BDP-12
Ampalex

MANUFACTURER
Cortex Pharmaceuticals

DESCRIPTION
Ampalex is an ampakine (AMPA) receptor enhancer being developed for the treatment of Alzheimer's disease and cognitive dysfunction associated with schizophrenia. The drug has completed a phase I/II trial.

INDICATION(S) AND RESEARCH PHASE
Alzheimer's Disease – Phase I/II completed
Schizophrenia and Schizoaffective Disorders – Phase I/II completed

CX-516, BDP-12
Ampakine

MANUFACTURER
Organon

DESCRIPTION
CX-516, BDP-12 is an ampakine (AMPA) receptor agonist used in the treatment of cognitive dysfunction associated with schizophrenia. The drug is in a phase I trial, with phase II planned for 2001. Organon is under exclusive worldwide licensing agreement with Cortex.

INDICATION(S) AND RESEARCH PHASE
Schizophrenia and Schizoaffective Disorders – Phase I

DAB-452
unknown

MANUFACTURER
Wyeth-Ayerst

DESCRIPTION
DAB-452 is a dopamine-2 partial agonist in phase II development for the treatment of schizophrenia.

INDICATION(S) AND RESEARCH PHASE
Schizophrenia and Schizoaffective Disorders – Phase II

EMD-57445
unknown

MANUFACTURER
Merck KgaA

DESCRIPTION
EMD-57445 is currently in a phase II trial for the treatment of schizophrenia.

INDICATION(S) AND RESEARCH PHASE
Schizophrenia and Schizoaffective Disorders – Phase II

iloperidone
Zomaril

MANUFACTURER
Titan Pharmaceuticals

DESCRIPTION
Zomaril (iloperidone) is a novel antipsychotic drug for schizophrenia and related mental diseases. Iloperidone has an antagonistic effect on dopamine and serotonin receptors in the brain. In phase III testing, Titan reported that subjects receiving Zomaril achieved a statistically significant reduction in the symptoms of schizophrenia, with little weight gain or extrapyramidal symptoms. Novartis Pharma is Titan's corporate partner for Zomaril.

INDICATION(S) AND RESEARCH PHASE
Schizophrenia and Schizoaffective Disorders – Phase III

M100907
unknown

MANUFACTURER
Aventis

DESCRIPTION
M100907 is serotonin type 2A (5-HT_{2A}) receptor antagonist that is being developed for the treatment of schizophrenia. The company reported that it is active against the positive and negative symptoms of schizophrenia, and the drug is well tolerated. Currently, M100907 is being tested in phase III studies.

INDICATION(S) AND RESEARCH PHASE
Schizophrenia and Schizoaffective Disorders – Phase III

neuroleptic
unknown

MANUFACTURER
Merck KgaA

DESCRIPTION
The company is developing a neuroleptic drug for the treatment of schizophrenia. Neuroleptics work through altering brain chemistry by stimulating and/or inhibiting neurotransmitters. Clinical trials are currently in phase II for this product.

INDICATION(S) AND RESEARCH PHASE
Schizophrenia and Schizoaffective Disorders – Phase II

NGD 94-4
unknown

MANUFACTURER
Schering-Plough Corporation

DESCRIPTION
NGD 94-4 is a dopamine D_4 receptor antagonist used in the treatment of schizophrenia. The drug is currently in a phase I trial in England.

INDICATION(S) AND RESEARCH PHASE
Schizophrenia and Schizoaffective Disorders – Phase I

NK-1
unknown

MANUFACTURER
Hoffmann-La Roche

DESCRIPTION
NK-1 is currently in a phase I trial for the treatment of depression and deficits associated with schizophrenia.

INDICATION(S) AND RESEARCH PHASE
Schizophrenia and Schizoaffective Disorders – Phase I
Depression – Phase I

olanzapine
Zyprexa

MANUFACTURER
Eli Lilly

DESCRIPTION
Zyprexa is an approved antipsychotic agent that may work by inhibiting receptors for several CNS neurotransmitters, including dopamine and serotonin type 2 (5-HT$_2$).

There was an NDA filed in June 2000 for Zyprexa in a short-acting intramuscular (SAIM) injectable formulation for the treatment of agitation in schizophrenia, bipolar I disorder, and dementia.

This drug is in phase II trials for treatment of depressive episodes associated with bipolar disorder and for the long-term relapse prevention in bipolar affective disorder, with NDA filing planned for late 2002. Zyprexa is also in a phase II trial in a four-week depot formulation.

INDICATION(S) AND RESEARCH PHASE
Bipolar Disorders – Phase II
Bipolar Disorders – NDA submitted
Schizophrenia and Schizoaffective Disorders – NDA submitted
Dementia – NDA submitted

ORG-23430
unknown

MANUFACTURER
Organon

DESCRIPTION
ORG-23430 is in a phase II trial for the treatment of schizophrenia.

INDICATION(S) AND RESEARCH PHASE
Schizophrenia and Schizoaffective Disorders – Phase II

ORG-5222
unknown

MANUFACTURER
Organon

DESCRIPTION
ORG-5222 is an anti-psychotic drug used for the treatment of schizophrenia. It is currently in a phase II trial.

INDICATION(S) AND RESEARCH PHASE
Schizophrenia and Schizoaffective Disorders – Phase II

quetiapine fumarate
Seroquel

MANUFACTURER
AstraZeneca

DESCRIPTION
Seroquel is an atypical antipsychotic medication, which belongs to a new chemical class, the dibenzothiazepine derivatives. Although the exact mechanism of action is unknown, scientists believe that Seroquel is a receptor antagonist for a combination of neurotransmitters, including dopamine type 2 (D$_2$) and serotonin type 2 (5-HT$_2$).

Seroquel is approved for the management of the manifestations of psychotic disorders. The antipsychotic effectiveness has been proven in schizophrenic subjects for a 6-week short-term usage.

Seroquel is being tested in phase III trials for the management of psychosis in Alzheimer's disease and line extension studies for the treatment of mania. Phase III trials for bipolar disorder and schizophrenia are also under way for the granule formulation of the drug as well as for schizophrenia in a sustained release formulation.

INDICATION(S) AND RESEARCH PHASE
Alzheimer's Disease – Phase III
Bipolar Disorders – Phase III
Manic Disorders – Phase III
Schizophrenia and Schizoaffective Disorders – Phase III

risperidone
Risperdal

MANUFACTURER
Janssen Pharmaceutica

DESCRIPTION
Risperdal is an antipsychotic medication that belongs to a new chemical class, the benzisoxazole derivatives. As with other antipsychotic drugs, the exact mechanism of action is unknown, but researchers believe that Risperdal works as a receptor antagonist for a combination of neurotransmitters, including dopamine type 2 (D$_2$) and serotonin type 2 (5-HT$_2$).

Risperdal has already been FDA approved in tablet and oral solutions to treat schizophrenia and schizoaffective disorder, though the company is conducting further studies for first-break treatment and relapse prevention for these indications.

Risperdal is currently in phase III trials for the treatment of conduct disorder in pediatric subjects ages five to 16 years old in both an oral and tablet formulation and for treatment of schizophrenia in I.M. depot formulation.

Janssen Pharmaceutica terminated their collaborative agreement for development and marketing with SmithKline Beecham in 1999.

INDICATION(S) AND RESEARCH PHASE
Bipolar Disorders – Phase III
Conduct Disorder – Phase III
Schizophrenia and Schizoaffective Disorders
 – Phase III
Pediatric – Phase III

SC-111
unknown

MANUFACTURER
Scotia Pharmaceuticals

DESCRIPTION
SC-111 is a phospholipase A_2 inhibitor used in the treatment of schizophrenia. This drug is currently in a phase II trial.

INDICATION(S) AND RESEARCH PHASE
Schizophrenia and Schizoaffective Disorders
 – Phase II

SR-141716
unknown

MANUFACTURER
Sanofi-Synthelabo Pharmaceuticals

DESCRIPTION
SR-141716 is a medication that may provide for the treatment of schizophrenia, obesity, and smoking addiction. It is in an oral formulation and is currently being tested in phase IIa clinical trials. Marijuana activates receptors in the body called cannabinoid (CB1) receptors. The human body itself makes a substance, anandamide, which also activates these receptors. It has long been observed that marijuana use increases appetite, probably through activation of these cannabinoid receptors. Scientists hope that by blocking these receptors with SR-141716, appetite will be reduced, leading to weight loss. Currently, this drug is being evaluated as a new weight loss therapy.

In addition, these cannabinoid receptors may play a role in drug and alcohol abuse, possibly by affecting the activity of brain reward systems. By lowering the "reward" (the pleasant sensation) that the brain experiences from smoking, drinking, or using mood altering drugs, blockage of these receptors may help control addictive behaviors.

The cannabinoid receptor also may contribute to schizophrenic behavior. The company reported that preliminary studies have shown that when these receptors were blocked with SR-141716, the hyperactive, psychotic behavior associated with schizophrenia was decreased. Overactivity or overproduction of cannabinoid receptors in the body may contribute to an imbalance in dopamine, the neurotransmitter most commonly associated with schizophrenia. Current clinical trials for all these indications are under way.

INDICATION(S) AND RESEARCH PHASE
Schizophrenia and Schizoaffective Disorders
 – Phase IIa
Obesity – Phase II
Smoking Cessation – Phase II

SR-142801, osanetant
unknown

MANUFACTURER
Sanofi-Synthelabo Pharmaceuticals

DESCRIPTION
Sanofi Laboratories is developing a new medication, SR-142801, that could become a new treatment for schizophrenia and major depression. It is currently in phase IIa clinical trials for the treatment of anxiety, psychosis, and schizophrenia and a phase II trial for major depressive disorder. It will be formulated as an oral medication. It is thought that both schizophrenia and depression are related to low serotonin levels in the brain. The molecule from which serotonin is made, 5-HT, is manufactured by enterochromaffin cells located in the gut. When these cells are stimulated, they release 5-HT into the circulation, spurring greater production of serotonin.

There are certain cell receptors (NK_3 receptors) found in the body that when activated, can prevent the release of 5-HT by the enterochromaffin cells, resulting in lower serotonin production. If the action of NK_3 receptors is blocked, then the levels of 5-HT and serotonin might increase. SR-142801, in preliminary studies, was shown to block the serotonin-lowering action of NK_3 receptors and thus may lead to increased 5-HT and serotonin levels in the body. Further study is necessary to determine the precise efficacy of this new compound.

INDICATION(S) AND RESEARCH PHASE
Schizophrenia and Schizoaffective Disorders
 – Phase IIa
Depression – Phase II
Anxiety Disorders – Phase IIa
Psychosis – Phase IIa

SR-31742
unknown

MANUFACTURER
Sanofi-Synthelabo Pharmaceuticals

DESCRIPTION
SR-31742 is a new medication being developed for the treatment of schizophrenia. It is to be given orally and is currently in phase IIa clinical trials.

This new drug acts by inhibiting the sigma receptor, which is found throughout the brain, and is most prevalent in the areas of the brain which regulate memory, movement, and pain sensation. Sigma receptors may be activated by many different substances, not only by neurotransmitters such as dopamine and serotonin, but also by hormones as well. A current hypothesis is that the psychotic symptoms of schizophrenia may be caused by prolonged activity of these sigma receptors—partly because their activation may stimulate the release of excess amounts of dopamine. It is believed that people with schizophrenia either have overactive sigma receptors, or they produce some substance or have some virus which overstimulates these receptors.

In any case, SR-31742 inhibits the action of the sigma receptor, thus decreasing the amount of free dopamine, and thus possibly reducing schizophrenic symptoms. Most current treatments for schizophrenia and depression already reduce sigma receptor action, but SR-31742 is one of a new group of drugs that acts on this receptor exclusively.

INDICATION(S) AND RESEARCH PHASE
Schizophrenia and Schizoaffective Disorders – Phase IIa

SR-46349
unknown

MANUFACTURER
Sanofi-Synthelabo Pharmaceuticals

DESCRIPTION
SR-46349 may prove to be an effective antidepressant medication. It blocks the action of 5-HT$_2$ receptors in the body. Normally, these receptors are responsible for absorbing 5-HT, a precursor of serotonin, back into neurons. Inadequate levels of serotonin outside nerve cells can lead to depressive states. The action of SR-46349 allows serotonin to circulate longer in the body and in greater amounts. Because this drug acts on a specific receptor, there may be fewer side effects associated with its use. Common antidepressant side effects include nausea, anorexia, and sexual dysfunction. Further study will determine whether these side effects are fewer with the use of SR-46349.

Additionally, SR-46349 is in trials for the treatment of sleep apnea and schizophrenia.

INDICATION(S) AND RESEARCH PHASE
Sleep Disorders – Phase IIb
Schizophrenia and Schizoaffective Disorders – Phase IIb
Depression – Phase IIb

SR-48692
unknown

MANUFACTURER
Sanofi-Synthelabo Pharmaceuticals

DESCRIPTION
SR-48692 is a neurotensin antagonist for treatment of colon cancer, prostate cancer, depression, psychosis, and schizophrenia. It is in an oral formulation.

INDICATION(S) AND RESEARCH PHASE
Colon Malignancies – Phase II
Prostate Cancer – Phase II
Schizophrenia and Schizoaffective Disorders – Phase IIa
Psychosis – Phase IIa
Depression – Phase II

Smoking Cessation

CP-526,555
unknown

MANUFACTURER
Pfizer

DESCRIPTION
CP-526,555 is an oral treatment for smoking cessation. As a partial agonist, CP-526-555 partially stimulates the nicotine receptor in the brain to satisfy a smoker's nicotine craving while, at the same time, blocking the nicotine receptor from the reinforcing value of nicotine in smoke.

INDICATION(S) AND RESEARCH PHASE
Smoking Cessation – Phase II

GW 468816
unknown

MANUFACTURER
GlaxoSmithKline

DESCRIPTION
GW 468816 is a glycine receptor antagonist in phase I development for migraine prophylaxis and for smoking cessation.

INDICATION(S) AND RESEARCH PHASE
Migraine and Cluster Headaches – Phase I
Smoking Cessation – Phase I

LY-354740
unknown

MANUFACTURER
Eli Lilly

DESCRIPTION
LY-354740 is a glutamate receptor agonist used as a smoking cessation aid and in the treatment of anxiety. This drug is currently in a phase II trial.

INDICATION(S) AND RESEARCH PHASE
Smoking Cessation – Phase II
Anxiety Disorders – Phase II

nicotine addiction product
unknown

MANUFACTURER
Algos Pharmaceutical

DESCRIPTION
This novel nicotine addiction product is being tested in a phase II trial for smoking cessation. It is made in an oral capsule formulation.

INDICATION(S) AND RESEARCH PHASE
Smoking Cessation – Phase II

SR-141716
unknown

MANUFACTURER
Sanofi-Synthelabo Pharmaceuticals

DESCRIPTION
SR-141716 is a medication that may provide for the treatment of schizophrenia, obesity, and smoking addiction. It is in an oral formulation and is currently being tested in phase IIa clinical trials. Marijuana activates receptors in the body called cannabinoid (CB1) receptors. The human body itself makes a substance, anandamide, which also activates these receptors. It has long been observed that marijuana use increases appetite, probably through activation of these cannabinoid receptors. Scientists hope that by blocking these receptors with SR-141716, appetite will be reduced, leading to weight loss. Currently, this drug is being evaluated as a new weight loss therapy.

In addition, these cannabinoid receptors may play a role in drug and alcohol abuse, possibly by affecting the activity of brain reward systems. By lowering the "reward" (the pleasant sensation) that the brain experiences from smoking, drinking, or using mood altering drugs, blockage of these receptors may help control addictive behaviors.

The cannabinoid receptor also may contribute to schizophrenic behavior. The company reported that preliminary studies have shown that when these receptors were blocked with SR-141716, the hyperactive, psychotic behavior associated with schizophrenia was decreased. Overactivity or overproduction of cannabinoid receptors in the body may contribute to an imbalance in dopamine, the neurotransmitter most commonly associated with schizophrenia. Current clinical trials for all these indications are under way.

INDICATION(S) AND RESEARCH PHASE
Schizophrenia and Schizoaffective Disorders – Phase IIa
Obesity – Phase II
Smoking Cessation – Phase II

Substance Abuse

lofexidine
unknown

MANUFACTURER
Britannia Pharmaceuticals Limited

DESCRIPTION
Lofexidine is an imidazoline derivative that belongs to a group of medicines that selectively stimulate alpha-2 adrenergic receptors. It is in phase III trials in the United States for detoxification and phase II trials for relapse.

INDICATION(S) AND RESEARCH PHASE
Substance Abuse – Phase III
Relapse – Phase II

methadone/dextromethorphan
unknown

MANUFACTURER
Algos Pharmaceutical

DESCRIPTION
A combination therapy using methadone and dextromethorphan is being tested in a phase II trial for opiate substance abuse. This dual therapy is a novel NMDA enhanced opiate addiction treatment. It is given as an oral capsule formulation.

INDICATION(S) AND RESEARCH PHASE
Substance Abuse – Phase II

naltrexone
Medisorb Naltrexone

MANUFACTURER
Alkermes

DESCRIPTION
Naltrexone is a narcotic antagonist approved by the FDA for the treatment of alcoholism and opiate abuse. It is currently available in a daily oral dosage form. Medisorb Naltrexone is a formulation of naltrexone utilizing Alkermes' Medisorb injectable sustained-release drug delivery technology. This technology is based on the encapsulation of drugs into small polymeric microspheres, which degrade slowly and release drugs at a controlled rate following injection.

Results of a randomized, placebo-controlled, dose-escalating phase I trial of Medisorb Naltrexone indicated that the formulation maintained therapeutic levels for a full month, while requiring less than 1/5th the total monthly oral dose.

INDICATION(S) AND RESEARCH PHASE
Substance Abuse – Phase I completed

therapeutic, substance abuse
unknown

MANUFACTURER
Elan Transdermal Technologies

DESCRIPTION
Elan Transdermal Technologies is developing a therapeutic treatment for substance abuse using a seven-day transdermal patch delivery formulation. Clinical testing is at the phase II stage.

INDICATION(S) AND RESEARCH PHASE
Substance Abuse – Phase II

vaccine, cocaine
TA-CD

MANUFACTURER
Cantab Pharmaceuticals plc

DESCRIPTION
TA-CD is a vaccine designed to generate drug-specific antibodies. These antibodies bind to cocaine and prevent it from traveling to the brain from the bloodstream, neutralizing its psychoactive effect. In a phase I trial, the vaccine was given to 34 subjects split into three cohorts to evaluate three different doses of the vaccine following 30 days of abstinence. Two subjects in each cohort received a placebo and the rest received active vaccine. The study's participants had to meet the criteria for cocaine dependence, including a three- to 10-year cocaine habit, and willingness to get treatment and participate in the study. Results indicated the vaccine was safe and produced cocaine antibodies. Clinical testing is currently in phase II.

INDICATION(S) AND RESEARCH PHASE
Substance Abuse – Phase II

5 | Oncology

Population with illnesses in this category	85 million
Drugs in the development pipeline	402

Source: Pharma

The American Cancer Society (ACS) estimates that cancer costs the United States economy an annual total of $107 billion. This amount includes all health expenditures and costs of lost productivity due to illness and premature death. In the United States today, 8.5 million people are suffering from cancer or are cancer survivors. In 2000, more than 1.2 million new cancer cases were diagnosed. This year more than half a million Americans will die from cancer, the second leading cause of death by disease. This disease is responsible for nearly one of every four deaths in the United States.

According to the ACS, in the U.S. men have a one in two lifetime risk of developing cancer and the risk for women is one in three. However, due to encouraging research in cancer treatment and prevention, death rates have been falling since 1991. Since 1995, there has been an even more rapid decline. The dream of conquering cancer will hopefully soon be a reality.

The progress of the past decade is due in part to the large number of drugs in clinical development for treatment of cancer. CenterWatch has identified close to 400 drugs involved in clinical trials for cancer treatment. The majority of these drugs are being tested for multiple cancer indications. The three most predominantly researched indications are lung, breast, and prostate cancer, with each accounting for approximately 70 drugs currently in trials. The ACS estimates that the annual direct medical costs of these three cancers is $20 billion and CenterWatch estimates the annual cost of clinical drug development to be between $900 million and $1 billion.

According to a survey from PhRMA, many of the drugs currently in the pipeline for treating malignancies use highly innovative techniques designed to target cancer cells without damaging healthy cells. Examples include: a compound that targets an abnormal protein that triggers chronic myelogenous leukemia; a medicine that recruits natural killer cells to attack pancreatic cancer cells; a vaccine made by combing the patient's own tumor cells with a "hapten", which is designed to trigger an immune response to treat advanced melanoma; a medication approved for the prevention and treatment of osteoporosis that shows promise in preventing breast cancer; a compound that inhibits a key enzyme involved in the replication of ovarian cancer cells; and a drug that blocks two key factors (anti-angiogenesis factors) that help create the blood vessels that cancer cells need to grow is being tested for multiple myeloma, kidney cancer, and lung cancer.

Lung cancer accounts for nearly 15% of all cancer cases in the United States, with an estimated 170,000 new cases diagnosed each year. There were an estimated 157,000 deaths from lung cancer in 2000. In the past ten years, lung cancer mortality rates in men have significantly declined, but have significantly increased in women. Since 1987, more women have died from lung cancer than breast cancer, which for over 40 years was the leading cause of cancer death in women. Declining lung cancer incidence and mortality rates most likely result from decreased cigarette smoking rates over the 30 previous years, which lag behind in women. Unfortunately, declines in tobacco use by adults have slowed and tobacco use by young people is rising. The five-year relative survival rate for lung cancer is only 14%, but increases to 49% in cases detected while the disease is still localized.

Lung cancer research is highly active due to the seriousness of the disease and the lack of a truly effective treatment. CenterWatch estimates that the industry will spend $300 million to $350 million this year researching the 70 identified potential treatments for lung cancer. In addition to chemotherapy treatments and vaccines, researchers are focusing on the use of monoclonal antibodies and anti-angiogenic therapy in the fight against lung cancer. Monoclonal antibodies are also being developed. ImClone is evaluating IMC-C225 in phase III trials for lung cancer in addition to a variety of other cancers. This biologic is a part mouse, part human monoclonal antibody that blocks the epidermal growth factor receptor, which may result in an inhibition of tumor growth by preventing tumor cells damaged by the effects of chemotherapy and radiotherapy from evading a pathway to cell death. Antiangiogenic therapy is being studied for adjunctive use with chemotherapy. This therapy cuts off the blood supply to tumor targets, thereby starving tumors of nutrients and preventing further growth. It may also help prevent cells from becoming progressively resistant to the effects of chemotherapy.

Breast cancer ranks second among cancer deaths in women in the U.S. In 2000, more than 40,000 women died from breast cancer and an estimated 183,000 new cases are expected to occur each year. Additionally, there will be about 1,400 new cases diagnosed in men. It is estimated that one in eight women will develop breast cancer in her lifetime. Approximately three million women in the United States today are living with breast cancer, including up to one million that have not yet been diagnosed. After increasing in the 1980s, breast cancer incidence rates in women have now leveled off and mortality rates have significantly declined, especially in younger women. These decreases are probably due to earlier detection and improved treatment. The five year survival rate for breast cancer is 96%, however if there are local metastases it drops to 77%, and declines to only 21% in women with distant metastases.

CenterWatch estimates that $320 million to $370 million will be spent this year on the clinical development of the approximately 70 drugs in the pipeline for treatment of breast cancer. New treatments currently being studied include aromatase inhibitors, monoclonal antibody therapies, and adjuvant therapies. Medications that block the activity of aromatase prevent further tumor growth by depriving breast cancer cells of estrogens that stimulate proliferation of tumor cells. In January 2000, Aromasin (exemenstane tablets), by Pharmacia & Upjohn, became the first oral aromatase inhibitor for the treatment of postmenopausal women with advanced breast cancer whose tumors stop responding to tamoxifen. A variety of monoclonal antibodies are being developed that target specific types of malignant breast cells, such as those that overexpress growth receptors. Adjuvant therapies use combinations of drugs that may be more effective or less toxic that just one drug. Phase II and III studies evaluating such therapies have shown promising results.

Prostate cancer is the most common cancer diagnosed in men in the United States and is the second leading cause of mortality due to cancer in men, after lung cancer. In 2000, an estimated 180,000 new cases were diagnosed and almost 32,000 deaths occurred. Between 1989 and 1992, incidence rates dramatically increased, but are now declining. This increase was most likely due to earlier diagnosis in men without any symptoms through the increased use of prostate-specific antigen (PSA) blood test screenings. In patients with localized prostate cancers with metastases only to regional structures, the five year survival rate is 100%. Even for all stages combined, the survival rate has now reached 92%.

These impressive survival rates are largely due to the numerous treatment options for men suffering from prostate cancer. This progress is evident from the close to 70 drugs currently in development. CenterWatch estimates that $300 million to $340 million will spent on this research. Current prostate cancer research focuses on hormone therapy, gene therapy, immunologic agents, vaccines, anti-angiogenesis, and drug delivery.

Most cancers treated with hormone therapy become resistant within months or years. Therefore, researchers are now focusing on intermittent or second line agents to decrease such resistance. Gene therapy is among the most active arenas in prostate cancer research, with several gene-directed biologics in the pipeline. Scientists have located the genes responsible for some forms of hereditary prostate cancer and now are determining in what way each one is responsible for cancer development and how to manipulate these genes to achieve prevention or cure. The potential of anti-angiogenesis drugs to arrest the growth of cancerous tissue is currently under intense investigation. By blocking blood vessel growth, these drugs may prevent the tissue from receiving nutrients and oxygen. With many new agents in the pipeline, prostate cancer treatment is progressing rapidly and the chance of survival is better than ever. More work is clearly needed, especially in the treatment of various brain and gastrointestinal tumors and other cancers that continue to exact high morbidity and mortality.

Adenomatous Polyposis Coli

exisulind
Aptosyn

MANUFACTURER
Cell Pathways

DESCRIPTION
Aptosyn (exisulind) belongs to a novel class of compounds called selective apoptotic anti-neoplastic drugs (SAANDs). SAANDs inhibit a form of cyclic GMP phosphodiesterase and selectively induce apoptosis in abnormally growing precancerous and cancerous cells. Aptosyn is being tested for several indications and is in five different trials for adenomatous polyposis coli (APC) and familial adenomatous polyposis coli; two of these trials are specifically for pediatric subjects.

The company received a non-approvable letter from the FDA in September 2000 for one of the trials for familial adenomatous polyposis. The company intends to amend the NDA and request a meeting to address the deficiencies and the possible requirement for additional clinical data.

Additionally, Aptosyn is being tested in trials for the treatment of prostate cancer, lung cancer, breast cancer, sporadic colonic polyps, and Barrett's esophagus disease.

INDICATION(S) AND RESEARCH PHASE
Adenomatous Polyposis Coli – Non-approvable letter
Pediatric, Familial Adenomatous Polyposis Coli – Phase II
Adenomatous Polyposis Coli – Phase I/II
Barrett's Esophagus Disease – Phase II
Prostate Cancer – Phase II/III
Breast Cancer – Phase II/III
Lung Cancer – Phase Ib
Colon Polyps – Phase II/III

Angiogenesis Inhibitor, Cancer

NM-3
unknown

MANUFACTURER
ILEX Oncology

DESCRIPTION
NM-3 is an orally active small molecule inhibitor of angiogenesis that appears to work by blocking one of the key factors that mediates angiogenesis, vascular endothelial growth factor (VEGF). A phase II trial was initiated in France in October 2000 and trials in the United States are expected to begin in early 2001.

INDICATION(S) AND RESEARCH PHASE
Angiogenesis Inhibitor, Cancer – Phase II

Bladder Cancer

arsenic trioxide (ATO)
Trisenox

MANUFACTURER
Cell Therapeutics

DESCRIPTION
Trisenox is believed to kill cancer cells through apoptosis. The mechanism of action of Trisenox is not fully understood, but the drug appears to induce apoptosis in a different manner than other anti-cancer agents such as retinoids.

Trisenox is FDA approved to treat acute promyelocytic leukemia (APL), and it is also in numerous trials in the United States for indications including other types of leukemia, prostate cancer, multiple myeloma, renal cell cancer, cervical cancer, and bladder cancer.

INDICATION(S) AND RESEARCH PHASE
Leukemia – Phase I
Lymphoma, Non-Hodgkin's – Phase II
Leukemia – Phase II
Multiple Myeloma – Phase II
Prostate Cancer – Phase II
Renal Cell Carcinoma – Phase II
Cervical Dysplasia/Cancer – Phase II
Bladder Cancer – Phase II

CI-1042, ONYX-015
unknown

MANUFACTURER
Onyx Pharmaceuticals

DESCRIPTION
CI-1042 (ONYX-015) is a tumor-selective, modified adenovirus that has been genetically engineered to replicate in and kill cancer cells that possess a mutated oncogene called p53, while sparing normal cells with functioning p53. p53 Is a tumor suppressor gene that is mutated in approximately 50% of all human cancers. CI-1042 is in development for several indications, including pancreatic cancer, liver metastases of colorectal cancer, and lung cancer.

In November 2000, results of a phase II trial demonstrated that CI-1042 administered as a single agent replicates and causes tumor regression in refractory head and neck cancer. CI-1042 was shown to selectively target cancer cells containing a mutant p53 gene, while sparing normal cells with a functioning p53 gene. Of the 19 subjects who received the standard dosing regimen, four (21%) had an objective response, including two complete responses and two partial responses. CI-1042 is being co-developed with Pfizer.

INDICATION(S) AND RESEARCH PHASE
Colorectal Cancer – Phase II
Pancreatic Cancer – Phase II
Head and Neck Cancer – Phase III
Cervical Dysplasia/Cancer – Phase I completed
Lung Cancer – Phase II
Bladder Cancer – Phase I completed
Brain Cancer – Phase I completed

cytostatics
unknown

MANUFACTURER
Bioenvision

DESCRIPTION
Cytostatics are a group of compounds that inhibit retinoic acid metabolizing enzyme, leading to an accumulation of retinoic acid.

Retinoic acid is important in maintaining differentiation of cells and has been shown to have an anti-proliferative effect on malignant cells. There are three potential products being developed in this group. One product, still unnamed, is currently being developed for the treatment of bladder cancer. A phase I trial for this indication is planned for 2001.

INDICATION(S) AND RESEARCH PHASE
Bladder Cancer – Phase I

eflornithine, DFMO (difluoromethylornydil)
unknown

MANUFACTURER
Aventis

DESCRIPTION
Eflornithine is a potent, irreversible inhibitor of ornithine decarboxylase (OCD), an enzyme that is elevated in most tumors and pre-malignant lesions. Eflornithine is currently in a phase III clinical trial to determine the effectiveness of the drug in treating subjects who have newly diagnosed or recurrent bladder cancer. The drug is administered orally in tablet form.

Eflornithine is also in trials for the prevention and treatment of HIV infections, skin cancer, breast cancer, prostate cancer, and cervical dysplasia/cancer.

INDICATION(S) AND RESEARCH PHASE
Bladder Cancer – Phase III
Breast Cancer – Phase II/III
Cervical Dysplasia/Cancer – Phase II
HIV Infection – Phase II
Prostate Cancer – Phase II
Skin Cancer – Phase III

EMD 82633
unknown

MANUFACTURER
Merck KgaA

DESCRIPTION
EMD 82633 is a humanized and bispecific monoclonal antibody derived from mice. These antibodies are altered in such a way that they no longer appear different from human antibodies. This genetic modification prevents immune reactions against foreign substances of animal origin used in humans. In this bispecific drug, one component binds to tumor cells, while the other activates the body's own CD8 "killer cells" to attack cancer cells.

This new drug is being given as an adjuvant therapy to subjects who have not been adequately helped by conventional forms of treatment, such as chemotherapy. EMD 82633 is being tested in trials for the treatment of renal cancer, head and neck cancer, breast cancer, bladder cancer, and ovarian cancer.

INDICATION(S) AND RESEARCH PHASE
Bladder Cancer – Phase II
Breast Cancer – Phase II
Cancer/Tumors (Unspecified) – Phase II
Head and Neck Cancer – Phase II
Ovarian Cancer – Phase II
Renal Cell Carcinoma – Phase II

gallium maltolate
unknown

MANUFACTURER
Titan Pharmaceuticals

DESCRIPTION
Gallium is a semi-metallic element that has shown some therapeutic activity in metabolic bone disease, hypercalcemia of malignancy and cancer. Gallium maltolate can displace divalent iron from the iron transporting protein, transferrin; thus gallium maltolate causes interference with iron metabolism with inhibition of enzymes requiring divalent iron. The most important of these in the cancer setting appears to be ribonucleotide reductase (RNR). Additionally, gallium appears to form salts with calcium and phosphate and become incorporated into bone. The bone that is created with incorporated gallium appears to be at least as strong as normal bone, and it appears to be more resistant to degradation by osteoclasts and tumor cells.

INDICATION(S) AND RESEARCH PHASE
Prostate Cancer – Phase I/II
Lymphomas – Phase I/II
Myeloma – Phase I/II
Bladder Cancer – Phase I/II
HIV Infection – Phase I/II

INGN-201, adenoviral p53
unknown

MANUFACTURER
Introgen Therapeutics

DESCRIPTION
INGN-201 is a p53 gene therapy product. It has been tested as a treatment for a variety of solid tumor cancers with administration via intratumoral injection. The drug was well tolerated according to the company, and additional trials are under way using an intravenous infusion in order to reach more types of cancers. The tumor-suppressing p53 gene encodes a protein that responds to damage involving cellular DNA by terminating cell division. Normal p53 genes are delivered into cancer cells of the subject through an adenoviral vector.

The developers of INGN-201 have signed a Cooperative Research and Development Agreement (CRADA) with the National Cancer Institute to evaluate the potential effectiveness and superiority of the drug over other treatments against breast, ovarian, bladder, prostate, and brain cancers in phase I and phase II trials. A phase III trial in head and neck cancer was initiated in March 2000.

INDICATION(S) AND RESEARCH PHASE
Head and Neck Cancer – Phase III
Bladder Cancer – Phase I
Brain Cancer – Phase I
Breast Cancer – Phase I
Bronchoalveolar Cancer – Phase I
Ovarian Cancer – Phase I
Prostate Cancer – Phase I
Lung Cancer – Phase II
Cancer/Tumors (Unspecified) – Phase I

MCC
unknown

MANUFACTURER
Bioniche Life Sciences

DESCRIPTION
MCC is a cell wall complex prepared from the non-pathogenic bacterium *Mycobacterium phlei* (*M. phlei*) that inhibits cancer cell division, induces apoptosis, and stimulates a profound immune response in a wide range of human cancer cells. Based on extensive preclinical research, the company believes these therapeutic activities are not affected by the presence of multidrug resistance in cancer cells. MCC is in a phase I/II trial for bladder cancer in Canada and Australia.

INDICATION(S) AND RESEARCH PHASE
Bladder Cancer – Phase I/II

MDX-447, H-447
unknown

MANUFACTURER
Medarex

DESCRIPTION
MDX-447 is a novel biological drug designed to stimulate an immune response against cancer cells. Certain cancer cells contain and express large amounts of unique proteins (such as epidermal growth factor receptors), which MDX-447 is directed to recognize. MDX-447 attaches itself both to these cancer proteins and to macrophages that specialize in killing foreign material.

The binding together of the cancer and the immune cells by MDX-447 signals the body to destroy the tumor. MDX-447 may offer a new therapeutic alternative to cancer subjects who have been unresponsive to conventional therapies. This agent is unique since it has two receptors on its surface, one that can attract the cancer cell, and the other that can attract a killer immune cell. This dual nature of the drug is why it is known as a "bispecific antibody."

This type of drug is designed to be more efficient than current anti-cancer therapies, and may have effects that last longer. This technology may also be useful in the development of an "anti-cancer vaccine" in the future. MDX-447 is currently being tested as an intravenous solution in phase II trials for multiple tumor indications, which include brain, bladder, breast, head and neck, and lung cancer.

INDICATION(S) AND RESEARCH PHASE
Brain Cancer – Phase II
Bladder Cancer – Phase II
Breast Cancer – Phase II
Head and Neck Cancer – Phase II
Lung Cancer – Phase II

---

unknown
BCI-Immune Activator

MANUFACTURER
INTRACEL Corporation

DESCRIPTION
BCI-Immune Activator is a non-specific immunotherapy for bladder cancer. The drug acts by inducing a non-specific inflammatory response in the bladder. In turn, this response stimulates macrophages and other immune cells to attack the site of the inflammation, thereby killing the tumor. BCI-Immune Activator is formulated as a liquid and delivered to the subject in two steps. First, a small amount of the drug is injected subcutaneously to stimulate or sensitize the immune system. Then, it is injected directly into the tumor.

Based on what the drug's developer believes to be positive results from a phase I/II study of the effects of increasing doses, a phase III clinical trial has begun to test the efficacy of BCI-Immune Activator for treatment of refractory bladder cancer.

INDICATION(S) AND RESEARCH PHASE
Bladder Cancer – Phase III

---

valrubicin
Valstar

MANUFACTURER
Anthra Pharmaceuticals

DESCRIPTION
Valstar Intravesical Solution is a lipophilic anthracycline-like chemotherapeutic agent. The drug acts by penetrating cells where it affects a variety of biological functions, most of which involve nucleic acid metabolism.

Previously approved for treatment of subjects with BCG-refractory carcinoma in situ (CIS) for whom surgical removal of the bladder would present unacceptable risks of morbidity or mortality, Valstar is in phase III trials for treatment of papillary bladder cancer.

Valstar is also in phase III trials for treatment of refractory ovarian cancer. For this indication, the drug is administered through the abdomen (intraperitoneal).

INDICATION(S) AND RESEARCH PHASE
Bladder Cancer – Phase III
Ovarian Cancer – Phase III

ZD-0473/AMD 473
unknown

MANUFACTURER
AstraZeneca

DESCRIPTION
ZD-0473 is a new platinum-based anti-cancer agent designed to deliver an extended spectrum of activity and overcome resistance to currently approved platinum drugs, such as cisplatin and carboplatin. It is being evaluated for the treatment of a range of solid-tumor cancers, including colorectal, non-small cell lung, and bladder cancer, which are resistant to carboplatin. ZD-0473 is formulated in both intravenous and oral forms. The intravenous formulation is in phase II trials and the oral form is in preclinical development.

INDICATION(S) AND RESEARCH PHASE
Bladder Cancer – Phase II
Cancer/Tumors (Unspecified) – Phase II
Colorectal Cancer – Phase II
Lung Cancer – Phase II
Ovarian Cancer – Phase II
Prostate Cancer – Phase II
Breast Cancer – Phase II
Cervical Dysplasia/Cancer – Phase II

Blood Cancer

LGD-1550
unknown

MANUFACTURER
Ligand Pharmaceuticals

DESCRIPTION
LGD-1550 is being formulated to limit the proliferation and spread of head, neck, and cervical cancers; it is to be given orally and is currently in phase II trials. Retinoids are a group of substances, one of which is vitamin A, that are thought to be responsible for growth, bone development, vision, and skin integrity. It is thought that retinoids act against cancer by regulating the process by which cells reproduce themselves (gene transcription regulation). Studies have shown that subjects with metastatic cancer have lower levels of retinoid activity in their bodies. LGD-1550 works by binding to retinoid receptors in cells, thereby stimulating retinoid activity.

Preliminary studies have shown that retinoids may inhibit cell proliferation and promote cell differentiation. Cancer arises when there is uncontrolled growth of immature cells. Retinoids act to slow cell division and stimulates cell maturation, making it less likely that these mature cells will be transformed into cancerous cells. Retinoids have also been shown in early studies to boost the effects of other anti-cancer medications.

Phase II trials of LGD-1550 for head and neck cancer, cervical cancer, and solid and hematological tumors are currently under way.

INDICATION(S) AND RESEARCH PHASE
Blood Cancer – Phase II
Cancer/Tumors (Unspecified) – Phase II
Cervical Dysplasia/Cancer – Phase II
Head and Neck Cancer – Phase II

Bone Marrow Transplant

anti B-7 humanized antibodies
unknown

MANUFACTURER
Wyeth-Ayerst

DESCRIPTION
Anti B-7 humanized antibodies are being developed for the prevention of graft versus host disease (GVHD) following haploidentical bone marrow transplant and for preventing kidney rejection. Clinical trials are currently in phase I/II development.

INDICATION(S) AND RESEARCH PHASE
Immunosuppressive – Phase I/II
Kidney Transplant Surgery – Phase I/II
Bone Marrow Transplant – Phase I/II

human immune globulin, intravenous solutions
Venoglobulin-S

MANUFACTURER
Alpha Therapeutic

DESCRIPTION
Venoglobulin-S is a solution of antibodies being tested for use in two indications. The first is to prevent infection from the hepatitis A virus, while the second is to prevent acute graft versus host disease (GVHD) in bone marrow transplant subjects.

This immune globulin product may replace missing antibodies, especially in subjects that have a compromised immune system or primary immunodeficiencies, which may be present at birth. This product is given by intramuscular injection.

INDICATION(S) AND RESEARCH PHASE
Bone Marrow Transplant – Phase III
Hepatitis – Phase III

keratinocyte growth gactor-2 (KGF-2)
Repifermin

MANUFACTURER
Human Genome Sciences

DESCRIPTION
Repifermin is a genomics-derived therapeutic protein drug, also known as keratinocyte growth factor-2 (KGF-2). It is in a phase II study for the treatment of mucositis associated with bone marrow transplantation for the treatment of cancer. This phase II trial is a randomized, double-blind, placebo-controlled, dose-escalation study that is being conducted at several sites in the United States. Additionally, Repifermin is in a phase IIb trial for topical wound healing treatment of venous ulcers and a phase II trial for inflammatory bowel disease (IBD).

The company reported that the results of phase I clinical trials showed that systemically administered Repifermin is safe and well tolerated in healthy human subjects at doses proposed for subsequent clinical studies. None of the subjects withdrew from the study or required dose modification because of adverse effects.

KGF-2 stimulates the growth of keratinocyte cells, which make up 95% of the epidermal cells. Together, keratinocyte and melanocyte cells form the epidermis of the body. The company claims that KGF-2 has demonstrated beneficial effects on both the dermal and epidermal tissues of the skin, healing full-thickness wounds in a short period of time. In mucositis, Repifermin may stimulate the creation of new mucosal tissue.

INDICATION(S) AND RESEARCH PHASE
Bone Marrow Transplant – Phase II
Effects of Chemotherapy – Phase II
Skin Wounds – Phase IIb
Inflammatory Bowel Disease – Phase II

recombinant human GM-CSF
Leucotropin

MANUFACTURER
Cangene Corporation

DESCRIPTION
Leucotropin is Cangene's brand of GM-CSF, a protein that stimulates the formation of mature white blood cells. It is produced recombinantly in *Streptomyces* bacteria using the company's Cangenus manufacturing system. At this time, development has been discontinued.

INDICATION(S) AND RESEARCH PHASE
Bone Marrow Transplant – Trial discontinued

Effects of Chemotherapy – Trial discontinued

tresperimus
unknown

MANUFACTURER
Fournier Research

DESCRIPTION
Tresperimus is a new immunosuppressive drug that is being formulated to protect bone marrow transplant subjects from graft versus host disease. In order to receive a bone marrow transplant, a subject's own immune system must be suppressed so that the subject's body will accept and not reject the new bone marrow. Graft versus host disease is a potentially lethal condition that arises when the immunologically active (competent) transplanted bone marrow cells attack the subject's immuno-compromised body. This complication can cause anorexia, diarrhea, low white cell and platelet counts, growth retardation, or death.

Tresperimus may prevent graft versus host disease by stimulating the production of CD4 suppressor cells that act to suppress the immunogenic activity of the donated bone marrow cells. This drug may also result in decreased amounts of CD8 cells, which act to destroy tissue that the immune cells see as foreign. In other words, tresperimus may act to reduce the amount of destructive, attacker immune cells, while increasing the immune cells, which act to suppress the potentially damaging immune reactions that lead to graft versus host disease. Further studies are needed to determine the precise clinical efficacy of this new immunosuppressive medication.

INDICATION(S) AND RESEARCH PHASE
Bone Marrow Transplant – Phase III

Bone Metastases

zoledronate
Zometa

MANUFACTURER
Novartis

DESCRIPTION
Zoledronate is an intravenous bisphosphonate osteoclast inhibitor. In September 2000, Novartis announced it had received an approvable letter from the FDA for Zometa for the treatment of hypercalcemia of malignancy (HCM), the most common life-threatening metabolic complication associated with cancer. Zometa is also in phase II development for the treatment of post-menopausal osteoporosis and phase III development for bone metastasis treatment and prevention.

INDICATION(S) AND RESEARCH PHASE
Osteoporosis – Phase II
Hypercalcemia – FDA recommend approval letter
Bone Metastases – Phase III

Brain Cancer

CI-1042, ONYX-015
unknown

MANUFACTURER
Onyx Pharmaceuticals

DESCRIPTION
CI-1042 (ONYX-015) is a tumor-selective, modified adenovirus (similar to the common cold virus) that has been genetically engineered to replicate in and kill cancer cells that possess a mutated oncogene called p53, while sparing normal cells with functioning p53. p53 Is a tumor suppressor gene that is mutated in approximately 50% of all human cancers. CI-1042 is in development for several indications, including pancreatic cancer, liver metastases of colorectal cancer, and lung cancer.

Results of a phase II trial demonstrated that CI-1042 administered as a single agent replicates and causes tumor regression in refractory head and neck cancer. CI-1042 was shown to selectively target cancer cells containing a mutant p53 gene, while sparing normal cells with a functioning p53 gene. Of the 19 subjects who received the standard dosing regimen, four (21%) had an objective response, including two complete responses and two partial responses. CI-1042 is being co-developed with Pfizer.

INDICATION(S) AND RESEARCH PHASE
Colorectal Cancer – Phase II
Pancreatic Cancer – Phase II
Head and Neck Cancer – Phase III
Cervical Dysplasia/Cancer – Phase I completed
Lung Cancer – Phase II
Bladder Cancer – Phase I completed
Brain Cancer – Phase I completed

docetaxel hydrate
Taxotere

MANUFACTURER
Aventis

DESCRIPTION
Many drugs for the treatment of cancer and other diseases originate in plants, many of them highly poisonous. Taxotere (docetaxel hydrate), an agent that inhibits the formation of new protoplasm, is derived from the renewable evergreen needles of the genus *Taxus* (Yew). Taxotere acts by disrupting the microtubular network in cells that is essential for cell division and many other cellular functions. The drug is approved for use in the United States for treatment of refractory breast cancer, refractory non-small cell lung cancer (NSCLC), and locally advanced or metastatic breast cancer.

New phase II/III trials are under way in head and neck, gastric, and ovarian cancers. Taxotere is also being tested either alone or in combination with other chemotherapy agents in the earlier stages of breast cancer, NSCLC and others tumors.

Phase I extension studies are under way for brain metastasis and lung cancer.

INDICATION(S) AND RESEARCH PHASE
Gastric Cancer – Phase II/III
Head and Neck Cancer – Phase II/III
Lung Cancer – Phase II/III
Ovarian Cancer – Phase II/III
Breast Cancer – Phase III/IV
Brain Cancer – Phase I
Lung Cancer – Phase I

INGN-201, adenoviral p53
unknown

MANUFACTURER
Introgen Therapeutics

DESCRIPTION
INGN-201 is a p53 gene therapy cancer product. It has been tested as a treatment for a variety of solid tumor cancers with administration via intratumoral injection. The drug was well tolerated according to the company, and additional trials are under way using an intravenous infusion in order to reach more types of cancers. The tumor-suppressing p53 gene encodes a protein that responds to damage involving cellular DNA by terminating cell division. Normal p53 genes are delivered into cancer cells of the subject through an adenoviral vector.

The developers of INGN-201 have signed a Cooperative Research and Development Agreement (CRADA) with the National Cancer Institute to evaluate the potential effectiveness and superiority of the drug over other treatments against breast, ovarian, bladder, prostate, and brain cancers in phase I and phase II trials. A phase III trial in head and neck cancer was initiated in March 2000.

INDICATION(S) AND RESEARCH PHASE
Head and Neck Cancer – Phase III
Bladder Cancer – Phase I
Brain Cancer – Phase I
Breast Cancer – Phase I
Bronchoalveolar Cancer – Phase I
Ovarian Cancer – Phase I
Prostate Cancer – Phase I
Lung Cancer – Phase II
Cancer/Tumors (Unspecified) – Phase I

interferon, beta-1a
Avonex

MANUFACTURER
Biogen

DESCRIPTION
Interferons are proteins naturally produced by the body to help fight viral infections and regulate the immune system. Avonex is a biosynthetic compound that contains the same arrangement of amino acids as the interferon-beta produced by the body. It is believed that Avonex regulates the body's immune response to decrease an attack against myelin, a possible mechanism for the nervous system destruction in multiple sclerosis.

Approved by the FDA for the treatment of relapsing forms of multiple sclerosis, Avonex is currently in phase II trials for the treatment of brain cancer and idiopathic pulmonary fibrosis (IPF). For IPF, treatment is aimed at minimizing the disease progression from inflammation to fibrosis.

Results of a phase III trial of Avonex for the treatment of secondary progressive multiple sclerosis (MS) demonstrated that the drug reduced the progression of disability by 27% versus treatment with placebo. IMPACT (International Multiple Sclerosis Secondary Progressive Avonex Controlled Trial) was a randomized, double-blind, placebo-controlled trial involving 436 subjects at 42 sites in the United States, Canada and Europe.

INDICATION(S) AND RESEARCH PHASE
Pulmonary Fibrosis – Phase II
Brain Cancer – Phase II
Multiple Sclerosis – Phase III

interleukin-4 (IL-4) fusion toxin, NBI-3001
unknown

MANUFACTURER
Neurocrine Biosciences

DESCRIPTION
IL-4 fusion toxin is being tested in a phase II trial for the treatment of glioblastoma multiforme (GBM). Preclinical data suggest that when infused directly into a glioblastoma, IL-4 fusion toxin kills tumor cells but not healthy brain cells. IL-4 fusion toxin is a protein in which a blood cell derived growth factor (IL-4) has been joined with a *Pseudomonas* exotoxin, a potent toxin that can destroy cancer cells. IL-4 has a very high affinity for binding to its receptors, which are highly expressed on malignant brain tumors, but not on normal brain cells. IL-4 binds tightly to the IL-4 receptors on the surface of the glioblastoma cells and delivers the exotoxin directly into the cell, resulting in cell death. IL-4 fusion toxin is administered via a special catheter that permits delivery directly into the brain tumor.

Additionally, results from a phase I/II testing IL-4 fusion toxin demonstrated 56% of the 31 subjects tested exhibited a reduction in tumor size. The phase I/II trial took place at nine leading neurosurgery centers in the United States and Germany. The 31 subjects being treated had end-stage (grade 4) recurrent glioblastoma and were treated with intratumoral infusions of IL-4 for up to four days.

The company claims that these findings show the drug to be safe and that it demonstrates anti-tumor effects in the majority of subjects receiving it. Phase III trials of IL-4 fusion toxin, which was granted fast-track designation by the FDA in 1999, are estimated to begin in 2001.

INDICATION(S) AND RESEARCH PHASE
Brain Cancer – Phase II

marimastat, BB-2516
unknown

MANUFACTURER
British Biotech plc

DESCRIPTION
Marimastat is an inhibitor of matrix metalloproteinase (MMP), a family of naturally occurring enzymes that are over-produced in a number of disease states. This is especially true of cancer, where MMPs are involved in the spread and local growth of tumors. Both angiogenesis and metastasis require MMPs during tumor invasion. Anti-angiogenic strategies, unlike other therapeutic approaches, do not aim to directly destroy or "kill" the tumor or cause tumor regression. Rather, they are designed to prevent the further growth of tumors by limiting their blood supply. Because peripheral tumor cells could theoretically survive on a diffusion-dependent basis, anti-angiogenic drugs may prove most effective when given in combination with other standard cytotoxic regimens. Marimastat is in phase III

development for the treatment of cancer.

In 1999, British Biotech and Schering-Plough Corporation signed an agreement to develop and commercialize British Biotech's metalloproteinase inhibitors, including merimastat.

INDICATION(S) AND RESEARCH PHASE
Pancreatic Cancer – Phase III
Lung Cancer – Phase III
Breast Cancer – Phase III
Brain Cancer – Phase III completed
Ovarian Cancer – Phase III

unknown
Prinomastat

MANUFACTURER
Agouron Pharmaceuticals

DESCRIPTION
Prinomastat is an orally active, synthetic molecule designed to potently and selectively inhibit certain members of a family of enzymes known as a matrix metalloproteases, which are believed to be involved in tumor angiogenesis, invasion, and metastasis. The drug is in trials for various indications, including osteoarthritis, brain cancer, and macular degeneration.

Two phase III trials for advanced non-small cell lung cancer and prostate cancer were halted in August 2000 due to the drug's lack of effectiveness in subjects with late-stage disease.

The most common side effects of Prinomastat have been observed in the joints, and include stiffness, joint swelling, and in a few subjects, some limits on the mobility of certain joints, most often in the shoulders and hands. All these effects were reported to be reversible and were effectively managed by treatment rests and dose reductions.

INDICATION(S) AND RESEARCH PHASE
Lung Cancer – Phase III halted
Prostate Cancer – Phase halted
Osteoarthritis – Phase II
Brain Cancer – Phase II
Macular Degeneration – Phase II

MDX-447, H-447
unknown

MANUFACTURER
Medarex

DESCRIPTION
MDX-447 is a novel biological drug designed to stimulate an immune response against cancer cells. Certain cancer cells contain and express large amounts of unique proteins (such as epidermal growth factor receptors), which MDX-447 is directed to recognize. MDX-447 attaches itself both to these cancer proteins and to macrophages that specialize in killing foreign material.

The binding together of the cancer cells and the immune cells by MDX-447 signals the body to destroy the tumor. MDX-447 may offer a new therapeutic alternative to cancer subjects who have been unresponsive to conventional therapies. This agent is unique since it has two receptors on its surface, one that can attract the cancer cell and one that can attract a killer immune cell. This dual nature of the drug is why it is known as a "bispecific antibody."

This type of drug is designed to be more efficient than current anti-cancer therapies, and may have effects that last longer. This technology may also be useful in the development of an "anti-cancer vaccine" in the future. MDX-447 is currently being tested as an intravenous solution in phase II trials for multiple tumor indications, which include brain, bladder, breast, head and neck, and lung cancer.

INDICATION(S) AND RESEARCH PHASE
Brain Cancer – Phase II
Bladder Cancer – Phase II
Breast Cancer – Phase II
Head and Neck Cancer – Phase II
Lung Cancer – Phase II

motexafing adolinium
Xcytrin

MANUFACTURER
Pharmacyclics

DESCRIPTION
Xcytrin (motexafing adolinium) injection is a novel drug that augments the activity of anti-cancer treatment. Preclinical and clinical data indicate that after repeated injections, Xcytrin accumulates selectively in tumors and increases the vulnerability of cancer cells to the effects of radiation or chemotherapy without increasing damage to surrounding healthy cells.

Positive results from the lead-in phase of an ongoing phase III trial of Xcytrin for brain metastases were announced in October 2000. Tumor response was observed in 68% of subjects evaluable by MRI scans, with a median reduction in tumor volume of 83%. Seventy-seven percent of the 25 subjects were free from neurologic progression.

INDICATION(S) AND RESEARCH PHASE
Brain Cancer – Phase III

prolifeprosan 20/carmustine
Gliadel

MANUFACTURER
Aventis

DESCRIPTION
One of the most common intravenous chemotherapy agents used to treat primary brain tumors is carmustine, which is also known as BCNU. BCNU can be useful in treating brain tumors like glioblastoma malignancies (GBM). However, when BCNU is given intravenously, it can cause serious side effects such as bone marrow damage, which interferes with new blood cell formation.

The Gliadel wafer was developed to deliver BCNU directly to the site of the recurrent brain tumor. After neurosurgical removal of GBM tissue, eight dime-sized Gliadel wafers are implanted in the space the tumor once occupied. Each wafer contains a precise amount of BCNU. Over the next two to three weeks, the wafers slowly dissolve, bathing the surrounding cells with BCNU. The goal of Gliadel wafer therapy is to kill the remaining small tumor cells that were previously undetectable during surgical removal, thereby extending subject survival.

Circumventing intravenous delivery by direct placement may decrease drug-related adverse events. The Gliadel wafers were being tested in phase III clinical trials as adjunctive therapy for the treatment of recurrent GBM. Currently, development of this drug therapy has been discontinued.

INDICATION(S) AND RESEARCH PHASE
Brain Cancer – Phase III discontinued

RSR13
unknown

MANUFACTURER
Allos Therapeutics

DESCRIPTION
RSR13 is a synthetic small molecule that increases the release of oxygen from hemoglobin, the oxygen carrying protein contained within red blood cells. The presence of oxygen in tumors is an essential part of the effectiveness of radiation therapy in cancer treatment. By increasing tumor oxygenation, RSR13 has the potential to enhance the effectiveness of standard radiation therapy.

In November 2000, positive preliminary phase II results of induction chemotherapy, followed by radiation therapy plus RSR13, for stage IIIA and IIIB non-small cell lung cancer were announced. Data from the first 30 of 47 subjects demonstrated that 87% had a complete or partial response of their tumors within the radiation therapy portal in the chest. Additionally, Allos Therapeutics is conducting a 408 subject, randomized, multicenter, international phase III trial to confirm that RSR13, when used in combination with radiation therapy, significantly improves the survival of subjects with brain metastases.

INDICATION(S) AND RESEARCH PHASE
Angina – Phase I completed
Myocardial Infarction – Phase II
Brain Cancer – Phase III
Lung Cancer – Phase II
Glomerulonephritis – Phase II completed

SU-101
unknown

MANUFACTURER
Sugen

DESCRIPTION
SU-101 is a synthetic, platelet-derived growth factor receptor, which blocks the essential enzyme tyrosine kinase. This drug may be helpful for the treatment of end-stage malignant glioma, a tumor of nerve tissue. The drug is being tested in phase III trials for refractory brain and prostate cancers, and phase II studies for non-small cell lung and ovarian cancers.

INDICATION(S) AND RESEARCH PHASE
Brain Cancer – Phase III
Prostate Cancer – Phase III
Lung Cancer – Phase II
Ovarian Cancer – Phase II

SU-101/BCNU
unknown

MANUFACTURER
Sugen

DESCRIPTION
SU-101 is a synthetic, platelet-derived growth factor receptor, which blocks the essential enzyme tyrosine kinase. This drug may be useful for the treatment of end-stage malignant glioma, a tumor of nerve tissue. SU-101 in combination with BCNU is being tested in phase II trials for the treatment of brain cancer.

INDICATION(S) AND RESEARCH PHASE
Brain Cancer – Phase II

T67
unknown

MANUFACTURER
Tularik

DESCRIPTION
T67 is an anti-cancer compound that binds irreversibly to tubulin and inhibits the growth of multi-drug resistant tumors. Tubulin is a protein that polymerizes into chains to form microtubules. Microtubules are essential for cell division, and by disrupting their function, T67 produces cell death and potentially causes tumor shrinkage.

The drug is currently in phase II trials in subjects with non-small cell lung cancer, glioma, colorectal cancer, and breast cancer. It is also in a phase I/II trial for the treatment of hepatocellular carcinoma. These trials are being conducted in the United States, the United Kingdom, Hong Kong, and Taiwan.

INDICATION(S) AND RESEARCH PHASE
Lung Cancer – Phase II
Brain Cancer – Phase II
Colorectal Cancer – Phase II
Breast Cancer – Phase II
Hepatocellular Carcinoma – Phase I/II

temozolomide
Temodar

MANUFACTURER
Schering-Plough Corporation

DESCRIPTION
Temodar is an oral cytotoxic chemotherapuetic agent that belongs to a class of compounds known as imidazotetrazines. Temodar has been approved by the FDA for the treatment of adults with anaplastic astrocytoma at the first relapse with disease progression on a nitrosourea- and procarbazine-containing drug regimen. It is currently in phase II trials for the treatment of a variety of solid tumors.

INDICATION(S) AND RESEARCH PHASE
Brain Cancer – FDA approved
Cancer/Tumors (Unspecified) – Phase II

thalidomide
Thalomid

MANUFACTURER
Celgene Corporation

DESCRIPTION
Thalomid is an oral formulation of the immunomodulatory agent thalidomide. Thalidomide has a notorious history of having caused birth defects when the medical

profession unsuspectingly prescribed it for pregnant women as a treatment for nausea and insomnia. Celgene is investigating new applications for the drug, while being particularly mindful of the potential risks of thalidomide treatment. Thalomid is currently being tested for numerous indications in the areas of oncology and immunology.

INDICATION(S) AND RESEARCH PHASE
Multiple Myeloma – Phase II
Myelodysplastic Syndrome – Phase II
Leukemia – Phase II
Brain Cancer – Phase II
Liver Cancer – Phase II
Kidney Cancer – Phase II
Prostate Cancer – Phase II
Kaposi's Sarcoma – Phase II
Cachexia – Phase II
Recurrent Aphthous Stomatitis – Phase III
Crohn's Disease – Phase II
Inflammatory Bowel Disease – Phase II
Sarcoidosis – Phase II
Scleroderma – Phase II

unknown
Cereport

MANUFACTURER
Alkermes

DESCRIPTION
Cereport is a bradykinin agonist, which temporarily increases the permeability of the blood-brain barrier by activating B2 receptors on these endothelial cells. The ability to transiently open the junctions between the tightly joined endothelial cells allows for the selective transport of drug molecules across the blood-brain barrier into the brain.

Cereport's safety, tolerability in combination with other drugs, and preliminary efficacy have been tested in a series of clinical trials in more than 600 subjects. Alkermes has completed four phase II trials of Cereport in combination with carboplatin in subjects with recurrent, malignant brain tumors. Additionally, Cereport is in a pediatric phase II trial for the treatment of brain tumors in children six to 18 years old. Alkermes is in a partnership with ALZA Corporation for the development and commercialization of Cereport.

INDICATION(S) AND RESEARCH PHASE
Brain Cancer – Phase II completed
Pediatric, Brain Tumors – Phase II

unknown
Lucanthone

MANUFACTURER
SuperGen

DESCRIPTION
Lucanthone is a topoisomerase II (topo II) inhibitor that appears to possess promising radio-sensitizing activity. Research has demonstrated that Lucanthone's mechanism of action is mediated via the inhibition of topo II, an enzyme involved in the replication of DNA, and the inhibition of the apurinic/apyrimidinic endonuclease, which contributes to the inhibition of DNA repair. Lucanthone is being tested in a multi-center phase II clinical trial, using a combination of Lucanthone and radiation therapy as a treatment for advanced brain tumors.

INDICATION(S) AND RESEARCH PHASE
Brain Cancer – Phase II

XR5000
unknown

MANUFACTURER
Xenova

DESCRIPTION
XR5000 is a topoisomerase I and II inhibitor being developed for the treatment of common solid tumors. Three phase II trials are under way at a number of European centers. The trials are being conducted on an "open-label" basis and target three cancer types—ovarian, non-small cell lung, and glioblastoma. The results of a fourth phase II trial, in which the efficacy of XR5000 was investigated in subjects with colorectal cancer, were announced in June 2000. No complete or partial responses to treatment were observed after two courses of treatment with XR5000. Two subjects showed stable disease and 13 subjects experienced disease progression. The company is not planning any further recruitment for this indication.

INDICATION(S) AND RESEARCH PHASE
Lung Cancer – Phase II
Ovarian Cancer – Phase II
Brain Cancer – Phase II

Breast Cancer

alitretinoin, ALRT-1057
Panretin

MANUFACTURER
Ligand Pharmaceuticals

DESCRIPTION
This product consists of 9-*cis*-retinoic acid and is chemically related to vitamin A. It activates all known retinoid receptors. Activation of retinoid receptors regulates the expression of genes controlling processes related to cell differentiation and proliferation. A topical gel formulation of Panretin has been on the market since February 1999 for the treatment of lesions associated with Kaposi's sarcoma.

These new trials are evaluating the effects of an oral capsule formulation for the following new indications: treatment of breast and pediatric cancers (phase II), myelodysplastic syndrome, bronchial metaplasia, and psoriasis and psoriatic disorders (phase II/III).

INDICATION(S) AND RESEARCH PHASE
Breast Cancer – Phase II
Lung Cancer – Phase II/III
Pediatric – Phase II
Psoriasis and Psoriatic Disorders – Phase II/III
White Blood Cell Disorders – Phase II/III

anastrozole, ZD-1033
Arimidex

MANUFACTURER
AstraZeneca

DESCRIPTION

Studies suggest that the female hormone estrogen stimulates the growth of some breast cancer tumors. Arimidex, a non-steroidal compound, is a selective oral inhibitor of the enzyme aromatase. Inhibition of aromatase reduces the production of estrogen. Thus, Arimidex reduces serum concentration of estrogen, an effect that has been shown to be of benefit in postmenopausal women with breast cancer.

Arimidex works differently from Tamoxifen, the most popularly prescribed first-line treatment for breast cancer. Tamoxifen works primarily by blocking estrogen receptors in tumor cells. Arimidex works by suppressing the synthesis of estrogen, such that less hormone is available to bind with estrogen receptors.

Arimidex is being tested in phase III trials for first-line treatment of advanced breast cancer in women who have never received hormonal therapy.

INDICATION(S) AND RESEARCH PHASE
Breast Cancer – Phase III
Pediatric, Pubertal Gynecomastia – Phase IV

anti-angiogenic ribozyme
Angiozyme

MANUFACTURER
Ribozyme Pharmaceuticals

DESCRIPTION
Angiozyme is an enzymatic nucleic acid that specifically inhibits formation of vascular endothelial growth factor receptor (VEGFr), a key component in the angiogenesis pathway. Angiogenesis is the formation of new blood vessels, which occurs with the growth of malignant tumors. Angiozyme is designed to be a broad spectrum cancer drug that cuts off the blood supply to solid tumors, thereby halting the growth and spread of the disease. In November 2000, results of a phase I/II trial of Angiozyme demonstrated the drug was well tolerated with good bioavailability, and supported daily subcutaneous injections for future trials. The company initiated a phase II trial in breast cancer in February 2001 and plans to initiate other trials in lung, colorectal, melanoma, and renal cancer subjects.

INDICATION(S) AND RESEARCH PHASE
Breast Cancer – Phase II

APC8024
unknown

MANUFACTURER
Dendreon Corporation

DESCRIPTION
APC8024 is a vaccine designed to elicit an antibody response to a protein antigen called HER-2/*neu*. HER-2/*neu* is overexpressed in approximately 25% of metastatic breast cancers, ovarian, pancreatic, and colon cancers. APC8024 is being tested in phase I trials.

INDICATION(S) AND RESEARCH PHASE
Breast Cancer – Phase I
Ovarian Cancer – Phase I
Colon Malignancies – Phase I

AR-522
Annamycin

MANUFACTURER
Aronex Pharmaceuticals

DESCRIPTION
Annamycin is an anthracycline analogue intended to overcome multi-drug resistance and irreversible cardiotoxicity associated with anthracycline agents. The compound is being tested in a phase II trial for treatment of refractory breast cancer. Other indications being evaluated include acute myelogenous leukemia (AML), acute lymphocytic leukemia (ALL), and chronic myelogenous leukemia (CML)—all of which are in phase I/II trials. Annamycin is made in a liposomal formulation.

INDICATION(S) AND RESEARCH PHASE
Breast Cancer – Phase II
Leukemia – Phase I/II
Leukemia – Phase I/II
Leukemia – Phase I/II

arcitumomab
CEA-Scan

MANUFACTURER
Immunomedics

DESCRIPTION
CEA-Scan is a monoclonal antibody attached to a carcinoembryonic (CEA) antigen that is radioactively labeled with technetium (Tc99m). CEA is an important cell surface marker expressed by certain tumor cells. This imaging agent can detect various cancer cells associated with CEA expressed tumors. CEA-Scan utilizes proprietary technetium (RAID) technology.

Currently, CEA-Scan is being tested in a phase II/III trial for breast cancer. It is being used to evaluate subjects with suspicious mammograms, palpable and non-palpable lesions.

Also, this agent is in a phase II trial for thyroid cancer. CEA-Scan is used for the diagnosis and localization of primary, residual, recurrent, and metastatic medullary thyroid carcinoma.

Additionally, CEA-Scan is in a phase III for lung cancer. It determines the presence, location and the extent of the metastatic disease in primary and recurrent lung cancer.

INDICATION(S) AND RESEARCH PHASE
Breast Cancer – Phase II/III
Lung Cancer – Phase III
Thyroid Cancer – Phase II

bexarotene
Targretin-capsule

MANUFACTURER
Ligand Pharmaceuticals

DESCRIPTION
Targretin, which selectively stimulates a retinoid subtype receptor, is being developed in an oral capsule formulation for the treatment of lung and breast cancer, head and neck cancer, cutaneous T-cell lymphoma (CTCL), and psoriasis and psoriatic disorders. The drug is in phase II trials for head and neck cancer, phase II/III trials for breast cancer, CTCL, and psoriasis and psoriatic disorders, and phase III trials for non-small cell lung cancer.

INDICATION(S) AND RESEARCH PHASE
Psoriasis and Psoriatic Disorders – Phase II/III
Lung Cancer – Phase III
Breast Cancer – Phase II/III
Head and Neck Cancer – Phase II
Lymphoma – Phase II/III

capecitabine/docetaxel
Xeloda/Taxotere

MANUFACTURER
Hoffmann-La Roche

DESCRIPTION
Xeloda and Taxotere, two established chemotherapies, are being tested as a combination therapy for the treatment of metastatic breast cancer. Xeloda is metabolized in the body to 5-fluorouracil, an active anti-metabolite that can cause cancer cell death and decrease tumor size. Taxotere acts by disrupting the microtubular network in cells, thereby interfering with cellular functions such as cell division.

Results of a phase III trial of Taxotere/Xeloda were announced in December 2000 at the San Antonio Breast Cancer Symposium. The trial indicated that combined treatment with Xeloda, an oral agent, and Taxotere, given by infusion, significantly extended survival in subjects with metastatic breast cancer for an average of three months compared to treatment with Taxotere alone. The Xeloda/Taxotere trial was conducted in the United States and Australia, among other locations, and involved subjects with metastatic breast cancer previously treated with anthracycline chemotherapy. The trial was sponsored by Roche; Xeloda is manufactured by Roche, and Taxotere is manufactured by Aventis.

INDICATION(S) AND RESEARCH PHASE
Breast Cancer – Phase III completed

CI-1033
unknown

MANUFACTURER
Pfizer

DESCRIPTION
CI-1033 is being investigated in clinical studies involving erbB positive cancers located in the breast, lung, head, and neck. The objective of the CI-1033 program is to achieve control of cancer via EGFR tyrosine kinase inhibition, without the side effect burden of cytotoxic agents.

INDICATION(S) AND RESEARCH PHASE
Breast Cancer – Phase I
Lung Cancer – Phase I
Head and Neck Cancer – Phase I

cisplatin/epinephrine
IntraDose

MANUFACTURER
Matrix Pharmaceutical

DESCRIPTION
IntraDose is a biodegradable collagen carrier matrix combined with a vasoconstrictor. The gel is injected directly into tumors where it localizes high concentrations of cisplatin, a widely used anticancer drug. It is currently being tested for several indications, including head and neck, breast, malignant melanoma, esophageal, and primary hepatocellular cancer.

A phase II trial of IntraDose Injectable Gel produced durable responses in subjects with colorectal cancer that had metastasized to the liver. Nine of 31 subjects who received IntraDose responded to therapy. Six subjects experienced a complete response (100% reduction in viable tumor volume of treated tumors) while the other three subjects demonstrated a partial response (at least a 50% reduction of viable tumor volume). Eight of the nine treatment responders have had durable responses with no relapse at the site of treatment. The average duration of response for the nine responders is now seven months with the longest response being one year. IntraDose was well tolerated by subjects.

INDICATION(S) AND RESEARCH PHASE
Breast Cancer – Phase II
Cancer/Tumors (Unspecified) – Phase II
Colorectal Cancer – Phase II completed
Esophageal Cancer – Phase II
Liver Cancer – Phase II
Malignant Melanoma – Phase II
Head and Neck Cancer – NDA submitted

CP-358,774
unknown

MANUFACTURER
OSI Pharmaceuticals

DESCRIPTION
CP-358,774 is a small molecule inhibitor of the epidermal growth factor receptor (EGFR)-tyrosine kinase. This drug targets the underlying molecular changes involving oncogenes and tumor suppressor genes, which play critical roles in the conversion of normal cells into cancerous cells. Increased expression of EGFR is an aberration frequently associated with a variety of cancers including ovarian, pancreatic, non-small cell lung cancers, and squamous cell cancers of the head and neck. The phase II clinical program is designed to assess CP-358,774 both as a single agent and in combination with existing chemotherapy regimens.

INDICATION(S) AND RESEARCH PHASE
Breast Cancer – Phase II
Lung Cancer – Phase II completed
Ovarian Cancer – Phase II
Head and Neck Cancer – Phase II

docetaxel hydrate
Taxotere

MANUFACTURER
Aventis

DESCRIPTION
Many drugs for the treatment of cancer and other diseases originate in plants, many of them highly poisonous. Taxotere (docetaxel hydrate), an agent that inhibits the formation of new protoplasm, is derived from the renewable evergreen needles of the genus *Taxus* (Yew). Taxotere acts by disrupting the microtubular network in cells that is essential for cell division and many other cellular functions. The drug is approved for use in the United States for treatment of refractory breast cancer, refractory non-small cell lung

cancer (NSCLC), and locally advanced or metastatic breast cancer.

New phase II/III trials are under way in head and neck, gastric, and ovarian cancers. Taxotere is also being tested either alone or in combination with other chemotherapy agents in the earlier stages of breast cancer, NSCLC, and others tumors.

Phase I extension studies are under way for brain metastasis and lung cancer.

INDICATION(S) AND RESEARCH PHASE
Gastric Cancer – Phase II/III
Head and Neck Cancer – Phase II/III
Lung Cancer – Phase II/III
Ovarian Cancer – Phase II/III
Breast Cancer – Phase III/IV
Brain Cancer – Phase I
Lung Cancer – Phase I

doxorubicin HCl
Doxil, Caelyx

MANUFACTURER
Alza (Sequus Pharmaceuticals)

DESCRIPTION
Doxil is a liposomal formulation of doxorubicin hydrochloride, an intravenous chemotherapy agent. This anthracycline anti-tumor agent is currently on the market for treatment of Kaposi's sarcoma. The drug uses a novel, targeted delivery system to help evade recognition and uptake by the immune system so that the liposomes can circulate in the body longer. A long circulation time increases the likelihood that the liposomes and their pharmaceutical contents will reach their targeted tumor site. Doxil may act through an ability to bind DNA and inhibit nucleic acid synthesis.

The company reported that Doxil is being tested in phase II/III trials for the additional indications of breast, liver, lung, and prostate cancers, as well as phase II for unspecified cancers and tumors.

Alza markets this product in the United States under the trade name Doxil; however, it is marketed under the name Caelyx in other areas. Schering-Plough has exclusive international marketing rights to Caelyx, excluding Japan and Israel, through a distribution agreement with Alza.

INDICATION(S) AND RESEARCH PHASE
Breast Cancer – Phase II/III
Liver Cancer – Phase II/III
Lung Cancer – Phase II/III
Prostate Cancer – Phase II/III
Cancer/Tumors (Unspecified) – Phase II

doxorubicin/docetaxel
Doxil/Taxotere

MANUFACTURER
Alza (Sequus Pharmaceuticals)

DESCRIPTION
Doxil and Taxotere are two chemotherapy agents being tested together to treat subjects with breast cancer. Doxil is a liposomal formulation of doxorubicin HCl, an intravenous chemotherapy agent. The drug uses a novel, targeted delivery system to help evade recognition and uptake by the immune system so that the liposomes can circulate in the body longer. A long circulation time increases the likelihood that the liposomes and their pharmaceutical contents will reach their targeted tumor site. Doxil may act through an ability to bind DNA and inhibit nucleic acid synthesis.

Drugs for the treatment of cancer and other diseases can originate in plants, many of them highly poisonous. Taxotere (docetaxel hydrate), an agent that inhibits the formation of new protoplasm, is derived from the renewable evergreen needles of the genus *Taxus* (Yew). Taxotere acts by disrupting the microtubular network in cells that is essential for cell division and many other cellular functions. The drug is approved for use in the United States for treatment of refractory breast, refractory non-small cell lung (NSCLC), and locally advanced or metastatic breast cancer.

This combination chemotherapy is being studied in phase II/III clinical trials for treating the earlier stages of breast cancer.

INDICATION(S) AND RESEARCH PHASE
Breast Cancer – Phase II/III

eflornithine, DFMO (difluoromethylornydil)
unknown

MANUFACTURER
Aventis

DESCRIPTION
Eflornithine is a potent, irreversible inhibitor of ornithine decarboxylase (OCD), an enzyme that is elevated in most tumors and pre-malignant lesions. Eflornithine is currently in a phase III clinical trial to determine the effectiveness of the drug in treating subjects who have newly diagnosed or recurrent bladder cancer. The drug is administered orally in tablet form.

Eflornithine is also in trials for the prevention and treatment of HIV infections, skin cancer, breast cancer, prostate cancer, and cervical dysplasia/cancer.

INDICATION(S) AND RESEARCH PHASE
Bladder Cancer – Phase III
Breast Cancer – Phase II/III
Cervical Dysplasia/Cancer – Phase II
HIV Infection – Phase II
Prostate Cancer – Phase II
Skin Cancer – Phase III

EMD 82633
unknown

MANUFACTURER
Merck KgaA

DESCRIPTION
EMD 82633 is a humanized and bispecific monoclonal antibody derived from mice. These antibodies are altered in such a way that they no longer appear different from human antibodies. This genetic modification prevents immune reactions against foreign substances of animal origin used in humans. In this bispecific drug, one component binds to tumor cells, while the other activates the body's own CD8 "killer cells" to attack cancer cells.

This new drug is being given as an adjuvant therapy to subjects who have not been adequately helped by conventional forms of treatment, such as chemotherapy. EMD 82633 is being tested in trials for the treatment of renal cancer, head and neck cancer, breast cancer, bladder cancer, and ovarian cancer.

Breast Cancer / 165

INDICATION(S) AND RESEARCH PHASE
Bladder Cancer – Phase II
Breast Cancer – Phase II
Cancer/Tumors (Unspecified) – Phase II
Head and Neck Cancer – Phase II
Ovarian Cancer – Phase II
Renal Cell Carcinoma – Phase II

ERA-923
unknown

MANUFACTURER
Wyeth-Ayerst

DESCRIPTION
ERA-923 is a novel tissue selective estrogen receptor (ER) modulator being evaluated for the treatment of advanced breast cancer. The drug is currently in phase II development.

INDICATION(S) AND RESEARCH PHASE
Breast Cancer – Phase II

exisulind
Aptosyn

MANUFACTURER
Cell Pathways

DESCRIPTION
Aptosyn (exisulind) belongs to a novel class of compounds called selective apoptotic anti-neoplastic drugs (SAANDs). SAANDs inhibit a form of cyclic GMP phosphodiesterase and selectively induce apoptosis in abnormally growing precancerous and cancerous cells. Aptosyn is being tested for several indications and is in five different trials for adenomatous polyposis coli (APC) and familial adenomatous polyposis coli; two of these trials are specifically for pediatric subjects.

The company received a non-approvable letter from the FDA in September 2000 for one of the trials for the treatment of familial adenomatous polyposis. The company intends to amend the NDA and request a meeting to address the deficiencies and the possible requirement for additional clinical data.

Additionally, Aptosyn is being tested in trials for the treatment of prostate cancer, lung cancer, breast cancer, sporadic colonic polyps, and Barrett's esophagus disease.

INDICATION(S) AND RESEARCH PHASE
Adenomatous Polyposis Coli – Non-approvable letter
Pediatric, Familial Adenomatous Polyposis Coli – Phase II
Adenomatous Polyposis Coli – Phase I/II
Barrett's Esophagus Disease – Phase II
Prostate Cancer – Phase II/III
Breast Cancer – Phase II/III
Lung Cancer – Phase Ib
Colon Polyps – Phase II/III

exisulind/capecitabine
Apotsyn/Xeloda

MANUFACTURER
Cell Pathways

DESCRIPTION
Aptosyn (exisulind) in combination with Roche Laboratories' Xeloda (capecitabine) is in a phase I/II trial for the treatment of breast cancer. Aptosyn, an oral anti-cancer medication with a unique mechanism of action, has none of the severe side effects seen with traditional chemotherapeutic agents, such as neutropenia, nausea, vomiting, hair loss, and weight loss. Xeloda is currently the only approved agent for the treatment of advanced breast cancer that has failed to respond to taxane- or anthracycline-based therapies. The combination of Aptosyn with Xeloda, a well tolerated oral chemotherapeutic agent, should provide enhanced activity with little toxicity and is an easy to use outsubject treatment because of its oral regime.

INDICATION(S) AND RESEARCH PHASE
Breast Cancer – Phase I/II

exisulind/docetaxel
Aposyn/Taxotere

MANUFACTURER
Cell Pathways

DESCRIPTION
Aptosyn is a sulfone derivative of sulindac, a non-steroidal anti-inflammatory compound being tested with Rhone-Poulenc Rorer's Taxotere for the treatment of prostate, lung, and breast cancer as well as for solid tumors. Aptosyn (exisulind) is the first product candidate from a novel class of compounds under development by Cell Pathways, called selective apoptotic anti-neoplastic drugs (SAANDs). SAANDs inhibit cyclic GMP phosphodiesterase and selectively induce apoptosis in abnormally growing precancerous and cancerous cells. Because SAANDs do not induce apoptosis in normal cells, they do not produce the serious side effects normally associated with traditional chemotherapeutic agents. They also do not inhibit cyclooxygenase (COX I or COX II) and have not exhibited the gastric and renal toxicities reported to be associated with non-steroidal anti-inflammatory drugs (NSAIDs), including the COX II inhibitors.

Both companies will jointly share the cost of the trials and will retain all marketing rights to its respective products.

INDICATION(S) AND RESEARCH PHASE
Prostate Cancer – Phase I/II
Breast Cancer – Phase I/II
Lung Cancer – Phase I/II
Lung Cancer – Phase III
Cancer/Tumors (Unspecified) – Phase I

FK-317
unknown

MANUFACTURER
Fujisawa Healthcare

DESCRIPTION
Fujisawa has developed a new anti-cancer medication, FK-317, that originally was developed as an antibiotic. The molecule, known as a dihydrobenzoxazine, underwent preliminary testing in 31 subjects with solid tumors that were refractory to other chemotherapeutic treatments. The company reported that tumor reduction was observed in four subjects, two of whom achieved complete remission. Side effects and other toxicities such as leukopenia (decreased white blood cells) and neutropenia were

modest in comparison to other established treatments.

It is unclear how exactly this compound works to limit the growth of cancer, but it seems to influence the process by which cells reproduce themselves. Currently, FK-317 is given at a dose of 24 mg/day intravenously and it is being evaluated in phase II trials. Scientists are testing it in a variety of solid tumors such as prostate, breast, and skin cancer.

INDICATION(S) AND RESEARCH PHASE
Breast Cancer – Phase II
Cancer/Tumors (Unspecified) – Phase II
Prostate Cancer – Phase II
Skin Cancer – Phase II

FLT3 ligand
Mobist

MANUFACTURER
ImClone Systems

DESCRIPTION
Mobist is a hematopoietic growth factor being tested exvivo. It is a stem cell mobilizer and potential anti-tumor agent. Mobist is being evaluated in phase II trials for treatment of breast cancer, solid tumors, non-Hodgkin's lymphoma, and ovarian cancer.

INDICATION(S) AND RESEARCH PHASE
Cancer/Tumors (Unspecified) – Phase II
Breast Cancer – Phase II
Lymphoma, Non-Hodgkin's – Phase II
Ovarian Cancer – Phase II

G3139/docetaxel
Genasense/Taxotere

MANUFACTURER
Genta

DESCRIPTION
Genasense (G3139) attacks Bcl-2, a protein that is over-expressed in many forms of cancer. Bcl-2 appears to contribute to the resistance of these diseases to standard treatment. Genta is using its proprietary antisense approach to first decrease the expression of Bcl-2, and then to administer state-of-the-art anticancer therapy in an effort to improve subject outcome. Genasense in combination with docetaxel is in trials for treatment of breast and prostate cancer.

INDICATION(S) AND RESEARCH PHASE
Breast Cancer – Phase I/II
Prostate Cancer – Phase II

gemcitabine HCl
Gemzar

MANUFACTURER
Eli Lilly

DESCRIPTION
Gemzar, a nucleoside analogue, is a novel chemotherapeutic agent that mimics a natural building block of DNA. Gemzar disrupts the process of cell replication and thereby slows or stops progression of the disease. The drug is administered intravenously.

Gemzar is currently indicated as first-line treatment of locally advanced or metastatic pancreatic cancer and, in combination with cisplatin, for locally advanced or metastatic non-small cell lung cancer.

INDICATION(S) AND RESEARCH PHASE
Breast Cancer – Phase III
Lung Cancer – FDA approved
Ovarian Cancer – Phase III
Pancreatic Cancer – FDA approved

goserelin acetate
Zoladex IVF

MANUFACTURER
AstraZeneca

DESCRIPTION
Zoladex IVF is a luteinizing hormone-releasing hormone (LHRH) analogue for use with in vitro fertilization. Currently, Zoladex IVF is being evaluated in a phase III clinical trial for infertility. It is also in phase III trials for premenopausal adjuvant breast cancer.

INDICATION(S) AND RESEARCH PHASE
Infertility – Phase III
Breast Cancer – Phase III

GPX-100
unknown

MANUFACTURER
Gem Pharmaceuticals

DESCRIPTION
GPX-100 is a noncardiotoxic version of the anticancer drug Adriamycin. Adriamycin, an anthracycline, is a commonly used drug in the treatment of cancers, including metastatic breast cancer. The cytotoxic effect of Adriamycin on malignant cells and its toxic effects on various organs are thought to be related to genetic insertion (nucleotide base intercalation) and cell membrane lipid binding activities. Intercalation inhibits both nucleotide replication and enzyme activity of DNA and RNA polymerases. The interaction of Adriamycin with topoisomerase II to form DNA-cleavable complexes appears to be an important mechanism of Adriamycin cell-killing activity. The drug's cellular membrane binding may affect a variety of cellular functions.

Unfortunately, Adriamycin and related drugs may produce irreversible damage to the heart if the subject receives too many doses. Thus, although Adriamycin may eliminate the tumor, if the cancer returns the drug often cannot be administered again because of the significant risk of heart failure and possible death. The company claims to have developed a platform technology that allows the chemical conversion of any standard anthracycline to a closely related analog that cannot be converted by the body to the cardiotoxic metabolite. GPX-100 is presently in phase II clinical trials in metastatic breast cancer as well as pediatric phase II trials for leukemia.

INDICATION(S) AND RESEARCH PHASE
Cancer/Tumors (Unspecified) – Phase II
Breast Cancer – Phase II
Pediatric, Leukemia – Phase II

HER-2/neu dendritic cell vaccine
unknown

MANUFACTURER
Corixa Corporation

DESCRIPTION
The HER-2/*neu* dendritic cell vaccine is currently undergoing phase I trials for breast and ovarian cancer.

INDICATION(S) AND RESEARCH PHASE
Breast Cancer – Phase I
Ovarian Cancer – Phase I
Vaccines – Phase I

ibandronate
Bonviva

MANUFACTURER
Hoffmann-La Roche

DESCRIPTION
Bonviva (ibandronate) belongs to the "third generation" of a relatively new class of drugs known as bisphosphonates. Bisphosphonates inhibit bone turnover by decreasing the resorption of bone. They work directly by inhibiting the recruitment and function of osteoclasts, which are bone-resorbing cells, and indirectly by stimulating osteoblasts, which are bone-forming cells. Other formulations of bisphosphonates have previously been approved for the treatment of Paget's disease and hypercalcemia of cancer.

INDICATION(S) AND RESEARCH PHASE
Osteoporosis – Phase III
Breast Cancer – Phase III

ICI-182,780
Faslodex

MANUFACTURER
AstraZeneca

DESCRIPTION
Studies suggest that the female hormone estrogen stimulates the growth of some breast cancer tumors. Faslodex is a synthetic estrogen blocker that works by down-regulating the activity of the estrogen receptor. If estrogen is unable to bind to a receptor then it cannot start the complex processes leading to cancer-cell growth. Formerly described as a pure anti-estrogen, Faslodex is now referred to as a selective estrogen receptor down-regulator (SERD).

Initial studies showed that SERDs appear to be more effective against breast cancer and showed less occurrence of secondary endometrial cancer as compared to tamoxifen.

The company expects to file an NDA for the second line treatment of advanced breast cancer in early 2001. The drug is in phase III trials as a first line treatment of advanced breast cancer. The NDA filing for this indication is expected in 2002.

INDICATION(S) AND RESEARCH PHASE
Breast Cancer – Phase III completed
Endometrial Cancer – Phase II
Breast Cancer – Phase III

IMC-C225, CPT-11
unknown

MANUFACTURER
ImClone Systems

DESCRIPTION
IMC-C225 is a chimerized (part mouse, part human) monoclonal antibody that may help fight cancer cells when used in conjunction with radiation therapy or other chemotherapy agents. This antibody selectively blocks the epidermal growth factor receptor (EGFr), which may be present in greater amounts on actively growing tumor cells. Since many cancers use specific growth factors to stimulate tumor cell growth, blocking this receptor may inhibit the cancer from increasing in size and spreading throughout the body.

The company is conducting phase III clinical trials evaluating IMC-C225 in combination with radiotherapy and with chemotherapy in subjects with advanced squamous cell head and neck carcinoma. IMC-C225 is in trials for several other indications in combination with various anti-cancer agents.

INDICATION(S) AND RESEARCH PHASE
Breast Cancer – Phase I/II
Head and Neck Cancer – Phase III
Lung Cancer – Phase III
Prostate Cancer – Phase I/II
Renal Cell Carcinoma – Phase II
Pancreatic Cancer – Phase II
Colorectal Cancer – Phase II

IMMU-MN14, anti-CEA
CEA-Cide

MANUFACTURER
Immunomedics

DESCRIPTION
Carcinoembryonic antigen (CEA) is a protein-polysaccharide complex released in the blood stream by certain cancers, especially colon carcinoma. This antigenic substance may provide early diagnosis when used as a therapeutic marker in immunologic tests. The CEA complex may also be targeted by specialized monoclonal antibodies in the design of a biologic therapeutic.

CEA-Cide is a novel monoclonal antibody that is designed for radioimmunotherapy (with 90 Y-labeled humanized MN-14). This drug is being tested in phase II trials for the treatment of advanced metastatic and CEA-producing cancers, particularly colorectal cancer. Other indications may include breast cancer, female reproductive system cancer, ovarian cancer, lung cancer, and pancreatic cancer.

INDICATION(S) AND RESEARCH PHASE
Breast Cancer – Phase II
Cancer/Tumors (Unspecified) – Phase II
Colorectal Cancer – Phase II
Lung Cancer – Phase II
Ovarian Cancer – Phase II
Pancreatic Cancer – Phase II

INGN 241 (mda-7)
unknown

MANUFACTURER
Introgen Therapeutics

DESCRIPTION
INGN 241 is the combination of Introgen's proprietary adenoviral delivery system with the mda-7 gene. INGN 241 is in a phase I trial for solid tumors in 15 subjects. Preclinical results with mda-7 demonstrate expression of mda-7 appears to be lost earlier in tumor progression and also indicate

that mda-7 may be easily combined with other tumor suppressor genes for additive effects. Additionally INGN 241 is in Preclinical development for lung and breast cancer.

INDICATION(S) AND RESEARCH PHASE
Breast Cancer – Preclinical
Lung Cancer – Preclinical
Cancer/Tumors (Unspecified) – Phase I

INGN-201, adenoviral p53
unknown

MANUFACTURER
Introgen Therapeutics

DESCRIPTION
INGN-201 is a p53 gene therapy cancer product. It has been tested as a treatment for a variety of solid tumor cancers with administration via intratumoral injection. The drug was well tolerated according to the company, and additional trials are under way using an intravenous infusion in order to reach more types of cancers. The tumor-suppressing p53 gene encodes a protein that responds to damage involving cellular DNA by terminating cell division. Normal p53 genes are delivered into cancer cells of the subject through an adenoviral vector.

The developers of INGN-201 have signed a Cooperative Research and Development Agreement (CRADA) with the National Cancer Institute to evaluate the potential effectiveness and superiority of the drug over other treatments against breast, ovarian, bladder, prostate, and brain cancers in phase I and phase II trials. A phase III trial in head and neck cancer was initiated in March 2000.

INDICATION(S) AND RESEARCH PHASE
Head and Neck Cancer – Phase III
Bladder Cancer – Phase I
Brain Cancer – Phase I
Breast Cancer – Phase I
Bronchoalveolar Cancer – Phase I
Ovarian Cancer – Phase I
Prostate Cancer – Phase I
Lung Cancer – Phase II
Cancer/Tumors (Unspecified) – Phase I

interleukin (IL)
MultiKine

MANUFACTURER
CEL-SCI Corporation

DESCRIPTION
MultiKine is a multiple combination therapy made from a natural, cytokine cocktail (which includes interleukin-2 (IL-2), IL-β, TNF-α, Gm-CSF and an IFN-γ/immunomodulator). It is being tested for the treatment of advanced head and neck cancer in subjects who have previously failed standard therapy, and for head and neck cancer treatment prior to surgery.

MultiKine has just completed two phase II trials for head and neck cancer. The first trial consisted of 16 subjects and tested four different doses of MultiKine in four subjects each. To qualify for the trial, the subjects must have had a recurrence of the cancer and failed conventional therapy.

The company reported that in an earlier and still ongoing study conducted in newly diagnosed head and neck cancer subjects, 10 subjects had tumor reductions prior to surgery within a short time period. Three of ten subjects had tumor reductions exceeding 50%, and one additional subject with a tumor that was nearly three inches in diameter had a complete clinical response. Lastly, two subjects refused surgery because they were satisfied with their condition after treatment with MultiKine.

A phase III trial to test MultiKine prior to surgery and/or radiation may reduce the fairly high recurrence rate of head and neck cancer. This drug is also in trials for prostate cancer, HIV, and breast cancer.

INDICATION(S) AND RESEARCH PHASE
Head and Neck Cancer – Phase II
HIV Infection – Phase II
Breast Cancer – Phase I
Prostate Cancer – Phase I/II

ISIS 2503
unknown

MANUFACTURER
Isis Pharmaceuticals

DESCRIPTION
ISIS 2503 is a potent, selective antisense inhibitor of H-ras gene expression. Antisense drugs inhibit the production of disease-causing proteins by altering the genetic information, which messenger RNA uses to produce new protein. H-ras is one of a family of ras genes that are involved in the process by which cells receive and send signals that affect their behavior. The company claims that substantial evidence exists to support a direct role for the ras gene products in the development and maintenance of human cancers.

In phase II trials, the compound is being evaluated as a single agent in subjects with colon, breast, pancreatic, and non-small cell lung cancers. These trials will provide preliminary data on the anti-tumor activity of ISIS 2503 against these common tumor types. Approximately ten sites in the United States and Europe will enroll 15 to 30 subjects per tumor type in these trials. The company plans future trials of ISIS 2503 in combination with approved cancer therapies.

INDICATION(S) AND RESEARCH PHASE
Breast Cancer – Phase II
Colon Malignancies – Phase II
Lung Cancer – Phase II
Pancreatic Cancer – Phase II

ISIS 3521
unknown

MANUFACTURER
Isis Pharmaceuticals

DESCRIPTION
ISIS 3521 is an antisense inhibitor of protein kinase C-alpha (PKC-α) expression. PKC-α is a member of a multigene family of signal transduction proteins that regulate information flow in and out of cells, and modulate cellular responses to the environment. ISIS 3521 is being tested in trials for the treatment of breast and lung cancer.

Results of a phase I/II trial indicated that ISIS 3521 in combination with standard chemotherapy agents has promising activity in subjects with stage IIIB or stage IV non-small cell lung cancer, based on both survival time and response rate. To date, the average survival time of subjects in the trial is 19 months. Two subjects have experienced complete responses and 18 subjects have experienced a partial response. Additionally, four of 48 (8%) subjects experienced a minor response, defined as a 25–50% reduction in tumor size measurements, and 16 (9%) subjects had a stabilization of their disease. Isis Pharmaceuticals initiated a phase III trial in October 2000.

INDICATION(S) AND RESEARCH PHASE
Breast Cancer – Phase II
Lung Cancer – Phase III

ISIS 5132, CGP 69846A
unknown

MANUFACTURER
Isis Pharmaceuticals

DESCRIPTION
ISIS 5132 is a potent antisense inhibitor of the enzyme c-Raf-1 kinase. Antisense drugs inhibit the production of disease-causing proteins by altering the genetic information, which messenger RNA uses to produce new protein. c-Raf kinase plays a role in signal processes that regulate cell growth and proliferation. It is one of a family of raf genes thought to play an important role in the development of some solid tumors. The company reports that activated-raf has also been detected in a substantial variety of human cancers including small cell lung carcinoma and breast cancer. For example, it has been reported that 60% of all lung carcinoma cells express unusually high levels of normal c-Raf mRNA and protein.

The sponsor companies reported that results from phase I studies, which examined subjects with a wide variety of solid tumors, demonstrated that the drug was well tolerated and that several subjects experienced disease stabilization. The companies are planning additional phase I safety studies involving the drug in combination with currently approved chemotherapies. Phase II clinical trials examining ISIS 5132 as a single agent therapy in subjects with breast, lung, colon, pancreatic, and prostate cancers are under way.

INDICATION(S) AND RESEARCH PHASE
Breast Cancer – Phase II
Cancer/Tumors (Unspecified) – Phase II
Colon Malignancies – Phase II
Lung Cancer – Phase II
Pancreatic Cancer – Phase II
Prostate Cancer – Phase II

letrozole
Femara

MANUFACTURER
Novartis

DESCRIPTION
Femara is an oral nonsteroidal aromatase inhibitor. Aromatase inhibitors bind to the enzyme aromatase, which is responsible for converting the precursor hormone androstenedione into estrogen in tissues such as fat, liver, and muscle.

Femara is currently being tested in a phase III trial as adjuvant therapy for breast cancer. In January 2001, the FDA approved a new indication for Femara as a first-line treatment for postmenopausal women with hormone receptor positive or hormone receptor unknown, advanced or metastatic breast cancer. Femara was approved for treatment of advanced breast cancer in 1997 in women whose cancer had not responded to antiestrogen drugs.

INDICATION(S) AND RESEARCH PHASE
Breast Cancer – Phase III
Breast Cancer – FDA approved

marimastat, BB-2516
unknown

MANUFACTURER
British Biotech plc

DESCRIPTION
Marimastat is an inhibitor of matrix metalloproteinase (MMP), a family of naturally occurring enzymes that are overproduced in a number of disease states. This is especially true of cancer, where MMPs are involved in the spread and local growth of tumors. Both angiogenesis and metastasis require MMPs during tumor invasion. Anti-angiogenic strategies, unlike other therapeutic approaches, do not aim to directly destroy or "kill" the tumor or cause tumor regression. Rather, they are designed to prevent the further growth of tumors by limiting their blood supply. Because peripheral tumor cells could theoretically survive on a diffusion-dependent basis, anti-angiogenic drugs may prove most effective when given in combination with other standard cytotoxic regimens. Marimastat is in phase III development for the treatment of cancer.

In 1999, British Biotech and Schering-Plough Corporation signed an agreement to develop and commercialize British Biotech's metalloproteinase inhibitors, including marimastat.

INDICATION(S) AND RESEARCH PHASE
Pancreatic Cancer – Phase III
Lung Cancer – Phase III
Breast Cancer – Phase III
Brain Cancer – Phase III completed
Ovarian Cancer – Phase III

MDX-210
unknown

MANUFACTURER
Medarex

DESCRIPTION
MDX-210 is a bispecific (target-trigger) monoclonal antibody (MAb)-based treatment being developed for cancers with specific markers (HER-2/neu positive), including renal cell, non-small cell lung, pancreatic, and kidney cancers. Phase II trials have been completed for kidney, prostate, and ovarian cancer. Phase III development for ovarian cancer has commenced in Europe.

INDICATION(S) AND RESEARCH PHASE
Prostate Cancer – Phase II completed
Renal Cell Carcinoma – Phase II completed
Colon Malignancies – Phase II
Breast Cancer – Phase II
Gastric Cancer – Phase II
Pancreatic Cancer – Phase II
Lung Cancer – Phase II
Ovarian Cancer – Phase III

MDX-447, H-447
unknown

MANUFACTURER
Medarex

DESCRIPTION
MDX-447 is a novel biological drug designed to stimulate an immune response against cancer cells. Certain cancer cells contain and express large amounts of unique proteins (such as epidermal growth factor receptors), which MDX-447 is directed to recognize. MDX-447 attaches itself both to these cancer proteins and to macrophages that specialize in killing foreign material.

The binding together of the cancer cells and the immune cells by MDX-447 signals the body to destroy the tumor. MDX-447 may offer a new therapeutic alternative to cancer subjects who have been unresponsive to conventional therapies. This agent is unique since it has two receptors on its surface, one that can attract the cancer cell and one that can attract a killer immune cell. This dual nature of the drug is why it is known as a "bispecific antibody."

This type of drug is designed to be more efficient than current anti-cancer therapies, and may have effects that last longer. This technology may also be useful in the development of an "anti-cancer vaccine" in the future. MDX-447 is currently being tested as an intravenous solution in phase II trials for multiple tumor indications, which include brain, bladder, breast, head and neck, and lung cancer.

INDICATION(S) AND RESEARCH PHASE
Brain Cancer – Phase II
Bladder Cancer – Phase II
Breast Cancer – Phase II
Head and Neck Cancer – Phase II
Lung Cancer – Phase II

MGI-114, hydroxymethylacylfulvene, HMAF
Irofulven

MANUFACTURER
MGI Pharma

DESCRIPTION
Irofulven (MGI-114) is the first product candidate being developed by MGI Pharma from its family of anti-cancer compounds called acylfulvenes. Early trials demonstrated that Irofulven is absorbed rapidly by tumor cells, and once inside binds to DNA and protein targets. The binding interferes with DNA replication and cell division, leading to tumor-specific apoptosis. The drug is being tested in a series of trials for a variety of cancers.

In November 2000, results from a phase II trial of Irofulven indicated that the drug produced anti-tumor activity in subjects with advanced pancreatic cancer who were refractory to gemcitabine (Gemzar). Ten of the 53 subjects enrolled achieved six-month survival and two subjects demonstrated objective responses: one subject experienced tumor shrinkage of 100% and another subject experienced an 84% decrease in tumor mass. A phase III trial was initiated in February 2001.

INDICATION(S) AND RESEARCH PHASE
Breast Cancer – Phase II
Colon Malignancies – Phase II
Renal Cell Carcinoma – Phase II
Cervical Dysplasia/Cancer – Phase II
Lung Cancer – Phase II
Ovarian Cancer – Phase I/II
Colorectal Cancer – Phase II
Prostate Cancer – Phase I/II
Cancer/Tumors (Unspecified) – Phase I/II
Pancreatic Cancer – Phase III
Liver Cancer – Phase II

MPI-5020
unknown

MANUFACTURER
Matrix Pharmaceutical

DESCRIPTION
MPI-5020, a locally injected gel containing the anticancer agent fluorouracil, is a radiopotentiator, which is designed to enhance the cytotoxic (cell-killing) effects of radiation therapy. Radiopotentiators are anticancer drugs that, when used in conjunction with radiation, lead to greater damage to tumor cells than would be possible using either drug or radiation alone. Establishing and maintaining high drug concentrations in the tumor can intensify the radiation effect at the tumor site, resulting in greater tumor control. This antitumor effect may be accomplished without any increased damage to the surrounding tissue. MPI-5020 is being tested in phase I/II trials for the treatment of recurrent and metastatic breast cancer.

INDICATION(S) AND RESEARCH PHASE
Breast Cancer – Phase I/II

paclitaxel/carboplatin/trastuzumab
Taxol/Paraplatin/Herceptin

MANUFACTURER
Bristol-Myers Squibb

DESCRIPTION
Taxol (paclitaxel) is a widely used chemotherapy agent originally developed from compounds found in the bark of the yew tree. The drug works on the microtubules of the cell preventing interphase and mitotic cell functions, thereby destroying the ability of cancer cells to divide. Paraplatin (carboplatin) is a platinum coordination compound used as a cancer chemotherapeutic agent. Herceptin (trastuzumab) is a recombinant DNA-derived humanized monoclonal antibody that selectively binds to the extracellular domain of the human epidermal growth factor receptor-2 protein, HER-2. Herceptin in combination with paclitaxel has been approved by the FDA for the treatment of subjects with metastatic breast cancer whose tumors overexpress the HER-2 protein and who have not received chemotherapy for their metastatic disease.

The addition of weekly Taxol plus Paraplatin to Herceptin (administered separately) is currently being evaluated for the treatment of metastatic breast cancer that overexpresses the HER-2/*neu* oncogene. Results of a phase II trial indicated that Taxol/Paraplatin/Herceptin improved subject response and disease control.

Taxol and Paraplatin are marketed by Bristol-Myers Squibb, and Herceptin is marketed by Genentech.

INDICATION(S) AND RESEARCH PHASE
Breast Cancer – Phase II completed

pure anti-estrogen
unknown

MANUFACTURER
Schering-Plough Corporation

DESCRIPTION
A novel, orally administered pure anti-estrogen agent for breast cancer is being developed in an attempt to provide more complete and longer-lasting regression of breast cancer and other estrogen sensitive tumors. Schering-Plough's pure anti-estrogen is currently in phase III trials.

INDICATION(S) AND RESEARCH PHASE
Breast Cancer – Phase III

r-hCG
Ovidrel

MANUFACTURER
Serono Laboratories

DESCRIPTION
Ovidrel is a sterile powder that contains recombinant human chorionic gonadotropin (r-hCG). The drug has been approved by the FDA for the induction of final follicular maturation and early luteinization in infertile women who have undergone pituitary desensitization and who have been appropriately pretreated with follicle stimulating hormones as part of an assisted reproductive technology (ART) program. Ovidrel is also indicated for the induction of ovulation and pregnancy in anovulatory infertile subjects in whom the cause of infertility is functional and not due to primary ovarian failure. Additionally, r-hCG is in phase II trials for the treatment of breast cancer.

INDICATION(S) AND RESEARCH PHASE
Infertility – FDA approved
Breast Cancer – Phase II

raloxifene, LY-139481
Evista

MANUFACTURER
Eli Lilly

DESCRIPTION
Evista is a selective estrogen receptor modulator for prevention of coronary events (heart attack or cardiac death) in postmenopausal women. A phase III trial is assessing Evista's effect on secondary prevention of coronary events. Evista is also being tested in a phase III study for the prevention of breast cancer.

INDICATION(S) AND RESEARCH PHASE
Coronary Artery Disease – Phase III
Breast Cancer – Phase III

RFS-2000
Rubitecan

MANUFACTURER
SuperGen

DESCRIPTION
Rubitecan is a novel drug in the late stages of phase III development for treating advanced pancreatic cancer. It works by inhibiting an enzyme called topoisomerase-I. This drug is made in an oral form that is an advantage for outpatient treatment compared to intravenous-type cancer drugs that may require a visit to a hospital setting.

In addition to treating pancreatic cancer, Rubitecan is being evaluated in treating a variety of solid tumors, such as in breast, colorectal, lung, ovarian, prostate cancers, metastatic melanoma, and advanced gastric carcinoma. Also, phase II trials in the United States and Europe are testing Rubitecan in blood cancers such as chronic myelomonocytic leukemia (CMML/myelodysplastic syndrome).

Clinical study results noted that Rubitecan was given to a group of end-stage pancreatic cancer subjects who failed all previous conventional therapies. Of the 60 subjects who completed Rubitecan treatment, 31.7% responded favorably with half of the subjects staying alive (the median survival) at 18.6 months. Additionally, 31.7% were stabilized with a 9.7 month median survival rate, and 36.6% were non-responders with a 6.8 month median survival rate.

INDICATION(S) AND RESEARCH PHASE
Pancreatic Cancer – Phase III
Breast Cancer – Phase II
Colorectal Cancer – Phase II
Gastric Cancer – Phase II
Leukemia – Phase II
Malignant Melanoma – Phase II
Ovarian Cancer – Phase II
Myelodysplastic Syndrome – Phase III

SD/01
unknown

MANUFACTURER
Amgen

DESCRIPTION
SD/01 is a sustained duration granulocyte colony stimulating factor (G-CSF) molecule being tested in chemotherapy induced neutropenia. Granulocytes and neutrophils are types of white blood cells that help the immune system protect the body from foreign substances. Amgen states that SD/01 consists of the protein G-CSF to which poly(ethylene) glycol (PEG) has been bound. PEGylated proteins stay circulating longer in the body, and it is thought that subjects may require fewer injections.

SD/01 is currently in a phase III study to evaluate its safety and efficacy in breast cancer subjects.

INDICATION(S) AND RESEARCH PHASE
Breast Cancer – Phase III
Effects of Chemotherapy – Phase III
White Blood Cell Disorders – Phase III

SERM III
unknown

MANUFACTURER
Eli Lilly

DESCRIPTION

A selective estrogen receptor modulator (SERM) is a substance that binds with high affinity to the estrogen receptor (ER) but has tissue specific effects distinct from estradiol. SERMs were originally developed for the treatment of osteoarthritis, as they have been shown to significantly affect bone density in post-menopausal women. SERMS are designed to act "selectively," eliminating some of the risks of estrogen such as undesirable effects on the uterus or breast tissue while supplementing inadequate estrogen supplies in post-menopausal women. Researchers have found that women in the SERM clinical trials for osteoporosis were contracting breast cancer at a rate lower than that of the general population. These phase II studies are evaluating the effects of SERMS specifically as a prophylactic treatment for breast cancer.

INDICATION(S) AND RESEARCH PHASE
Breast Cancer – Phase II

SGN-15/Taxotere
unknown

MANUFACTURER
Seattle Genetics

DESCRIPTION
SGN-15 is an antibody drug conjugate composed of the chimeric monoclonal antibody BR96 chemically linked to the drug doxorubicin with an average of eight drug molecules per each mAb molecule. SGN-15 works by binding to a cell surface Ley-related antigen expressed on many tumor types, rapidly internalizing, and then releasing its payload of drug at the low pH present within the cell through acid catalyzed hydrolysis in the endosome. This mechanism of targeted drug delivery allows for relative sparing of tissues normally affected by non-specific chemotherapy, and represents an attractive strategy for the treatment of tumors expressing the BR96 antigen.

SGN-15 is being tested in a combination therapy with Aventis' drug Taxotere in a phase I/II trial in subjects with breast or colon cancer. This trial is being co-funded by Aventis. Additionally, a phase II trial is testing SGN/Taxotere in hormone refractory prostate cancer.

INDICATION(S) AND RESEARCH PHASE
Breast Cancer – Phase I/II
Prostate Cancer – Phase II
Colon Malignancies – Phase I/II

squalamine
unknown

MANUFACTURER
Magainin Pharmaceuticals

DESCRIPTION
Squalamine is an aminosterol compound isolated from the tissues of the dogfish shark. This drug inhibits salt-and-acid-regulating pumps on endothelial cells that normally line blood vessels, which prevents growth factors from stimulating the cells to form capillaries. It is thought that this activity results in anti-angiogenesis, anti-inflammatory, and anti-tumor effects.

The company is conducting several phase II trials testing squalamine against certain cancers, such as breast cancer and ovarian cancer. Also, there is a phase IIa study against stage IIIB and IV non-small cell lung cancer, conducted at the University of Wisconsin and M.D. Anderson, Houston, TX.

Additional studies are being planned for ovarian cancer, pediatric neuroblastoma, and other solid tumors.

INDICATION(S) AND RESEARCH PHASE
Breast Cancer – Phase II
Lung Cancer – Phase IIa
Ovarian Cancer – Phase II
Cancer/Tumors (Unspecified) – Phase II

T64
unknown

MANUFACTURER
Tularik

DESCRIPTION
T64 is an antifolate that disrupts DNA synthesis through the inhibition of purine biosynthesis. The compound is currently in phase II trials in subjects with head and neck cancer, soft tissue sarcoma, melanoma, breast cancer, and non-small cell lung cancer. Additionally, T64 is in phase I combination trials with gemcitabine, doxorubicin, and paclitaxel. Tularik expects to initiate two additional T64 phase I combination trials with carboplatin and temozolamide in the first quarter of 2001. The T64 trials are being conducted in the United States, the United Kingdom, the Netherlands, and Australia.

INDICATION(S) AND RESEARCH PHASE
Head and Neck Cancer – Phase II
Sarcoma – Phase II
Melanoma – Phase II
Breast Cancer – Phase II
Lung Cancer – Phase II
Cancer/Tumors (Unspecified) – Phase I

T67
unknown

MANUFACTURER
Tularik

DESCRIPTION
T67 is an anti-cancer compound that binds irreversibly to tubulin and inhibits the growth of multi-drug resistant tumors. Tubulin is a protein that polymerizes into chains to form microtubules. Microtubules are essential for cell division, and by disrupting their function, T67 produces cell death and potentially causes tumor shrinkage.

The drug is currently in phase II trials in subjects with non-small cell lung cancer, glioma, colorectal cancer, and breast cancer. It is also in a phase I/II trial for the treatment of hepatocellular carcinoma. These trials are being conducted in the United States, the United Kingdom, Hong Kong, and Taiwan.

INDICATION(S) AND RESEARCH PHASE
Lung Cancer – Phase II
Brain Cancer – Phase II
Colorectal Cancer – Phase II
Breast Cancer – Phase II
Hepatocellular Carcinoma – Phase I/II

tgDCC-E1A, RGG 0853
unknown

MANUFACTURER
Targeted Genetics

DESCRIPTION
The drug E1A may possess multiple cancer-fighting effects, such as reducing expression (also called "down-regulation") of the oncogene HER-2/*neu*. Overexpression of HER-2/*neu* occurs in substantial percentages of ovarian and breast cancer subjects, as well as in cancers of the lung, prostate, and bladder. Furthermore, HER-2/*neu* correlates with poor prognosis, including metastasis—the process by which cancer spreads to other sites in the body.

Clinical phase I trials for breast, ovarian, and head and neck cancers are complete, as well as a phase II trial for head and neck cancer as a single agent. A second phase II has been initiated to test tgDCC-E1A in combination with radiation therapy for the treatment of head and neck squamous cell carcinoma. The phase II trial expects to treat up to 50 subjects who will receive twice-weekly injections of tgDCC-E1A throughout 6-7 weeks of radiation therapy.

INDICATION(S) AND RESEARCH PHASE
Breast Cancer – Phase I completed
Head and Neck Cancer – Phase II
Ovarian Cancer – Phase I completed

trastuzumab
Herceptin

MANUFACTURER
Genentech

DESCRIPTION
Herceptin (trastuzumab) is currently on the market for the treatment of metastatic breast cancer. The Herceptin monoclonal antibody works by binding to HER-2 (human epidermal growth factor receptor-2) present in excessive amounts on the surface of the cancer cells, slowing the growth of HER-2 breast cancer cells.

In collaboration with Hoffmann-La Roche and United States national cooperative groups, Genentech is conducting trials for potential adjuvant treatment of early-stage breast cancer in subjects who overexpress the HER-2 protein.

INDICATION(S) AND RESEARCH PHASE
Breast Cancer – Phase III

unknown
TheraFab

MANUFACTURER
Antisoma plc

DESCRIPTION
TheraFab is the F(ab)(2) fragment of the monoclonal antibody, HMFG1, which is covalently linked to yttrium-90 via CITC-DTPA. Therafab will be used in conjunction with the proprietary RACER technology (Radiolabelled Antibody Combined with External Radiotherapy). The radioactivity labeled monoclonal antibody is used in conjunction with conventional radiation therapy, thereby increasing the radiation exposure of malignant tissue, while relatively sparing the normal surrounding tissue. Initial trials are under way in the treatment of breast cancer.

INDICATION(S) AND RESEARCH PHASE
Breast Cancer – Phase I

unknown
MARstem

MANUFACTURER
Maret Pharmaceuticals

DESCRIPTION
MARstem is a peptide that resembles the human hormone angiotensin. The compound has shown promise as a therapy to stimulate the formation of red blood cells, white blood cells, and platelets when they are below normal levels. In preclinical studies, the drug was shown to minimize neutropenia (decreased number of white blood cells) following chemotherapy or radiation. It is a common effect of chemotherapy to lower the blood levels of neutrophils, which are a specialized type of granular white blood cells. Since neutrophils serve as the first line of defense for the immune system, decreased numbers may predispose individuals to certain infections.

As of November 2000, MARstem is in phase I development as a multilineage hematopoietic therapy (multiple blood cell stimulant) to treat or prevent pancytopenia (a reduction in different types of blood cells) following chemotherapy in breast cancer subjects. It is also in phase I/II trials for the treatment of anemia in chronic renal failure subjects.

INDICATION(S) AND RESEARCH PHASE
Breast Cancer – Phase I
Anemia – Phase I/II

unknown
Detox

MANUFACTURER
Corixa Corporation

DESCRIPTION
Detox is a novel vaccine adjuvant contained in Melacine and Biomira's Theratope vaccines. It is currently in phase III trials for breast cancer.

INDICATION(S) AND RESEARCH PHASE
Breast Cancer – Phase III
Vaccines – Phase III

unknown
Combidex

MANUFACTURER
Advanced Magnetics

DESCRIPTION
Combidex MRI contrast agent was developed to help in the detection, diagnosis and staging of various cancers. The first indication is for the diagnosis of metastatic cancer to assist in directing biopsy and surgery as well as to aid in the staging of a variety of cancers, including breast and prostate cancer. In clinical studies, Combidex significantly reduced the number of false diagnoses (both false positive and false negative nodes) compared to unenhanced MRI

exams. The second indication is for the detection, diagnosis and characterization of benign versus malignant lesions of the liver and spleen.

In phase III clinical trials, post-Combidex MRI showed clear differentiation between normal and metastatic lymph nodes, while a post-gadolinium image showed no differentiation in normal and metastatic nodes when compared with pre-dose images.

INDICATION(S) AND RESEARCH PHASE
Breast Cancer – Phase III/IV
Liver Cancer – Phase III
Prostate Cancer – Phase III/IV

unknown
GnRH Pharmaccine

MANUFACTURER
Aphton Corporation

DESCRIPTION
Aphton's novel GnRH Pharmaccine is an anti-gonadotropin releasing hormone (GnRH) immunogen, which neutralizes the hormone GnRH. Study results indicate that it induces and maintains castration levels of testosterone and reduced levels of prostate-specific antigen (PSA). Chemical castration of this type is a standard therapy to extend the survival of subjects with advanced prostate cancer. GnRH Pharmaccine is also involved in trials for breast cancer, endometrial cancer, endometriosis and prostate cancer.

INDICATION(S) AND RESEARCH PHASE
Prostate Cancer – Phase I/II
Breast Cancer – Phase I/II
Endometrial Cancer – Phase I/II
Endometriosis – Phase I/II

vaccine, anti-cancer
TriAb

MANUFACTURER
Titan Pharmaceuticals

DESCRIPTION
TriAb is an anti-cancer monoclonal antibody based product designed to help the subject's immune system recognize and kill tumor cells. Preliminary results with TriAb have shown that the drug consistently generated an active immune response in both advanced and earlier stage breast cancer subjects. TriAb is currently in phase II trials for the treatment of breast cancer.

INDICATION(S) AND RESEARCH PHASE
Breast Cancer – Phase II

vaccine, breast cancer
Theratope

MANUFACTURER
Biomira

DESCRIPTION
Theratope vaccine works by inducing the body to mount an effective immune response against cancerous cells using a synthetic antigen. Cancer cells secrete substances, known as mucins, which suppress the immune response to cancer and render the body's own cancer-fighting mechanisms ineffective. Scientists found that the cancer antigen called MUC-1 mucin, which is secreted by most cancer cells, inhibits T-cells and causes the immune system to ignore the presence of disease. By producing synthetic mimics of cancer-associated antigens, scientists found a way to sensitize the body into recognizing the cancerous cells as abnormalities.

The aim of this vaccine is to induce appropriate immune responses, which will control the growth of cancers by preventing or delaying metastasis. Theratope vaccine is made as an injectable formulation. The phase III trial is designed to enroll 900 subjects at approximately 75 sites worldwide to test the vaccine for the treatment of recurrent or metastatic breast cancer.

INDICATION(S) AND RESEARCH PHASE
Breast Cancer – Phase III

vaccine, cancer
B-vax

MANUFACTURER
AVAX Technologies

DESCRIPTION
B-Vax is a therapeutic cancer vaccine being developed as a non-toxic, post-surgical experimental treatment for breast cancer. It is in a phase I/II at the University of Tokyo in Japan.

INDICATION(S) AND RESEARCH PHASE
Breast Cancer – Phase I/II

vaccine, cancer
GeneVax

MANUFACTURER
Centocor

DESCRIPTION
GeneVax is a DNA-based vaccine technology in phase I development for the treatment of breast and prostate cancer.

INDICATION(S) AND RESEARCH PHASE
Vaccines – Phase I
Breast Cancer – Phase I
Prostate Cancer – Phase I

votumumab
HumaSPECT/BR

MANUFACTURER
INTRACEL Corporation

DESCRIPTION
HumaSPECT is the trade name for votumumab, which is being tested in different formulations for a variety of indications. HumaSPECT/BR uses a fully human tumor-specific monoclonal antibody (MAb) as a diagnostic imaging agent for breast cancer. The antibody, labeled with radioactive 99-technetium, discloses the tumor location. The drug, given by intramammary injection, is in phase I/II trials as an imaging agent for breast cancer.

INDICATION(S) AND RESEARCH PHASE
Breast Cancer – Phase I/II

YM-511
unknown

MANUFACTURER
Yamanouchi Pharmaceutical

DESCRIPTION
YM-511 is an aromatase inhibitor that is administered in an oral formulation. The drug is being developed in Europe and is currently in phase II trials for the treatment of breast cancer. It is also part of the company's domestic pipeline, where it is in phase II trials for breast cancer, endometriosis and uterine fibroids.

INDICATION(S) AND RESEARCH PHASE
Breast Cancer – Phase II
Endometriosis – Phase II
Uterine Fibroids – Phase II

YM-529, minodronate
unknown

MANUFACTURER
Yamanouchi Pharmaceutical

DESCRIPTION
YM-529 is a bisphosphonate being evaluated for the treatment of multiple myeloma and bone metastasis with breast cancer. The drug is manufactured in both oral and injectable formulations. It is in phase III trials and is part of Yamanouchi's domestic pipeline.

INDICATION(S) AND RESEARCH PHASE
Multiple Myeloma – Phase III
Breast Cancer – Phase III

ZD-0473/AMD 473
unknown

MANUFACTURER
AstraZeneca

DESCRIPTION
ZD-0473 is a new platinum-based anticancer agent designed to deliver an extended spectrum of activity and overcome resistance to currently approved platinum drugs, such as cisplatin and carboplatin. It is being evaluated for the treatment of a range of solid-tumor cancers, including colorectal, non-small cell lung, and bladder cancer, which are resistant to carboplatin. ZD-0473 is formulated in both intravenous and oral forms. The intravenous formulation is in phase II trials and the oral form is in preclinical development.

INDICATION(S) AND RESEARCH PHASE
Bladder Cancer – Phase II
Cancer/Tumors (Unspecified) – Phase II
Colorectal Cancer – Phase II
Lung Cancer – Phase II
Ovarian Cancer – Phase II
Prostate Cancer – Phase II
Breast Cancer – Phase II
Cervical Dysplasia/Cancer – Phase II

Cancer/Tumors (Unspecified)

A4, prodrug
Combretastatin

MANUFACTURER
Bristol-Myers Squibb

DESCRIPTION
Combretastatin is one of a new class of anti-cancer therapies that act by directly reducing a tumor's blood supply. CA4P is different from angiogenic inhibitors now in clinical development in that it attacks pre-existent tumor vasculature, as opposed to anti-angiogenic agents that inhibit the formation of new tumor-associated vasculature. Two phase I/II clinical studies are being conducted in the United States. Interim results from these studies have demonstrated significant reduction in blood flow to existing solid tumors including certain instances of total tumor regression. Bristol-Myers Squibb licensed the technology for the systemic use of CA4P from OXiGENE in December 1999.

INDICATION(S) AND RESEARCH PHASE
Cancer/Tumors (Unspecified) – Phase I/II

ABX-EGF
unknown

MANUFACTURER
Abgenix

DESCRIPTION
ABX-EGF is a fully human monoclonal antibody being developed for the treatment of several malignancies. ABX-EGF targets the receptor for human epidermal growth factor (EGFr), which is overexpressed on some of the most prevalent human tumor types including lung, prostate, pancreatic, colorectal, renal cell, and esophageal. It has been demonstrated that cancer cells can become dependent on growth signals mediated through the EGFr. ABX-EGF in mouse models can both eradicate established human tumors and block the growth of human tumors. ABX-EGF is being co-developed with Immunex.

INDICATION(S) AND RESEARCH PHASE
Cancer/Tumors (Unspecified) – Phase I

AE-941
Neovastat

MANUFACTURER
AEterna Laboratories

DESCRIPTION
Neovastat is an angiogenesis inhibitor being tested for the treatment of non-small cell lung cancer, psoriasis, multiple myeloma, and kidney cancer, among other indications.

A phase II trial for multiple myeloma was initiated in October 2000 and will treat 120 subjects and include approximately 20 sites across North America and Europe. Trial results are expected in the summer of 2002.

Additionally, a phase III trial was initiated in May 2000 for kidney cancer, which will include 270 subjects at sites in North America and Europe.

INDICATION(S) AND RESEARCH PHASE
Lung Cancer – Phase III
Psoriasis and Psoriatic Disorders – Phase I/II completed
Cancer/Tumors (Unspecified) – Phase I/II completed
Multiple Myeloma – Phase II
Renal Cell Carcinoma – Phase III
Macular Degeneration – Phase I completed

AZD3409
unknown

MANUFACTURER
AstraZeneca

DESCRIPTION
AZD3409 is a farnesyl-transferase inhibitor (FAR) indicated for the treatment of solid tumors. It is currently in phase I trials.

INDICATION(S) AND RESEARCH PHASE
Cancer/Tumors (Unspecified) – Phase I

AZD6474
unknown

MANUFACTURER
AstraZeneca

DESCRIPTION
AZD6474 is an anti-angiogenic vascular endothelial cell growth factor receptor tyrosine kinase inhibitor indicated for the treatment of solid tumors. It is currently in phase I trials.

INDICATION(S) AND RESEARCH PHASE
Cancer/Tumors (Unspecified) – Phase I

BB-3644
unknown

MANUFACTURER
British Biotech plc

DESCRIPTION
BB-3644 is a second-generation metalloproteinase inhibitor (MMPI), which is under development as an anti-cancer agent. Results of a phase I trial in cancer subjects showed that BB-3644 was safe and well tolerated up to doses of 20 mg twice daily, but at doses of 30 mg twice daily it caused musculoskeletal pain similar to that seen with marimastat. It has been determined that at its maximum tolerated dose of 20 mg twice daily, BB-3644 does not appear to have any advantage over marimastat in the cancer setting. British Biotech is reviewing arrangements with Schering-Plough, which has licensed worldwide rights to develop marimastat and other British Biotech MMPIs in cancer, excluding Japan and certain Far Eastern territories.

INDICATION(S) AND RESEARCH PHASE
Cancer/Tumors (Unspecified) – Phase I

BNP 1350
Karenitecin

MANUFACTURER
BioNumerik Pharmaceuticals

DESCRIPTION
BMP 1350 belongs to a novel class of orally active highly lipophilic topoisomerase I inhibitors called karenitecins. The compound has demonstrated potent antitumor activity in several preclinical models including human cancer cell lines and animal bearing human tumor models.

BioNumerik is planning to proceed with phase II trials in solid tumors and leukemias. Additionally, a pediatric phase I trial has been initiated in individuals ages 1-20 years of age with solid tumors.

INDICATION(S) AND RESEARCH PHASE
Cancer/Tumors (Unspecified) – Phase I completed
Pediatric, Solid Tumors – Phase I

Carn 750
CarraVex

MANUFACTURER
Carrington Laboratories

DESCRIPTION
CarraVex is one of many drugs derived from plants, in this instance, from *Aloe barbadensis*. This complex carbohydrate contains certain acetylated mannans (polymers occurring in a variety of plants) that have demonstrated the ability to interact with and modulate a subject's immune response. The company claims that these acetylated mannans stimulate the subject's immune response to help destroy or contain various cancers, including benign and malignant tumors such as sarcomas, carcinomas, and lymphomas. This proprietary investigational anticancer product will be developed as an adjuvant in conjunction with other cancer therapies. CarraVex is in phase I/II trials for treatment of a variety of cancers. The drug is given as an intravenous formulation.

INDICATION(S) AND RESEARCH PHASE
Cancer/Tumors (Unspecified) – Phase I/II

CCI-779
unknown

MANUFACTURER
Wyeth-Ayerst

DESCRIPTION
CCI-779 is a derivative of rapamycin, an agent that exhibits antifungal, immunosuppressant, and antitumor activities. CCI-779 appears to block the effect of mTOR, an enzyme that has an important role in regulating the synthesis of proteins that control cell division. Therefore, CCI-779 may stop the production of proteins essential for cancer cell proliferation and possibly the survival of cancer cells. Early clinical trials of CCI-779, alone or in combination with other cancer drugs, will investigate effectiveness against a number of solid tumor types.

INDICATION(S) AND RESEARCH PHASE
Cancer/Tumors (Unspecified) – Phase II

cisplatin/epinephrine
IntraDose

MANUFACTURER
Matrix Pharmaceutical

DESCRIPTION
IntraDose is a biodegradable collagen carrier matrix combined with a vasoconstrictor. The gel is injected directly into tumors where it localizes high concentrations of cisplatin, a widely used anticancer drug. It is currently being tested for several indications, including head and neck, breast, malignant melanoma, esophageal, and primary hepatocellular cancer.

A phase II trial of IntraDose Injectable Gel produced durable responses in subjects with colorectal cancer that had metastasized to the liver. Nine of 31 subjects who received IntraDose responded to therapy. Six subjects experienced a complete response (100% reduction in viable tumor volume of treated tumors) while the other three subjects demonstrated a partial response (at least a 50% reduction of viable tumor volume). Eight of the nine treatment responders have had durable responses with no relapse at the site of treatment. IntraDose was well tolerated by subjects.

INDICATION(S) AND RESEARCH PHASE
Breast Cancer – Phase II
Cancer/Tumors (Unspecified) – Phase II
Colorectal Cancer – Phase II completed
Esophageal Cancer – Phase II
Liver Cancer – Phase II
Malignant Melanoma – Phase II
Head and Neck Cancer – NDA submitted

CP-461
unknown

MANUFACTURER
Cell Pathways

DESCRIPTION
CP-461 is a novel anti-cancer compound, which belongs to a new class of pro-apoptotic drugs termed selective apoptotic anti-neoplastic drugs (SAANDs). SAAND compounds inhibit a particular cyclic GMP phosphodiesterase and induce apoptosis in abnormally growing precancerous and cancerous cells. Because SAANDs do not induce apoptosis in normal cells, they do not produce the serious side effects normally associated with traditional chemotherapeutic agents. Nor do they inhibit cyclooxygenase (COX) and therefore do not produce the gastric and renal toxicities reported to be associated with non-steroidal anti-inflammatory drugs (NSAIDs) including the COX II inhibitors. CP-461 is in a phase Ib trial for the treatment of advanced solid tumors.

Results from a phase Ia trial conducted in healthy volunteers demonstrated excellent tolerability in all subjects following oral administration. Plasma levels of CP-461 exceeded those predicted to be necessary to achieve anti-cancer effects, based on preclinical studies. No clinically significant drug-related side effects were observed at any dose.

INDICATION(S) AND RESEARCH PHASE
Cancer/Tumors (Unspecified) – Phase Ib

D1927
unknown

MANUFACTURER
Bristol-Myers Squibb

DESCRIPTION
Matrix metalloproteinases (MMP) are a family of enzymes that are over-expressed in tumor tissues and have been found to support the growth, invasion, and metastatic process of developing tumors. D1927 is an orally formulated drug that inhibits these enzymes. This drug was being tested for arthritis and cancer indications in phase II clinical trials, but development is currently on hold.

INDICATION(S) AND RESEARCH PHASE
Arthritis and Arthritic Pain – Phase II on hold
Cancer/Tumors (Unspecified) – Phase II on hold

D2163, BMS 275291
unknown

MANUFACTURER
Celltech Chiroscience plc

DESCRIPTION
D2163 is a small molecule MMP inhibitor for the treatment of various tumors. It is currently being tested in phase I trials under an agreement with Bristol-Meyer-Squibb.

INDICATION(S) AND RESEARCH PHASE
Cancer/Tumors (Unspecified) – Phase I

darbepoetin alfa
Aranesp

MANUFACTURER
Amgen

DESCRIPTION
Aranesp (darbepoetin alfa) is a sustained-release form of Epogen (epoetin alfa), a drug developed by Amgen for the treatment of anemia in subjects with kidney disease and other conditions. Chronic kidney disease is characterized by decreased levels of erythropoietin, a hormone that stimulates the production of red blood cells. Aranesp is a novel erythropoiesis stimulating protein developed to treat anemia with less frequent administration than recombinant epoetin alfa.

Trial results for Aranesp indicated that the drug was effective given once every three weeks to anemic cancer subjects with solid tumors. In a double-blind, placebo-controlled, dose-finding phase I/II trial of 163 subjects, a dose response was seen between four different doses of Aranesp as demonstrated by increases in hemoglobin as well as a decrease in transfusions.

INDICATION(S) AND RESEARCH PHASE
Kidney Disease – NDA submitted
Cancer/Tumors (Unspecified) – Phase II

doxorubicin HCl
Doxil, Caelyx

MANUFACTURER
Alza (Sequus Pharmaceuticals)

DESCRIPTION
Doxil is a liposomal formulation of doxorubicin hydrochloride, an intravenous chemotherapy agent. This anthracycline anti-tumor agent is currently on the market for treatment of Kaposi's sarcoma. The drug uses a novel, targeted delivery system to help evade recognition and uptake by the immune system so that the liposomes can circulate in the body longer. A long circulation time increases the likelihood that the liposomes and their pharmaceutical contents will reach their targeted tumor site. Doxil may act through an ability to bind DNA and inhibit nucleic acid synthesis.

The company reported that Doxil is being tested in phase II/III trials for the additional indications of breast, liver, lung, and prostate cancers, as well as phase II for unspecified cancers and tumors.

Alza markets this product in the United States under the trade name Doxil; however, it is marketed under the name Caelyx in other areas. Schering-Plough has exclusive international marketing rights to Caelyx, excluding Japan and Israel, through a distribution agreement with Alza.

INDICATION(S) AND RESEARCH PHASE
Breast Cancer – Phase II/III
Liver Cancer – Phase II/III
Lung Cancer – Phase II/III
Prostate Cancer – Phase II/III
Cancer/Tumors (Unspecified) – Phase II

DX-8951
unknown

MANUFACTURER
Daiichi Pharmaceutical

DESCRIPTION
Many drugs for the treatment of cancer and other diseases originate in plants. Camptothecin, the primary active ingredient in DX-8951, was discovered in the bark of the *Camptotheca acuminata* tree native only to China and Tibet, where the compound was used to treat leukemia and cancers of the stomach and liver. The primary anti-cancer ingredient, a quinoline alkaloid called camptothecin, has been modified to create a host of other anti-cancer drugs. These analogs are being investigated to treat a wide variety of cancers, but the compounds are quite toxic. To reduce toxicity, camptothecin is synthesized as in the case of DX-8951. Several chemically different camptothecin compounds are on the market in the United States and other countries for treatment of refractory ovarian cancer, non-small cell lung cancer, and metastatic colorectal cancer. DX-8951 is being tested in phase I/II trials against a variety of solid tumor cancers. This camptothecin compound is administered intravenously.

DX-8951 inhibits the enzyme topoisomerase I, which is involved in DNA transcription and replication. Topoisomerases adjust DNA winding by making temporary cuts in the DNA strands. Chromosomes must be unwound in order for the cell to use the genetic information to synthesize proteins; camptothecin keeps the chromosomes wound tight, and as a result the cell stops growing. Because cancer cells grow and reproduce at a much faster rate than normal cells, they are more vulnerable to topoisomerase inhibition.

INDICATION(S) AND RESEARCH PHASE
Cancer/Tumors (Unspecified) – Phase I/II

E21R
unknown

MANUFACTURER
British Biotech plc

DESCRIPTION
E21R is in phase I development for the treatment of solid tumors.

INDICATION(S) AND RESEARCH PHASE
Cancer/Tumors (Unspecified) – Phase I

E7010
unknown

MANUFACTURER
Eisai

DESCRIPTION
E7010 is an orally active sulfonamide antitumor agent that inhibits mitosis. It is currently in phase I trials.

INDICATION(S) AND RESEARCH PHASE
Cancer/Tumors (Unspecified) – Phase I

ecteinascidin, ET-743
unknown

MANUFACTURER
PharmaMar

DESCRIPTION
Tunicates are a class of marine animals that are encased by tough membranes; one tunicate found in the Caribbean and Mediterranean Seas, a sea squirt designated *Ecteinascidia turbinata*, provides the compound ET-743. This compound, administered in a 24-hour intravenous infusion, seems to shrink tumors and control disease in subjects with soft-tissue sarcomas. Its interaction with the DNA of tumor cells is not perfectly understood but appears to be effective.

Three phase II trials were conducted at Harvard for ET-743. The first trial included subjects with advanced soft-tissue sarcomas who had received one or two prior chemotherapy regimens for metastatic disease. The second trial was the first time that ET-743 was tried as a first-line therapy in advanced soft-tissue sarcoma subjects who had not received prior chemotherapy. Eighteen subjects were enrolled in the less successful third trial, with only 6% finding ET-743 helpful with their hard-to-treat gastrointestinal stromal tumors.

INDICATION(S) AND RESEARCH PHASE
Cancer/Tumors (Unspecified) – Phase II completed

EGF-receptor specific monoclonal antibody
unknown

MANUFACTURER
Merck KgaA

DESCRIPTION
This monoclonal antibody is being developed for supplemental (adjuvant) therapy of endothelial growth factor (EGF)-receptor carrying tumors. This specific biological drug product is being tested in phase II trials in these EGF-receptor typed cancers.

INDICATION(S) AND RESEARCH PHASE
Cancer/Tumors (Unspecified) – Phase II

EMD 82633
unknown

MANUFACTURER
Merck KgaA

DESCRIPTION
EMD 82633 is a humanized and bispecific monoclonal antibody derived from mice.

These antibodies are altered in such a way that they no longer appear different from human antibodies. This genetic modification prevents immune reactions against foreign substances of animal origin used in humans. In this bispecific drug, one component binds to tumor cells, while the other activates the body's own CD8 "killer cells" to attack cancer cells.

This new drug is being given as an adjuvant therapy to subjects who have not been adequately helped by conventional forms of treatment, such as chemotherapy. EMD 82633 is being tested in trials for the treatment of renal cancer, head and neck cancer, breast cancer, bladder cancer, and ovarian cancer.

INDICATION(S) AND RESEARCH PHASE
Bladder Cancer – Phase II
Breast Cancer – Phase II
Cancer/Tumors (Unspecified) – Phase II
Head and Neck Cancer – Phase II
Ovarian Cancer – Phase II
Renal Cell Carcinoma – Phase II

exisulind/docetaxel
Aposyn/Taxotere

MANUFACTURER
Cell Pathways

DESCRIPTION
Aptosyn is a sulfone derivative of sulindac, a non-steroidal anti-inflammatory compound being tested with Rhone-Poulenc Rorer's Taxotere for the treatment of prostate, lung, and breast cancer as well as for solid tumors. Aptosyn (exisulind) is the first product candidate from a novel class of compounds under development by Cell Pathways, called selective apoptotic anti-neoplastic drugs (SAANDs). SAANDs inhibit cyclic GMP phosphodiesterase and selectively induce apoptosis in abnormally growing precancerous and cancerous cells. Because SAANDs do not induce apoptosis in normal cells, they do not produce the serious side effects normally associated with traditional chemotherapeutic agents. They also do not inhibit cyclooxygenase (COX I or COX II) and have not exhibited the gastric and renal toxicities reported to be associated with non-steroidal anti-inflammatory drugs (NSAIDs), including the COX II inhibitors.

Both companies will jointly share the cost of the trials and will retain all marketing rights to its respective products.

INDICATION(S) AND RESEARCH PHASE
Prostate Cancer – Phase I/II
Breast Cancer – Phase I/II
Lung Cancer – Phase I/II
Lung Cancer – Phase III
Cancer/Tumors (Unspecified) – Phase I

farnesyl protein transferase inhibitor
unknown

MANUFACTURER
Schering-Plough Corporation

DESCRIPTION
Farnesyl protein transferase (FPT) inhibitor is an oral drug being tested for the treatment of a variety of solid tumors. This anticancer agent works by blocking the FPT enzyme that may be involved in the growth of organ cancers such as bladder, colon, pancreas, and lung. It is in phase II testing.

INDICATION(S) AND RESEARCH PHASE
Cancer/Tumors (Unspecified) – Phase II

FK-317
unknown

MANUFACTURER
Fujisawa Healthcare

DESCRIPTION
Fujisawa has developed a new anti-cancer medication, FK-317, that originally was developed as an antibiotic. The molecule, known as a dihydrobenzoxazine, underwent preliminary testing in thirty-one subjects with solid tumors that were refractory to other chemotherapeutic treatments. The company reported that tumor reduction was observed in four subjects, two of whom achieved complete remission. Side effects and other toxicities such as leukopenia (decreased white blood cells) and neutropenia were modest in comparison to other established treatments.

It is unclear how exactly this compound works to limit the growth of cancer, but it seems to influence the process by which cells reproduce themselves. Currently, FK-317 is given at a dose of 24 mg/day intravenously and it is being evaluated in phase II trials. Scientists are testing it in a variety of solid tumors such as prostate, breast, and skin cancer.

INDICATION(S) AND RESEARCH PHASE
Breast Cancer – Phase II
Cancer/Tumors (Unspecified) – Phase II
Prostate Cancer – Phase II
Skin Cancer – Phase II

FLT3 ligand
Mobist

MANUFACTURER
ImClone Systems

DESCRIPTION
Mobist is a hematopoietic growth factor being tested exvivo. It is a stem cell mobilizer and potential anti-tumor agent. Mobist is being evaluated in phase II trials for treatment of breast cancer, solid tumors, non-Hodgkin's lymphoma, and ovarian cancer.

INDICATION(S) AND RESEARCH PHASE
Cancer/Tumors (Unspecified) – Phase II
Breast Cancer – Phase II
Lymphoma, Non-Hodgkin's – Phase II
Ovarian Cancer – Phase II

fluoropyrimidine, S-1
unknown

MANUFACTURER
Bristol-Myers Squibb

DESCRIPTION
Fluoropyrimidine is a combination medication that is being tested in subjects with solid tumors. The drug is given orally at 80 mg twice a day, and it is currently being tested in phase II clinical trials. One of the active components in fluoropyrimidine is tegafur, which is a type of a chemotherapeu-

tic drug known as 5-fluorouracil (5-FU). 5-FU prevents the metabolic activities of cancer cells, thus limiting their ability to grow and replicate. In clinical use for over forty years, 5-FU has been used to treat gastrointestinal, breast, head and neck, and bladder cancers. Problems associated with 5-FU use include subject tolerance to its anti-cancer effects, serious side effects, and toxicity to the digestive tract when taken orally.

Fluoropyrimidine may be an improvement over 5-FU alone because it also contains the molecule otastat potassium, which protects the GI tract from toxic effects, and the substance gimestat, which increases the action of 5-FU by inhibiting the enzyme in the body that breaks it down. Studies will demonstrate whether these two molecules will allow the drug to be given orally, producing fewer resultant adverse effects. This may mean that subjects will be able to tolerate the drug for longer periods of time, thus increasing subject compliance and potentially the effectiveness of the drug. It also may reduce the variability of clinical response to the drug among subjects, allowing doctors to better predict the effect its administration will have on their subjects' condition and what doses would be optimal for them. Preliminary studies have shown that fluoropyrimidine produces greater efficacy and less toxicity than conventional chemotherapeutic agents.

INDICATION(S) AND RESEARCH PHASE
Cancer/Tumors (Unspecified) – Phase II
Gastric Cancer – Phase II

GEM-231
unknown

MANUFACTURER
Hybridon

DESCRIPTION
GEM-231 is a genetically engineered (hybridized) antisense drug being developed for the treatment of refractory solid tumors. Antisense technology uses synthetic segments of DNA that stop the production of disease-related proteins by interacting with target strands of messenger RNA. GEM-231 binds to the Ria-regulatory subunit of the enzyme protein kinase-A (PKA), which has been associated with the unregulated growth of cancer. By inhibiting the production of excessive PKA, GEM-231 may prove a useful anticancer agent. The drug is being tested in phase II trials.

INDICATION(S) AND RESEARCH PHASE
Cancer/Tumors (Unspecified) – Phase II

GPX-100
unknown

MANUFACTURER
Gem Pharmaceuticals

DESCRIPTION
GPX-100 is noncardiotoxic version of the anticancer drug Adriamycin. Adriamycin, an anthracycline, is a commonly used drug in the treatment of cancers, including metastatic breast cancer. The cytotoxic effect of Adriamycin on malignant cells and its toxic effects on various organs are thought to be related to genetic insertion (nucleotide base intercalation) and cell membrane lipid binding activities. Intercalation inhibits both nucleotide replication and enzyme activity of DNA and RNA polymerases. The interaction of Adriamycin with topoisomerase II to form DNA-cleavable complexes appears to be an important mechanism of Adriamycin cell-killing activity. The drug's cellular membrane binding may affect a variety of cellular functions.

Unfortunately, Adriamycin and related drugs may produce irreversible damage to the heart if the subject receives too many doses. Thus, although Adriamycin may eliminate the tumor, if the cancer returns the drug often cannot be administered again because of the significant risk of heart failure and possible death. The company claims to have developed a platform technology that allows the chemical conversion of any standard anthracycline to a closely related analog that cannot be converted by the body to the cardiotoxic metabolite. GPX-100 is presently in phase II clinical trials in metastatic breast cancer and pediatric trials for leukemia.

INDICATION(S) AND RESEARCH PHASE
Cancer/Tumors (Unspecified) – Phase II
Breast Cancer – Phase II
Pediatric, Leukemia – Phase II

GW 572016
unknown

MANUFACTURER
GlaxoSmithKline

DESCRIPTION
GW 572016 is an Erb-B2 and epidermal growth factor receptor (EGFR) dual kinase inhibitor. It is currently in phase I development for the treatment of solid tumors.

INDICATION(S) AND RESEARCH PHASE
Cancer/Tumors (Unspecified) – Phase I

HP-4
unknown

MANUFACTURER
Milkhaus Laboratory

DESCRIPTION
HP-4 is currently being tested for the treatment of benign hyperstatic hyperplasia (BHH), which is a type of abnormal growth. HP-4 is made in an oral formulation and its presumed mechanism of action causes induces apoptosis. Clinical testing has completed phase II and the company is seeking a licensing partner for further development.

INDICATION(S) AND RESEARCH PHASE
Cancer/Tumors (Unspecified) – Phase II Completed

human endostatin protein
rhEndostatin

MANUFACTURER
EntreMed

DESCRIPTION
RhEndostatin is an angiogenic agent that has been shown to inhibit both the formation of new blood vessels and the growth of primary and metastatic tumors. EntreMed

announced data from three phase I trials in November 2000, which indicated the drug was well tolerated with no serious adverse events. Additionally, encouraging results were observed in terms of clinical effectiveness. Using an MRI scan to measure the size of tumors, one subject with sarcoma in the jawbone, after two months at 300 mg/m^2 a day of rhEndostatin, experienced an over 50% decrease in tumor measurements. One subject with a neuroendocrine tumor had a minor response and participated in the study for one year. Twelve subjects received between four and twelve months of rhEndostatin therapy; of these, at least five subjects had stable disease for a minimum of four months, with two of the subjects receiving one year of therapy.

INDICATION(S) AND RESEARCH PHASE
Cancer/Tumors (Unspecified) – Phase I completed

ILX-651
unknown

MANUFACTURER
ILEX Oncology

DESCRIPTION
ILX-651 is a synthetic pentapeptide analog of dolastatin, with a mechanism of action that is analogous to taxanes such as Taxol and Taxotere. A tublin interactive, antimitotic compound, ILX-651 appears to be active in taxane-resistant tumors in animal models of human breast carcinoma. Additionally, it appears to be active for a variety of invitro solid tumor cell models, including breast, ovarian, and lung carcinomas, and melanoma and leukemia.

Two phase I trials are expected to begin during the first quarter of 2001 as well as one other phase I trial anticipated for the second half of the year.

INDICATION(S) AND RESEARCH PHASE
Cancer/Tumors (Unspecified) – Phase I

IMMU-MN14, anti-CEA
CEA-Cide

MANUFACTURER
Immunomedics

DESCRIPTION
Carcinoembryonic antigen (CEA) is a protein-polysaccharide complex released in the bloodstream by certain cancers, especially colon carcinoma. This antigenic substance may provide early diagnosis when used as a therapeutic marker in immunologic tests. The CEA complex may also be targeted by specialized monoclonal antibodies in the design of a biologic therapeutic.

CEA-Cide is a novel monoclonal antibody that is designed for radioimmunotherapy (with 90 Y-labeled humanized MN-14). This drug is being tested in phase II trials for the treatment of advanced metastatic and CEA-producing cancers, particularly colorectal cancer. Other indications may include breast cancer, female reproductive system cancer, ovarian cancer, lung cancer, and pancreatic cancer.

INDICATION(S) AND RESEARCH PHASE
Breast Cancer – Phase II
Cancer/Tumors (Unspecified) – Phase II
Colorectal Cancer – Phase II
Lung Cancer – Phase II
Ovarian Cancer – Phase II
Pancreatic Cancer – Phase II

INGN 241 (mda-7)
unknown

MANUFACTURER
Introgen Therapeutics

DESCRIPTION
INGN 241 is the combination of Introgen's proprietary adenoviral delivery system with the mda-7 gene. INGN 241 is in a phase I trial for solid tumors in 15 subjects. Preclinical results with mda-7 demonstrate expression of mda-7 appears to be lost earlier in tumor progression and also indicate that mda-7 may be easily combined with other tumor suppressor genes for additive effects. Additionally, INGN 241 is in preclinical development for lung and breast cancer.

INDICATION(S) AND RESEARCH PHASE
Breast Cancer – Preclinical
Lung Cancer – Preclinical
Cancer/Tumors (Unspecified) – Phase I

INGN-201, adenoviral p53
unknown

MANUFACTURER
Introgen Therapeutics

DESCRIPTION
INGN-201 is a p53 gene therapy cancer product. It has been tested as a treatment for a variety of solid tumor cancers with administration via intratumoral injection. The drug was well tolerated according to the company, and additional trials are under way using an intravenous infusion in order to reach more types of cancers. The tumor-suppressing p53 gene encodes a protein that responds to damage involving cellular DNA by terminating cell division. Normal p53 genes are delivered into cancer cells of the subject through an adenoviral vector.

The developers of INGN-201 have signed a Cooperative Research and Development Agreement (CRADA) with the National Cancer Institute to evaluate the potential effectiveness and superiority of the drug over other treatments against breast, ovarian, bladder, prostate, and brain cancers in phase I and phase II trials. A phase III trial in head and neck cancer was initiated in March 2000.

INDICATION(S) AND RESEARCH PHASE
Head and Neck Cancer – Phase III
Bladder Cancer – Phase I
Brain Cancer – Phase I
Breast Cancer – Phase I
Bronchoalveolar Cancer – Phase I
Ovarian Cancer – Phase I
Prostate Cancer – Phase I
Lung Cancer – Phase II
Cancer/Tumors (Unspecified) – Phase I

interferon alfa-2b
PEG-Intron

MANUFACTURER
Schering-Plough Corporation

DESCRIPTION

PEG-Intron is a long-acting antiviral/biological response modifier. Clinical trials include testing for the treatment of chronic myelogenous leukemia, solid tumors, and malignant melanoma.

PEG-Intron was developed by Enzon for Schering-Plough who owns the exclusive rights. The drug was approved by the FDA for the treatment of hepatitis C in January 2001.

INDICATION(S) AND RESEARCH PHASE

Cancer/Tumors (Unspecified) – Phase II
Hepatitis – FDA approved
Leukemia – Phase III
Malignant Melanoma – Phase III

ISIS 5132, CGP 69846A
unknown

MANUFACTURER
Isis Pharmaceuticals

DESCRIPTION

ISIS 5132 is a potent antisense inhibitor of the enzyme c-Raf-1 kinase. Antisense drugs inhibit the production of disease-causing proteins by altering the genetic information, which messenger RNA uses to produce new protein. c-Raf kinase plays a role in signal processes that regulate cell growth and proliferation. It is one of a family of raf genes thought to play an important role in the development of some solid tumors. The company reports that activated-raf has also been detected in a substantial variety of human cancers including small cell lung carcinoma and breast cancer. For example, it has been reported that 60% of all lung carcinoma cells express unusually high levels of normal c-Raf mRNA and protein.

The sponsor companies reported that results from phase I studies, which examined subjects with a wide variety of solid tumors, demonstrated that the drug was well tolerated and that several subjects experienced disease stabilization. The companies are planning additional phase I safety studies involving the drug in combination with currently approved chemotherapies. Phase II clinical trials examining ISIS 5132 as a single agent therapy in subjects with breast, lung, colon, pancreatic, and prostate cancers are under way.

INDICATION(S) AND RESEARCH PHASE

Breast Cancer – Phase II
Cancer/Tumors (Unspecified) – Phase II
Colon Malignancies – Phase II
Lung Cancer – Phase II
Pancreatic Cancer – Phase II
Prostate Cancer – Phase II

L-glutathione
Cachexon

MANUFACTURER
Telluride Pharmaceutical

DESCRIPTION

Cachexon is an oral capsule formulation of glutathione, an antioxidant produced naturally by the body. Glutathione levels in individuals decrease with the onset of age-related conditions. Adding glutathione to disintegrating cells that have lost their immune activity revives the cells and causes them to become immuno-efficient again.

Cancer and AIDS subjects have lowered levels of glutathione. This capsule is designed as replacement therapy for glutathione in order to provide direct protection to intestinal epithelial cells (enterocytes) against oxidative stress. Oxidative stress leads to activation of HIV replication, resulting in damage to enterocytes, malabsorption and cachexia. Cachexon is in phase III trials for AIDS and AIDS-related infections, unspecified cancer and tumors, and diet and nutrition.

INDICATION(S) AND RESEARCH PHASE

Acquired Immune Deficiency Syndrome (AIDS) and AIDS-Related Infections – Phase III
Cancer/Tumors (Unspecified) – Phase III
Diet and Nutrition – Phase III

LDP-341, PS-341
unknown

MANUFACTURER
Millennium Pharmaceuticals

DESCRIPTION

LDP-341 is a proteasome inhibitor being developed for the treatment of cancer. In tumor cells, proteasome inhibition produces cellular stress by stabilizing cell cycle regulatory proteins and disrupting cell proliferation, ultimately leading to apoptosis. In preclinical studies, LDP-341 has shown activity against multiple myeloma cells, resulting in the inducement of apoptosis. The anti-tumor action of LDP-341 on multiple myeloma cells in these studies appears to involve both direct (apoptosis) and indirect inhibition of growth factors that promote tumor growth. Additionally, LDP-341 appears to increase the effectiveness of other anti-cancer drugs by overcoming cellular resistance, which in humans is a major cause of chemotherapy failure.

Among other programs, LDP-341 is currently in a phase I trial in subjects with advanced hematological malignancies. Preliminary results for this trial were presented in December 2000. LDP-341 reduced serum myeloma protein levels and myeloma cell numbers in bone marrow in two of three subjects with advanced multiple myeloma. The drug was well tolerated by these subjects and in addition appears to have induced a complete response in one subject and a reduction in bone marrow plasma cells in another.

INDICATION(S) AND RESEARCH PHASE

Cancer/Tumors (Unspecified) – Phase I
Multiple Myeloma – Phase I

LGD-1550
unknown

MANUFACTURER
Ligand Pharmaceuticals

DESCRIPTION

LGD-1550 is being formulated to limit the proliferation and spread of head, neck, and cervical cancers; it is to be given orally and is currently in phase II trials. Retinoids are a group of substances, one of which is vitamin A, that are thought to be responsible for growth, bone development, vision, and skin integrity. It is thought that retinoids act against cancer by regulating the process by which cells reproduce themselves (gene transcription regulation). Studies have shown that subjects with metastatic cancer have lower levels of retinoid activity in their bodies. LGD-1550 works by binding to retinoid receptors in cells, thereby stimulating retinoid activity.

Preliminary studies have shown that retinoids may inhibit cell proliferation and promote cell differentiation. Cancer arises when there is uncontrolled growth of immature cells. Retinoids act to slow cell division and stimulate cell maturation, making it less likely that these mature cells will be transformed into cancerous cells. Retinoids have also been shown in early studies to boost the effects of other anti-cancer medications.

Phase II trials of LGD-1550 for head and neck cancer, blood cancer, cervical cancer, and solid and hematological tumors are currently under way.

INDICATION(S) AND RESEARCH PHASE
Blood Cancer – Phase II
Cancer/Tumors (Unspecified) – Phase II
Cervical Dysplasia/Cancer – Phase II
Head and Neck Cancer – Phase II

LY231514, antifolate
unknown

MANUFACTURER
Eli Lilly

DESCRIPTION
LY231514 is a new drug that is being developed to treat various forms of cancer, including late-stage breast, colon, non-small cell lung, and head and neck. It is administered intravenously for eight days every three weeks, and it is currently being tested in phase III trials for the treatment of solid tumors.

Part of cancer cell replication is the copying of DNA. Anti-folate medications block this formation of new DNA by preventing the synthesis of DNA building blocks known as nucleotides. LY231514 is a combination of three different anti-folate medications: thymidylate synthase inhibitor, dihydrofolate reductase inhibitor, and glycinamide ribonucleotide formyl transferase inhibitor. These three substances may work synergistically to arrest the growth of cancer cells, possibly producing a more potent anti-cancer effect than an individual anti-folate medication alone.

The company reported that in a phase II trial in subjects with metastatic cancer, nine (of 32 evaluable) subjects achieved partial responses while fourteen subjects achieved stable, nonprogressive disease. Further study is necessary to delineate the exact potency and side effects of this new cancer treatment.

INDICATION(S) AND RESEARCH PHASE
Cancer/Tumors (Unspecified) – Phase III

MDAM (y-methylene-10-deazaaminopterin)
unknown

MANUFACTURER
BioNumerik Pharmaceuticals

DESCRIPTION
MDAM (y-methylene-10-deazaaminopterin) is an antifolate structurally similar to the widely used cancer drug, methotrexate. In preclinical studies, it has shown promising activity against human solid malignancies. MDAM is in phase I trials in the United States.

INDICATION(S) AND RESEARCH PHASE
Cancer/Tumors (Unspecified) – Phase I

MGI-114, hydroxymethylacylfulvene, HMAF
Irofulven

MANUFACTURER
MGI Pharma

DESCRIPTION
Irofulven (MGI-114) is the first product candidate being developed by MGI Pharma from its family of anti-cancer compounds called acylfulvenes. Early trials demonstrated that Irofulven is absorbed rapidly by tumor cells, and once inside binds to DNA and protein targets. The binding interferes with DNA replication and cell division, leading to tumor-specific cell death. The drug is being tested in a series of trials for a variety of cancers.

In November 2000, results from a phase II trial of Irofulven indicated that the drug produced anti-tumor activity in subjects with advanced pancreatic cancer who were refractory to gemcitabine (Gemzar). Ten of the 53 subjects enrolled achieved six-month survival and two subjects demonstrated objective responses: one subject experienced tumor shrinkage of 100% and another subject experienced an 84% decrease in tumor mass. A phase III trial was initiated in February 2001.

INDICATION(S) AND RESEARCH PHASE
Breast Cancer – Phase II
Colon Malignancies – Phase II
Renal Cell Carcinoma – Phase II
Cervical Dysplasia/Cancer – Phase II
Lung Cancer – Phase II
Ovarian Cancer – Phase I/II
Colorectal Cancer – Phase II
Prostate Cancer – Phase I/II
Cancer/Tumors (Unspecified) – Phase I/II
Pancreatic Cancer – Phase III
Liver Cancer – Phase II

MGV
unknown

MANUFACTURER
Progenics Pharmaceuticals

DESCRIPTION
The MGV vaccine is designed to stimulate a subject's immune system to control or eradicate residual cancer cells after surgery, radiation, or chemotherapy. The vaccine is based on the GM2 and GD2 gangliosides, cancer antigens that are present in many of the most common types of cancers, including colorectal and gastric cancers, small cell lung cancer, lymphoma, sarcoma, and neuroblastoma. MGV contains the GM2 and GD2 antigens separately coupled to the carrier protein keyhole limpet hemocyanin (KLH) and mixed with QS-21 adjuvant. Vaccination of subjects with MGV is designed to destroy cancer cells without damaging healthy tissue by stimulating the

formation of antibodies to GM2 and GD2.

Results for MGV demonstrated that the cancer vaccine was free of significant toxicity and induced antibodies against two different targets on cancer cells. The trial evaluated 31 subjects with malignant melanoma or sarcoma. MGV induced antibodies to the GM2 ganglioside in 97% of subjects. Additionally, 91% of subjects who received an optimal dose of the vaccine also developed antibodies to GD2. The trial results have been published in *Clinical Cancer Research* (Vol. 6, No. 12). Progenics is currently planning tumor-specific phase II trials with clinical endpoints to be initiated in 2001. MGV is being developed under a collaboration with Bristol-Myers Squibb.

INDICATION(S) AND RESEARCH PHASE
Cancer/Tumors (Unspecified) – Phase I completed

monoclonal antibody (Mab), anti-VEGF
unknown

MANUFACTURER
Genentech

DESCRIPTION
This humanized monoclonal anti-VEGF antibody is a novel inhibitor of angiogenesis. It is being tested in trials for the treatment of solid tumors and coronary artery disease.

INDICATION(S) AND RESEARCH PHASE
Cancer/Tumors (Unspecified) – Phase II
Coronary Artery Disease – Phase II

O6-Benzylguanine (BG)
unknown

MANUFACTURER
Procept

DESCRIPTION
O6-Benzylguanine (BG) is a chemosensitizer designed to overcome tumor resistance to a significant class of commonly used chemotherapeutic agents known as 0-6-alkylating agents. BG inactivates tumor AGT, a DNA repair protein, which interferes with the effectiveness of these agents.

BG is being tested in combination with the chemotherapeutic drug carmustine for the treatment of cerebral anaplastic gliomas. This is one of several phase II trials that will be sponsored by the NCI in various cancer indications including, but not limited to, colon cancer, glioma, melanoma, and sarcomas.

INDICATION(S) AND RESEARCH PHASE
Cancer/Tumors (Unspecified) – Phase II

OC144-093
unknown

MANUFACTURER
Ontogen Corporation

DESCRIPTION
OC144-093 is a P-glycoprotein (P-gp) inhibitor and multidrug resistance modulator. An IND for the drug has been filed in Canada, and the company plans to begin phase I testing in cancer subjects in the first quarter of 2001.

INDICATION(S) AND RESEARCH PHASE
Cancer/Tumors (Unspecified) – Phase I

DHA-paclitaxel
Taxoprexin

MANUFACTURER
Protarga

DESCRIPTION
DHA-paclitaxel is a patented new anticancer agent in the class of taxane drugs that includes Taxol (from Bristol-Myers Squibb) and Taxotere (from Aventis), both of which are currently approved for the treatment of non-small cell lung cancer. DHA-paclitaxel is a synthetic small molecule made by chemically linking paclitaxel, the active ingredient in Taxol, to the natural fatty acid docosahexaenoic acid (DHA), an approved nutritional additive.

In March 2001, Protarga announced the commencement of phase II clinical studies of DHA-paclitaxel. This program involves separate clinical studies for eight types of cancers and is being conducted at twenty hospitals in the United States and the United Kingdom.

INDICATION(S) AND RESEARCH PHASE
Cancer/Tumors (Unspecified) – Phase II

PEG-camptothecin
Prothecan

MANUFACTURER
Enzon

DESCRIPTION
Prothecan (PEG-camptothecin) is a polyethylene glycol (PEG)-modified version of a small molecule called camptothecin, which is an anticancer compound in a class of drugs called topoisomerase inhibitors. Camptothecin is believed to be a potent topoisomerase inhibitor, interfering with the essential function of topoisomerase in DNA replication.

In November 2000, results of an ongoing phase I trial indicated that Prothecan has been well tolerated at doses up to 7,000 mg/m^2. Myelosuppression (depression of bone marrow function, such as the formation of red blood cells and platelets) was found to be the principal dose-limiting factor. Additionally, antitumor activity has been observed. Dose escalation is continuing in this and a second phase I trial of Prothecan in order to establish the maximum tolerated dose for use in phase II trials, planned to begin in early 2001.

INDICATION(S) AND RESEARCH PHASE
Cancer/Tumors (Unspecified) – Phase I

perfluorohexane emulsion
Imagent

MANUFACTURER
Alliance Pharmaceutical

DESCRIPTION
Imagent is a perfluorochemical-based microbubble intravenous contrast agent. It is used along with an ultrasound for the

evaluation of cardiac function, myocardial perfusion, detection of organ lesions, and blood flow abnormalities.

INDICATION(S) AND RESEARCH PHASE
Cardiac Surgery – Phase III
Cancer/Tumors (Unspecified) – Phase III

phenoxodiol
unknown

MANUFACTURER
Novogen

DESCRIPTION
Phenoxodiol is a novel cytotoxic, anti-cancer drug that arrests cancer cell growth and restores apoptosis. It acts through a variety of mechanisms including the inhibition of a number of cellular enzyme systems, including topoisomerase 2 and protein tyrosine kinases, which are integral to the development of cancer. Inhibiting these enzyme systems is recognized as a key factor in preventing the growth of cancerous cells. Additionally, the novelty of phenoxodiol lies in its ability to combine a high degree of potency with no known adverse effects on normal cells. Phenoxodiol also possesses a number of other anti-cancer mechanisms that appear to contribute to the overall anti-cancer effect.

Phenoxodiol is currently undergoing a phase Ib trial in an Australian hospital in subjects with solid malignant tumors, including prostate cancer. This study, which commenced in the final quarter of 2000, is investigating the safety and anti-cancer efficacy of phenoxodiol when injected intravenously once weekly for 12 weeks.

Novogen has received approval to commence a second phase Ib trial, which will be conducted at a major Sydney teaching hospital. This new study will measure the safety and anti-cancer effectiveness of phenoxodiol when administered by continuous intravenous infusion over seven days. The study will involve subjects with solid cancers whose cancers have become unresponsive to standard treatment.

INDICATION(S) AND RESEARCH PHASE
Cancer/Tumors (Unspecified) – Phase Ib
Prostate Cancer – Phase Ib

PI-88
unknown

MANUFACTURER
Progen Industries

DESCRIPTION
PI-88 will be entering phase II trials for the prevention of blood clots in thromboembolic diseases and angioplasty induced restenosis in 2001. Results from previous trials have shown that PI-88 is a potent antithrombotic and anticoagulant with a unique mode of action. PI-88 inhibits growth of vascular smooth muscle cells (restenosis) in animal models that are analogues to balloon angioplasty.

Balloon angioplasty is a surgical procedure where a balloon-tipped catheter is used to widen blocked arteries. Local vascular irritation occurs in 30% of people who have received the angioplasty procedure. This irritation induces rapid growth of smooth muscle cells surrounding the artery, causing arterial re-blockage.

In addition to trials for restenosis and other indications, PI-88 will be entering phase II trials for cancer in early 2001.

INDICATION(S) AND RESEARCH PHASE
Thrombocytopenia – Phase II
Cancer/Tumors (Unspecified) – Phase II

PKC 412
unknown

MANUFACTURER
Novartis

DESCRIPTION
PKC 412, an oral anti-sense drug, inhibits the action of protein kinase C (PKC). Anti-sense technology is a method for disrupting the expression of a specific protein or proteins within cells. This technology involves the introduction of an anti-sense DNA that is complementary to the messenger RNA (mRNA) that encodes the target protein. This anti-sense DNA binds specifically to the mRNA and inhibits its translation into protein. Thus, this technology may disrupt the specific production of a single protein within cells. PKC plays a role in signal processes that regulate cell growth and differentiation. It is one of a family of enzymes thought to have an important function in the development of some solid tumors. An oral formulation of PKC 412 is being tested in phase II trials for a variety of solid tumors and for diabetic macular edema.

INDICATION(S) AND RESEARCH PHASE
Cancer/Tumors (Unspecified) – Phase II
Eye Disorders/Infections – Phase II

R115777
unknown

MANUFACTURER
Janssen Pharmaceutica

DESCRIPTION
R115777 is an anticancer drug that inhibits the transformation of normal cells to cancer cells. It is belongs to a group of drugs called farnesyl transferase inhibitors (FTIs), which are signal transduction inhibitors that may suppress Ras function. Ras proteins play key roles in cell growth and survival, and activating mutations of the proteins are common in human cancer. R115777 is currently in phase III trials for the treatment of solid tumors in adults and is in phase I pediatric studies for refractory solid tumors in children two to 18 years of age.

INDICATION(S) AND RESEARCH PHASE
Cancer/Tumors (Unspecified) – Phase III
Pediatric, Cancer/Tumors (Unspecified) – Phase I

raltitrexed, ZD-1694
Tomudex

MANUFACTURER
AstraZeneca

DESCRIPTION
Tomudex is a cytotoxic enzyme inhibitor of thymidylate synthase. It is administered as a single agent infusion. Tomudex is in trials for colorectal cancer, other unspecified

Ras pathway inhibitor
unknown

MANUFACTURER
Onyx Pharmaceuticals

DESCRIPTION
This Ras pathway inhibitor is an anti-cancer agent being tested in a phase I trial in Germany. The major function of the Ras pathway inhibitor is inhibition of cell proliferation. In normal cells the Ras pathway is transiently activated. When a gene in the pathway is mutated, the signal may not stop, which causes the cell to continuously reproduce. Scientists believe inhibiting the Ras pathway will have an effect on controlling the tumor growth.

The Ras pathway inhibitor is being developed in partnership with the Bayer Corporation. The companies filed an IND in May 2000 in the United States and additional phase I trials are planned in Canada and Belgium.

INDICATION(S) AND RESEARCH PHASE
Cancer/Tumors (Unspecified) – Phase I

S-8184
unknown

MANUFACTURER
Sonus Pharmaceuticals

DESCRIPTION
S-8184 is an injectable form of paclitaxel emulsion being tested in a phase I trial in 25 subjects with advanced cancers, who have failed to respond to other therapies. S-8184 will be administered as a single injection instead of three- to 24-hour infusions typically required with other paclitaxel formulations. Additionally, the trial will evaluate whether premedications, which are used to suppress allergic-type reactions to the currently marketed formulation of paclitaxel, may be eliminated with S-8184. The company expects the phase I trial to be finished in late 2001.

Preclinical results demonstrated S-8184, using the company's Tocosol drug delivery system, to be less toxic than the currently marketed formulation of paclitaxel.

INDICATION(S) AND RESEARCH PHASE
Cancer/Tumors (Unspecified) – Phase I

SB 596168
unknown

MANUFACTURER
GlaxoSmithKline

DESCRIPTION
SB 596168 is a selective RNA polymerase inhibitor. It is in phase II trials for the treatment of solid tumors.

INDICATION(S) AND RESEARCH PHASE
Cancer/Tumors (Unspecified) – Phase II

squalamine
unknown

MANUFACTURER
Magainin Pharmaceuticals

DESCRIPTION
Squalamine is an aminosterol compound isolated from the tissues of the dogfish shark. This drug inhibits salt-and-acid-regulating pumps on endothelial cells that normally line blood vessels, which prevents growth factors from stimulating the cells to form capillaries. It is thought that this activity results in anti-angiogenesis, anti-inflammatory, and anti-tumor effects.

The company is conducting several phase II trials testing squalamine against certain cancers, such as breast and ovarian. Additionally, there is a phase IIa study for stage IIIB and IV non-small cell lung cancer being conducted at the University of Wisconsin and M.D. Anderson, Houston, Texas.

Additional studies are being planned for ovarian cancer, pediatric neuroblastoma and other solid tumors.

INDICATION(S) AND RESEARCH PHASE
Breast Cancer – Phase II
Lung Cancer – Phase IIa
Ovarian Cancer – Phase II
Cancer/Tumors (Unspecified) – Phase II

T607
unknown

MANUFACTURER
Tularik

DESCRIPTION
T607 is an analog of T67 that also binds irreversibly to tubulin and disrupts microtubule function. Preclinical studies indicate that T607 has a reduced propensity to enter the brain compared to T67. The compound is in phase I trials in the United States, the United Kingdom, and Canada. Tularik expects to establish the phase II dosing schedule in the first half of 2001 and commence phase II trials in selected tumor types in the second half of 2001.

INDICATION(S) AND RESEARCH PHASE
Cancer/Tumors (Unspecified) – Phase I

T64
unknown

MANUFACTURER
Tularik

DESCRIPTION
T64 is an antifolate that disrupts DNA synthesis through the inhibition of purine biosynthesis. The compound is currently in phase II trials in subjects with head and neck cancer, soft tissue sarcoma, melanoma, breast cancer, and non-small cell lung cancer. Additionally, T64 is in phase I combination trials with gemcitabine, doxorubicin, and paclitaxel. Tularik expects to initiate two additional T64 phase I combination trials with carboplatin and temozolamide in the first quarter of 2001. The T64 trials are being conducted in the United States, the United Kingdom, the Netherlands, and Australia.

Cancer/Tumors (Unspecified)/187

INDICATION(S) AND RESEARCH PHASE
Head and Neck Cancer – Phase II
Sarcoma – Phase II
Melanoma – Phase II
Breast Cancer – Phase II
Lung Cancer – Phase II
Cancer/Tumors (Unspecified) – Phase I

temozolomide
Temodar

MANUFACTURER
Schering-Plough Corporation

DESCRIPTION
Temodar is an oral cytotoxic chemotherapeutic agent belonging to a class of compounds known as imidazotetrazines. Temodar has been approved by the FDA for the treatment of adult subjects with anaplastic astrocytoma at the first relapse with disease progression on a nitrosourea- and procarbazine-containing drug regimen. It is currently in phase II trials for the treatment of a variety of solid tumors.

INDICATION(S) AND RESEARCH PHASE
Brain Cancer – FDA approved
Cancer/Tumors (Unspecified) – Phase II

thalidomide
Thalomid

MANUFACTURER
Celgene Corporation

DESCRIPTION
Thalomid is an oral formulation of the immunomodulatory agent thalidomide. Thalidomide has a notorious history of having caused birth defects when the medical profession unsuspectingly prescribed it for pregnant women as a treatment for nausea and insomnia. Celgene is investigating new applications for the drug, while being particularly mindful of the potential risks of thalidomide treatment. Thalomid is currently being tested for numerous indications in the areas of oncology and immunology.

INDICATION(S) AND RESEARCH PHASE
Multiple Myeloma – Phase II
Myelodysplastic Syndrome – Phase II
Leukemia – Phase II
Brain Cancer – Phase II
Liver Cancer – Phase II
Kidney Cancer – Phase II
Prostate Cancer – Phase II
Kaposi's Sarcoma – Phase II
Cachexia – Phase II
Recurrent Aphthous Stomatitis – Phase III
Crohn's Disease – Phase II
Inflammatory Bowel Disease – Phase II
Sarcoidosis – Phase II
Scleroderma – Phase II

TNP-470
unknown

MANUFACTURER
Takeda Chemical Industries

DESCRIPTION
TNP-470 is a synthetically modified form of the antibiotic fumagillin. This drug inhibits new blood vessel growth and is being tested in phase II trials for treatment of adults with malignant solid tumors. It is also being evaluated in a phase I trial in children with solid tumors, lymphomas, and acute leukemias.

INDICATION(S) AND RESEARCH PHASE
Cancer/Tumors (Unspecified) – Phase II
Pediatric, Solid Tumors, Lymphoma, Leukemia – Phase I

troxacitabine, BCH-4556
Troxatyl

MANUFACTURER
BioChem Pharma

DESCRIPTION
Troxatyl is a dioxolane nucleoside analog being investigated as an anticancer agent. The drug is a complete DNA chain terminator and DNA polymerase inhibitor. It acts by incorporating itself into the growing DNA chain of cancer cells, interfering with their ability to replicate further. Currently, Troxatyl is being evaluated as a single agent or in combination therapy in a number of ongoing single and multi-center trials in hematologic malignancies, including acute myeloid leukemia and chronic myeloid leukemia (blastic phase), and in lymphoproliferative disorders such as lymphoma, chronic lymphocytic leukemia, and myeloma. It is also being evaluated as a single agent in pancreatic cancer and in combination therapy in a number of solid tumors. Troxatyl is currently in phase II development.

INDICATION(S) AND RESEARCH PHASE
Cancer/Tumors (Unspecified) – Phase II
Colorectal Cancer – Phase II
Head and Neck Cancer – Phase II
Leukemia – Phase II
Lung Cancer – Phase II
Malignant Melanoma – Phase II
Ovarian Cancer – Phase II
Pancreatic Cancer – Phase II
Prostate Cancer – Phase II
Renal Cell Carcinoma – Phase II

unknown
Angiostatin with radiation therapy

MANUFACTURER
EntreMed

DESCRIPTION
Angiostatin is a potent, naturally occurring inhibitor of angiogenesis. Angiostatin combined with radiation therapy is in a phase I trial for advanced cancer.

INDICATION(S) AND RESEARCH PHASE
Cancer/Tumors (Unspecified) – Phase I

unknown
Reolysin

MANUFACTURER
Oncolytics Biotech

DESCRIPTION
Reolysin is a reovirus in phase I development for the treatment of cancer. Reovirus is able to infect and kill malignant cells in which the Ras pathway is activated. In an activated pathway, the cellular protein PKR cannot be activated due to an element of the Ras signal transduction pathway. This allows

the replication of the reovirus in these cancer cells, which eventually leads to cell death.

A phase I trial of Reolysin as a potential cancer therapeutic is under way in Canada. The goal of the trial is to determine the dose limiting toxicity and maximum tolerated dose of intralesional administration of Reolysin in oncology subjects.

INDICATION(S) AND RESEARCH PHASE
Cancer/Tumors (Unspecified) – Phase I

unknown
Palonosetron

MANUFACTURER
Helsinn Healthcare SA

DESCRIPTION
Palonosetron is an intravenously administered anti-emetic designed to combat the nausea and vomiting that often arise after the administration of chemotherapy. A single dose of Palonosetron offers extended coverage. It also appears to have no major side effects involving the gastrointestinal, respiratory, CNS, renal, or cardiovascular systems.

An estimated 75% of cancer subjects who undergo chemotherapy experience nausea; the problem can be so severe it can lead a subject to refuse or delay further treatments. Palonosetron is a selective $5HT_3$ receptor agonist that prevents these symptoms.

Approximately 1,800 cancer subjects are expected to be enrolled in the phase III trials, which will be conducted at 80 medical centers in the United States and Europe. Helsinn expects to receive FDA approval in 2002 and is currently seeking an American marketing partner.

INDICATION(S) AND RESEARCH PHASE
Cancer/Tumors (Unspecified) – Phase III

unknown
SGN-10

MANUFACTURER
Seattle Genetics

DESCRIPTION
SGN-10 is a genetically engineered single-chain immunotoxin (SCIT) comprised of the cloned binding site from the BR96 mAb and PE40 (a binding-defective form of the protein toxin *Pseudomonas exotoxin* (PE) A). The concept of SGN-10 is to redirect the potent cell-killing activity of PE from its normal target to cancer cells. This can be achieved by genetically deleting the natural binding domain of PE and replacing it with the binding domain of the cancer reactive BR96 mAb. The portion of PE that results in catalytic inhibition of protein synthesis and cell death is retained. BR96 reacts with the Lewis-Y (Ley) related carbohydrate antigen that is expressed at high levels on carcinoma including those of the breast, lung, colon, pancreas, ovary, and prostate, and at lower levels on epithelial cells from the gastrointestinal tract. The resulting agent, SGN-10, identifies cancer cells that display the BR96 antigen and cell death ensues after the delivery of the PE portion of the drug by halting cellular protein synthesis.

SGN-10 is being tested in two separate phase I trials in subjects with lung, breast, colon, ovarian, pancreatic, or prostate cancer. The first trial is with SGN-10 as a single-agent. The objective of this study is to evaluate the toxicities associated with incrementally increasing doses of SGN-10 and to establish its pharmacokinetic profile. The second phase I trial utilizes SGN-10 in combination with the widely used chemotherapeutic drug Taxotere in cancer subjects. This clinical trial is based on data demonstrating that the combination of SGN-10 and taxanes may result in greater (and potentially synergistic) antitumor activity than can be achieved by either agent alone. The objective of this combination study is to determine the optimal dose of SGN-10 to use with Taxotere (at its standard dose), define the toxicity profile of the combination and rapidly translate the results into disease-specific phase II efficacy.

INDICATION(S) AND RESEARCH PHASE
Cancer/Tumors (Unspecified) – Phase I

unknown
Vitaxin

MANUFACTURER
MedImmune

DESCRIPTION
During angiogenesis, growth factors are secreted, which cause blood vessel-forming endothelial cells to multiply and extend toward a solid tumor. These cells use a family of proteins called integrins to adhere to the surrounding tissue, allowing them to continue their extension toward the tumor. Vitaxin has been shown to bind to the integrin found on newly sprouting blood vessels and to stop the growth of these vessels through an apoptotic signaling mechanism. This inhibition of new blood vessel formation has been shown to block the growth and spread of solid tumors in various animal models.

INDICATION(S) AND RESEARCH PHASE
Cancer/Tumors (Unspecified) – Phase I

unknown
Triapine

MANUFACTURER
Vion Pharmaceuticals

DESCRIPTION
Triapine is a potent ribonucleotide reductase inhibitor that blocks a critical step in the synthesis of DNA, thereby preventing the replication of tumor cells. The maximum tolerated dose of two different single-agent regimens administered to subjects with advanced cancer was determined in trials conducted in 2000. Testing of a more compressed, every other week schedule for both regimens is in progress, since more frequent administration is expected to have the greatest effect on subjects' tumors. In 2001, the company expects to initiate phase II trials as well as a number of phase I combination trials of Triapine in conjunction with standard chemotherapy treatments.

INDICATION(S) AND RESEARCH PHASE
Cancer/Tumors (Unspecified) – Phase I

unknown
Angiocol

MANUFACTURER
BioStratum

DESCRIPTION
Angiocol is a recombinant type IV collagen-derived anti-angiogenesis compound that inhibits new blood vessel growth by targeting the assembly and organization of the basal lamina. Without an increased blood supply, the growth of a tumor is substantially limited. Therapies that inhibit new blood vessel growth are a promising approach for the treatment of cancer. Angiocol has demonstrated anti-angiogenic and anti-tumor activity in a wide range of test systems and animal models of cancer. Preclinical toxicology studies are under way and phase I clinical trials are scheduled to begin in 2001

INDICATION(S) AND RESEARCH PHASE
Cancer/Tumors (Unspecified) – Phase I

vincristine
Onco TCS

MANUFACTURER
Inex Pharmaceuticals

DESCRIPTION
Onco TCS is a proprietary drug comprised of the widely used, off-patent cancer drug vincristine encapsulated in the company's patented drug delivery technology, Transmembrane Carrier Systems (TCS). The drug is being evaluated for treatment of non-Hodgkin's lymphoma (NHL). The TCS technology provides prolonged blood circulation, tumor accumulation, and extended-drug release at the cancer site and is designed to increase the effectiveness and reduce the toxicity of the encapsulated drug.

The company reported that phase IIa trials achieved over a 40% response rate with mild and manageable toxicity in relapsed aggressive and transformed NHL subjects. The investigators reported results from 68 total evaluable NHL subjects, 50 of whom suffered from the aggressive or transformed type of the disease. Analysis of 38 subjects with aggressive NHL and 12 subjects with transformed NHL provided a 45% and 42% response rate, respectively. The additional 18 subjects had other types of NHL and did not experience significant response rates to the treatment.

The FDA has given the company permission to proceed with the pivotal phase II/III trial of Onco TCS for NHL. Phase II trials have begun for small cell lung cancer and solid tumors. Additional indications for this drug may include colon cancer, lymph cancer, lymphoma, and pancreatic cancer.

INDICATION(S) AND RESEARCH PHASE
Lymphoma, Non-Hodgkin's – Phase II/III
Lung Cancer – Phase II
Cancer/Tumors (Unspecified) – Phase II

VNP 20009
Tapet

MANUFACTURER
Vion Pharmaceuticals

DESCRIPTION
Tapet (tumor amplified protein expression therapy) is the designation for attenuated *Salmonella typhimurium* that have been shown to accumulate preferentially in solid tumors, reaching high tumor to normal tissue ratios. Accumulation of the bacterial vector, VNP 20009, in tumors provides a platform for preferential delivery of anti-cancer agents to tumors, which can be accomplished through genetic modification of the bacteria. The base (unarmed) vector VNP 20009 also inhibits tumor growth in animal models.

Phase I trials of Tapet administered by direct injection into tumors or by intravenous infusion have been initiated in subjects with advanced cancer. Intratumoral administration has been well tolerated, and viable bacteria can be detected in injected tumors for an extended time period beyond the initial treatment. Additionally, phase I intravenous trials remain open with the objective of optimizing tumor colonization by modifications of dose and schedule and administration of VNP 20009 in combination with methods to reduce dose-limiting toxicities.

INDICATION(S) AND RESEARCH PHASE
Cancer/Tumors (Unspecified) – Phase I

VX-853
unknown

MANUFACTURER
Vertex Pharmaceuticals

DESCRIPTION
VX-853 is an inhibitor of two major cellular drug pumps (P-glycoprotein [MDR-1] and multidrug resistance associated protein [MRP]), which are responsible for manifesting multidrug resistance to cancer chemotherapy. The drug is administered orally and is given with traditional chemotherapeutic agents. As of January 2001, VX-853 is in phase I/II development.

INDICATION(S) AND RESEARCH PHASE
Cancer/Tumors (Unspecified) – Phase I/II

XR9576
unknown

MANUFACTURER
Xenova

DESCRIPTION
XR9576 is an agent designed to overcome P-gp (P-glycoprotein), a protein produced in the cancer cell membrane that forces anti-cancer drugs out of the cell. When taken in conjunction with common chemotherapeutic drugs, XR9576 should increase their effectiveness. The first intravenous formulation of XR9576 is a combination therapy with paclitaxel in phase II/III development. The second intravenous formulation is a combination of XR9576 with doxorubicin in phase II development. The third is a combination therapy with vinorelbine also in phase II development. XR9576 in an oral formulation by itself is currently in phase I/II development.

INDICATION(S) AND RESEARCH PHASE
Cancer/Tumors (Unspecified) – Phase II/III
Cancer/Tumors (Unspecified) – Phase II
Cancer/Tumors (Unspecified) – Phase I/II

ZD-0101, CM-101
unknown

MANUFACTURER
AstraZeneca

DESCRIPTION
ZD-0101 is an anti-angiogenesis agent that is being tested against solid tumors. By preventing new blood vessel formation that is essential to growing cancers, ZD-0101 may inhibit tumor expansion and possibly kill the aberrant growth. This anti-cancer drug is being tested in phase II trials.

INDICATION(S) AND RESEARCH PHASE
Cancer/Tumors (Unspecified) – Phase II

ZD-0473/AMD 473
unknown

MANUFACTURER
AstraZeneca

DESCRIPTION
ZD-0473 is a new platinum-based anti-cancer agent designed to deliver an extended spectrum of activity and overcome resistance to currently approved platinum drugs, such as cisplatin and carboplatin. It is being evaluated for the treatment of a range of solid-tumor cancers, including colorectal, non-small cell lung, and bladder cancer, which are resistant to carboplatin. ZD-0473 is formulated in both intravenous and oral forms. The intravenous formulation is in phase II trials and the oral form is in preclinical development.

INDICATION(S) AND RESEARCH PHASE
Bladder Cancer – Phase II
Cancer/Tumors (Unspecified) – Phase II
Colorectal Cancer – Phase II
Lung Cancer – Phase II
Ovarian Cancer – Phase II
Prostate Cancer – Phase II
Breast Cancer – Phase II
Cervical Dysplasia/Cancer – Phase II

ZD-1839
Iressa

MANUFACTURER
AstraZeneca

DESCRIPTION
Iressa binds to the epidermal growth factor receptor (EGFR) and inhibits tyrosine kinase, thereby blocking signals for cancer growth and survival. The company reported encouraging results from phase I trials in a variety of tumors, but particularly in non-small cell lung cancer (NSCLC). Iressa is being investigated both as a monotherapy and in combination with other anti-tumor drugs in NSCLC, gastric, colorectal, and hormone-resistant prostate cancers. In 1999, the FDA gave Iressa fast-track status. The drug is currently in phase III studies for solid tumors.

INDICATION(S) AND RESEARCH PHASE
Cancer/Tumors (Unspecified) – Phase III
Colorectal Cancer – Phase III
Gastric Cancer – Phase III
Lung Cancer – Phase III
Prostate Cancer – Phase III

ZD-9331
unknown

MANUFACTURER
AstraZeneca

DESCRIPTION
ZD-9331 inhibits the formation of thymidine triphosphate, an essential molecule for both DNA and RNA synthesis. As a result of the pathway disruption, tumor cells are unable to reproduce. In earlier phase I studies, oral and intravenous formulations were investigated, including a dose-escalation trial with 71 subjects. The company reported that the results were encouraging with anti-tumor activity seen in a wide range of tumor types. In phase II trials, ZD-9331 showed anti-cancer activity in a number of solid cancer types such as colorectal, breast, ovarian, and melanomas. This drug may provide a therapeutic alternative for subjects with late stage cancers who have not been successfully treated using standard therapies. BTG International has a licensing agreement with AstraZeneca for development of ZD-9331.

INDICATION(S) AND RESEARCH PHASE
Cancer/Tumors (Unspecified) – Phase II

Cervical Dysplasia/ Cancer

arsenic trioxide (ATO)
Trisenox

MANUFACTURER
Cell Therapeutics

DESCRIPTION
Trisenox is believed to kill cancer cells through apoptosis. The mechanism of action of Trisenox is not fully understood, but the drug appears to induce apoptosis in a different manner than other anti-cancer agents such as retinoids.

Trisenox is FDA approved to treat acute promyelocytic leukemia (APL), and it is also in numerous trials in the United States for indications including other types of leukemias, prostate cancer, multiple myeloma, renal cell cancer, cervical cancer, and bladder cancer.

INDICATION(S) AND RESEARCH PHASE
Leukemia – Phase I
Lymphoma, Non-Hodgkin's – Phase II
Leukemia – Phase II
Multiple Myeloma – Phase II
Prostate Cancer – Phase II
Renal Cell Carcinoma – Phase II
Cervical Dysplasia/Cancer – Phase II
Bladder Cancer – Phase II

CI-1042, ONYX-015
unknown

MANUFACTURER
Onyx Pharmaceuticals

DESCRIPTION
CI-1042 (ONYX-015) is a tumor-selective, modified adenovirus (similar to the common cold virus) that has been genetically engineered to replicate in and kill cancer cells that possess a mutated oncogene called p53, while sparing normal cells with functioning p53. p53 Is a tumor suppressor gene that is mutated in approximately 50% of all human cancers. CI-1042 is in development for several indications, including pancreatic

cancer, liver metastases of colorectal cancer, and lung cancer.

Results of a phase II trial demonstrated that CI-1042 administered as a single agent replicates and causes tumor regression in refractory head and neck cancer. CI-1042 was shown to selectively target cancer cells containing a mutant p53 gene, while sparing normal cells with a functioning p53 gene. Of the 19 subjects who received the standard dosing regimen, four (21%) had an objective response, including two complete responses and two partial responses. CI-1042 is being co-developed with Pfizer.

INDICATION(S) AND RESEARCH PHASE
Colorectal Cancer – Phase II
Pancreatic Cancer – Phase II
Head and Neck Cancer – Phase III
Cervical Dysplasia/Cancer – Phase I completed
Lung Cancer – Phase II
Bladder Cancer – Phase I completed
Brain Cancer – Phase I completed

eflornithine, DFMO (difluoromethylornydil)
unknown

MANUFACTURER
Aventis

DESCRIPTION
Eflornithine is a potent, irreversible inhibitor of ornithine decarboxylase (OCD), an enzyme that is elevated in most tumors and pre-malignant lesions. Eflornithine is currently in a phase III clinical trial to determine the effectiveness of the drug in treating subjects who have newly diagnosed or recurrent bladder cancer. The drug is administered orally in tablet form.

Eflornithine is also in trials for the prevention and treatment of HIV infections, skin cancer, breast cancer, prostate cancer, and cervical dysplasia/cancer.

INDICATION(S) AND RESEARCH PHASE
Bladder Cancer – Phase III
Breast Cancer – Phase II/III
Cervical Dysplasia/Cancer – Phase II
HIV Infection – Phase II
Prostate Cancer – Phase II
Skin Cancer – Phase III

HspE7
unknown

MANUFACTURER
StressGen

DESCRIPTION
HspE7 is a recombinant fusion product composed of the heat shock protein 65 (Hsp65) from *M. bovis* BCG and the protein E7. The E7 protein is derived from the human papillomavirus (HPV) and is involved in the malignant transformation of anal and cervical epithelial cells. E7 is a tumor-specific antigen and represents a precise target for immune system attack on abnormal cells.

StressGen has initiated treatment in a phase III trial to investigate HspE7 as a novel immunotherapeutic for anal dysplasia (AIN) caused by HPV. Phase II trials are also under way in women with HPV-related cervical dysplasia and cervical cancer. In January 2001, a phase II trial was initiated to test HspE7 on 52 subjects suffering from genital warts caused by HPV.

INDICATION(S) AND RESEARCH PHASE
Cervical Dysplasia/Cancer – Phase II
Anal Dysplasia – Phase III
Genital Warts – Phase II

LGD-1550
unknown

MANUFACTURER
Ligand Pharmaceuticals

DESCRIPTION
LGD-1550 is being formulated to limit the proliferation and spread of head, neck, and cervical cancers; it is to be given orally and is currently in phase II trials. Retinoids are a group of substances, one of which is vitamin A, that are thought to be responsible for growth, bone development, vision, and skin integrity. It is thought that retinoids act against cancer by regulating the process by which cells reproduce themselves (gene transcription regulation). Studies have shown that subjects with metastatic cancer have lower levels of retinoid activity in their bodies. LGD-1550 works by binding to retinoid receptors in cells, thereby stimulating retinoid activity.

Preliminary studies have shown that retinoids may inhibit cell proliferation and promote cell differentiation. Cancer arises when there is uncontrolled growth of immature cells. Retinoids act to slow cell division and stimulates cell maturation, making it less likely that these mature cells will be transformed into cancerous cells. Retinoids have also been shown in early studies to boost the effects of other anti-cancer medications.

Phase II trials of LGD-1550 for head and neck cancer, cervical cancer, and solid and hematological tumors are currently under way.

INDICATION(S) AND RESEARCH PHASE
Blood Cancer – Phase II
Cancer/Tumors (Unspecified) – Phase II
Cervical Dysplasia/Cancer – Phase II
Head and Neck Cancer – Phase II

MEDI-517
unknown

MANUFACTURER
MedImmune

DESCRIPTION
MEDI-517 is a virus-like particle vaccine designed to elicit an immune response against the human papillomavirus (HPV). HPVs have been implicated in the development of genital warts and cervical cancer, with specific types of HPV associated with each condition. HPV-6 and HPV-11 cause the majority of genital warts, while HPV-16 and HPV-18 cause the majority of cervical cancers. MEDI-517 is currently in phase II trials for the prevention of cervical cancer.

INDICATION(S) AND RESEARCH PHASE
Viral Infection – Phase II
Cervical Dysplasia/Cancer – Phase II

MGI-114, hydroxymethylacylfulvene,

HMAF
Irofulven

MANUFACTURER
MGI Pharma

DESCRIPTION
Irofulven (MGI-114) is the first product candidate being developed by MGI Pharma from its family of anti-cancer compounds called acylfulvenes. Early trials demonstrated that Irofulven is absorbed rapidly by tumor cells, and once inside binds to DNA and protein targets. The binding interferes with DNA replication and cell division, leading to tumor specific cell death. The drug is being tested in a series of trials for a variety of cancers.

In November 2000, results from a phase II trial of Irofulven indicated that the drug produced anti-tumor activity in subjects with advanced pancreatic cancer who were refractory to gemcitabine (Gemzar). Ten of the 53 subjects enrolled achieved six-month survival and two subjects demonstrated objective responses: one subject experienced tumor shrinkage of 100% and another subject experienced an 84% decrease in tumor mass. A phase III trial was initiated in February 2001.

INDICATION(S) AND RESEARCH PHASE
Breast Cancer – Phase II
Colon Malignancies – Phase II
Renal Cell Carcinoma – Phase II
Cervical Dysplasia/Cancer – Phase II
Lung Cancer – Phase II
Ovarian Cancer – Phase I/II
Colorectal Cancer – Phase II
Prostate Cancer – Phase I/II
Cancer/Tumors (Unspecified) – Phase I/II
Pancreatic Cancer – Phase III
Liver Cancer – Phase II

MX6
unknown

MANUFACTURER
Maxia Pharmaceuticals

DESCRIPTION
MX6 is a naphthoic acid derivative that inhibits cancer cell proliferation and promotes cell apoptosis. The drug is in phase III trials for treatment of cervical dysplasia using a topical gel formulation.

INDICATION(S) AND RESEARCH PHASE
Cervical Dysplasia/Cancer – Phase III

TA-CIN
unknown

MANUFACTURER
Cantab Pharmaceuticals plc

DESCRIPTION
TA-CIN is a novel vaccine in phase I trials for the treatment of cervical dysplasia—an abnormality of the cervix associated with human papillomavirus (HPV) infection that can lead to cervical cancer if left untreated. TA-CIN is based on a genetically engineered fusion protein derived from HPV, and it is designed to stimulate the immune system to destroy cervical cells infected with HPV-16, the most common HPV type found in advanced stages of cervical dyplasia. A phase I trial is being conducted in 40 subjects at a center in the Netherlands.

INDICATION(S) AND RESEARCH PHASE
Cervical Dysplasia/Cancer – Phase I

TA-HPV
unknown

MANUFACTURER
Cantab Pharmaceuticals plc

DESCRIPTION
TA-HPV is a vaccine for the treatment of cervical cancer. It is designed to initiate a natural immune response to cancer cells, eliminating tumor growth or metastatic spread. A phase II study held by the company in collaboration with the European Organization for the Research and Treatment of Cancer (EORTC) showed efficacy in treating subjects with cervical cancer. Two additional phase II studies are under way in Europe.

INDICATION(S) AND RESEARCH PHASE
Cervical Dysplasia/Cancer – Phase II

vaccine, cervical cancer
unknown

MANUFACTURER
MediGene AG

DESCRIPTION
MediGene's HPV16-L1E7-CVLP vaccine is being developed for the treatment of pre-cancerous lesions of the cervix (CIN) caused by human papillomaviruses (HPV). The company's CVLP technology is based on chimeric virus-like particles (CVLPs), which induce an immune response against HPV, both preventing infection and killing already infected cells. Phase I/II testing is under way.

INDICATION(S) AND RESEARCH PHASE
Cervical Dysplasia/Cancer – Phase I/II

ZD-0473/AMD 473
unknown

MANUFACTURER
AstraZeneca

DESCRIPTION
ZD-0473 is a new platinum-based anti-cancer agent designed to deliver an extended spectrum of activity and overcome resistance to currently approved platinum drugs, such as cisplatin and carboplatin. It is being evaluated for the treatment of a range of solid-tumor cancers, including colorectal, non-small cell lung and bladder cancer, which are resistant to carboplatin. ZD-0473 is formulated in both intravenous and oral forms. The intravenous formulation is in phase II trials and the oral form is in preclinical development.

INDICATION(S) AND RESEARCH PHASE
Bladder Cancer – Phase II
Cancer/Tumors (Unspecified) – Phase II
Colorectal Cancer – Phase II
Lung Cancer – Phase II
Ovarian Cancer – Phase II
Prostate Cancer – Phase II
Breast Cancer – Phase II
Cervical Dysplasia/Cancer – Phase II

Chemotherapy

MK-663
unknown

MANUFACTURER
Merck & Co.

DESCRIPTION
MK-663 belongs to a class of non-steroidal anti-inflammatory drugs (NSAIDs) called Cox-2 inhibitors. MK-663 is designed to specifically inhibit cyclooxygenase-2 (Cox-2), an enzyme that leads to the production of substances that cause acute or chronic discomfort in joints with the associated pain and inflammation of arthritis.

Clinical studies have shown that Cox-2 inhibitors work with the body to help it strengthen the system and prevent activation of several enzymes of arachidonic acid metabolism. Consequently, the inhibitors prevent the formation of eicosanoids, which are short-lived chemical agents that control a large number of physiological functions. Cox-2 inhibitors counteract the formation of at least two undesired biochemicals: prostaglandins that are responsible for short-term joint discomfort, and also leukotrienes that are responsible for long-term joint discomfort. By inhibiting prostaglandin synthesis and counteracting the destructive changes in healthy joints caused by leukotrienes, the extract Cox-2 is the first dual inhibitor available.

The company reported favorable results from a phase II trial that showed MK-663 relieved pain better than the placebo in 617 subjects with osteoarthritis of the knee. MK-663 is being tested in trials for the treatment and relief of pain associated with rheumatoid arthritis and for the treatment of chemotherapy induced emesis.

INDICATION(S) AND RESEARCH PHASE
Pain, Acute or Chronic – Phase III
Rheumatoid Arthritis – Phase III
Chemotherapy – Phase III

polymer platinate, AP5280
unknown

MANUFACTURER
Access Pharmaceuticals

DESCRIPTION
AP5280 is a chemotherapeutic agent that uses platinum bound to a new polymer to improve the concentration of the treatment at the tumor and reduce side effects. This therapy is currently in phase I trials.

INDICATION(S) AND RESEARCH PHASE
Chemotherapy – Phase I

Colon Malignancies

APC8024
unknown

MANUFACTURER
Dendreon Corporation

DESCRIPTION
APC8024 is a vaccine designed to elicit an antibody response to a protein antigen called HER-2/*neu*. HER-2/*neu* is overexpressed in approximately 25% of metastatic breast cancers, ovarian, pancreatic, and colon cancers. APC8024 is being tested in phase I trials.

INDICATION(S) AND RESEARCH PHASE
Breast Cancer – Phase I
Ovarian Cancer – Phase I
Colon Malignancies – Phase I

GL-331
unknown

MANUFACTURER
Genelabs Technologies

DESCRIPTION
GL-331 is an inhibitor of topoisomerase II. It is a semi-synthetic derivative of podophyllotoxin, which is a chemotherapeutic agent designed to overcome multi-drug resistant (MDR) cancers. At this time, trials have been discontinued.

INDICATION(S) AND RESEARCH PHASE
Colon Malignancies – Trial discontinued
Leukemia – Trial discontinued
Lung Cancer – Trial discontinued
Renal Cell Carcinoma – Trial discontinued

ISIS 2503
unknown

MANUFACTURER
Isis Pharmaceuticals

DESCRIPTION
ISIS 2503 is a potent, selective antisense inhibitor of H-ras gene expression. Antisense drugs inhibit the production of disease-causing proteins by altering the genetic information, which messenger RNA uses to produce new protein. H-ras is one of a family of ras genes that are involved in the process by which cells receive and send signals that affect their behavior. The company claims that substantial evidence exists to support a direct role for the ras gene products in the development and maintenance of human cancers.

In phase II trials, the compound is being evaluated as a single agent in subjects with colon, breast, pancreatic, and non-small cell lung cancers. These trials will provide preliminary data on the anti-tumor activity of ISIS 2503 against these common tumor types. Approximately ten sites in the United States and Europe will enroll 15-30 subjects per tumor type in these trials. The company plans future trials of ISIS 2503 in combination with approved cancer therapies.

INDICATION(S) AND RESEARCH PHASE
Breast Cancer – Phase II
Colon Malignancies – Phase II
Lung Cancer – Phase II
Pancreatic Cancer – Phase II

ISIS 5132, CGP 69846A
unknown

MANUFACTURER
Isis Pharmaceuticals

DESCRIPTION
ISIS 5132 is a potent antisense inhibitor of the enzyme c-Raf-1 kinase. Antisense drugs inhibit the production of disease-causing

proteins by altering the genetic information, which messenger RNA uses to produce new protein. c-Raf kinase plays a role in signal processes that regulate cell growth and proliferation. It is one of a family of raf genes thought to play an important role in the development of some solid tumors. The company reports that activated-raf has also been detected in a substantial variety of human cancers including small cell lung carcinoma and breast cancer. For example, it has been reported that 60% of all lung carcinoma cells express unusually high levels of normal c-Raf mRNA and protein.

The sponsor companies reported that results from phase I studies, which examined subjects with a wide variety of solid tumors, demonstrated that the drug was well tolerated and that several subjects experienced disease stabilization. The companies are planning additional phase I safety studies involving the drug in combination with currently approved chemotherapies. Phase II clinical trials examining ISIS 5132 as a single-agent therapy in subjects with breast, lung, colon, pancreatic, and prostate cancers are under way.

INDICATION(S) AND RESEARCH PHASE
Breast Cancer – Phase II
Cancer/Tumors (Unspecified) – Phase II
Colon Malignancies – Phase II
Lung Cancer – Phase II
Pancreatic Cancer – Phase II
Prostate Cancer – Phase II

MDX-210
unknown

MANUFACTURER
Medarex

DESCRIPTION
MDX-210 is a bispecific (target-trigger) monoclonal antibody (MAb)-based treatment being developed for cancers with specific markers (HER-2/*neu* positive), including renal cell, non-small cell lung, pancreatic, and kidney cancers. Phase II trials have been completed for kidney, prostate, and ovarian cancer. Phase III development for ovarian cancer has commenced in Europe.

INDICATION(S) AND RESEARCH PHASE
Prostate Cancer – Phase II completed
Renal Cell Carcinoma – Phase II completed
Colon Malignancies – Phase II
Breast Cancer – Phase II
Gastric Cancer – Phase II
Pancreatic Cancer – Phase II
Lung Cancer – Phase II
Ovarian Cancer – Phase III

MGI-114, hydroxymethylacylfulvene, HMAF
Irofulven

MANUFACTURER
MGI Pharma

DESCRIPTION
Irofulven (MGI-114) is the first product candidate being developed by MGI Pharma from its family of anti-cancer compounds called acylfulvenes. Early trials demonstrated that Irofulven is absorbed rapidly by tumor cells, and once inside binds to DNA and protein targets. The binding interferes with DNA replication and cell division, leading to tumor-specific cell death. The drug is being tested in a series of trials for a variety of cancers.

In November 2000, results from a phase II trial of Irofulven indicated that the drug produced anti-tumor activity in subjects with advanced pancreatic cancer who were refractory to gemcitabine (Gemzar). Ten of the 53 subjects enrolled achieved six-month survival and two subjects demonstrated objective responses: one subject experienced tumor shrinkage of 100% and another subject experienced an 84% decrease in tumor mass. A phase III trial was initiated in February 2001.

INDICATION(S) AND RESEARCH PHASE
Breast Cancer – Phase II
Colon Malignancies – Phase II
Renal Cell Carcinoma – Phase II
Cervical Dysplasia/Cancer – Phase II
Lung Cancer – Phase II
Ovarian Cancer – Phase I/II
Colorectal Cancer – Phase II
Prostate Cancer – Phase I/II
Cancer/Tumors (Unspecified) – Phase I/II
Pancreatic Cancer – Phase III
Liver Cancer – Phase II

SGN-15/Taxotere
unknown

MANUFACTURER
Seattle Genetics

DESCRIPTION
SGN-15 is an antibody drug conjugate composed of the chimeric monoclonal antibody BR96 chemically linked to the drug doxorubicin with an average of eight drug molecules per mAb molecule. SGN-15 works by binding to a cell surface Ley-related antigen expressed on many tumor types, rapidly internalizing, and then releasing its payload of drug at the low pH present within the cell through acid catalyzed hydrolysis in the endosome. This mechanism of targeted drug delivery allows for relative sparing of tissues normally affected by non-specific chemotherapy, and represents an attractive strategy for the treatment of tumors expressing the BR96 antigen.

SGN-15 is being tested in a combination therapy with Aventis' drug Taxotere in a phase I/II trial in subjects with breast or colon cancer. This trial is being co-funded by Aventis. Additionally, a phase II trial is testing SGN/Taxotere in hormone refractory prostate cancer.

INDICATION(S) AND RESEARCH PHASE
Breast Cancer – Phase I/II
Prostate Cancer – Phase II
Colon Malignancies – Phase I/II

SR-48692
unknown

MANUFACTURER
Sanofi-Synthelabo Pharmaceuticals

DESCRIPTION
SR-48692 is an orally formulated neurotensin antagonist being tested for several indications, including colon cancer, prostate cancer, and schizophrenia.

INDICATION(S) AND RESEARCH PHASE
Colon Malignancies – Phase II
Prostate Cancer – Phase II
Schizophrenia and Schizoaffective Disorders – Phase IIa
Psychosis – Phase IIa
Depression – Phase II

Colon Polyps

exisulind
Aptosyn

MANUFACTURER
Cell Pathways

DESCRIPTION
Aptosyn (exisulind) belongs to a novel class of compounds called selective apoptotic anti-neoplastic drugs (SAANDs). SAANDs inhibit a form of cyclic GMP phosphodiesterase and selectively induce apoptosis in abnormally growing precancerous and cancerous cells. Aptosyn is being tested for several indications and is in five different trials for adenomatous polyposis coli (APC) and familial adenomatous polyposis coli; two of these trials are specifically for pediatric subjects.

The company received a non-approvable letter from the FDA in September 2000 for one of the trials for the treatment of familial adenomatous polyposis. The company intends to amend the NDA and request a meeting to address the deficiencies and the possible requirement for additional clinical data.

Additionally, Aptosyn is being tested in trials for the treatment of prostate cancer, lung cancer, breast cancer, sporadic colonic polyps, and Barrett's Esophagus disease.

INDICATION(S) AND RESEARCH PHASE
Adenomatous Polyposis Coli – Non-approvable letter
Pediatric, Familial Adenomatous Polyposis Coli – Phase II
Adenomatous Polyposis Coli – Phase I/II
Barrett's Esophagus Disease – Phase II
Prostate Cancer – Phase II/III
Breast Cancer – Phase II/III
Lung Cancer – Phase Ib
Colon Polyps – Phase II/III

ursodiol
Urso

MANUFACTURER
Axcan Pharma

DESCRIPTION
Urso is an oral tablet composed of a bile acid (ursodeoxycholic acid) found in small amounts in normal human bile and in larger quantities in the bile of certain bears. This drug has been marketed in the United States for the treatment of primary biliary cirrhosis (PBC) since 1998. It is also approved in Canada for the treatment of cholestatic liver diseases such as PBC and the dissolution of gallstones. Additionally, Urso is being tested in trials for at least five other indications: the treatment of hypercholesterolemia, treatment with chemo-prevention of colorectal polyps, treatment of colorectal cancer, treatment of non-alcoholic steatohepatitis, and treatment of viral hepatitis. The drug is licensed by Sanofi-Synthelabo to Axcan Pharma in a joint venture with Schwarz Pharma.

INDICATION(S) AND RESEARCH PHASE
Cholesterol - high levels – Phase II
Colon Polyps – Phase II
Colorectal Cancer – Phase II
Gallbladder Disorders – Phase III/IV
Hepatitis – Phase II

Colorectal Cancer

capecitabine
Xeloda

MANUFACTURER
Hoffmann-La Roche

DESCRIPTION
Xeloda is an anticancer agent and the prodrug of 5-fluorouracil (5-FU). 5-FU is a pyrimidine analog that works by interfering with the synthesis of DNA and RNA. An NDA has been submitted for the treatment of colorectal cancer.

INDICATION(S) AND RESEARCH PHASE
Colorectal Cancer – NDA submitted

CI-1042, ONYX-015
unknown

MANUFACTURER
Onyx Pharmaceuticals

DESCRIPTION
CI-1042 (ONYX-015) is a tumor-selective, modified adenovirus (similar to the common cold virus) that has been genetically engineered to replicate in and kill cancer cells that possess a mutated oncogene called p53, while sparing normal cells with functioning p53. p53 Is a tumor suppressor gene that is mutated in approximately 50% of all human cancers. CI-1042 is in development for several indications, including pancreatic cancer, liver metastases of colorectal cancer, and lung cancer.

In November 2000, results of a phase II trial demonstrated that CI-1042 administered as a single agent replicates and causes tumor regression in refractory head and neck cancer. CI-1042 was shown to selectively target cancer cells containing a mutant p53 gene, while sparing normal cells with a functioning p53 gene. Of the 19 subjects who received the standard dosing regimen, four (21%) had an objective response, including two complete responses and two partial responses. CI-1042 is being co-developed with Pfizer.

INDICATION(S) AND RESEARCH PHASE
Colorectal Cancer – Phase II
Pancreatic Cancer – Phase II
Head and Neck Cancer – Phase III
Cervical Dysplasia/Cancer – Phase I completed
Lung Cancer – Phase II
Bladder Cancer – Phase I completed
Brain Cancer – Phase I completed

cisplatin/epinephrine
IntraDose

MANUFACTURER
Matrix Pharmaceutical

DESCRIPTION

IntraDose is a biodegradable collagen carrier matrix combined with a vasoconstrictor. The gel is injected directly into tumors where it localizes high concentrations of cisplatin, a widely used anticancer drug. It is currently being tested for several indications, including head and neck, breast, malignant melanoma, esophageal, and primary hepatocellular cancer.

A phase II trial of IntraDose Injectable Gel produced durable responses in subjects with colorectal cancer that has metastasized to the liver. Nine of 31 subjects who received IntraDose responded to therapy. Six subjects experienced a complete response (100% reduction in viable tumor volume of treated tumors) while the other three subjects demonstrated a partial response (at least a 50% reduction of viable tumor volume). Eight of the nine treatment responders have had durable responses with no relapse at the site of treatment.

INDICATION(S) AND RESEARCH PHASE

Breast Cancer – Phase II
Cancer/Tumors (Unspecified) – Phase II
Colorectal Cancer – Phase II completed
Esophageal Cancer – Phase II
Liver Cancer – Phase II
Malignant Melanoma – Phase II
Head and Neck Cancer – NDA submitted

CTP-37
Avicine

MANUFACTURER
AVI BioPharma

DESCRIPTION

Avicine is a hormone vaccine derived from human chorionic gonadotropin peptide that is being tested for prevention of colorectal, pancreatic, and prostate cancer. The drug is in phase II trials for prostate cancer, and phase III trials for colorectal and pancreatic cancer. AVI BioPharma has partnered with SuperGen and under the terms of the agreement, SuperGen will be responsible for U.S. marketing and sales of Avicine, and AVI will be responsible for product manufacturing.

INDICATION(S) AND RESEARCH PHASE

Colorectal Cancer – Phase III
Pancreatic Cancer – Phase III
Prostate Cancer – Phase II

declopramide
unknown

MANUFACTURER
OXiGENE

DESCRIPTION

Declopramide is a DNA repair inhibitor in development for the treatment of various cancers. DNA repair inhibitors may increase the effectiveness of standard treatment by inhibiting the ability of tumor cells to repair damaged DNA, leading to apoptosis. Two phase I trials showed that declopramide increases the vulnerability of cancer cells to conventional forms of chemotherapy and radiation. The two trials took place at the Ireland Cancer Center in Cleveland, Ohio, and at St. John's Mercy Medical Center in St. Louis, Missouri. Subjects were given declopramide with either 5-fluorouracil or cisplatin. Results determined the recommended combination dose for the phase II trial that was initiated in January 2001 for colon cancer.

INDICATION(S) AND RESEARCH PHASE

Colorectal Cancer – Phase II

FMdC
unknown

MANUFACTURER
Matrix Pharmaceutical

DESCRIPTION

FMdC is a nucleoside analogue being tested for the treatment of cancer. Nucleoside analogues are a class of drugs that affect DNA synthesis, and they have long been used to treat hematologic cancers such as leukemia. The early members of this drug class were minimally effective against solid tumors.

DNA synthesis occurs during cell division and is critical to successful replication. FMdC enters cells where it is metabolized into two active forms: FMdC diphosphate and FMdC triphosphate. These two active metabolites of FMdC interrupt the process of DNA synthesis, which leads to cell death. FMdC is being evaluated in phase II studies for the treatment of non-small cell lung cancer, colorectal, and ovarian cancer.

INDICATION(S) AND RESEARCH PHASE

Colorectal Cancer – Phase II
Lung Cancer – Phase II
Ovarian Cancer – Phase II

G3139/irinotecan
Genasense/Irinotecan

MANUFACTURER
Genta

DESCRIPTION

Genasense (G3139) is designed to reduce levels of bcl-2, a protein that contributes to resistance of cancer cells to current forms of cancer treatment. Treatment with Genasense may markedly improve the effectiveness of standard anticancer therapies. Genasense in combination with irinotecan is in phase II trials for the treatment of colorectal cancer.

INDICATION(S) AND RESEARCH PHASE

Colorectal Cancer – Phase II

G3139/mitoxantrone
Genasense/Mitoxantrone

MANUFACTURER
Genta

DESCRIPTION

Genasense (G3139) is designed to reduce levels of bcl-2, a protein that contributes to resistance of cancer cells to current forms of cancer treatment. Treatment with Genasense may markedly improve the effectiveness of standard anticancer therapies. G-3139 in combination with mitoxantrone is in trials for treatment of prostate and colorectal cancers.

INDICATION(S) AND RESEARCH PHASE

Colorectal Cancer – Phase II
Prostate Cancer – Phase I/II

GBC-590
unknown

MANUFACTURER
Safe Sciences

DESCRIPTION
GBC-590 belongs to a new class of drugs called lectin inhibitors that specifically interfere with cellular interactions. GBC-590 competitively binds to unique lectins (special protein cell-surface receptors) on cancer cells and disrupts the metastatic process. GBC-590's affinity for cancer lectins is the core reason for its significant biological activity and specificity.

GBC-590 is being tested in phase II studies for pancreatic and colorectal cancer, and the company plans to test it in phase II trials for prostate cancer.

INDICATION(S) AND RESEARCH PHASE
Colorectal Cancer – Phase II
Pancreatic Cancer – Phase II
Prostate Cancer – Phase I/II

HSPPC-96
Oncophage

MANUFACTURER
Antigenics

DESCRIPTION
Oncophage cancer vaccine is an injectable protein that contains the unique profile ("antigenic fingerprint") of each subject's cancer. The antigens activate the immune system to elicit an anti-tumor response. Oncophage is in clinical trials for several indications, including renal cell carcinoma (phase III), melanoma (phase II), colorectal cancer (phase II), gastric cancer (phase I/II), pancreatic cancer (phase I/II completed), and non-Hodgkin's lymphoma (phase II).

In October 2000, Antigenics announced that it had initiated a phase II trial of Oncophage in subjects who have been diagnosed with sarcoma, also known as soft tissue cancer. The study is expected to initially enroll 20 subjects diagnosed with recurrent metastatic or unresectable soft tissue sarcoma and may be expanded to include an additional 15 subjects depending on preliminary results.

INDICATION(S) AND RESEARCH PHASE
Renal Cell Carcinoma – Phase III
Malignant Melanoma – Phase II
Colorectal Cancer – Phase II
Gastric Cancer – Phase I/II
Pancreatic Cancer – Phase I/II completed
Lymphoma, Non-Hodgkin's – Phase II
Sarcoma – Phase II

HuC242-DM1/SB-408075
unknown

MANUFACTURER
ImmunoGen

DESCRIPTION
HuC242-DM1/SB-408075 is a tumor-activated prodrug (TAP) designed for the treatment of colorectal, pancreatic, and certain non-small cell lung cancers. Tumor-activated prodrugs consist of chemically linked monoclonal antibodies and potent, cell-killing chemicals. HuC242-DM1, in particular, is created by joining the cytotoxic maytansinoid drug DM1 with the humanized monoclonal antibody C242. The attached chemical remains inactive until the monoclonal antibody reaches its targeted tumor cell and the TAP is drawn inside. Once inside, DM1 is able to kill the tumor cell without affecting surrounding healthy cells. HuC242-DM1 is currently in phase I/II trials.

INDICATION(S) AND RESEARCH PHASE
Colorectal Cancer – Phase I/II
Pancreatic Cancer – Phase I/II
Lung Cancer – Phase I/II

IMC-1C11
unknown

MANUFACTURER
ImClone Systems

DESCRIPTION
IMC-1C11 is a chimerized monoclonal antibody that inhibits the KDR report, also known as vascular endothelial growth factor receptor (VEGFr), on vascular endothelial cells by blocking the binding of VEGF to the receptor. In animal models, IMC-1C11 demonstrated it inhibited new blood vessels and by doing this, IMC-1C11 deprived tumors of required nutrients. IMC-1C11 is currently being tested in a phase I trial for the treatment of metastatic colorectal cancer.

INDICATION(S) AND RESEARCH PHASE
Colorectal Cancer – Phase I

IMC-C225, CPT-11
unknown

MANUFACTURER
ImClone Systems

DESCRIPTION
IMC-C225 is a chimerized (part mouse, part human) monoclonal antibody that may help fight cancer cells when used in conjunction with radiation therapy or other chemotherapy agents. This antibody selectively blocks the epidermal growth factor receptor (EGFr), which may be present in greater amounts on actively growing tumor cells. Since many cancers use specific growth factors to stimulate tumor cell growth, blocking this receptor may inhibit the cancer from increasing in size and spreading throughout the body.

The company is conducting phase III clinical trials evaluating IMC-C225 in combination with radiotherapy and with chemotherapy in subjects with advanced squamous cell head and neck carcinoma. IMC-C225 is in trials for several other indications in combination with various anti-cancer agents.

INDICATION(S) AND RESEARCH PHASE
Breast Cancer – Phase I/II
Head and Neck Cancer – Phase III
Lung Cancer – Phase III
Prostate Cancer – Phase I/II
Renal Cell Carcinoma – Phase II
Pancreatic Cancer – Phase II
Colorectal Cancer – Phase II

IMMU-MN14, anti-CEA

Colorectal Cancer

CEA-Cide

MANUFACTURER
Immunomedics

DESCRIPTION
Carcinoembryonic antigen (CEA) is a protein-polysaccharide complex released in the bloodstream by certain cancers, especially colon carcinoma. This antigenic substance may provide early diagnosis when used as a therapeutic marker in immunologic tests. The CEA complex may also be targeted by specialized monoclonal antibodies in the design of a biologic therapeutic.

CEA-Cide is a novel monoclonal antibody that is designed for radioimmunotherapy (with 90 Y-labeled humanized MN-14). This drug is being tested in phase II trials for the treatment of advanced metastatic and CEA-producing cancers, particularly colorectal cancer. Other indications may include breast cancer, female reproductive system cancer, ovarian cancer, lung cancer, and pancreatic cancer.

INDICATION(S) AND RESEARCH PHASE
Breast Cancer – Phase II
Cancer/Tumors (Unspecified) – Phase II
Colorectal Cancer – Phase II
Lung Cancer – Phase II
Ovarian Cancer – Phase II
Pancreatic Cancer – Phase II

MDX-220
unknown

MANUFACTURER
Medarex

DESCRIPTION
MDX-220 is a bispecific (target-trigger) monoclonal antibody (MAb) that targets Tag-72 in the treatment of a variety of cancers, including lung, colon, prostate, ovarian, endometrial, pancreatic, and gastric cancer.

INDICATION(S) AND RESEARCH PHASE
Endometrial Cancer – Phase I/II
Gastric Cancer – Phase I/II
Lung Cancer – Phase I/II
Ovarian Cancer – Phase I/II
Pancreatic Cancer – Phase I/II
Prostate Cancer – Phase II
Colorectal Cancer – Phase II

MGI-114, hydroxymethylacylfulvene, HMAF
Irofulven

MANUFACTURER
MGI Pharma

DESCRIPTION
Irofulven (MGI-114) is the first product candidate being developed by MGI Pharma from its family of anti-cancer compounds called acylfulvenes. Early trials demonstrated that Irofulven is absorbed rapidly by tumor cells, and once inside binds to DNA and protein targets. The binding interferes with DNA replication and cell division, leading to tumor-specific cell death. The drug is being tested in a series of trials for a variety of cancers.

In November 2000, results from a phase II trial of Irofulven indicated that the drug produced anti-tumor activity in subjects with advanced pancreatic cancer who were refractory to gemcitabine (Gemzar). Ten of the 53 subjects enrolled achieved six-month survival and two subjects demonstrated objective responses: one subject experienced tumor shrinkage of 100% and another subject experienced an 84% decrease in tumor mass. A phase III trial was initiated in February 2001.

INDICATION(S) AND RESEARCH PHASE
Breast Cancer – Phase II
Colon Malignancies – Phase II
Renal Cell Carcinoma – Phase II
Cervical Dysplasia/Cancer – Phase II
Lung Cancer – Phase II
Ovarian Cancer – Phase I/II
Colorectal Cancer – Phase II
Prostate Cancer – Phase I/II
Cancer/Tumors (Unspecified) – Phase I/II
Pancreatic Cancer – Phase III
Liver Cancer – Phase II

raltitrexed, ZD-1694
Tomudex

MANUFACTURER
AstraZeneca

DESCRIPTION
Tomudex is a cytotoxic enzyme inhibitor of thymidylate synthase. It is administered as a single agent infusion. Tomudex is in trials for colorectal cancer, other unspecified tumors, and as a cancer vaccine.

INDICATION(S) AND RESEARCH PHASE
Colorectal Cancer – Phase II
Cancer/Tumors (Unspecified) – Phase II/III
Vaccines – Phase III

RFS-2000
Rubitecan

MANUFACTURER
SuperGen

DESCRIPTION
Rubitecan is a novel drug in the late stages of phase III development for treating advanced pancreatic cancer. It works by inhibiting an enzyme called topoisomerase-I. This drug is made in an oral form that is an advantage for outpatient treatment compared to intravenous type cancer drugs that may require a visit to a hospital setting.

In addition to treating pancreatic cancer, Rubitecan is being evaluated in treating a variety of solid tumors, such as in breast, colorectal, lung, ovarian, and prostate cancers, as well as metastatic melanoma and advanced gastric carcinoma. Also, phase II trials in the United States and Europe are testing Rubitecan in blood cancers such as chronic myelomonocytic leukemia (CMML/myelodysplastic syndrome).

Clinical study results reported in the May 1999 issue of the *International Journal of Oncology* noted that Rubitecan was given to a group of end-stage pancreatic cancer subjects who failed all previous conventional therapies. Of the 60 subjects who completed Rubitecan treatment, 31.7% responded favorably with half of the subjects staying alive (the median survival) at 18.6 months. Additionally, 31.7% were stabilized with a 9.7 month median survival rate, and 36.6% were non-responders with a 6.8 month median survival rate.

Colorectal Cancer

INDICATION(S) AND RESEARCH PHASE
Pancreatic Cancer – Phase III
Breast Cancer – Phase II
Colorectal Cancer – Phase II
Gastric Cancer – Phase II
Leukemia – Phase II
Malignant Melanoma – Phase II
Ovarian Cancer – Phase II
Myelodysplastic Syndrome – Phase III

SB 408075
unknown

MANUFACTURER
GlaxoSmithKline

DESCRIPTION
SB 408075 is a tumor activated pro-drug (maytansine-antibody conjugate) in phase I trials. It is being tested as a second line therapy for the treatment of colorectal cancer.

INDICATION(S) AND RESEARCH PHASE
Colorectal Cancer – Phase I

T67
unknown

MANUFACTURER
Tularik

DESCRIPTION
T67 is an anti-cancer compound that binds irreversibly to tubulin and inhibits the growth of multi-drug resistant tumors. Tubulin is a protein that polymerizes into chains to form microtubules. Microtubules are essential for cell division, and by disrupting their function, T67 produces cell death and potentially causes tumor shrinkage.

The drug is currently in phase II trials in subjects with non-small cell lung cancer, glioma, colorectal cancer, and breast cancer. It is also in a phase I/II trial for the treatment of hepatocellular carcinoma. These trials are being conducted in the United States, the United Kingdom, Hong Kong, and Taiwan.

INDICATION(S) AND RESEARCH PHASE
Lung Cancer – Phase II
Brain Cancer – Phase II
Colorectal Cancer – Phase II
Breast Cancer – Phase II
Hepatocellular Carcinoma – Phase I/II

TBA-CEA
unknown

MANUFACTURER
Therion Biologics

DESCRIPTION
TBA-CEA is being developed for the treatment of colorectal cancer. This biological drug targets carcinoembryonic antigen, which is a marker of colorectal cancer. Clinical trials are in phase II development.

INDICATION(S) AND RESEARCH PHASE
Colorectal Cancer – Phase II

topotecan HCl
Hycamtin

MANUFACTURER
GlaxoSmithKline

DESCRIPTION
Hycamtin (topotecan HCl) is a topoisomerase I inhibitor administered by injection. It is currently indicated for the treatment of metastatic carcinoma of the ovary after failure of initial or subsequent chemotherapy. Hycamtin is also indicated for the treatment of small cell lung cancer sensitive disease after failure of first-line chemotherapy.

Hycamtin is being evaluated in a variety of phase II and III trials. It is being tested as a second-line therapy for the treatment of colorectal cancer (phase II), as first-line therapy for small cell and non-small cell lung cancer (phase II), as oral second-line therapy for small cell lung cancer (phase III), and as first-line therapy for ovarian cancer (phase III). Lastly, Hycamtin is in phase III trials for the treatment of myelodysplastic syndrome.

INDICATION(S) AND RESEARCH PHASE
Colorectal Cancer – Phase II
Lung Cancer – Phase II
Lung Cancer – Phase III
Ovarian Cancer – Phase III
Myelodysplastic Syndrome – Phase III

trimetrexate glucuronate/ leucovorin
NeuTrexin

MANUFACTURER
MedImmune

DESCRIPTION
NeuTrexin, a product already approved in 13 countries for the management of moderate-to-severe *Pneumocystis carinii* pneumonia (PCP), one of the most serious complications of HIV infection, may have potential oncologic applications. NeuTrexin disrupts DNA, RNA, and protein synthesis, causing cell death. The drug may prove effective as a pharmacologic modulator of the combination of 5-fluorouracil and leucovorin, which is a current standard therapy.

Data from a phase II study at Memorial Sloan-Kettering Cancer Center demonstrated that the combination resulted in a 20% response rate and a 14 month median survival in subjects who had previously failed 5-fluorouracil based treatment regimens.

Phase III trials are under way for the treatment of colorectal cancer. Additional indications may include gastrointestinal cancer, advanced non-small cell lung cancer (orphan indication), prostate cancer, pancreatic cancer, and sarcomas. NeuTrexin is given in an oral formulation.

INDICATION(S) AND RESEARCH PHASE
Colorectal Cancer – Phase III

troxacitabine, BCH-4556
Troxatyl

MANUFACTURER
BioChem Pharma

DESCRIPTION
Troxatyl is a dioxolane nucleoside analog being investigated as an anticancer agent. The drug is a complete DNA chain terminator and DNA polymerase inhibitor. It acts

by incorporating itself into the growing DNA chain of cancer cells, interfering with their ability to replicate further. Currently, Troxatyl is being evaluated as a single agent or in combination therapy in a number of ongoing single and multicenter trials in hematologic malignancies, including acute myeloid leukemia, chronic myeloid leukemia—blastic phase, and in lymphoproliferative disorders such as lymphoma, chronic lymphocytic leukemia, and myeloma. It is also being evaluated as a single agent in pancreatic cancer and in combination therapy in a number of solid tumors. Troxatyl is currently in phase II development.

INDICATION(S) AND RESEARCH PHASE
Cancer/Tumors (Unspecified) – Phase II
Colorectal Cancer – Phase II
Head and Neck Cancer – Phase II
Leukemia – Phase II
Lung Cancer – Phase II
Malignant Melanoma – Phase II
Ovarian Cancer – Phase II
Pancreatic Cancer – Phase II
Prostate Cancer – Phase II
Renal Cell Carcinoma – Phase II

unknown
Cea-Tricom

MANUFACTURER
Therion Biologics

DESCRIPTION
Cea-Tricom is a recombinant pox virus-based vaccine that targets carcinoembryonic antigen (CEA), a protein found on the surface of colorectal, pancreatic, breast, and lung cancer cells. Cea-Tricom will be administered using two pox virus vectors, rV-Cea-Tricom and rF-Cea-Tricom. The Tricom component of the vaccine consists of three co-stimulatory molecules known to elicit strong cellular immune responses necessary for complete tumor destruction. A phase I trial testing Cea-Tricom will treat 42 subjects who have advanced metastatic colorectal cancer. This trial is being co-sponsored by NCI.

INDICATION(S) AND RESEARCH PHASE
Colorectal Cancer – Phase I

ursodiol
Urso

MANUFACTURER
Axcan Pharma

DESCRIPTION
Urso is an oral tablet composed of a bile acid (ursodeoxycholic acid) found in small amounts in normal human bile and in larger quantities in the bile of certain bears. This drug has been marketed in the United States for the treatment of primary biliary cirrhosis (PBC) since 1998. It is also approved in Canada for the treatment of cholestatic liver diseases such as PBC and the dissolution of gallstones. Urso is being tested in trials for at least five other indications: the treatment of hypercholesterolemia, treatment with chemo-prevention of colorectal polyps, treatment of colorectal cancer, treatment of non-alcoholic steatohepatitis, and treatment of viral hepatitis. The drug is licensed by Sanofi-Synthelabo to Axcan Pharma in a joint venture with Schwarz Pharma.

INDICATION(S) AND RESEARCH PHASE
Cholesterol - high levels – Phase II
Colon Polyps – Phase II
Colorectal Cancer – Phase II
Gallbladder Disorders – Phase III/IV
Hepatitis – Phase II

vaccine
Onyvax CR

MANUFACTURER
Onyvax

DESCRIPTION
Onyvax CR is an allogenic whole-cell colorectal cancer vaccine. It is currently in a phase I/II trial in subjects with advanced metastatic disease at St. George's Hospital in London and is designed to principally examine the safety and immunogenicity of the vaccine. The vaccine is initially administered every two weeks for six weeks, and then monthly for up to a year.

INDICATION(S) AND RESEARCH PHASE
Colorectal Cancer – Phase I/II
Vaccines – Phase I/II

vaccine, anti-cancer
CeaVac

MANUFACTURER
Titan Pharmaceuticals

DESCRIPTION
CeaVac is an anti-cancer monoclonal antibody based product designed to help the subject's immune system recognize and kill tumor cells. Titan announced early phase I/II results of CeaVac in subjects with colorectal cancer that suggested a positive clinical effect, with nine of 15 subjects continuing without disease. Phase III trials are under way.

INDICATION(S) AND RESEARCH PHASE
Colorectal Cancer – Phase III

vaccine, anti-cancer
CeaVac/TriAb

MANUFACTURER
Titan Pharmaceuticals

DESCRIPTION
Both CeaVac and TriAb are anti-cancer monoclonal antibody based products designed to help the subject's immune system recognize and kill tumor cells. They are being tested in a combined therapy for the treatment of non-small cell lung cancer and colorectal cancer.

INDICATION(S) AND RESEARCH PHASE
Lung Cancer – Phase II
Colorectal Cancer – Phase II

vaccine, anti-gastrin
Gastrimmune

MANUFACTURER
Aphton Corporation

DESCRIPTION
Gastrimmune is a therapeutic vaccine that

neutralizes specific hormones (G17 & Gly-extended G17). The drug is in phase III trials for the treatment of cancers of the gastrointestinal tract, including gastric cancer and colorectal cancer. It is also in trials for liver cancer, esophageal cancer and two phase III trials for advanced pancreatic cancer—one in the the United States and one in Europe.

INDICATION(S) AND RESEARCH PHASE
Colorectal Cancer – Phase III
Esophageal Cancer – Phase III
Gastric Cancer – Phase III
Liver Cancer – Phase II/III
Pancreatic Cancer – Phase III

vaccine, 105AD7
Onyvax 105

MANUFACTURER
Onyvax

DESCRIPTION
Onyvax 105 is a human monoclonal antibody being developed for the treatment of colorectal cancer. The drug works by inducing immune responses against the widespread tumor antigen CD55. CD55 is overexpressed in numerous cancers, including those of the prostate, colon and pancreas. Onyvax 105 is currently in phase I/II trials.

INDICATION(S) AND RESEARCH PHASE
Colorectal Cancer – Phase I/II
Vaccines – Phase I/II

VNP 40101M
unknown

MANUFACTURER
Vion Pharmaceuticals

DESCRIPTION
Sulfonyl hydrazine prodrugs (SHPs) are a series of unique, small molecule antitumor alkylating agents that prevent cell division upon interaction with DNA. VNP 40101M has been identified as the lead candidate of these compounds for clinical development. The drug has demonstrated broad antitumor activity in animal models including tumors resistant to standard alkylating agents. A phase I trial was initiated in February 2001 for the treatment of colorectal cancer in 42 subjects.

INDICATION(S) AND RESEARCH PHASE
Colorectal Cancer – Phase I

XR5000
unknown

MANUFACTURER
Xenova

DESCRIPTION
XR5000 is a topoisomerase I and II inhibitor being developed for the treatment of common solid tumors. Three phase II trials are under way at a number of European centers. The trials are being conducted on an "open-label" basis and target three cancer types—ovarian, non-small cell lung, and glioblastoma. The results of a fourth phase II trial, in which the efficacy of XR5000 was investigated in subjects with colorectal cancer, were announced in June 2000. No complete or partial responses to treatment were observed after two courses of treatment with XR5000. Two subjects showed stable disease and 13 subjects experienced disease progression. The company is not planning any further recruitment for this indication.

INDICATION(S) AND RESEARCH PHASE
Brain Cancer – Phase II
Colorectal Cancer – Phase II completed
Lung Cancer – Phase II
Ovarian Cancer – Phase II

YMB-6H9
unknown

MANUFACTURER
YM Biosciences

DESCRIPTION
YMB-6H9 is an anti-CEA super high affinity monoclonal antibody (SHMAs). Phase I/II development is planned for 2001 for the treatment of colorectal cancer.

INDICATION(S) AND RESEARCH PHASE
Colorectal Cancer – Phase I

ZD-0473/AMD 473
unknown

MANUFACTURER
AstraZeneca

DESCRIPTION
ZD-0473 is a new platinum-based anticancer agent designed to deliver an extended spectrum of activity and overcome resistance to currently approved platinum drugs, such as cisplatin and carboplatin. It is being evaluated for the treatment of a range of solid-tumor cancers, including colorectal, non-small cell lung, and bladder cancer, which are resistant to carboplatin. ZD-0473 is being tested in both intravenous and oral formulations. The intravenous formulation is in phase II trials, and the oral formulation is in preclinical development.

INDICATION(S) AND RESEARCH PHASE
Bladder Cancer – Phase II
Cancer/Tumors (Unspecified) – Phase II
Colorectal Cancer – Phase II
Lung Cancer – Phase II
Ovarian Cancer – Phase II
Prostate Cancer – Phase II
Breast Cancer – Phase II
Cervical Dysplasia/Cancer – Phase II

ZD-1839
Iressa

MANUFACTURER
AstraZeneca

DESCRIPTION
Iressa binds to the epidermal growth factor receptor (EGFR) and inhibits tyrosine kinase, thereby blocking signals for cancer growth and survival. The company reported encouraging results from phase I trials in a variety of tumors, but particularly in non-small cell lung cancer (NSCLC). Iressa is being investigated both as a monotherapy and in combination with other anti-tumor drugs in NSCLC, gastric, colorectal, and hormone-resistant prostate cancers. In 1999,

the FDA gave Iressa fast track status. The drug is currently in phase III studies for solid tumors.

INDICATION(S) AND RESEARCH PHASE
Cancer/Tumors (Unspecified) – Phase III
Colorectal Cancer – Phase III
Gastric Cancer – Phase III
Lung Cancer – Phase III
Prostate Cancer – Phase III

Effects of Chemotherapy

amifostine
Ethyol

MANUFACTURER
MedImmune

DESCRIPTION
Ethyol is a prodrug that is dephosphorylated by alkaline phosphatase in tissues to a pharmacologically active free thiol metabolite. Ethyol is currently undergoing phase II development via subcutaneous administration in subjects with head and neck cancer and non-small cell lung cancer, with reduction in mucositis and xerostomia endpoints. It is also in phase II development for myelodysplastic syndromes (MDS), a group of bone marrow disorders for which treatment alternatives are very limited.

INDICATION(S) AND RESEARCH PHASE
Myelodysplastic Syndromes – Phase II
Effects of Chemotherapy – Phase II

amlexanox liquid
OraRinse

MANUFACTURER
Access Pharmaceuticals

DESCRIPTION
OraRinse is an oral liquid formulation of amlexanox for the treatment of mucositis, a severe side effect of chemotherapy and radiation therapy. It is currently in phase II trials.

INDICATION(S) AND RESEARCH PHASE
Effects of Chemotherapy – Phase II

CP-99142
unknown

MANUFACTURER
Sanofi-Synthelabo Pharmaceuticals

DESCRIPTION
CP-99142 is a new drug that may prevent one of the potentially lethal complications of cancer therapy—high uric acid levels in the blood (hyperuricemia). The compound is actually an enzyme called urate oxidase, which changes uric acid into a harmless molecule that can be excreted by the kidneys. This is crucial, as uric acid cannot be destroyed and eliminated by the human body, and thus can produce a toxic accumulation in the system.

When cancer chemotherapy causes the destruction of huge numbers of tumor cells, these dead cells release enormous amounts of uric acid into the subject's body. If the uric acid levels are high enough, serious kidney failure can result. Urate oxidase has been difficult to purify and produce in the amount necessary for therapy, but Sanofi Laboratory uses biotechnological methods to manufacture it in sufficient quantities. CP-99142 is currently is phase III clinical trials. This drug may prove a useful adjunct to any cancer chemotherapy, limiting the chance of the development of hyperuricemia.

INDICATION(S) AND RESEARCH PHASE
Effects of Chemotherapy – Phase III

dimethyl sulfoxide, DMSO
unknown

MANUFACTURER
Topical Technologies

DESCRIPTION
Dimethyl sulfoxide (DMSO) is a topical medication being developed for the treatment of two indications: palmar-plantar dystensia syndrome caused by anti-cancer drugs (phase III) and soft-tissue injury following extravasation of cytotoxic drugs (phase II). An orphan drug status has been granted for both of these indications.

Dimethyl sulfoxide has a history of use in the wood industry as a commercial solvent since 1953. Since it penetrates the skin deeply and quickly without apparent damage, DMSO can carry other drugs with it across membranes. It is more successful ferrying some drugs, such as morphine sulfate, penicillin, steroids, and cortisone, than others, such as insulin. What DMSO can carry depends on the molecular weight, shape, and electrochemistry of the molecule. This property may enable DMSO to act as a new drug delivery system with a lower risk of infection compared to when the skin is penetrated.

Phase II and III trials of DMSO are under way. While approved for topical use over much of the world, the drug has had a long and controversial history with the FDA due to concerns regarding eye problems and other issues.

INDICATION(S) AND RESEARCH PHASE
Connective Tissue Diseases – Phase II
Effects of Chemotherapy – Phase III

keratinocyte growth factor (KGF)
unknown

MANUFACTURER
Amgen

DESCRIPTION
Keratinocyte growth factor (KGF) is a recombinant form of a naturally occurring epithelial tissue growth factor that stimulates the growth of cells comprising the surface lining of the gastrointestinal tract. Phase II trials are ongoing to determine whether KGF can reduce the incidence, severity, and duration of oral and gastrointestinal mucositis in cancer subjects receiving some forms of chemotherapy and radiation therapy. KGF is administered by intravenous injection.

INDICATION(S) AND RESEARCH PHASE
Effects of Chemotherapy – Phase II
Gastrointestinal Diseases and Disorders,

miscellaneous – Phase II

keratinocyte growth factor-2 (KGF-2)
Repifermin

MANUFACTURER
Human Genome Sciences

DESCRIPTION
Repifermin is a genomics-derived therapeutic protein drug, also known as keratinocyte growth factor-2 (KGF-2). It is in a phase II study for the treatment of mucositis associated with bone marrow transplantation for the treatment of cancer. This trial is a randomized, double-blind, placebo-controlled, dose-escalation study being conducted at several sites in the United States. Additionally, Repifermin is in a phase IIb trial for topical wound healing treatment of venous ulcers and a phase II trial for inflammatory bowel disease (IBD).

The company reported that results of phase I clinical trials showed that systemically administered Repifermin is safe and well tolerated in healthy human subjects at doses proposed for subsequent clinical studies. None of the subjects withdrew from the study or required dose modification because of adverse effects.

KGF-2 stimulates the growth of keratinocyte cells, which make up 95% of the epidermal (skin) cells. Together, keratinocyte and melanocyte cells form the epidermis of the body. The company claims that KGF-2 has demonstrated beneficial effects on both the dermal and epidermal tissues of the skin, healing full-thickness wounds in a short period of time. In mucositis, Repifermin may stimulate the creation of new mucosal tissue.

INDICATION(S) AND RESEARCH PHASE
Bone Marrow Transplant – Phase II
Effects of Chemotherapy – Phase II
Skin Wounds – Phase IIb
Inflammatory Bowel Disease – Phase II

MK-869
unknown

MANUFACTURER
Merck & Co.

DESCRIPTION
MK-869 is a substance P receptor antagonist for the treatment of chemotherapy induced emesis, anxiety and bipolar disorders, and depression. Substance P acts on neurokinin-1 (NK_1) receptors in areas of the brain stem associated with vomiting.

Results from a phase II trial showed that MK-869 prevented nausea and vomiting induced by cisplatin. The phase II trial included 150 subjects who received granisetron and dexamethasone followed by therapy with cisplatin.

INDICATION(S) AND RESEARCH PHASE
Anxiety Disorders – Phase III
Bipolar Disorders – Phase III
Depression – Phase III
Effects of Chemotherapy – Phase III

myeloid progenitor inhibitory factor (MPIF)
unknown

MANUFACTURER
Human Genome Sciences

DESCRIPTION
Myeloid progenitor inhibitory factor (MPIF), a novel human protein, shields hematopoietic progenitor (blood cell forming) cells in the bone marrow from the effects of a number of chemotherapeutic agents. MPIF may work by inhibiting the proliferation and differentiation of the progenitor cells.

Double-blind, placebo-controlled studies are being conducted at several leading medical centers in the United States involving established chemotherapy regimens used to treat breast and ovarian cancers. These studies may help to identify appropriate doses and regimens for future studies.

INDICATION(S) AND RESEARCH PHASE
Effects of Chemotherapy – Phase II

Protegrin IB-367, Rinse, Gel
unknown

MANUFACTURER
IntraBiotics Pharmaceuticals

DESCRIPTION
Protegrin IB-367 is a synthetic antimicrobial peptide molecule that belongs to a new class of agents called protegrins. Studies suggest that Protegrin IB-367 kills bacteria by integrating with and disrupting the integrity of bacterial cell membranes. This antibiotic has a broad spectrum of microbicidal activity against gram-positive and gram-negative bacteria, which are frequent pathogens in ventilator-associated pneumonia.

Results of a single-dose phase I trial indicated that Protegrin IB-367 safely reduces bacterial levels in the mouths of subjects at risk of experiencing ventilator-associated pneumonia. A rinse and gel formulation of Protegrin IB-367 was topically applied to the mouth to reduce the number of oral and oropharyngeal bacteria of intubated subjects. A single administration of 9 mg of the rinse formulation safely and rapidly reduced the total bacteria in orally intubated subjects compared to placebo. The magnitude and duration of effect after a single 9 mg dose of Protegrin IB-367 rinse similar to the response measured after a single 30 mg dose. IntraBiotics has begun subject enrollment in a phase IIa trial.

The rinse formulation of Protegrin IB-367 is also undergoing evaluation in two phase III trials for the prevention of oral mucositis. One trial has completed enrollment of subjects receiving high-dose chemotherapy, while the other continues to enroll subjects receiving radiotherapy.

INDICATION(S) AND RESEARCH PHASE
Effects of Chemotherapy – Phase III
Bacterial Infection – Phase IIa
Pneumonia – Phase IIa

recombinant human GM-CSF
Leucotropin

MANUFACTURER
Cangene Corporation

DESCRIPTION
Leucotropin is Cangene's brand of GM-CSF, a protein that stimulates the formation

of mature white blood cells, which are key components of the immune system. At this time, phase III trials have been discontinued.

INDICATION(S) AND RESEARCH PHASE
Bone Marrow Transplant – Trial discontinued
Effects of Chemotherapy – Trial discontinued

RF-1012
unknown

MANUFACTURER
SuperGen

DESCRIPTION
SuperGen is developing RF-1012 to counteract the anemia and leukopenia (white cell depletion) often associated with chemotherapy and radiotherapy treatments. This drug is currently being evaluated in phase II trials, and it is to be given in an intravenous formulation.

RF-1012 is a protective agent that may potentially limit the effect of chemotherapy and radiotherapy on normal, growing blood cells. This protective ability is crucial since cancer treatment regimens are frequently stopped because of severe anemia or leukopenia. This agent may also prevent life-threatening infections secondary to white blood cell depletion, as well as congestive heart failure and other organ damage resulting from a decline in red blood cells. Further study is necessary to evaluate the efficacy of this new medication.

INDICATION(S) AND RESEARCH PHASE
Anemia – Phase II
Effects of Chemotherapy – Phase II
White Blood Cell Disorders – Phase II

rhIL-11
unknown

MANUFACTURER
Wyeth-Ayerst

DESCRIPTION
Recombinant human interleukin-11 (rhIL-11) is a pleiotropic cytokine with effects on multiple cell types. IL-11 is currently marketed in the United States as Neumega—a thrombopoietic growth factor for preventing severe thrombocytopenia and the corresponding need for platelet transfusions following chemotherapy. rhIL-11 is currently in trials for mucositis and Crohn's disease.

INDICATION(S) AND RESEARCH PHASE
Effects of Chemotherapy – Phase II/III
Crohn's Disease – Phase II/III

SB 251353
unknown

MANUFACTURER
GlaxoSmithKline

DESCRIPTION
SB 251353 is a CXC chemokine in phase I trials for the prevention of chemotherapy-induced cytopenias and stem cell mobilization.

INDICATION(S) AND RESEARCH PHASE
Effects of Chemotherapy – Phase I

SD/01
unknown

MANUFACTURER
Amgen

DESCRIPTION
SD/01 is a sustained duration granulocyte colony stimulating factor (G-CSF) molecule being tested for chemotherapy induced neutropenia. Granulocytes and neutrophils are types of white blood cells that help the immune system protect the body from foreign substances. Amgen states that SD/01 consists of the protein G-CSF to which poly(ethylene) glycol (PEG) has been bound. PEGylated proteins stay circulating longer in the body, and it is thought that subjects may require fewer injections.

SD/01 is currently in a phase III study to evaluate its safety and efficacy in breast cancer subjects.

INDICATION(S) AND RESEARCH PHASE
Breast Cancer – Phase III
Effects of Chemotherapy – Phase III
White Blood Cell Disorders – Phase III

VML-670
unknown

MANUFACTURER
Vernalis

DESCRIPTION
VML-670 is being tested for the treatment of nausea and vomiting in subjects receiving chemotherapy treatment. Early stage evaluation of the efficacy of VML-670 for nausea has commenced in Europe.

INDICATION(S) AND RESEARCH PHASE
Effects of Chemotherapy – Phase II

Wobe-Mugos-E
unknown

MANUFACTURER
Mucos Pharma GmbH

DESCRIPTION
Wobe-Mugos-E is an enzyme combination of papain, trypsin, and chymotrypsin being tested for its ability to improve the general health of cancer subjects. It may reduce the need for additional medications (such as pain relievers and antiemetics) during or after chemotherapy.

Wobe-Mugos-E is an alpha-macroglobulin that binds interleukins, TGF-β, TNF receptor I and II, hyperactive T-cells, and CRP. Given orally, the general health of cancer subjects was reported to increase (appetite improvement, weight gain, and reduction in fatigue and depression were observed). Leukopenia and thrombopenia induced by cancer cytostatic agents and radiation were reduced.

Clinical trials in phase II/III are evaluating this enzyme combination for multiple myeloma and effects of chemotherapy.

INDICATION(S) AND RESEARCH PHASE
Multiple Myeloma – Phase II/III
Effects of Chemotherapy – Phase II/III

Endometrial Cancer

aminopterin
unknown

MANUFACTURER
ILEX Oncology

DESCRIPTION
Aminopterin is an anti-folate in the same family as methotrexate, a widely used anti-cancer drug. Aminopterin kills tumor cells by interfering with their ability to synthesize DNA. Although the drug has been around for many years, it moved out of common use because it was difficult to synthesize and there were concerns about its toxicity. It is currently being tested for the treatment of metastatic endometrial cancer resistant to methotrexate and other drugs, as well as for acute lymphocytic leukemia. Aminopterin has received an orphan drug status for acute lymphocytic leukemia.

INDICATION(S) AND RESEARCH PHASE
Endometrial Cancer – Phase II
Leukemia – Phase II

ICI-182,780
Faslodex

MANUFACTURER
AstraZeneca

DESCRIPTION
Studies suggest that the female hormone estrogen stimulates the growth of some breast cancer tumors. Faslodex is a synthetic estrogen blocker that works by down-regulating the activity of the estrogen receptor. If estrogen is unable to bind to a receptor, it cannot start the complex processes leading to cancer-cell growth. Formerly described as a pure anti-estrogen, Faslodex is now referred to as a selective estrogen receptor down-regulator (SERD).

Initial studies indicated that SERDs are more effective against breast cancer and showed less occurrence of secondary endometrial cancer than tamoxifen.

The company expects to file an NDA for the second line treatment of advanced breast cancer in early 2001. The drug is in phase III trials as a first line treatment of advanced breast cancer. The NDA filing for this indication is expected in 2002.

INDICATION(S) AND RESEARCH PHASE
Breast Cancer – Phase III completed
Endometrial Cancer – Phase II
Breast Cancer – Phase III

MDX-220
unknown

MANUFACTURER
Medarex

DESCRIPTION
MDX-220 is a bispecific (target-trigger) monoclonal antibody (MAb) that targets Tag-72 in the treatment of a variety of cancers, including lung, colon, prostate, ovarian, endometrial, pancreatic, and gastric cancer.

INDICATION(S) AND RESEARCH PHASE
Endometrial Cancer – Phase I/II
Gastric Cancer – Phase I/II
Lung Cancer – Phase I/II
Ovarian Cancer – Phase I/II
Pancreatic Cancer – Phase I/II
Prostate Cancer – Phase II
Colorectal Cancer – Phase II

unknown
GnRH Pharmaccine

MANUFACTURER
Aphton Corporation

DESCRIPTION
Aphton's novel GnRH Pharmaccine is an anti-gonadotropin releasing hormone (GnRH) immunogen. Study results indicate that it induces and maintains castration levels of testosterone and reduced levels of prostate-specific antigen (PSA). Chemical castration of this type is a standard therapy to extend the survival of subjects with advanced prostate cancer. GnRH Pharmaccine is also involved in trials for breast cancer, endometrial cancer, and endometriosis, in addition to prostate cancer.

INDICATION(S) AND RESEARCH PHASE
Prostate Cancer – Phase I/II
Breast Cancer – Phase I/II
Endometrial Cancer – Phase I/II
Endometriosis – Phase I/II

Esophageal Cancer

cisplatin/epinephrine
IntraDose

MANUFACTURER
Matrix Pharmaceutical

DESCRIPTION
IntraDose is a biodegradable collagen carrier matrix combined with a vasoconstrictor. The gel is injected directly into tumors where it localizes high concentrations of cisplatin, a widely used anticancer drug. It is currently being tested for several indications, including head and neck, breast, malignant melanoma, esophageal, and primary hepatocellular cancer.

A phase II trail of IntraDose Injectable Gel produced durable responses in subjects with colorectal cancer that had metastasized to the liver. Nine of 31 subjects who received IntraDose responded to therapy. Six subjects experienced a complete response (100% reduction in viable tumor volume of treated tumors) while the other three subjects demonstrated a partial response (at least a 50% reduction of viable tumor volume). Eight of the nine treatment responders have had durable responses with no relapse at the site of treatment. IntraDose was well tolerated by subjects.

INDICATION(S) AND RESEARCH PHASE
Breast Cancer – Phase II
Cancer/Tumors (Unspecified) – Phase II
Colorectal Cancer – Phase II completed
Esophageal Cancer – Phase II
Liver Cancer – Phase II
Malignant Melanoma – Phase II
Head and Neck Cancer – NDA submitted

flavopiridol, HMR-1275
unknown

MANUFACTURER
Aventis

DESCRIPTION
Flavopiridol belongs to a new class of drugs for cancer therapy called cyclin-dependent kinase (CDK) inhibitors. It is being tested in phase II trials as a treatment for chronic lymphatic leukemia, esophageal cancer, and non-small cell lung cancer.

INDICATION(S) AND RESEARCH PHASE
Esophageal Cancer – Phase II
Leukemia – Phase II
Lung Cancer – Phase II

---

vaccine, anti-gastrin
Gastrimmune

MANUFACTURER
Aphton Corporation

DESCRIPTION
Gastrimmune is a therapeutic vaccine that neutralizes specific hormones (G17 & Gly-extended G17). The drug is in phase III trials for the treatment of cancers of the gastrointestinal tract, including gastric cancer and colorectal cancer. It is also in trials for liver cancer, esophageal cancer and two phase III trials for advanced pancreatic cancer—one in the the United States and one in Europe.

INDICATION(S) AND RESEARCH PHASE
Colorectal Cancer – Phase III
Esophageal Cancer – Phase III
Gastric Cancer – Phase III
Liver Cancer – Phase II/III
Pancreatic Cancer – Phase III

Gastric Cancer

docetaxel hydrate
Taxotere

MANUFACTURER
Aventis

DESCRIPTION
Drugs for the treatment of cancer and other diseases often originate in plants, many of them highly poisonous. Taxotere (docetaxel hydrate), an agent that inhibits the formation of new protoplasm, is derived from the renewable evergreen needles of the genus *Taxus* (Yew). Taxotere acts by disrupting the microtubular network in cells that is essential for cell division and other cellular functions. The drug is approved for use in the United States for treatment of refractory breast cancer, refractory non-small cell lung cancer (NSCLC), and locally advanced or metastatic breast cancer.

New phase II/III trials are under way in head and neck, gastric, and ovarian cancers. Taxotere is also being tested either alone or in combination with other chemotherapy agents in the earlier stages of breast cancer, NSCLC, and others tumors.

Phase I extension studies are under way for brain metastasis and lung cancer.

INDICATION(S) AND RESEARCH PHASE
Gastric Cancer – Phase II/III
Head and Neck Cancer – Phase II/III
Lung Cancer – Phase II/III
Ovarian Cancer – Phase II/III
Breast Cancer – Phase III/IV
Brain Cancer – Phase I
Lung Cancer – Phase I

---

fluoropyrimidine, S-1
unknown

MANUFACTURER
Bristol-Myers Squibb

DESCRIPTION
Fluoropyrimidine is a combination medication that is being tested in subjects with solid tumors. The drug is given orally at 80 mg twice a day, and it is currently being tested in phase II clinical trials. One of the active components in fluoropyrimidine is tegafur, which is a type of chemotherapeutic drug known as 5-fluorouracil (5-FU). 5-FU prevents the metabolic activities of cancer cells, thus limiting their ability to grow and replicate. In clinical use for over forty years, 5-FU has been used to treat gastrointestinal, breast, head and neck, and bladder cancers. Problems associated with 5-FU use include subject tolerance to its anti-cancer effects, serious side effects, and toxicity to the digestive tract when taken orally.

Fluoropyrimidine may be an improvement over 5-FU alone because it also contains the molecule otastat potassium, which protects the GI tract from toxic effects, and the substance gimestat, which increases the action of 5-FU by inhibiting the enzyme in the body that breaks it down. Studies will demonstrate whether these two molecules will allow the drug to be given orally, producing fewer resultant adverse effects. This may mean that subjects will be able to tolerate the drug for longer periods of time, thus increasing subject compliance and potentially the effectiveness of the drug. It also may reduce the variability of clinical response to the drug among subjects, allowing doctors to better predict the effect its administration will have on their subjects' condition and what doses would be optimal for them. Preliminary studies have shown that fluoropyrimidine produces greater efficacy and less toxicity than conventional chemotherapeutic agents.

INDICATION(S) AND RESEARCH PHASE
Cancer/Tumors (Unspecified) – Phase II
Gastric Cancer – Phase II

HSPPC-96
Oncophage

MANUFACTURER
Antigenics

DESCRIPTION
Oncophage cancer vaccine is an injectable protein that contains the unique profile ("antigenic fingerprint") of each subject's cancer. The antigens activate the immune system to elicit an anti-tumor response. Oncophage is in clinical trials for several indications, including renal cell carcinoma (phase III), melanoma (phase II), colorectal cancer (phase II), gastric cancer (phase I/II), pancreatic cancer (phase I/II completed), and non-Hodgkin's lymphoma (phase II).

In October 2000, Antigenics announced

that it had initiated a phase II trial of Oncophage in subjects who have been diagnosed with sarcoma, also known as soft tissue cancer. The study is expected to initially enroll 20 subjects diagnosed with recurrent metastatic or unresectable soft tissue sarcoma and may be expanded to include an additional 15 subjects depending on preliminary results.

INDICATION(S) AND RESEARCH PHASE
Renal Cell Carcinoma – Phase III
Malignant Melanoma – Phase II
Colorectal Cancer – Phase II
Gastric Cancer – Phase I/II
Pancreatic Cancer – Phase I/II completed
Lymphoma, Non-Hodgkin's – Phase II
Sarcoma – Phase II

MDX-210
unknown

MANUFACTURER
Medarex

DESCRIPTION
MDX-210 is a bispecific (target-trigger) monoclonal antibody (MAb)-based treatment being developed for cancers with specific markers (HER-2/*neu* positive), including renal cell, non-small cell lung, pancreatic and kidney cancers. Phase II trials have been completed for kidney, prostate, and ovarian cancer. Phase III development for ovarian cancer has commenced in Europe.

INDICATION(S) AND RESEARCH PHASE
Prostate Cancer – Phase II completed
Renal Cell Carcinoma – Phase II completed
Colon Malignancies – Phase II
Breast Cancer – Phase II
Gastric Cancer – Phase II
Pancreatic Cancer – Phase II
Lung Cancer – Phase II
Ovarian Cancer – Phase III

MDX-220
unknown

MANUFACTURER
Medarex

DESCRIPTION
MDX-220 is a bispecific (target-trigger) monoclonal antibody (MAb) that targets Tag-72. It is being developed for the treatment of a variety of cancers, including lung, colon, prostate, ovarian, endometrial, pancreatic and gastric cancer.

INDICATION(S) AND RESEARCH PHASE
Endometrial Cancer – Phase I/II
Gastric Cancer – Phase I/II
Lung Cancer – Phase I/II
Ovarian Cancer – Phase I/II
Pancreatic Cancer – Phase I/II
Prostate Cancer – Phase II
Colorectal Cancer – Phase II

murine monoclonal antibody
Theragyn

MANUFACTURER
Antisoma plc

DESCRIPTION
Theragyn is composed of a mouse monoclonal antibody (HMFG1) linked to a radioactive isotope. It is thought that small numbers of residual tumor cells remaining in the abdomen after surgery and chemotherapy are one of the main causes of relapse. These residual tumor cells are the targets of Theragyn. Theragyn uses the natural targeting ability of antibodies to selectively deliver radioactivity to tumor cells.

Theragyn is being tested as an adjuvant treatment in trials for gastric cancer and also in phase III trials for ovarian cancer.

INDICATION(S) AND RESEARCH PHASE
Gastric Cancer – Phase II
Ovarian Cancer – Phase III

RFS-2000
Rubitecan

MANUFACTURER
SuperGen

DESCRIPTION
Rubitecan is a novel drug in the late stages of phase III development for treating advanced pancreatic cancer. It works by inhibiting an enzyme called topoisomerase-I. This drug is made in an oral form that is an advantage for outpatient treatment compared to intravenous type cancer drugs that may require a visit to a hospital setting.

In addition to treating pancreatic cancer, Rubitecan is being evaluated in treating a variety of solid tumors, such as in breast, colorectal, lung, ovarian, and prostate cancers, as well as metastatic melanoma and advanced gastric carcinoma. Also, phase II trials in the United States and Europe are testing Rubitecan in blood cancers such as chronic myelomonocytic leukemia (CMML/myelodysplastic syndrome).

Clinical study results reported in the May 1999 issue of the International Journal of Oncology noted that Rubitecan was given to a group of end-stage pancreatic cancer subjects who failed all previous conventional therapies. Of the 60 subjects who completed Rubitecan treatment, 31.7% responded favorably with half of the subjects staying alive (the median survival) at 18.6 months. Additionally, 31.7% were stabilized with a 9.7 month median survival rate, and 36.6% were non-responders with a 6.8 month median survival rate.

INDICATION(S) AND RESEARCH PHASE
Pancreatic Cancer – Phase III
Breast Cancer – Phase II
Colorectal Cancer – Phase II
Gastric Cancer – Phase II
Leukemia – Phase II
Malignant Melanoma – Phase II
Ovarian Cancer – Phase II
Myelodysplastic Syndrome – Phase III

vaccine, anti-gastrin
Gastrimmune

MANUFACTURER
Aphton Corporation

DESCRIPTION
Gastrimmune is a therapeutic vaccine that neutralizes specific hormones (G17 & Gly-extended G17). The drug is in phase III trials for the treatment of cancers of the gastrointestinal tract, including gastric cancer and colorectal cancer. It is also in trials for liver cancer, esophageal cancer,

and two phase III trials for advanced pancreatic cancer—one in the the United States and one in Europe.

INDICATION(S) AND RESEARCH PHASE
Colorectal Cancer – Phase III
Esophageal Cancer – Phase III
Gastric Cancer – Phase III
Liver Cancer – Phase II/III
Pancreatic Cancer – Phase III

ZD-1839
Iressa

MANUFACTURER
AstraZeneca

DESCRIPTION
Iressa binds to the epidermal growth factor receptor (EGFR) and inhibits tyrosine kinase, thereby blocking signals for cancer growth and survival. The company reported encouraging results from phase I trials in a variety of tumors, but particularly in non-small cell lung cancer (NSCLC). Iressa is being investigated both as a monotherapy and in combination with other anti-tumor drugs in NSCLC, gastric, colorectal, and hormone-resistant prostate cancers. In 1999, the FDA gave Iressa fast track status. The drug is currently in phase III development.

INDICATION(S) AND RESEARCH PHASE
Cancer/Tumors (Unspecified) – Phase III
Colorectal Cancer – Phase III
Gastric Cancer – Phase III
Lung Cancer – Phase III
Prostate Cancer – Phase III

Head and Neck Cancer

bexarotene
Targretin-capsule

MANUFACTURER
Ligand Pharmaceuticals

DESCRIPTION
Targretin, which selectively stimulates a retinoid subtype receptor, is being developed in an oral capsule formulation for the treatment of lung and breast cancer, head and neck cancer, cutaneous T-cell lymphoma (CTCL), and psoriasis and psoriatic disorders. The drug is in phase II trials for head and neck cancer, phase II/III trials for breast cancer, CTCL, and psoriasis and psoriatic disorders, and phase III trials for non-small cell lung cancer.

INDICATION(S) AND RESEARCH PHASE
Psoriasis and Psoriatic Disorders – Phase II/III
Lung Cancer – Phase III
Breast Cancer – Phase II/III
Head and Neck Cancer – Phase II
Lymphoma – Phase II/III

CI-1033
unknown

MANUFACTURER
Pfizer

DESCRIPTION
CI-1033 is being investigated in clinical studies involving erbB positive cancers located in the breast, lung, and head and neck. The objective of the CI-1033 program is to achieve control of cancer via EGFR tyrosine kinase inhibition, without the side effect burden of cytotoxic agents.

INDICATION(S) AND RESEARCH PHASE
Breast Cancer – Phase I
Lung Cancer – Phase I
Head and Neck Cancer – Phase I

CI-1042, ONYX-015
unknown

MANUFACTURER
Onyx Pharmaceuticals

DESCRIPTION
CI-1042 (ONYX-015) is a tumor-selective, modified adenovirus (similar to the common cold virus) that has been genetically engineered to replicate in and kill cancer cells that possess a mutated oncogene called p53, while sparing normal cells with functioning p53. p53 Is a tumor suppressor gene that is mutated in approximately 50% of all human cancers. CI-1042 is in development for several indications, including pancreatic cancer, liver metastases of colorectal cancer, and lung cancer.

In November 2000, results of a phase II trial demonstrated that CI-1042 administered as a single-agent replicates and causes tumor regression in refractory head and neck cancer. CI-1042 was shown to selectively target cancer cells containing a mutant p53 gene, while sparing normal cells with a functioning p53 gene. Of the 19 subjects who received the standard dosing regimen, four (21%) had an objective response, including two complete responses and two partial responses. CI-1042 is being co-developed with Pfizer.

INDICATION(S) AND RESEARCH PHASE
Colorectal Cancer – Phase II
Pancreatic Cancer – Phase II
Head and Neck Cancer – Phase III
Cervical Dysplasia/Cancer – Phase I completed
Lung Cancer – Phase II
Bladder Cancer – Phase I completed
Brain Cancer – Phase I completed

cisplatin/epinephrine
IntraDose

MANUFACTURER
Matrix Pharmaceutical

DESCRIPTION
IntraDose is a biodegradable collagen carrier matrix combined with a vasoconstrictor. The gel is injected directly into tumors where it localizes high concentrations of cisplatin, a widely used anticancer drug. It is currently being tested for several indications, including head and neck, breast, malignant melanoma, esophageal, and primary hepatocellular cancer.

A phase II trail of IntraDose Injectable Gel produced durable responses in subjects with colorectal cancer that had metastasized to the liver. Nine of 31 subjects who received IntraDose responded to therapy. Six subjects experienced a complete response (100% reduction in viable tumor volume of treated tumors) while the other three subjects demonstrated a partial response (at least a

50% reduction of viable tumor volume). Eight of the nine treatment responders have had durable responses with no relapse at the site of treatment. IntraDose was well tolerated by subjects.

INDICATION(S) AND RESEARCH PHASE
Breast Cancer – Phase II
Cancer/Tumors (Unspecified) – Phase II
Colorectal Cancer – Phase II completed
Esophageal Cancer – Phase II
Liver Cancer – Phase II
Malignant Melanoma – Phase II
Head and Neck Cancer – NDA submitted

CP-358,774
unknown

MANUFACTURER
OSI Pharmaceuticals

DESCRIPTION
CP-358,774 is a small molecule inhibitor of the epidermal growth factor receptor (EGFR)-tyrosine kinase. This drug targets the underlying molecular changes involving oncogenes and tumor suppressor genes, which play critical roles in the conversion of normal cells into cancerous cells. Increased expression of EGFR is an aberration frequently associated with a variety of cancers including ovarian, pancreatic, and non-small cell lung cancers. The phase II clinical program is designed to assess CP-358,774 both as a single agent and in combination with existing chemotherapy regimens.

INDICATION(S) AND RESEARCH PHASE
Breast Cancer – Phase II
Lung Cancer – Phase II completed
Ovarian Cancer – Phase II
Head and Neck Cancer – Phase II

diclofenac
Oralease

MANUFACTURER
Skye Pharma

DESCRIPTION
Oralease (diclofenac) is an anti-inflammatory being evaluated for the treatment of oral lesions in AIDS subjects. It is also being developed for the treatment of mucositis in cancer subjects undergoing head and neck radiation. This orally formulated drug is in phase II trials.

INDICATION(S) AND RESEARCH PHASE
Acquired Immune Deficiency Syndrome (AIDS) and AIDS-Related Infections – Phase II
Head and Neck Cancer – Phase II
Oral Medicine – Phase II

docetaxel hydrate
Taxotere

MANUFACTURER
Aventis

DESCRIPTION
Many drugs for the treatment of cancer and other diseases originate in plants, many of them highly poisonous. Taxotere (docetaxel hydrate), an agent that inhibits the formation of new protoplasm, is derived from the renewable evergreen needles of the genus *Taxus* (Yew). Taxotere acts by disrupting the microtubular network in cells that is essential for cell division and many other cellular functions. The drug is approved for use in the United States for treatment of refractory breast cancer, refractory non-small cell lung cancer (NSCLC), and locally advanced or metastatic breast cancer.

New phase II/III trials are under way in head and neck, gastric, and ovarian cancers. Taxotere is also being tested either alone or in combination with other chemotherapy agents in the earlier stages of breast cancer, NSCLC, and others tumors.

Phase I extension studies are under way for brain metastasis and lung cancer.

INDICATION(S) AND RESEARCH PHASE
Gastric Cancer – Phase II/III
Head and Neck Cancer – Phase II/III
Lung Cancer – Phase II/III
Ovarian Cancer – Phase II/III
Breast Cancer – Phase III/IV
Brain Cancer – Phase I
Lung Cancer – Phase I

EMD 82633
unknown

MANUFACTURER
Merck KgaA

DESCRIPTION
EMD 82633 is a humanized and bispecific monoclonal antibody derived from mice. These antibodies are altered in such a way that they no longer appear different from human antibodies. This genetic modification prevents immune reactions against foreign substances of animal origin used in humans. In this bispecific drug, one component binds to tumor cells, while the other activates the body's own CD8 "killer cells" to attack cancer cells.

This new drug is being given as an adjuvant therapy to subjects who have not been adequately helped by conventional forms of treatment, such as chemotherapy. EMD 82633 is being tested in trials for the treatment of renal cancer, head and neck cancer, breast cancer, bladder cancer, and ovarian cancer.

INDICATION(S) AND RESEARCH PHASE
Bladder Cancer – Phase II
Breast Cancer – Phase II
Cancer/Tumors (Unspecified) – Phase II
Head and Neck Cancer – Phase II
Ovarian Cancer – Phase II
Renal Cell Carcinoma – Phase II

gene therapy, interleukin-2
unknown

MANUFACTURER
Valentis

DESCRIPTION
This cancer therapeutic encodes the human IL-2 gene and a proprietary cationic lipid gene in a plasmid delivery system. Plasmids are self-replicating structures outside the chromosomes in a bacterial cell that carry genes for functions not essential to growth, such as the production of enzymes, toxins, and antigens. This gene therapy is in trials for the treatment of head and neck cancer and malignant melanoma.

INDICATION(S) AND RESEARCH PHASE
Head and Neck Cancer – Phase II
Malignant Melanoma – Phase I

IMC-C225, CPT-11
unknown

MANUFACTURER
ImClone Systems

DESCRIPTION
IMC-C225 is a chimerized (part mouse, part human) monoclonal antibody that may help fight cancer cells when used in conjunction with radiation therapy or other chemotherapy agents. This antibody selectively blocks the rpidermal growth factor receptor (EGFr), which may be present in greater amounts on actively growing tumor cells. Since many cancers use specific growth factors to stimulate tumor cell growth, blocking this receptor may inhibit the cancer from increasing in size and spreading throughout the body.

The company is conducting phase III clinical trials evaluating IMC-C225 in combination with radiotherapy and with chemotherapy in subjects with advanced squamous cell head and neck carcinoma. IMC-C225 is in trials for several other indications in combination with various anticancer agents.

INDICATION(S) AND RESEARCH PHASE
Breast Cancer – Phase I/II
Head and Neck Cancer – Phase III
Lung Cancer – Phase III
Prostate Cancer – Phase I/II
Renal Cell Carcinoma – Phase II
Pancreatic Cancer – Phase II
Colorectal Cancer – Phase II

INGN-201, adenoviral p53
unknown

MANUFACTURER
Introgen Therapeutics

DESCRIPTION
INGN-201 is a p53 gene therapy cancer product. It has been tested as a treatment for a variety of solid tumor cancers with administration via intratumoral injection. The drug was well tolerated according to the company, and additional trials are under way using an intravenous infusion in order to reach more types of cancers. The tumor-suppressing p53 gene encodes a protein that responds to damage involving cellular DNA by terminating cell division. Normal p53 genes are delivered into cancer cells of the subject through an adenoviral vector.

The developers of INGN-201 have signed a Cooperative Research and Development Agreement (CRADA) with the National Cancer Institute to evaluate the potential effectiveness and superiority of the drug over other treatments against breast, ovarian, bladder, prostate, and brain cancers in phase I and phase II trials. A phase III trial in head and neck cancer was initiated in March 2000.

INDICATION(S) AND RESEARCH PHASE
Head and Neck Cancer – Phase III
Bladder Cancer – Phase I
Brain Cancer – Phase I
Breast Cancer – Phase I
Bronchoalveolar Cancer – Phase I
Ovarian Cancer – Phase I
Prostate Cancer – Phase I
Lung Cancer – Phase II
Cancer/Tumors (Unspecified) – Phase I

interleukin (IL)
MultiKine

MANUFACTURER
CEL-SCI Corporation

DESCRIPTION
MultiKine is a multiple combination therapy made from a natural, cytokine cocktail (which includes interleukin-2 (IL-2), IL-β, TNF-α, Gm-CSF and an IFN-γ/immunomodulator). It is being tested for the treatment of advanced head and neck cancer in subjects who have previously failed standard therapy, and for head and neck cancer treatment prior to surgery.

MultiKine has just completed two phase II trials for head and neck cancer. The first trial consisted of 16 subjects and tested four different doses of MultiKine in four subjects each. To qualify for the trial, the subjects must have had a recurrence of the cancer and failed conventional therapy.

The company reported that in an earlier and still ongoing study conducted in newly diagnosed head and neck cancer subjects, 10 subjects had tumor reductions prior to surgery within a short time period. Three of ten subjects had tumor reductions exceeding 50%, and one additional subject with a tumor that was nearly three inches in diameter had a complete clinical response. Lastly, two subjects refused surgery because they were satisfied with their condition after treatment with MultiKine.

A phase III trial to test MultiKine prior to surgery and/or radiation may reduce the fairly high recurrence rate of head and neck cancer. This drug is also in trials for prostate cancer, HIV, and breast cancer.

INDICATION(S) AND RESEARCH PHASE
Head and Neck Cancer – Phase II
HIV Infection – Phase II
Breast Cancer – Phase I
Prostate Cancer – Phase I/II

interleukin-12 gene therapy
unknown

MANUFACTURER
Valentis

DESCRIPTION
Interleukin-12 (IL-12) is a hormone-like substance that regulates the activity of cells involved in an immune response. IL-12 is made by a select group of immune cells that normally are the first to encounter disease-causing organisms in the body and react to them. IL-12 activates other immune cells such as T-cells, B-cells, dendritic cells, and natural killer (NK) cells. Together, T-cells and NK cells seek out and destroy tumor cells. Additionally, IL-12 increases the production of interferon-gamma, which in turn augments the killing ability of immune cells. IL-12 also promotes antibody production by B-cells and stimulates dendritic cells to multiply. Lastly, IL-12 inhibits angiogenesis, the development of new blood vessels within tumors.

The company has initiated a multi-center phase IIa trial for the treatment of squamous cell carcinoma of the head and neck.

INDICATION(S) AND RESEARCH PHASE
Head and Neck Cancer – Phase IIa
Skin Cancer – Phase IIa

LGD-1550
unknown

MANUFACTURER
Ligand Pharmaceuticals

DESCRIPTION
LGD-1550 is being formulated to limit the proliferation and spread of head, neck, and cervical cancers; it is to be given orally and is currently in phase II trials. Retinoids are a group of substances, one of which is vitamin A, that are thought to be responsible for growth, bone development, vision, and skin integrity. It is thought that retinoids act against cancer by regulating gene transcription. Studies have shown that subjects with metastatic cancer have lower levels of retinoid activity in their bodies. LGD-1550 binds to retinoid receptors in cells, thereby stimulating retinoid activity.

Preliminary studies have shown that retinoids may inhibit cell proliferation and promote cell differentiation. Cancer arises when there is uncontrolled growth of immature cells. Retinoids act to slow cell division and stimulate cell maturation, making it less likely that these mature cells will be transformed into cancerous cells. Retinoids have also been shown in early studies to boost the effects of other anti-cancer medications.

Phase II trials of LGD-1550 for head and neck cancer, cervical cancer, and solid and hematological tumors are currently under way.

INDICATION(S) AND RESEARCH PHASE
Blood Cancer – Phase II
Cancer/Tumors (Unspecified) – Phase II
Cervical Dysplasia/Cancer – Phase II
Head and Neck Cancer – Phase II

MDX-447, H-447
unknown

MANUFACTURER
Medarex

DESCRIPTION
MDX-447 is a novel biological drug designed to stimulate an immune response against cancer cells. Certain cancer cells contain and express large amounts of unique proteins (such as epidermal growth factor receptors), which MDX-447 is directed to recognize. MDX-447 attaches itself both to these cancer proteins and to macrophages that specialize in killing foreign material.

The binding together of the cancer cells and the immune cells by MDX-447 signals the body to destroy the tumor. MDX-447 may offer a new therapeutic alternative to cancer subjects who have been unresponsive to conventional therapies. This agent is unique since it has two receptors on its surface, one that can attract the cancer cell and one that can attract a killer immune cell. This dual nature of the drug is why it is known as a "bispecific antibody."

This type of drug is designed to be more efficient than current anti-cancer therapies, and may have effects that last longer. This technology may also be useful in the development of an "anti-cancer vaccine" in the future. MDX-447 is currently being tested as an intravenous solution in phase II trials for multiple tumor indications, which include brain, bladder, breast, head and neck, and lung cancer.

INDICATION(S) AND RESEARCH PHASE
Brain Cancer – Phase II
Bladder Cancer – Phase II
Breast Cancer – Phase II
Head and Neck Cancer – Phase II
Lung Cancer – Phase II

MG98
unknown

MANUFACTURER
MGI Pharma

DESCRIPTION
MG98 inhibits the production of DNA methyltransferase by binding to its messenger ribonucleic acid (mRNA). Hypermethylation, which leads to the inhibition of tumor suppressor genes, has been associated with overproduction of DNA methyltransferase in a variety of cancers, such as colon, kidney, prostate, and head and neck cancers. In particular, the p16 tumor suppressor gene is reportedly hypermethylated, and therefore inactivated, in approximately 50% of head and neck cancers.

Preclinical results demonstrated that MG98 has the potential to reduce the methylation of the p16 gene, which allows the restoration of normal tumor suppressor gene expression. The company plans to initiate phase II trials with MG98 in other cancers—its currently being tested for head and neck cancer. MGI Pharma is co-developing MG98 with the company MethylGene.

INDICATION(S) AND RESEARCH PHASE
Head and Neck Cancer – Phase II

monoclonal antibody
TheraCIM

MANUFACTURER
YM Biosciences

DESCRIPTION
TheraCIM is a humanized monoclonal antibody designed to target the epidermal growth factor receptor (EGFr). It is currently in phase I/II trials for head and neck cancer.

INDICATION(S) AND RESEARCH PHASE
Head and Neck Cancer – Phase I/II

OSI-774
unknown

MANUFACTURER
OSI Pharmaceuticals

DESCRIPTION
OSI-774 is a potent, selective, and orally active inhibitor of the epidermal growth factor receptor (EGFR), tyrosine kinase. EGFR is an oncogene that is produced during the aberrant growth of certain cancer cells.

OSI Pharmaceuticals has announced updated findings from two ongoing phase II trials of OSI-774 as a single agent. In a trial consisting of 56 subjects with advanced, refractory non-small cell lung cancer, OSI-774 was given orally on a once-a-day dosing schedule. Results showed that 48% of the subjects had either a partial response or stable disease at 12 weeks and continued on the drug. Intermediate data were presented from the second trial, which consisted of 113 subjects with advanced squamous cell carcinoma of the head and neck. Results for the first 78 evaluable subjects showed that 42% had either a partial response or demonstrated evidence of disease stabilization at 12 weeks.

INDICATION(S) AND RESEARCH PHASE
Lung Cancer – Phase II
Head and Neck Cancer – Phase II

p53 gene therapy
unknown

MANUFACTURER
Aventis

DESCRIPTION
Aventis' p53 gene therapy is an anti-cancer treatment that produces an increased expression of the p53 protein. The p53 protein has the ability to activate other proteins to stop the cell cycle until damage to the cell may be repaired. Additionally, the p53 protein may stop growth in response to additional stimuli, such as reduced nutritional resources or high cell density.

According to scientists, the p53 gene is one of the most frequently altered genes in human cancer, with 50% of all cancers having distorted forms of p53. This p53 gene therapy is delivered by an intraprostatic injection that may result in the suppression of prostate cancer growth. It is currently being tested in a phase I/II trial. Additionally, p53 gene therapy is being tested in phase III trials for head and neck cancer.

INDICATION(S) AND RESEARCH PHASE
Prostate Cancer – Phase I/II
Head and Neck Cancer – Phase III

porfiromycin
Promycin

MANUFACTURER
Vion Pharmaceuticals

DESCRIPTION
Promycin is a bioreductive, alkylating agent with chemical and metabolic properties that are selectively toxic to hypoxic tumor cells. Interim results of a phase III trial of Promycin combined with radiation therapy in subjects with non-resectable head and neck cancer did not meet the predetermined criteria that would warrant continuation of the study.

INDICATION(S) AND RESEARCH PHASE
Head and Neck Cancer – Phase III discontinued

T64
unknown

MANUFACTURER
Tularik

DESCRIPTION
T64 is an antifolate that disrupts DNA synthesis through the inhibition of purine biosynthesis. The compound is currently in phase II trials in subjects with head and neck cancer, soft tissue sarcoma, melanoma, breast cancer, and non-small cell lung cancer. Additionally, T64 is in phase I combination trials with gemcitabine, doxorubicin, and paclitaxel. Tularik expects to initiate two additional T64 phase I combination trials with carboplatin and temozolamide in the first quarter of 2001. The T64 trials are being conducted in the United States, the United Kingdom, the Netherlands, and Australia.

INDICATION(S) AND RESEARCH PHASE
Head and Neck Cancer – Phase II
Sarcoma – Phase II
Melanoma – Phase II
Breast Cancer – Phase II
Lung Cancer – Phase II
Cancer/Tumors (Unspecified) – Phase I

tgDCC-E1A, RGG 0853
unknown

MANUFACTURER
Targeted Genetics

DESCRIPTION
The drug E1A may possess multiple cancer-fighting effects, such as reducing expression (also called "down-regulation") of the oncogene HER-2/*neu*. Overexpression of HER-2/*neu* occurs in substantial percentages of ovarian and breast cancer subjects, as well as in cancers of the lung, prostate, and bladder. Furthermore, HER-2/*neu* correlates with poor prognosis, including metastasis - the process by which cancer spreads to other sites in the body.

Clinical phase I trials for breast, ovarian, and head and neck cancers are complete, as well as a phase II trial for head and neck cancer as a single agent. A second phase II has been initiated to test tgDCC-E1A in combination with radiation therapy for the treatment of head and neck squamous cell carcinoma. The phase II trial expects to treat up to 50 subjects who will receive twice-weekly injections of tgDCC-E1A throughout 6-7 weeks of radiation therapy.

INDICATION(S) AND RESEARCH PHASE
Breast Cancer – Phase I completed
Head and Neck Cancer – Phase II
Ovarian Cancer – Phase I completed

troxacitabine, BCH-4556
Troxatyl

MANUFACTURER
BioChem Pharma

DESCRIPTION
Troxatyl is a dioxolane nucleoside analog being investigated as an anticancer agent. The drug is a complete DNA chain terminator and DNA polymerase inhibitor. It acts by incorporating itself into the growing DNA chain of cancer cells, interfering with their ability to replicate further. Troxatyl is being evaluated as a single agent or in combination therapy in a number of ongoing trials in hematologic malignancies, includ-

ing acute myeloid leukemia and chronic myeloid leukemia (blastic phase), and in lymphoproliferative disorders such as lymphoma, chronic lymphocytic leukemia, and myeloma. It is also being evaluated as a single agent in pancreatic cancer and in combination therapy in a number of solid tumors. Troxatyl is currently in phase II development.

INDICATION(S) AND RESEARCH PHASE
Cancer/Tumors (Unspecified) – Phase II
Colorectal Cancer – Phase II
Head and Neck Cancer – Phase II
Leukemia – Phase II
Lung Cancer – Phase II
Malignant Melanoma – Phase II
Ovarian Cancer – Phase II
Pancreatic Cancer – Phase II
Prostate Cancer – Phase II
Renal Cell Carcinoma – Phase II

unknown
Allovectin-7

MANUFACTURER
Vical

DESCRIPTION
Allovectin-7 is a DNA/lipid complex containing the human gene that encodes HLA-B7 antigen. The drug is designed to be injected directly into a tumor, where malignant cells absorb it and express the HLA-B7 antigen. This antigen alerts the immune system to the presence of foreign tissue, inducing an immune response.

Allovectin-7 is in clinical testing for subjects with metastatic melanoma and for subjects with tumors of the head and neck. For metastatic melanoma, a phase I/II trial is under way in subjects who have failed conventional therapies, and a phase III trial is being conducted in subjects who have never been treated with chemotherapy. In the phase I/II trial, Allovectin-7 will be administered in addition to low-dose interleukin-2. Subjects in the phase III trial will receive intravenous DTIC in addition to Allovectin-7. Additionally, a trial was initiated in February 2001 for the surgical treatment of early-stage cancer of the oral cavity and oropharynx.

INDICATION(S) AND RESEARCH PHASE
Melanoma – Phase III
Head and Neck Cancer – Phase II
Melanoma – Phase I/II
Oral Cavity Cancer – Phase II

unknown
HumaRAD-HN

MANUFACTURER
Intracel Corporation

DESCRIPTION
HumaRAD is a fully human antibody linked to a radioisotope that has potential applications in several areas of oncology. It is designed to deliver radiation at higher doses to solid tumors than external radiation without systemic toxicity. Intracel is targeting HumaRAD to compartmentalized tumors, where the product can be administered locally or regionally. The company has two HumaRAD products in development—HumaRAD-HN is in phase II trials for the treatment of head and neck cancer.

INDICATION(S) AND RESEARCH PHASE
Head and Neck Cancer – Phase II

ZD0473
unknown

MANUFACTURER
AstraZeneca

DESCRIPTION
ZD0473 is a new generation platinum agent designed to deliver an extended spectrum of anti-cancer activity and overcome platinum resistance for the treatment of cisplatin and carboplatin-resistant tumors, including non-small cell lung, ovarian, colorectal, and bladder cancer. AnorMED has a licensing agreement with AstraZeneca who is conducting the phase II development of ZD0473.

INDICATION(S) AND RESEARCH PHASE
Bladder Cancer – Phase II
Colorectal Cancer – Phase II
Head and Neck Cancer – Phase II
Lung Cancer – Phase II
Ovarian Cancer – Phase II

Histiocytoma

piritrexim
unknown

MANUFACTURER
ILEX Oncology

DESCRIPTION
Piritrexim is a lipid-soluble antifolate drug that works by interrupting a cancer cell's ability to replicate. Specifically, this drug inhibits the enzyme dihydrofolate reductase, which causes an interruption of DNA synthesis. ILEX is currently evaluating the efficacy of orally administered piritrexim in malignant fibrous histiocytoma (MFH), a tumor of the connective tissue. This trial is a phase II research study testing piritrexim in subjects with MFH whose disease progressed after one prior standard chemotherapy regimen.

INDICATION(S) AND RESEARCH PHASE
Histiocytoma – Phase II

Hypercalcemia

zoledronate
Zometa

MANUFACTURER
Novartis

DESCRIPTION
Zoledronate is an intravenous bisphosphonate osteoclast inhibitor. In September 2000, Novartis announced it had received an approvable letter from the FDA for Zometa for the treatment of hypercalcemia of malignancy (HCM), the most common life-threatening metabolic complication associated with cancer. Zometa is also in trials for post-menopausal osteoporosis and bone metastasis treatment and prevention.

INDICATION(S) AND RESEARCH PHASE
Osteoporosis – Phase II

Hypercalcemia – FDA recommend approval letter
Bone Metastases – Phase III

Hyponatremia

YM-087, conivaptan
unknown

MANUFACTURER
Yamanouchi Pharmaceutical

DESCRIPTION
YM-087 is a receptor antagonist to the peptide hormone vasopressin, which is released by the hypothalamus to regulate water balance in the body. The drug is currently in phase III trials for the treatment of hyponatremia, and phase II trials for the treatment of heart failure. It is being developed in both Europe and the United States. The drug is also part of Yamanouchi's domestic pipeline, where it is in phase II trials for both hyponatremia and heart failure. YM-087 is manufactured in oral and injectable formulations.

INDICATION(S) AND RESEARCH PHASE
Congestive Heart Failure – Phase II
Hyponatremia – Phase III
Hyponatremia – Phase II

Kaposi's Sarcoma

Col-3
Metastat

MANUFACTURER
CollaGenex Pharmaceuticals

DESCRIPTION
Metastat is an anti-angiogenesis compound being developed to treat subjects with HIV-related Kaposi's sarcoma. It is an anti-tumor agent that reduces the amount of inflammatory cytokines involved in metastasis and cell proliferation. The compound has been well tolerated in phase I clinical trials.

INDICATION(S) AND RESEARCH PHASE
Kaposi's Sarcoma – Phase I

IM862
unknown

MANUFACTURER
Cytran

DESCRIPTION
IM862 is a small peptide comprised of two amino acids that may inhibit new blood vessel formation (angiogenesis). When there is excessive growth of new blood vessels, a number of pathological conditions may result, including malignant tumors, age-related macular degeneration, and vascular diseases. Limiting the growth of new blood vessels deprives tumors of nourishment necessary for their growth and survival. This drug is being developed in phase III trials for Kaposi's sarcoma and phase I/II trials for ovarian cancer.

INDICATION(S) AND RESEARCH PHASE
Kaposi's Sarcoma – Phase III
Ovarian Cancer – Phase I/II

thalidomide
Thalomid

MANUFACTURER
Celgene Corporation

DESCRIPTION
Thalomid is an oral formulation of the immunomodulatory agent thalidomide. Thalidomide has a notorious history of having caused birth defects when the medical profession unsuspectingly prescribed it for pregnant women as a treatment for nausea and insomnia. Celgene is investigating new applications for the drug, while being particularly mindful of the potential risks of thalidomide treatment. Thalomid is currently being tested for numerous indications in the areas of oncology and immunology.

INDICATION(S) AND RESEARCH PHASE
Multiple Myeloma – Phase II
Myelodysplastic Syndrome – Phase II
Leukemia – Phase II
Brain Cancer – Phase II
Liver Cancer – Phase II
Kidney Cancer – Phase II
Prostate Cancer – Phase II
Kaposi's Sarcoma – Phase II
Cachexia – Phase II
Recurrent Aphthous Stomatitis – Phase III
Crohn's Disease – Phase II
Inflammatory Bowel Disease – Phase II
Sarcoidosis – Phase II
Scleroderma – Phase II

Laryngeal Tumors/Disorders

cidofovir
Vistide

MANUFACTURER
Gilead Sciences

DESCRIPTION
Vistide is being tested in an injectable formulation for the treatment of central nervous system infections, and hepatitis B virus (HBV) respiratory tumors, in addition to tumors or disorders of the larynx. The drug is in phase I/II trials for HBV respiratory tumors, laryngeal papillomatosis, and progressive multifocal leukoencephalopathy.

INDICATION(S) AND RESEARCH PHASE
Hepatitis – Phase I/II
Laryngeal Tumors/Disorders – Phase I/II
Viral Infection – Phase I/II

Leukemia

aldesleukin, interleukin-2 (IL-2)
Proleukin

MANUFACTURER
Chiron Corporation

DESCRIPTION
Proleukin is a genetically engineered (recombinant) form of interleukin-2, which is a naturally occurring immune modulator. Proleukin is being evaluated in phase III trials for acute myelogenous leukemia, non-Hodgkin's lymphoma, and HIV infection.

Additionally, Proleukin was approved in July 2000 for advanced-stage kidney cancer and melanoma.

INDICATION(S) AND RESEARCH PHASE
HIV Infection – Phase III
Leukemia – Phase III
Lymphoma, Non-Hodgkin's – Phase III
Renal Cell Carcinoma – FDA approved
Melanoma – FDA approved

aminopterin
unknown

MANUFACTURER
ILEX Oncology

DESCRIPTION
Aminopterin is an anti-folate in the same family as methotrexate, a widely used anti-cancer drug. Aminopterin kills tumor cells by interfering with their ability to synthesize DNA. Although the drug has been around for many years, it moved out of common use because it was difficult to synthesize and there were concerns about its toxicity. It is currently being tested for the treatment of metastatic endometrial cancer resistant to methotrexate and other drugs, as well as for acute lymphocytic leukemia. Aminopterin has received an orphan drug status for acute lymphocytic leukemia.

INDICATION(S) AND RESEARCH PHASE
Endometrial Cancer – Phase II
Leukemia – Phase II

AR-522
Annamycin

MANUFACTURER
Aronex Pharmaceuticals

DESCRIPTION
Annamycin is an anthracycline analogue intended to overcome multi-drug resistance and irreversible cardiotoxicity associated with anthracycline agents. The compound is being tested in a phase II trial for treatment of refractory breast cancer. Other indications being evaluated include acute myelogenous leukemia (AML), acute lymphocytic leukemia (ALL), and chronic myelogenous leukemia (CML)—all of which are in phase I/II trials. Annamycin is made in a liposomal formulation.

INDICATION(S) AND RESEARCH PHASE
Breast Cancer – Phase II
Leukemia – Phase I/II

arsenic trioxide (ATO)
Trisenox

MANUFACTURER
Cell Therapeutics

DESCRIPTION
Trisenox is believed to kill cancer cells through apoptosis. The mechanism of action of Trisenox is not fully understood, but the drug appears to induce apoptosis in a different manner than other anti-cancer agents such as retinoids.

Trisenox is FDA approved to treat acute promyelocytic leukemia (APL), and it is also in numerous trials in the United States for indications including other types of leukemia, prostate cancer, multiple myeloma, renal cell cancer, cervical cancer, and bladder cancer.

INDICATION(S) AND RESEARCH PHASE
Leukemia – Phase I
Lymphoma, Non-Hodgkin's – Phase II
Leukemia – Phase II
Multiple Myeloma – Phase II
Prostate Cancer – Phase II
Renal Cell Carcinoma – Phase II
Cervical Dysplasia/Cancer – Phase II
Bladder Cancer – Phase II

BCX-34
unknown

MANUFACTURER
BioCryst Pharmaceuticals

DESCRIPTION
BCX-34 is an inhibitor of the enzyme purine nucleoside phosphorylase (PNP), which may be essential for T-cell replication. T-cells normally attack invading bacteria and viruses as part of normal immune function. Proliferative diseases, such as cutaneous T-cell lymphoma (CTCL) and T-cell leukemia, occur when T-cells multiply abnormally or attack healthy body tissue. BCX-34 is currently in trials for the treatment of lymphomas and HIV infection.

INDICATION(S) AND RESEARCH PHASE
HIV Infection – Phase I/II
Leukemia – Trial discontinued
Lymphomas – Phase I/II

CTLA4-Ig
unknown

MANUFACTURER
Repligen Corporation

DESCRIPTION
CTLA4 is a key regulator that signals the immune system to "turn off." CTLA4-Ig, an injectable form of CTLA4, is a T-cell regulatory protein that may prevent graft vs. host disease (GVHD) by down regulating the immune response. CTLA4-Ig has the potential to inactivate only those cells that are initiating an unwanted immune response without compromising the body's ability to fight infections.

Results of a phase I trial demonstrated that CTLA4-Ig prevented the development of GVHD in eight of 11 evaluable subjects receiving a stem cell transplantation for leukemia. In October 2000, Repligen received approval from the FDA to initiate a phase II clinical trial with CTLA4-Ig. The trial will evaluate the safety and efficacy of CTLA4-Ig in subjects receiving stem cell transplantation for leukemia or other malignancies. The primary objective of the study is to determine if CTLA4-Ig, in combination with T-cell depletion, can reduce the incidence or severity of GVHD in subjects receiving a stem cell transplant from a "genetically mismatched" donor.

INDICATION(S) AND RESEARCH PHASE
Leukemia – Phase I completed

daunorubicin citrate
DaunoXome

MANUFACTURER
Gilead Sciences

DESCRIPTION
DaunoXome is a liposome anticancer product that has received approval as a first-line chemotherapy agent for advanced HIV-associated Kaposi's sarcoma (KS). DaunoXome's active ingredient is daunorubicin, a member of the anthracycline family of compounds, a potent group of antibiotics. Liposomes are microscopic fat bubbles that can be used to encase a drug. In animal studies, daunorubicin has been shown to accumulate in tumors to a greater extent when administered as DaunoXome than when administered as conventional daunorubicin. This anticancer drug is being tested in phase II trials for leukemias and the treatment of non-Hodgkin's lymphoma.

INDICATION(S) AND RESEARCH PHASE
Leukemia – Phase II
Lymphoma, Non-Hodgkin's – Phase II

decitabine
unknown

MANUFACTURER
SuperGen

DESCRIPTION
Decitabine is an investigational chemotherapeutic agent in development for the treatment of sickle cell anemia and a variety of solid tumors and hematological malignancies, including myelodysplastic syndrome, non-small cell lung cancer, and chronic myelogenous leukemia. Decitabine inhibits DNA methyltransferase activity, and in this manner presumably reactivates tumor suppressor genes.

Results of a phase I/II trial of decitabine for sickle cell anemia demonstrated that it produced a response in 100% of subjects tested. The trial enrolled a total of eight subjects: five of whom had shown no response to hydroxyurea (HU) after one year of treatment; two of whom had a moderate but unsustained response to HU; and one subject who was not treated with HU. After administration of decitabine, the five subjects previously treated with HU experienced an average 35-fold increase of fetal hemoglobin levels compared to levels during HU treatment. The two subjects who responded briefly to HU experienced an average fetal hemoglobin level increase of 52% with decitabine, and the one subjects who had not received HU treatment experienced more than a 50% increase in fetal hemoglobin levels.

INDICATION(S) AND RESEARCH PHASE
Myelodysplastic Syndrome – Phase III
Lung Cancer – Phase II
Anemia – Phase I/II completed
Leukemia – Phase II

denileukin diftitox
Ontak

MANUFACTURER
Ligand Pharmaceuticals

DESCRIPTION
Ontak, previously known as DAB389IL-2, is a novel targeted cytotoxic biologic. The cytotoxic diphtheria toxin is fused to a subunit of IL-2 and therefore is delivered only to cells that express the IL-2 receptor (IL-2R). IL-2R may be expressed in a variety of malignant cells, including those of chronic lymphocytic leukemia. A phase II trial was initiated in January 2001 in subjects diagnosed with fludarabine-refractory, CD25-positive B-cell chronic lymphocytic leukemia.

The FDA has granted Seragen, a subsidiary of Ligand, marketing approval for Ontak for the treatment of subjects with persistent or recurrent cutaneous T-cell lymphoma whose malignant cells express the CD25 component of the IL-2 receptor.

INDICATION(S) AND RESEARCH PHASE
Leukemia – Phase II
Lymphomas – FDA approved

flavopiridol, HMR-1275
unknown

MANUFACTURER
Aventis

DESCRIPTION
Flavopiridol belongs to a new class of drugs for cancer therapy known as cyclin-dependent kinase (CDK) inhibitors. It is being tested in phase II trials as a treatment for chronic lymphatic leukemia, esophageal cancer and non-small cell lung cancer.

INDICATION(S) AND RESEARCH PHASE
Esophageal Cancer – Phase II
Leukemia – Phase II
Lung Cancer – Phase II

G3139/gemtuzumab ozogamicin
Genasense/Mylotarg

MANUFACTURER
Genta

DESCRIPTION
Genasense (G3139) attacks Bcl-2, a protein that is over-expressed in many forms of cancer. Bcl-2 appears to contribute to the resistance of these diseases to standard treatment. Genta is using its proprietary antisense approach to first decrease the expression of Bcl-2, and then to administer anticancer therapy in an effort to improve subject outcome. A phase II trial was initiated in January 2001 using Genasense in combination with Mylotarg (gemtuzumab ozogamicin) from Wyeth/Genetics Institute for the treatment of acute myeloid leukemia.

INDICATION(S) AND RESEARCH PHASE
Leukemia – Phase II

G3139
Genasense

MANUFACTURER
Genta

DESCRIPTION
Genasense (G3139) attacks Bcl-2, a protein that is over-expressed in many forms of cancer. Bcl-2 appears to contribute to the resistance of these diseases to standard treatment. Genta is using its proprietary antisense approach to first decrease the expression of Bcl-2, and then to administer anti-

cancer therapy in an effort to improve subject outcome. A phase III trial was initiated in March 2001 testing Genasense as a single agent in subjects suffering from chronic lymphocytic leukemia.

INDICATION(S) AND RESEARCH PHASE
Leukemia – Phase III

gene therapy, leukemia
unknown

MANUFACTURER
Bioenvision

DESCRIPTION
Bioenvision's gene therapy product for the treatment of leukemia is currently in clinical development.

INDICATION(S) AND RESEARCH PHASE
Leukemia – Phase I/II

GL-331
unknown

MANUFACTURER
Genelabs Technologies

DESCRIPTION
GL-331 is an inhibitor of topoisomerase II. It is a semi-synthetic derivative of podophyllotoxin, which is a chemotherapeutic agent designed to overcome multi-drug resistant (MDR) cancers. At this time, development has been discontinued.

INDICATION(S) AND RESEARCH PHASE
Colon Malignancies – Trial discontinued
Leukemia – Trial discontinued
Lung Cancer – Trial discontinued
Renal Cell Carcinoma – Trial discontinued

GPX-100
unknown

MANUFACTURER
Gem Pharmaceuticals

DESCRIPTION
GPX-100 is noncardiotoxic version of the anticancer drug adriamycin. Adriamycin, an anthracycline, is a commonly used drug in the treatment of cancers, including metastatic breast cancer. The cytotoxic effect of adriamycin on malignant cells and its toxic effects on various organs are thought to be related to genetic insertion (nucleotide base intercalation) and cell membrane lipid binding activities. Intercalation inhibits both nucleotide replication and enzyme activity of DNA and RNA polymerases. The interaction of adriamycin with topoisomerase II to form DNA-cleavable complexes appears to be an important mechanism of adriamycin cell-killing activity. The drug's cellular membrane binding may affect a variety of cellular functions.

Unfortunately, adriamycin and related drugs may produce irreversible damage to the heart if the subject receives too many doses. Thus, although adriamycin may eliminate the tumor, if the cancer returns the drug often cannot be administered again because of the significant risk of heart failure and possible death. The company claims to have developed a platform technology that allows the chemical conversion of any standard anthracycline to a closely related analog that cannot be converted by the body to the cardiotoxic metabolite. GPX-100 is presently in trials for metastatic breast cancer and pediatric trials for leukemia.

INDICATION(S) AND RESEARCH PHASE
Cancer/Tumors (Unspecified) – Phase II
Breast Cancer – Phase II
Pediatric, Leukemia – Phase II

histamine dihydrochloride
Ceplene

MANUFACTURER
Maxim Pharmaceuticals

DESCRIPTION
Ceplene (formally Maxamine) is a histamine-2 (H-2) receptor stimulator that is being co-administered with immunotherapies, including cytokines and interleukin-2 (IL-2). Clinical testing includes treatment of acute myelogenous leukemia (AML), chronic hepatitis C, malignant melanoma, multiple myeloma, and renal cell carcinoma. Results from a phase III trial in stage-IV malignant melanoma subjects indicated that Ceplene used in combination with a lower dose of interleukin-2 (IL-2) improved survival rates compared to treatment with the same doses of IL-2 alone. Treatment with Ceplene and IL-2 improved overall survival, increased survival rates at 12, 18, and 24 months, and improved time-to-disease progression compared to treatment with IL-2 alone. Twenty-five percent of subjects treated with Ceplene and lower-dose IL-2 survived for a 24-month period. Overall response was achieved in 38% of the subjects treated with Ceplene and lower-dose IL-2. The company received an NDA non-approvable letter in January 2001 because the FDA stated that the phase III trial forming the basis of the NDA would not be adequate as a single study to support approval.

INDICATION(S) AND RESEARCH PHASE
Hepatitis – Phase II
Leukemia – Phase III completed
Malignant Melanoma – NDA denied
Multiple Myeloma – Phase II
Renal Cell Carcinoma – Phase II

imatinib, STI 571
Glivec

MANUFACTURER
Novartis

DESCRIPTION
Glivec is an oral signal transduction inhibitor (specifically, a Bcr-Abl tyrokinase inhibitor). Glivec works by blocking signals within cancer cells that express the Bcr-Abl protein, thus preventing a series of chemical reactions that elicit cell proliferation. Glivec is currently in phase III trials for acute lymphoic leukemia and chronic myeloid leukemia. It is also in a phase I trial for Philadelphia-positive leukemia for ages newborn to 16 years.

INDICATION(S) AND RESEARCH PHASE
Leukemia – Phase III
Pediatric, Leukemia – Phase I

interferon alfa-2b

PEG-Intron

MANUFACTURER
Schering-Plough Corporation

DESCRIPTION
PEG-Intron is a long-acting antiviral/biological response modifier. Clinical trials include testing for the treatment of chronic myelogenous leukemia, solid tumors, and malignant melanoma.

PEG-Intron was developed by Enzon for Schering-Plough who owns the exclusive rights. The drug was approved by the FDA for the treatment of hepatitis C in January 2001.

INDICATION(S) AND RESEARCH PHASE
Cancer/Tumors (Unspecified) – Phase II
Hepatitis – FDA approved
Leukemia – Phase III
Malignant Melanoma – Phase III

LDI-200
unknown

MANUFACTURER
Milkhaus Laboratory

DESCRIPTION
Clinical trials are testing a subcutanous formulation of LDI-200 for at least three indications: leukemia, myelodysplastic syndrome, and prostate cancer. Results demonstrated that LDI-200 showed both efficacy and safety in a small phase II/III open label crossover trial in subjects with myelodysplastic syndrome. The control consisted of subjects given supportive therapy, consisting of transfusions and antibiotics, who became eligible for treatment if their disease progressed more rapidly than anticipated. A total of 23 subjects were treated using LDI-200, and seven showed significant clinical response.

INDICATION(S) AND RESEARCH PHASE
Leukemia – Phase II completed
Prostate Cancer – Phase II/III
White Blood Cell Disorders – Phase II/III
Myelodysplastic Syndrome – Phase III completed

LDP-03
Campath

MANUFACTURER
BTG International

DESCRIPTION
Campath is a genetically engineered monoclonal antibody targeted to the CD52 antigen, which is a surface marker on abnormal human lymphocytes. This biological drug therapy is being tested for the treatment of chronic lymphocytic leukemia (CLL) that has not responded to conventional chemotherapy. It works by attacking these cancerous white blood cells and tagging them for immune system disposal. BTG International is developing Campath in a joint venture with LeukoSite.

INDICATION(S) AND RESEARCH PHASE
Leukemia – NDA submitted

liposomal ether lipid
TLC ELL-12

MANUFACTURER
The Liposome Company

DESCRIPTION
TLC ELL-12 is a liposomal ether lipid that may have efficacy in the treatment of several cancers. This drug has exhibited significant anti-tumor activity, but did not have the hemolytic side effects common to this type of ether lipid when therapeutic doses were used in experimental models. It does not appear to be myelosuppressive.

TLC ELL-12 is currently being developed in phase I trials for the treatment of lung cancer, multiple myeloma, leukemia, and prostate cancer.

INDICATION(S) AND RESEARCH PHASE
Lung Cancer – Phase I
Multiple Myeloma – Phase I
Leukemia – Phase I
Prostate Cancer – Phase I

MDX-22
unknown

MANUFACTURER
Medarex

DESCRIPTION
MDX-22 is used to purge leukemia cells from the bone marrow of acute myeloid leukemia (AML) subjects who are undergoing a transplant of their own bone marrow. This therapy uses a monoclonal antibody to attack the abnormal leukemia cells.

INDICATION(S) AND RESEARCH PHASE
Leukemia – Phase II

peginterferon alfa-2a
Pegasys

MANUFACTURER
Hoffmann-La Roche

DESCRIPTION
Pegasys is a longer-lasting form of interferon, which is a naturally produced immune boosting substance. It is in clinical trials for the treatment of hepatitis B and C, malignant melanoma, renal cell carcinoma, and chronic myelogenous leukemia.

INDICATION(S) AND RESEARCH PHASE
Hepatitis – Phase III
Malignant Melanoma – Phase II
Renal Cell Carcinoma – Phase II
Leukemia – Phase III

pentostatin
Nipent

MANUFACTURER
SuperGen

DESCRIPTION
Nipent (pentostatin) belongs to a group of drugs called antimetabolites. Pentostatin inhibits the enzyme adenosine deaminase, which leads to cytotoxicity and cell death. This drug is in trials for rheumatoid arthritis, chronic lymphocytic leukemia, and non-Hodgkin's lymphoma, among other indications.

In December 2000, results of a phase II trial of Nipent indicated the drug has significant activity (75% overall response rate) in the treatment of graft versus host disease (GVHD). Twelve subjects with steroid refractory GVHD received Nipent as "salvage therapy" because each had previously failed all other treatments.

INDICATION(S) AND RESEARCH PHASE
Leukemia – Phase III
Lymphoma, Non-Hodgkin's – Phase II
Rheumatoid Arthritis – Phase II
Immunosuppressive – Phase III
Cutaneous T-cell Lymphoma (CTCL)/Peripheral T-cell Lymphoma (PTCL) – NDA submitted

RFS-2000
Rubitecan

MANUFACTURER
SuperGen

DESCRIPTION
Rubitecan is a novel drug that works by inhibiting an enzyme called topoisomerase I. This drug is made in an oral formulation, which is an advantage for outpatient treatment compared to intravenous cancer drugs that may require a visit to a hospital setting.

In addition to treating pancreatic cancer, Rubitecan is being evaluated in treating a variety of solid tumors, such as in breast, colorectal, lung, ovarian, and prostate cancers, as well as metastatic melanoma and advanced gastric carcinoma. Additionally, phase II trials in the United States and Europe are testing Rubitecan in blood cancers such as chronic myelomonocytic leukemia (CMML/myelodysplastic syndrome).

INDICATION(S) AND RESEARCH PHASE
Pancreatic Cancer – Phase III
Breast Cancer – Phase II
Colorectal Cancer – Phase II
Gastric Cancer – Phase II
Leukemia – Phase II
Malignant Melanoma – Phase II
Ovarian Cancer – Phase II
Myelodysplastic Syndrome – Phase III

SMART M195
unknown

MANUFACTURER
Protein Design Labs

DESCRIPTION
SMART M195 is a radioactive compound that is linked to a humanized monoclonal antibody. Radiotherapy using alpha-particle emitting isotopes (bismuth-213) has been used for some years to treat different forms of cancer. This combination therapy is a specialized targeting method that allows the monoclonal antibody to attach itself to the cancer cell, giving the adjoining radioactive isotope a greater chance by proximity to kill the cancer.

SMART M195 is currently in a phase III trial for the treatment of acute myeloid leukemia using radiotherapy. This biologic product is also being tested in two other Phase II studies for the indications of acute promyelocytic leukemia and myelodysplastic syndrome.

INDICATION(S) AND RESEARCH PHASE
Leukemia – Phase III
Leukemia – Phase II
White Blood Cell Disorders – Phase II

tiazofurin
Tiazole

MANUFACTURER
ICN Pharmaceuticals

DESCRIPTION
Tiazole is a nucleoside analogue being assessed in phase II/III testing for the treatment of acute myelogenous leukemia and chronic myelogenous leukemia. ICN Pharmaceuticals and the National Cancer Institute are sponsoring this clinical study.

INDICATION(S) AND RESEARCH PHASE
Leukemia – Phase II/III

tretinoin
Atragen

MANUFACTURER
Aronex Pharmaceuticals

DESCRIPTION
Atragen is a liposomal, intravenous formulation of tretinoin or all-trans-retinoic acid. Tretinoin induces cell differentiation in rapidly proliferating cells, such as those observed in malignant diseases. Additionally, Atragen appears to affect the cellular signaling mechanisms that become unbalanced in cancer cells. Results of a phase II trial of Atragen monotherapy for acute promyelocytic leukemia (APL) indicated its potential to induce complete remission. The trial was conducted in Peru, and included 16 subjects with newly diagnosed or previously untreated APL who were treated with Atragen every other day as a single agent for a maximum of 28 doses. Fourteen subjects (87.5%) achieved morphologic remission, and 28.6% of these subjects also attained molecular remission. The safety profile observed in the subject population is similar to that reported with the currently approved oral formulation of Atra.

In addition to investigating the safety and efficacy of Atragen as a treatment for APL, the company is conducting trials to evaluate the compound for the treatment of non-Hodgkin's lymphoma, hormone-resistant prostate cancer, acute myelogenous leukemia (AML), and renal cell carcinoma in combination with interferon alpha.

In January 2001, Aronex announced that the FDA has denied approval of the company's NDA for Atragen as a treatment for subjects with APL, for whom therapy with tretinoin (all-trans-retinoic acid or Atra) is necessary but for whom an intravenous administration is required.

INDICATION(S) AND RESEARCH PHASE
Lymphoma, Non-Hodgkin's – Phase II
Prostate Cancer – Phase II
Renal Cell Carcinoma – Phase I/II
Leukemia, APL (intravenous) – NDA denied
Leukemia, APL (monotherapy) – Phase II
Leukemia, AML – Phase II

troxacitabine, BCH-4556
Troxatyl

MANUFACTURER
BioChem Pharma

DESCRIPTION

Troxatyl is a dioxolane nucleoside analog being investigated as an anticancer agent. The drug is a complete DNA chain terminator and DNA polymerase inhibitor. It acts by incorporating itself into the growing DNA chain of cancer cells, interfering with their ability to replicate further. Currently, Troxatyl is being evaluated as a single agent or in combination therapy in a number of ongoing single and multicenter trials in hematologic malignancies, including acute myeloid leukemia, chronic myeloid leukemia—blastic phase, and in lymphoproliferative disorders such as lymphoma, chronic lymphocytic leukemia, and myeloma. It is also being evaluated as a single agent in pancreatic cancer and in combination therapy in a number of solid tumors. Troxatyl is currently in phase II development.

INDICATION(S) AND RESEARCH PHASE

Cancer/Tumors (Unspecified) – Phase II
Colorectal Cancer – Phase II
Head and Neck Cancer – Phase II
Leukemia – Phase II
Lung Cancer – Phase II
Malignant Melanoma – Phase II
Ovarian Cancer – Phase II
Pancreatic Cancer – Phase II
Prostate Cancer – Phase II
Renal Cell Carcinoma – Phase II

unknown
Vasogen IMT

MANUFACTURER
Vasogen

DESCRIPTION

Vasogen immune modulation therapy (IMT) is being developed for the treatment of chronic lymphocytic leukemia (CLL). The company's immune modulation therapies target the destructive inflammatory processes that lead to disease. This inhibition of inflammatory responses is thought to be mediated by anti-inflammatory cytokines, including interleukin-10, produced by the activation of regulatory immune cells. Vasogen IMT is currently in phase II development.

INDICATION(S) AND RESEARCH PHASE
Leukemia – Phase II

unknown
Clofarabine

MANUFACTURER
Bioenvision

DESCRIPTION

Clofarabine is currently in a phase II trial at the M.D. Anderson Cancer Center in Houston. The drug is being given to fludarabine-resistant subjects with chronic lymphocytic leukemia and to subjects with acute leukemia. The company is currently looking for a development partner to help fund further trials with Clofarabine.

INDICATION(S) AND RESEARCH PHASE
Leukemia – Phase II

unknown
L-Vax

MANUFACTURER
AVAX Technologies

DESCRIPTION

L-Vax is a cancer vaccine being tested in 40 subjects with acute myelogenous leukemia (AML) in a phase I/II trial. L-Vax will be prepared from blood samples of the subjects obtained after their first relapse. AVAX uses a process known as "haptenization," which alters the tumor cells and makes them appear foreign to the subject's immune system. When the hapten-modified cells are injected into subjects, they stimulate the immune system to recognize the cancer cells and destroy them. Additionally, subjects in second remission will receive seven weekly L-Vax vaccinations. The company plans to evaluate whether or not L-Vax induces an immune response against leukemia cells and if it prevents or delays another response.

INDICATION(S) AND RESEARCH PHASE
Leukemia – Phase I/II

vaccine, cancer
Gvax

MANUFACTURER
Cell Genesys

DESCRIPTION

Gvax is an allogenic compound that involves the genetic modification of prostate cancer cell lines. These cancer cells have been irradiated and modified to secrete granulocyte-macrophage colony stimulating factor (GM-CSF), a hormone which plays a key role in stimulating the body's immune response to vaccines. The compound is in trials for prostate cancer, pancreatic cancer, lung cancer, leukemia, and malignant melanoma.

The Gvax prostate cancer vaccine demonstrated anti-tumor activity in an initial phase II trial in subjects with advanced metastatic prostate cancer who have not responded to hormone therapy. Prior to initiating a phase III trial, Cell Genesys plans to initiate further trials of Gvax prostate cancer vaccine in 2001 that will employ a higher potency version of the same product. Additionally, future phase III trials in hormone refractory prostate cancer subjects may compare Gvax vaccine in combination with chemotherapy to chemotherapy alone.

INDICATION(S) AND RESEARCH PHASE

Prostate Cancer – Phase II
Lung Cancer – Phase I/II completed
Malignant Melanoma – Phase I/II
Vaccines – Phase I/II
Pancreatic Cancer – Phase II
Leukemia – Phase I/II

Liver Cancer

cisplatin/epinephrine
IntraDose

MANUFACTURER
Matrix Pharmaceutical

DESCRIPTION

IntraDose is a biodegradable collagen carrier matrix combined with a vasoconstrictor. The gel is injected directly into tumors where it localizes high concentrations of cisplatin, a widely used anticancer drug. It is currently being tested for several indications, including head and neck, breast, malignant melanoma, esophageal, and primary hepatocellular cancer.

A phase II trail of IntraDose Injectable Gel produced durable responses in subjects with colorectal cancer that had metastasized to the liver. Nine of 31 subjects who received IntraDose responded to therapy. Six subjects experienced a complete response (100% reduction in viable tumor volume of treated tumors) while the other three subjects demonstrated a partial response (at least a 50% reduction of viable tumor volume). Eight of the nine treatment responders have had durable responses with no relapse at the site of treatment. IntraDose was well tolerated by subjects.

INDICATION(S) AND RESEARCH PHASE
Breast Cancer – Phase II
Cancer/Tumors (Unspecified) – Phase II
Colorectal Cancer – Phase II completed
Esophageal Cancer – Phase II
Liver Cancer – Phase II
Malignant Melanoma – Phase II
Head and Neck Cancer – NDA submitted

doxorubicin HCl
Doxil, Caelyx

MANUFACTURER
Alza (Sequus Pharmaceuticals)

DESCRIPTION
Doxil is a liposomal formulation of doxorubicin hydrochloride, an intravenous chemotherapy agent. This anthracycline anti-tumor agent is currently on the market for treatment of Kaposi's sarcoma. The drug uses a novel, targeted delivery system to help evade recognition and uptake by the immune system so that the liposomes can circulate in the body longer. A long circulation time increases the likelihood that the liposomes and their pharmaceutical contents will reach their targeted tumor site. Doxil may act through an ability to bind DNA and inhibit nucleic acid synthesis.

The company reported that Doxil is being tested in phase II/III trials for the additional indications of breast, liver, lung, and prostate cancers, as well as phase II for unspecified cancers and tumors.

Alza markets this product in the United States under the tradename Doxil; however, it is marketed under the name Caelyx in other areas. Schering-Plough has exclusive international marketing rights to Caelyx, excluding Japan and Israel, through a distribution agreement with Alza.

INDICATION(S) AND RESEARCH PHASE
Breast Cancer – Phase II/III
Liver Cancer – Phase II/III
Lung Cancer – Phase II/III
Prostate Cancer – Phase II/III
Cancer/Tumors (Unspecified) – Phase II

imaging agent
AFP-Scan

MANUFACTURER
Immunomedics

DESCRIPTION
AFP-Scan, a nuclear imaging diagnostic tool, can reveal the location and extent of alpha-fetoprotein (AFP) germ cell tumors or infections. The active agent consists of a mouse-derived AFP antibody fragment directly labeled with technetium-99m (Tc-99m), a widely available, inexpensive radioisotope. Tc-99m enhances imaging, particularly in the liver, which is the first site of metastasis or spread for many cancers. The labeling of the antibody with Tc-99m is performed in a one-vial, 5-minute proprietary procedure. After administration to the subject, a conventional nuclear medicine camera is used to display radioisotope concentrations. This instant imaging diagnostic kit is being tested in phase II trials for liver cancer.

INDICATION(S) AND RESEARCH PHASE
Liver Cancer – Phase II

MGI-114, hydroxymethylacylfulvene, HMAF
Irofulven

MANUFACTURER
MGI Pharma

DESCRIPTION
Irofulven (MGI-114) is the first product candidate being developed by MGI Pharma from its family of anti-cancer compounds called acylfulvenes. Early trials demonstrated that Irofulven is absorbed rapidly by tumor cells, and once inside binds to DNA and protein targets. The binding interferes with DNA replication and cell division, leading to tumor-specific cell death. The drug is being tested in a series of trials for a variety of cancers.

Results from a phase II trial of Irofulven indicated that the drug produced anti-tumor activity in subjects with advanced pancreatic cancer who were refractory to gemcitabine (Gemzar). Ten of the 53 subjects enrolled achieved six-month survival and two subjects demonstrated objective responses: one subject experienced tumor shrinkage of 100% and another subject experienced an 84% decrease in tumor mass. A phase III trial was initiated in February 2001.

INDICATION(S) AND RESEARCH PHASE
Breast Cancer – Phase II
Colon Malignancies – Phase II
Renal Cell Carcinoma – Phase II
Cervical Dysplasia/Cancer – Phase II
Lung Cancer – Phase II
Ovarian Cancer – Phase I/II
Colorectal Cancer – Phase II
Prostate Cancer – Phase I/II
Cancer/Tumors (Unspecified) – Phase I/II
Pancreatic Cancer – Phase III
Liver Cancer – Phase II

MTC-DOX
unknown

MANUFACTURER
FeRx

DESCRIPTION
MTC-DOX is a drug delivery vehicle for doxorubicin, a widely used anti-cancer drug. Magnetic targeted carriers (MTCs) are microparticles composed of elemental iron and activated carbon that serve as delivery vehicles for site-specific targeting, retentionc

and sustained release of pharmaceuticals. With MTC-DOX, doxorubicin is absorbed into the MTC and delivered to the tumor so that the drug will remain in the tumor rather than spreading throughout the body. FeRX, the company developing MTC-DOX, hopes that this system will reduce complications of chemotherapy, as well as improve response rates of anti-cancer drugs. The company has initiated a phase II trial.

INDICATION(S) AND RESEARCH PHASE
Liver Cancer – Phase II

nolatrexed dihydrochloride
Thymitaq

MANUFACTURER
Zarix

DESCRIPTION
Thymitaq is a thymidylate synthase inhibitor. It is a novel compound with the potential to treat several cancers including liver cancer, head and neck cancer, non-small cell lung cancer, adenocarcinoma of the colon, prostate cancer, and pancreatic cancer. It is currently in phase III trials for unresectable hepatocellular carcinoma, which are taking place in the United States, Canada, Europe and South Africa.

INDICATION(S) AND RESEARCH PHASE
Liver Cancer – Phase III

pivaloyloxymethylbutyrate
Pivanex

MANUFACTURER
Titan Pharmaceuticals

DESCRIPTION
Pivanex, an analog of butyric acid, is a small molecule drug that attacks cancer cells through the mechanism of cellular differentiation. It is being tested for the treatment of advanced stages of non-small cell lung cancer that have not responded well to other drug therapy. Results of a phase I/II trial testing Pivanex for the treatment of liver metastases are pending.

INDICATION(S) AND RESEARCH PHASE
Lung Cancer – Phase II
Liver Cancer – Phase I/II

thymalfasin
Zadaxin

MANUFACTURER
SciClone Pharmaceuticals

DESCRIPTION
Zadaxin is a twenty-eight amino acid peptide originally isolated from the thymus gland now produced synthetically. The compound has been shown to promote the maturation of T-cells, which are involved in the control of various immune responses. Zadaxin has been administered to over 3,000 subjects in over 70 clinical trials without serious drug related side effects.

Zadaxin is presently in phase II trials in the United States in combination with lamivudine for the treatment of hepatitis B. SciClone plans to initiate additional U.S. phase II Zadaxin clinical programs in liver cancer and malignant melanoma. Pivotal phase III hepatitis B studies are currently ongoing in Japan. SciClone plans to start a pivotal phase III hepatitis C trial in the United States, which will be complemented by a pivotal phase III hepatitis C trial in Europe to be conducted by Sigma-Tau S.p.A., SciClone's European partner.

INDICATION(S) AND RESEARCH PHASE
Hepatitis – Phase II
Hepatitis – Phase III
Viral Infection – Phase III
Liver Cancer – Phase II
Malignant Melanoma – Phase II

unknown
Combidex

MANUFACTURER
Advanced Magnetics

DESCRIPTION
Combidex MRI contrast agent was developed to help in the detection, diagnosis, and staging of various cancers. The first indication is for the diagnosis of metastatic cancer to assist in directing biopsy and surgery as well as to aid in the staging of a variety of cancers, including breast and prostate cancer. In clinical studies, Combidex significantly reduced the number of false diagnoses (both false positive and false negative nodes) compared to unenhanced MRI exams. The second indication is for the detection, diagnosis, and characterization of benign versus malignant lesions of the liver and spleen.

In phase III clinical trials, post-Combidex MRI showed clear differentiation between normal and metastatic lymph nodes, while a post-gadolinium image showed no differentiation in normal and metastatic nodes when compared with pre-dose images.

INDICATION(S) AND RESEARCH PHASE
Breast Cancer – Phase III/IV
Liver Cancer – Phase III
Prostate Cancer – Phase III/IV

vaccine, anti-gastrin
Gastrimmune

MANUFACTURER
Aphton Corporation

DESCRIPTION
Gastrimmune is a therapeutic vaccine that neutralizes specific hormones (G17 & Gly-extended G17). The drug is in phase III trials for the treatment of cancers of the gastrointestinal tract, including gastric cancer and colorectal cancer. It is also in trials for liver cancer, esophageal cancer and two phase III trials for advanced pancreatic cancer—one in the the United States and one in Europe.

INDICATION(S) AND RESEARCH PHASE
Colorectal Cancer – Phase III
Esophageal Cancer – Phase III
Gastric Cancer – Phase III
Liver Cancer – Phase II/III
Pancreatic Cancer – Phase III

Lung Cancer

AE-941

Neovastat

MANUFACTURER
AEterna Laboratories

DESCRIPTION
Neovastat is an angiogenesis inhibitor being tested for the treatment of non-small cell lung cancer, psoriasis, multiple myeloma and kidney cancer, among other indications.

A phase II trial for multiple myeloma was initiated in October 2000 and will treat 120 subjects and include approximately 20 sites across North America and Europe. Trial results are expected in the summer of 2002.

Additionally, a phase III trial was initiated in May 2000 for kidney cancer, which will include 270 subjects at sites in North America and Europe.

INDICATION(S) AND RESEARCH PHASE
Lung Cancer – Phase III
Psoriasis and Psoriatic Disorders – Phase I/II completed
Cancer/Tumors (Unspecified) – Phase I/II completed
Multiple Myeloma – Phase II
Renal Cell Carcinoma – Phase III
Macular Degeneration – Phase I completed

alitretinoin, ALRT-1057
Panretin

MANUFACTURER
Ligand Pharmaceuticals

DESCRIPTION
This product consists of 9-*cis*-retinoic acid and is chemically related to vitamin A. It activates all known retinoid receptors. Activation of retinoid receptors regulates the expression of genes controlling processes related to cell differentiation and proliferation. A topical gel formulation of Panretin has been on the market since February 1999 for the treatment of lesions associated with Kaposi's sarcoma.

These new trials are evaluating the effects of an oral capsule formulation for the following new indications: treatment of breast and pediatric cancers (phase II), myelodysplastic syndrome, bronchial metaplasia, and psoriasis and psoriatic disorders (phase II/III).

INDICATION(S) AND RESEARCH PHASE
Breast Cancer – Phase II
Lung Cancer – Phase II/III
Pediatric – Phase II
Psoriasis and Psoriatic Disorders – Phase II/III
White Blood Cell Disorders – Phase II/III

arcitumomab
CEA-Scan

MANUFACTURER
Immunomedics

DESCRIPTION
CEA-Scan is a monoclonal antibody attached to carcinoembryonic (CEA) antigen that is radioactively labeled with technetium (Tc99m). CEA is an important cell surface marker expressed by certain tumor cells. This imaging agent can detect various cancer cells associated with CEA expressed tumors. CEA-Scan utilizes proprietary technetium (RAID) technology.

Currently, CEA-Scan is being tested in a phase II/III trial for breast cancer. It is being used to evaluate subjects with suspicious mammograms, as well as palpable and non-palpable lesions.

This agent is also in a phase II trial for thyroid cancer. CEA-Scan is used for the diagnosis and localization of primary, residual, recurrent, and metastatic medullary thyroid carcinoma.

Lastly, CEA-Scan is in a phase III for lung cancer. It determines the presence, location, and the extent of the metastatic disease in primary and recurrent lung cancer.

INDICATION(S) AND RESEARCH PHASE
Breast Cancer – Phase II/III
Lung Cancer – Phase III
Thyroid Cancer – Phase II

BAM-002
unknown

MANUFACTURER
Novelos Therapeutics

DESCRIPTION
BAM-002 is a proprietary form of a peptide found in all cells of the human body. BAM-002 stablizes the peptide in its oxidized form, which allows it to exert direct and indirect anti-tumor effects, protect normal cells from the effects of toxic agents, promote hematopoiesis, and stimulate the immune system. Furthermore, according to the company, BAM-002 is believed to increase tolerance of the highly toxic drugs used in chemotherapeutic regimens, potentiate a chemotherapeutic impact on tumor cells, as well as stimulate recovery of the immune and blood systems.

A phase II trial of BAM-002 in non-small cell lung cancer has been initiated. The trial consists of 84 subjects and is examining the effects of BAM-002 plus chemotherapy to BAM-002 alone. Two different delivery combinations are being evaluated (intravenous/intramuscular delivery versus intravenous/subcutaneous delivery), and trial endpoints include tumor response, one-year survival, and hematopoietic recovery following chemotherapy.

BAM-002 was approved in Russia in September 1998. Results from the 2,000 subjects treated demonstrated that BAM-002 was safe, well tolerated, and efficacious.

INDICATION(S) AND RESEARCH PHASE
Lung Cancer – Phase II

BAY 12-9566
unknown

MANUFACTURER
Bayer Corporation

DESCRIPTION
Scientists believe that cancer cells produce enzymes called matrix metalloproteinases (MMPs) to break down the body's natural protective barriers, allowing cancer to grow and spread. MMP inhibitors, such as BAY 12-9566, are designed to interfere with this process.

Bayer Corporation was conducting phase III clinical trials of BAY 12-9566 for the treatment of arthritis, pancreatic cancer, ovarian cancer, and small and non-small cell lung cancer. However, the company announced that it has halted all clinical trials of its BAY 12-9566 in cancer and osteoarthritis. This action follows a recommendation from an independent Data Safety Monitoring Board that trials in small cell lung cancer be stopped.

INDICATION(S) AND RESEARCH PHASE
Lung Cancer – Trial discontinued
Pancreatic Cancer – Trial discontinued
Ovarian Cancer – Trial discontinued
Osteoarthritis – Trial discontinued

BEC2
unknown

MANUFACTURER
ImClone Systems

DESCRIPTION
BEC2, a cancer vaccine, is a monoclonal anti-idiotypic antibody. These antibodies are "custom-made" to mimic a specific antigen in an individual subject. This induces the body to produce an immune response to that specific antigen. The anti-idiotypic antibody seems to stimulate a stronger immune response than the antigen itself. The BEC2 vaccine is given to the subject after an initial treatment of the tumor. The antibody resembles an antigen (GD3 ganglioside) on the tumor, thus inducing the immune system to attack the cancer cells. GD3 is overexpressed on a number of cancers including small cell lung carcinoma, melanoma and soft tissue sarcomas.

The company reported that in preclinical studies BEC2 was shown to eliminate tumor metastases and prevent cancer reccurrence. Also reported, was a trial of 15 subjects with small cell lung cancer who showed significantly increased survival. Median survival was 20.5 months versus a reference group with median survival of 17.9 months.

BEC2 is currently in a phase III clinical trial for the treatment of limited disease in small cell lung carcinoma. The trial will evaluate the antitumor effect in approximately 800 subjects. Future trials may investigate malignant melanoma.

INDICATION(S) AND RESEARCH PHASE
Lung Cancer – Phase III

bexarotene
Targretin-capsule

MANUFACTURER
Ligand Pharmaceuticals

DESCRIPTION
Targretin, which selectively stimulates a retinoid subtype receptor, is being developed in an oral capsule formulation for the treatment of lung cancer, breast cancer, head and neck cancer, cutaneous T-cell lymphoma (CTCL), and psoriasis and psoriatic disorders. The drug is in phase II trials for head and neck cancer, phase II/III trials for breast cancer, CTCL and psoriasis and psoriatic disorders, and phase III trials for non-small cell lung cancer.

INDICATION(S) AND RESEARCH PHASE
Psoriasis and Psoriatic Disorders – Phase II/III
Lung Cancer – Phase III
Breast Cancer – Phase II/III
Head and Neck Cancer – Phase II

biricodar dicitrate, VX-710
Incel

MANUFACTURER
Vertex Pharmaceuticals

DESCRIPTION
Incel is a novel intravenous compound designed to treat multidrug resistance of malignant cells, which occurs with cancer chemotherapy regimens. Incel may potentially resensitize drug-resistant tumors to chemotherapy by inhibiting molecular pumps that expel chemotherapy drugs. Vertex is developing compounds that block two major drug pumps or multidrug resistance mechanisms: P-glycoprotein (MDR-1) and multidrug resistance-associated protein (MRP).

Phase II trials investigating the activity of Incel in combination with other agents for the treatment of advanced refractory ovarian cancer and small cell lung cancer are currently under way.

INDICATION(S) AND RESEARCH PHASE
Lung Cancer – Phase II
Ovarian Cancer – Phase II

blood substitute
Hemolink

MANUFACTURER
Hemosol

DESCRIPTION
Hemolink is a type of artificial blood or blood substitute. It is a human hemoglobin-based oxygen carrier for use in coronary artery bypass grafting (CABG) surgery.

As of December 2000, Hemosol has completed eight clinical trials of Hemolink, three in cardiovascular surgery (including a pivotal Phase III Canada/United Kingdom study in CABG), three in orthopedic surgery, one in anemia, and one in normal volunteers. A Phase III CABG trial is currently under way in the United States.

Additionally, a phase I/II trial was initiated in December 2000 in 18 subjects with non-small cell lung cancer who are experiencing chemotherapy associated anemia. The trial is expected to be complete by the fourth quarter of 2001.

INDICATION(S) AND RESEARCH PHASE
Cardiac Surgery – Phase III
Lung Cancer – Phase I/II

BLP-25
unknown

MANUFACTURER
Biomira

DESCRIPTION
BLP25 is a vaccine designed to induce an immune response to cancer cells. This vaccine incorporates a 25-amino acid sequence of the MUC-1 cancer mucin, encapsulated in a liposomal delivery system that enhances recognition by the immune system and provides better delivery to the tumor.

The company has initiated a phase IIb trial for advanced non-small cell lung cancer at the Cross Cancer Institute in Edmonton, Alberta, which involves seven to ten subjects. The purpose of this trial is to determine whether a higher dose and more frequent administration of the vaccine will enhance its effect. A randomized and comparative phase IIb trial is currently under way.

The company reported that the results of the phase I trial showed the product was well tolerated and excited a cytotoxic T-lymphocyte (CTL) immune response against cancer cells. Additionally, BLP25 has shown an early subjective indication of improved quality of life compared to that seen in chemotherapy subjects in previous trials for non-small cell lung cancer.

INDICATION(S) AND RESEARCH PHASE
Lung Cancer – Phase IIb
Vaccines – Phase IIb

BMS-182751, JM-216
unknown

MANUFACTURER
Bristol-Myers Squibb

DESCRIPTION
In order for cancer cells to replicate, the double-stranded DNA has to separate or "unzip." Platinum (BMS-182751) appears to cause permanent links to form so that the DNA cannot unzip and the cell cannot reproduce. Intrastrand links permanently seal the two edges of the DNA zipper, while interstrand links seal two different parts of the zipper together, as in a loop. Recent evidence indicates that platinum causes more interstrand than intrastrand DNA links to form.

Additionally, the cell's built-in DNA-repair mechanism has trouble fixing the platinum links. Platinum may bind directly to the proteins that are involved in the repair mechanism, essentially making them inactive. This binding results in more damage to the cancer cell and more efficient tumor death. BMS-182751 is being tested in phase III trials for the treatment of lung and ovarian cancer.
Lung Cancer – Phase III
Ovarian Cancer – Phase III

CI-1033
unknown

MANUFACTURER
Pfizer

DESCRIPTION
CI-1033 is being investigated in clinical studies involving erbB positive cancers located in the breast, lung, and head and neck. The objective of the CI-1033 program is to achieve control of cancer via EGFR tyrosine kinase inhibition, without the side effect burden of cytotoxic agents.

INDICATION(S) AND RESEARCH PHASE
Breast Cancer – Phase I
Lung Cancer – Phase I
Head and Neck Cancer – Phase I

CI-1042, ONYX-015
unknown

MANUFACTURER
Onyx Pharmaceuticals

DESCRIPTION
CI-1042 (ONYX-015) is a tumor-selective, modified adenovirus (similar to the common cold virus) that has been genetically engineered to replicate in and kill cancer cells that possess a mutated oncogene called p53, while sparing normal cells with functioning p53. p53 Is a tumor suppressor gene that is mutated in approximately 50% of all human cancers. CI-1042 is in development for several indications, including pancreatic cancer, liver metastases of colorectal cancer, and lung cancer.

In November 2000, results of a phase II trial demonstrated that CI-1042 administered as a single-agent replicates and causes tumor regression in refractory head and neck cancer. CI-1042 was shown to selectively target cancer cells containing a mutant p53 gene, while sparing normal cells with a functioning p53 gene. Of the 19 subjects who received the standard dosing regimen, four (21%) had an objective response, including two complete responses and two partial responses. CI-1042 is being co-developed with Pfizer.

INDICATION(S) AND RESEARCH PHASE
Colorectal Cancer – Phase II
Pancreatic Cancer – Phase II
Head and Neck Cancer – Phase III
Cervical Dysplasia/Cancer – Phase I completed
Lung Cancer – Phase II
Bladder Cancer – Phase I completed
Brain Cancer – Phase I completed

cisplatin/vinblastine/amifostine
unknown

MANUFACTURER
MedImmune

DESCRIPTION
Cisplatin and vinblastine are chemotherapeutic agents that interfere with tumor cell growth. The heavy metal platinum, a component of cisplatin, binds to certain plasma proteins and is highly cytotoxic. Vinblastine interferes with the process of cell division. MedImmune has conducted a phase III trial in subjects with Stage IIIb or IVb non-small cell lung cancer, in which 50% of the subjects were given a cisplatin/vinblastine combination, and the other 50% were given the combination plus Ethyol (amifostine), which reduces the toxic effects of platinum more strongly in normal cells than in tumor cells.

INDICATION(S) AND RESEARCH PHASE
Lung Cancer – Phase III completed

CP-358,774
unknown

MANUFACTURER
OSI Pharmaceuticals

DESCRIPTION
CP-358,774 is a small molecule inhibitor of the epidermal growth factor receptor (EGFR) tyrosine kinase. This drug targets the underlying molecular changes involving oncogenes and tumor suppressor genes, which play critical roles in the conversion of normal cells into cancerous cells. Increased expression of EGFR is an aberration frequently associated with a variety of cancers including ovarian, pancreatic, and non-

small cell lung cancers. The phase II clinical program is designed to assess CP-358,774 both as a single agent and in combination with existing chemotherapy regimens.

INDICATION(S) AND RESEARCH PHASE
Breast Cancer – Phase II
Lung Cancer – Phase II completed
Ovarian Cancer – Phase II
Head and Neck Cancer – Phase II

decitabine
unknown

MANUFACTURER
SuperGen

DESCRIPTION
Decitabine is an investigational chemotherapeutic agent in development for the treatment of sickle cell anemia and a variety of solid tumors and hematological malignancies, including myelodysplastic syndrome, non-small cell lung cancer, and chronic myelogenous leukemia. Decitabine inhibits DNA methyltransferase activity, and in this manner presumably reactivates tumor suppressor genes.

In October 2000, results of a phase I/II trial of decitabine for sickle cell anemia demonstrated that it produced a response in 100% of subjects tested. The trial enrolled a total of eight subjects: five of whom had shown no response to hydroxyurea (HU) after one year of treatment; two of whom had a moderate but unsustained response to HU; and one subject who was not treated with HU. After administration of decitabine, the five subjects previously treated with HU experienced an average 35-fold increase of fetal hemoglobin levels compared to levels during HU treatment. The two subjects who responded briefly to HU experienced an average fetal hemoglobin level increase of 52% with decitabine, and the one subject who had not received HU treatment experienced more than a 50% increase in fetal hemoglobin levels.

INDICATION(S) AND RESEARCH PHASE
Myelodysplastic Syndrome – Phase III
Lung Cancer – Phase II
Anemia – Phase I/II completed
Leukemia – Phase II

diarysulfonylurea, ILX-295501
unknown

MANUFACTURER
ILEX Oncology

DESCRIPTION
ILX-295501 belongs to a novel class of antitumor compounds called diarysulfonylureas. This orally formulated drug is in phase II trials for renal cell carcinoma, malignant melanoma, lung, and ovarian cancers.

INDICATION(S) AND RESEARCH PHASE
Renal Cell Carcinoma – Phase II
Malignant Melanoma – Phase II
Lung Cancer – Phase II
Ovarian Cancer – Phase II

diethylnorspermine
DENSPM

MANUFACTURER
GelTex Pharmaceuticals

DESCRIPTION
DENSPM (diethylnorspermine) is similar to a naturally produced polyamine, except that it may interrupt the rapid growth of tumor cells that need polyamines for growth. The drug is in phase II trials for renal cell carcinoma, pancreatic cancer, malignant melanoma, and non-small cell lung cancer. Additional indications may include ovarian and colon cancers.

INDICATION(S) AND RESEARCH PHASE
Renal Cell Carcinoma – Phase II
Pancreatic Cancer – Phase II
Malignant Melanoma – Phase II
Lung Cancer – Phase II

docetaxel hydrate
Taxotere

MANUFACTURER
Aventis

DESCRIPTION
Many drugs for the treatment of cancer and other diseases originate in plants, many of them highly poisonous. Taxotere (docetaxel hydrate), an agent that inhibits the formation of new protoplasm, is derived from the renewable evergreen needles of the genus *Taxus* (Yew). Taxotere acts by disrupting the microtubular network in cells that is essential for cell division and many other cellular functions. The drug is approved for use in the United States for treatment of refractory breast cancer, refractory non-small cell lung cancer (NSCLC), and locally advanced or metastatic breast cancer.

New phase II/III trials are under way in head and neck, gastric, and ovarian cancers. Taxotere is also being tested either alone or in combination with other chemotherapy agents in the earlier stages of breast cancer, NSCLC, and other tumors.

Phase I extension studies are under way for brain metastasis and lung cancer.

INDICATION(S) AND RESEARCH PHASE
Gastric Cancer – Phase II/III
Head and Neck Cancer – Phase II/III
Lung Cancer – Phase II/III
Ovarian Cancer – Phase II/III
Breast Cancer – Phase III/IV
Brain Cancer – Phase I
Lung Cancer – Phase I

doxorubicin HCl
Doxil, Caelyx

MANUFACTURER
Alza (Sequus Pharmaceuticals)

DESCRIPTION
Doxil is a liposomal formulation of doxorubicin hydrochloride, an intravenous chemotherapy agent. This anthracycline anti-tumor agent is currently on the market for the treatment of Kaposi's sarcoma. The drug uses a novel, targeted delivery system to help evade recognition and uptake by the immune system so that the liposomes can circulate in the body longer. A long circulation time increases the likelihood that the liposomes and their pharmaceutical contents will reach their targeted tumor site. Doxil may act through its ability to bind

DNA and inhibit nucleic acid synthesis.

Doxil is being tested in trials for the treatment of breast, liver, lung, and prostate cancers, as well as for unspecified cancers and tumors.

Alza markets this product in the United States under the tradename Doxil; however, it is marketed under the name Caelyx in other areas. Schering-Plough has exclusive international marketing rights to Caelyx, excluding Japan and Israel, through a distribution agreement with Alza.

INDICATION(S) AND RESEARCH PHASE
Breast Cancer – Phase II/III
Liver Cancer – Phase II/III
Lung Cancer – Phase II/III
Prostate Cancer – Phase II/III
Cancer/Tumors (Unspecified) – Phase II

exisulind
Aptosyn

MANUFACTURER
Cell Pathways

DESCRIPTION
Aptosyn (exisulind) belongs to a novel class of compounds called selective apoptotic anti-neoplastic drugs (SAANDs). SAANDs inhibit a form of cyclic GMP phosphodiesterase and selectively induce apoptosis in abnormally growing precancerous and cancerous cells. Aptosyn is being tested for several indications and is in five different trials for adenomatous polyposis coli (APC) and familial adenomatous polyposis coli; two of these trials are specifically for pediatric subjects.

The company received a non-approval letter from the FDA in September 2000 for one of the trials for familial adenomatous polyposis. The company intends to amend the NDA and request a meeting to address the deficiencies and the possible requirement for additional clinical data.

Additionally, Aptosyn is being tested in trials for the treatment of prostate cancer, lung cancer, breast cancer, sporadic colonic polyps, and Barrett's esophagus disease.

INDICATION(S) AND RESEARCH PHASE
Adenomatous Polyposis Coli – Non-approvable letter
Pediatric, Familial Adenomatous Polyposis coli – Phase II
Adenomatous Polyposis Coli – Phase I/II
Barrett's Esophagus Disease – Phase II
Prostate Cancer – Phase II/III
Breast Cancer – Phase II/III
Lung Cancer – Phase Ib
Colon Polyps – Phase II/III

exisulind/docetaxel
Aposyn/Taxotere

MANUFACTURER
Cell Pathways

DESCRIPTION
Aptosyn is a sulfone derivative of sulindac, a non-sterodial anti-inflammatory compound being tested with Rhone-Poulenc Rorer's Taxotere for the treatment of prostate, lung, and breast cancer as well as for solid tumors. Aptosyn (exisulind) is the first product candidate from a novel class of compounds under development by Cell Pathways, called selective apoptotic anti-neoplastic drugs (SAANDs). SAANDs inhibit cyclic GMP phosphodiesterase and selectively induce apoptosis in abnormally growing precancerous and cancerous cells. Because SAANDs do not induce apoptosis in normal cells, they do not produce the serious side effects normally associated with traditional chemotherapeutic agents. They also do not inhibit cyclooxygenase (COX I or COX II) and have not exhibited the gastric and renal toxicities reported to be associated with non-steroidal anti-inflammatory drugs (NSAIDs), including the COX II inhibitors.

Both companies will jointly share the cost of the trials and will retain all marketing rights to its respective products.

INDICATION(S) AND RESEARCH PHASE
Prostate Cancer – Phase I/II
Breast Cancer – Phase I/II
Lung Cancer – Phase I/II
Lung Cancer – Phase III
Cancer/Tumors (Unspecified) – Phase I

exisulind/gemcitabine HCl
Aptosyn/Gemzar

MANUFACTURER
Cell Pathways

DESCRIPTION
Aptosyn (exisulind) belongs to a novel class of compounds called selective apoptotic anti-neoplastic drugs (SAANDs). SAANDs inhibit a form of cyclic GMP phosphodiesterase and selectively induce apoptosis in abnormally growing precancerous and cancerous cells.

Aptosyn is being tested with Eli Lilly's Gemzar to evaluate time-to-progression in subjects with non-small cell lung cancer who have progressed through first-line therapy (refractory) or who have developed progressive disease more than three months from completion of first-line therapy (recurrent). The response rate, overall survival, and toxicity profile will also be determined in this phase II trial. Gemzar is currently approved for the treatment of pancreatic cancer and non-small cell lung cancer (the latter in combination with cisplatin).

INDICATION(S) AND RESEARCH PHASE
Lung Cancer – Phase II

exisulind/vinorelbine tartrate injection
Aptosyn/Navelbine

MANUFACTURER
Cell Pathways

DESCRIPTION
Aptosyn/Navelbine is in a phase I/II trial for the first line treatment of elderly subjects with non-small cell lung cancer at the University of Wisconsin. Both Aptosyn from Cell Pathways and Navelbine from GlaxoSmithKline are approved drugs for lung cancer, and their combined use may demonstrate additive anticancer effects over either drug alone. The two companies will share the costs of the clinical trials.

INDICATION(S) AND RESEARCH PHASE
Lung Cancer – Phase I/II

flavopiridol, HMR-1275
unknown

MANUFACTURER
Aventis

DESCRIPTION
Flavopiridol belongs to a new class of drugs for cancer therapy known as cyclin-dependent kinase (CDK) inhibitors. It is being tested in phase II trials as a treatment for chronic lymphatic leukemia, esophageal cancer, and non-small cell lung cancer.

INDICATION(S) AND RESEARCH PHASE
Esophageal Cancer – Phase II
Leukemia – Phase II
Lung Cancer – Phase II

FMdC
unknown

MANUFACTURER
Matrix Pharmaceutical

DESCRIPTION
FMdC is a nucleoside analogue being tested for the treatment of cancer. Nucleoside analogues are a class of drugs that affect DNA synthesis, and they have long been used to treat hematologic cancers such as leukemia. The early members of this drug class were minimally effective against solid tumors.

DNA synthesis occurs during cell division and is critical to successful cell replication. FMdC enters cells and is metabolized into two active forms: FMdC diphosphate and FMdC triphosphate. These two active metabolites of FMdC interrupt the process of DNA synthesis, which leads to cell death. FMdC is being evaluated in phase II studies for the treatment of non-small cell lung cancer, colorectal, and ovarian cancer.

INDICATION(S) AND RESEARCH PHASE
Colorectal Cancer – Phase II
Lung Cancer – Phase II
Ovarian Cancer – Phase II

gemcitabine HCl
Gemzar

MANUFACTURER
Eli Lilly

DESCRIPTION
Gemzar, a nucleoside analogue, is a novel chemotherapeutic agent that mimics a natural building block of DNA. Gemzar disrupts the process of cell replication and thereby slows or stops progression of the disease. The drug is administered intravenously.

Gemzar is currently indicated as first-line treatment of locally advanced or metastatic pancreatic cancer and, in combination with cisplatin, for locally advanced or metastatic non-small cell lung cancer.

INDICATION(S) AND RESEARCH PHASE
Breast Cancer – Phase III
Lung Cancer – FDA approved
Ovarian Cancer – Phase III
Pancreatic Cancer – FDA approved

GL-331
unknown

MANUFACTURER
Genelabs Technologies

DESCRIPTION
GL-331 is an inhibitor of topoisomerase II. It is a semi-synthetic derivative of podophyllotoxin, which is a chemotherapeutic agent designed to overcome multi-drug resistant (MDR) cancers. At this time, development has been discontinued.

INDICATION(S) AND RESEARCH PHASE
Colon Malignancies – Trial discontinued
Leukemia – Trial discontinued
Lung Cancer – Trial discontinued
Renal Cell Carcinoma – Trial discontinued

HuC242-DM1/SB-408075
unknown

MANUFACTURER
ImmunoGen

DESCRIPTION
HuC242-DM1/SB-408075 is a tumor-activated prodrug (TAP) designed for the treatment of colorectal, pancreatic, and certain non-small cell lung cancers. Tumor-activated prodrugs consist of chemically linked monoclonal antibodies and potent, cell-killing chemicals. HuC242-DM1, in particular, is created by joining the cytotoxic maytansinoid drug DM1 with the humanized monoclonal antibody C242. The attached chemical remains inactive until the monoclonal antibody reaches its targeted tumor cell and the TAP is drawn inside. Once inside, DM1 is able to kill the tumor cell without affecting surrounding healthy cells. HuC242-DM1 is currently in phase I/II trials.

INDICATION(S) AND RESEARCH PHASE
Colorectal Cancer – Phase I/II
Pancreatic Cancer – Phase I/II
Lung Cancer – Phase I/II

HuN901-DM1
unknown

MANUFACTURER
ImmunoGen

DESCRIPTION
HuN901-DM1 is a tumor-activated prodrug (TAP) consisting of a humanized monoclonal antibody (huN901) targeting small cell lung cancer, coupled with a highly potent cytotoxic agent (DM1). Preclinical results demonstrated that HuN901-DM1 was successful in eradicating small cell lung cancer tumors.

British Biotech has exclusive rights to commercialize HuN901-DM1 in the European Union and Japan, whereas ImmunoGen has the rights in the United States and the rest of the world.

INDICATION(S) AND RESEARCH PHASE
Lung Cancer – Phase I

IMC-C225, CPT-11
unknown

MANUFACTURER
ImClone Systems

DESCRIPTION
IMC-C225 is a chimerized (part mouse,

part human) monoclonal antibody that may help fight cancer cells when used in conjunction with radiation therapy or other chemotherapy agents. This antibody selectively blocks the epidermal growth factor receptor (EGFr), which may be present in greater amounts on actively growing tumor cells. Since many cancers use specific growth factors to stimulate tumor cell growth, blocking this receptor may inhibit the cancer from increasing in size and spreading throughout the body.

The company is conducting phase III clinical trials evaluating IMC-C225 in combination with radiotherapy and with chemotherapy in subjects with advanced squamous cell head and neck carcinoma. IMC-C225 is in trials for several other indications in combination with various anti-cancer agents.

INDICATION(S) AND RESEARCH PHASE
Breast Cancer – Phase I/II
Head and Neck Cancer – Phase III
Lung Cancer – Phase III
Prostate Cancer – Phase I/II
Renal Cell Carcinoma – Phase II
Pancreatic Cancer – Phase II
Colorectal Cancer – Phase II

IMMU-MN14, anti-CEA
CEA-Cide

MANUFACTURER
Immunomedics

DESCRIPTION
Carcinoembryonic antigen (CEA) is a protein-polysaccharide complex released in the bloodstream by certain cancers, especially colon carcinoma. This antigenic substance may provide early diagnosis when used as a therapeutic marker in immunologic tests. The CEA complex may also be targeted by specialized monoclonal antibodies in the design of a biologic therapeutic.

CEA-Cide is a novel monoclonal antibody that is designed for radioimmunotherapy (with 90 Y-labeled humanized MN-14). This drug is being tested in phase II trials for the treatment of advanced metastatic and CEA-producing cancers, particularly colorectal cancer. Other indications may include breast cancer, female reproductive system cancer, ovarian cancer, lung cancer, and pancreatic cancer.

INDICATION(S) AND RESEARCH PHASE
Breast Cancer – Phase II
Cancer/Tumors (Unspecified) – Phase II
Colorectal Cancer – Phase II
Lung Cancer – Phase II
Ovarian Cancer – Phase II
Pancreatic Cancer – Phase II

INGN 241 (mda-7)
unknown

MANUFACTURER
Introgen Therapeutics

DESCRIPTION
INGN 241 is the combination of Introgen's proprietary adenoviral delivery system with the mda-7 gene. INGN 241 is in a phase I trial in 15 subjects for the treatment of solid tumors. Preclinical results demonstrated that expression of mda-7 appears to be lost earlier in tumor progression, and that mda-7 may be easily combined with other tumor suppressor genes for additive effects. INGN 241 is also in preclinical development for lung and breast cancer.

INDICATION(S) AND RESEARCH PHASE
Breast Cancer – Preclinical
Lung Cancer – Preclinical
Cancer/Tumors (Unspecified) – Phase I

INGN-201, adenoviral p53
unknown

MANUFACTURER
Introgen Therapeutics

DESCRIPTION
INGN-201 is a p53 gene therapy product. It has been tested as a treatment for a variety of solid tumor cancers with administration via intratumoral injection. The drug was well tolerated according to the company, and additional trials are under way using an intravenous infusion in order to reach more types of cancers. The tumor-suppressing p53 gene encodes a protein that responds to damage involving cellular DNA by terminating cell division. Normal p53 genes are delivered into cancer cells of the subject through an adenoviral vector.

The developers of INGN-201 have signed a Cooperative Research and Development Agreement (CRADA) with the National Cancer Institute to evaluate the potential effectiveness and superiority of the drug over other treatments against breast, ovarian, bladder, prostate, and brain cancers in phase I and phase II trials. A phase III trial in head and neck cancer was initiated in March 2000.

INDICATION(S) AND RESEARCH PHASE
Head and Neck Cancer – Phase III
Bladder Cancer – Phase I
Brain Cancer – Phase I
Breast Cancer – Phase I
Bronchoalveolar Cancer – Phase I
Ovarian Cancer – Phase I
Prostate Cancer – Phase I
Lung Cancer – Phase II
Cancer/Tumors (Unspecified) – Phase I

INS316
unknown

MANUFACTURER
Inspire Pharmaceuticals

DESCRIPTION
INS316 is a sterile proprietary formulation of uridine 5'-triphosphate (UTP). It is an acute-use agent being developed to enhance the production of deep-lung sputum specimens suitable for any diagnostic testing purposes, for example, lung cancer or respiratory infection. INS316 applied by a nebulized formulation acts to stimulate P2Y2 receptors on the airway surface to enhance the natural mucociliary process.

INDICATION(S) AND RESEARCH PHASE
Lung Cancer – Phase III

ISIS 2503
unknown

MANUFACTURER
Isis Pharmaceuticals

DESCRIPTION

ISIS 2503 is a potent, selective antisense inhibitor of H-ras gene expression. Antisense drugs inhibit the production of disease-causing proteins by altering the genetic information that messenger RNA uses to produce new protein. H-ras is one of a family of ras genes that are involved in the process by which cells receive and send signals that affect their behavior. The company claims that substantial evidence exists to support a direct role for the ras gene products in the development and maintenance of human cancers.

In phase II trials, the compound is being evaluated as a single agent in subjects with colon, breast, pancreatic, and non-small cell lung cancers. These trials will provide preliminary data on the anti-tumor activity of ISIS 2503 against these common tumor types. Approximately ten sites in the United States and Europe will enroll 15-30 subjects per tumor type in these trials. The company plans future trials of ISIS 2503 in combination with approved cancer therapies.

INDICATION(S) AND RESEARCH PHASE
Breast Cancer – Phase II
Colon Malignancies – Phase II
Lung Cancer – Phase II
Pancreatic Cancer – Phase II

ISIS 3521
unknown

MANUFACTURER
Isis Pharmaceuticals

DESCRIPTION

ISIS 3521 is an antisense inhibitor of protein kinase C-alpha (PKC-α) expression. PKC-α is a member of a multigene family of signal transduction proteins that regulate information flow in and out of cells and modulate cellular responses to the environment. It is being tested in trials for the treatment of breast and lung cancer.

Results of a phase I/II trial indicated that ISIS 3521 in combination with standard chemotherapy agents has promising activity in subjects with stage IIIB or stage IV non-small cell lung cancer, based on both survival time and response rate. Two subjects have experienced complete responses and 18 subjects have experienced a partial response. Additionally, four of 48 (8%) subjects experienced a minor response, defined as a 25-50% reduction in tumor size measurements, and 16 (9%) subjects had a stabilization of their disease. Isis Pharmaceuticals initiated a phase III trial in October 2000.

INDICATION(S) AND RESEARCH PHASE
Breast Cancer – Phase II
Lung Cancer – Phase III

ISIS 5132, CGP 69846A
unknown

MANUFACTURER
Isis Pharmaceuticals

DESCRIPTION

ISIS 5132 is a potent antisense inhibitor of the enzyme c-Raf-1 kinase. Antisense drugs inhibit the production of disease-causing proteins by altering the genetic information that messenger RNA uses to produce new protein. c-Raf kinase plays a role in signal processes that regulate cell growth and proliferation. It is one of a family of raf genes thought to play an important role in the development of some solid tumors. The company reports that activated-raf has also been detected in a substantial variety of human cancers including small cell lung carcinoma and breast cancer. For example, it has been reported that 60% of all lung carcinoma cells express unusually high levels of normal c-Raf mRNA and protein.

The sponsor companies reported that results from phase I studies, which examined subjects with a wide variety of solid tumors, demonstrated that the drug was well tolerated and that several subjects experienced disease stabilization. The companies are planning additional phase I safety studies involving the drug in combination with currently approved chemotherapies. Phase II clinical trials examining ISIS 5132 as a single agent therapy in subjects with breast, lung, colon, pancreatic, and prostate cancers are under way.

INDICATION(S) AND RESEARCH PHASE
Breast Cancer – Phase II
Cancer/Tumors (Unspecified) – Phase II
Colon Malignancies – Phase II
Lung Cancer – Phase II
Pancreatic Cancer – Phase II
Prostate Cancer – Phase II

liposomal ether lipid
TLC ELL-12

MANUFACTURER
The Liposome Company

DESCRIPTION

TLC ELL-12 is a liposomal ether lipid that may have efficacy in the treatment of several cancers. This drug has exhibited significant anti-tumor activity, but did not have the hemolytic side effects common to this type of ether lipid when therapeutic doses were used in experimental models. It does not appear to be myelosuppressive.

TLC ELL-12 is currently being developed in phase I trials for the treatment of lung cancer, multiple myeloma, leukemia, and prostate cancer.

INDICATION(S) AND RESEARCH PHASE
Lung Cancer – Phase I
Multiple Myeloma – Phase I
Leukemia – Phase I
Prostate Cancer – Phase I

marimastat, BB-2516
unknown

MANUFACTURER
British Biotech plc

DESCRIPTION

Marimastat is an inhibitor of matrix metalloproteinase (MMP), a family of naturally occurring enzymes that are over-produced in a number of disease states. This is especially true of cancer, where MMPs are involved in the spread and local growth of tumors. Both angiogenesis and metastasis require MMPs during tumor invasion. Anti-angiogenic strategies, unlike other therapeutic approaches, do not aim to directly destroy or "kill" the tumor or cause tumor regression. Rather, they are designed to prevent the further growth of tumors by limiting their blood supply. Because peripheral tumor cells could theoretically survive on a diffusion-dependent basis, anti-angiogenic drugs may prove most effective when given in combination with other standard cytotoxic regimens. As of October 2000, marimastat is in phase III development for the treatment of cancer.

In 1999, British Biotech and Schering-Plough Corporation signed an agreement to develop and commercialize British Biotech's metalloproteinase inhibitors, including marimastat.

INDICATION(S) AND RESEARCH PHASE
Pancreatic Cancer – Phase III
Lung Cancer – Phase III
Breast Cancer – Phase III
Brain Cancer – Phase III completed
Ovarian Cancer – Phase III

unknown
Prinomastat

MANUFACTURER
Agouron Pharmaceuticals

DESCRIPTION
Prinomastat is an orally active, synthetic molecule designed to potently and selectively inhibit certain members of a family of enzymes known as a matrix metalloproteases, which are believed to be involved in tumor angiogenesis, invasion, and metastasis. The drug is in trials for various indications, including osteoarthritis, brain cancer, and macular degeneration.

Two phase III trials for advanced non-small cell lung cancer and prostate cancer were halted in August 2000 due to the drug's lack of effectiveness in subjects with late-stage disease.

The most common side effects of Prinomastat have been observed in the joints, and include stiffness, joint swelling, and in a few subjects, some limits on the mobility of certain joints, most often in the shoulders and hands. All these effects were reported to be reversible and were effectively managed by treatment rests and dose reductions.

INDICATION(S) AND RESEARCH PHASE
Lung Cancer – Phase halted
Prostate Cancer – Phase halted
Osteoarthritis – Phase II
Brain Cancer – Phase II
Macular Degeneration – Phase II

MDX-210
unknown

MANUFACTURER
Medarex

DESCRIPTION
MDX-210 is a bispecific (target-trigger) monoclonal antibody (MAb)-based treatment being developed for cancers with specific markers (HER-2/*neu* positive), including renal cell, non-small cell lung, pancreatic, and prostate cancer. Phase II trials have been completed for kidney, prostate, and ovarian cancer. Phase III trials for ovarian cancer have commenced in Europe.

INDICATION(S) AND RESEARCH PHASE
Prostate Cancer – Phase II completed
Renal Cell Carcinoma – Phase II completed
Colon Malignancies – Phase II
Breast Cancer – Phase II
Gastric Cancer – Phase II
Pancreatic Cancer – Phase II
Lung Cancer – Phase II
Ovarian Cancer – Phase III

MDX-220
unknown

MANUFACTURER
Medarex

DESCRIPTION
MDX-220 is a bispecific (target-trigger) monoclonal antibody (MAb) that targets Tag-72 in the treatment of a variety of cancers, including lung, colon, prostate, ovarian, endometrial, pancreatic, and gastric.

INDICATION(S) AND RESEARCH PHASE
Endometrial Cancer – Phase I/II
Gastric Cancer – Phase I/II
Lung Cancer – Phase I/II
Ovarian Cancer – Phase I/II
Pancreatic Cancer – Phase I/II
Prostate Cancer – Phase II
Colorectal Cancer – Phase II

MDX-447, H-447
unknown

MANUFACTURER
Medarex

DESCRIPTION
MDX-447 is a novel biological drug designed to stimulate an immune response against cancer cells. Certain cancer cells contain and express large amounts of unique proteins (such as epidermal growth factor receptors), which MDX-447 is directed to recognize. MDX-447 attaches itself both to these cancer proteins and to macrophages that specialize in killing foreign material.

The binding together of the cancer cells and the immune cells by MDX-447 signals the body to destroy the tumor. MDX-447 may offer a new therapeutic alternative to cancer subjects who have been unresponsive to conventional therapies. This agent is unique since it has two receptors on its surface, one that can attract the cancer cell and one that can attract a killer immune cell. This dual nature of the drug is why it is known as a "bispecific antibody."

This type of drug is designed to be more efficient than current anti-cancer therapies, and may have effects that last longer. This technology may also be useful in the development of an "anti-cancer vaccine" in the future. MDX-447 is currently being tested as an intravenous solution in phase II trials for multiple tumor indications, which include brain, bladder, breast, head and neck, and lung cancer.

INDICATION(S) AND RESEARCH PHASE
Brain Cancer – Phase II
Bladder Cancer – Phase II
Breast Cancer – Phase II
Head and Neck Cancer – Phase II
Lung Cancer – Phase II

MGI-114, hydroxymethylacylfulvene,

HMAF
Irofulven

MANUFACTURER
MGI Pharma

DESCRIPTION
Irofulven (MGI-114) is the first product candidate being developed by MGI Pharma from its family of anti-cancer compounds called acylfulvenes. Early trials demonstrated that Irofulven is absorbed rapidly by tumor cells, and once inside binds to DNA and protein targets. The binding interferes with DNA replication and cell division, leading to tumor-specific cell death. The drug is being tested in a series of trials for a variety of cancers.

Results from a phase II trial of Irofulven indicated that the drug produced anti-tumor activity in subjects with advanced pancreatic cancer who were refractory to gemcitabine (Gemzar). Ten of the 53 subjects enrolled achieved six-month survival and two subjects demonstrated objective responses: one subject experienced tumor shrinkage of 100% and another subject experienced an 84% decrease in tumor mass. A phase III trial was initiated in February 2001.

INDICATION(S) AND RESEARCH PHASE
Breast Cancer – Phase II
Colon Malignancies – Phase II
Renal Cell Carcinoma – Phase II
Cervical Dysplasia/Cancer – Phase II
Lung Cancer – Phase II
Ovarian Cancer – Phase I/II
Colorectal Cancer – Phase II
Prostate Cancer – Phase I/II
Cancer/Tumors (Unspecified) – Phase I/II
Pancreatic Cancer – Phase III
Liver Cancer – Phase II

NX 211
unknown

MANUFACTURER
Gilead Sciences

DESCRIPTION
NX 211 is a liposomal formulation of a novel topoisomerase I inhibitor for the treatment of various solid tumors. A phase II trial has been initiated at five sites in the United States. It includes 58 subjects with ovarian cancer who have progressed or relapsed within six months of treatment with a regimen including topotecan. The trial will evaluate the efficacy and safety of NX 211 as determined by response rate, time to disease progression, and subject tolerance. Subjects will be treated with NX 211 on days one and eight, to be repeated every 21 days.

Additionally, a phase II trial was also initiated to test NX 211 in 87 subjects with recurrent small cell lung cancer at numerous sites in the United States.

INDICATION(S) AND RESEARCH PHASE
Ovarian Cancer – Phase II
Lung Cancer – Phase II

OSI-774
unknown

MANUFACTURER
OSI Pharmaceuticals

DESCRIPTION
OSI-774 is a potent, selective and orally active inhibitor of the epidermal growth factor receptor (EGFR) tyrosine kinase. EGFR is an oncogene that is produced during the aberrant growth of certain cancer cells.

OSI Pharmaceuticals has announced updated findings from two ongoing phase II trials of OSI-774 as a single agent. In a trial consisting of 56 subjects with advanced, refractory non-small cell lung cancer, OSI-774 was given orally on a once-a-day dosing schedule. Results showed that 48% of the subjects had either a partial response or stable disease at 12 weeks and continued on the drug. Intermediate data were presented from the second trial, which consisted of 113 subjects with advanced squamous cell carcinoma of the head and neck. Results for the first 78 evaluable subjects showed that 42% had either a partial response or demonstrated evidence of disease stabilization at 12 weeks.

INDICATION(S) AND RESEARCH PHASE
Lung Cancer – Phase II
Head and Neck Cancer – Phase II

paclitaxel/carboplatin/amifostine
unknown

MANUFACTURER
MedImmune

DESCRIPTION
Taxol (paclitaxel) and carboplatin are both chemotherapeutic agents that interfere with tumor cell growth. Paclitaxel, which is derived from the Yew plant *Taxus baccata*, interferes with the process of cell division. The heavy metal platinum, a component of carboplatin, binds to certain plasma proteins and is highly cytotoxic.

The company has conducted a phase III trial consisting of 300 subjects diagnosed with Stage IIIb or IVb non-small cell lung cancer. Half of the subjects received a paclitaxel/carboplatin combination, and the other half received the combination plus Ethyol (amifostine). Ethyol is noted to reduce the toxic effects of platinum more strongly in normal cells than in tumor cells.

INDICATION(S) AND RESEARCH PHASE
Lung Cancer – Phase III completed

pivaloyloxymethylbutyrate
Pivanex

MANUFACTURER
Titan Pharmaceuticals

DESCRIPTION
Pivanex, an analog of butyric acid, is a small molecule drug that attacks cancer cells through the mechanism of cellular differentiation. It is being tested for the treatment of advanced stages of non-small cell lung cancer that have not responded well to other drug therapy. Results of a phase I/II trial testing Pivanex for the treatment of liver metastases are pending.

INDICATION(S) AND RESEARCH PHASE
Lung Cancer – Phase II
Liver Cancer – Phase I/II

recombinant human interferon beta-1a
Rebif

MANUFACTURER
Serono Laboratories

DESCRIPTION
Rebif is an interferon beta-1a product being developed for a variety of indications. These include non-small cell lung cancer, chronic hepatitis C, Crohn's disease, ulcerative colitis, Guillain-Barré syndrome, and rheumatoid arthritis. Rebif has been approved in several countries for the treatment of relapsing-remitting multiple sclerosis. It is currently being evaluated as an early treatment of multiple sclerosis and as a treatment for secondary-progressive multiple sclerosis.

INDICATION(S) AND RESEARCH PHASE
Multiple Sclerosis – Phase III
Lung Cancer – Phase II
Hepatitis – Phase II
Crohn's Disease – Phase II
Inflammatory Bowel Disease – Phase II
Guillain-Barré syndrome – Phase II
Rheumatoid Arthritis – Phase II

RSR13
unknown

MANUFACTURER
Allos Therapeutics

DESCRIPTION
RSR13 is a synthetic small molecule that increases the release of oxygen from hemoglobin, the oxygen carrying protein contained within red blood cells. The presence of oxygen in tumors is an essential part of the effectiveness of radiation therapy in cancer treatment. By increasing tumor oxygenation, RSR13 has the potential to enhance the effectiveness of standard radiation therapy.

In November 2000, positive preliminary phase II results of induction chemotherapy, followed by radiation therapy plus RSR13, for Stage IIIA and IIIB non-small cell lung cancer were announced. Data from the first 30 of 47 subjects demonstrated that 87% had a complete or partial response of their tumors within the radiation therapy portal in the chest. Additionally, Allos Therapeutics is conducting a 408 subject, randomized, multicenter, international phase III trial to confirm that RSR13, when used in combination with radiation therapy, significantly improves the survival of subjects with brain metastases.

INDICATION(S) AND RESEARCH PHASE
Angina – Phase I completed
Myocardial Infarction – Phase II
Brain Cancer – Phase III
Lung Cancer – Phase II
Glomerulonephritis – Phase II completed

SB 249553
unknown

MANUFACTURER
GlaxoSmithKline

DESCRIPTION
SB 249553 is a recombinant pharmaccine in phase II development for the treatment of lung cancer and melanoma.

INDICATION(S) AND RESEARCH PHASE
Lung Cancer – Phase II
Melanoma – Phase II

squalamine
unknown

MANUFACTURER
Magainin Pharmaceuticals

DESCRIPTION
Squalamine is an aminosterol compound isolated from the tissues of the dogfish shark. This drug inhibits salt and acid regulating pumps on endothelial cells that normally line blood vessels, which prevents growth factors from stimulating the cells to form capillaries. It is thought that this activity results in anti-angiogenisis, anti-inflammatory, and anti-tumor effects.

The company is conducting several phase II trials testing squalamine against certain cancers, such as breast cancer and ovarian cancer. Additionally, there is a phase IIa study for the treatment of stage IIIB and IV non-small cell lung cancer being conducted at the University of Wisconsin and M.D. Anderson, Houston, Texas.

Additional studies are being planned for ovarian cancer, pediatric neuroblastoma, and other solid tumors.

INDICATION(S) AND RESEARCH PHASE
Breast Cancer – Phase II
Lung Cancer – Phase IIa
Ovarian Cancer – Phase II
Cancer/Tumors (Unspecified) – Phase II

SU-101
unknown

MANUFACTURER
Sugen

DESCRIPTION
SU-101 is a synthetic, platelet-derived growth factor receptor, which blocks the essential enzyme, tyrosine kinase. This drug may be helpful for the treatment of end-stage malignant glioma, a tumor of nerve tissue. The drug is being tested in phase III trials for refractory brain and prostate cancers, and phase II studies for non-small cell lung and ovarian cancers.

INDICATION(S) AND RESEARCH PHASE
Brain Cancer – Phase III
Prostate Cancer – Phase III
Lung Cancer – Phase II
Ovarian Cancer – Phase II

T64
unknown

MANUFACTURER
Tularik

DESCRIPTION
T64 is an antifolate that disrupts DNA synthesis through the inhibition of purine biosynthesis. The compound is currently in phase II trials in subjects with head and neck cancer, soft tissue sarcoma, melanoma, breast cancer, and non-small cell lung cancer. Additionally, T64 is in phase I combination trials with gemcitabine, doxorubicin, and paclitaxel. Tularik expects to initiate two

additional T64 phase I combination trials with carboplatin and temozolamide in the first quarter of 2001. The T64 trials are being conducted in the United States, the United Kingdom, the Netherlands, and Australia.

INDICATION(S) AND RESEARCH PHASE
Head and Neck Cancer – Phase II
Sarcoma – Phase II
Melanoma – Phase II
Breast Cancer – Phase II
Lung Cancer – Phase II
Cancer/Tumors (Unspecified) – Phase I

T67
unknown

MANUFACTURER
Tularik

DESCRIPTION
T67 is an anti-cancer compound that binds irreversibly to tubulin and inhibits the growth of multi-drug resistant tumors. Tubulin is a protein that polymerizes into chains to form microtubules. Microtubules are essential for cell division, and by disrupting their function, T67 produces cell death and potentially causes tumor shrinkage.

The drug is currently in phase II trials in subjects with non-small cell lung cancer, glioma, colorectal cancer, and breast cancer. It is also in a phase I/II trial for the treatment of hepatocellular carcinoma. These trials are being conducted in the United States, the United Kingdom, Hong Kong, and Taiwan.

INDICATION(S) AND RESEARCH PHASE
Lung Cancer – Phase II
Brain Cancer – Phase II
Colorectal Cancer – Phase II
Breast Cancer – Phase II
Hepatocellular Carcinoma – Phase I/II

tirapazamine/cisplatin
Tirazone

MANUFACTURER
Sanofi-Synthelabo Pharmaceuticals

DESCRIPTION
Tirazone (tirapazamine) is a novel anti-cancer drug that is inactive in normal tissues that are well oxygenated, but becomes active at the low oxygen levels found in solid tumors. As a result, the drug kills these poorly oxygenated or hypoxic cells.

Tirazone is being investigated for new uses in combination with chemotherapy (particularly cisplatin) for the treatment of a variety of cancers, including non-small cell lung cancer, melanoma, refractory cancers, and cervical cancers. Results with non-small cell lung cancer and melanoma were encouraging, which has led to the initiation of phase III studies in which treatment with tirapazamine plus cisplatin is being compared with cisplatin alone. In another trial, the tirapazamine/cisplatin combination is being compared to cisplatin plus etoposide for stages IIIb and IV non-small cell lung cancer.

INDICATION(S) AND RESEARCH PHASE
Lung Cancer – Phase III

topotecan HCl
Hycamtin

MANUFACTURER
GlaxoSmithKline

DESCRIPTION
Hycamtin (topotecan HCl) is a topoisomerase I inhibitor administered by injection. It is currently indicated for the treatment of metastatic carcinoma of the ovary after failure of initial or subsequent chemotherapy. Hycamtin is also indicated for the treatment of small cell lung cancer sensitive disease after failure of first-line chemotherapy.

Hycamtin is being evaluated in a variety of phase II and III trials. It is being tested as a second-line therapy for the treatment of colorectal cancer, as first-line therapy for small cell and non-small cell lung cancer, as oral second-line therapy for small cell lung cancer, as first-line therapy for ovarian cancer and for the treatment of myelodysplastic syndrome.

INDICATION(S) AND RESEARCH PHASE
Colorectal Cancer – Phase II
Lung Cancer – Phase II
Lung Cancer – Phase III
Ovarian Cancer – Phase III
Myelodysplastic Syndrome – Phase III

troxacitabine, BCH-4556
Troxatyl

MANUFACTURER
BioChem Pharma

DESCRIPTION
Troxatyl is a dioxolane nucleoside analog being investigated as an anticancer agent. The drug is a complete DNA chain terminator and DNA polymerase inhibitor. It acts by incorporating itself into the growing DNA chain of cancer cells, interfering with their ability to further replicate. Troxatyl is being evaluated as a single agent or in combination therapy in a number of trials in hematologic malignancies, including acute myeloid leukemia and chronic myeloid leukemia (blastic phase), and in lymphoproliferative disorders such as lymphoma, chronic lymphocytic leukemia, and myeloma. It is also being evaluated as a single agent in pancreatic cancer and in combination therapy in a number of solid tumors. Troxatyl is currently in phase II development.

INDICATION(S) AND RESEARCH PHASE
Cancer/Tumors (Unspecified) – Phase II
Colorectal Cancer – Phase II
Head and Neck Cancer – Phase II
Leukemia – Phase II
Lung Cancer – Phase II
Malignant Melanoma – Phase II
Ovarian Cancer – Phase II
Pancreatic Cancer – Phase II
Prostate Cancer – Phase II
Renal Cell Carcinoma – Phase II

unknown
Aptosyn/Taxotere/carboplatin

MANUFACTURER
Cell Pathways

DESCRIPTION
Aptosyn is Cell Pathways' lead drug from

a novel class of compounds called selective apoptotic anti-neoplastic drugs (SAANDs). SAANDs inhibit a form of cyclic GMP phosphodiesterase and selectively induce apoptosis in abnormally growing precancerous and cancerous cells.

Cell Pathways is conducting clinical studies with this compound as a single agent and in combination with conventional chemotherapeutic drugs in a variety of cancer and precancerous indications. Aptosyn is being tested in a phase I/II trial in combination with Taxotere (docetaxel) and carboplatin in subjects with metastatic non-small cell lung cancer (NSCLC).

INDICATION(S) AND RESEARCH PHASE
Lung Cancer – Phase I/II

unknown
TriAb/TriGem

MANUFACTURER
Titan Pharmaceuticals

DESCRIPTION
Both TriAb and TriGem are anti-cancer monoclonal antibody based products designed to elicit an immune response to malignant cells. They are being tested as a combined therapy for the treatment of small cell lung cancer.

INDICATION(S) AND RESEARCH PHASE
Lung Cancer – Phase II

vaccine, anti-cancer
CeaVac/TriAb

MANUFACTURER
Titan Pharmaceuticals

DESCRIPTION
Both CeaVac and TriAb are anti-cancer monoclonal antibody based products designed to help the subject's immune system recognize and kill tumor cells. They are being tested as a combined therapy for the treatment of non-small cell lung cancer and colorectal cancer.

INDICATION(S) AND RESEARCH PHASE
Lung Cancer – Phase II
Colorectal Cancer – Phase II

vaccine, cancer
Gvax

MANUFACTURER
Cell Genesys

DESCRIPTION
Gvax is an allogenic compound that involves the genetic modification of prostate cancer cell lines. These cancer cells have been irradiated and modified to secrete granulocyte-macrophage colony stimulating factor (GM-CSF), a hormone which plays a key role in stimulating the body's immune response to vaccines. The compound is in trials for prostate cancer, pancreatic cancer, lung cancer, leukemia, and malignant melanoma.

The Gvax prostate cancer vaccine demonstrated anti-tumor activity in an initial phase II trial in subjects with advanced metastatic prostate cancer who have not responded to hormone therapy. Prior to initiating a phase III trial, Cell Genesys plans to initiate further trials of Gvax prostate cancer vaccine in 2001 that will employ a higher potency version of the same product. Additionally, future phase III trials in hormone refractory prostate cancer subjects may compare Gvax vaccine in combination with chemotherapy to chemotherapy alone.

INDICATION(S) AND RESEARCH PHASE
Prostate Cancer – Phase II
Lung Cancer – Phase I/II completed
Malignant Melanoma – Phase I/II
Vaccines – Phase I/II
Pancreatic Cancer – Phase II
Leukemia – Phase I/II

vaccine, EGF cancer
unknown

MANUFACTURER
YM Biosciences

DESCRIPTION
EGF cancer vaccine contains recombinant human epidermal growth factor (EGF) conjugated to a highly immunogenic recombinant bacterial protein, P64K. The vaccine is designed to stimulate the immune system to produce anti-EGF antibodies to inhibit the growth of cancer cells over-expressing EGF receptors. The EGF cancer vaccine is in a phase II trial in Canada and the United Kingdom for the treatment of non-small cell lung cancer.

INDICATION(S) AND RESEARCH PHASE
Lung Cancer – Phase II

vincristine
Onco TCS

MANUFACTURER
Inex Pharmaceuticals

DESCRIPTION
Onco TCS is a proprietary drug comprised of the widely used, off-patent cancer drug vincristine encapsulated in the company's patented drug delivery technology, Transmembrane Carrier Systems (TCS). The drug is being evaluated for treatment of non-Hodgkin's lymphoma (NHL). The TCS technology provides prolonged blood circulation, tumor accumulation, and extended-drug release at the cancer site and is designed to increase the effectiveness and reduce the toxicity of the encapsulated drug.

The company reported that phase IIa trials achieved over a 40% response rate with mild and manageable toxicity in relapsed aggressive and transformed NHL subjects. The investigators reported results from 68 total evaluable NHL subjects, 50 of whom suffered from the aggressive or transformed type of the disease. Analysis of 38 subjects with aggressive NHL and 12 subjects with transformed NHL provided a 45% and 42% response rate, respectively. The additional 18 subjects had other types of NHL and did not experience significant response rates to the treatment.

The FDA has given the company permission to proceed with the pivotal phase II/III trial of Onco TCS for NHL. Phase II trials have begun for small cell lung cancer and solid tumors. Additional indications for this drug may include colon cancer, lymph cancer, lymphoma, and pancreatic cancer.

INDICATION(S) AND RESEARCH PHASE
Lymphoma, Non-Hodgkin's – Phase II
Lung Cancer – Phase II
Cancer/Tumors (Unspecified) – Phase II

VX-710
Incel

MANUFACTURER
Vertex Pharmaceuticals

DESCRIPTION
Incel blocks two major multi-drug resistance mechanisms: P-glycoprotein (MDR-1) and multi-drug resistance-associated protein (MRP). Administered intravenously, Incel is to be used in combination with cancer chemotherapy agents. Vertex's research shows that Incel can enhance the accumulation of chemotherapy agents in tumor cells by blocking the drug pumps P-gp and MRP, and that it is capable of restoring the sensitivity of tumors to treatment with chemotherapeutic agents. Phase II trials investigating the activity of Incel in combination with other agents for the treatment of advanced refractory ovarian cancer, soft tissue sarcoma, and small cell lung cancer are under way.

INDICATION(S) AND RESEARCH PHASE
Lung Cancer – Phase II
Ovarian Cancer – Phase II
Sarcoma – Phase II

XR5000
unknown

MANUFACTURER
Xenova

DESCRIPTION
XR5000 is a topoisomerase I and II inhibitor being developed for the treatment of common solid tumors. Three phase II trials are under way at a number of European centers. The trials are being conducted on an "open-label" basis and target three cancer types—ovarian, non-small cell lung, and glioblastoma. The results of a fourth phase II trial, in which the efficacy of XR5000 was investigated in subjects with colorectal cancer, were announced in June 2000. No complete or partial responses to treatment were observed after two courses of treatment with XR5000. Two subjects showed stable disease and 13 subjects experienced disease progression. The company is not planning any further recruitment for this indication.

INDICATION(S) AND RESEARCH PHASE
Brain Cancer – Phase II
Colorectal Cancer – Phase II completed
Lung Cancer – Phase II
Ovarian Cancer – Phase II

ZD-0473/AMD 473
unknown

MANUFACTURER
AstraZeneca

DESCRIPTION
ZD-0473 is a new platinum-based anti-cancer agent designed to deliver an extended spectrum of activity and overcome resistance to currently approved platinum drugs, such as cisplatin and carboplatin. It is being evaluated for the treatment of a range of solid-tumor cancers, including colorectal, non-small cell lung and bladder cancer, which are resistant to carboplatin. ZD-0473 is formulated in both intravenous and oral forms. The intravenous formulation is in phase II trials and the oral form is in preclinical development. AnorMED has a licensing agreement with AstraZeneca who is conducting the phase II study development of ZD-0473.

INDICATION(S) AND RESEARCH PHASE
Bladder Cancer – Phase II
Cancer/Tumors (Unspecified) – Phase II
Colorectal Cancer – Phase II
Lung Cancer – Phase II
Ovarian Cancer – Phase II
Prostate Cancer – Phase II
Breast Cancer – Phase II
Cervical Dysplasia/Cancer – Phase II

ZD-1839
Iressa

MANUFACTURER
AstraZeneca

DESCRIPTION
Iressa binds to the epidermal growth factor receptor (EGFR) and inhibits tyrosine kinase, thereby blocking signals for cancer growth and survival. The company reported encouraging results from phase I trials in a variety of tumors, but particularly in non-small cell lung cancer (NSCLC). Iressa is being investigated both as a monotherapy and in combination with other anti-tumor drugs in NSCLC, gastric, colorectal, and hormone-resistant prostate cancers. In 1999, the FDA gave Iressa fast track status. The drug is currently in phase III development.

INDICATION(S) AND RESEARCH PHASE
Cancer/Tumors (Unspecified) – Phase III
Colorectal Cancer – Phase III
Gastric Cancer – Phase III
Lung Cancer – Phase III
Prostate Cancer – Phase III

Lymphoma, non-Hodgkin's

aldesleukin, interleukin-2 (IL-2)
Proleukin

MANUFACTURER
Chiron Corporation

DESCRIPTION
Proleukin is a genetically engineered (recombinant) form of interleukin-2, which is a naturally occurring immune modulator. Proleukin is being evaluated in phase III trials for acute myelogenous leukemia, non-Hodgkin's lymphoma, and HIV infection. Additionally, Proleukin was approved in July 2000 for advanced-stage kidney cancer and melanoma.

INDICATION(S) AND RESEARCH PHASE
HIV Infection – Phase III
Leukemia – Phase III
Lymphoma, Non-Hodgkin's – Phase III
Renal Cell Carcinoma – FDA approved
Melanoma – FDA approved

arsenic trioxide (ATO)
Trisenox

MANUFACTURER
Cell Therapeutics

DESCRIPTION
Trisenox is believed to kill cancer cells through apoptosis. The mechanism of action of Trisenox is not fully understood, but the drug appears to induce apoptosis in a different manner than other anti-cancer agents such as retinoids.

Trisenox is FDA approved to treat acute promyelocytic leukemia (APL), and it is also in numerous trials in the United States for indications including other types of leukemia, prostate cancer, multiple myeloma, renal cell cancer, cervical cancer, and bladder cancer.

INDICATION(S) AND RESEARCH PHASE
Leukemia – Phase I
Lymphoma, Non-Hodgkin's – Phase II
Leukemia – Phase II
Multiple Myeloma – Phase II
Prostate Cancer – Phase II
Renal Cell Carcinoma – Phase II
Cervical Dysplasia/Cancer – Phase II
Bladder Cancer – Phase II

bectumomab
LymphoScan

MANUFACTURER
Immunomedics

DESCRIPTION
LymphoScan is a diagnostic agent that combines genetic engineering with the ability to trace radioactivity in the body. Using a mouse-derived monoclonal antibody labeled with technetium-99m (Tc-99m), a widely available, inexpensive radioisotope, medical professionals can determine through nuclear imaging the extent of CD22-expressing lymphomas. LymphoScan is in a phase III clinical trial to evaluate its utility in determining the location and stage of the disease in subjects with non-Hodgkin's lymphoma.

INDICATION(S) AND RESEARCH PHASE
Lymphoma, Non-Hodgkin's – Phase III

CpG 7909
unknown

MANUFACTURER
Coley Pharmaceutical

DESCRIPTION
CpG 7909 is from a synthetic DNA sequence that naturally activates the human immune system to fight disease. CpG 7909 is being tested in three phase I/II trials for the treatment of cancer. The first trial has been initiated at the University of Iowa Cancer Center and is testing 24 subjects with refractory or relapsed non-Hodgkin's lymphoma. Subjects in this trial will receive weekly infusions of CpG 7909 for three weeks. Two other trials have been initiated in Europe. The first trial includes subjects with melanoma, while the second includes subjects with metastatic melanoma or basal cell carcinoma.

INDICATION(S) AND RESEARCH PHASE
Lymphoma, Non-Hodgkin's – Phase I/II
Melanoma – Phase I/II
Skin Cancer – Phase I/II

daunorubicin citrate
DaunoXome

MANUFACTURER
Gilead Sciences

DESCRIPTION
DaunoXome is a liposome anticancer product that has received approval as a first-line chemotherapy agent for advanced HIV-associated Kaposi's sarcoma (KS). DaunoXome's active ingredient is daunorubicin, a member of the anthracycline family of compounds, a potent group of antibiotics. Liposomes are microscopic fat bubbles that can be used to encase a drug. In animal studies, daunorubicin has been shown to accumulate in tumors to a greater extent when administered as DaunoXome than when administered as conventional daunorubicin. This anticancer drug is being tested in phase II trials for leukemias and the treatment of non-Hodgkin's lymphoma.

INDICATION(S) AND RESEARCH PHASE
Leukemia – Phase II
Lymphoma, Non-Hodgkin's – Phase II

epratuzumab
LymphoCide

MANUFACTURER
Immunomedics

DESCRIPTION
LymphoCide is a humanized monoclonal antibody that targets the CD22 receptor of non-Hodgkin's lymphoma (NHL) cells. LymphoCide is currently being studied in both an unlabeled and a radiolabeled (yttrium-90 [90Y]) form. The unlabeled epratuzumab is in phase III trials for the treatment of NHL, while the 90Y-version is in phase I trials.

INDICATION(S) AND RESEARCH PHASE
Lymphoma, Non-Hodgkin's – Phase III
Lymphoma, Non-Hodgkin's – Phase I

FLT3 ligand
Mobist

MANUFACTURER
ImClone Systems

DESCRIPTION
Mobist is a hematopoietic growth factor being tested exvivo. It is a stem cell mobilizer and potential anti-tumor agent. Mobist is being evaluated in phase II trials for the treatment of breast cancer, solid tumors, non-Hodgkin's lymphoma, and ovarian cancer.

INDICATION(S) AND RESEARCH PHASE
Cancer/Tumors (Unspecified) – Phase II
Breast Cancer – Phase II
Lymphomas, Non-Hodgkin's – Phase II
Ovarian Cancer – Phase II

fludarabine phosphate
Fludara

MANUFACTURER
Berlex Laboratories

DESCRIPTION
Fludara belongs to a class of anticancer drugs known as antimetabolites, which kill cells by blocking essential growth inside the cell. Administered intravenously, Fludara takes on the properties of certain enzymes necessary for cell growth. Cancer cells are fooled into accepting these false enzymes that are devoid of the crucial ingredients found in genuine enzymes. Fludara also interferes with the production of new DNA in cancer cells and helps other drugs work more effectively when used in combination therapy. Approved by the FDA for the treatment of recurrent chronic lymphocytic leukemia, Fludara is currently being tested in a phase III trial for the treatment of non-Hodgkin's lymphoma.

INDICATION(S) AND RESEARCH PHASE
Lymphoma, Non-Hodgkin's – Phase III

G3139/cyclophosphamide
Genasense/cyclophosphamide

MANUFACTURER
Genta

DESCRIPTION
Genasense (G3139) is designed to reduce levels of Bcl-2, a protein that contributes to resistance of cancer cells to current forms of cancer treatment. Treatment with Genasense may markedly improve the effectiveness of standard anticancer therapies. G3139 in combination with cyclophosphamide is in phase II trials for the treatment of non-Hodgkin's lymphoma.

INDICATION(S) AND RESEARCH PHASE
Lymphoma, Non-Hodgkin's – Phase II

HSPPC-96
Oncophage

MANUFACTURER
Antigenics

DESCRIPTION
Oncophage cancer vaccine is an injectable protein that contains the unique profile ("antigenic fingerprint") of each subject's cancer. The antigens activate the immune system to elicit an anti-tumor response. Oncophage is in clinical trials for several indications, including renal cell carcinoma (phase III), melanoma (phase II), colorectal cancer (phase II), gastric cancer (phase I/II), pancreatic cancer (phase I/II completed), and non-Hodgkin's lymphoma (phase II).

In October 2000, Antigenics announced that it had initiated a phase II trial of Oncophage in subjects who have been diagnosed with sarcoma, also known as soft tissue cancer. The study is expected to initially enroll 20 subjects diagnosed with recurrent metastatic or unresectable soft tissue sarcoma and may be expanded to include an additional 15 subjects depending on preliminary results.

INDICATION(S) AND RESEARCH PHASE
Renal Cell Carcinoma – Phase III
Malignant Melanoma – Phase II
Colorectal Cancer – Phase II
Gastric Cancer – Phase I/II
Pancreatic Cancer – Phase I/II completed
Lymphoma, Non-Hodgkin's – Phase II
Sarcoma – Phase II

IDEC-Y2B8, In2B8
Zevalin

MANUFACTURER
IDEC Pharmaceuticals

DESCRIPTION
Zevalin is an investigational immunotherapy being developed for the treatment of low grade or follicular, relapsed or refractory, CD20-positive B-cell non-Hodgkin's lymphoma (NHL) and Rituximab-refractory NHL. Zevalin is a monoclonal antibody that targets the CD20 antigen (similar to the drug Rituxan). In the case of Zevalin, a chelating agent links the antibody to the radioisotope yttrium-90. The radioactive component attached to the antibody will potentially kill cells that bind the antibody.

In December 2000, final results of two pivotal phase III trials were presented at the 42nd Annual Meeting of the American Society of Hematology. The first randomized, controlled trial involved 143 subjects with relapsed or refractory low-grade, follicular, or CD20-positive transformed B-cell NHL. Zevalin combined with Rituxan showed an overall response rate of 80%, while a Rituxan control showed an overall response rate of 56%. The second phase III trial of Zevalin included 54 follicular NHL subjects who were refractory to Rituxan. Zevalin treated subjects showed an overall response rate of 74%, and 15% achieved complete responses.

INDICATION(S) AND RESEARCH PHASE
Lymphoma, Non-Hodgkin's – Phase III completed

subject-specific immunotherapy
unknown

MANUFACTURER
Genitope Corporation

DESCRIPTION
Genitope Corporation is developing a subject-specific immunotherapy for the treatment of indolent B-cell non-Hodgkin's lymphoma (NHL). The company genetically engineered the tumor-derived protein using their patented High Throughput Gene Expression Technology (Hi-GET) to recruit the subject's immune cells to act against the tumor, leaving other cells unharmed.

Phase II trial results indicated that the subject-specific immunotherapy stimulated a positive immune response against the subject's tumor. As of December 2000, ten of 25 subjects had received injections of a custom-made protein derived from each subject's tumor cells and coupled to a carrier protein, keyhole limpet hemocyanin. The immunotherapy appeared to be safe and non-toxic, with minor side effects limited to local injection-site inflammation and flu-like symptoms. Genitope has initiated a multicenter phase III trial.

INDICATION(S) AND RESEARCH PHASE
Lymphoma, Non-Hodgkin's – Phase III

pentostatin

Nipent

MANUFACTURER
SuperGen

DESCRIPTION
Nipent (pentostatin) belongs to a group of drugs called antimetabolites. Pentostatin inhibits the enzyme adenosine deaminase, which leads to cytotoxicity and cell death. This drug is in trials for rheumatoid arthritis, chronic lymphocytic leukemia and non-Hodgkin's lymphoma, among other indications.

In December 2000, results of a phase II trial of Nipent indicated the drug has significant activity (75% overall response rate) in the treatment of graft versus host disease (GVHD). Twelve subjects with steroid refractory GVHD received Nipent as "salvage therapy" because each had previously failed all other treatments.

INDICATION(S) AND RESEARCH PHASE
Leukemia – Phase III
Lymphoma, Non-Hodgkin's – Phase II
Rheumatoid Arthritis – Phase II
Immunosuppressive – Phase III
Cutaneous T-cell Lymphoma (CTCL)/Peripheral T-cell Lymphoma (PTCL) – NDA submitted

ribozyme gene therapy
unknown

MANUFACTURER
Ribozyme Pharmaceuticals

DESCRIPTION
Gene therapies represent a promising direction for the treatment of retroviral and other diseases. Ribozymes are RNA enzymes that perform numerous functions, including the cleavage of ribonucleic acid (RNA) molecules. Ribozymes can be designed to selectively recognize, bind, and cleave any mRNA sequence. As human therapeutics, ribozymes can be chemically synthesized to selectively inhibit disease-causing proteins through the specific cleavage of the disease-causing mRNA. The company has made proprietary chemical modifications to ribozymes that allow them to be stable and active in human serum for several days, thus broadening their potential therapeutic applications.

INDICATION(S) AND RESEARCH PHASE
Acquired Immune Deficiency Syndrome (AIDS) and AIDS-Related Infections – Phase II
HIV Infection – Phase II
Lymphoma, Non-Hodgkin's – Phase II

rituximab/chemotherapy
Rituxan

MANUFACTURER
Genentech

DESCRIPTION
Rituxan is a monoclonal antibody in trials for the treatment of intermediate- and high-grade non-Hodgkin's lymphoma. Rituxan has been approved by the FDA for the treatment of relapsed or refractory low-grade or follicular, CD20-positive B-cell non-Hodgkin's lymphoma. This drug is being developed in collaboration with IDEC.

Results from phase II trials showed that adding Rituxan to CHOP chemotherapy may have the potential to provide durable remissions for subjects with NHL. Adverse events of Rituxan plus CHOP were similar to those observed with CHOP chemotherapy alone. Hematologic toxicity included Grade III and IV neutropenia. Neutropenia (decreased numbers of neutrophil immune cells), fever, and dehydration were the most common causes of hospitalization.

INDICATION(S) AND RESEARCH PHASE
Lymphoma, Non-Hodgkin's – Phase III

SMART 1D10 antibody
unknown

MANUFACTURER
Protein Design Labs

DESCRIPTION
SMART 1D10 is a monoclonal humanized mouse antibody that induces apoptosis of malignant B-cells. SMART 1D10 binds to an HLA-DR determinant found on many pre-B and B-cell lymphomas. The interaction between SMART 1D10 and its target causes the SMART 1D10-HLA-DR complex to move into a portion of the cell membrane called a membrane raft. In this location, the linked HLA-DR molecules trigger a variety of signaling molecules that lead to the death of the malignant B-cell by apoptosis. SMART 1D10 is currently in a phase II trial for the treatment of non-Hodgkin's B-cell lymphoma in 60 subjects.

INDICATION(S) AND RESEARCH PHASE
Lymphoma, Non-Hodgkin's – Phase II

tositumomab
Bexxar

MANUFACTURER
Coulter Pharmaceuticals

DESCRIPTION
Bexxar, an antibody conjugated to iodine 131, attaches to a protein found only on the surface of B-cells, including both non-Hodgkin's lymphoma B-cells and some normal B-cell tissues. The company believes that a dual mechanism of action consisting of apoptosis from the attachment of the monoclonal antibody plus the DNA-damaging effects of the iodine (I-131) radioisotope is responsible for Bexxar's promising safety and efficacy results as demonstrated in clinical trials.

Coulter Pharmaceuticals and GlaxoSmithKline held a phase II trial testing Bexxar in combination with CVP, a commonly used chemotherapy for the treatment of previously untreated low-grade non-Hodgkin's lymphoma (NHL). This trial included 30 subjects who had never been treated for NHL. Subjects received six cycles of CVP (cyclophosphamide, vincristine, and prednisone), followed within 56 days by Bexxar. An NDA has been submitted for the treatment of NHL.

INDICATION(S) AND RESEARCH PHASE
Lymphoma, Non-Hodgkin's – NDA submitted

tretinoin

Lymphoma, non-Hodgkin's

Atragen

MANUFACTURER
Aronex Pharmaceuticals

DESCRIPTION
Atragen is a liposomal, intravenous formulation of tretinoin or all-trans-retinoic acid. Tretinoin induces cell differentiation in rapidly proliferating cells, such as those observed in malignant diseases. Additionally, Atragen appears to affect the cellular signaling mechanisms that become unbalanced in cancer cells. Results of a phase II trial of Atragen monotherapy for acute promyelocytic leukemia (APL) indicated its potential to induce complete remission. The trial was conducted in Peru, and included 16 subjects with newly diagnosed or previously untreated APL who were treated with Atragen every other day as a single agent for a maximum of 28 doses. Fourteen subjects (87.5%) achieved morphologic remission, and 28.6% of these subjects also attained molecular remission. The safety profile observed in the subject population is similar to that reported with the currently approved oral formulation of Atra.

In addition to investigating the safety and efficacy of Atragen as a treatment for APL, the company is conducting trials to evaluate the compound for the treatment of non-Hodgkin's lymphoma, hormone-resistant prostate cancer, acute myelogenous leukemia (AML), and renal cell carcinoma in combination with interferon alpha.

In January 2001, Aronex announced that the FDA has denied approval of the company's NDA for Atragen as a treatment for subjects with APL, for whom therapy with tretinoin (all-trans-retinoic acid or Atra) is necessary but for whom an intravenous administration is required.

INDICATION(S) AND RESEARCH PHASE
Lymphoma, Non-Hodgkin's – Phase II
Prostate Cancer – Phase II
Renal Cell Carcinoma – Phase I/II
Leukemia, APL (intravenous) – NDA denied
Leukemia, APL (monotherapy) – Phase II
Leukemia, AML – Phase II

unknown
Pretarget

MANUFACTURER
NeoRx Corporation

DESCRIPTION
Pretarget is a proprietary method of radioimmunotherapy, in which an antibody and radionuclide are separately injected and subsequently joined at the tumor. Because a radionuclide is a small, drug-sized molecule, its circulation time is short, which helps to avoid subject exposure to large amounts of radiation that are not targeted directly to the tumor. The company has treated seven late-stage non-Hodgkin's lymphoma subjects using a prototype Pretarget product. Six of the seven showed evidence of tumor regression and three had complete remissions, according to the company.

INDICATION(S) AND RESEARCH PHASE
Lymphoma, Non-Hodgkin's – Phase II

unknown
Oncolym

MANUFACTURER
Berlex Laboratories

DESCRIPTION
Oncolym is in a phase I trial for the treatment of non-Hodgkin's lymphoma, which will enroll 18 subjects at four sites. After completing a successful phase I trial, the company plans to initiate phase II/III trials treating 100 subjects.

INDICATION(S) AND RESEARCH PHASE
Lymphoma, Non-Hodgkin's – Phase I

vincristine
Onco TCS

MANUFACTURER
Inex Pharmaceuticals

DESCRIPTION
Onco TCS is a proprietary drug comprised of the widely used, off-patent cancer drug vincristine encapsulated in the company's patented drug delivery technology, Transmembrane Carrier Systems (TCS). The drug is being evaluated for treatment of non-Hodgkin's lymphoma (NHL). The TCS technology provides prolonged blood circulation, tumor accumulation, and extended-drug release at the cancer site and is designed to increase the effectiveness and reduce the toxicity of the encapsulated drug.

The company reported that phase IIa trials achieved over a 40% response rate with mild and manageable toxicity in relapsed aggressive and transformed NHL subjects. The investigators reported results from 68 total evaluable NHL subjects, 50 of whom suffered from the aggressive or transformed type of the disease. Analysis of 38 subjects with aggressive NHL and 12 subjects with transformed NHL provided a 45% and 42% response rate, respectively. The additional 18 subjects had other types of NHL and did not experience significant response rates to the treatment.

The FDA has given the company permission to proceed with a pivotal phase II/III trial of Onco TCS for NHL. Phase II trials have begun for small cell lung cancer and solid tumors. Additional indications for this drug may include colon cancer, lymph cancer, lymphoma, and pancreatic cancer.

INDICATION(S) AND RESEARCH PHASE
Lymphoma, Non-Hodgkin's – Phase II
Lung Cancer – Phase II
Cancer/Tumors (Unspecified) – Phase II

Lymphomas

APL400-020 V-B
Genevax-TCR

MANUFACTURER
Wyeth-Lederle Vaccines

DESCRIPTION
Genevax-TCR is a novel DNA-based vaccine that is in early clinical testing for T-cell lymphomas and other autoimmune diseases. Treatment of cutaneous T-cell lymphoma is an orphan indication currently is being evaluated in a phase I/II trial.

INDICATION(S) AND RESEARCH PHASE
Autoimmune Diseases – Phase I/II
Lymphomas – Phase I/II

BCX-34
unknown

MANUFACTURER
BioCryst Pharmaceuticals

DESCRIPTION
BCX-34 is an inhibitor of the enzyme purine nucleoside phosphorylase (PNP), which may be essential for T-cell replication. T-cells normally attack invading bacteria and viruses as part of normal immune function. Proliferative diseases, such as cutaneous T-cell lymphoma (CTCL) and T-cell leukemia, occur when T-cells multiply abnormally or attack healthy body tissue. BCX-34 is currently in trials for the treatment of lymphomas and HIV infection. Trials for leukemia, however, were discontinued.

INDICATION(S) AND RESEARCH PHASE
HIV Infection – Phase I/II
Leukemia – Trial discontinued
Lymphomas – Phase I/II

bexarotene
Targretin-capsule

MANUFACTURER
Ligand Pharmaceuticals

DESCRIPTION
Targretin, which selectively stimulates a retinoid subtype receptor, is being developed in an oral capsule formulation for the treatment of lung cancer, breast cancer, head and neck cancer, cutaneous T-cell lymphoma (CTCL), and psoriasis and psoriatic disorders. The drug is in phase II trials for head and neck cancer, phase II/III trials for breast cancer, CTCL and psoriasis and psoriatic disorders, and phase III trials for non-small cell lung cancer.

INDICATION(S) AND RESEARCH PHASE
Psoriasis and Psoriatic Disorders – Phase II/III
Lung Cancer – Phase III
Breast Cancer – Phase II/III
Head and Neck Cancer – Phase II
Lymphomas – Phase II/III

denileukin diftitox
Ontak

MANUFACTURER
Ligand Pharmaceuticals

DESCRIPTION
Ontak, previously known as DAB389IL-2, is a novel targeted cytotoxic biologic. The cytotoxic diphtheria toxin is fused to a subunit of IL-2 and therefore is delivered only to cells that express the IL-2 receptor (IL-2R). IL-2R may be expressed in a variety of malignant cells, including those of chronic lymphocytic leukemia. A phase II trial was initiated in January 2001 at the Comprehensive Cancer Center of the Wake Forest University School of Medicine in Winston-Salem, NC in subjects diagnosed with fludarabine-refractory, CD25-positive B-cell chronic lymphocytic leukemia.

Results of a phase III trial showed that Ontak induced substantial and durable partial and complete responses (30% response overall) in subjects with persistent or refractory cutaneous T-cell lymphoma (CTCL). Overall, 21 of 71 CTCL subjects treated with Ontak had an objective response. There was a trend suggesting a dose-effect for those subjects with more advanced disease: an objective response was seen in 2/21 (10%) and 9/24 (38%) subjects with at least stage IIb disease treated with 9 or 18(u)kg/d, respectively. Fifty-three of the 71 subjects entered had significant pruritus at baseline and 36 (68%) of these experienced clinically significant improvements.

The FDA has granted Seragen, a subsidiary of Ligand, marketing approval for Ontak for the treatment of subjects with persistent or recurrent CTCL whose malignant cells express the CD25 component of the IL-2 receptor.

INDICATION(S) AND RESEARCH PHASE
Leukemia – Phase II
Lymphomas – FDA approved

gallium maltolate
unknown

MANUFACTURER
Titan Pharmaceuticals

DESCRIPTION
Gallium is a semi-metallic element that has shown some therapeutic activity in metabolic bone disease, hypercalcemia of malignancy and cancer. Gallium maltolate can displace divalent iron from the iron transporting protein, transferrin; thus gallium maltolate causes interference with iron metabolism with inhibition of enzymes requiring divalent iron. The most important of these in the cancer setting appears to be ribonucleotide reductase (RNR). Additionally, gallium appears to form salts with calcium and phosphate that become incorporated into bone. The bone that is created with incorporated gallium appears to be at least as strong as normal bone, and it appears to be more resistant to degradation by osteoclasts and tumor cells.

INDICATION(S) AND RESEARCH PHASE
Prostate Cancer – Phase I/II
Lymphomas – Phase I/II
Myeloma – Phase I/II
Bladder Cancer – Phase I/II
HIV Infection – Phase I/II

organ transplantion system
AlloMune

MANUFACTURER
BioTransplant

DESCRIPTION
AlloMune is an organ transplantation system for the creation of specific immune tolerance in solid organ transplants from human donor organs using a novel anti-CD2 antibody/immunosuppressive monoclonal antibody (MAb). The drug is designed to re-educate the recipient's immune system to recognize the foreign tissue as "self." The AlloMune System for cancer applications is designed to attack tumor cells more aggressively than the subject's own immune defenses. Phase I/II trials are

being conducted for kidney transplant surgery, for use as an immunosuppressant and refractory lymphoma. Additional indications may include other types of cancer.

INDICATION(S) AND RESEARCH PHASE
Immunosuppressive – Phase I/II
Kidney Transplant Surgery – Phase I/II
Lymphomas – Phase I/II

---

unknown
Beta LT

MANUFACTURER
LifeTime Pharmaceuticals

DESCRIPTION
Beta LT is an anti-cancer agent designed to stimulate the immune system. Positive results were noted in two phase I/II trials testing Beta LT. The 14 subjects treated received the target dose for up to one year with no serious side effects except for mild bowel habit changes in one subject. The trial took place at McGill University, Jewish General Hospital in Montreal, Canada.

The FDA has cleared Beta LT for testing in subjects with progressing pre-malignant myeloma-related disease (MGUS), as well as testing the drug to decrease cancer in subjects with advanced disease. Beta LT is also being tested for the treatment of lymphoma.

INDICATION(S) AND RESEARCH PHASE
Lymphomas – Phase I/II completed
Multiple Myeloma – Phase I/II completed

---

vaccine, cancer
unknown

MANUFACTURER
Genzyme Genetics Division

DESCRIPTION
This cancer vaccine is made from proteins associated with tumors taken from the individual subject. Phase I/II clinical trials are testing the vaccine in subjects with B-cell lymphoma and multiple myeloma.

INDICATION(S) AND RESEARCH PHASE
Lymphomas – Phase I/II
Multiple Myeloma – Phase I/II

---

vaccine, lymphoma
Vaxid

MANUFACTURER
Vical

DESCRIPTION
Vaxid is a DNA protective vaccine being developed for the treatment of B-cell lymphoma. Immunization of post-chemotherapy subjects with Vaxid could result in the elimination of residual disease and the prevention of relapse. The vaccine was developed using Vical's proprietary naked DNA delivery technology. It is manufactured in an intramuscular injection formulation.

INDICATION(S) AND RESEARCH PHASE
Lymphomas – Phase I/II

Malignant Melanoma

CancerVax, C-VAX
unknown

MANUFACTURER
John Wayne Cancer Institute

DESCRIPTION
C-VAX is a polyvalent melanoma vaccine containing three irradiated melanoma cell lines. Currently, C-VAX is in a phase III trial for the treatment of malignant melanoma. The trial is split into two studies to separately test C-VAX in subjects with stage III and IV melanoma.

INDICATION(S) AND RESEARCH PHASE
Malignant Melanoma – Phase III

---

cisplatin/epinephrine
IntraDose

MANUFACTURER
Matrix Pharmaceutical

DESCRIPTION
IntraDose is a biodegradable collagen carrier matrix combined with a vasoconstrictor. The gel is injected directly into tumors where it localizes high concentrations of cisplatin, a widely used anticancer drug. It is currently being tested for several indications, including head and neck, breast, malignant melanoma, esophageal, and primary hepatocellular cancer.

A phase II trail of IntraDose Injectable Gel produced durable responses in subjects with colorectal cancer that had metastasized to the liver. Nine of 31 subjects who received IntraDose responded to therapy. Six subjects experienced a complete response (100% reduction in viable tumor volume of treated tumors) while the other three subjects demonstrated a partial response (at least a 50% reduction of viable tumor volume). IntraDose was well tolerated by subjects.

INDICATION(S) AND RESEARCH PHASE
Breast Cancer – Phase II
Cancer/Tumors (Unspecified) – Phase II
Colorectal Cancer – Phase II completed
Esophageal Cancer – Phase II
Liver Cancer – Phase II
Malignant Melanoma – Phase II
Head and Neck Cancer – NDA submitted

---

diarysulfonylurea, ILX-295501
unknown

MANUFACTURER
ILEX Oncology

DESCRIPTION
ILX-295501 belongs to a novel class of anti-tumor compounds known as diarysulfonylureas. This orally formulated drug is in phase II trials for renal cell carcinoma, malignant melanoma, and lung and ovarian cancers.

INDICATION(S) AND RESEARCH PHASE
Renal Cell Carcinoma – Phase II
Malignant Melanoma – Phase II
Lung Cancer – Phase II
Ovarian Cancer – Phase II

---

diethylnorspermine
DENSPM

MANUFACTURER
GelTex Pharmaceuticals

DESCRIPTION
DENSPM (diethylnorspermine) resembles a naturally produced polyamine, except that it may interrupt the rapid growth of tumor cells that need polyamines for growth. The drug is in phase II trials for renal cell carcinoma, pancreatic cancer, malignant melanoma, and non-small cell lung cancer. Additional indications may include ovarian and colon cancers.

INDICATION(S) AND RESEARCH PHASE
Renal Cell Carcinoma – Phase II
Pancreatic Cancer – Phase II
Malignant Melanoma – Phase II
Lung Cancer – Phase II

gene therapy, IL-2 and superantigen gene (SEB)
unknown

MANUFACTURER
Valentis

DESCRIPTION
A phase IIa trial is under way for the treatment of malignant melanoma using a combination of cytokine gene (IL-2) and superantigen gene (SEB). The vaccine is injected directly into the tumor, producing an anticancer immune response.

INDICATION(S) AND RESEARCH PHASE
Malignant Melanoma – Phase IIa
Vaccines – Phase IIa

gene therapy, interleukin-2
unknown

MANUFACTURER
Valentis

DESCRIPTION
This cancer therapeutic encodes the human IL-2 gene and a proprietary cationic lipid gene in a plasmid delivery system. Plasmids are self-replicating structures outside the chromosomes in a bacterial cell that carry genes for functions not essential to growth, such as the production of enzymes, toxins, and antigens. This gene therapy is in trials for the treatment of head and neck cancer and malignant melanoma.

INDICATION(S) AND RESEARCH PHASE
Head and Neck Cancer – Phase II
Malignant Melanoma – Phase I

histamine dihydrochloride
Ceplene

MANUFACTURER
Maxim Pharmaceuticals

DESCRIPTION
Ceplene (formally Maxamine) is a histamine-2 (H-2) receptor stimulator that is being co-administered with immunotherapies, including cytokines and interleukin-2 (IL-2). Clinical testing includes treatment of acute myelogenous leukemia (AML), chronic hepatitis C, malignant melanoma, multiple myeloma, and renal cell carcinoma.

Results from a phase III trial in stage IV malignant melanoma subjects indicated that Ceplene used in combination with a lower dose of interleukin-2 (IL-2) improved survival rates compared to treatment with the same doses of IL-2 alone. Treatment with Ceplene and IL-2 improved overall survival, increased survival rates at 12, 18, and 24 months, and improved time-to-disease progression compared to treatment with IL-2 alone. Twenty-five percent of subjects treated with Ceplene and lower-dose IL-2 survived for a 24-month period. Overall response was achieved in 38% of the subjects treated with Ceplene and lower-dose IL-2. The company received an NDA non-approvable letter in January 2001 because the FDA stated that the phase III trial forming the basis of the NDA would not be adequate as a single study to support approval.

INDICATION(S) AND RESEARCH PHASE
Hepatitis – Phase II
Leukemia – Phase III completed
Malignant Melanoma – NDA denied
Multiple Myeloma – Phase II
Renal Cell Carcinoma – Phase II

HSPPC-96
Oncophage

MANUFACTURER
Antigenics

DESCRIPTION
Oncophage cancer vaccine is an injectable protein that contains the unique profile ("antigenic fingerprint") of each subject's cancer. The antigens activate the immune system to elicit an anti-tumor response. Oncophage is in clinical trials for several indications, including renal cell carcinoma (phase III), melanoma (phase II), colorectal cancer (phase II), gastric cancer (phase I/II), pancreatic cancer (phase I/II completed), and non-Hodgkin's lymphoma (phase II).

In October 2000, Antigenics announced that it had initiated a phase II trial of Oncophage in subjects who have been diagnosed with sarcoma, also known as soft tissue cancer. The study is expected to initially enroll 20 subjects diagnosed with recurrent metastatic or unresectable soft tissue sarcoma and may be expanded to include an additional 15 subjects depending on preliminary results.

INDICATION(S) AND RESEARCH PHASE
Renal Cell Carcinoma – Phase III
Malignant Melanoma – Phase II
Colorectal Cancer – Phase II
Gastric Cancer – Phase I/II
Pancreatic Cancer – Phase I/II completed
Lymphoma, Non-Hodgkin's – Phase II
Sarcoma – Phase II

IM862
unknown

MANUFACTURER
Cytran

DESCRIPTION
IM862 is a small peptide comprised of two amino acids that may inhibit new blood vessel formation (angiogenesis). When there is excessive growth of new blood vessels, a number of pathological conditions result, including malignant tumors, age-related macular degeneration, and vascular diseases.

Limiting the growth of new blood vessels in tumors deprives them of nourishment and can ultimately kill these cancers. This drug is being developed in phase III trials for Kaposi's sarcoma and phase I/II trials for ovarian cancer.

INDICATION(S) AND RESEARCH PHASE
Kaposi's Sarcoma – Phase III
Ovarian Cancer – Phase I/II
Malignant Melanoma – Preclinical
Prostate Cancer – Preclinical

interferon alfa-2b
PEG-Intron

MANUFACTURER
Schering-Plough Corporation

DESCRIPTION
PEG-Intron is a long-acting antiviral/biological response modifier. Clinical trials include testing for the treatment of chronic myelogenous leukemia, solid tumors, and malignant melanoma.

PEG-Intron was developed by Enzon for Schering-Plough who owns the exclusive rights. The drug was approved by the FDA for the treatment of hepatitis C in January 2001.

INDICATION(S) AND RESEARCH PHASE
Cancer/Tumors (Unspecified) – Phase II
Hepatitis – FDA approved
Leukemia – Phase III
Malignant Melanoma – Phase III

peginterferon alfa-2a
Pegasys

MANUFACTURER
Hoffmann-La Roche

DESCRIPTION
Pegasys is a longer-lasting form of interferon, which is a naturally produced immune boosting substance. It is in clinical trials for the treatment of hepatitis B and C, malignant melanoma, renal cell carcinoma, and chronic myelogenous leukemia.

INDICATION(S) AND RESEARCH PHASE
Hepatitis – Phase III
Malignant Melanoma – Phase II
Renal Cell Carcinoma – Phase II
Leukemia – Phase III

poly I:poly C-12-U
Ampligen

MANUFACTURER
Hemispherx Biopharma

DESCRIPTION
Ampligen is a novel therapeutic composed of genetic building blocks (polyribonucleotide and synthetic nucleic acid). This intravenous drug is being evaluated in phase II/III trials for renal cell carcinoma, phase I/II trials for malignant melanoma, and phase III trials for chronic fatigue syndrome and HIV.

INDICATION(S) AND RESEARCH PHASE
Renal Cell Carcinoma – Phase II/III
Malignant Melanoma – Phase I/II
Chronic Fatigue Syndrome – Phase III
HIV Infection – Phase III

RFS-2000
Rubitecan

MANUFACTURER
SuperGen

DESCRIPTION
Rubitecan is a novel drug that works by inhibiting an enzyme called topoisomerase I. This drug is made in an oral formulation, which is an advantage for outpatient treatment compared to intravenous cancer drugs that may require a visit to a hospital setting.

In addition to treating pancreatic cancer, Rubitecan is being evaluated in treating a variety of solid tumors, such as in breast, colorectal, lung, ovarian, and prostate cancers, as well as metastatic melanoma and advanced gastric carcinoma. Additionally, phase II trials in the United States and Europe are testing Rubitecan in blood cancers such as chronic myelomonocytic leukemia (CMML/myelodysplastic syndrome).

INDICATION(S) AND RESEARCH PHASE
Pancreatic Cancer – Phase III
Breast Cancer – Phase II
Colorectal Cancer – Phase II
Gastric Cancer – Phase II
Leukemia – Phase II
Malignant Melanoma – Phase II
Ovarian Cancer – Phase II
Myelodysplastic Syndrome – Phase III

thymalfasin
Zadaxin

MANUFACTURER
SciClone Pharmaceuticals

DESCRIPTION
Zadaxin is a twenty-eight amino acid peptide originally isolated from the thymus gland now produced synthetically. The compound has been shown to promote the maturation of T-cells, which are involved in the control of various immune responses. Zadaxin has been administered to over 3,000 subjects in over 70 clinical trials without serious drug related side effects.

Zadaxin is presently in phase II trials in the United States in combination with lamivudine for the treatment of hepatitis B. SciClone plans to initiate additional U.S. phase II Zadaxin clinical programs in liver cancer and malignant melanoma. Pivotal phase III hepatitis B studies are currently ongoing in Japan. SciClone plans to start a pivotal phase III hepatitis C trial in the United States, which will be complemented by a pivotal phase III hepatitis C trial in Europe to be conducted by Sigma-Tau S.p.A., SciClone's European partner.

INDICATION(S) AND RESEARCH PHASE
Hepatitis – Phase II
Hepatitis – Phase III
Viral Infection – Phase III
Liver Cancer – Phase II
Malignant Melanoma – Phase II

troxacitabine, BCH-4556
Troxatyl

MANUFACTURER
BioChem Pharma

DESCRIPTION
Troxatyl is a dioxolane nucleoside analog being investigated as an anticancer agent. This drug is a complete DNA chain terminator and DNA polymerase inhibitor. It acts by incorporating itself into the growing DNA chain of cancer cells, interfering with their ability to replicate further. Troxatyl is being evaluated as a single agent or in combination therapy in a number of trials in hematologic malignancies, including acute myeloid leukemia and chronic myeloid leukemia (blastic phase), and in lymphoproliferative disorders such as lymphoma, chronic lymphocytic leukemia, and myeloma. It is also being evaluated as a single agent in pancreatic cancer and in combination therapy in a number of solid tumors. Troxatyl is currently in phase II development.

INDICATION(S) AND RESEARCH PHASE
Cancer/Tumors (Unspecified) – Phase II
Colorectal Cancer – Phase II
Head and Neck Cancer – Phase II
Leukemia – Phase II
Lung Cancer – Phase II
Malignant Melanoma – Phase II
Ovarian Cancer – Phase II
Pancreatic Cancer – Phase II
Prostate Cancer – Phase II
Renal Cell Carcinoma – Phase II

vaccine, anti-cancer
TriGem

MANUFACTURER
Titan Pharmaceuticals

DESCRIPTION
TriGem is an anti-cancer monoclonal antibody based product designed to help the subject's immune system recognize and kill tumor cells. Preliminary results of TriGem demonstrated that 100% of 12 subjects with metastatic melanoma developed an immune response following therapy. TriGem is in phase II trials for the treatment of malignant melanoma.

INDICATION(S) AND RESEARCH PHASE
Malignant Melanoma – Phase II

vaccine, cancer
Gvax

MANUFACTURER
Cell Genesys

DESCRIPTION
Gvax is an allogenic compound that involves the genetic modification of prostate cancer cell lines. These cancer cells have been irradiated and modified to secrete granulocyte-macrophage colony stimulating factor (GM-CSF), a hormone which plays a key role in stimulating the body's immune response to vaccines. The compound is in trials for prostate cancer, pancreatic cancer, lung cancer, leukemia, and malignant melanoma.

The Gvax prostate cancer vaccine demonstrated anti-tumor activity in an initial phase II trial in subjects with advanced metastatic prostate cancer who have not responded to hormone therapy. Prior to initiating a phase III trial, Cell Genesys plans to initiate further trials of Gvax prostate cancer vaccine in 2001 that will employ a higher potency version of the same product. Additionally, future phase III trials in hormone refractory prostate cancer subjects may compare Gvax vaccine in combination with chemotherapy to chemotherapy alone.

INDICATION(S) AND RESEARCH PHASE
Prostate Cancer – Phase II
Lung Cancer – Phase I/II completed
Malignant Melanoma – Phase I/II
Vaccines – Phase I/II
Pancreatic Cancer – Phase II
Leukemia – Phase I/II

vaccine, GMK
unknown

MANUFACTURER
Progenics Pharmaceuticals

DESCRIPTION
GMK targets the GM2 ganglioside on the surface of malignant melanoma cells. The vaccine combines a GM2 molecule with an immunogenic carrier protein, keyhole limpet hemocyanin (KLH), and Aquila Biopharmaceuticals lead Stimulon adjuvant. The vaccine induces the immune system to produce antibodies, which bind to GM2 molecules on cancer cells and catalyze cellular destruction.

GMK is being tested in a phase III trial for melanoma in subjects who are at risk of relapse after surgery. This vaccine is administered on an outpatient basis, and it is being tested at hundreds of sites throughout the United States.

INDICATION(S) AND RESEARCH PHASE
Malignant Melanoma – Phase III
Vaccines – Phase III

vaccine, melanoma
M-Vax

MANUFACTURER
AVAX Technologies

DESCRIPTION
M-Vax is an autologous cell vaccine being tested for the treatment of metastatic melanoma. In phase II studies, subjects with stage III melanoma demonstrated a five-year survival rate of 55%. The vaccine is currently in phase I development for stage III melanoma, and phase II development for Stage IV melanoma. M-Vax was approved in Australia in July 2000.

INDICATION(S) AND RESEARCH PHASE
Malignant Melanoma – Phase I
Malignant Melanoma – Phase II

vaccine, melanoma
Melacine

MANUFACTURER
Schering-Plough Corporation

DESCRIPTION
Melacine is a melanoma vaccine in phase III trials for the treatment of late-stage (III & IV) melanoma. Previous phase III trials demonstrated that the vaccine provided a survival rate equal to the standard four-drug chemotherapy.

Melacine consists of lysed cells from two human melanoma cell lines combined with the company's proprietary Detox adjuvant. Detox adjuvant includes MPL immunostimulant (monophosphoryl lipid A) and mycobacterial cell wall skeleton, both of which have a powerful effect in terms of activating the human immune system.

Melacine is being developed under a collaborative agreement between Schering-Plough and Corixa.

INDICATION(S) AND RESEARCH PHASE
Malignant Melanoma – Phase III
Vaccines – Phase III

Melanoma

aldesleukin, interleukin-2 (IL-2)
Proleukin

MANUFACTURER
Chiron Corporation

DESCRIPTION
Proleukin is a genetically engineered (recombinant) form of interleukin-2, which is a naturally occurring immune modulator. Proleukin is being evaluated in trials for the treatment of acute myelogenous leukemia, non-Hodgkin's lymphoma, and HIV infection. Additionally, Proleukin was approved in July 2000 for advanced-stage kidney cancer and melanoma.

INDICATION(S) AND RESEARCH PHASE
HIV Infection – Phase III
Leukemia – Phase III
Lymphoma, Non-Hodgkin's – Phase III
Renal Cell Carcinoma – FDA approved
Melanoma – FDA approved

CpG 7909
unknown

MANUFACTURER
Coley Pharmaceutical

DESCRIPTION
CpG 7909 is from a synthetic DNA sequence that naturally activates the human immune system to fight disease. CpG 7909 is being tested in three phase I/II trials for the treatment of cancer. The first trial has been initiated at the University of Iowa Cancer Center and is testing 24 subjects with refractory or relapsed non-Hodgkin's lymphoma. Subjects in this trial will receive weekly infusions of CpG 7909 for three weeks. Two other trials have been initiated in Europe. The first trial includes subjects with melanoma, while the second includes subjects with metastatic melanoma or basal cell carcinoma.

INDICATION(S) AND RESEARCH PHASE
Lymphoma, Non-Hodgkin's – Phase I/II
Melanoma – Phase I/II
Skin Cancer – Phase I/II

DISC GM-CSF
unknown

MANUFACTURER
Cantab Pharmaceuticals plc

DESCRIPTION
This new cancer therapy combines the immunostimulator GM-CSF with the DISC HsV delivery vector to create an anti-tumor/anti-cancer therapy with the potential to eliminate tumor growth, as well as target metastases that may have spread to other parts of body. This therapy may also provide the body with "immunological memory" to prevent recurrent tumors. DISC GM-CSF is currently in phase I trials for melanoma.

INDICATION(S) AND RESEARCH PHASE
Melanoma – Phase I

G3139/dacarbazine
Genasense/dacarbazine

MANUFACTURER
Genta

DESCRIPTION
Bcl-2, the target of Genasense (G3139) therapy, is a protein that appears to be a major contributing factor to cancer treatment resistance. Conversely, depletion of Bcl-2 may overcome both inherent and clinically acquired resistance to anticancer therapy, including chemotherapy, radiation, and monoclonal antibodies.

In November 2000, phase I/II trial results indicated that the compound reduced levels of bcl-2 protein, produced major antitumor responses, and possibly extended the life of subjects when used in combination with dacarbazine. The trial involved 14 subjects with advanced stage IV melanoma. A phase III trial has been initiated.

INDICATION(S) AND RESEARCH PHASE
Melanoma – Phase III

Novovac-M1
unknown

MANUFACTURER
Viventia Biotech

DESCRIPTION
Novovac-M1, otherwise known as 4B5, is a monoclonal human anti-idiotype antibody targeted to the ganglioside GD2, a molecule that is overexpressed in certain malignant cells. In January 2001, results of a phase I/II trial indicated that immunization with 4B5 led to a specific antibody response to the tumor cell target GD2 on the surface of melanoma cells. Sixteen subjects with metastatic melanoma were enrolled in the trial to establish the safety and immunogenicity of 4B5 alone and in combination with the adjuvants GM-CSF or Alum. Immunization with 4B5 was able to induce a low but specific immune response in 20% of subjects immunized with 4B5 without adjuvant and in 60% of subjects in the Alum group.

INDICATION(S) AND RESEARCH PHASE
Melanoma – Phase I/II completed

SB 249553
unknown

MANUFACTURER
GlaxoSmithKline

DESCRIPTION
SB 249553 is a recombinant pharmaccine in

phase II development for the treatment of lung cancer and melanoma.

INDICATION(S) AND RESEARCH PHASE
Lung Cancer – Phase II
Melanoma – Phase II

T64
unknown

MANUFACTURER
Tularik

DESCRIPTION
T64 is an antifolate that disrupts DNA synthesis through the inhibition of purine biosynthesis. The compound is currently in phase II trials in subjects with head and neck cancer, soft tissue sarcoma, melanoma, breast cancer, and non-small cell lung cancer. Additionally, T64 is in phase I combination trials with gemcitabine, doxorubicin, and paclitaxel. Tularik expects to initiate two additional T64 phase I combination trials with carboplatin and temozolamide in the first quarter of 2001. The T64 trials are being conducted in the United States, the United Kingdom, the Netherlands, and Australia.

INDICATION(S) AND RESEARCH PHASE
Head and Neck Cancer – Phase II
Sarcoma – Phase II
Melanoma – Phase II
Breast Cancer – Phase II
Lung Cancer – Phase II
Cancer/Tumors (Unspecified) – Phase I

unknown
Allovectin-7

MANUFACTURER
Vical

DESCRIPTION
Allovectin-7 is a DNA/lipid complex containing the human gene that encodes HLA-B7 antigen. The drug is to be injected directly into a tumor, where malignant cells absorb it and express the HLA-B7 antigen. This antigen alerts the immune system to the presence of foreign tissue, inducing an immune response.

Allovectin-7 is in clinical testing for subjects with metastatic melanoma and for subjects with tumors of the head and neck. For metastatic melanoma, a phase I/II trial is under way in subjects who have failed conventional therapies, and a phase III trial is being conducted in subjects who have never been treated with chemotherapy. In the phase I/II trial, Allovectin-7 will be administered in addition to low-dose interleukin-2. Subjects in the phase III trial will receive intravenous DTIC in addition to Allovectin-7. Additionally, a trial was initiated in February 2001 for the surgical treatment of early-stage cancer of the oral cavity and oropharynx.

INDICATION(S) AND RESEARCH PHASE
Melanoma – Phase III
Head and Neck Cancer – Phase II
Melanoma – Phase I/II
Oral Cavity Cancer – Phase II

vaccine, melanoma
unknown

MANUFACTURER
Genzyme Molecular Oncology

DESCRIPTION
This melanoma cancer vaccine utilizes a novel technology called dendritic/cancer cell fusion. This cell fusion technology combines a subject's dendritic cells with their inactivated tumor cells in a chemical fusion procedure. The fused cells are then injected back into the subject. A phase I/II trial testing this vaccine is under way in subjects with advanced stage metastatic melanoma.

INDICATION(S) AND RESEARCH PHASE
Melanoma – Phase I/II

Mesothelioma

ranpirnase
Onconase

MANUFACTURER
Alfacell

DESCRIPTION
Onconase (ranpirnase) is a novel ribonuclease that is unique among the superfamily of pancreatic ribonuclease. Over 700 subjects have been treated with Onconase, and the treatment was associated with only modest side effects. Additionally, in conjunction with the studies performed by the National Cancer Institute, Developmental Therapeutics Program, Onconase has shown significant anti-cancer activity in several animal tumor models. Currently, Onconase is being investigated in phase III trials in subjects with unresectable malignant mesothelioma.

INDICATION(S) AND RESEARCH PHASE
Mesothelioma – Phase III

unknown
Aroplatin

MANUFACTURER
Aronex Pharmaceuticals

DESCRIPTION
Platinum is a chemotherapeutic agent widely used in the treatment of solid tumors. Aroplatin is a liposomal formulation of a novel platinum product designed to overcome the toxicity and drug resistance associated with platinum use. It is currently in phase II trials for both mesothelioma and renal cell carcinoma.

INDICATION(S) AND RESEARCH PHASE
Mesothelioma – Phase II
Renal Cell Carcinoma – Phase II

Multiple Myeloma

AE-941
Neovastat

MANUFACTURER
AEterna Laboratories

DESCRIPTION
Neovastat is an angiogenesis inhibitor being tested for the treatment of non-small cell lung cancer, psoriasis, multiple myeloma

and kidney cancer, among other indications.

A phase II trial for multiple myeloma was initiated in October 2000. The trial will treat 120 subjects and include approximately 20 sites across North America and Europe. Trial results are expected in the summer of 2002.

Additionally, a phase III trial was initiated in May 2000 for kidney cancer, which will include 270 subjects at sites in North America and Europe.

INDICATION(S) AND RESEARCH PHASE
Lung Cancer – Phase III
Psoriasis and Psoriatic Disorders – Phase I/II completed
Cancer/Tumors (Unspecified) – Phase I/II completed
Multiple Myeloma – Phase II
Renal Cell Carcinoma – Phase III
Macular Degeneration – Phase I completed

APC8020
Mylovenge

MANUFACTURER
Dendreon Corporation

DESCRIPTION
Mylovenge is a therapeutic vaccine designed to trigger the immune system to recognize and destroy cancer cells. It involves isolating dendritic cells from a subject's blood and activating them with a protein, called an M component or idiotype, that is specific for each subject. The activated dendritic cells are infused back into the subject to stimulate an immune response.

Long-term follow-up data from phase II trials involving multiple myeloma and amyloidosis subjects were presented in December 2000. The trials indicated that Mylovenge caused disease regression or stabilization in more than 30% of subjects. In some subjects, these benefits were found to extend more than 18 months following treatment.

INDICATION(S) AND RESEARCH PHASE
Amyloidosis – Phase II completed
Multiple Myeloma – Phase II completed

arsenic trioxide (ATO)
Trisenox

MANUFACTURER
Cell Therapeutics

DESCRIPTION
Trisenox is believed to kill cancer cells through apoptosis. The mechanism of action of Trisenox is not fully understood, but the drug appears to induce apoptosis in a different manner than other anti-cancer agents such as retinoids.

Trisenox is FDA approved to treat acute promyelocytic leukemia (APL), and it is also in numerous trials in the United States for indications including other types of leukemia, prostate cancer, multiple myeloma, renal cell cancer, cervical cancer, and bladder cancer.

INDICATION(S) AND RESEARCH PHASE
Leukemia – Phase I
Lymphoma, Non-Hodgkin's – Phase II
Leukemia – Phase II
Multiple Myeloma – Phase II
Prostate Cancer – Phase II
Renal Cell Carcinoma – Phase II
Cervical Dysplasia/Cancer – Phase II
Bladder Cancer – Phase II

CDC 801
SelCIDs

MANUFACTURER
Celgene Corporation

DESCRIPTION
SelCIDs (selective cytokine inhibitory drugs) are oral immunotherapeutic agents that treat various inflammatory diseases by inhibiting phosphodiesterase type-4 enzyme (PDE-4). The inhibition of PDE-4 decreases production of tumor necrosis factor-alpha (TNF-α), a protein manufactured by cells of the immune system. This inhibition reduces the level of circulating TNF-α and, therefore, its ability to cause inflammation in cells. At normal levels, the protein is essential for effective immune function. However, overproduction of TNF as a result of age, genetic, and other influences contributes to the pathology of numerous diseases.

SelCIDs are in phase II trials for the following indications: inflammatory bowel disease, rheumatoid arthritis, multiple sclerosis, tuberculosis, autoimmune diseases, multiple myeloma, and mycobacterial infections such as leprosy.

INDICATION(S) AND RESEARCH PHASE
Inflammatory Bowel Disease – Phase II
Rheumatoid Arthritis – Phase II
Multiple Sclerosis – Phase II
Asthma – Phase discontinued
Tuberculosis – Phase II
Autoimmune Diseases – Phase II
Bacterial Infection – Phase II
Multiple Myeloma – Phase II

histamine dihydrochloride
Ceplene

MANUFACTURER
Maxim Pharmaceuticals

DESCRIPTION
Ceplene (formally Maxamine) is a histamine-2 (H-2) receptor stimulator that is being co-administered with immunotherapies, including cytokines and interleukin-2 (IL-2). Clinical testing includes treatment of acute myelogenous leukemia (AML), chronic hepatitis C, malignant melanoma, multiple myeloma, and renal cell carcinoma.

Results from a phase III trial in stage-IV malignant melanoma subjects indicated that Ceplene used in combination with a lower dose of interleukin-2 (IL-2) improved survival rates compared to treatment with the same doses of IL-2 alone. Treatment with Ceplene and IL-2 improved overall survival, increased survival rates at 12, 18, and 24 months, and improved time-to-disease progression compared to treatment with IL-2 alone. Twenty-five percent of subjects treated with Ceplene and lower-dose IL-2 survived for a 24-month period. Overall response was achieved in 38% of the subjects treated with Ceplene and lower-dose IL-2. The company received an NDA non-approvable letter in January 2001 because the FDA stated that the phase III trial forming the basis of the NDA would not be adequate as a single study to support approval.

INDICATION(S) AND RESEARCH PHASE
Hepatitis – Phase II
Leukemia – Phase III completed
Malignant Melanoma – NDA denied
Multiple Myeloma – Phase II
Renal Cell Carcinoma – Phase II

LDP-341, PS-341
unknown

MANUFACTURER
Millennium Pharmaceuticals

DESCRIPTION
LDP-341 is a proteasome inhibitor being developed for the treatment of cancer. In tumor cells, proteasome inhibition produces cellular stress by stabilizing cell cycle regulatory proteins and disrupting cell proliferation, ultimately leading to apoptosis. In preclinical studies, LDP-341 has shown activity against multiple myeloma cells. Additionally, LDP-341 appears to increase the effectiveness of other anti-cancer drugs by overcoming cellular resistance, which is a major cause of chemotherapy failure.

Among other programs, LDP-341 is currently in a phase I trial in subjects with advanced hematological malignancies. Preliminary results for this trial were presented in December 2000. LDP-341 reduced serum myeloma protein levels and myeloma cell numbers in bone marrow in two of three subjects with advanced multiple myeloma. The drug was well tolerated by these subjects and appears to have induced a complete response in one subject and a reduction in bone marrow plasma cells in another.

INDICATION(S) AND RESEARCH PHASE
Cancer/Tumors (Unspecified) – Phase I
Multiple Myeloma – Phase I

liposomal ether lipid
TLC ELL-12

MANUFACTURER
The Liposome Company

DESCRIPTION
TLC ELL-12 is a liposomal ether lipid that may have efficacy in the treatment of several cancers. This drug has exhibited significant anti-tumor activity, but did not have the hemolytic side effects common to this type of ether lipid when therapeutic doses were used in experimental models. It does not appear to be myelosuppressive.

TLC ELL-12 is currently being developed in phase I trials for the treatment of lung cancer, multiple myeloma, leukemia, and prostate cancer.

INDICATION(S) AND RESEARCH PHASE
Lung Cancer – Phase I
Multiple Myeloma – Phase I
Leukemia – Phase I
Prostate Cancer – Phase I

monoclonal antibody
BrevaRex MAb

MANUFACTURER
AltaRex

DESCRIPTION
BrevaRex MAb is a cancer immunotherapeutic being developed for the treatment of MUC1 expressing cancers. Multiple myeloma cells express tumor associated antigens that are ideal targets for immunotherapy. One such antigen is the core protein of MUC1. The ability of an antibody to bind to MUC1 is largely dependent on the extent of "mutation" of the antigen. In contrast to breast and certain more common cancers, MUC1 is highly mutated in virtually every multiple myeloma subject, thereby making antibody therapy targeting the core peptide more promising.

Results of a phase I trial in late-stage cancer subjects with substantial tumor burden indicated that BrevaRex MAb was well tolerated and without significant adverse effects. Also, immune responses were induced to both the antibody and MUC1, to which BrevaRex MAb is targeted.

Due to the limited therapy options for multiple myeloma, the BrevaRex clinical development program could possibly be accelerated under U.S. regulations. AltaRex expects to conduct the next trial in the second half of 2001, and if favorable results are obtained, a phase II/IIb trial may be initiated for registration.

INDICATION(S) AND RESEARCH PHASE
Multiple Myeloma – Phase I/II

skeletal targeted radiotherapy (STR)
unknown

MANUFACTURER
NeoRx Corporation

DESCRIPTION
Skeletal targeted radiotherapy (STR) uses a bone-targeting molecule as a means of administering radiation to the bone and bone marrow for the treatment of multiple myeloma. The molecule tightly binds Holmium-166, a beta emitting radionuclide.

The company reported that a completed phase I/II trial of this STR product resulted in an acceptable safety profile in the 28 subjects who had been monitored for safety, and that nine of 17 subjects achieved completed regression of their tumors.

INDICATION(S) AND RESEARCH PHASE
Multiple Myeloma – Phase III

unknown
Beta LT

MANUFACTURER
LifeTime Pharmaceuticals

DESCRIPTION
Beta LT is a new anti-cancer agent designed to stimulate the immune system, therefore having an anti-cancer effect. Positive results were noted in two phase I/II trials testing Beta LT as a treatment for progressing pre-malignant myeloma-related disease (MGUS) and for cancer treatment in subjects having the advanced disease. The 14 subjects treated received the target dose for up to one year with no serious side effects except for mild bowel habit changes in one subject. The trial took place at McGill University Jewish General Hospital in Montreal, Canada.

INDICATION(S) AND RESEARCH PHASE

Multiple Myeloma

Lymphomas – Phase I/II completed
Multiple Myeloma – Phase I/II completed

vaccine, cancer
unknown

MANUFACTURER
Genzyme Genetics Division

DESCRIPTION
This cancer vaccine is made from proteins associated with tumors taken from the individual subject. Phase I/II clinical trials are testing the vaccine in subjects suffering from B-cell lymphoma and multiple myeloma.

INDICATION(S) AND RESEARCH PHASE
Lymphomas – Phase I/II
Multiple Myeloma – Phase I/II

Wobe-Mugos-E
unknown

MANUFACTURER
Mucos Pharma GmbH

DESCRIPTION
Wobe-Mugos-E is an enzyme combination of papain, trypsin, and chymotrypsin being tested for its ability to improve the general health of cancer subjects. It may reduce the need for additional medications (such as pain relievers and antiemetics) during or after chemotherapy.

Wobe-Mugos-E is an alpha-macroglobulin that binds interleukins, TGF-β, TNF receptor I and II, hyperactive T-cells, and CRP. Given orally, the general health of cancer subjects was reported to increase (appetite improvement, weight gain, and reduction in fatigue and depression were observed). Leukopenia and thrombopenia induced by cancer cytostatic agents and radiation were reduced.

Clinical trials in phase II/III are evaluating this enzyme combination for multiple myeloma and effects of chemotherapy.

INDICATION(S) AND RESEARCH PHASE
Multiple Myeloma – Phase II/III
Effects of Chemotherapy – Phase II/III

YM-529, minodronate
unknown

MANUFACTURER
Yamanouchi Pharmaceutical

DESCRIPTION
YM-529 is a bisphosphonate being evaluated for the treatment of multiple myeloma and bone metastasis with breast cancer. The drug is manufactured in both oral and injectable formulations. It is in phase III trials and is part of Yamanouchi's domestic pipeline.

INDICATION(S) AND RESEARCH PHASE
Multiple Myeloma – Phase III
Breast Cancer – Phase III

Mycosis Fungoides

HOE-351
unknown

MANUFACTURER
Aventis

DESCRIPTION
HOE-351 is a novel compound designed for the treatment of superficial fungal infections of the skin (dermatomycoses). The company discontinued testing of the drug for mycosis fungoides in phase II trials.

INDICATION(S) AND RESEARCH PHASE
Mycosis Fungoides – Phase II discontinued

terbinafine
Lamisil

MANUFACTURER
Novartis

DESCRIPTION
Lamasil inhibits squalene epoxidase, a key enzyme in sterol biosynthesis, causing a decrease in ergosterol and a corresponding accumulation of sterol within fungal cells. The drug is being evaluated in phase III trials in an oral formulation for the treatment of both systemic mycoses and tinea capitis. Additionally, Lamisil is being tested in phase II trials for tinea capitis in children ages four years and younger.

INDICATION(S) AND RESEARCH PHASE
Pediatric, Tinea Capitis – Phase II
Tinea Capitis – Phase III
Mycosis Fungoides – Phase III

Myeloma

gallium maltolate
unknown

MANUFACTURER
Titan Pharmaceuticals

DESCRIPTION
Gallium is a semi-metallic element that has shown some therapeutic activity in metabolic bone disease, hypercalcemia of malignancy, and cancer. Gallium maltolate can displace divalent iron from the iron transporting protein, transferrin; thus gallium maltolate causes interference with iron metabolism with inhibition of enzymes requiring divalent iron. The most important of these in the cancer setting appears to be ribonucleotide reductase (RNR). Additionally, gallium appears to form salts with calcium and phosphate and become incorporated into bone. The bone that is created with incorporated gallium appears to be at least as strong as normal bone, and it appears to be more resistant to degradation by osteoclasts and tumor cells.

INDICATION(S) AND RESEARCH PHASE
Prostate Cancer – Phase I/II
Lymphomas – Phase I/II
Myeloma – Phase I/II
Bladder Cancer – Phase I/II
HIV Infection – Phase I/II

Neuroblastoma

vaccine, allogenic and autologous neuroblastoma cells
unknown

MANUFACTURER
St. Jude Children's Research Hospital

DESCRIPTION
Currently, phase II/III clinical trials are evaluating gene-modified cancer vaccines using autologous and allogenic (transplants from self and same species, respectively) tumor cells from interleukin-2 (IL-2) secreting neuroblastomas after autologous bone marrow transplant in first remission. Researchers are conducting parallel clinical trials in children with recurrent neuroblastoma who are receiving either allogenic or autologous tumor cells that are modified to secrete small amounts of IL-2.

In the autologous trial, one subject had a complete tumor response, one had a partial response and three had stable disease following the tumor immunogen alone. Four of the five subjects with tumor responses had co-existing neuroblastoma-specific cytotoxic T-lymphocyte activity, as opposed to only one of the subjects with non-responsive disease. These results show a promising correlation between immune response and clinical outcome with autologous vaccines.

In the allogenic group, one child had a partial response, five had stable disease, and four had progressive disease. Although immunization with autologous vaccine produced superior immune responses, these results offer encouragement for the continued pursuit of allogenic vaccine strategies in human cancer.

INDICATION(S) AND RESEARCH PHASE
Pediatric, Neuroblastoma – Phase II/III
Pediatric, Vaccines – Phase II/III

Oral Cavity Cancer

unknown
Allovectin-7

MANUFACTURER
Vical

DESCRIPTION
Allovectin-7 is a DNA/lipid complex containing the human gene that encodes HLA-B7 antigen. The drug is to be injected directly into a tumor, where malignant cells absorb it and express the HLA-B7 antigen. This antigen alerts the immune system to the presence of foreign tissue, inducing an immune response.

Allovectin-7 is in clinical testing for subjects with metastatic melanoma and for subjects with tumors of the head and neck. For metastatic melanoma, a phase I/II trial is under way in subjects who have failed conventional therapies, and a phase III trial is being conducted in subjects who have never been treated with chemotherapy. In the phase I/II trial, Allovectin-7 will be administered in addition to low-dose interleukin-2. Subjects in the phase III trial will receive intravenous DTIC in addition to Allovectin-7. Additionally, a phase II trial was initiated in February 2001 for the surgical treatment of early-stage cancer of the oral cavity and oropharynx.

INDICATION(S) AND RESEARCH PHASE
Melanoma – Phase III
Head and Neck Cancer – Phase II
Melanoma – Phase I/II
Oral Cavity Cancer – Phase II

Ovarian Cancer

APC8024
unknown

MANUFACTURER
Dendreon Corporation

DESCRIPTION
APC8024 is a vaccine designed to elicit an antibody response to a protein antigen called HER-2/*neu*. HER-2/*neu* is overexpressed in approximately 25% of metastatic breast cancers, ovarian, pancreatic, and colon cancers. APC8024 is being tested in phase I trials.

INDICATION(S) AND RESEARCH PHASE
Breast Cancer – Phase I
Ovarian Cancer – Phase I
Colon Malignancies – Phase I

BAY 12-9566
unknown

MANUFACTURER
Bayer Corporation

DESCRIPTION
Scientists believe that cancer cells produce enzymes called matrix metalloproteinases (MMPs) to break down the body's natural protective barriers, allowing cancer to grow and spread. MMP inhibitors, such as BAY 12-9566, are designed to interfere with this process.

Bayer Corporation was conducting phase III clinical trials of BAY 12-9566 for the treatment of arthritis, pancreatic cancer, ovarian cancer, and small and non-small cell lung cancer. However, the company announced that it has halted all clinical trials of its BAY 12-9566 in cancer and osteoarthritis. This action follows a recommendation from an independent Data Safety Monitoring Board that trials in small cell lung cancer be stopped.

INDICATION(S) AND RESEARCH PHASE
Lung Cancer – Trial discontinued
Pancreatic Cancer – Trial discontinued
Ovarian Cancer – Trial discontinued
Osteoarthritis – Trial discontinued

biricodar dicitrate, VX-710
Incel

MANUFACTURER
Vertex Pharmaceuticals

DESCRIPTION
Incel is a novel intravenous compound designed to treat multi-drug resistance of malignant cells. Incel may potentially resensitize drug-resistant tumors to chemotherapy by inhibiting molecular pumps that expel chemotherapy drugs. Vertex is developing compounds that block two major drug pumps or multi-drug resistance mechanisms: P-glycoprotein (MDR-1) and multidrug resistance-associated protein (MRP). Phase II trials investigating the activity of Incel in combination with other agents for the treatment of advanced refractory ovari-

an cancer and small cell lung cancer are currently under way.

INDICATION(S) AND RESEARCH PHASE
Lung Cancer – Phase II
Ovarian Cancer – Phase II

BMS-182751, JM-216
unknown

MANUFACTURER
Bristol-Myers Squibb

DESCRIPTION
In order for cancer cells to replicate, the double-stranded DNA has to separate or "unzip." Platinum (BMS-182751) appears to cause permanent links to form so that the DNA cannot unzip and the cell cannot reproduce. Intrastrand links permanently seal the two edges of the DNA zipper, while interstrand links seal two different parts of the zipper together, as in a loop. Recent evidence indicates that platinum causes more interstrand than intrastrand DNA links to form.

Additionally, the cell's built-in DNA-repair mechanism has trouble fixing the platinum links. Platinum may bind directly to the proteins that are involved in the repair mechanism, essentially making them inactive. This binding results in more damage to the cancer cell and more efficient tumor death. BMS-182751 is being tested in phase III trials for the treatment of lung and ovarian cancer.

INDICATION(S) AND RESEARCH PHASE
Lung Cancer – Phase III
Ovarian Cancer – Phase III

CP-358,774
unknown

MANUFACTURER
OSI Pharmaceuticals

DESCRIPTION
CP-358,774 is a small molecule inhibitor of the epidermal growth factor receptor (EGFR) tyrosine kinase. This drug targets the underlying molecular changes involving oncogenes and tumor suppressor genes, which play critical roles in the conversion of normal cells into cancerous cells. Increased expression of EGFR is an aberration frequently associated with a variety of cancers including ovarian, pancreatic, and non-small cell lung. The phase II clinical program is designed to assess CP-358,774 both as a single agent and in combination with existing chemotherapy regimens.

INDICATION(S) AND RESEARCH PHASE
Breast Cancer – Phase II
Lung Cancer – Phase II completed
Ovarian Cancer – Phase II
Head and Neck Cancer – Phase II

diarysulfonylurea, ILX-295501
unknown

MANUFACTURER
ILEX Oncology

DESCRIPTION
ILX-295501 belongs to a novel class of anti-tumor compounds called diarysulfonylureas. This orally formulated drug is in phase II trials for renal cell carcinoma, malignant melanoma, and lung and ovarian cancers.

INDICATION(S) AND RESEARCH PHASE
Renal Cell Carcinoma – Phase II
Malignant Melanoma – Phase II
Lung Cancer – Phase II
Ovarian Cancer – Phase II

docetaxel hydrate
Taxotere

MANUFACTURER
Aventis

DESCRIPTION
Many drugs for the treatment of cancer and other diseases originate in plants, many of them highly poisonous. Taxotere (docetaxel hydrate), an agent that inhibits the formation of new protoplasm, is derived from the renewable evergreen needles of the genus *Taxus* (Yew). Taxotere acts by disrupting the microtubular network in cells that is essential for cell division and many other cellular functions. The drug is approved for use in the United States for treatment of refractory breast cancer, refractory non-small cell lung cancer (NSCLC), and locally advanced or metastatic breast cancer.

New phase II/III trials are under way in head and neck, gastric, and ovarian cancers. Taxotere is also being tested either alone or in combination with other chemotherapy agents in the earlier stages of breast cancer, NSCLC, and other tumors.

Phase I extension studies are under way for brain metastasis and lung cancer.

INDICATION(S) AND RESEARCH PHASE
Gastric Cancer – Phase II/III
Head and Neck Cancer – Phase II/III
Lung Cancer – Phase II/III
Ovarian Cancer – Phase II/III
Breast Cancer – Phase III/IV
Brain Cancer – Phase I
Lung Cancer – Phase I

EMD 82633
unknown

MANUFACTURER
Merck KgaA

DESCRIPTION
EMD 82633 is a humanized and bispecific monoclonal antibody derived from mice. These antibodies are altered in such a way that they no longer appear different from human antibodies. This genetic modification prevents immune reactions against foreign substances of animal origin used in humans. In this bispecific drug, one component binds to tumor cells, while the other activates the body's own CD8 "killer cells" to attack cancer cells.

This new drug is being given as an adjuvant therapy to subjects who have not been adequately helped by conventional forms of treatment, such as chemotherapy. EMD 82633 is being tested in trials for the treatment of renal cancer, head and neck cancer, breast cancer, bladder cancer and ovarian cancer.

INDICATION(S) AND RESEARCH PHASE
Bladder Cancer – Phase II

Breast Cancer – Phase II
Cancer/Tumors (Unspecified) – Phase II
Head and Neck Cancer – Phase II
Ovarian Cancer – Phase II
Renal Cell Carcinoma – Phase II

FLT3 ligand
Mobist

MANUFACTURER
ImClone Systems

DESCRIPTION
Mobist is a hematopoietic growth factor being tested exvivo. It is a stem cell mobilizer and potential anti-tumor agent. Mobist is being evaluated in phase II trials for treatment of breast cancer, solid tumors, non-Hodgkin's lymphoma, and ovarian cancer.

INDICATION(S) AND RESEARCH PHASE
Cancer/Tumors (Unspecified) – Phase II
Breast Cancer – Phase II
Lymphoma, Non-Hodgkin's – Phase II
Ovarian Cancer – Phase II

FMdC
unknown

MANUFACTURER
Matrix Pharmaceutical

DESCRIPTION
FMdC is a nucleoside analogue being tested for the treatment of cancer. Nucleoside analogues are a class of drugs that affect DNA synthesis, and they have long been used to treat hematologic cancers such as leukemia. The early members of this drug class were minimally effective against solid tumors.

DNA synthesis occurs during cell division and is critical to successful cell replication. FMdC enters cells and is metabolized into two active forms: FMdC diphosphate and FMdC triphosphate. These two active metabolites interrupt the process of DNA synthesis, which leads to cell death. FMdC is being evaluated in phase II studies for the treatment of non-small cell lung cancer, colorectal, and ovarian cancer.

INDICATION(S) AND RESEARCH PHASE
Colorectal Cancer – Phase II
Lung Cancer – Phase II
Ovarian Cancer – Phase II

gemcitabine HCl
Gemzar

MANUFACTURER
Eli Lilly

DESCRIPTION
Gemzar, a nucleoside analogue, is a novel chemotherapeutic agent that mimics a natural building block of DNA. Gemzar disrupts the process of cell replication and thereby slows or stops progression of the disease. The drug is administered intravenously.

Gemzar is currently indicated as first-line treatment of locally advanced or metastatic pancreatic cancer and, in combination with cisplatin, for locally advanced or metastatic non-small cell lung cancer.

INDICATION(S) AND RESEARCH PHASE
Breast Cancer – Phase III
Lung Cancer – FDA approved
Ovarian Cancer – Phase III
Pancreatic Cancer – FDA approved

HER-2/neu dendritic cell vaccine
unknown

MANUFACTURER
Corixa Corporation

DESCRIPTION
The HER-2/*neu* dendritic cell vaccine is currently in phase I trials for breast and ovarian cancer.

INDICATION(S) AND RESEARCH PHASE
Breast Cancer – Phase I
Ovarian Cancer – Phase I
Vaccines – Phase I

hyperteria/doxorubicin
unknown

MANUFACTURER
BSD Medical

DESCRIPTION
Hyperteria/doxorubicin is being evaluated for the treatment of ovarian cancer in a phase I/II trial.

INDICATION(S) AND RESEARCH PHASE
Ovarian Cancer – Phase I/II

IM862
unknown

MANUFACTURER
Cytran

DESCRIPTION
IM862 is a small peptide comprised of two amino acids that may inhibit new blood vessel formation (angiogenesis). When there is excessive growth of new blood vessels, a number of pathological conditions can result, including malignant tumors, age-related macular degeneration, and vascular diseases. Limiting the growth of new blood vessels deprives tumors of nourishment essential for their survival. This drug is being developed in phase III trials for Kaposi's sarcoma and phase I/II trials for ovarian cancer.

INDICATION(S) AND RESEARCH PHASE
Kaposi's Sarcoma – Phase III
Ovarian Cancer – Phase I/II
Malignant Melanoma – Preclinical
Prostate Cancer – Preclinical

IMMU-MN14, anti-CEA
CEA-Cide

MANUFACTURER
Immunomedics

DESCRIPTION
Carcinoembryonic antigen (CEA) is a protein-polysaccharide complex released in the bloodstream by certain cancers, especially colon carcinoma. This antigenic substance may provide early diagnosis when used as a therapeutic marker in immunologic tests. The CEA complex may also be targeted by specialized monoclonal antibodies in the design of a biologic therapeutic.

CEA-Cide is a novel monoclonal antibody

that is designed for radioimmunotherapy (with 90 Y-labeled humanized MN-14). This drug is being tested in phase II trials for the treatment of advanced metastatic and CEA-producing cancers, particularly colorectal cancer. Other indications may include breast cancer, female reproductive system cancer, ovarian cancer, lung cancer, and pancreatic cancer.

INDICATION(S) AND RESEARCH PHASE
Breast Cancer – Phase II
Cancer/Tumors (Unspecified) – Phase II
Colorectal Cancer – Phase II
Lung Cancer – Phase II
Ovarian Cancer – Phase II
Pancreatic Cancer – Phase II

INGN-201, adenoviral p53
unknown

MANUFACTURER
Introgen Therapeutics

DESCRIPTION
INGN-201 is a p53 gene therapy product. It has been tested as a treatment for a variety of solid tumor cancers with administration via intratumoral injection. The drug was well tolerated according to the company, and additional trials are under way using an intravenous infusion in order to reach more types of cancers. The tumor-suppressing p53 gene encodes a protein that responds to damage involving cellular DNA by terminating cell division. Normal p53 genes are delivered into cancer cells of the subject through an adenoviral vector.

The developers of INGN-201 have signed a Cooperative Research and Development Agreement (CRADA) with the National Cancer Institute to evaluate the potential effectiveness and superiority of the drug over other treatments against breast, ovarian, bladder, prostate, and brain cancers in phase I and phase II trials. A phase III trial in head and neck cancer was initiated in March 2000.

INDICATION(S) AND RESEARCH PHASE
Head and Neck Cancer – Phase III
Bladder Cancer – Phase I
Brain Cancer – Phase I
Breast Cancer – Phase I
Bronchoalveolar Cancer – Phase I
Ovarian Cancer – Phase I
Prostate Cancer – Phase I
Lung Cancer – Phase II
Cancer/Tumors (Unspecified) – Phase I

marimastat, BB-2516
unknown

MANUFACTURER
British Biotech plc

DESCRIPTION
Marimastat is an inhibitor of matrix metalloproteinase (MMP), a family of naturally occurring enzymes that are over-produced in a number of disease states. This is especially true of cancer, where MMPs are involved in the spread and local growth of tumors. Both angiogenesis and metastasis require MMPs during tumor invasion. Anti-angiogenic strategies, unlike other therapeutic approaches, do not aim to directly destroy or "kill" the tumor or cause tumor regression. Rather, they are designed to prevent the further growth of tumors by limiting their blood supply. Because peripheral tumor cells could theoretically survive on a diffusion-dependent basis, anti-angiogenic drugs may prove most effective when given in combination with other standard cytotoxic regimens. As of October 2000, marimastat is in phase III development for the treatment of cancer.

In 1999, British Biotech and Schering-Plough Corporation signed an agreement to develop and commercialize British Biotech's metalloproteinase inhibitors, including marimastat.

INDICATION(S) AND RESEARCH PHASE
Pancreatic Cancer – Phase III
Lung Cancer – Phase III
Breast Cancer – Phase III
Brain Cancer – Phase III completed
Ovarian Cancer – Phase III

MDX-210
unknown

MANUFACTURER
Medarex

DESCRIPTION
MDX-210 is a bispecific (target-trigger) monoclonal antibody (MAb)-based treatment being developed for cancers with specific markers (HER-2/*neu* positive), including renal cell, non-small cell lung, pancreatic and prostate cancer. Phase II trials have been completed for kidney, prostate, and ovarian cancer. Phase III trials for ovarian cancer have commenced in Europe.

INDICATION(S) AND RESEARCH PHASE
Prostate Cancer – Phase II completed
Renal Cell Carcinoma – Phase II completed
Colon Malignancies – Phase II
Breast Cancer – Phase II
Gastric Cancer – Phase II
Pancreatic Cancer – Phase II
Lung Cancer – Phase II
Ovarian Cancer – Phase III

MDX-220
unknown

MANUFACTURER
Medarex

DESCRIPTION
MDX-220 is a bispecific (target-trigger) monoclonal antibody (MAb) that targets Tag-72 in the treatment of a variety of cancers, including lung, colon, prostate, ovarian, endometrial, pancreatic, and gastric cancer.

INDICATION(S) AND RESEARCH PHASE
Endometrial Cancer – Phase I/II
Gastric Cancer – Phase I/II
Lung Cancer – Phase I/II
Ovarian Cancer – Phase I/II
Pancreatic Cancer – Phase I/II
Prostate Cancer – Phase II
Colorectal Cancer – Phase II

MGI-114, hydroxymethylacylfulvene, HMAF
Irofulven

MANUFACTURER

MGI Pharma

DESCRIPTION

Irofulven (MGI-114) is the first product candidate being developed by MGI Pharma from its family of anti-cancer compounds called acylfulvenes. Early trials demonstrated that Irofulven is absorbed rapidly by tumor cells, and once inside binds to DNA and protein targets. The binding interferes with DNA replication and cell division, leading to tumor-specific cell death. The drug is being tested in a series of trials for a variety of cancers.

In November 2000, results from a phase II trial of Irofulven indicated that the drug produced anti-tumor activity in subjects with advanced pancreatic cancer who were refractory to gemcitabine (Gemzar). Ten of the 53 subjects enrolled achieved six-month survival and two subjects demonstrated objective responses: one subject experienced tumor shrinkage of 100% and another subject experienced an 84% decrease in tumor mass. A phase III trial was initiated in February 2001.

INDICATION(S) AND RESEARCH PHASE
Breast Cancer – Phase II
Colon Malignancies – Phase II
Renal Cell Carcinoma – Phase II
Cervical Dysplasia/Cancer – Phase II
Lung Cancer – Phase II
Ovarian Cancer – Phase I/II
Colorectal Cancer – Phase II
Prostate Cancer – Phase I/II
Cancer/Tumors (Unspecified) – Phase I/II
Pancreatic Cancer – Phase III
Liver Cancer – Phase II

murine monoclonal antibody
Theragyn

MANUFACTURER
Antisoma plc

DESCRIPTION

Theragyn is composed of a mouse monoclonal antibody (HMFG1) linked to a radioactive isotope. It is thought small numbers of residual tumor cells remaining in the abdomen after surgery and chemotherapy are one of the main causes of relapse. These residual tumor cells are the targets of Theragyn. Theragyn uses the natural targeting ability of antibodies to selectively deliver radioactivity to tumor cells.

Theragyn is being tested as an adjuvant treatment in phase II trials for gastric cancer and in phase III trials for ovarian cancer.

INDICATION(S) AND RESEARCH PHASE
Gastric Cancer – Phase II
Ovarian Cancer – Phase III

NX 211
unknown

MANUFACTURER
Gilead Sciences

DESCRIPTION

NX 211 is a liposomal formulation of a novel topoisomerase I inhibitor for the treatment of various solid tumors. A phase II trial has been initiated at five sites in the United States. It includes 58 subjects with ovarian cancer who have progressed or relapsed within six months of treatment with a regimen including topotecan. The trial will evaluate the efficacy and safety of NX 211 as determined by response rate, time to disease progression, and subject tolerance. Subjects will be treated with NX 211 on days one and eight, to be repeated every 21 days.

Additionally, a phase II trial was also initiated to test NX 211 in 87 subjects with recurrent small cell lung cancer at numerous sites in the United States.

INDICATION(S) AND RESEARCH PHASE
Ovarian Cancer – Phase II
Lung Cancer – Phase II

p53 tumor suppressor gene
unknown

MANUFACTURER
Schering-Plough Corporation

DESCRIPTION

This gene therapy is being developed in an injectable formulation for the treatment of ovarian cancer. Phase II trials are testing its effectiveness on a variety of solid tumors that carry the p53 gene mutation or deletion. Preclinical studies have shown that when a normal p53 gene is inserted into a malignant cell where the gene is either absent or mutated, this new agent suppresses or kills the abnormal tumor cell. This type of p53 transgene expression may offer cancer subjects with solid tumors another avenue of therapy if trials prove this agent to be safe and effective.

INDICATION(S) AND RESEARCH PHASE
Ovarian Cancer – Phase II

PSC 833, valspodar
Amdray

MANUFACTURER
Novartis

DESCRIPTION

Amdray, a multi-drug resistance (MDR) modulator, is a non-immunosuppressive and non-nephrotoxic derivative of cyclosporine. One mechanism through which MDR occurs is P-glycoprotein (P-gp) overexpression. P-gp is a protein within the cancer cell membrane that "pumps" cytotoxic drugs from the cell, thereby preventing these drugs from reaching toxic levels and causing cell death. Amdray works as a potent inhibitor of P-gp. It is currently being tested in phase III trials in an oral formulation for the treatment of ovarian cancer.

INDICATION(S) AND RESEARCH PHASE
Ovarian Cancer – Phase III

RFS-2000
Rubitecan

MANUFACTURER
SuperGen

DESCRIPTION

Rubitecan is a novel drug that works by inhibiting an enzyme called topoisomerase I. This drug is made in an oral formulation, which is an advantage for outpatient treatment compared to intravenous cancer drugs that may require a visit to a hospital setting.

In addition to treating pancreatic cancer, Rubitecan is being evaluated in treating a variety of solid tumors, such as in breast, colorectal, lung, ovarian, and prostate cancers, as well as metastatic melanoma and advanced gastric carcinoma. Additionally, phase II trials in the United States and Europe are testing Rubitecan in blood cancers such as chronic myelomonocytic leukemia (CMML/myelodysplastic syndrome).

INDICATION(S) AND RESEARCH PHASE
Pancreatic Cancer – Phase III
Breast Cancer – Phase II
Colorectal Cancer – Phase II
Gastric Cancer – Phase II
Leukemia – Phase II
Malignant Melanoma – Phase II
Ovarian Cancer – Phase II
Myelodysplastic Syndrome – Phase III

squalamine
unknown

MANUFACTURER
Magainin Pharmaceuticals

DESCRIPTION
Squalamine is an aminosterol compound isolated from the tissues of the dogfish shark. This drug inhibits salt and acid regulating pumps on endothelial cells that normally line blood vessels, which prevents growth factors from stimulating the cells to form capillaries. It is thought that this activity results in anti-angiogenisis, anti-inflammatory, and anti-tumor effects.

The company is conducting several phase II trials testing squalamine for the treatment of certain cancers, such as breast and ovarian. Additionally, there is a phase IIa trial for stage IIIB and IV non-small cell lung cancer being conducted at the University of Wisconsin and M.D. Anderson, Houston, Texas.

Additional studies are being planned for ovarian cancer, pediatric neuroblastoma, and other solid tumors.

INDICATION(S) AND RESEARCH PHASE
Breast Cancer – Phase II
Lung Cancer – Phase IIa
Ovarian Cancer – Phase II
Cancer/Tumors (Unspecified) – Phase II

SU-101
unknown

MANUFACTURER
Sugen

DESCRIPTION
SU-101 is a synthetic, platelet-derived, growth factor receptor, which blocks the essential enzyme, tyrosine kinase. This drug may be helpful for the treatment of end-stage malignant glioma, a tumor of nerve tissue. The drug is being tested in phase III trials for refractory brain and prostate cancers, and phase II trials for non-small cell lung and ovarian cancers.

INDICATION(S) AND RESEARCH PHASE
Brain Cancer – Phase III
Prostate Cancer – Phase III
Lung Cancer – Phase II
Ovarian Cancer – Phase II

tgDCC-E1A, RGG 0853
unknown

MANUFACTURER
Targeted Genetics

DESCRIPTION
The drug E1A may possess multiple cancer-fighting effects, such as reducing expression (also called "down-regulation") of the oncogene HER-2/*neu*. Overexpression of HER-2/*neu* occurs in substantial percentages of ovarian and breast cancer subjects, as well as in cancers of the lung, prostate, and bladder. Furthermore, HER-2/*neu* correlates with poor prognosis, including metastasis—the process by which cancer spreads to other sites in the body.

Clinical phase I trials for breast, ovarian, and head and neck cancers are complete, as well as a phase II trial for head and neck cancer as a single agent. A second phase II has been initiated to test tgDCC-E1A in combination with radiation therapy for the treatment of head and neck squamous cell carcinoma. The phase II trial expects to treat up to 50 subjects who will receive twice-weekly injections of tgDCC-E1A throughout six to seven weeks of radiation therapy.

INDICATION(S) AND RESEARCH PHASE
Breast Cancer – Phase I completed
Head and Neck Cancer – Phase II
Ovarian Cancer – Phase I completed

topotecan HCl
Hycamtin

MANUFACTURER
GlaxoSmithKline

DESCRIPTION
Hycamtin (topotecan HCl) is a topoisomerase I inhibitor administered by injection. It is currently indicated for the treatment of metastatic carcinoma of the ovary after failure of initial or subsequent chemotherapy. Hycamtin is also indicated for the treatment of small cell lung cancer sensitive disease after failure of first-line chemotherapy.

Hycamtin is being evaluated in a variety of phase II and III trials. It is being tested as a second-line therapy for the treatment of colorectal cancer, as first-line therapy for small cell and non-small cell lung cancer, as oral second-line therapy for small cell lung cancer, and as first-line therapy for ovarian cancer and myelodysplastic syndrome.

INDICATION(S) AND RESEARCH PHASE
Colorectal Cancer – Phase II
Lung Cancer – Phase II
Lung Cancer – Phase III
Ovarian Cancer – Phase III
Myelodysplastic Syndrome – Phase III

troxacitabine, BCH-4556
Troxatyl

MANUFACTURER
BioChem Pharma

DESCRIPTION
Troxatyl is a dioxolane nucleoside analog being investigated as an anticancer agent. The drug is a complete DNA chain termina-

tor and DNA polymerase inhibitor. It acts by incorporating itself into the growing DNA chain of cancer cells, interfering with their ability to replicate further. Troxatyl is being evaluated as a single agent or in combination therapy in a number of ongoing trials for hematologic malignancies, including acute myeloid leukemia, and chronic myeloid leukemia (blastic phase), and in lymphoproliferative disorders such as lymphoma, chronic lymphocytic leukemia and myeloma. It is also being evaluated as a single agent in pancreatic cancer and in combination therapy in a number of solid tumors. Troxatyl is currently in phase II development.

INDICATION(S) AND RESEARCH PHASE
Cancer/Tumors (Unspecified) – Phase II
Colorectal Cancer – Phase II
Head and Neck Cancer – Phase II
Leukemia – Phase II
Lung Cancer – Phase II
Malignant Melanoma – Phase II
Ovarian Cancer – Phase II
Pancreatic Cancer – Phase II
Prostate Cancer – Phase II
Renal Cell Carcinoma – Phase II

unknown
OvaRex

MANUFACTURER
AltaRex

DESCRIPTION
OvaRex contains a murine monoclonal antibody that binds to a specific tumor associated antigen (CA 125). This antigen is over-expressed by ovarian cancer cells in most subjects with the disease. OvaRex is an immunotherapeutic agent that increases the natural immune response to ovarian cancer cells. Preliminary phase II results indicated that OvaRex induced a tumor-specific cellular immune response in the first ovarian cancer subject from the prospective, open-label trial.

INDICATION(S) AND RESEARCH PHASE
Ovarian Cancer – Phase III

unknown
HMFG1

MANUFACTURER
Abbott Laboratories

DESCRIPTION
HMFG1 (Human Milk Fat Globule 1) is being tested in phase III trials for the treatment of ovarian cancer. HMFG1 will be given through a single injection, and it is designed to attach to and destroy cancer cells. Subject follow up will last two years and study visits will be required once a week for the first eight weeks following treatment. HMFG1 is being co-developed by Abbott Laboratories and Antisoma.

INDICATION(S) AND RESEARCH PHASE
Ovarian Cancer – Phase III

vaccine, tumor cell suspension
O-Vax

MANUFACTURER
AVAX Technologies

DESCRIPTION
O-Vax is a vaccine composed of an immunogenic (haptenized) tumor cell suspension that was developed for the treatment of stage III ovarian cancer subjects. Currently, O-Vax is being tested in a phase II clinical trial that will enroll 400 subjects.

The company reported that results from two previous studies treating 17 women showed O-Vax to induce an immunological (DTH) response to the subject's own tumor cells. O-Vax prepared from the subject's tumor tissue taken at the time of surgical debulking was administered following standard chemotherapy.

About 80% of women initially respond to standard chemotherapy; however, the majority of these women will subsequently develop recurrent disease. Currently, there are limited therapies available for subjects who initially respond to chemotherapy, but are at high risk of having their cancer return.

INDICATION(S) AND RESEARCH PHASE
Ovarian Cancer – Phase II

valrubicin
Valstar

MANUFACTURER
Anthra Pharmaceuticals

DESCRIPTION
Valstar Intravesical Solution is a lipophilic anthracycline-like chemotherapeutic agent. The drug acts by penetrating cells where it affects a variety of biological functions, most of which involve nucleic acid metabolism.

Previously approved for treatment of subjects with BCG-refractory carcinoma in situ (CIS) for whom surgical removal of the bladder would present unacceptable risks of morbidity or mortality, Valstar is in phase III trials for treatment of papillary bladder cancer.

Valstar is also in phase III trials for treatment of refractory ovarian cancer. For this indication, the drug is administered through the abdomen (intraperitoneal).

INDICATION(S) AND RESEARCH PHASE
Bladder Cancer – Phase III
Ovarian Cancer – Phase III

VX-710
Incel

MANUFACTURER
Vertex Pharmaceuticals

DESCRIPTION
Incel blocks two major multi-drug resistance mechanisms: P-glycoprotein (MDR-1) and multi-drug resistance-associated protein (MRP). Administered intravenously, Incel is to be used in combination with cancer chemotherapy agents. Vertex's research shows that Incel can enhance the accumulation of chemotherapy agents in tumor cells by blocking the drug pumps P-gp and MRP, and that it is capable of restoring the sensitivity of tumors to treatment with chemotherapeutic agents. Phase II trials investigating the activity of Incel in combination with other agents for the

treatment of advanced refractory ovarian cancer, soft tissue sarcoma, and small cell lung cancer are under way.

INDICATION(S) AND RESEARCH PHASE
Lung Cancer – Phase II
Ovarian Cancer – Phase II
Sarcoma – Phase II

XR5000
unknown

MANUFACTURER
Xenova

DESCRIPTION
XR5000 is a topoisomerase I and II inhibitor being developed for the treatment of common solid tumors. Three phase II trials are under way at a number of European centers. The trials are being conducted on an "open-label" basis and target three cancer types—ovarian, non-small cell lung, and glioblastoma. The results of a fourth phase II trial, in which the efficacy of XR5000 was investigated in subjects with colorectal cancer, were announced in June 2000. No complete or partial responses to treatment were observed after two courses of treatment with XR5000. Two subjects showed stable disease and 13 subjects experienced disease progression. The company is not planning any further recruitment for this indication.

INDICATION(S) AND RESEARCH PHASE
Brain Cancer – Phase II
Colorectal Cancer – Phase II completed
Lung Cancer – Phase II
Ovarian Cancer – Phase II

ZD-0473/AMD 473
unknown

MANUFACTURER
AstraZeneca

DESCRIPTION
ZD-0473 is a new platinum-based anti-cancer agent designed to deliver an extended spectrum of activity and overcome resistance to currently approved platinum drugs, such as cisplatin and carboplatin. It is being evaluated for the treatment of a range of solid-tumor cancers, including colorectal, non-small cell lung, and bladder cancer, which are resistant to carboplatin. ZD-0473 is formulated in both intravenous and oral forms. The IV formulation is in phase II trials and the oral form is in pre-clinical development. AnorMED has a licensing agreement with AstraZeneca who is conducting the phase II study development of ZD-0473.

INDICATION(S) AND RESEARCH PHASE
Bladder Cancer – Phase II
Cancer/Tumors (Unspecified) – Phase II
Colorectal Cancer – Phase II
Lung Cancer – Phase II
Ovarian Cancer – Phase II
Prostate Cancer – Phase II
Breast Cancer – Phase II
Cervical Dysplasia/Cancer – Phase II

Pancreatic Cancer

BAY 12-9566
unknown

MANUFACTURER
Bayer Corporation

DESCRIPTION
Scientists believe that cancer cells produce enzymes called matrix metalloproteinases (MMPs) to break down the body's natural protective barriers, allowing cancer to grow and spread. MMP inhibitors, such as BAY 12-9566, are designed to interfere with this process.

Bayer Corporation was conducting phase III clinical trials of BAY 12-9566 for the treatment of arthritis, pancreatic cancer, ovarian cancer, and small and non-small cell lung cancer. However, the company announced that it has halted all clinical trials of its BAY 12-9566 in cancer and osteoarthritis. This action follows a recommendation from an independent Data Safety Monitoring Board that trials in small cell lung cancer be stopped.

INDICATION(S) AND RESEARCH PHASE
Lung Cancer – Trial discontinued
Pancreatic Cancer – Trial discontinued
Ovarian Cancer – Trial discontinued
Osteoarthritis – Trial discontinued

CEP-701
unknown

MANUFACTURER
Cephalon

DESCRIPTION
CEP-701 is an orally active inhibitor of the enzyme tyrosine kinase. It works as a signal transduction modulator for the treatment of various cancers. CEP-701 is being evaluated in phase II studies for prostate cancer and pancreatic ductal adenocarcinoma.

INDICATION(S) AND RESEARCH PHASE
Pancreatic Cancer – Phase II
Prostate Cancer – Phase II

CI-1042, ONYX-015
unknown

MANUFACTURER
Onyx Pharmaceuticals

DESCRIPTION
CI-1042 (ONYX-015) is a tumor-selective, modified adenovirus (similar to the common cold virus) that has been genetically engineered to replicate in and kill cancer cells that possess a mutated oncogene called p53, while sparing normal cells with functioning p53. p53 Is a tumor suppressor gene that is mutated in approximately 50% of all human cancers. CI-1042 is in development for several indications, including pancreatic cancer, liver metastases of colorectal cancer, and lung cancer.

In November 2000, results of a phase II trial demonstrated that CI-1042 administered as a single-agent replicates and causes tumor regression in refractory head and neck cancer. CI-1042 was shown to selectively target cancer cells containing a mutant p53 gene, while sparing normal cells with a functioning p53 gene. Of the 19 subjects who received the standard dosing regimen, four (21%) had an objective response, including two complete responses and two partial responses. CI-1042 is being co-developed with Pfizer.

INDICATION(S) AND RESEARCH PHASE
Colorectal Cancer – Phase II
Pancreatic Cancer – Phase II
Head and Neck Cancer – Phase III
Cervical Dysplasia/Cancer – Phase I completed
Lung Cancer – Phase II
Bladder Cancer – Phase I completed
Brain Cancer – Phase I completed

CTP-37
Avicine

MANUFACTURER
AVI BioPharma

DESCRIPTION
Avicine is a hormone vaccine derived from human chorionic gonadotropin peptide that is being tested for prevention of colorectal, pancreatic, and prostate cancer. The drug is in phase II trials for prostate cancer, and phase III trials for colorectal and pancreatic cancer. AVI BioPharma has partnered with SuperGen and under the terms of the agreement, SuperGen will be responsible for U.S. marketing and sales of Avicine, and AVI will be responsible for product manufacturing.

INDICATION(S) AND RESEARCH PHASE
Colorectal Cancer – Phase III
Pancreatic Cancer – Phase III
Prostate Cancer – Phase II

diethylnorspermine
DENSPM

MANUFACTURER
GelTex Pharmaceuticals

DESCRIPTION
DENSPM (diethylnorspermine) is similar to a naturally produced polyamine, except that it may interrupt the rapid growth of tumor cells that need polyamines for growth. The drug is in phase II trials for renal cell carcinoma, pancreatic cancer, malignant melanoma, and non-small cell lung cancer. Additional indications may include ovarian and colon cancers.

INDICATION(S) AND RESEARCH PHASE
Renal Cell Carcinoma – Phase II
Pancreatic Cancer – Phase II
Malignant Melanoma – Phase II
Lung Cancer – Phase II

GBC-590
unknown

MANUFACTURER
Safe Sciences

DESCRIPTION
GBC-590 belongs to a new class of drugs called lectin inhibitors that specifically interfere with cellular interactions. GBC-590 competitively binds to unique lectins (special protein cell-surface receptors) on cancer cells and disrupts the metastatic process. GBC-590's affinity for cancer lectins is the core reason for its significant biological activity and specificity.

GBC-590 is being tested in phase II trials for pancreatic and colorectal cancer, and the company plans to test the drug in phase II trials for prostate cancer.

INDICATION(S) AND RESEARCH PHASE
Colorectal Cancer – Phase II
Pancreatic Cancer – Phase II
Prostate Cancer – Phase I/II

gemcitabine HCl
Gemzar

MANUFACTURER
Eli Lilly

DESCRIPTION
Gemzar, a nucleoside analogue, is a novel chemotherapeutic agent that mimics a natural building block of DNA. Gemzar disrupts the process of cell replication and thereby slows or stops progression of the disease. The drug is administered intravenously.

Gemzar is currently indicated as first-line treatment of locally advanced or metastatic pancreatic cancer and, in combination with cisplatin, for locally advanced or metastatic non-small cell lung cancer.

INDICATION(S) AND RESEARCH PHASE
Bladder Cancer – Phase III
Lung Cancer – FDA approved
Pancreatic Cancer – Phase II completed

HSPPC-96
Oncophage

MANUFACTURER
Antigenics

DESCRIPTION
Oncophage cancer vaccine is an injectable protein that contains the unique profile ("antigenic fingerprint") of each subject's cancer. The antigens activate the immune system to elicit an anti-tumor response. Oncophage is in clinical trials for several indications, including renal cell carcinoma (phase III), melanoma (phase II), colorectal cancer (phase II), gastric cancer (phase I/II), pancreatic cancer (phase I/II completed), and non-Hodgkin's lymphoma (phase II).

In October 2000, Antigenics announced that it had initiated a phase II trial of Oncophage in subjects who have been diagnosed with sarcoma, also known as soft tissue cancer. The study is expected to initially enroll 20 subjects diagnosed with recurrent metastatic or unresectable soft tissue sarcoma and may be expanded to include an additional 15 subjects depending on preliminary results.

INDICATION(S) AND RESEARCH PHASE
Renal Cell Carcinoma – Phase III
Malignant Melanoma – Phase II
Colorectal Cancer – Phase II
Gastric Cancer – Phase I/II
Pancreatic Cancer – Phase I/II completed
Lymphoma, Non-Hodgkin's – Phase II
Sarcoma – Phase II

HuC242-DM1/SB-408075
unknown

MANUFACTURER
ImmunoGen

DESCRIPTION

HuC242-DM1/SB-408075 is a tumor-activated prodrug (TAP) designed for the treatment of colorectal, pancreatic, and certain non-small cell lung cancers. Tumor-activated prodrugs consist of chemically linked monoclonal antibodies and potent, cell-killing chemicals. HuC242-DM1, in particular, is created by joining the cytotoxic maytansinoid drug DM1 with the humanized monoclonal antibody C242. The attached chemical remains inactive until the monoclonal antibody reaches its targeted tumor cell and the TAP is drawn inside. Once inside, DM1 is able to kill the tumor cell without affecting surrounding healthy cells. HuC242-DM1 is currently in phase I/II trials.

INDICATION(S) AND RESEARCH PHASE
Colorectal Cancer – Phase I/II
Pancreatic Cancer – Phase I/II
Lung Cancer – Phase I/II

IMC-C225, CPT-11
unknown

MANUFACTURER
ImClone Systems

DESCRIPTION
IMC-C225 is a chimerized (part mouse, part human) monoclonal antibody that may help fight cancer cells when used in conjunction with radiation therapy or other chemotherapy agents. This antibody selectively blocks the epidermal growth factor receptor (EGFr), which may be present in greater amounts on actively growing tumor cells. Since many cancers use specific growth factors to stimulate tumor cell growth, blocking this receptor may inhibit the cancer from increasing in size and spreading throughout the body.

The company is conducting phase III clinical trials evaluating IMC-C225 in combination with radiotherapy and with chemotherapy in subjects with advanced squamous cell head and neck carcinoma. IMC-C225 is in trials for several other indications in combination with various anti-cancer agents.

INDICATION(S) AND RESEARCH PHASE
Breast Cancer – Phase I/II
Head and Neck Cancer – Phase III
Lung Cancer – Phase III
Prostate Cancer – Phase I/II
Renal Cell Carcinoma – Phase II
Pancreatic Cancer – Phase II
Colorectal Cancer – Phase II

IMMU-MN14, anti-CEA
CEA-Cide

MANUFACTURER
Immunomedics

DESCRIPTION
Carcinoembryonic antigen (CEA) is a protein-polysaccharide complex released in the bloodstream by certain cancers, especially colon carcinoma. This antigenic substance may provide early diagnosis when used as a therapeutic marker in immunologic tests. The CEA complex may also be targeted by specialized monoclonal antibodies in the design of a biologic therapeutic.

CEA-Cide is a novel monoclonal antibody that is designed for radioimmunotherapy (with 90 Y-labeled humanized MN-14). This drug is being tested in phase II trials for the treatment of advanced metastatic and CEA-producing cancers, particularly colorectal cancer. Other indications may include breast cancer, female reproductive system cancer, ovarian cancer, lung cancer, and pancreatic cancer.

INDICATION(S) AND RESEARCH PHASE
Breast Cancer – Phase II
Cancer/Tumors (Unspecified) – Phase II
Colorectal Cancer – Phase II
Lung Cancer – Phase II
Ovarian Cancer – Phase II
Pancreatic Cancer – Phase II

ISIS 2503
unknown

MANUFACTURER
Isis Pharmaceuticals

DESCRIPTION
ISIS 2503 is a potent, selective antisense inhibitor of H-ras gene expression. Antisense drugs inhibit the production of disease-causing proteins by altering the genetic information, which messenger RNA uses to produce new protein. H-ras is one of a family of ras genes that are involved in the process by which cells receive and send signals that affect their behavior. The company claims that substantial evidence exists to support a direct role for the ras gene products in the development and maintenance of human cancers.

In phase II trials, the compound is being evaluated as a single-agent in subjects with colon, breast, pancreatic, and non-small cell lung cancers. These trials will provide preliminary data on the anti-tumor activity of ISIS 2503 against these common tumor types. Approximately ten sites in the United States and Europe will enroll 15-30 subjects per tumor type in these trials. The company plans future trials of ISIS 2503 in combination with approved cancer therapies.

INDICATION(S) AND RESEARCH PHASE
Breast Cancer – Phase II
Colon Malignancies – Phase II
Lung Cancer – Phase II
Pancreatic Cancer – Phase II

ISIS 5132, CGP 69846A
unknown

MANUFACTURER
Isis Pharmaceuticals

DESCRIPTION
ISIS 5132 is a potent antisense inhibitor of the enzyme c-Raf-1 kinase. Antisense drugs inhibit the production of disease-causing proteins by altering the genetic information that messenger RNA uses to produce new protein. c-Raf kinase plays a role in signal processes that regulate cell growth and proliferation. It is one of a family of raf genes thought to play an important role in the development of some solid tumors. The company reports that activated raf has also been detected in a substantial variety of human cancers including small cell lung carcinoma and breast cancer. For example, it has been reported that 60% of all lung carcinoma cells express unusually high levels of normal c-Raf mRNA and protein.

The sponsor companies reported that results from phase I studies, which examined subjects with a wide variety of solid tumors, demonstrated that the drug was well tolerated and that several subjects experienced disease stabilization. The companies are planning additional phase I safety studies involving the drug in combination with currently approved chemotherapies. Phase II clinical trials examining ISIS 5132 as a single agent therapy in subjects with breast, lung, colon, pancreatic, and prostate cancers are under way.

INDICATION(S) AND RESEARCH PHASE
Breast Cancer – Phase II
Cancer/Tumors (Unspecified) – Phase II
Colon Malignancies – Phase II
Lung Cancer – Phase II
Pancreatic Cancer – Phase II
Prostate Cancer – Phase II

marimastat, BB-2516
unknown

MANUFACTURER
British Biotech plc

DESCRIPTION
Marimastat is an inhibitor of matrix metalloproteinase (MMP), a family of naturally occurring enzymes that are over-produced in a number of diseases. This is especially true of cancer, where MMPs are involved in the spread and local growth of tumors. Both angiogenesis and metastasis require MMPs during tumor invasion. Anti-angiogenic strategies, unlike other therapeutic approaches, do not aim to directly destroy or "kill" the tumor or cause tumor regression. Rather, they are designed to prevent the further growth of tumors by limiting their blood supply. Because peripheral tumor cells could theoretically survive on a diffusion-dependent basis, anti-angiogenic drugs may prove most effective when given in combination with other standard cytotoxic regimens.

Marimastat is in phase III development for the treatment of cancer. In 1999, British Biotech and Schering-Plough Corporation signed an agreement to develop and commercialize British Biotech's metalloproteinase inhibitors, including marimastat.

INDICATION(S) AND RESEARCH PHASE
Pancreatic Cancer – Phase III
Lung Cancer – Phase III
Breast Cancer – Phase III
Brain Cancer – Phase III completed
Ovarian Cancer – Phase III

MDX-210
unknown

MANUFACTURER
Medarex

DESCRIPTION
MDX-210 is a bispecific (target-trigger) monoclonal antibody (MAb)-based treatment being developed for cancers with specific markers (HER-2/*neu* positive), including renal cell, non-small cell lung, pancreatic and kidney cancers. Phase II trials have been completed for kidney, prostate, and ovarian cancer. Phase III development for ovarian cancer has commenced in Europe.

INDICATION(S) AND RESEARCH PHASE
Prostate Cancer – Phase II completed
Renal Cell Carcinoma – Phase II completed
Colon Malignancies – Phase II
Breast Cancer – Phase II
Gastric Cancer – Phase II
Pancreatic Cancer – Phase II
Lung Cancer – Phase II
Ovarian Cancer – Phase III

MDX-220
unknown

MANUFACTURER
Medarex

DESCRIPTION
MDX-220 is a bispecific (target-trigger) monoclonal antibody (MAb) that targets Tag-72. It is being developed for the treatment of a variety of cancers, including lung, colon, prostate, ovarian, endometrial, pancreatic, and gastric cancer.

INDICATION(S) AND RESEARCH PHASE
Endometrial Cancer – Phase I/II
Gastric Cancer – Phase I/II
Lung Cancer – Phase I/II
Ovarian Cancer – Phase I/II
Pancreatic Cancer – Phase I/II
Prostate Cancer – Phase II
Colorectal Cancer – Phase II

MGI-114, hydroxymethylacylfulvene, HMAF
Irofulven

MANUFACTURER
MGI Pharma

DESCRIPTION
Irofulven (MGI-114) is the first product candidate being developed by MGI Pharma from its family of anti-cancer compounds called acylfulvenes. Early trials demonstrated that Irofulven is absorbed rapidly by tumor cells, and once inside binds to DNA and protein targets. The binding interferes with DNA replication and cell division, leading to tumor-specific cell death. The drug is being tested in a series of trials for a variety of cancers.

In November 2000, results from a phase II trial of Irofulven indicated that the drug produced anti-tumor activity in subjects with advanced pancreatic cancer who were refractory to gemcitabine (Gemzar). Ten of the 53 subjects enrolled achieved six-month survival and two subjects demonstrated objective responses: one subject experienced tumor shrinkage of 100% and another subject experienced an 84% decrease in tumor mass. A phase III trial was initiated in February 2001.

INDICATION(S) AND RESEARCH PHASE
Breast Cancer – Phase II
Colon Malignancies – Phase II
Renal Cell Carcinoma – Phase II
Cervical Dysplasia/Cancer – Phase II
Lung Cancer – Phase II
Ovarian Cancer – Phase I/II
Colorectal Cancer – Phase II
Prostate Cancer – Phase I/II
Cancer/Tumors (Unspecified) – Phase I/II
Pancreatic Cancer – Phase III
Liver Cancer – Phase II

RFS-2000
Rubitecan

MANUFACTURER
SuperGen

DESCRIPTION
Rubitecan is a novel drug that works by inhibiting an enzyme called topoisomerase I. This drug is made in an oral formulation, which is an advantage for outpatient treatment compared to intravenous cancer drugs that may require a visit to a hospital setting.

In addition to treating pancreatic cancer, Rubitecan is being evaluated in treating a variety of solid tumors, such as in breast, colorectal, lung, ovarian, and prostate cancers, as well as metastatic melanoma and advanced gastric carcinoma. Additionally, phase II trials in the United States and Europe are testing Rubitecan in blood cancers such as chronic myelomonocytic leukemia (CMML/myelodysplastic syndrome).

INDICATION(S) AND RESEARCH PHASE
Pancreatic Cancer – Phase III
Breast Cancer – Phase II
Colorectal Cancer – Phase II
Gastric Cancer – Phase II
Leukemia – Phase II
Malignant Melanoma – Phase II
Ovarian Cancer – Phase II
Myelodysplastic Syndrome – Phase III

SR-27897B
unknown

MANUFACTURER
Sanofi-Synthelabo Pharmaceuticals

DESCRIPTION
CCK-A (cholecystokinin-A) is a molecule that is present in the central nervous system and also secreted from the lining of the small intestine. It causes many different actions throughout the body, including gallbladder contraction, release of pancreatic digestive enzymes, and promotion of the feeling of digestive fullness. CCK also promotes cell growth and division, especially in the pancreas, and it has a regulating effect on the amount of dopamine and serotonin present in the body.

SR-27897 is a potent substance that blocks the receptors to which CCK would ordinarily bind, thus blocking CCK's effects on the body. By negating the action of CCK, people may lose their sense of satiety, making SR-27897 a potential therapy for anorexia. Additionally, CCK's probable role in the pathogenesis of pancreatic cancer (because it can cause abnormal pancreatic cell division) may also be reduced with the use of SR-27897.

INDICATION(S) AND RESEARCH PHASE
Pancreatic Cancer – Phase II
Anorexia – Phase II

troxacitabine, BCH-4556
Troxatyl

MANUFACTURER
BioChem Pharma

DESCRIPTION
Troxatyl is a dioxolane nucleoside analog being investigated as an anticancer agent. The drug is a complete DNA chain terminator and DNA polymerase inhibitor. It acts by incorporating itself into the growing DNA chain of cancer cells, interfering with their ability to replicate further. Troxatyl is being evaluated as a single agent or in combination therapy in a number of ongoing trials for hematologic malignancies, including acute myeloid leukemia and chronic myeloid leukemia (blastic phase), and in lymphoproliferative disorders such as lymphoma, chronic lymphocytic leukemia and myeloma. It is also being evaluated as a single agent in pancreatic cancer and in combination therapy in a number of solid tumors. Troxatyl is currently in phase II development.

INDICATION(S) AND RESEARCH PHASE
Cancer/Tumors (Unspecified) – Phase II
Colorectal Cancer – Phase II
Head and Neck Cancer – Phase II
Leukemia – Phase II
Lung Cancer – Phase II
Malignant Melanoma – Phase II
Ovarian Cancer – Phase II
Pancreatic Cancer – Phase II
Prostate Cancer – Phase II
Renal Cell Carcinoma – Phase II

vaccine, anti-gastrin
Gastrimmune

MANUFACTURER
Aphton Corporation

DESCRIPTION
Gastrimmune is a therapeutic vaccine that neutralizes specific hormones (G17 & Gly-extended G17). The drug is in phase III trials for the treatment of cancers of the gastrointestinal tract, including gastric cancer and colorectal cancer. It is also in trials for liver cancer, esophageal cancer, and two phase III trials for advanced pancreatic cancer—one in the the United States and one in Europe.

INDICATION(S) AND RESEARCH PHASE
Colorectal Cancer – Phase III
Esophageal Cancer – Phase III
Gastric Cancer – Phase III
Liver Cancer – Phase II/III
Pancreatic Cancer – Phase III

vaccine, cancer
Gvax

MANUFACTURER
Cell Genesys

DESCRIPTION
Gvax is an allogenic compound that involves the genetic modification of prostate cancer cell lines. These cancer cells have been irradiated and modified to secrete granulocyte-macrophage colony stimulating factor (GM-CSF), a hormone which plays a key role in stimulating the body's immune response to vaccines. The compound is in trials for prostate cancer, pancreatic cancer, lung cancer, leukemia, and malignant melanoma.

The Gvax prostate cancer vaccine demonstrated anti-tumor activity in an initial phase II trial in subjects with advanced metastatic prostate cancer who have not responded to hormone therapy. Prior to initiating a phase III trial, Cell Genesys plans to initiate further trials of Gvax prostate cancer vaccine in 2001 that will employ a higher potency version of the same product. Additionally, future phase III trials in hormone refractory prostate cancer subjects may compare Gvax vaccine in combination with chemotherapy to chemotherapy alone.

INDICATION(S) AND RESEARCH PHASE
Prostate Cancer – Phase II
Lung Cancer – Phase I/II completed
Malignant Melanoma – Phase I/II
Vaccines – Phase I/II
Pancreatic Cancer – Phase II
Leukemia – Phase I/II

virulizin
unknown

MANUFACTURER
Lorus Therapeutics

DESCRIPTION
Virulizin, which is isolated from bovine bile, is a potent activator of monocytes and macrophages. The compound has demonstrated significant antitumor activity against several tumor types including pancreatic cancer, melanoma, and AIDS related lymphoma.

In a phase I/II study, 26 patients with advanced pancreatic cancer who previously failed standard therapies were enrolled. A total of 19 evaluable patients were treated with different doses of Virulizin (1.5, 3.0, 6.0 ml, 3 times per week and 3.0 ml, 5 times per week) for at least 4 weeks. The maximum dose level was well-tolerated. Seven patients (37%) achieved stable disease and one patient in the last cohort achieved a complete response. The patients treated with Virulizin had a median survival of 6.7 months with a 6-month survival rate of 58% and showed a significant improvement in quality of life. The company initiated phase III trials for pancreatic cancer in early 2001.

INDICATION(S) AND RESEARCH PHASE
Pancreatic cancer – Phase III

Prostate Cancer

abarelix depot, PPI-149
unknown

MANUFACTURER
Praecis Pharmaceuticals

DESCRIPTION
Approximately 85% of newly diagnosed prostate cancers are hormone-dependent tumors that require the male hormone testosterone for their continued growth. Lowering the body's normal production of testosterone, therefore, is the primary goal of hormonal treatment. However, available hormonal therapies may cause an initial surge or increase in the level of testosterone before the desired effect of lowering testosterone occurs. Abarelix depot is designed to rapidly block the production of testosterone and avoid the initial testosterone level surge. An NDA was submitted in December 2000.

Additionally, a multisite, blinded phase II/III trial of abarelix depot for the treatment of endometriosis is under way. Subject enrollment in this study is complete, with 365 subjects enrolled. Praecis is developing abarelix depot under an agreement with Amgen and Sanofi-Synthelabo.

INDICATION(S) AND RESEARCH PHASE
Prostate Cancer – NDA submitted
Endometriosis – Phase II/III

abiraterone acetate
unknown

MANUFACTURER
BTG International

DESCRIPTION
Abiraterone acetate, an approved drug in the United Kingdom, inhibits both testicular and adrenal androgen production by selective inhibition of 17 alpha-hydroxylase/C17-20 lyase, the key enzyme in the androgen biosynthetic pathway. Due to abiraterone acetate's high inhibitory potency, a phase I trial for the treatment of prostate cancer was conducted. The trial examined the effects of single or multiple doses of abiraterone acetate in chemically castrated or untreated subjects. Results indicated that the drug is a potent inhibitor of testosterone production and can itself reduce testosterone to sub-castrate levels.

INDICATION(S) AND RESEARCH PHASE
Prostate Cancer – Phase I completed

ABT-627
unknown

MANUFACTURER
Abbott Laboratories

DESCRIPTION
ABT-627 is a drug that is being developed to halt the progression of late-stage, metastatic prostate cancer. Cancer requires the growth of blood vessels that will nourish the cancer cells as they grow and divide. If there is a limited blood supply, the cancer cells will die and the growth of the tumor will be slowed. ABT-627 acts to restrict the blood supply to newly forming cancer cells.

ABT-627 blocks the action of a potent substance in the body (endothelin-A). This substance is a strong constrictor of blood vessels that also stimulates cell proliferation. By preventing the action of endothelin-A, it is thought that blood vessel and cancer cell growth will be slowed or halted altogether. In initial trials, ABT-627 decreased the amount of a prostate protein (PSA) that is used to monitor the progression of prostate cancer therapy. Additionally, the drug decreased pain resulting from cancerous spread to the bone, and it enabled subjects to decrease their narcotic use.

This new medication has shown that it can stabilize the progression of prostate cancer for up to fifteen months and improve the quality of life of prostate cancer subjects. Phase II studies are currently under way.

INDICATION(S) AND RESEARCH PHASE
Prostate Cancer – Phase II

APC8015
Provenge

MANUFACTURER
Dendreon Corporation

DESCRIPTION
Provenge is a dendritic exvivo cell therapy being tested for the treatment of advanced prostate cancer. The aim of the therapy is to heighten the immunologic response to cancer cells by removing dendritic cells from a subject, pulsing them with a prostate cancer antigen, and reinjecting them into the subject. The dendritic cells help the immune system by attaching pieces of the tumor proteins to their own surface and presenting them to lymphocytes, which then learn to recognize the antigens as foreign matter and attack them.

Phase II trial results published in December 2000 indicated that Provenge was safe, well tolerated, and stimulated an immune response in subjects with prostate cancer. Phase III trials are under way throughout the United States.

INDICATION(S) AND RESEARCH PHASE
Prostate Cancer – Phase III

---

arsenic trioxide (ATO)
Trisenox

MANUFACTURER
Cell Therapeutics

DESCRIPTION
Trisenox is believed to kill cancer cells through apoptosis. The mechanism of action of Trisenox is not fully understood, but the drug appears to induce apoptosis in a different manner than other anti-cancer agents such as retinoids.

Trisenox is FDA approved to treat acute promyelocytic leukemia (APL), and it is also in numerous trials in the United States for indications including other types of leukemia, prostate cancer, multiple myeloma, renal cell cancer, cervical cancer, and bladder cancer.

INDICATION(S) AND RESEARCH PHASE
Leukemia – Phase I
Lymphoma, Non-Hodgkin's – Phase II
Leukemia – Phase II
Multiple Myeloma – Phase II
Prostate Cancer – Phase II
Renal Cell Carcinoma – Phase II
Cervical Dysplasia/Cancer – Phase II
Bladder Cancer – Phase II

---

bicalutimide
Casodex

MANUFACTURER
AstraZeneca

DESCRIPTION
Casodex is a non-steroidal anti-androgen for the treatment of advanced prostate cancer. Prostate cancer is known to be sensitive to androgen—it responds to treatment that counteracts the effects of androgen and/or removes the source of androgen. Data suggest that this oral hormonal medication shows no statistical difference in overall survival or time-to-progression when compared to castration in subjects with non-metastatic, locally advanced prostate cancer. The company has submitted a supplemental NDA for this indication. Casodex is given in an oral tablet form.

INDICATION(S) AND RESEARCH PHASE
Prostate Cancer – Phase sNDA submitted

CEP-2563
unknown

MANUFACTURER
Cephalon

DESCRIPTION
CEP-2563 is an orally active inhibitor of tyrosine kinase. It is currently in phase I development for the treatment of prostate cancer. Cephalon has CEP-2563 development agreements with TAP Pharmaceuticals and Abbott Laboratories.

INDICATION(S) AND RESEARCH PHASE
Prostate Cancer – Phase I

CEP-701
unknown

MANUFACTURER
Cephalon

DESCRIPTION
CEP-701 is an orally active inhibitor of the enzyme tyrosine kinase. It is being evaluated in phase II studies for prostate cancer and pancreatic ductal adenocarcinoma.

INDICATION(S) AND RESEARCH PHASE
Pancreatic Cancer – Phase II
Prostate Cancer – Phase II

CT-2584
Apra

MANUFACTURER
Cell Therapeutics

DESCRIPTION
Apra is a novel synthetic inhibitor of phosphatidic acid metabolism in tumor cells. This antineoplastic agent kills cancer cells without having to depend on cell division to exert its effect. Additionally, Apra may also help inhibit multi-drug resistance of certain cancers. The drug is in trials for the treatment of prostate cancer and sarcomas. Additional indications may include cancers of the colon, breast, and female reproductive system including the ovaries.

INDICATION(S) AND RESEARCH PHASE
Prostate Cancer – Phase II
Sarcoma – Phase II

CTP-37
Avicine

MANUFACTURER
AVI BioPharma

DESCRIPTION
Avicine is a hormone vaccine derived from human chorionic gonadotropin peptide that is being tested for prevention of colorectal, pancreatic, and prostate cancer. The drug is in phase II trials for prostate cancer, and phase III trials for colorectal and pancreatic cancer. AVI BioPharma has partnered with SuperGen and under the terms of the agreement, SuperGen will be responsible for U.S. marketing and sales of Avicine, and AVI will

be responsible for product manufacturing.

INDICATION(S) AND RESEARCH PHASE
Colorectal Cancer – Phase III
Pancreatic Cancer – Phase III
Prostate Cancer – Phase II

CV706
unknown

MANUFACTURER
Calydon

DESCRIPTION
CV706 is an oncolytic virus that is able to replicate in and kill targeted cancer cells, leaving non-cancer cells unharmed. It is currently in development for the treatment of prostate cancer. In October 2000, phase I/II trial results indicated that CV706 displayed anti-tumor activity and that the drug was well tolerated. Subjects showing the greatest anti-tumor response were treated at one of the top two doses evaluated; four of these 11 subjects exhibited a prostate specific antigen (PSA) partial response, defined as a 50% or greater reduction in serum PSA for at least four weeks. In three of the subjects, their partial response lasted at least nine months. PSA levels decreased from baseline in nine of the 11 subjects (80%) treated in the top two dose groups. A study of post-treatment biopsy samples demonstrated that adenoviral replication—the mechanism upon which CV706 has been designed to both target and kill prostate cancer cells—had occurred in subjects.

INDICATION(S) AND RESEARCH PHASE
Prostate Cancer – Phase I/II completed

CV787
unknown

MANUFACTURER
Calydon

DESCRIPTION
CV787 is a genetically engineered adenovirus type 5 that is cytolytic to cells expressing prostate specific antigen (PSA). It is being evaluated in a phase I/II trial in subjects with locally recurrent prostate cancer following definitive radiotherapy and/or brachytherapy. The phase I/II trial is an open-label, dose finding study designed to determine the safety and tolerance of an injection of CV787 directly into the prostate. The trial is being conducted at six hospitals in the United States.

INDICATION(S) AND RESEARCH PHASE
Prostate Cancer – Phase I/II

cVax-Pr
unknown

MANUFACTURER
Jenner BioTherapies

DESCRIPTION
cVax-Pr is a vaccine designed from DNA pieces from a protein (prostate-specific antigen, PSA) found in both healthy and cancerous prostate cancer cells. Scientists add molecules to this DNA that stimulate the body's immune system. In this manner, the body is manipulated into recognizing PSA-DNA as foreign material. Consequently, this immune response attacks both normal and cancerous prostate cells.

In preliminary studies, administration of cVax-Pr stimulated antibody and white blood cell production. cVax-Pr is being tested in phase II trials.

INDICATION(S) AND RESEARCH PHASE
Prostate Cancer – Phase II

doxorubicin HCl
Doxil, Caelyx

MANUFACTURER
Alza (Sequus Pharmaceuticals)

DESCRIPTION
Doxil is a liposomal formulation of doxorubicin hydrochloride, an intravenous chemotherapy agent. This anthracycline anti-tumor agent is currently on the market for the treatment of Kaposi's sarcoma. The drug uses a novel, targeted delivery system to help evade recognition and uptake by the immune system so that the liposomes can circulate in the body longer. A long circulation time increases the likelihood that the liposomes and their pharmaceutical contents will reach their targeted tumor site. Doxil may act through its ability to bind DNA and inhibit nucleic acid synthesis.

Doxil is being tested in trials for the treatment of breast, liver, lung, and prostate cancers, as well as for unspecified cancers and tumors.

Alza markets this product in the United States under the trade name Doxil; however, it is marketed under the name Caelyx in other areas. Schering-Plough has exclusive international marketing rights to Caelyx, excluding Japan and Israel, through a distribution agreement with Alza.

INDICATION(S) AND RESEARCH PHASE
Breast Cancer – Phase II/III
Liver Cancer – Phase II/III
Lung Cancer – Phase II/III
Prostate Cancer – Phase II/III
Cancer/Tumors (Unspecified) – Phase II

DPPE
unknown

MANUFACTURER
Bristol-Myers Squibb

DESCRIPTION
DPPE is being developed to potentiate the effects of chemotherapy in subjects with late-stage prostate cancer. There are many substances in the body that play a role in the regulation of cell growth. When there is an imbalance or problem with one of these regulatory substances, uncontrolled cell growth or cancer may result.

An example of one such substance is histamine, which acts as a growth factor in both normal and cancer cells. It spurs cell growth by stimulating growth receptors located within the cell.

DPPE is a drug designed to block these receptors for histamine. By blocking the effects of histamine, it is proposed that unregulated cell growth will decrease. When given with standard chemotherapy agents, DPPE may help these agents better destroy cancer cells.

INDICATION(S) AND RESEARCH PHASE
Prostate Cancer – Phase II

eflornithine, DFMO (difluoromethylornydil)
unknown

MANUFACTURER
Aventis

DESCRIPTION
Eflornithine is a potent, irreversible inhibitor of ornithine decarboxylase (OCD), an enzyme that is elevated in most tumors and pre-malignant lesions. Eflornithine is currently in a phase III clinical trial to determine the effectiveness of the drug in treating subjects who have newly diagnosed or recurrent bladder cancer. The drug is administered orally in tablet form.

Eflornithine is also in trials for the prevention and treatment of HIV infections, skin cancer, breast cancer, prostate cancer, and cervical dysplasia/cancer.

INDICATION(S) AND RESEARCH PHASE
Bladder Cancer – Phase III
Breast Cancer – Phase II/III
Cervical Dysplasia/Cancer – Phase II
HIV Infection – Phase II
Prostate Cancer – Phase II
Skin Cancer – Phase III

exisulind
Aptosyn/LHRH agonist

MANUFACTURER
Cell Pathways

DESCRIPTION
Aptosyn (exisulind) belongs to a novel class of compounds called selective apoptotic anti-neoplastic drugs (SAANDs). SAANDs inhibit a form of cyclic GMP phosphodiesterase and selectively induce apoptosis in abnormally growing precancerous and cancerous cells. Aptosyn is being tested with LHRH agonist hormone therapy for the treatment of prostate cancer. The objective of this study is to determine the preliminary efficacy of Aptosyn in subjects who are receiving LHRH agonist hormone therapy and have rising prostate specific antigen (PSA) levels. This open-label, 12-month phase II trial will include 15 subjects.

INDICATION(S) AND RESEARCH PHASE
Prostate Cancer – Phase II

exisulind
Aptosyn

MANUFACTURER
Cell Pathways

DESCRIPTION
Aptosyn (exisulind) belongs to a novel class of compounds called selective apoptotic anti-neoplastic drugs (SAANDs). SAANDs inhibit a form of cyclic GMP phosphodiesterase and selectively induce apoptosis in abnormally growing precancerous and cancerous cells. Aptosyn is being tested for several indications and is in five different trials for adenomatous polyposis coli (APC) and familial adenomatous polyposis coli; two of these trials are specifically for pediatric subjects.

The company received a non-approvable letter from the FDA in September 2000 for one of the trials for familial adenomatous polyposis. The company intends to amend the NDA and request a meeting to address the deficiencies and the possible requirement for additional clinical data.

Additionally, Aptosyn is being tested in trials for the treatment of prostate cancer, lung cancer, breast cancer, sporadic colonic polyps and Barrett's esophagus disease.

INDICATION(S) AND RESEARCH PHASE
Adenomatous Polyposis Coli – Phase Non-approvable letter
Pediatric, Familial Adenomatous Polyposis Coli – Phase II
Adenomatous Polyposis Coli – Phase I/II
Barrett's Esophagus Disease – Phase II
Prostate Cancer – Phase II/III
Breast Cancer – Phase II/III
Lung Cancer – Phase Ib
Colon Polyps – Phase II/III

exisulind/docetaxel
Aposyn/Taxotere

MANUFACTURER
Cell Pathways

DESCRIPTION
Aptosyn (exisulind) belongs to a novel class of compounds called selective apoptotic anti-neoplastic drugs (SAANDs). SAANDs inhibit a form of cyclic GMP phosphodiesterase and selectively induce apoptosis in abnormally growing precancerous and cancerous cells. Because SAANDs do not induce apoptosis in normal cells, they do not produce the serious side effects normally associated with traditional chemotherapeutic agents. They also do not inhibit cyclooxygenase (COX I or COX II) and have not exhibited the gastric and renal toxicities associated with non-steroidal anti-inflammatory drugs (NSAIDs), including the COX II inhibitors.

Aptosyn is being tested with Rhone-Poulenc Rorer's Taxotere for the treatment of prostate, lung, and breast cancer as well as for solid tumors. Both companies will jointly share the cost of the trials and will retain all marketing rights to its respective products.

INDICATION(S) AND RESEARCH PHASE
Prostate Cancer – Phase I/II
Breast Cancer – Phase I/II
Lung Cancer – Phase I/II
Lung Cancer – Phase III
Cancer/Tumors (Unspecified) – Phase I

FK-317
unknown

MANUFACTURER
Fujisawa Healthcare

DESCRIPTION
Fujisawa has developed a new anti-cancer medication, FK-317, that originally was developed as an antibiotic. The molecule, known as a dihydrobenzoxazine, underwent preliminary testing in thirty-one subjects with solid tumors that were refractory to other chemotherapeutic treatments. The company reported that tumor reduction was observed in four subjects, two of whom achieved complete remission. Side effects and other toxicities such as leukopenia

(decreased white blood cells) and neutropenia were modest in comparison to other established treatments.

It is unclear how exactly this compound works to limit the growth of cancer, but it seems to influence the process by which cells reproduce themselves. Currently, FK-317 is given at a dose of 24 mg/day intravenously and it is being evaluated in phase II trials. Scientists are testing it in a variety of solid tumors such as prostate, breast, and skin cancer.

INDICATION(S) AND RESEARCH PHASE
Breast Cancer – Phase II
Cancer/Tumors (Unspecified) – Phase II
Prostate Cancer – Phase II
Skin Cancer – Phase II

G3139/mitoxantrone
Genasense/mitoxantrone

MANUFACTURER
Genta

DESCRIPTION
Genasense (G3139) is designed to reduce levels of bcl-2, a protein that contributes to the resistance of cancer cells to current forms of cancer treatment. Treatment with Genasense may markedly improve the effectiveness of standard anticancer therapies; it is being tested in combination with mitoxantrone for treatment of prostate and colorectal cancers.

INDICATION(S) AND RESEARCH PHASE
Colorectal Cancer – Phase II
Prostate Cancer – Phase I/II

G3139/docetaxel
Genasense/Taxotere

MANUFACTURER
Genta

DESCRIPTION
Genasense (G3139) attacks Bcl-2, a protein that is over-expressed in many forms of cancer. Bcl-2 appears to contribute to the resistance of these diseases to standard treatment. Genta is using its proprietary antisense approach to first decrease the expression of Bcl-2, and then to administer state-of-the-art anticancer therapy in an effort to improve subject outcome. Genasense in combination with docetaxel is in trials for treatment of breast and prostate cancer.

INDICATION(S) AND RESEARCH PHASE
Breast Cancer – Phase I/II
Prostate Cancer – Phase II

G3139/androgen blockade
Genasense/androgen blockade

MANUFACTURER
Genta

DESCRIPTION
Genasense (G3139) is designed to reduce levels of bcl-2, a protein that contributes to the resistance of cancer cells to current forms of cancer treatment. Genasense in combination with androgen blockade is in phase I/II trials for the treatment of androgen-insensitive metastatic prostate cancer.

INDICATION(S) AND RESEARCH PHASE
Prostate Cancer – Phase I/II

GBC-590
unknown

MANUFACTURER
Safe Sciences

DESCRIPTION
GBC-590 belongs to a new class of drugs called lectin inhibitors that specifically interfere with cellular interactions. GBC-590 competitively binds to unique lectins (special protein cell-surface receptors) on cancer cells and disrupts the metastatic process. GBC-590's affinity for cancer lectins is the core reason for its significant biological activity and specificity.

GBC-590 is being tested in phase II studies for pancreatic and colorectal cancer, and the company plans to test it in phase II trials for prostate cancer.

INDICATION(S) AND RESEARCH PHASE
Colorectal Cancer – Phase II
Pancreatic Cancer – Phase II
Prostate Cancer – Phase I/II

gallium maltolate
unknown

MANUFACTURER
Titan Pharmaceuticals

DESCRIPTION
Gallium is a semi-metallic element that has shown some therapeutic activity in metabolic bone disease, hypercalcemia of malignancy and cancer. Gallium maltolate can displace divalent iron from the iron transporting protein, transferrin; thus gallium maltolate causes interference with iron metabolism with inhibition of enzymes requiring divalent iron. The most important of these in the cancer setting appears to be ribonucleotide reductase (RNR). Additionally, gallium appears to form salts with calcium and phosphate and become incorporated into bone. The bone that is created with incorporated gallium appears to be at least as strong as normal bone, and it appears to be more resistant to degradation by osteoclasts and tumor cells.

INDICATION(S) AND RESEARCH PHASE
Prostate Cancer – Phase I/II
Lymphomas – Phase I/II
Myeloma – Phase I/II
Bladder Cancer – Phase I/II
HIV Infection – Phase I/II

IM862
unknown

MANUFACTURER
Cytran

DESCRIPTION
IM862 is a small peptide comprised of two amino acids that may inhibit new blood vessel formation (angiogenesis). When there is excessive growth of new blood vessels, a number of pathological conditions result, including malignant tumors, age-related macular degeneration, and vascular diseases. Limiting the growth of new blood vessels in tumors deprives them of nourishment and

can ultimately kill these cancers. This drug is being developed in phase III trials for Kaposi's sarcoma and phase I/II trials for ovarian cancer.

INDICATION(S) AND RESEARCH PHASE
Kaposi's Sarcoma – Phase III
Ovarian Cancer – Phase I/II
Malignant Melanoma – Preclinical
Prostate Cancer – Preclinical

IMC-C225, CPT-11
unknown

MANUFACTURER
ImClone Systems

DESCRIPTION
IMC-C225 is a chimerized (part mouse, part human) monoclonal antibody that may help fight cancer cells when used in conjunction with radiation therapy or other chemotherapy agents. This antibody selectively blocks the epidermal growth factor receptor (EGFr), which may be present in greater amounts on actively growing tumor cells. Since many cancers use specific growth factors to stimulate tumor cell growth, blocking this receptor may inhibit the cancer from increasing in size and spreading throughout the body.

The company is conducting phase III clinical trials evaluating IMC-C225 in combination with radiotherapy and with chemotherapy in subjects with advanced squamous cell head and neck carcinoma. IMC-C225 is in trials for several other indications in combination with various anti-cancer agents.

INDICATION(S) AND RESEARCH PHASE
Breast Cancer – Phase I/II
Head and Neck Cancer – Phase III
Lung Cancer – Phase III
Prostate Cancer – Phase I/II
Renal Cell Carcinoma – Phase II
Pancreatic Cancer – Phase II
Colorectal Cancer – Phase II

INGN-201, adenoviral p53
unknown

MANUFACTURER
Introgen Therapeutics

DESCRIPTION
INGN-201 is a p53 gene therapy product. It has been tested as a treatment for a variety of solid tumor cancers with administration via intratumoral injection. The drug was well tolerated according to the company, and additional trials are under way using an intravenous infusion in order to reach more types of cancers. The tumor-suppressing p53 gene encodes a protein that responds to damage involving cellular DNA by terminating cell division. Normal p53 genes are delivered into cancer cells of the subject through an adenoviral vector.

The developers of INGN-201 have signed a Cooperative Research and Development Agreement (CRADA) with the National Cancer Institute to evaluate the potential effectiveness and superiority of the drug over other treatments against breast, ovarian, bladder, prostate, and brain cancers in phase I and phase II trials. A phase III trial in head and neck cancer was initiated in March 2000.

INDICATION(S) AND RESEARCH PHASE
Head and Neck Cancer – Phase III
Bladder Cancer – Phase I
Brain Cancer – Phase I
Breast Cancer – Phase I
Bronchoalveolar Cancer – Phase I
Ovarian Cancer – Phase I
Prostate Cancer – Phase I
Lung Cancer – Phase II
Cancer/Tumors (Unspecified) – Phase I

interleukin (IL)
MultiKine

MANUFACTURER
CEL-SCI Corporation

DESCRIPTION
MultiKine is a multiple combination therapy made from a natural, cytokine cocktail (which includes interleukin-2 (IL-2), IL-β, TNF-α, Gm-CSF and an IFN-γ/immunomodulator). It is being tested for the treatment of advanced head and neck cancer in subjects who have previously failed standard therapy, and for head and neck cancer treatment prior to surgery.

MultiKine has just completed two phase II trials for head and neck cancer. The first trial consisted of 16 subjects and tested four different doses of MultiKine in four subjects each. To qualify for the trial, the subjects must have had a recurrence of the cancer and failed conventional therapy.

The company reported that in an earlier and still ongoing study conducted in newly diagnosed head and neck cancer subjects, 10 subjects had tumor reductions prior to surgery within a short time period. Three of ten subjects had tumor reductions exceeding 50%, and one additional subject with a tumor that was nearly three inches in diameter had a complete clinical response. Lastly, two subjects refused surgery because they were satisfied with their condition after treatment with MultiKine.

INDICATION(S) AND RESEARCH PHASE
Head and Neck Cancer – Phase II
HIV Infection – Phase II
Breast Cancer – Phase I
Prostate Cancer – Phase I/II

ISIS 5132, CGP 69846A
unknown

MANUFACTURER
Isis Pharmaceuticals

DESCRIPTION
ISIS 5132 is a potent antisense inhibitor of the enzyme c-Raf-1 kinase. Antisense drugs inhibit the production of disease-causing proteins by altering the genetic information that messenger RNA uses to produce new protein. c-Raf kinase plays a role in signal processes that regulate cell growth and proliferation. It is one of a family of raf genes thought to play an important role in the development of some solid tumors. The company reports that activated-raf has also been detected in a substantial variety of human cancers including small cell lung carcinoma and breast cancer. For example, it has been reported that 60% of all lung carcinoma cells express unusually high levels of normal c-Raf mRNA and protein.

The sponsor companies reported that

results from phase I studies, which examined subjects with a wide variety of solid tumors, demonstrated that the drug was well tolerated and that several subjects experienced disease stabilization. The companies are planning additional phase I safety studies involving the drug in combination with currently approved chemotherapies. Phase II clinical trials examining ISIS 5132 as a single agent therapy in subjects with breast, lung, colon, pancreatic, and prostate cancers are under way.

INDICATION(S) AND RESEARCH PHASE
Breast Cancer – Phase II
Cancer/Tumors (Unspecified) – Phase II
Colon Malignancies – Phase II
Lung Cancer – Phase II
Pancreatic Cancer – Phase II
Prostate Cancer – Phase II

LDI-200
unknown

MANUFACTURER
Milkhaus Laboratory

DESCRIPTION
Clinical trials are testing a subcutaneous formulation of LDI-200 for at least three indications: leukemia, myelodysplastic syndrome, and prostate cancer. Results demonstrated that LDI-200 showed both efficacy and safety in a small phase II/III open label crossover trial in subjects with myelodysplastic syndrome. The control consisted of subjects given supportive therapy, consisting of transfusions and antibiotics, who became eligible for treatment if their disease progressed more rapidly than anticipated. A total of 23 subjects were treated using LDI-200, and seven showed significant clinical response.

INDICATION(S) AND RESEARCH PHASE
Leukemia – Phase II completed
Prostate Cancer – Phase II/III
White Blood Cell Disorders – Phase II/III
Myelodysplastic Syndrome – Phase III completed

leuprolide acetate
30-day Leuprogel

MANUFACTURER
Atrix Laboratories

DESCRIPTION
30-Day Leuprogel is a new Atrigel formulation that contains leuprolide acetate. The product is injected subcutaneously as a liquid, where it solidifies and releases a predetermined amount of leuprolide. The sustained levels of leuprolide result in decreased testosterone levels, which in turn suppress tumor growth in subjects with hormone-responsive prostate cancer. Leuprogel has an advantage over current treatments due to its delivery by subcutaneous injection and small volume (compared to commonly used large volume intramuscular injection).

INDICATION(S) AND RESEARCH PHASE
Prostate Cancer – Phase III

leuprolide acetate
3-month Leuprogel

MANUFACTURER
Atrix Laboratories

DESCRIPTION
Atrix recently announced the early completion of enrollment for a Leuprogel 3-month 22.5 mg phase III trial. This drug is in development for the treatment of prostate cancer.

INDICATION(S) AND RESEARCH PHASE
Prostate Cancer – Phase III

liposomal ether lipid
TLC ELL-12

MANUFACTURER
The Liposome Company

DESCRIPTION
TLC ELL-12 is a liposomal ether lipid that may have efficacy in the treatment of several cancers. This drug has exhibited significant anti-tumor activity, but did not have the hemolytic side effects common to this type of ether lipid when therapeutic doses were used in experimental models. It does not appear to be myelosuppressive.

TLC ELL-12 is currently being developed in phase I trials for the treatment of lung cancer, multiple myeloma, leukemia, and prostate cancer.

INDICATION(S) AND RESEARCH PHASE
Lung Cancer – Phase I
Multiple Myeloma – Phase I
Leukemia – Phase I
Prostate Cancer – Phase I

unknown
Prinomastat

MANUFACTURER
Agouron Pharmaceuticals

DESCRIPTION
Prinomastat is an orally active, synthetic molecule designed to potently and selectively inhibit certain members of a family of enzymes known as a matrix metalloproteases, which are believed to be involved in tumor angiogenesis, invasion and metastasis. The drug is in trials for various indications, including osteoarthritis, brain cancer and macular degeneration.

Two phase III trials for advanced non-small cell lung cancer and prostate cancer were halted in August 2000 due to the drug's lack of effectiveness in subjects with late-stage disease.

The most common side effects of Prinomastat have been observed in the joints, and include stiffness, joint swelling, and in a few subjects, some limits on the mobility of certain joints, most often in the shoulders and hands. All these effects were reported to be reversible and were effectively managed by treatment rests and dose reductions.

INDICATION(S) AND RESEARCH PHASE
Lung Cancer – Phase III halted
Prostate Cancer – Phase III halted
Osteoarthritis – Phase II
Brain Cancer – Phase II
Macular Degeneration – Phase II

MDX-210

unknown

MANUFACTURER
Medarex

DESCRIPTION
MDX-210 is a bispecific (target-trigger) monoclonal antibody (MAb)-based treatment being developed for cancers with specific markers (HER-2/*neu* positive), including renal cell, non-small cell lung, pancreatic, and prostate cancer. Phase II trials have been completed for kidney, prostate, and ovarian cancer. Phase III trials for ovarian cancer have have commenced in Europe.

INDICATION(S) AND RESEARCH PHASE
Prostate Cancer – Phase II completed
Renal Cell Carcinoma – Phase II completed
Colon Malignancies – Phase II
Breast Cancer – Phase II
Gastric Cancer – Phase II
Pancreatic Cancer – Phase II
Lung Cancer – Phase II
Ovarian Cancer – Phase III

MDX-220
unknown

MANUFACTURER
Medarex

DESCRIPTION
MDX-220 is a bispecific (target-trigger) monoclonal antibody (MAb) that targets Tag-72 in the treatment of a variety of cancers, including lung, colon, prostate, ovarian, endometrial, pancreatic, and gastric cancer.

INDICATION(S) AND RESEARCH PHASE
Endometrial Cancer – Phase I/II
Gastric Cancer – Phase I/II
Lung Cancer – Phase I/II
Ovarian Cancer – Phase I/II
Pancreatic Cancer – Phase I/II
Prostate Cancer – Phase II
Colorectal Cancer – Phase II

MGI-114, hydroxymethylacylfulvene, HMAF
Irofulven

MANUFACTURER
MGI Pharma

DESCRIPTION
Irofulven (MGI-114) is the first product candidate being developed by MGI Pharma from its family of anti-cancer compounds called acylfulvenes. Early trials demonstrated that Irofulven is absorbed rapidly by tumor cells, and once inside binds to DNA and protein targets. The binding interferes with DNA replication and cell division, leading to tumor-specific cell death. The drug is being tested in a series of trials for a variety of cancers.

In November 2000, results from a phase II trial of Irofulven indicated that the drug produced anti-tumor activity in subjects with advanced pancreatic cancer who were refractory to gemcitabine (Gemzar). Ten of the 53 subjects enrolled achieved six-month survival and two subjects demonstrated objective responses: one subject experienced tumor shrinkage of 100% and another subject experienced an 84% decrease in tumor mass. A phase III trial was initiated in February 2001.

INDICATION(S) AND RESEARCH PHASE
Breast Cancer – Phase II
Colon Malignancies – Phase II
Renal Cell Carcinoma – Phase II
Cervical Dysplasia/Cancer – Phase II
Lung Cancer – Phase II
Ovarian Cancer – Phase I/II
Colorectal Cancer – Phase II
Prostate Cancer – Phase I/II
Cancer/Tumors (Unspecified) – Phase I/II
Pancreatic Cancer – Phase III
Liver Cancer – Phase II

phenoxodiol
unknown

MANUFACTURER
Novogen

DESCRIPTION
Phenoxodiol is a novel, cytotoxic, anit-cancer drug that arrests cancer cell growth and restores apoptosis. It acts through a variety of mechanisms including the inhibition of a number of cellular enzyme systems, including topoisomerase 2 and protein tyrosine kinases, which are integral to the development of cancer. Inhibiting these enzyme systems is recognized as a key factor in preventing the growth of cancerous cells. Additionally, the novelty of phenoxodiol lies in its ability to combine a high degree of potency with no known adverse effects on normal cells. Phenoxodiol also possesses a number of other anti-cancer mechanisms that appear to contribute to the overall anti-cancer effect.

Phenoxodiol is currently undergoing a phase Ib trial in an Australian hospital in subjects with solid malignant tumors, including prostate cancer. This study, which commenced in the final quarter of 2000, is investigating the safety and anti-cancer efficacy of phenoxodiol when injected intravenously once weekly for 12 weeks.

Novogen has received approval to commence a second phase Ib trial, which will be conducted at a major Sydney teaching hospital. This new study will measure the safety and anti-cancer effectiveness of phenoxodiol when administered by continuous intravenous infusion over seven days. The study will involve subjects with solid cancers whose cancers have become unresponsive to standard treatment.

INDICATION(S) AND RESEARCH PHASE
Cancer/Tumors (Unspecified) – Phase Ib
Prostate Cancer – Phase Ib

p53 gene therapy
unknown

MANUFACTURER
Aventis

DESCRIPTION
Aventis' p53 gene therapy is an anti-cancer treatment that produces an increased expression of the p53 protein. The p53 protein has the ability to activate other proteins to stop the cell cycle until damage to the cell may be repaired. Additionally, the p53 protein may stop growth in response to additional stimuli, such as reduced nutritional

resources or high cell density.

According to scientists, the p53 gene is one of the most frequently altered genes in human cancer, with 50% of all cancers having distorted forms of p53. This p53 gene therapy is delivered by an intraprostatic injection that may result in the suppression of prostate cancer growth. It is currently being tested in a phase I/II trial. Additionally, p53 gene therapy is being tested in phase III trials for head and neck cancer.

INDICATION(S) AND RESEARCH PHASE
Prostate Cancer – Phase I/II
Head and Neck Cancer – Phase III

PSMA - P1/P2
unknown

MANUFACTURER
Northwest Biotherapeutics

DESCRIPTION
Prostate specific membrane antigen (PSMA) is a substance found on a high proportion of prostate cancer cells. PSMA—P1/P2 is in phase I development.

INDICATION(S) AND RESEARCH PHASE
Prostate Cancer – Phase I

samarium Sm 153 lexidronam pentasodium
Quadramet

MANUFACTURER
Cytogen Corporation

DESCRIPTION
Quadramet is a radiopharmaceutical agent containing the radioisotope samarium-153. It is currently in phase II development for the treatment of prostate cancer that has metastasized.

INDICATION(S) AND RESEARCH PHASE
Prostate Cancer – Phase II

SGN-15/Taxotere
unknown

MANUFACTURER
Seattle Genetics

DESCRIPTION
SGN-15 is an antibody drug conjugate composed of the chimeric monoclonal antibody BR96 chemically linked to the drug doxorubicin with an average of eight drug molecules per mAb molecule. SGN-15 works by binding to a cell surface Ley-related antigen expressed on many tumor types, rapidly internalizing, and then releasing its payload of drug at the low pH present within the cell through acid catalyzed hydrolysis in the endosome. This mechanism of targeted drug delivery allows for relative sparing of tissues normally affected by non-specific chemotherapy, and represents an attractive strategy for the treatment of tumors expressing the BR96 antigen.

SGN-15 is being tested in a combination therapy with Aventis' drug Taxotere in a phase I/II trial in subjects with breast or colon cancer. This trial is being co-funded by Aventis. Additionally, a phase II trial is testing SGN/Taxotere in hormone refractory prostate cancer.

INDICATION(S) AND RESEARCH PHASE
Breast Cancer – Phase I/II
Prostate Cancer – Phase II
Colon Malignancies – Phase I/II

SPD 424
unknown

MANUFACTURER
Shire Pharmaceuticals

DESCRIPTION
SPD 424 (previously RL0903) is a subcutaneous implant that contains a gonadotropin releasing hormone (GnRH) agonist for the treatment of prostate cancer. The hydrogel implant delivers therapeutic agents at a controlled constant release for over one year. Phase III trials are under way.

INDICATION(S) AND RESEARCH PHASE
Prostate Cancer – Phase III

SR-48692
unknown

MANUFACTURER
Sanofi-Synthelabo Pharmaceuticals

DESCRIPTION
SR-48692 is an orally formulated neurotensin antagonist being tested for several indications, including colon cancer, prostate cancer, and schizophrenia.

INDICATION(S) AND RESEARCH PHASE
Colon Malignancies – Phase II
Prostate Cancer – Phase II
Schizophrenia and Schizoaffective Disorders – Phase IIa
Psychosis – Phase IIa
Depression – Phase II

strontium-89 chloride injection
Metastron

MANUFACTURER
Nycomed Amersham Imaging

DESCRIPTION
Metastron is an injectable radiopharmaceutical currently indicated for the relief of bone pain in subjects with painful skeletal metastases. Results of a phase II trial demonstrated that subjects with advanced prostate cancer treated with bone-targeted therapy consisting of Metastron in combination with chemotherapy survived longer than those who did not receive the Metastron therapy.

INDICATION(S) AND RESEARCH PHASE
Prostate Cancer – Phase II completed

SU-101
unknown

MANUFACTURER
Sugen

DESCRIPTION
SU-101 is a synthetic, platelet-derived growth factor receptor, which blocks the essential enzyme tyrosine kinase. This drug may be helpful for the treatment of end-stage malignant glioma, a tumor of nerve

tissue. The drug is being tested in phase III trials for refractory brain and prostate cancers, and phase II studies for non-small cell lung and ovarian cancers.

INDICATION(S) AND RESEARCH PHASE
Brain Cancer – Phase III
Prostate Cancer – Phase III
Lung Cancer – Phase II
Ovarian Cancer – Phase II

tretinoin
Atragen

MANUFACTURER
Aronex Pharmaceuticals

DESCRIPTION
Atragen is a liposomal, intravenous formulation of tretinoin or all-trans-retinoic acid. Tretinoin induces cell differentiation in rapidly proliferating cells, such as those observed in malignant diseases. Additionally, Atragen appears to affect the cellular signaling mechanisms that become unbalanced in cancer cells. Results of a phase II trial of Atragen monotherapy for acute promyelocytic leukemia (APL) indicated its potential to induce complete remission. The trial was conducted in Peru, and included 16 subjects with newly diagnosed or previously untreated APL who were treated with Atragen every other day as a single agent for a maximum of 28 doses. Fourteen subjects (87.5%) achieved morphologic remission, and 28.6% of these subjects also attained molecular remission. The safety profile observed in the subject population is similar to that reported with the currently approved oral formulation of Atra.

In addition to investigating the safety and efficacy of Atragen as a treatment for APL, the company is conducting trials to evaluate the compound for the treatment of non-Hodgkin's lymphoma, hormone-resistant prostate cancer, acute myelogenous leukemia (AML), and renal cell carcinoma in combination with interferon alpha.

In January 2001, Aronex announced that the FDA has denied approval of the company's NDA for Atragen as a treatment for subjects with APL, for whom therapy with tretinoin (all-trans-retinoic acid or Atra) is necessary but for whom an intravenous administration is required.

INDICATION(S) AND RESEARCH PHASE
Lymphoma, Non-Hodgkin's – Phase II
Prostate Cancer – Phase II
Renal Cell Carcinoma – Phase I/II
Leukemia, APL (intravenous) – NDA denied
Leukemia, APL (monotherapy) – Phase II
Leukemia, AML – Phase II

troxacitabine, BCH-4556
Troxatyl

MANUFACTURER
BioChem Pharma

DESCRIPTION
Troxatyl is a dioxolane nucleoside analog being investigated as an anticancer agent. The drug is a complete DNA chain terminator and DNA polymerase inhibitor. It acts by incorporating itself into the growing DNA chain of cancer cells, interfering with their ability to replicate further. Troxatyl is being evaluated as a single agent or in combination therapy in a number of ongoing trials in hematologic malignancies, including acute myeloid leukemia and chronic myeloid leukemia (blastic phase), and in lymphoproliferative disorders such as lymphoma, chronic lymphocytic leukemia and myeloma. It is also being evaluated as a single agent in pancreatic cancer and in combination therapy in a number of solid tumors. Troxatyl is currently in phase II development.

INDICATION(S) AND RESEARCH PHASE
Cancer/Tumors (Unspecified) – Phase II
Colorectal Cancer – Phase II
Head and Neck Cancer – Phase II
Leukemia – Phase II
Lung Cancer – Phase II
Malignant Melanoma – Phase II
Ovarian Cancer – Phase II
Pancreatic Cancer – Phase II
Prostate Cancer – Phase II
Renal Cell Carcinoma – Phase II

unknown
CyPat

MANUFACTURER
Barr Laboratories

DESCRIPTION
CyPat is a prostate cancer therapy in a phase III clinical trial. The trial is expected to include over 1,000 subjects and more than 40 sites. The drug is expected to be indicated for the treatment of hot flashes experienced by prostate cancer subjects with surgical or chemical castration.

INDICATION(S) AND RESEARCH PHASE
Prostate Cancer – Phase III

unknown
Leuvectin

MANUFACTURER
Vical

DESCRIPTION
The active ingredient in the DNA-based drug Leuvectin is a gene encoding interleukin-2 (IL-2), a naturally occurring protein that stimulates the immune system. Administration occurs by direct injection into a tumor, leading to uptake by the tumor cells and subsequent expression of the IL-2 protein. The company anticipates that local expression of IL-2 by cancer cells may stimulate the subject's immune system to attack and destroy the tumor cells. Leuvectin is being evaluated in phase II trials in subjects with kidney and prostate cancer.

INDICATION(S) AND RESEARCH PHASE
Renal Cell Carcinoma – Phase II
Prostate Cancer – Phase II

unknown
Abetafen

MANUFACTURER
Bioenvision

DESCRIPTION

Abetafen is a derivative of Modrefen, the company's marketed drug for breast cancer. Modrefen acts on the second estrogen receptor, which may be present in breast cancer and prostate cancer cells. This estrogen receptor is known to play some part in controlling normal prostate growth and may also influence growth of prostate cancer. New trials are under way to test effects of the drug on ERb in prostate cancer. Preclinical tests have shown that Modrefen decreases prostate growth in animals and modulates ligand binding to ERb in prostate cancer cell lines. Abetafen is currently in phase II trials for prostate cancer.

INDICATION(S) AND RESEARCH PHASE
Prostate Cancer – Phase II

unknown
Norelin

MANUFACTURER
YM Biosciences

DESCRIPTION
Norelin is an immunopharmaceutical product based on a proprietary recombinant antigen. It utilizes the subject's immune system to stimulate the development of antibodies to gonadotropin-releasing hormone (GnRH). The antibodies block the action of GnRH, which has therapeutic benefits for certain hormone-dependent cancers, such as prostate, breast, ovarian, and uterine cancer. The cancer vaccine has been shown to induce an immune response to GnRH in preclinical models, and a significant anti-tumor effect has been demonstrated.

A formulation with an aluminum-salt based adjuvant was shown to be safe in a phase I/II trial in subjects with hormone-sensitive prostate cancer; however, this formulation did not elicit a satisfactory immune response to GnRH. The company is in the process of commencing immunogenicity studies and testing a variety of formulations, following which it intends to resume clinical testing—phase I/II trials are expected in 2001 for the treatment of prostate cancer.

INDICATION(S) AND RESEARCH PHASE
Prostate Cancer – Phase I/II

unknown
Combidex

MANUFACTURER
Advanced Magnetics

DESCRIPTION
Combidex MRI contrast agent was developed to help in the detection, diagnosis, and staging of various cancers. The first indication is for the diagnosis of metastatic cancer to assist in directing biopsy and surgery as well as to aid in the staging of a variety of cancers, including breast and prostate cancer. In clinical studies, Combidex significantly reduced the number of false diagnoses (both false positive and false negative nodes) compared to unenhanced MRI exams. The second indication is for the detection, diagnosis, and characterization of benign versus malignant lesions of the liver and spleen.

In phase III clinical trials, post-Combidex MRI showed clear differentiation between normal and metastatic lymph nodes, while a post-gadolinium image showed no differentiation in normal and metastatic nodes when compared with pre-dose images.

INDICATION(S) AND RESEARCH PHASE
Breast Cancer – Phase III/IV
Liver Cancer – Phase III
Prostate Cancer – Phase III/IV

unknown
Tesmilifene

MANUFACTURER
YM Biosciences

DESCRIPTION
Tesmilifene is an intracellular histamine antagonist being developed as a chemopotentiator for the treatment of malignant solid tumors. The compound is cytotoxic to tumor cells and cytoprotective to the gut and normal bone marrow progenitor cells. Studies have indicated its ability to augment the in vivo anti-tumor activity of cytotoxic drugs routinely used in the treatment of cancer, such as doxorubicin, cyclophosphamide, 5-fluorouracil (5-FU), cisplatin, and mitoxantrone.

Interim analysis of data from a North American phase II pilot study in hormone refractory metastatic prostate cancer has shown promising results. The company hopes to conclude this phase II trial in 2001 and initiate a randomized pivotal study.

INDICATION(S) AND RESEARCH PHASE
Prostate Cancer – Phase II

unknown
GnRH Pharmaccine

MANUFACTURER
Aphton Corporation

DESCRIPTION
Aphton's novel GnRH Pharmaccine is an anti-gonadotropin releasing hormone (GnRH) immunogen, which neutralizes the hormone GnRH. Study results indicate that it induces and maintains castration levels of testosterone and reduced levels of prostate-specific antigen (PSA). Chemical castration of this type is a standard therapy to extend the survival of subjects with advanced prostate cancer. GnRH Pharmaccine is also involved in trials for breast cancer, endometrial cancer, and endometriosis, in addition to prostate cancer.

INDICATION(S) AND RESEARCH PHASE
Prostate Cancer – Phase I/II
Breast Cancer – Phase I/II
Endometrial Cancer – Phase I/II
Endometriosis – Phase I/II

unknown
Leuplin 3M DPS

MANUFACTURER
Takeda Chemical Industries

DESCRIPTION
Leuplin 3M DPS is a luteinizing hormone releasing factor being developed for the treatment of prostate cancer. It is currently in phase II trials in Japan.

INDICATION(S) AND RESEARCH PHASE
Prostate Cancer – Phase II

unknown
Apomine

MANUFACTURER
ILEX Oncology

DESCRIPTION
Apomine is a potent, orally active bisphosphonate estrogen derivative being developed to treat prostate cancer. Apomine induces apoptosis, which is a normal biological process involving a genetically programmed series of events that leads to cell death. Apomine activates the farnesoid X receptor (FXR) and a cascade of biological signals within the cell that rapidly induces apoptosis without affecting normal cells.

Apomine is being tested in phase II clinical trials in Lyon, France. It is currently being developed by ILEX and Symphar S.A. of Geneva, Switzerland.

INDICATION(S) AND RESEARCH PHASE
Prostate Cancer – Phase II

unknown
DCVax

MANUFACTURER
Northwest Biotherapeutics

DESCRIPTION
DCVAx is Northwest Biotherapeutics' proprietary dendritic cell-based immunotherapy. In October 2000, the company announced that no serious side effects had been reported following the first 40 injections of DCVax, and that company immunologists were encouraged by early immunology and PSA data from treated subjects. DCVax is being evaluated as a treatment for late-stage prostate cancer at M.D. Anderson Cancer Center, Houston, and the University of California, Los Angeles (UCLA).

INDICATION(S) AND RESEARCH PHASE
Prostate Cancer – Phase I/II

vaccine
Onyvax P

MANUFACTURER
Onyvax

DESCRIPTION
Onyvax P is an allogeneic whole-cell vaccine being developed for the treatment of prostate cancer. Phase I/II trials have been completed, and the vaccine is scheduled to enter phase II development in the first quarter of 2001. The phase I/II trial involved 60 subjects with advanced disease. Results showed the vaccine to be safe and capable of generating cancer-specific immune responses.

INDICATION(S) AND RESEARCH PHASE
Prostate Cancer – Phase I/II completed
Vaccines – Phase I/II completed

vaccine, adjuvant
AdjuVax-100a

MANUFACTURER
Jenner BioTherapies

DESCRIPTION
AdjuVax-100a is a proprietary emulsion formulation being tested with OncoVax-P prostate cancer vaccine. The combination therapy is in phase II trials.

INDICATION(S) AND RESEARCH PHASE
Prostate Cancer – Phase II
Vaccines – Phase II

vaccine, cancer
Gvax

MANUFACTURER
Cell Genesys

DESCRIPTION
Gvax is an allogeneic compound that involves the genetic modification of prostate cancer cell lines. These cancer cells have been irradiated and modified to secrete granulocyte-macrophage colony stimulating factor (GM-CSF), a hormone which plays a key role in stimulating the body's immune response to vaccines. The compound is in trials for prostate cancer, pancreatic cancer, lung cancer, leukemia, and malignant melanoma.

The Gvax prostate cancer vaccine demonstrated anti-tumor activity in an initial phase II trial in subjects with advanced metastatic prostate cancer who have not responded to hormone therapy. Prior to initiating a phase III trial, Cell Genesys plans to initiate further trials of Gvax prostate cancer vaccine in 2001 that will employ a higher potency version of the same product. Additionally, future phase III trials in hormone refractory prostate cancer subjects may compare Gvax vaccine in combination with chemotherapy to chemotherapy alone.

INDICATION(S) AND RESEARCH PHASE
Prostate Cancer – Phase II
Lung Cancer – Phase I/II completed
Malignant Melanoma – Phase I/II
Vaccines – Phase I/II
Pancreatic Cancer – Phase II
Leukemia – Phase I/II

vaccine, cancer
GeneVax

MANUFACTURER
Centocor

DESCRIPTION
GeneVax is a DNA-based vaccine technology in phase I development for the treatment of breast and prostate cancer.

INDICATION(S) AND RESEARCH PHASE
Vaccines – Phase I
Breast Cancer – Phase I
Prostate Cancer – Phase I

vaccine, prostate cancer (rV-psa)
Prostvac

MANUFACTURER
Therion Biologics

DESCRIPTION
Prostvac is a genetically engineered vaccine that is derived from the poxvirus. This

immunotherapeutic is being tested in phase II trials for the treatment of prostate cancer.

INDICATION(S) AND RESEARCH PHASE
Prostate Cancer – Phase II
Vaccines – Phase II

YM-598
unknown

MANUFACTURER
Yamanouchi Pharmaceutical

DESCRIPTION
YM-598 is an orally administered endothelin type A receptor (ETA) antagonist being evaluated for the treatment of advanced prostate cancer. It is being developed in Europe and has reached phase II trials.

INDICATION(S) AND RESEARCH PHASE
Prostate Cancer – Phase II

ZD-0473/AMD 473
unknown

MANUFACTURER
AstraZeneca

DESCRIPTION
ZD-0473 is a new platinum-based anticancer agent designed to deliver an extended spectrum of activity and overcome resistance to currently approved platinum drugs, such as cisplatin and carboplatin. It is being evaluated for the treatment of a range of solid-tumor cancers, including colorectal, non-small cell lung, and bladder cancer, which are resistant to carboplatin. ZD-0473 is being tested in both intravenous and oral formulations. The intravenous formulation is in phase II trials and the oral formulation is in preclinical development.

INDICATION(S) AND RESEARCH PHASE
Bladder Cancer – Phase II
Cancer/Tumors (Unspecified) – Phase II
Colorectal Cancer – Phase II
Lung Cancer – Phase II
Ovarian Cancer – Phase II
Prostate Cancer – Phase II
Breast Cancer – Phase II

Cervical Dysplasia/Cancer – Phase II

ZD-1839
Iressa

MANUFACTURER
AstraZeneca

DESCRIPTION
Iressa binds to the epidermal growth factor receptor (EGFR) and inhibits tyrosine kinase, thereby blocking signals for cancer growth and survival. The company reported encouraging results from phase I trials in a variety of tumors, but particularly in non-small cell lung cancer (NSCLC). Iressa is being investigated both as a monotherapy and in combination with other anti-tumor drugs in NSCLC, gastric, colorectal, and hormone-resistant prostate cancers. In 1999, the FDA gave Iressa fast-track status. The drug is currently in phase III studies for solid tumors.

INDICATION(S) AND RESEARCH PHASE
Cancer/Tumors (Unspecified) – Phase III
Colorectal Cancer – Phase III
Gastric Cancer – Phase III
Lung Cancer – Phase III
Prostate Cancer – Phase III

Renal Cell Carcinoma

AE-941
Neovastat

MANUFACTURER
AEterna Laboratories

DESCRIPTION
Neovastat is an angiogenesis inhibitor being tested for the treatment of non-small cell lung cancer, psoriasis, multiple myeloma, and kidney cancer, among other indications.

A phase II trial for multiple myeloma was initiated in October 2000 and will treat 120 subjects and include approximately 20 sites across North America and Europe. Trial results are expected in the summer of 2002.

Additionally, a phase III trial was initiated in May 2000 for kidney cancer, which will include 270 subjects at sites in North America and Europe.

INDICATION(S) AND RESEARCH PHASE
Lung Cancer – Phase III
Psoriasis and Psoriatic Disorders – Phase I/II completed
Cancer/Tumors (Unspecified) – Phase I/II completed
Multiple Myeloma – Phase II
Renal Cell Carcinoma – Phase III
Macular Degeneration – Phase I completed

aldesleukin, interleukin-2 (IL-2)
Proleukin

MANUFACTURER
Chiron Corporation

DESCRIPTION
Proleukin is a genetically engineered (recombinant) form of interleukin-2, which is a naturally occurring immune modulator. Proleukin is being evaluated in trials for acute myelogenous leukemia, non-Hodgkin's lymphoma, and HIV infection. Additionally, Proleukin was approved in July 2000 for advanced-stage kidney cancer and melanoma.

INDICATION(S) AND RESEARCH PHASE
HIV Infection – Phase III
Leukemia – Phase III
Lymphoma, Non-Hodgkin's – Phase III
Renal Cell Carcinoma – FDA approved
Melanoma – FDA approved

arsenic trioxide (ATO)
Trisenox

MANUFACTURER
Cell Therapeutics

DESCRIPTION
Trisenox is believed to kill cancer cells through apoptosis, or programmed cell death. The mechanism of action of Trisenox is not fully understood, but the drug appears to induce apoptosis in a different manner than other anti-cancer agents such as retinoids.

Trisenox is FDA approved to treat acute

promyelocytic leukemia (APL), and it is also in numerous trials in the United States for indications including other types of leukemia, prostate cancer, multiple myeloma, renal cell cancer, cervical cancer, and bladder cancer.

INDICATION(S) AND RESEARCH PHASE
Leukemia – Phase I
Lymphoma, Non-Hodgkin's – Phase II
Leukemia – Phase II
Multiple Myeloma – Phase II
Prostate Cancer – Phase II
Renal Cell Carcinoma – Phase II
Cervical Dysplasia/Cancer – Phase II
Bladder Cancer – Phase II

CD40 ligand
Avrend

MANUFACTURER
Immunex Corporation

DESCRIPTION
Avrend is a man-made CD40 ligand product. CD40 ligand is a glycoprotein found primarily on the surface of activated T cells, while its receptor (CD40) is found on immune system cells and cancer cells. Avrend binds directly to CD40 on many tumor cell types, generating a signal for the tumor cell to either stop growing or undergo apoptosis. Avrend also works by stimulating specific immune responses to the tumor.

INDICATION(S) AND RESEARCH PHASE
Renal Cell Carcinoma – Phase II

diarysulfonylurea, ILX-295501
unknown

MANUFACTURER
ILEX Oncology

DESCRIPTION
ILX-295501 belongs to a novel class of anti-tumor compounds known as diarysulfonylureas. This orally formulated drug is in phase II trials for renal cell carcinoma, malignant melanoma, lung, and ovarian cancers.

INDICATION(S) AND RESEARCH PHASE
Renal Cell Carcinoma – Phase II
Malignant Melanoma – Phase II
Lung Cancer – Phase II
Ovarian Cancer – Phase II

diethylnorspermine
DENSPM

MANUFACTURER
GelTex Pharmaceuticals

DESCRIPTION
DENSPM (diethylnorspermine) is similar to a naturally produced polyamine, except that it may interrupt the rapid growth of tumor cells that need polyamines for growth. The drug is in phase II trials for renal cell carcinoma, pancreatic cancer, malignant melanoma, and non-small cell lung cancer. Additional indications may include ovarian and colon cancers.

INDICATION(S) AND RESEARCH PHASE
Renal Cell Carcinoma – Phase II
Pancreatic Cancer – Phase II
Malignant Melanoma – Phase II
Lung Cancer – Phase II

EMD 82633
unknown

MANUFACTURER
Merck KgaA

DESCRIPTION
EMD 82633 is a humanized and bispecific monoclonal antibody derived from mice. These antibodies are altered in such a way that they no longer appear different from human antibodies. This genetic modification prevents immune reactions against foreign substances of animal origin used in humans. In this bispecific drug, one component binds to tumor cells, while the other activates the body's own CD8 "killer cells" to attack cancer cells.

This new drug is being given as an adjuvant therapy to subjects who have not been adequately helped by conventional forms of treatment, such as chemotherapy. EMD 82633 is being tested in trials for the treatment of renal cancer, head and neck cancer, breast cancer, bladder cancer, and ovarian cancer.

INDICATION(S) AND RESEARCH PHASE
Bladder Cancer – Phase II
Breast Cancer – Phase II
Cancer/Tumors (Unspecified) – Phase II
Head and Neck Cancer – Phase II
Ovarian Cancer – Phase II
Renal Cell Carcinoma – Phase II

GL-331
unknown

MANUFACTURER
Genelabs Technologies

DESCRIPTION
GL-331 is an inhibitor of topoisomerase II. It is a semi-synthetic derivative of podophyllotoxin, which is a chemotherapeutic agent designed to overcome multi-drug resistant (MDR) cancers. At this time, development has been discontinued.

INDICATION(S) AND RESEARCH PHASE
Colon Malignancies – Trial discontinued
Leukemia – Trial discontinued
Lung Cancer – Trial discontinued
Renal Cell Carcinoma – Trial discontinued

histamine dihydrochloride
Ceplene

MANUFACTURER
Maxim Pharmaceuticals

DESCRIPTION
Ceplene (formally Maxamine) is a histamine-2 (H-2) receptor stimulator that is being co-administered with immunotherapies, including cytokines and interleukin-2 (IL-2). Clinical testing includes treatment of acute myelogenous leukemia (AML), chronic hepatitis C, malignant melanoma, multiple myeloma, and renal cell carcinoma.

Results from a phase III trial in stage IV malignant melanoma subjects indicated that Ceplene used in combination with a lower dose of interleukin-2 (IL-2) improved survival rates compared to treatment with the same doses of IL-2 alone. Treatment with Ceplene and IL-2 improved overall survival, increased survival rates at 12, 18, and 24 months, and improved time-to-disease progression compared to treatment with IL-2 alone. Twenty-five percent of subjects treated with Ceplene and lower-dose IL-2 survived for a 24-month period. Overall response was achieved in 38% of the subjects treated with Ceplene and lower-dose IL-2. The company received an NDA non-approvable letter in January 2001 because the FDA stated that the phase III trial forming the basis of the NDA would not be adequate as a single study to support approval.

INDICATION(S) AND RESEARCH PHASE
Hepatitis – Phase II
Leukemia – Phase III completed
Malignant Melanoma – NDA denied
Multiple Myeloma – Phase II
Renal Cell Carcinoma – Phase II

HSPPC-96
Oncophage

MANUFACTURER
Antigenics

DESCRIPTION
Oncophage cancer vaccine is an injectable protein that contains the unique profile ("antigenic fingerprint") of each subject's cancer. The antigens activate the immune system to elicit an anti-tumor response. Oncophage is in clinical trials for several indications, including renal cell carcinoma (phase III), melanoma (phase II), colorectal cancer (phase II), gastric cancer (phase I/II), pancreatic cancer (phase I/II completed), and non-Hodgkin's lymphoma (phase II).

In October 2000, Antigenics announced that it had initiated a phase II trial of Oncophage in subjects who have been diagnosed with sarcoma, also known as soft tissue cancer. The study is expected to initially enroll 20 subjects diagnosed with recurrent metastatic or unresectable soft tissue sarcoma and may be expanded to include an additional 15 subjects depending on preliminary results.

INDICATION(S) AND RESEARCH PHASE
Renal Cell Carcinoma – Phase III
Malignant Melanoma – Phase II
Colorectal Cancer – Phase II
Gastric Cancer – Phase I/II
Pancreatic Cancer – Phase I/II completed
Lymphoma, Non-Hodgkin's – Phase II
Sarcoma – Phase II

IMC-C225, CPT-11
unknown

MANUFACTURER
ImClone Systems

DESCRIPTION
IMC-C225 is a chimerized (part mouse, part human) monoclonal antibody that may help fight cancer cells when used in conjunction with radiation therapy or other chemotherapy agents. This antibody selectively blocks the epidermal growth factor receptor (EGFr), which may be present in greater amounts on actively growing tumor cells. Since many cancers use specific growth factors to stimulate tumor cell growth, blocking this receptor may inhibit the cancer from increasing in size and spreading throughout the body.

The company is conducting phase III clinical trials evaluating IMC-C225 in combination with radiotherapy and with chemotherapy in subjects with advanced squamous cell head and neck carcinoma. IMC-C225 is in trials for several other indications in combination with various anti-cancer agents.

INDICATION(S) AND RESEARCH PHASE
Breast Cancer – Phase I/II
Head and Neck Cancer – Phase III
Lung Cancer – Phase III
Prostate Cancer – Phase I/II
Renal Cell Carcinoma – Phase II
Pancreatic Cancer – Phase II
Colorectal Cancer – Phase II

interleukin-12 (IL-12)
unknown

MANUFACTURER
Genetics Institute

DESCRIPTION
Interleukin-12 (IL-12) is a novel, genetically engineered human immune modulator. It is being tested in phase II trials for the treatment of hepatitis-C, chronic liver disease due to hepatitis infection, AIDS, and renal cell carcinoma.

INDICATION(S) AND RESEARCH PHASE
Acquired Immune Deficiency Syndrome (AIDS) and AIDS-Related Infections – Phase II
Hepatitis – Phase II
Renal Cell Carcinoma – Phase II

MDX-210
unknown

MANUFACTURER
Medarex

DESCRIPTION
MDX-210 is a bispecific (target-trigger) monoclonal antibody (MAb)-based treatment being developed for cancers with specific markers (HER-2/*neu* positive), including renal cell, non-small cell lung, pancreatic and prostate cancer. Phase II trials have been completed for kidney, prostate, and ovarian cancer. Phase III trials for ovarian cancer have have commenced in Europe.

INDICATION(S) AND RESEARCH PHASE
Prostate Cancer – Phase II completed
Renal Cell Carcinoma – Phase II completed
Colon Malignancies – Phase II
Breast Cancer – Phase II
Gastric Cancer – Phase II
Pancreatic Cancer – Phase II
Lung Cancer – Phase II
Ovarian Cancer – Phase III

MGI-114, hydroxymethylacylfulvene, HMAF
Irofulven

MANUFACTURER
MGI Pharma

DESCRIPTION
Irofulven (MGI-114) is the first product

candidate being developed by MGI Pharma from its family of anti-cancer compounds called acylfulvenes. Early trials demonstrated that Irofulven is absorbed rapidly by tumor cells, and once inside binds to DNA and protein targets. The binding interferes with DNA replication and cell division, leading to tumor-specific cell death. The drug is being tested in a series of trials for a variety of cancers.

In November 2000, results from a phase II trial of Irofulven indicated that the drug produced anti-tumor activity in subjects with advanced pancreatic cancer who were refractory to gemcitabine (Gemzar). Ten of the 53 subjects enrolled achieved six-month survival and two subjects demonstrated objective responses: one subject experienced tumor shrinkage of 100% and another subject experienced an 84% decrease in tumor mass. A phase III trial was initiated in February 2001.

INDICATION(S) AND RESEARCH PHASE
Breast Cancer – Phase II
Colon Malignancies – Phase II
Renal Cell Carcinoma – Phase II
Cervical Dysplasia/Cancer – Phase II
Lung Cancer – Phase II
Ovarian Cancer – Phase I/II
Colorectal Cancer – Phase II
Prostate Cancer – Phase I/II
Cancer/Tumors (Unspecified) – Phase I/II
Pancreatic Cancer – Phase III
Liver Cancer – Phase II

peginterferon alfa-2a
Pegasys

MANUFACTURER
Hoffmann-La Roche

DESCRIPTION
Pegasys is a longer-lasting form of interferon, which is a naturally produced immune boosting substance. This drug is in trials for hepatitis B and C, malignant melanoma, renal cell carcinoma, and chronic myelogenous leukemia.

INDICATION(S) AND RESEARCH PHASE
Hepatitis – Phase III
Malignant Melanoma – Phase II
Renal Cell Carcinoma – Phase II
Leukemia – Phase III

poly I:poly C-12-U
Ampligen

MANUFACTURER
Hemispherx Biopharma

DESCRIPTION
Ampligen is a novel therapeutic treatment composed of polyribonucleotide and synthetic nucleic acid. This intravenous drug is being evaluated in trials for renal carcinoma, malignant melanoma, chronic fatigue syndrome, and HIV.

INDICATION(S) AND RESEARCH PHASE
Renal Cell Carcinoma – Phase II/III
Malignant Melanoma – Phase I/II
Chronic Fatigue Syndrome – Phase III
HIV Infection – Phase III

T-cells/Xcellerate technology
unknown

MANUFACTURER
Xcyte Therapies

DESCRIPTION
Xcellerate is a new technology that activates helper T-cells exvivo and causes them to proliferate. T-cells are isolated from the subject's blood, activated with the Xcellerate technology, and eventually injected back into the subject. Phase I trials are under way for the treatment of metastatic kidney cancer. Other indications may include various cancers and infectious disease.

INDICATION(S) AND RESEARCH PHASE
Renal Cell Carcinoma – Phase I

tretinoin
Atragen

MANUFACTURER
Aronex Pharmaceuticals

DESCRIPTION
Atragen is a liposomal, intravenous formulation of tretinoin or all-trans-retinoic acid. Tretinoin induces cell differentiation in rapidly proliferating cells, such as those observed in malignant diseases.

Additionally, Atragen appears to affect the cellular signaling mechanisms that become unbalanced in cancer cells. Results of a phase II trial of Atragen monotherapy for acute promyelocytic leukemia (APL) indicated its potential to induce complete remission. The trial was conducted in Peru, and included 16 subjects with newly diagnosed or previously untreated APL who were treated with Atragen every other day as a single agent for a maximum of 28 doses. Fourteen subjects (87.5%) achieved morphologic remission, and 28.6% of these subjects also attained molecular remission. The safety profile observed in the subject population is similar to that reported with the currently approved oral formulation of Atra.

In addition to investigating the safety and efficacy of Atragen as a treatment for APL, the company is conducting trials to evaluate the compound for the treatment of non-Hodgkin's lymphoma, hormone-resistant prostate cancer, acute myelogenous leukemia (AML), and renal cell carcinoma in combination with interferon alpha.

In January 2001, Aronex announced that the FDA has denied approval of the company's NDA for Atragen as a treatment for subjects with APL, for whom therapy with tretinoin (all-trans-retinoic acid or Atra) is necessary but for whom an intravenous administration is required.

INDICATION(S) AND RESEARCH PHASE
Lymphoma, Non-Hodgkin's – Phase II
Prostate Cancer – Phase II
Renal Cell Carcinoma – Phase I/II
Leukemia, APL (intravenous) – NDA denied
Leukemia, APL (monotherapy) – Phase II
Leukemia, AML – Phase II

troxacitabine, BCH-4556
Troxatyl

MANUFACTURER
BioChem Pharma

DESCRIPTION
Troxatyl is a dioxolane nucleoside analog being investigated as an anticancer agent. The drug is a complete DNA chain terminator and DNA polymerase inhibitor. It acts by incorporating itself into the growing DNA chain of cancer cells, interfering with their ability to replicate further. Troxatyl is being evaluated as a single agent or in combination therapy in a number of ongoing trials in hematologic malignancies, including acute myeloid leukemia and chronic myeloid leukemia (blastic phase), and in lymphoproliferative disorders such as lymphoma, chronic lymphocytic leukemia, and myeloma. It is also being evaluated as a single agent in pancreatic cancer and in combination therapy in a number of solid tumors. Troxatyl is currently in phase II development.

INDICATION(S) AND RESEARCH PHASE
Cancer/Tumors (Unspecified) – Phase II
Colorectal Cancer – Phase II
Head and Neck Cancer – Phase II
Leukemia – Phase II
Lung Cancer – Phase II
Malignant Melanoma – Phase II
Ovarian Cancer – Phase II
Pancreatic Cancer – Phase II
Prostate Cancer – Phase II
Renal Cell Carcinoma – Phase II

unknown
Leuvectin

MANUFACTURER
Vical

DESCRIPTION
The active ingredient in the DNA-based drug Leuvectin is a gene encoding interleukin-2 (IL-2), a naturally occurring protein that stimulates the immune system. Administration occurs by direct injection into a tumor, leading to uptake by the tumor cells and subsequent expression of the IL-2 protein. The company anticipates that local expression of IL-2 by cancer cells may stimulate the subject's immune system to attack and destroy the tumor cells. Leuvectin is being evaluated in phase II trials in subjects with kidney and prostate cancer.

INDICATION(S) AND RESEARCH PHASE
Renal Cell Carcinoma – Phase II
Prostate Cancer – Phase II

unknown
Aroplatin

MANUFACTURER
Aronex Pharmaceuticals

DESCRIPTION
Platinum is a chemotherapeutic agent widely used in the treatment of solid tumors. Aroplatin is a liposomal formulation of a novel platinum product designed to overcome the toxicity and drug resistance associated with platinum use. It is currently in phase II trials for both mesothelioma and renal cell carcinoma.

INDICATION(S) AND RESEARCH PHASE
Mesothelioma – Phase II
Renal Cell Carcinoma – Phase II

vaccine, kidney cancer
unknown

MANUFACTURER
Genzyme Molecular Oncology

DESCRIPTION
This kidney cancer vaccine is currently in a phase I/II trial using proprietary cell fusion technology licensed to Genzyme Molecular Oncology from the Dana-Farber Cancer Institute.

INDICATION(S) AND RESEARCH PHASE
Renal Cell Carcinoma – Phase I/II

Sarcoma

CT-2584
Apra

MANUFACTURER
Cell Therapeutics

DESCRIPTION
Apra is a novel synthetic inhibitor of phosphatidic acid metabolism in tumor cells. This antineoplastic agent kills cancer cells without having to depend on cell division to exert its effect. Additionally, Apra may also help inhibit multi-drug resistance of certain cancers. The drug is in trials for the treatment of prostate cancer and sarcomas. Additional indications may include cancers of the colon, breast, and female reproductive system including the ovaries.

INDICATION(S) AND RESEARCH PHASE
Prostate Cancer – Phase II
Sarcoma – Phase II

disaccharide tripeptide glycerol dipalmitoyl
ImmTher

MANUFACTURER
Endorex Corporation

DESCRIPTION
ImmTher, a bone cancer drug candidate, stimulates human macrophages to exhibit broad tumoricidal activity against a variety of human cancer cells. ImmTher is a novel muramyl dipeptide immunomodulator formulated in liposomes. The drug acts by activating macrophages to attack micrometastatic cancer cells that have evaded chemotherapy or surgery. These activated macrophages kill cancer cells by engulfing them or by secreting lethal factors.

Trials are under way for the treatment of subjects with osteosarcoma and Ewing's sarcoma. Additionally, a phase II trial is under way for children six to 18 years of age for the treatment of Ewing's sarcoma. The FDA has designated ImmTher as an Orphan Drug for the treatment of the primary types of bone cancers, Ewing's sarcoma and osteosarcoma.

INDICATION(S) AND RESEARCH PHASE
Pediatric, Sarcoma – Phase II
Sarcoma – Phase II

HSPPC-96
Oncophage

MANUFACTURER
Antigenics

DESCRIPTION
Oncophage cancer vaccine is an injectable protein that contains the unique profile ("antigenic fingerprint") of each subject's cancer. The antigens activate the immune system to elicit an anti-tumor response. Oncophage is in clinical trials for several indications, including renal cell carcinoma (phase III), melanoma (phase II), colorectal cancer (phase II), gastric cancer (phase I/II), pancreatic cancer (phase I/II completed), and non-Hodgkin's lymphoma (phase II).

In October 2000, Antigenics announced that it had initiated a phase II trial of Oncophage in subjects who have been diagnosed with sarcoma, also known as soft tissue cancer. The study is expected to initially enroll 20 subjects diagnosed with recurrent metastatic or unresectable soft tissue sarcoma and may be expanded to include an additional 15 subjects depending on preliminary results.

INDICATION(S) AND RESEARCH PHASE
Renal Cell Carcinoma – Phase III
Malignant Melanoma – Phase II
Colorectal Cancer – Phase II
Gastric Cancer – Phase I/II
Pancreatic Cancer – Phase I/II completed
Lymphoma, Non-Hodgkin's – Phase II
Sarcoma – Phase II

T64
unknown

MANUFACTURER
Tularik

DESCRIPTION
T64 is an antifolate that disrupts DNA synthesis through the inhibition of purine biosynthesis. The compound is currently in phase II trials in subjects with head and neck cancer, soft tissue sarcoma, melanoma, breast cancer, and non-small cell lung cancer. Additionally, T64 is in phase I combination trials with gemcitabine, doxorubicin, and paclitaxel. Tularik expects to initiate two additional T64 phase I combination trials with carboplatin and temozolamide in the first quarter of 2001. The T64 trials are being conducted in the United States, the United Kingdom, the Netherlands, and Australia.

INDICATION(S) AND RESEARCH PHASE
Head and Neck Cancer – Phase II
Sarcoma – Phase II
Melanoma – Phase II
Breast Cancer – Phase II
Lung Cancer – Phase II
Cancer/Tumors (Unspecified) – Phase I

VX-710
Incel

MANUFACTURER
Vertex Pharmaceuticals

DESCRIPTION
Incel blocks two major multi-drug resistance mechanisms: P-glycoprotein (MDR-1) and multi-drug resistance-associated protein (MRP). Administered intravenously, Incel is to be used in combination with cancer chemotherapy agents. Vertex's research shows that Incel can enhance the accumulation of chemotherapy agents in tumor cells by blocking the drug pumps P-gp and MRP, and that it is capable of restoring the sensitivity of tumors to treatment with chemotherapeutic agents. Phase II trials investigating the activity of Incel in combination with other agents for the treatment of advanced refractory ovarian cancer, soft tissue sarcoma, and small cell lung cancer are under way.

INDICATION(S) AND RESEARCH PHASE
Lung Cancer – Phase II
Ovarian Cancer – Phase II
Sarcoma – Phase II

Skin Cancer

CpG 7909
unknown

MANUFACTURER
Coley Pharmaceutical

DESCRIPTION
CpG 7909 is from a synthetic DNA sequence that naturally activates the human immune system to fight disease. This drug is being tested in three phase I/II trials for the treatment of cancer. The first trial has been initiated at the University of Iowa Cancer Center and is testing 24 subjects with refractory or relapsed non-Hodgkin's lymphoma. Subjects in this trial will receive weekly infusions of CpG 7909 for three weeks. Two other trials have been initiated in Europe. The first trial includes subjects with melanoma, while the second includes subjects with metastic melanoma or basal cell carcinoma.

INDICATION(S) AND RESEARCH PHASE
Lymphoma, Non-Hodgkin's – Phase I/II
Melanoma – Phase I/II
Skin Cancer – Phase I/II

eflornithine, DFMO (difluoromethylornydil)
unknown

MANUFACTURER
Aventis

DESCRIPTION
Eflornithine is a potent, irreversible inhibitor of ornithine decarboxylase (OCD), an enzyme that is elevated in most tumors and pre-malignant lesions. Eflornithine is currently in a phase III clinical trial to determine the effectiveness of the drug in treating subjects who have newly diagnosed or recurrent bladder cancer. The drug is administered orally in tablet form.

Eflornithine is also in trials for the prevention and treatment of HIV infections, skin cancer, breast cancer, prostate cancer, and cervical dysplasia/cancer.

INDICATION(S) AND RESEARCH PHASE
Bladder Cancer – Phase III
Breast Cancer – Phase II/III
Cervical Dysplasia/Cancer – Phase II
HIV Infection – Phase II
Prostate Cancer – Phase II
Skin Cancer – Phase III

FK-317
unknown

MANUFACTURER
Fujisawa Healthcare

DESCRIPTION
Fujisawa has developed a new anti-cancer medication, FK-317, that originally was developed as an antibiotic. The molecule, known as a dihydrobenzoxazine, underwent preliminary testing in thirty-one subjects with solid tumors that were refractory to other chemotherapeutic treatments. The company reported that tumor reduction was observed in four subjects, two of whom achieved complete remission. Side effects and other toxicities such as leukopenia (decreased white blood cells) and neutropenia were modest in comparison to other established treatments.

It is unclear how exactly this compound works to limit the growth of cancer, but it seems to influence the process by which cells reproduce themselves. Currently, FK-317 is given at a dose of 24 mg/day intravenously and it is being evaluated in phase II trials. Scientists are testing it in a variety of solid tumors such as prostate, breast, and skin cancer.

INDICATION(S) AND RESEARCH PHASE
Breast Cancer – Phase II
Cancer/Tumors (Unspecified) – Phase II
Prostate Cancer – Phase II
Skin Cancer – Phase II

interleukin-12 gene therapy
unknown

MANUFACTURER
Valentis

DESCRIPTION
Interleukin-12 (IL-12) is a hormone-like substance that regulates the activity of cells involved in an immune response. IL-12 is made by a select group of immune cells that normally are the first to encounter disease-causing organisms in the body and react to them. IL-12 activates other immune cells such as T-cells, B-cells, dendritic cells and natural killer (NK) cells. Together, T-cells, and NK cells seek out and destroy tumor cells. Additionally, IL-12 increases the production of interferon-gamma, which in turn augments the killing ability of immune cells. IL-12 also promotes antibody production by B-cells and stimulates dendritic cells to multiply. Lastly, IL-12 inhibits angiogenesis, the development of new blood vessels within tumors.

The company has initiated a multi-center phase IIa trial for the treatment of squamous cell carcinoma of the head and neck.

INDICATION(S) AND RESEARCH PHASE
Head and Neck Cancer – Phase IIa
Skin Cancer – Phase IIa

unknown
Metvix PDT

MANUFACTURER
PhotoCure ASA

DESCRIPTION
Metvix photodynamic therapy (PDT) is a topical cream being developed for the treatment of high-risk basal cell carcinoma (BCC), primary BCC, and pre-cancerous skin lesions known as actinic keratosis. The cream is applied to a lesion and left to stand so that the active ingredient can be absorbed into target cells. The active ingredient in Metvix is an ALA ester, which is converted into a photosensitizer inside the cancerous cells. After a period of time has elapsed, the area of skin selected for treatment is illuminated by red light, which excites the photosensitizer and produces cytotoxic singlet oxygen.

In January 2001, results of a phase III trial of topical Metvix PDT for the treatment of primary superficial basal cell carcinoma indicated that more than 90% of skin cancer lesions were completely cured three months after treatment with the drug. Results from the initial response evaluation demonstrated that topical Metvix PDT was as effective as cryotherapy in removing this type of skin lesion. Additionally, the trial indicated that Metvix PDT provided a better cosmetic outcome than cryotherapy. A total of 120 subjects were enrolled in the trial, which involved 13 clinical centers in seven European countries.

PhotoCure completed phase III trials for Metvix for the treatment of actinic keratosis and filed an application for European marketing approval in May 2000. Pivotal trials for BCC are ongoing and the company plans to file an application for marketing approval first quarter 2001.

INDICATION(S) AND RESEARCH PHASE
Skin Cancer – Phase III
Actinic Keratosis – MAA Filed

Thrombocytopenia

5c8
Antova

MANUFACTURER
Biogen

DESCRIPTION
Biogen has engineered 5c8 (anti CD-40 ligand antibody), a humanized monoclonal antibody for the treatment of a number of autoimmune disorders, including idiopathic thrombocytopenia purpura (ITP), systemic lupus erythematosus, kidney transplantation, and factor VIII antibody inhibition.

In these autoimmune diseases, it is thought that activated white blood cells (T-cell lymphocytes) bind to other tissue cells through a cell surface receptor called the CD-40 ligand. In turn, abnormal antibodies are produced that now recognize healthy body tissues as foreign, and thereby cause an inflammatory response. The 5c8 antibody may stop this abnormal immune cycle by binding to the CD-40 ligand inhibiting its ability to bind with its receptor on a variety of normal cells.

INDICATION(S) AND RESEARCH PHASE
Thrombocytopenia – Phase II
Systemic Lupus Erythematosus – Phase II
Kidney Transplant Surgery – Phase II

CBP-1011
Colirest

Thrombocytopenia

MANUFACTURER
Inkine Pharmaceutical Company

DESCRIPTION
CBP-1011 is an oral steroid-like drug in development for the treatment of idiopathic thrombocytopenic purpura (ITP). ITP is a disorder in which the immune system attacks its own platelets, targeting them with antibodies and then destroying the resulting immune complexed platelets. Preliminary studies have indicated CBP-1011 may help increase platelet counts. The drug is currently in phase III trials for ITP.

Additionally, phase II trials for the treatment of Crohn's disease have been completed, and the drug is also in development for ulcerative colitis. In December 2000, positive results were announced for a multicenter open-label phase II trial of Colirest in subjects with mild or moderate active ulcerative colitis. Nine of 11 evaluable subjects completed eight weeks of Colirest treatment. Seven of the nine (78%) subjects responded to Colirest treatment in the Disease Activity Index (DAI) and Investigator Global Assessment (IGA) evaluations. Inkine Pharmaceutical Company plans to move Colirest into later stage pivotal trials.

INDICATION(S) AND RESEARCH PHASE
Thrombocytopenia – Phase III
Crohn's Disease – Phase II completed
Inflammatory Bowel Disease – Phase II completed

MDX-33
unknown

MANUFACTURER
Medarex

DESCRIPTION
MDX-33 is a humanized monoclonal antibody being evaluated for its ability to decrease the activity of monocytes, macrophages, or other white blood cells that can destroy healthy platelets or red blood cells. It is in trials for the treatment of autoimmune blood disorders such as idiopathic thrombocytopenia purpura (ITP) and autoimmune hemolytic anemia.

Results of a phase II trial of MDX-33 suggested the drug was well tolerated in adult subjects with chronic ITP. Additionally, a single dose of MDX-33 appeared to substantially elevate platelet counts in all subjects treated with the optimal dose. The dose-escalating, double-blind, placebo-controlled trial consisted of 30 adults with chronic ITP. MDX-33 is being developed through a corporate alliance between Medarex and Aventis Behring.

INDICATION(S) AND RESEARCH PHASE
Anemia – Phase II
Thrombocytopenia – Phase II completed

PI-88
unknown

MANUFACTURER
Progen Industries

DESCRIPTION
PI-88 will be entering phase II trials for the prevention of blood clots in thromboembolic diseases and angioplasty induced restenosis in 2001. Results from previous trials have shown that PI-88 is a potent antithrombotic and anti-coagulant with a unique mode of action. PI-88 inhibits growth of vascular smooth muscle cells (restenosis) in animal models that are analogues to balloon angioplasty.

Balloon angioplasty is a surgical procedure where a balloon-tipped catheter is used to widen blocked arteries. Local vascular irritation occurs in 30% of people who have received the angioplasty procedure. This irritation induces rapid growth of smooth muscle cells surrounding the artery, causing arterial re-blockage.

In additional to trials for restenosis and other indications, PI-88 will be entering phase II trials for cancer in early 2001.

INDICATION(S) AND RESEARCH PHASE
Thrombocytopenia – Phase II
Cancer/Tumors (Unspecified) – Phase II

psoralen, S-59
unknown

MANUFACTURER
Cerus Corporation

DESCRIPTION
S-59 is a light-activated psoralen compound being developed to target and inactivate blood-borne pathogens without damaging the therapeutic properties of platelets and plasma solutions. A phase III thrombocytopenia program is under way in the United States, and a European phase III study will involve four sites attempting to recruit 100 subjects.

Additionally, a pathogen inactivation system for fresh frozen plasma (FFP) also started a phase III program in the United States. Subjects will include those with congenital or acquired coagulation factor deficiencies, and those with thrombocytopenic purpura who need large volume FFP transfusions. Cerus Corporation is developing psoralen in collaboration with Baxter Healthcare.

INDICATION(S) AND RESEARCH PHASE
Bacterial Infection – Phase III
Red Blood Cell Disorders – Phase III
Thrombocytopenia – Phase III
Viral Infection – Phase III

YM-294, oprelvekin
unknown

MANUFACTURER
Yamanouchi Pharmaceutical

DESCRIPTION
YM-294 is an injectable thrombocytopoietic factor (rhIL-11) being evaluated for its effectiveness in preventing chemotherapy-induced thrombocytopenia. The drug is in phase III trials and is part of Yamanouchi's domestic pipeline. The company is developing the drug with Genetics Institute.

INDICATION(S) AND RESEARCH PHASE
Thrombocytopenia – Phase III

Thyroid Cancer

arcitumomab
CEA-Scan

MANUFACTURER
Immunomedics

DESCRIPTION
CEA-Scan is a monoclonal antibody attached to carcinoembryonic (CEA) antigen that is radioactively labeled with technetium (Tc99m). CEA is an important cell surface marker expressed by certain tumor cells. This imaging agent can detect various cancer cells associated with CEA expressed tumors. CEA-Scan utilizes proprietary technetium (RAID) technology.

Currently, CEA-Scan is being tested in a phase II/III trial for breast cancer. It is being used to evaluate subjects with suspicious mammograms, as well as palpable and nonpalpable lesions.

This agent is also in a phase II trial for thyroid cancer. CEA-Scan is used for the diagnosis and localization of primary, residual, recurrent, and metastatic medullary thyroid carcinoma.

Lastly, CEA-Scan is in a phase III for lung cancer. It determines the presence, location, and extent of the metastatic disease in primary and recurrent lung cancer.

INDICATION(S) AND RESEARCH PHASE
Breast Cancer – Phase II/III
Lung Cancer – Phase III
Thyroid Cancer – Phase II

6 | Infectious Disease and Immunology

Drugs in the development pipeline	455*
Number of drugs in preclinical testing	261
Number of drugs in clinical testing	171

Source: Parexel

According to Pharmaceutical Research and Manufacturers of America (PhRMA), infectious diseases are responsible for more than 100,000 deaths each year in the United States and cost more than $30 billion in direct treatment expenses. Immunologic disorders also have a significant impact, and as a result, the combined therapeutic area of infectious disease and immunology encompasses a considerable market share for clinical trials in all phases of development.

CenterWatch has identified approximately 30 to 40 drugs on trials for various bacterial infections and estimates that $180 million to $200 million will be spent in investigator grants this year. The need for new treatments is in part due to the growing problem of multi-drug resistant bacterial infections. While the discovery and widespread use of antibiotics has considerably aided the treatment of infectious disease, bacteria and other organisms have proven remarkably adaptive in developing resistance to existing therapies. Furthermore, the treatment of antimicrobial resistant infection is associated with a significant cost. According to the US Department of Health and Human Services (HHS), it has been estimated that the in-hospital cost of hospital-acquired infections caused by just six common kinds of resistant bacteria is at least $1.3 billion per year, in 1992 dollars.

The problem of resistance has not gone unnoticed. Infection control programs are a disease management strategy to reduce the number of infections. Additionally, HHS recently unveiled an action plan, developed by an interdepartmental task force, designed to combat antimicrobial resistance. The plan has four major components: surveillance, prevention and control, research, and product development—initiatives now underway or planned to begin by 2002. Consumers have also become more aware of the problem and realize that the overuse of antibiotics encourages the development of bacterial resistance.

Other events in the field of bacterial infection include the approval of a drug from the first completely new class of antibiotics to reach hospitals in 35 years. Pharmacia's Zyvox (linezolid) is the first of a new class of synthetic antibiotics called the oxazolidinones, which inhibit bacterial protein synthesis at a very early step. Individuals in the public health and infectious disease communities have identified infections caused by Gram-positive bacteria as one of the greatest challenges in hospital infections. Clinical studies have shown that Zyvox is effective in treating infections caused by Gram-positive bacteria, including some that are resistant to all other antibiotics.

Viral infections are also a major target of research and emerging products. For hepatitis C virus (HCV) infection, promising therapies include the newer forms of long-acting interferons, alpha interferons modified by polyethylene glycol (PEG) so that they can be given once a week and yet provide a sustained level of interferon. These pegylated formulations may avoid the peaks and troughs of interferon levels and may reduce interferon side effects that occur when the drug is given three times a week. Other promising approaches are the use of other cytokines and the development of newer antivirals, such as RNA polymerase, helicase or protease inhibitors. A major focus for HCV infection is developing a tissue culture system that will enable researchers to study HCV in a more efficient manner. Animal models and molecular approaches to the study of HCV are also important and advances in these areas have been made. Understanding how the virus replicates and how it injures cells will be helpful in developing additional strategies of controlling the virus and in screening for new drugs effective in HCV infection.

Research in the area of immunology primarily centers on acquired immunodeficiency syndrome or AIDS. With more than 33 million people worldwide infected with the HIV virus, including a million people in North America, it is no surprise that billions of dollars are spent on medications to combat this disease. It is also clear that more money, resources, and energies are being focused toward developing new pharmacological therapies to treat HIV than ever before. According to CenterWatch, approximately 55 to 65 drugs are in development for AIDS/HIV and related complications at an annual cost of about $290 million to $320 million in investigator grants.

There are three principle classes of drugs that target HIV replication. Already, in clinical practice, the standard of care is to combine several drugs from these different classes. The first major class of drugs is one that blocks an enzyme crucial for viral replication—reverse transcriptase. Within this reverse transcriptase group, there are two subclasses: nucleoside reverse transcriptase inhibitors (NRTI) and non-nucleoside reverse transcriptase inhibitors (NNRTI). NNRTI drugs do not physically interrupt the DNA chain like the NRTIs; instead, they bind to the reverse transcriptase enzyme itself, changing its shape so that the enzyme becomes inactivated. The first effective antiretrovirals (e.g., zidovudine, didanosine, etc.) are NRTIs.

A second focus in the field of HIV/AIDS treatment is the inhibition of the protease enzyme. HIV protease cuts the new viral protein into smaller, active protein strands. Inhibition of protease effectively inhibits the release of viable viral particles from the infected cells. One of the new protease inhibitors recently approved by the FDA is Kaletra, a combination of lopinavir and low dose ritonavir. Ritonavir inhibits the metabolism of lopinavir, which results in higher blood levels of lopinavir than if it were given alone, thus enhancing its efficacy against the HIV virus and improving the dosing regimen so that the drug can be given twice daily.

According to the National Institute of Allergy and Infectious Diseases (NIAID) 2000 annual vaccine report, since 1987 more than 3,000 non-HIV-infected volunteers have enrolled in 52 NIAID-supported preventive vaccine studies involving 27 vaccines. Such immune-based therapies are another rapidly growing area of HIV/AIDS drug development. An experimental vaccine in phase III trials is composed of synthetic proteins patterned after an HIV virus surface protein, gp120, which binds to human T-cells and allows viral entry into the cells. Early trials indicated that individuals given the vaccine produced antibodies that neutralized a particular strain of the HIV virus. Other strategies focus on boosting macrophage function, which is reduced in patients with AIDS. By restoring macrophage activity, the rate of disease progression may be reduced.

Finally, additional new compounds for the treatment of invasive fungal infections are under development, including new triazole compounds such as voriconazole, posaconazole, and ravuconazole; new echinocandins, which inhibit the synthase of beta-glucan in the fungal cell wall, FK463 (norfungin); liposomal nystatin; and a variety of inhibitors of various stages of intermediary metabolism of the fungus.

Acquired Immune Deficiency Syndrome (AIDS) and AIDS-Related Infections

dOTC
unknown

MANUFACTURER
BioChem Pharma

DESCRIPTION
dOTC is a novel nucleoside substitute (analogue) that inhibits the AIDS virus from multiplying. It works by slowing down or inhibiting the enzyme, reverse transcriptase, from copying the genetic code of the virus. This drug is being tested on HIV strains that have developed resistance to AZT and 3TC and to certain protease inhibitors.

INDICATION(S) AND RESEARCH PHASE
Acquired Immune Deficiency Syndrome (AIDS) and AIDS-Related Infections – Phase II
HIV Infection – Phase II

AIDS gene therapy
unknown

MANUFACTURER
Aventis

DESCRIPTION
This gene therapy for AIDS involves genetically engineered T-cells that may target and eliminate residual virus in HIV-infected cells. The AIDS virus can remain dormant as reservoirs for future infection even after treatment with the best available antiviral drugs. This therapy was being tested in phase II trials for the treatment of AIDS. Future therapeutic studies may include cancer.

INDICATION(S) AND RESEARCH PHASE
Acquired Immune Deficiency Syndrome (AIDS) and AIDS-Related Infections – Phase II
HIV Infection – Phase II

ALVAC-HIV 1
unknown

MANUFACTURER
Aventis Pasteur

DESCRIPTION
ALVAC-HIV 1 is a vaccine that uses live canary poxvirus, which does not infect human beings. The poxvirus is acting as a carrier or vector to deliver a preparation of genetically engineered HIV surface glycoproteins (gp 160). This complex was developed to stimulate the body's production of HIV-neutralizing antibodies to protect against AIDS. This vaccine is being tested in phase II trials.

INDICATION(S) AND RESEARCH PHASE
Acquired Immune Deficiency Syndrome (AIDS) and AIDS-Related Infections – Phase II
HIV Infection – Phase II

AMD-3100
unknown

MANUFACTURER
AnorMED

DESCRIPTION
AMD-3100, a fusion inhibitor for the treatment of human immunodeficiency virus (HIV) acts by blocking the binding of the virus's CXCR4 receptor with a human host cell. The drug is being tested in phase II trials in an intravenous infusion formulation. AMD-3100 is also in phase I trials for the mobilization of white blood cells.

INDICATION(S) AND RESEARCH PHASE
Acquired Immune Deficiency Syndrome (AIDS) and AIDS-Related Infections – Phase II
HIV Infection – Phase II
Mobilization of White Blood Cells – Phase I

BMS-232632
unknown

MANUFACTURER
Bristol-Myers Squibb

DESCRIPTION
BMS-232632 is a new protease inhibitor that may enable HIV subjects to take their medication once a day, rather than taking multiple pills several times a day. Protease inhibitors act against the HIV virus by inhibiting the action of the protease enzyme that the virus needs in order to reproduce. When this enzyme is blocked, HIV makes copies of itself that cannot infect new cells. Because these drugs reduce HIV production, they help to decrease the total amount of virus in a subject's system.

Among the many challenges that face subjects with HIV is the necessity of having to take up to eighty pills throughout the day. In preclinical studies, BMS-232632 has been shown to be effective against the HIV virus when administered only once a day. This frequency of dosing represents a more convenient way for subjects to take their antiviral medication, and it could enhance subject compliance and therefore, improve the effective outcome. Early research has demonstrated that the reason BMS-232632 is effective in once daily administration is because it is one of the more potent protease inhibitors. Further study is necessary to confirm preliminary animal findings. BMS-232632 is currently being tested in phase II clinical trials.

INDICATION(S) AND RESEARCH PHASE
Acquired Immune Deficiency Syndrome (AIDS) and AIDS-Related Infections – Phase II
HIV Infection – Phase II

C319-14/6
Oramed

MANUFACTURER
Biosyn

DESCRIPTION
Oramed is an antifungal oral rinse for treatment of azole-resistant strains of oral candidiasis in HIV positive subjects. The drug completed phase II trials. Testing for other indications may include acquired immune deficiency syndrome Syndrome (AIDS)

related diseases, infectious diseases and viral diseases, antifungal applications, and candidiasis.

INDICATION(S) AND RESEARCH PHASE
Acquired Immune Deficiency Syndrome (AIDS) and AIDS-Related Infections – Phase II completed
Fungal Infections – Phase II completed

capravirine
unknown

MANUFACTURER
Pfizer

DESCRIPTION
The compound capravirine is a member of an important class of anti-HIV agents called non-nucleoside reverse transcriptase inhibitors (NNRTIs). In January 2001, Pfizer announced that it has restricted use of capravirine for some subjects in clinical trials based on results of a 12-month animal toxicology study, which demonstrated an unexpected finding of vasculitis in animals that received very high doses of capravirine. The drug is presently the subject of phase II and III trials to determine its safety and efficacy in people living with HIV. The FDA is permitting treatment-experienced subjects who previously have failed NNRTIs, but are responding well to capravirine, to continue their current capravirine drug regimens. The remaining subjects will discontinue use of capravirine but will remain on study protocols.

INDICATION(S) AND RESEARCH PHASE
Acquired Immune Deficiency Syndrome (AIDS) and AIDS-Related Infections – Phase III
HIV Infection – Phase III

CPI-1189
unknown

MANUFACTURER
Centaur Pharmaceuticals

DESCRIPTION
CPI-1189 is being tested for the treatment of AIDS and Parkinson's disease. Results from a phase IIa trial for AIDS dementia complex (ADC) in May included 64 HIV subjects with cognitive and motor impairment. Subjects either received 100 mg a day or 50 mg a day of CPI-1189 or the placebo over 10 weeks, with a 12 week open label follow-on for those who volunteered.

INDICATION(S) AND RESEARCH PHASE
Acquired Immune Deficiency Syndrome (AIDS) and AIDS-Related Infections – Phase IIa completed
Parkinson's Disease – Phase IIa

diclofenac
Oralease

MANUFACTURER
Skye Pharma

DESCRIPTION
Oralease (diclofenac) is an anti-inflammatory being evaluated for the treatment of mouth lesions in AIDS subjects and mucositis in cancer subjects undergoing head and neck radiation.

INDICATION(S) AND RESEARCH PHASE
Acquired Immune Deficiency Syndrome (AIDS) and AIDS-Related Infections – Phase II
Head and Neck Cancer – Phase II
Oral Medicine – Phase II

dihydrotestosterone
Andractim

MANUFACTURER
Unimed Pharmaceuticals

DESCRIPTION
Andractim is a hormone replacement therapy for the treatment of male testosterone deficiency. It is a clear, odorless, non-irritating, topical gel that delivers dihydrotestosterone transdermally to the bloodstream. It is being tested in phase III trials for geriatric hypogonadism, a condition characterized by abnormally decreased sexual function of the testes in elderly males.

Additionally, this anabolic steroid is being tested in phase II trials for the treatment of weight loss associated with HIV wasting in AIDS subjects. Dihydrotestosterone is a natural male hormone that can assist in building muscle mass. Unimed Pharmaceuticals has a collaborative agreement with BioChem Pharma to develop Andractim, which is licensed from Laboratoires Besins Iscovesco S. A., France.

INDICATION(S) AND RESEARCH PHASE
Acquired Immune Deficiency Syndrome (AIDS) and AIDS-Related Infections – Phase II
Male Hormonal Deficiencies/Abnormalities – Phase III

DMP-450
unknown

MANUFACTURER
Du Pont

DESCRIPTION
DMP-450, a second-generation protease inhibitor, belongs to a class of chemicals that are novel for the treatment of HIV infections: the cyclic ureas. The company completed a phase I study and plans phase I/II studies outside the United States. The initiation of potential efficacy studies in the United States awaits the outcome of further discussions with the FDA who have placed the DMP-450 program on partial clinical hold.

INDICATION(S) AND RESEARCH PHASE
Acquired Immune Deficiency Syndrome (AIDS) and AIDS-Related Infections – Phase I/II
HIV Infection – Phase I/II

emivirine
Coactinon

MANUFACTURER
Triangle Pharmaceuticals

DESCRIPTION
Coactinon is a nucleoside analogue derivative that functions as a non-nucleoside reverse transcriptase inhibitor (NNRTI). In

August 2000, the company announced its intention to continue developing Coactinon for the treatment of HIV infection, following notification in 1999 that additional phase III trials may be necessary to prove that regimens containing Coactinon are equivalent or superior to current first-line therapies. MKC-401 is currently ongoing and has been amended to enroll an additional 280 subjects.

INDICATION(S) AND RESEARCH PHASE
Acquired Immune Deficiency Syndrome (AIDS) and AIDS-Related Infections – Phase III
HIV Infection – Phase III
Pediatric, AIDS/HIV – Phase III

EWBH Treatment
unknown

MANUFACTURER
First Circle Medical

DESCRIPTION
Extracorporeal whole body hyperthermia (EWBH) is being developed to treat HIV and AIDS subjects who have not responded to standard therapies. EWBH is a technique in which the core body temperature is raised by removing blood from the subject, heating it, and then returning it to the subject. Special equipment designed by First Circle Medical is being developed to carry out this process.

Ever since the ancient Greeks, the concept of elevating body temperature to fight disease has been present in medicine. Raising the temperature of the body actually simulates the body's own fever response as part of its immune reaction to disease. The artificial "fever" state created by EWBH may increase the rate of viral killing in subjects with HIV and AIDS.

A phase I study demonstrated lower levels of the HIV virus in subjects' blood after EWBH, as well as improvement in overall functioning. Using the blood, in effect, to warm the body from the inside out may result in greater control of desired temperatures, higher uniformity of heat distribution throughout the body, and fewer side effects, since the process is carried out at a slow, monitored rate. If results from further studies confirm phase I safety and effectiveness findings, hyperthermia centers would be set up where subjects could receive this therapy outside of the hospital.

INDICATION(S) AND RESEARCH PHASE
Acquired Immune Deficiency Syndrome (AIDS) and AIDS-Related Infections – Phase II
HIV Infection – Phase II

GEM-92
unknown

MANUFACTURER
Hybridon

DESCRIPTION
GEM-92 is not being actively developed for the treatment of HIV/AIDS at this time. Further development is pending the availablility of a partner to contribute to the expenses of further trials. A pilot study has been completed, while phase I has been initiated but not completed.

INDICATION(S) AND RESEARCH PHASE
Acquired Immune Deficiency Syndrome (AIDS) and AIDS-Related Infections – Phase I
HIV Infection – Phase I

HMR-4004
unknown

MANUFACTURER
Aventis

DESCRIPTION
CD4 cells are specific types of immune cells that the HIV virus targets and destroys. Hoechst Marion Roussel was developing a genetically resistant variety of CD4 cells that cannot be infected by the HIV virus. CD4 cells, once stimulated by foreign material, signal the production of other immune cells to attack the incoming pathogen. Therefore, with a decreased number of these cells, a person's immune system is severely compromised.

There is a protein found on the outer surface of the HIV molecule (gp 120) that binds to CD4 cells. This specialized binding site allows the virus to infiltrate these CD4 cells and destroy them. This systematic decimation of a person's CD4 immune cells may lead to the serious symptoms of AIDS since the body cannot protect itself from infection. It is thought that if HIV or AIDS subjects could be supplied with these cells, the severity of the disease could potentially be mitigated and subjects' lifespan may be prolonged.

Scientists were modifying a CD4 cell gene in order to make it more resistant to HIV infection. This modification could make it more difficult for the HIV virus to bind to the CD4 cell or prevent its replication once the virus gains access to the interior of the cell. According to the company phase II trials using HMR-4004 have stopped and all further development has been discontinued.

INDICATION(S) AND RESEARCH PHASE
Acquired Immune Deficiency Syndrome (AIDS) and AIDS-Related Infections – Phase II discontinued
HIV Infection – Phase II discontinued

interleukin-12 (IL-12)
unknown

MANUFACTURER
Genetics Institute

DESCRIPTION
Interleukin-12 (IL-12) is a novel genetically engineered, human immune modulator being tested in phase II trials for the treatment of hepatitis C, chronic liver disease due to hepatitis infection, and AIDS. There is an additional indication for renal carcinoma, which may have an orphan drug status.

INDICATION(S) AND RESEARCH PHASE
Acquired Immune Deficiency Syndrome (AIDS) and AIDS-Related Infections – Phase II
Hepatitis – Phase II
Renal Cell Carcinoma – Phase II

L-glutathione
Cachexon

MANUFACTURER
Telluride Pharmaceutical

DESCRIPTION
Cachexon is an oral capsule formulation of glutathione, an antioxidant produced naturally by the body. Cachexon consists of a tripeptide, composed of three amide-linked amino acids. Glutathione levels in individuals decrease with the onset of age-related conditions. Glutathione helps to regenerate immune cells. Adding glutathione to disintegrating cells that have lost their immune activity revives the cell and causes it to become immuno-efficient again.

Cancer and AIDS subjects have very lowered levels of glutathione. This capsule is designed as replacement therapy for glutathione in order to provide direct protection to intestinal epithelial cells (enterocytes) against oxidative stress. Oxidative stress leads to activation of HIV replication, resulting in damage to enterocytes, malabsorption, and cachexia (general ill health). Cachexon is in phase III trials for AIDS and AIDS-related infections, unspecified cancer and tumors, and diet and nutrition.

INDICATION(S) AND RESEARCH PHASE
Acquired Immune Deficiency Syndrome (AIDS) and AIDS-Related Infections – Phase III
Cancer/Tumors (Unspecified) – Phase III
Diet and Nutrition – Phase III

memantine
unknown

MANUFACTURER
Neurobiological Technologies

DESCRIPTION
Memantine is an orally available compound that appears to restore the function of damaged nerve cells and reduce abnormal excitatory signals. This is accomplished by the modulation of N-methyl-D-aspartate (NMDA) receptor activity.

Memantine is in trials for diabetic neuropathy (phase II completed), AIDS-related dementia and neurological function (phase II), and moderate to severe dementia and Alzheimer's disease (phase III). Forest Laboratories intends to prepare an NDA for submission around the end of 2001 for the treatment of Alzheimer's disease, but will also begin additional phase III trials in both mild to moderate and moderately severe to severe Alzheimer's disease.

Forest Laboratories has entered into an agreement with Merz & Co. (collaborator of Neurobiological Technologies), for the development and marketing of memantine in the United States.

INDICATION(S) AND RESEARCH PHASE
Alzheimer's Disease – Phase III
Acquired Immune Deficiency Syndrome (AIDS) and AIDS-Related Infections – Phase II
Neuropathy, Diabetic – Phase II completed

nelfinavir, AG1661
Remune

MANUFACTURER
Agouron Pharmaceuticals

DESCRIPTION
Results from a clinical study suggest that Remune, an immune-based therapy for the treatment of HIV, may significantly enhance an HIV-specific immune response. When combination anti-viral drug therapy is accompanied by quarterly injections of Remune, immunologic markers and positive trends in virologic markers of the response to HIV improved. In this universal drug-target interaction, the drug molecule inserts itself into a functionally important crevice of its target protein, like a key in a lock, and can then promote or inhibit the protein's normal function. Remune is in phase III trials.

INDICATION(S) AND RESEARCH PHASE
Acquired Immune Deficiency Syndrome (AIDS) and AIDS-Related Infections – Phase III
HIV Infection – Phase III

nitazoxanide (NTZ)
unknown

MANUFACTURER
BioChem Pharma

DESCRIPTION
Nitazoxanide (NTZ) is a medication that is being developed to treat diarrhea caused by cryptosporidial parasites in immunocompromised people, such as AIDS subjects. Currently this drug is in phase III trials and it is to be given orally. Cryptosporidiosis is an infection of the intestinal lining with the parasite *Cryptosporidium parvum* that can be found in contaminated food and water. Forty-five million people each year may be exposed to this parasite through municipal water systems. This parasite is found in up to twenty percent of people with AIDS.

Symptoms of this infection include watery diarrhea, with up to twenty bowel movements each day. NTZ is a molecule (thiazolide derivative) that acts not only against parasites such as protozoa and helminths (worms), but against bacteria as well. This drug is already available in developing countries where parasitic infections are common. People who are immunocompromised due to AIDS, steroid treatment, or cancer treatment are the most susceptible to infection by the *Cryptosporidium* organism and these subjects may potentially derive the greatest benefit from this new therapy.

INDICATION(S) AND RESEARCH PHASE
Diarrhea – Phase III
Parasites and Protozoa – Phase III
Acquired Immune Deficiency Syndrome (AIDS) and AIDS-Related Infections – Phase III

nitrone radical trap (NRT)
unknown

MANUFACTURER
Centaur Pharmaceuticals

DESCRIPTION
Nitrone radical trap (NRT) is an oxidative stress reducing neuroprotective compound for the treatment of Parkinson's disease and stroke. NRT is also being tested in a phase IIa trial for AIDS dementia complex. NRTs are designed to combine with free radicals to create a less reactive molecule.

INDICATION(S) AND RESEARCH PHASE
Acquired Immune Deficiency Syndrome (AIDS) and AIDS-Related Infections – Phase IIa
Parkinson's Disease – Phase IIa
Strokes – Phase IIb/III

oxymetholone
Anadrol-50

MANUFACTURER
Unimed Pharmaceuticals

DESCRIPTION
Anadrol-50 is an oral anabolic (constructive metabolism) steroid that helps build muscle mass in AIDS subjects afflicted with cachexia (general ill health and malnutrition). The phase II trials for this indication are in progress. Another formulation of Anadrol-50 is currently being sold under that name to treat red blood cell deficiency anemias. The company says it plans related studies of this drug for use in the frail elderly.

INDICATION(S) AND RESEARCH PHASE
Acquired Immune Deficiency Syndrome (AIDS) and AIDS-Related Infections – Phase II

perthon/abavca
Perthon

MANUFACTURER
Advanced Plant Pharmaceuticals

DESCRIPTION
Perthon (formally known as Abavca), derived exclusively from eleven different plants, is being evaluated for use as an immune system booster for AIDS subjects. The manufacturer, Advanced Plant Pharmaceuticals, claims that Perthon has clinically demonstrated the ability to overcome many of the debilitating symptoms of HIV, the AIDS virus, while enhancing the immune system.

INDICATION(S) AND RESEARCH PHASE
Acquired Immune Deficiency Syndrome (AIDS) and AIDS-Related Infections – Phase I/II

PRO 367
unknown

MANUFACTURER
Progenics Pharmaceuticals

DESCRIPTION
PRO 367, a fusion protein, binds to gp120 (a glycoprotein receptor on the surface of HIV-infected cells) via an engineered molecule linked to a therapeutic radioisotope. This targeted complex releases a low but lethal dose of radiation, killing the cell and halting the spread of viral infection. This proprietary technology models the fusion of HIV cells in a way that makes the use of a live virus unnecessary.

INDICATION(S) AND RESEARCH PHASE
Acquired Immune Deficiency Syndrome (AIDS) and AIDS-Related Infections – Phase I/II
HIV Infection – Phase I/II

PRO 542
unknown

MANUFACTURER
Progenics Pharmaceuticals

DESCRIPTION
PRO 542, a novel fusion protein, incorporates the HIV-binding region of the human cell surface receptor (CD4) into a human antibody molecule. This complex binds to the HIV surface glycoprotein (gp120) and blocks the virus from attaching itself to human host cells. This mechanism of action is unique among antiretrovirals that are either approved or in late stage clinical development.

Results from a phase I trial demonstrated PRO 542 had strong antiviral effects and was considered safe and effective in subjects who were infected with HIV. The subjects received a single injection of PRO 542 at one of four dose levels. Subjects receiving high doses of PRO 542 showed a statistically significant acute reduction in plasma HIV RNA or viral load, which is considered an accepted clinical endpoint for antiretroviral therapies.

INDICATION(S) AND RESEARCH PHASE
Acquired Immune Deficiency Syndrome (AIDS) and AIDS-Related Infections – Phase II
HIV Infection – Phase II
Pediatric, HIV – Phase II

procaine HCl
Anticort

MANUFACTURER
Samaritan Pharmaceuticals

DESCRIPTION
Cortisol is the primary steroid hormone involved in carbohydrate metabolism and the body's response to stress. It is known that high cortisol levels play a major role in destroying the immune system in such diseases as AIDS and cancer. Anticort is an oral anti-cortisol, steroidogenesis inhibitor drug being tested for the treatment of immune deficiency in AIDS/HIV infection and other diseases. Procaine (the active ingredient of Anticort) has been used clinically for more than 40 years, primarily as the injectable local anesthetic Novocaine.

INDICATION(S) AND RESEARCH PHASE
Acquired Immune Deficiency Syndrome (AIDS) and AIDS-Related Infections – Phase Ib/IIa
HIV Infection – Phase Ib/IIa

Proleukin Interleukin-2 and standard anti-HIV therapy
unknown

MANUFACTURER
Chiron Corporation

DESCRIPTION
Proleukin is a genetically engineered (recombinant) form of interleukin-2, which is a naturally occurring immune modulator. The use of Proleukin may represent a new approach to treat HIV because this drug is designed to bolster and help rebuild the compromised immune system rather than target the virus specifically like other treatments. This combination therapy has produced increases in CD4+ counts and an

improvement in other immune function parameters that appear to be sustained over the course of one year.

An international phase III study is evaluating the safety and effectiveness of Proleukin (aldesleukin) Interleukin-2 in combination with standard anti-HIV therapy in 1,400 subjects living with HIV with low CD4+ T-cell counts. The objective of this study is to determine if intermittent cycles of Proleukin delay the progression of HIV disease compared to what is observed with anti-HIV therapy alone in people with advanced HIV infection.

INDICATION(S) AND RESEARCH PHASE
Acquired Immune Deficiency Syndrome (AIDS) and AIDS-Related Infections – Phase III
HIV Infection – Phase III

ribozyme gene therapy
unknown

MANUFACTURER
Ribozyme Pharmaceuticals

DESCRIPTION
Gene therapies represent a promising direction for treatment of retrovitral and other diseases. This therapeutic construct is based on the ability of ribozymes to alter RNA molecules.

Ribozymes are RNA enzymes that perform numerous functions, including the cleavage of ribonucleic acid (RNA) molecules. Ribozymes can be designed to selectively recognize, bind, and cleave any mRNA sequence. As human therapeutics, ribozymes can be chemically synthesized to selectively inhibit disease-causing proteins through the specific cleavage of the disease-causing mRNA. The company has made proprietary chemical modifications to ribozymes that allow them to be stable and active in human serum for several days, thus broadening their potential therapeutic applications.

INDICATION(S) AND RESEARCH PHASE
Acquired Immune Deficiency Syndrome (AIDS) and AIDS-Related Infections – Phase II
HIV Infection – Phase II
Lymphoma, Non-Hodgkin's – Phase II

rifapentine, MDL-473
Priftin

MANUFACTURER
Aventis

DESCRIPTION
Phase III trials of Priftin, an antibiotic prophylactic, for the treatment of *Mycobacterium avium* complex in subjects with AIDS and bacterial infections were discontinued.

INDICATION(S) AND RESEARCH PHASE
Acquired Immune Deficiency Syndrome (AIDS) and AIDS-Related Infections – Phase discontinued
Bacterial Infection – Phase discontinued

somatropin, r-hGH
Serostim

MANUFACTURER
Serono Laboratories

DESCRIPTION
Serostim is a recombinant human growth hormone in trials for several indications. The drug is currently marketed for the treatment of AIDS wasting (cachexia), and it is in development for growth hormone deficiency in adults, short bowel syndrome, lipodystrophy, and congestive heart failure.

INDICATION(S) AND RESEARCH PHASE
Acquired Immune Deficiency Syndrome (AIDS) and AIDS-Related Infections – FDA approved
Hormone Deficiencies – Phase III
Gastrointestinal Diseases and Disorders, miscellaneous – Phase III
Lipodystrophy – Phase II
Congestive Heart Failure – Phase II

SP-303
Provir

MANUFACTURER
Shaman Pharmaceuticals

DESCRIPTION
Provir is a naturally occurring compound derived from the red, viscous latex of the Croton tree (Croton lechlerli) that grows in the Amazonian jungles of South America. Provir is an oral drug that acts as a specific inhibitor of fluid loss via an antisecretory mechanism to treat diarrhea. Provir has entered phase III trials for the treatment of AIDS-associated diarrhea, and the treatment of acute watery and traveler's diarrhea.

INDICATION(S) AND RESEARCH PHASE
Acquired Immune Deficiency Syndrome (AIDS) and AIDS-Related Infections – Phase III
Diarrhea – Phase III

SPC3
Advantage-S

MANUFACTURER
Columbia Laboratories

DESCRIPTION
SPC3 is a synthetic eight-chain peptide/HIV co-receptor for prevention of progression of AIDS in late stage HIV. Phase III trials were discontinued because SPC3 did not prevent transmission of HIV.

INDICATION(S) AND RESEARCH PHASE
Acquired Immune Deficiency Syndrome (AIDS) and AIDS-Related Infections – Trial discontinued

T-1249
unknown

MANUFACTURER
Trimeris

DESCRIPTION
T-1249 is a rationally designed proprietary peptide, which blocks fusion of HIV with host cells. T-1249 has demonstrated potent HIV suppression in animal models and is highly active against a wide range of HIV strains in culture.

In January 2001, results of a phase I/II dose escalation trial of the second-generation fusion inhibitor, T-1249, indicated that the drug was well tolerated over 14 days, had pharmacokinetic characteristics that support once-daily dosing, and conferred dose-related suppression of plasma HIV RNA. The trial assessed 72 HIV positive, treatment-experienced adults with no concomitant antiretroviral therapy. Based on the favorable tolerability and activity observed with T-1249, Trimeris and Roche will continue to explore higher doses in subsequent cohorts of this trial.

INDICATION(S) AND RESEARCH PHASE
HIV Infection – Phase I/II
Acquired Immune Deficiency Syndrome (AIDS) and AIDS-Related Infections – Phase I/II

tenofovir disoproxil fumarate
Tenofovir DF

MANUFACTURER
Gilead Sciences

DESCRIPTION
Tenofovir disproxil fumarate (tenofovir DF) is a nucleotide analogue formulated as an oral pill taken once daily as part of combination antiretroviral regimens. It is being tested in a phase III study for HIV that plans to enroll a total of 600 subjects at nearly 70 sites in the United States, Europe, and Australia.

Based on results from the phase II study, subjects will be randomized to receive a dose of tenofovir DF 300 mg or placebo in addition to their antiretroviral regimen for 24 weeks of blinded dosing. After 24 weeks, subjects in the trial receiving tenofovir DF 300 mg may make changes in their background antiretroviral therapy, and subjects assigned to receive placebo will cross over to open label active tenofovir DF for the remainder of the 48 week study period.

INDICATION(S) AND RESEARCH PHASE
Acquired Immune Deficiency Syndrome (AIDS) and AIDS-Related Infections – Phase III
HIV Infection – Phase III

testosterone
unknown

MANUFACTURER
Watson Pharmaceuticals

DESCRIPTION
Testosterone is a naturally produced hormone responsible for proper development of male secondary sex characteristics. It is an anabolic steroid that may help build up muscle mass in subjects suffering from AIDS. This hormone, which has been formulated in the MTX transdermal patch, is being tested in phase II trials for the treatment of sexual dysfunction in surgically menopausal subjects, menopause associated hormone replacement therapy, and osteoporosis. Additionally, this drug is in phase III clinical trials for male hormonal deficiencies and abnormalities.

This hormone regime is also being evaluated in phase II trials for treatment of female AIDS wasting.

INDICATION(S) AND RESEARCH PHASE
Acquired Immune Deficiency Syndrome (AIDS) and AIDS-Related Infections – Phase II
Hormone Replacement Therapy: Menopause – Phase II
Male Hormonal Deficiencies/Abnormalities – Phase III
Osteoporosis – Phase II
Sexual Dysfunction – Phase II completed

thalidomide
Thalomid

MANUFACTURER
Celgene Corporation

DESCRIPTION
Thalomid is an oral formulation of the immunomodulatory agent thalidomide. Thalidomide has a notorious history of having caused birth defects when the medical profession unsuspectingly prescribed it for pregnant women as a treatment for nausea and insomnia. Celgene is investigating new applications for the drug, while being particularly mindful of the potential risks of thalidomide treatment. Thalomid is currently being tested for numerous indications in the areas of oncology and immunology.

INDICATION(S) AND RESEARCH PHASE
Multiple Myeloma – Phase II
Myelodysplastic Syndrome – Phase II
Leukemia – Phase II
Brain Cancer – Phase II
Liver Cancer – Phase II
Kidney Cancer – Phase II
Prostate Cancer – Phase II
Kaposi's Sarcoma – Phase II
Cachexia – Phase II
Recurrent Aphthous Stomatitis – Phase III
Crohn's Disease – Phase II
Inflammatory Bowel Disease – Phase II
Sarcoidosis – Phase II
Scleroderma – Phase II

unknown
Protectaid

MANUFACTURER
Axcan Pharma

DESCRIPTION
Protectaid is a new contraceptive sponge which is being developed both to provide effective contraception and to prevent the contraction of sexually transmitted diseases (STDs), including HIV. The Protectaid sponge is made of a foam material that is saturated with a formulation called F-5 Gel which is a combination of three sperm-killing (spermicidal) chemicals. This sponge acts in three ways: it creates a physical barrier against sperm entering the uterus it absorbs the semen, preventing its progression; and it destroys sperm because of its spermicidal chemicals. The company reported that initial studies demonstrated high contraceptive efficacy with few side effects.

The sponge may cause less vaginal irritation because instead of using large amounts of one potentially irritating spermicidal ingredient, it contains smaller amounts of three synergistically acting spermicidal compounds. Its sperm-killing ingredients and the gel that composes the sponge's structure all contribute to limiting the amount of vaginal irritation. Therefore, this product has the potential to limit the transmission of sexually transmitted diseases that are more easily spread when there is vaginal lining irritation.

Early studies also show that the spermicidal components in Protectaid could destroy STDs such as viruses, fungi, and HIV. The F-5 Gel has been shown to destroy organisms such as HIV, *Chlamydia*, and *Neisseria gonorrhea*. From a contraceptive standpoint, Protectaid has been demonstrated to be 90% effective when used correctly in preventing pregnancy. The sponge can be inserted any time prior to sexual intercourse and should not be removed for at least six hours after intercourse. Protectaid is currently being evaluated in phase II trials.

INDICATION(S) AND RESEARCH PHASE
Acquired Immune Deficiency Syndrome (AIDS) and AIDS-Related Infections – Phase II
HIV Infection – Phase II
Pregnancy, Labor, and Delivery – Phase II

vaccine, HIV
Aidsvax

MANUFACTURER
VaxGen

DESCRIPTION
Aidsvax is a genetically engineered, aluminum-adjuvanted subunit vaccine cloned from a protein (gp120) found on the surface of the HIV virus. Because it is a subunit vaccine it does not contain viral DNA, and therefore, no participant in the trial can become infected by HIV due to the vaccination.

Aidsvax is currently being tested in phase III trials. The subjects are between the ages of 18 and 60 and do not have HIV-1 infection, but they are at risk of acquiring HIV-1 infection through sexual contact.

INDICATION(S) AND RESEARCH PHASE
Acquired Immune Deficiency Syndrome (AIDS) and AIDS-Related Infections – Phase III
HIV Infection – Phase III
Vaccines – Phase III

vaccine, HIV
GeneVax-HIV-Px

MANUFACTURER
Wyeth-Lederle Vaccines

DESCRIPTION
GeneVax-HIV-Px is a novel prophylactic DNA vaccine for the treatment of HIV infection. It is an injectable therapeutic that uses the proprietary GeneVax delivery technology. The drug is in phase II trials.

INDICATION(S) AND RESEARCH PHASE
Acquired Immune Deficiency Syndrome (AIDS) and AIDS-Related Infections – Phase II
HIV Infection – Phase II

vaccine, HIV-1 gp-120 prime-boost
unknown

MANUFACTURER
Chiron Corporation

DESCRIPTION
Chiron Corporation is developing a vaccine for AIDS that works in two ways. There is a protein found on the outer surface of the HIV molecule (gp 120) that binds to important human immune cells (CD4). This specialized binding site allows the virus to infiltrate these CD4 cells and destroy them. This systematic decimation of a person's CD4 immune cells leads to the serious symptoms of AIDS since the body cannot adequately compensate for the loss in immune protection.

This new vaccine is composed of synthetically made proteins that closely resemble the gp 120 proteins of the AIDS virus. Scientists believe that, upon immunization, the body makes antibodies to these synthetic proteins, and these antibodies will act against the real HIV molecule as well. This vaccine also contains another protein that enhances the immune response. This protein (MF59) is known as an adjuvant because it causes the body to produce a stronger and longer lasting immune reaction than would occur with the vaccine alone. These two mechanisms may potentially immunize people against this pervasive and serious disease. Phase II trials are currently taking place using this intravenous vaccination.

INDICATION(S) AND RESEARCH PHASE
Acquired Immune Deficiency Syndrome (AIDS) and AIDS-Related Infections – Phase II
HIV Infection – Phase II
Vaccines – Phase II

WF10
unknown

MANUFACTURER
OXO Chemie

DESCRIPTION
WF10 is an immune therapeutic that targets macrophage function. The active ingredient in WF10 is a chemically stabilized chlorite matrix called tetrachlorodecaoxygen (TDCO). WF10 has completed phase III trials for HIV.

Results from phase II trials showed WF10 lowered frequency of infections, required fewer hospitalizations and increased survival rates for subjects who had AIDS.

Additionally, WF10 is in phase III trials for chronic inflammatory diseases.

INDICATION(S) AND RESEARCH PHASE
Acquired Immune Deficiency Syndrome (AIDS) and AIDS-Related Infections – Phase III
HIV Infection – Phase III

Allergy

brompheniramine/ pseudoephedrine HCl
Conquer-A

MANUFACTURER
Verex Laboratories

DESCRIPTION
Conquer-A is a once daily tablet formulation of brompheniramine/pseudoephedrine,

which is a combination of an antihistamine plus a vasoconstrictor. This drug was being developed for the treatment of allergies and other minor respiratory problems. However, Conquer-A has stalled in a phase II trial due to low interest from the industry, but the company hopes it will soon be restarted. They believe that Conquer-A is unique compared to other antihistamines because only the low dosage of 12-16 mg of brompheniramine appears to be needed to provide relief of allergies.

INDICATION(S) AND RESEARCH PHASE
Allergy – Phase II on hold

CpG compound
unknown

MANUFACTURER
Coley Pharmaceutical

DESCRIPTION
CpG compound is a novel immune modulator designed to redirect hypersensitivity reactions (allergic and asthmatic) into more normal responses, thereby eliminating or reducing the appearance of symptoms. CpG molecules simultaneously suppress Th2-type (allergic) immune responses that can result in airway inflammation and bronchial spasm, and induce Th1-type (normal) immune responses that promote antibody and cellular responses. A phase II trial for the treatment of allergic asthma is being conducted in the United Kingdom, and is designed to evaluate the safety and efficacy of CpG.

INDICATION(S) AND RESEARCH PHASE
Asthma – Phase II
Allergy – Phase I

desloratadine, descarboethoxyloratadine
unknown

MANUFACTURER
Sepracor

DESCRIPTION
Desloratadine is an active metabolite of Claritin, a non-sedating antihistamine, for the treatment of seasonal allergic rhinitis. The drug selectively blocks histamine-1 receptors in the bloodstream, and thereby prevents the release of histamine by inflammatory cells. Desloratadine is being developed under an agreement between Sepracor and Schering-Plough Corporation.

INDICATION(S) AND RESEARCH PHASE
Allergy – NDA submitted
Rhinitis – NDA submitted

Hu-901
unknown

MANUFACTURER
Tanox

DESCRIPTION
Hu-901 is an anti-IgE monoclonal antibody currently being tested for the prevention of anaphylactic reactions to peanuts (PIA). Anti-IgE is a genetically engineered humanized monoclonal antibody that has been developed to target the source of allergy symptoms for all allergens. Anti-IgE inhibits the allergic response by binding to IgE, thereby blocking the consequent release of inflammatory mediators such as histamine, prostaglandins, and leukotrienes. In general, these inflammatory mediators play a role in the pathology of a variety of allergic diseases including allergic asthma, allergic rhinitis, atopic dermatitis, and anaphylactic shock.

INDICATION(S) AND RESEARCH PHASE
Allergy – Phase I/II

IDEC-152
unknown

MANUFACTURER
IDEC Pharmaceuticals

DESCRIPTION
IDEC-152 is an anti-CD23 monoclonal antibody, which targets the CD23 receptor on immune cells. The anti-CD23 antibody is part of IDEC's "Primatized Antibody" technology that may be useful in treating allergic condition such as allergic asthma, allergic rhinitis, and atopic conditions. This antibody enables the treatment of specific allergy conditions because it combines with the CD23 factor to regulate the production of the allergy-triggering immunoglobulin (IgE), and generates no further immunoglobulin production. IDEC-152 is in a phase I trial for the treatment of allergic asthma to evaluate safety, tolerability, and pharmacokinetics. IDEC-152 is being developed by IDEC Pharmaceuticals and Seikagaku Corporation of Japan.

INDICATION(S) AND RESEARCH PHASE
Asthma – Phase I
Allergy – Phase I

ketotifen fumarate
Zaditen

MANUFACTURER
Novartis

DESCRIPTION
Zaditen is a topical selective H1-receptor antagonist, mast cell stabilizer, eosinophil infiltration inhibitor. An application has been filed overseas and the drug is in registration as an anti-allergic eyedrop.

INDICATION(S) AND RESEARCH PHASE
Allergy – MAA submitted
Eye Disorders/Infections – MAA submitted

levocetirizine
xyzal, xusal

MANUFACTURER
Sepracor

DESCRIPTION
Levocetirizine is the single-isomer version of Zyrtec, which contains both isomers of cetirizine. This isomer offers the possibility of an improved treatment for subjects with allergies. All development and marketing rights have been licensed to UCB Pharma for Europe. Levocetrizine has obtained marketing approval from the German Health Authorities, and has been submitted for approval in other European countries.

INDICATION(S) AND RESEARCH PHASE
Allergy – Filed

unknown
AIC

MANUFACTURER
Dynavax

DESCRIPTION
AIC is Dynavax's proprietary conjugate of purified ragweed allergen. ISS (immunostimulatory DNA) administered with allergens is thought to enhance immune response. ISS is attached to specific allergens so that they are presented to the immune system simultaneously. ISS, when linked to an allergen, "hides" the allergen from the immune system, thereby preventing the symptoms of an allergy attack. AIC ragweed immunotherapy is currently in phase II development.

INDICATION(S) AND RESEARCH PHASE
Skin Infections/Disorders – Phase II
Allergy – Phase II

unknown
MPL vaccine adjuvant

MANUFACTURER
Corixa Corporation

DESCRIPTION
MPL, a vaccine adjuvant, is currently undergoing III trials in Europe for use in allergy vaccines marketed by Allergy Therapeutics.

Allergies caused by grasses, trees, and house dust mites afflict an estimated 20% of the population in developed countries. While most allergy medications offer some relief to sufferers, the company believes that adding MPL adjuvant may allow the development of more effective and easily administered allergy treatments.

INDICATION(S) AND RESEARCH PHASE
Allergy – Phase III
Vaccines – Phase III

Aspergillosis

FK463, echinocandin
unknown

MANUFACTURER
Fujisawa Healthcare

DESCRIPTION
Echinocandin is a novel antifungal agent for the treatment of systemic fungal infections. The drug is used as prophylaxis, empirical therapy, and second line treatment for candidiasis and aspergillosis. Echinocandin is in phase II/III trials for these indications and other fungal infections.

INDICATION(S) AND RESEARCH PHASE
Aspergillosis – Phase II/III
Candidiasis – Phase II/III
Fungal Infections – Phase II/III

nystatin, AR-121
Nyotran

MANUFACTURER
Aronex Pharmaceuticals

DESCRIPTION
Nyotran is an intravenous liposomal formulation of nystatin being developed for the treatment of serious systemic, opportunistic fungal infections. Phase III trials have been completed for systemic fungal infections and confirmed cryptococcal meningitis. Additionally, phase II trials have been completed for candidiasis and aspergillosis.

Nyotran is under agreement with Abbott Laboratories for worldwide commercialization. Abbott will fund clinical development and will submit marketing registration outside the United States.

INDICATION(S) AND RESEARCH PHASE
Aspergillosis – Phase II completed
Candidiasis – Phase II completed
Systemic Fungal Infections – Phase III completed
Meningitis – Phase III completed

Atopic Dermatitis

ADL 2-1294
unknown

MANUFACTURER
Adolor

DESCRIPTION
ADL2-1294 is a peripheral opiate (synthetic narcotic) being tested for the treatment of pain and itching associated with burns, abrasions, eczema, and dermatitis. The drug, in a topical formulation, is in phase II trials for atopic dermatitis, burns and burn infections, herpes zoster infections, psoriasis and psoriatic disorders, as well as for eye disorders and infections.

INDICATION(S) AND RESEARCH PHASE
Atopic Dermatitis – Phase II
Burns and Burn Infections – Phase II
Herpes Zoster Infections – Phase II
Psoriasis and Psoriatic Disorders – Phase II
Eye Disorders/Infections – Phase II
Skin Infections/Disorders – Phase II

LDP-392
unknown

MANUFACTURER
LeukoSite

DESCRIPTION
LDP-392 is formulated as a topical product designed to block two biochemical pathways involving inflammation. LDP-392 is a small-molecule alternative to steroids for the treatment of inflammatory skin disorders. It is a dual function, 5-lipoxygenase (5-LO) inhibitor and platelet activating factor (PAF) antagonist. It treats inflammation by targeting the two critical pathways that form leukotrienes and mediate PAF activity, respectively. These pro-inflammatory pathways have been implicated in dermatological conditions such as psoriasis and atopic dermatitis. Early trials indicate that LDP-392 may help subjects to avoid the toxicities associated with steroid treatment. This drug is being tested in phase II trials for the treatment of atopic dermatitis in children and psoriasis and psoriatic disorders.

INDICATION(S) AND RESEARCH PHASE
Atopic Dermatitis – Phase II
Psoriasis and Psoriatic Disorders – Phase II
Pediatric, Atopic Dermatitis – Phase II

pimecrolimus, ASM 981
Elidel

MANUFACTURER
Novartis

DESCRIPTION
Elidel is an ascomycin derivative being studied for the treatment of inflammatory skin disease. It produces a therapeutic effect through the inhibition of T-cells and mast cells. Elidel is being developed in both an oral and topical (cream) formulation. The oral formulation is in phase II trials, while an NDA has been filed for the cream formulation. Phase III trials involving more than 2,000 subjects ages three months to adult have recently been completed. The majority of the subjects in the phase III studies were pediatric.

Data presented from two previous vehicle-controlled trials demonstrated that ASM 981 cream was safe and effective for the treatment of atopic dermatitis. The two trials involved a total of 403 (267 ASM 981 and 136 vehicle) pediatric subjects ages two to 17 years old with mild to moderate atopic dermatitis. Both studies consisted of a six-week randomized, multicenter, double-blind, parallel-group phase followed by a 20-week open-label phase to assess safety and efficacy. Thirty-seven percent of ASM subjects were clear or almost clear of the signs of atopic dermatitis, significantly more than in the vehicle-control group. Over 65% of subjects achieved some degree of improvement. Of those who showed improvement, over 85% were cleared of the disease.

INDICATION(S) AND RESEARCH PHASE
Atopic Dermatitis – Phase II
Pediatric, Atopic Dermatitis – Phase III completed
Atopic Dermatitis – NDA submitted

tacrolimus hydrate
Prograf

MANUFACTURER
Fujisawa Healthcare

DESCRIPTION
Prograf is a novel immunosuppressant for the treatment of dermatological (skin) autoimmune diseases, including atopic dermatitis. The drug is administered as a topical ointment and it is being tested in phase III trials.

INDICATION(S) AND RESEARCH PHASE
Atopic Dermatitis – Phase III
Rheumatoid Arthritis – Phase III

Autoimmune Diseases

AGT-1
unknown

MANUFACTURER
Advanced Biotherapy

DESCRIPTION
Researchers have found an overproduction of cytokines in people with certain autoimmune diseases, such as rheumatoid arthritis. Within these cytokines, alpha interferon, tumor necrosis factor, and gamma interferon are soluble components of the immune system that are largely responsible for regulating the immune response and inflammation.

AGT-1, composed of a combination of antibody preparations, removes or neutralizes the cytokines' alpha interferon, gamma interferon, and tumor necrosis factor, thereby alleviating the autoimmune activity of these cells. Early phase I/II clinical trials are testing AGT-1 for the treatment of autoimmune diseases.

INDICATION(S) AND RESEARCH PHASE
Autoimmune Diseases – Phase I/II
Rheumatoid Arthritis – Phase I/II

APL400-020 V-B
Genevax-TCR

MANUFACTURER
Wyeth-Lederle Vaccines

DESCRIPTION
Genevax-TCR is a novel DNA-based vaccine that is in early clinical testing for T-cell lymphomas and other autoimmune diseases. Treatment of cutaneous T-cell lymphoma is an orphan indication currently being evaluated in a phase I/II trial.

INDICATION(S) AND RESEARCH PHASE
Autoimmune Diseases – Phase I/II
Lymphomas – Phase I/II

CDC 801
SelCID

MANUFACTURER
Celgene Corporation

DESCRIPTION
SelCIDs (selective cytokine inhibitory drugs) are oral immunotherapeutic agents that treat various inflammatory diseases by inhibiting phosphodiesterase type-4 enzyme (PDE-4). The inhibition of PDE-4 decreases production of tumor necrosis factor-alpha (TNF-α), a protein manufactured by cells of the immune system. This inhibition reduces the level of circulating TNF-α and, therefore, its ability to cause inflammation in cells. At normal levels, the protein is essential for effective immune function. However, overproduction of TNF as a result of age, genetic, and other influences contributes to the pathology of numerous diseases.

SelCIDs are in phase II trials for the following indications: inflammatory bowel disease, rheumatoid arthritis, multiple sclerosis, asthma, tuberculosis, autoimmune diseases, and mycobacteriosis such as leprosy.

INDICATION(S) AND RESEARCH PHASE
Inflammatory Bowel Disease – Phase II
Rheumatoid Arthritis – Phase II
Multiple Sclerosis – Phase II
Asthma – Trial discontinued
Tuberculosis – Phase II
Autoimmune Diseases – Phase II
Bacterial Infection – Phase II
Multiple Myeloma – Phase II

VX-148
unknown

MANUFACTURER
Vertex Pharmaceuticals

DESCRIPTION
VX-148 is an inhibitor of inosine monophosphate dehydrogenase (IMPDH), a cellular enzyme essential for production of guanine nucleotides, one of the building blocks of RNA and DNA. Inhibiting IMPDH may be an effective strategy for blocking the growth of lymphocytes and the replication of viruses, since both depend on nucleotide synthesis for replication. Vertex's IMPDH inhibitors have the potential to treat viral infections, autoimmune diseases, and psoriasis. These three indications are currently being tested in phase I trials.

INDICATION(S) AND RESEARCH PHASE
Viral Infection – Phase I
Autoimmune Diseases – Phase I
Psoriasis and Psoriatic Disorders – Phase I

Bacterial Infection

ABT-773
unknown

MANUFACTURER
Abbott Laboratories

DESCRIPTION
ABT-773 is a novel ketolide antibiotic, which has the potential to fight drug resistant respiratory infections. ABT-773 is in a phase II trial treating subjects two years and older.

INDICATION(S) AND RESEARCH PHASE
Pediatric, Bacterial Infection – Phase II

amikacin
Mikasome

MANUFACTURER
Gilead Sciences

DESCRIPTION
Mikasome, an aminoglycoside antibiotic, is in phase II trials for treatment of serious bacterial and mycobacterial infections including nosocomial *Pseudomonas pneumonia*, complicated urinary tract infections and *Pseudomonas*-colonized subjects with cystic fibrosis. The drug is delivered in a liposomal formulation.

INDICATION(S) AND RESEARCH PHASE
Bacterial Infection – Phase II
Pneumonia – Phase II
Urinary Tract Infections – Phase II

amikacin
DepoAmikacin

MANUFACTURER
Skye Pharma

DESCRIPTION
DepoAmikacin broad-spectrum antibiotic is being tested in the prevention and treatment of local and regional bacterial infections. The drug combines the antibiotic with a proprietary delivery system using an encapsulated injectable sustained-release lipid-based medium (DepoFoam). The company has completed phase I trials and is seeking a development partner before proceeding with phase II trials.

INDICATION(S) AND RESEARCH PHASE
Bacterial Infection – Phase I/II

amoxicillin/clavulante potassium
Augmentin SR

MANUFACTURER
GlaxoSmithKline

DESCRIPTION
Augmentin SR is a beta lactam antibiotic. It is currently being developed for the treatment of respiratory tract infections, including penicillin-resistant *S. pneumoniae*, in a modified release formulation. An NDA and MAA have been submitted to the appropriate regulatory agencies.

INDICATION(S) AND RESEARCH PHASE
Bacterial Infection – NDA submitted
Bacterial Infection – MAA submitted

AZD2563
unknown

MANUFACTURER
AstraZeneca

DESCRIPTION
AZD2563 is an oxazolidinone antibiotic for the treatment of gram-positive infections, including multiresistant strains. It is currently in phase I trials.

INDICATION(S) AND RESEARCH PHASE
Bacterial Infection – Phase I

C. difficile vaccine, CdVax
unknown

MANUFACTURER
Acambis

DESCRIPTION
CdVax is a vaccine being developed for the prevention of antibiotic-associated colitis caused by *Clostridium difficile* (*C. difficile*). The *C. difficile* bacteria produce A and B toxins that cause intestinal inflammation and fluid secretion. CdVax contains chemically inactivated A and B toxins, which could potentially stimulate high-level antitoxin antibodies in plasma donors. These plasma donations could then be used to prepare an immune globulin product (IVIG) for use in the short-term prophylaxis and therapy of *C. difficile* infection.

INDICATION(S) AND RESEARCH PHASE
Bacterial Infection – Phase I/II completed
Vaccines – Phase I/II completed
Gastrointestinal Diseases and Disorders, miscellaneous – Phase I/II completed

CDC 801
SelCID

MANUFACTURER
Celgene Corporation

DESCRIPTION

SelCIDs (selective cytokine inhibitory drugs) are oral immunotherapeutic agents that treat various inflammatory diseases by inhibiting phosphodiesterase type-4 enzyme (PDE-4). The inhibition of PDE-4 decreases production of tumor necrosis factor-alpha (TNF-α), a protein manufactured by cells of the immune system. This inhibition reduces the level of circulating TNF-α and, therefore, its ability to cause inflammation in cells. At normal levels, the protein is essential for effective immune function. However, overproduction of TNF as a result of age, genetic, and other influences contributes to the pathology of numerous diseases.

SelCIDs are in phase II trials for the following indications: inflammatory bowel disease, rheumatoid arthritis, multiple sclerosis, asthma, tuberculosis, autoimmune diseases, and mycobacteriosis such as leprosy.

INDICATION(S) AND RESEARCH PHASE

Inflammatory Bowel Disease – Phase II
Rheumatoid Arthritis – Phase II
Multiple Sclerosis – Phase II
Asthma – Phase discontinued
Tuberculosis – Phase II
Autoimmune Diseases – Phase II
Bacterial Infection – Phase II
Multiple Myeloma – Phase II

daptomycin
Cidecin

MANUFACTURER
Cubist Pharmaceuticals

DESCRIPTION
Daptomycin is a novel antibiotic lipopeptide for the treatment of skin and soft tissue infections, urinary tract infections in hospitalized subjects, and bacteremia. The drug is made in an intravenous formulation. Daptomycin is being tested for the treatment of skin infections, urinary tract infections, and bacterial infections.

INDICATION(S) AND RESEARCH PHASE
Skin Infections/Disorders – Phase III
Bacterial Infection – Phase II
Urinary Tract Infections – Phase II/III
Heart Disease – Phase II/III

ETEC vaccine
unknown

MANUFACTURER
Acambis

DESCRIPTION
This is an oral live attenuated vaccine being developed for the prevention of traveler's diarrhea. The vaccine is designed to be orally administered and to induce mucosal immune responses against the predominant disease-causing strains of ETEC. The vaccine is currently in phase I testing.

INDICATION(S) AND RESEARCH PHASE
Diarrhea – Phase I
Vaccines – Phase I
Bacterial Infection – Phase I

evernimicin
Ziracin

MANUFACTURER
Schering-Plough Corporation

DESCRIPTION
Ziracin (evernimicin) is an intravenous antibiotic designed for restricted use in hospitalized subjects with resistant gram-positive infections. Schering-Plough has voluntarily discontinued clinical development.

INDICATION(S) AND RESEARCH PHASE
Bacterial Infection – Trial discontinued

galasomite
Synsorb PK

MANUFACTURER
Synsorb Biotech

DESCRIPTION
Synsorb Pk is an orally delivered gastroenteric product designed for the prevention of hemolytic uremic syndrome (HUS) caused by *E. coli* toxins in children. Development of Synsorb Pk has been discontinued as of the first quarter of 2001. The company intends to concentrate resources on aggressive development of its lead product, Synsorb Cd, which management believes offers a more significant market opportunity.

INDICATION(S) AND RESEARCH PHASE
Pediatric, Bacterial Infection – Trial discontinued

GAR-936
unknown

MANUFACTURER
Wyeth-Ayerst

DESCRIPTION
GAR-936, a novel tetracycline, is being developed as an injectable antibiotic for the treatment of polymicrobic infections in hospitalized subjects where resistant pathogens are known or suspected.

INDICATION(S) AND RESEARCH PHASE
Bacterial Infection – Phase II

gatifloxacin
Tequin

MANUFACTURER
Bristol-Myers Squibb

DESCRIPTION
Tequin is a broad-spectrum 8-methoxy fluoroquinolone antibiotic in a phase II trial for the treatment of recurrent otitis media in subjects six months to 17 years old. Tequin is primarily excreted through the kidneys and less than 1% is metabolized by the liver. Tequim has been approved by the FDA for the treatment of certain infections in adults.

INDICATION(S) AND RESEARCH PHASE
Pediatric, Bacterial Infection – Phase II

gemifloxacin mesylate
Factive

MANUFACTURER
GlaxoSmithKline

DESCRIPTION
Factive is a broad spectrum fluoroquinolone

being developed for the treatment of various bacterial infections. It is in phase III trials in an intravenous formulation for the treatment of respiratory tract infections. Additionally, Factive has been developed in an oral formulation for the treatment of respiratory and urinary tract infections. An NDA and MAA have been submitted for the latter indications.

INDICATION(S) AND RESEARCH PHASE
Bacterial Infection – Phase III
Bacterial Infection – NDA submitted
Bacterial Infection – MAA submitted
Urinary Tract Infections – MAA submitted

H. pylori vaccine
unknown

MANUFACTURER
Acambis

DESCRIPTION
Acambis is developing vaccines designed to prevent and treat peptic ulcers and chronic gastritis caused by *H. pylori*. The vaccines would be used to treat *H. pylori* infection, to prevent reinfection in previously infected persons, and to stimulate immunity in uninfected persons. The vaccines are being developed under a joint venture with Aventis Pasteur.

INDICATION(S) AND RESEARCH PHASE
Vaccines – Phase II
Bacterial Infection – Phase II
Gastrointestinal Diseases and Disorders, miscellaneous – Phase II

HMR-3647, RU-64,004
unknown

MANUFACTURER
Aventis

DESCRIPTION
HMR-3647 is an anti-infective drug, which was being tested against a broad range of bacteria, including drug-resistant, susceptible strains of *Streptococcus pneumoniae* and other common pathogens. The company reported that development of this antibiotic was discontinued.

INDICATION(S) AND RESEARCH PHASE
Bacterial Infection – Phase discontinued
Pneumonia – Phase discontinued

immune globulin (IG-IV)
unknown

MANUFACTURER
Massachusetts Biologic Laboratories

DESCRIPTION
Immune globulin (a class of proteins involved in producing an immune response) or IG-IV is in phase II for the treatment of pertussis (whooping cough), using an intravenous formulation.

INDICATION(S) AND RESEARCH PHASE
Bacterial Infection – Phase II on hold
Pediatric, Pertussis – Phase II on hold

immune globulin (IgG)
DiffGAM

MANUFACTURER
ImmuCell Corporation

DESCRIPTION
DiffGAM is a hyperimmune bovine antibody, immunoglobulin-G (IgG) that uses cow's milk-derived passive antibody technology as an alternative to antibiotics in the treatment and/or prevention of *Clostridium difficile*-associated diarrhea and other bacterial infections. The development of this drug is currently on hold until the company can find a development partner.

INDICATION(S) AND RESEARCH PHASE
Bacterial Infection – Phase I/II
Diarrhea – Phase I/II

LY333328
Oritavancin

MANUFACTURER
Eli Lilly

DESCRIPTION
Bacterial resistance to current drug therapy has become an increasingly difficult dilemma in the design of newer antibiotics. LY333328 is a new chemical entity, structured similarly to vancomycin, which may be able to eradicate many bacteria already resistant to most of the major antibiotics in use today. Thousands of people each year die of resistant bacterial infections. People most at risk for these infections include the elderly, individuals with severe underlying disease, and subjects who have experienced prolonged hospitalization.

Bacteria fight antibiotics in different ways, but one of the most common methods is the production of chemicals (enzymes) that destroy the activity of antibiotics. One of the most lethal of these virulent bacteria is *Enterococcus faecium*, which is resistant to vancomycin, one of the most powerful antibiotics currently in use by doctors today. These bacteria can rapidly change their genetic makeup in order to quickly produce new enzymes to attack antibiotics. They most commonly cause infections of the blood, abdomen, and urinary tract. About forty percent of people with enterococcal blood infection may die from the infection.

LY-333328 is a promising antibiotic that may eradicate enterococcal infection. It is a synthetic protein that shares many of the same bacteria killing qualities of vancomycin but has been shown to be up to one thousand times more potent. Scientists believe that LY-333328 may be more efficacious in treating infection than other antibiotics because of its stronger binding action to the bacteria.

INDICATION(S) AND RESEARCH PHASE
Bacterial Infection – Phase II

lomefloxacin HCl
Maxaquin

MANUFACTURER
Unimed Pharmaceuticals

DESCRIPTION
Maxaquin is currently on the market for the treatment of subjects with uncomplicated urinary tract infections and lower respiratory tract infections. The antibiotic drug is in

phase III trials for a new indication, chronic bacterial prostatitis. Maxaquin is given in an oral tablet. Additional indications may include metabolic disorders and benign prostatic hypertrophy.

INDICATION(S) AND RESEARCH PHASE
Bacterial Infection – Phase III
Prostate Disorders – Phase III

MBI 226
unknown

MANUFACTURER
Micrologix

DESCRIPTION
An estimated 200,000 hospital subjects contract bloodstream infections each year in the United States of whom 50,000 subjects die annually. Central venous catheters (CVCs) cause more than 90% of these infections. Micrologix is hoping to conquer this serious problem by testing MBI 226 to prevent bloodstream infections.

Results from phase I trials showed that MBI 226 was safe and well tolerated. The drug eliminated 99.9% of bacteria commonly found on the skin. In addition, it prevented bacterial growth on catheters. This level of killing and suppression was maintained for three days following a single application of MBI 226. According to the company, this was very significant because physicians do not routinely change the dressing on intravenous catheters more than once every two or three days. By stopping the flora at catheter insertion sites, MBI 226 limits the microbial growth that will be able to develop on the skin, and the risk of catheter-related bloodstream infection is decreased.

INDICATION(S) AND RESEARCH PHASE
Bacterial Infection – Phase III

MK-826, carbapenem
unknown

MANUFACTURER
Merck & Co.

DESCRIPTION
Carbapenem is a broad-spectrum antibiotic being developed for the treatment of bacterial infections including pneumonia, intra-abdominal infections, skin and skin structure infections, urinary tract infection, and obstetric and gynecologic infections. Phase III trials are in progress for pneumonia, skin infections and disorders, urinary tract infections, gynecological infections, bacterial infection, and gastrointestinal diseases and disorders.

INDICATION(S) AND RESEARCH PHASE
Pneumonia – Phase III
Skin Infections/Disorders – Phase III
Urinary Tract Infections – Phase III
Gynecological Infections – Phase III
Bacterial Infection – Phase III
Gastrointestinal Diseases and Disorders, miscellaneous – Phase III

moxifloxacin
Avelox

MANUFACTURER
Bayer Corporation

DESCRIPTION
At the end of 1999, the Food and Drug Administration (FDA) approved Bayer's respiratory antibiotic Avelox (moxifloxacin) for the treatment of acute exacerbations of chronic bronchitis, community-acquired pneumonia, and acute sinusitis. The company is evaluating the drug in phase III trials for additional indications of respiratory tract infections and lung disease.

INDICATION(S) AND RESEARCH PHASE
Bacterial Infection – Phase III
Lung Disease – Phase III

opebecan, rBPI-21, recombinant human bactericidal/permeability-increasing protein
Neuprex

MANUFACTURER
XOMA Corporation

DESCRIPTION
Neuprex is a systemic formulation of recombinant bactericidal/permeability-increasing protein; rBPI-21, for the treatment of severe meningococcemia, a rare systemic gram-negative bacterial infection that primarily affects children. The active molecule in Neuprex, rBPI-21, binds to endotoxin molecules (LOS and LPS, lipopolysaccharide) in living bacteria, disrupting their cell walls, killing the bacteria or making them more susceptible to antibiotics. Phase III data were released in September 2000 for both pediatric and adult trials.

XOMA is pursuing various indications for Neuprex: One indication is severe meningococcemia in children who become infected with these harmful bacteria that attack their brain and spinal cord's protective sheathing after entering the bloodstream. The gram-negative bacteria, called *Neisseria meningitidis*, cause meningococcemia and produce spiking high fever and a classic rigid stiff neck. Shock and death may occur in just a few hours after infection. Additionally, Neuprex is being tested in trials for the treatment of serious lung complications (pneumonia and acute respiratory distress syndrome (ARDS)), in combination with other antibiotics and subjects who had their liver removed during surgery.

INDICATION(S) AND RESEARCH PHASE
Bacterial Infection – Phase III
Pediatric, Meningococcemia – Phase III completed
Meningitis – Phase III
Acute Respiratory Distress Syndrome (ARDS) – Phase III
Pneumonia – Phase III
Liver Disease – Phase II
Intra-Abdominal Infection – Phase I/II

Protegrin IB-367, rinse, gel
unknown

MANUFACTURER
IntraBiotics Pharmaceuticals

DESCRIPTION
Protegrin IB-367 is a synthetic antimicrobial peptide molecule that belongs to a new class of agents called protegrins. Studies suggest

that Protegrin IB-367 kills bacteria by integrating with and disrupting the integrity of bacterial cell membranes. The antibiotic has a broad spectrum of microbicidal activity against gram-positive and gram-negative bacteria that are frequent pathogens in ventilator-associated pneumonia.

Results of a single-dose phase I trial indicated that Protegrin IB-367 safely reduces bacterial levels in the mouths of subjects at risk of experiencing ventilator-associated pneumonia. A rinse and gel formulation of Protegrin IB-367 was topically applied to the mouth to reduce the number of oral and oropharyngeal bacteria of intubated subjects. A single administration of 9 mg of the rinse formulation safely and rapidly reduced the total bacteria in orally intubated subjects compared to placebo. The magnitude and duration of effect after a single 9 mg dose of Protegrin IB-367 rinse was similar to the response measured after a single 30 mg dose. In November 2000, IntraBiotics began subject enrollment in a phase IIa trial.

The rinse formulation of Protegrin IB-367 is also undergoing evaluation in two phase III trials for the prevention of oral mucositis. As of February 2001, one trial had completed enrollment of subjects receiving high-dose chemotherapy, while the other continues to enroll subjects receiving radiotherapy.

INDICATION(S) AND RESEARCH PHASE
Effects of Chemotherapy – Phase III
Bacterial Infection – Phase IIa
Pneumonia – Phase IIa

psoralen, S-59
unknown

MANUFACTURER
Cerus Corporation

DESCRIPTION
Psoralen uses ultraviolet-A light to initiate a platelet pathogen inactivation system. This invitro process works on blood temporarily drawn outside of the body for sterilization of viruses, bacteria, and other pathogens that may be present. Psoralen is being tested in phase III trials with blood components (platelets, fresh frozen plasma (FFP), and red blood cells) used in transfusions. The purpose is to enhance the safety of blood transfusions by inactivating pathogens in the blood components.

Also, psoralen may help inactivate white blood cells, which are responsible for a variety of adverse transfusion reactions. This therapy may be useful for treatment of thrombocytopenia, and red and white blood cell disorders.

Phase III trials are under way in the United States and Europe for the treatment of thrombocytopenia.

Cerus Corporation is developing psoralen in collaboration with Baxter Healthcare.

INDICATION(S) AND RESEARCH PHASE
Bacterial Infection – Phase III
Red Blood Cell Disorders – Phase III
Thrombocytopenia – Phase III
Viral Infection – Phase III

quinupristin/dalfopristin
Synercid

MANUFACTURER
Aventis

DESCRIPTION
Synercid is a combination therapy of two semi-synthetic antibacterial agents, quinupristin and dalfopristen. The antibiotic blocks bacterial protein synthesis.

Synercid has been FDA approved for the treatment of bloodstream infections due to vancomycin-resistant *Enterococcus faecium* (VREF) and skin and skin structure infections (SSTI) caused by methicillin-susceptible *Staphylococcus aureus* or *Streptococcus pyogenes*. It is in intravenous formulation. Additionally, it is in pediatric trials for pneumonia.

INDICATION(S) AND RESEARCH PHASE
Bacterial Infection – FDA approved
Skin Infections/Disorders – FDA approved
Pediatric, Pneumonia – Phase III
Pneumonia – Phase III

rifapentine, MDL-473
Priftin

MANUFACTURER
Aventis

DESCRIPTION
Phase III trials of Priftin, an antibiotic prophylactic for the treatment of *Mycobacterium avium* complex in subjects with AIDS and bacterial infections, were discontinued.

INDICATION(S) AND RESEARCH PHASE
Acquired Immune Deficiency Syndrome (AIDS) and AIDS-Related Infections – Phase III discontinued
Bacterial Infection – Phase III discontinued

rifaximin
unknown

MANUFACTURER
Salix Pharmaceuticals

DESCRIPTION
Rifaximin is a novel broad-spectrum antibiotic for treatment of gastrointestinal infections, including bacterial infectious diarrhea, antibiotic-associated colitis, and inflammatory bowel syndrome. The drug is chemically designed to be active in the gastrointestinal tract while remaining minimally absorbed.

INDICATION(S) AND RESEARCH PHASE
Bacterial Infection – Phase III
Diarrhea – Phase III
Gastrointestinal Diseases and Disorders, miscellaneous – Phase III
Inflammatory Bowel Disease – Phase III

roxithromycine, RU-28,965
unknown

MANUFACTURER
Aventis

DESCRIPTION
Roxithromycine is a new antibiotic similar in action and composition to existing antibiotics such as erythromycin and clarithromycin. It is being developed to treat a wide array of bacterial infections including those of the lungs, genitals, urinary tract,

skin, and soft tissues. It also may have potent action against parasitic infections from parasites such as cryptosporidium, *Pneumocystis carinii* (PCP), and *Toxoplasma gondii*. Many of these parasites infect people with compromised immune systems, such as AIDS subjects. Roxithromycine, if proved effective, may help improve quality of life and decrease mortality in these subjects.

Roxithromycine was being tested in phase III trials. Development has been discontinued.

INDICATION(S) AND RESEARCH PHASE
Bacterial Infection – Phase III discontinued
Parasites and Protozoa – Phase III discontinued

Saccharomyces boulardii
unknown

MANUFACTURER
Biocodex

DESCRIPTION
Saccharomyces boulardii is a yeast that appears to have an inhibitory effect against a type of bacteria (*Clostridium difficile*) that causes severe diarrhea in a variety of subjects. Sixty-one percent of neonates are colonized with this bacteria, and in a study at the Children's Hospital in Philadelphia, one-third of the children tested were found to have the destructive chemicals (toxins) made by *C. difficile* bacteria in their stools.

Scientists are not certain how exactly this yeast exerts its destructive effect against bacterial infection, but it might produce an enzyme that destroys one of the toxins produced by the bacteria. It also may prevent invading bacteria from binding to the intestinal walls, or it might stimulate the production of immune cells by the body that helps attack the invading bacteria. One French study showed that subjects who were producing four to eight liters of diarrhea a day had normal stools after an eight-day course of *Saccharomyces boulardii*.

People taking antibiotics for infections are susceptible to *C. difficile* infection, since antibiotics strip the intestinal walls of normal bacteria that are protective against infection. In a study of people taking antibiotics for various reasons, the group receiving *Saccharomyces boulardii* experienced a lower incidence of *C. difficile* diarrhea than those receiving other anti-diarrheal therapies. Further study is under way to determine exactly how effective this yeast may be in treating infection and what subjects might receive the most benefit from it.

INDICATION(S) AND RESEARCH PHASE
Bacterial Infection – Phase II
Diarrhea – Phase II
Pediatric, Clostridium difficile – Phase II

streptogamin
unknown

MANUFACTURER
Aventis

DESCRIPTION
Streptogamin is an antibiotic treatment for community-acquired (non-hospital) infections, including those due to multi-resistant gram-positive bacteria. The drug was being evaluated in phase II/III trials against bacterial infections in an oral formulation for adult and pediatric subjects. Development has been discontinued.

INDICATION(S) AND RESEARCH PHASE
Bacterial Infection – Phase discontinued
Pediatric, Bacterial Infection – Phase discontinued

telithromycin
Ketek

MANUFACTURER
Aventis

DESCRIPTION
Ketek is a novel antibiotic that fights resistant bacteria by inhibiting the protein synthesis necessary for bacterial reproduction. Invitro data suggest that it has a low propensity to induce bacterial resistance. Phase III data from ten multinational studies found that Ketek tablets may provide a convenient, once-daily, short-course treatment option for select respiratory tract infections (RTIs), including those infections caused by bacteria resistant to available therapies. The ten phase III studies were comprised of data from almost 2,500 subjects treated with Ketek and almost 1,800 subjects treated with comparator antibiotics. Ketek showed a high level of activity against *Streptococcus pneumoniae*, *Streptococcus pyogenes*, *Staphylococcus aureus*, *Haemophilus influenzae*, and *Moraxella catarrhalis*, as well as against atypical bacteria such as *Chlamydia pneumoniae*, *Mycoplasma pneumoniae*, and *Legionella pneumoniae*. An NDA was submitted in March 2000 for adults. A phase III trial for pediatric subjects is ongoing in the United States.

INDICATION(S) AND RESEARCH PHASE
Bacterial Infection – NDA submitted
Pediatric, Bacterial Infection – Phase III

typhoid vaccine
unknown

MANUFACTURER
Acambis

DESCRIPTION
This is an oral, live vaccine for the prevention of typhoid that consists of attenuated *S. typhi* bacteria. The vaccine contains bacteria that have been weakened enough to not cause the disease, but they are still capable of inducing an immune response. A phase II trial was successfully completed. The company is currently seeking a partner for the remainder of development.

INDICATION(S) AND RESEARCH PHASE
Vaccines – Phase II completed
Bacterial Infection – Phase II completed

unknown
Synsorb Cd

MANUFACTURER
Synsorb Biotech

DESCRIPTION
Synsorb Cd is an oral tablet being developed for the prevention of recurrent *Clostridium*

difficile associated disease (CDAD), a condition often associated with antibiotic use, AIDS, and chemotherapy. The product is based on the company's proprietary platform technology, consisting of synthetically produced carbohydrates designed to bind to targeted toxins. These carbohydrates are stabilized by being chemically linked to an inert silica-like substrate. The complex binds to potentially damaging bacterial toxins so they can be excreted from the body. Synsorb Cd is in phase III development.

INDICATION(S) AND RESEARCH PHASE
Bacterial Infection – Phase III

V-Glycopeptide, BI-397
unknown

MANUFACTURER
Versicor

DESCRIPTION
V-Glycopeptide is a novel intravenous glycopeptide antibiotic being developed for the treatment of serious gram-positive infections. Versicor is developing V-Glycopeptide as an improved alternative to Vancomycin, which is currently used to treat staphylococcal infections. Preclinical studies indicated that V-Glycopeptide produced a rapid and long-lasting killing effect invivo against *Staphylococcus aureus*. Single doses of BI-397 were sufficient to induce dramatic and sustained reductions of bacterial loads. BI-397 is in a phase I trial being conducted in the United States. Phase II trials are planned to begin in early 2001. Versicor and Biosearch Italia have established the "Biocor Alliance" for the optimization of novel lead molecules. Biosearch contributes leads, while Versicor provides chemistry technology to optimize the leads and identify product candidates.

INDICATION(S) AND RESEARCH PHASE
Bacterial Infection – Phase I

vaccine, Campylobacter
Campyvax

MANUFACTURER
Antex Biologics

DESCRIPTION
This vaccine, developed under a Cooperative Research and Development Agreement (CRADA) with the U.S. Navy and Army, is designed to prevent gastroenteritis and diarrhea (traveler's diarrhea), caused by the enteropathogenic (causing intestinal disease) *Campylobacter jejuni*. A novel proprietary technology combines the vaccine, consisting of inactivated whole cells, with an adjuvant. While vaccines typically provide protection after bacteria enter the body, this new genetic engineering technology is the platform for vaccines that prevent infection before bacteria can penetrate tissue. The vaccine is given orally in liquid form.

According to the companies involved, the phase II trials showed encouraging results to continue development of the vaccine.

INDICATION(S) AND RESEARCH PHASE
Bacterial Infection – Phase II completed
Diarrhea – Phase II completed
Gastroenteritis – Phase II completed
Pediatric, Campylobacter Infection – Phase II completed

vaccine, DPT/ Haemophilus influenzae tyype B
unknown

MANUFACTURER
Chiron Corporation

DESCRIPTION
Chiron Corporation has formulated a combination vaccine that might effectively immunize children against four serious diseases: *Haemophilus influenzae* type B, diphtheria, pertussis, and tetanus—with a single injection. This vaccine has the potential to simplify pediatric vaccination schedules, thereby lowering costs, increasing convenience and improving compliance. The vaccine is composed of inactive molecules of diptheria toxin, pertussis toxin, and tetanus toxin. Toxins are the destructive molecules that cause most of the pathology seen in these diseases. The vaccine also contains inactivated *H. influenzae* proteins. Diphtheria is an infection that can cause upper respiratory symptoms, heart problems, or nerve damage. Five to ten percent of cases are fatal. Tetanus causes nerve and muscle destruction as a result of the toxin that the bacterium *Clostridium tetani* releases. Affected subjects can experience muscular rigidity and spasms, and if untreated, have difficulty breathing and subsequent death. Pertussis (whooping cough) affects the respiratory tract and can progress to cause pneumonia, seizures, and brain damage. *Haemophilus influenzae* type B is a bacterium that is responsible for a significant percentage of bacterial sepsis (blood poisoning) in infants under four months of age. It can also cause upper airway, lung, skin, and joint infections. The combination vaccine given as an intramuscular injection is currently in phase III trials.

INDICATION(S) AND RESEARCH PHASE
Bacterial Infection – Phase III
Pediatric, Influenza – Phase III
Pediatric, Vaccines – Phase III
Viral Infection – Phase III

vaccine, Pseudomonas infection
Pseudostat

MANUFACTURER
Provalis

DESCRIPTION
Pseudostat is an oral (mucosal) therapeutic vaccine against *Pseudomonas aeruginosa* infections in cystic fibrosis subjects and subjects with chronic bronchitis, bronchiectasis, and influenza. The company intended to re-enter phase II trials in Australia in late 1999, and, if successful, plans to initiate phase II trials in the United States, where it has been in discussion with the National Institute of Health and the Cystic Fibrosis Foundation. In addition, the developer has filed for Orphan Drug Designation in the United States

INDICATION(S) AND RESEARCH PHASE
Bronchitis – Phase I/II
Bacterial Infection – Phase I/II
Cystic Fibrosis – Phase I/II
Influenza – Phase I/II

Vaccines – Phase I/II

vaccine, S. pneumoniae
unknown

MANUFACTURER
GlaxoSmithKline

DESCRIPTION
This conjugated vaccine is currently in phase III trials for *S. pneumoniae* disease prophylaxis.

INDICATION(S) AND RESEARCH PHASE
Bacterial Infection – Phase I
Pediatric, Bacterial Infection – Phase III

vaccine, Shigella flexneri and sonneii
unknown

MANUFACTURER
Intellivax International

DESCRIPTION
Shigella infections cause 200 million cases of dysentery and diarrhea worldwide every year. Shigellosis, infectious dysentery caused by bacteria of the genus *Shigella*, is marked by intestinal pain, tenesmus, diarrhea with mucus and blood in the stools, and toxemia. This novel vaccine, in a nasal spray formulation, is expected to complete phase II trials.

INDICATION(S) AND RESEARCH PHASE
Bacterial Infection – Phase II
Diarrhea – Phase II
Vaccines – Phase II

vaccine, Streptococcus pneumoniae
unknown

MANUFACTURER
GlaxoSmithKline

DESCRIPTION
This conjugated pediatric vaccine is currently in phase III trials for Streptococcus pneumoniae disease prophylaxis. The vaccine contains antigens for prevention of pneumonia, middle ear infections, and meningitis in pediatric patients.

INDICATION(S) AND RESEARCH PHASE
Pediatric, Bacterial Infection—Phase III
Pediatric, Ear Infections —Phase III
Pediatric, Meningitis —Phase III
Pediatric, Pneumonia— Phase III

Candidiasis

FK463, echinocandin
unknown

MANUFACTURER
Fujisawa Healthcare

DESCRIPTION
Echinocandin is a novel antifungal agent for the treatment of systemic fungal infections. The drug is used as prophylaxis, empirical therapy, and second line treatment for candidiasis and aspergillosis. Echinocandin is in phase II/III trials for these indications and other fungal infections.

INDICATION(S) AND RESEARCH PHASE
Aspergillosis – Phase II/III
Candidiasis – Phase II/III
Fungal Infections – Phase II/III

nystatin, AR-121
Nyotran

MANUFACTURER
Aronex Pharmaceuticals

DESCRIPTION
Nyotran is an intravenous liposomal formulation of nystatin being developed for the treatment of serious systemic, opportunistic fungal infections. Phase III trials have been completed for systemic fungal infections and confirmed cryptococcal meningitis. Additionally, phase II trials have been completed for candidiasis and aspergillosis.

Nyotran is under agreement with Abbott Laboratories for worldwide commercialization. Abbott will fund clinical development and will submit marketing registration outside the United States.

INDICATION(S) AND RESEARCH PHASE
Aspergillosis – Phase II completed
Candidiasis – Phase II completed
Systemic Fungal Infections – Phase III completed
Meningitis – Phase III completed

Chronic Fatigue Syndrome

2CVV
unknown

MANUFACTURER
Milkhaus Laboratory

DESCRIPTION
2CVV is an orally formulated therapy that was being tested for chronic fatigue syndrome. Trials have completed phase II and are suspended indefinitely from further development.

INDICATION(S) AND RESEARCH PHASE
Chronic Fatigue Syndrome – Phase II discontinued

galantamine hydrobromide
Reminyl

MANUFACTURER
Janssen Research Foundation

DESCRIPTION
Reminyl (galantamine) is a nicotinic modulator that is being developed for the treatment of both chronic fatigue syndrome (CFS) and Alzheimer's disease. This drug works by slowing down or reversibly inhibiting acetylcholinesterase, which is the enzyme responsible for degrading the neurotransmitter acetylcholine. It is produced in an oral tablet formulation.

Study results show that volunteers with Alzheimer's treated with Reminyl exhibited improved memory, behavior, and ability to perform activities of daily living. In addition, a second study suggested that the cognitive and functional benefits of galantamine may be sustained for at least 12 months. Reminyl is being developed by the

Janssen Research Foundation under a co-development agreement with Shire Pharmaceuticals.

INDICATION(S) AND RESEARCH PHASE
Alzheimer's Disease – FDA approved
Chronic Fatigue Syndrome – Phase II
Dementia – Phase III

poly I:poly C-12-U
Ampligen

MANUFACTURER
Hemispherx Biopharma

DESCRIPTION
Ampligen is a novel therapeutic treatment composed of genetic building blocks (polyribonucleotide and synthetic nucleic acid) for the treatment of metastatic renal carcinoma, as an orphan indication. This intravenous drug is being evaluated in phase II/III trials for renal carcinoma, phase I/II for malignant melanoma, and phase III for chronic fatigue syndrome and HIV.

INDICATION(S) AND RESEARCH PHASE
Renal Cell Carcinoma – Phase II/III
Malignant Melanoma – Phase I/II
Chronic Fatigue Syndrome – Phase III
HIV Infection – Phase III

Cytomegalovirus (CMV) Retinitis

ganciclovir
Cytovene

MANUFACTURER
Hoffmann-La Roche

DESCRIPTION
Cytovene is currently on the market for treatment and prevention of cytomegalovirus (CMV) retinitis in AIDS subjects. This drug is in phase III trials for a new indication: treatment and prevention of cytomegalovirus in transplant subjects. Additional indications may include infectious diseases and viral diseases.

INDICATION(S) AND RESEARCH PHASE
Cytomegalovirus (CMV) Retinitis – Phase III

ISIS-13312
unknown

MANUFACTURER
Isis Pharmaceuticals

DESCRIPTION
ISIS-13312 is a genetically engineered complex (second-generation antisense compound). This drug is being tested in phase I/II trials for the treatment of cytomegalovirus (CMV) retinitis.

INDICATION(S) AND RESEARCH PHASE
Cytomegalovirus (CMV) Retinitis – Phase I/II

vaccine, cytomegalovirus
unknown

MANUFACTURER
Aviron

DESCRIPTION
A cytomegalovirus (CMV) vaccine is in a phase I trial and will test four live attenuated injectable vaccine candidates developed by Aviron. The trial is being conducted by the National Insititute of Allergy and Infectious Disease and is taking place at Saint Louis University and will include 25 subjects. Currently, there is no vaccine available for CMV.

INDICATION(S) AND RESEARCH PHASE
Cytomegalovirus (CMV) Retinitis – Phase I

valganciclovir
Cymeval

MANUFACTURER
Hoffmann-La Roche

DESCRIPTION
Cymeval is an antiviral agent being evaluated for the prevention of cytomegalovirus (CMV) retinitis in subjects with AIDS. Valganciclovir is a pro-drug of Roche's existing anti-CMV treatment, ganciclovir (Cytovene) and is manufactured by adding a valine amino acid to ganciclovir. This allows the drug to be given orally, rather than intravenously. In addition, absorption is much better than that of the present compound, ganciclovir. The company submitted an NDA in October 2000.

In addition, a phase III trial is comparing valganciclovir to oral Cytovene for prevention of cytomegalovirus disease in solid organ transplant recipients.

INDICATION(S) AND RESEARCH PHASE
Cytomegalovirus (CMV) Retinitis – NDA submitted
Organ Transplantation – Phase II

Genital Herpes

APL400-024Px
Genevax-HSV-Px

MANUFACTURER
Wyeth-Lederle Vaccines

DESCRIPTION
HSV-Px is a novel facilitated DNA vaccine for prevention of herpes simplex virus-2 (HSV-2) infection that causes genital herpes. This vaccine uses injected Genevax delivery technology and it is in phase II trials.

INDICATION(S) AND RESEARCH PHASE
Genital Herpes – Phase II

GW 419458, DISC-HSV
unknown

MANUFACTURER
GlaxoSmithKline

DESCRIPTION
DISC (disabled infectious single cycle)-HSV is an immunotherapeutic vaccine using a disabled live virus for treatment and prevention of genital herpes. Since the drug therapy induces a natural immune response and may promote "immunologic memory," the

chance of disease recurrence is drastically reduced. It also eliminates the need for constant dosing, thereby increasing subject compliance and improving lifestyle. The drug is in phase II trials for genital herpes. GlaxoSmithKline has worldwide development and marketing rights.

INDICATION(S) AND RESEARCH PHASE
Genital Herpes – Phase II

resiquimod
unknown

MANUFACTURER
3M Pharmaceuticals

DESCRIPTION
Resiquimod is in phase III trials for recurrent genital herpes in both the United States and Europe. In November 2000, positive phase II results of a double-blind, placebo-controlled trial were reported. In the six month follow-up, the time to the first recurrence was significantly increased and the total number of recurrences was significantly decreased for subjects on active study medication compared to a placebo gel.

INDICATION(S) AND RESEARCH PHASE
Genital Herpes – Phase III

TA-HSV
unknown

MANUFACTURER
Cantab Pharmaceuticals plc

DESCRIPTION
TA-HSV (therapeutic antigen-herpes simplex virus) is a genetically disabled vaccine containing HSV that allows only a single cycle of replication within a host cell. It is in phase II trials for the treatment of genital herpes.

INDICATION(S) AND RESEARCH PHASE
Genital Herpes – Phase II

unknown
Docosanol

MANUFACTURER
AVANIR Pharmaceuticals

DESCRIPTION
Docosanol is approved as a treatment for cold sores and fever blisters. It is in phase III trials for the treatment of genital herpes. Docosanol works by inhibiting fusion between the plasma membrane and the herpes simplex virus (HSV) envelope, thereby preventing viral entry into cells and subsequent viral replication. Since the compound doesn't act directly on the virus, it is unlikely it will produce drug resistant mutants of HSV. All known competitive Rx products work by inhibition of viral DNA replication and, as such, carry risk of mutating the virus.

INDICATION(S) AND RESEARCH PHASE
Genital Herpes – Phase III

vaccine, genital herpes
Simplirix

MANUFACTURER
GlaxoSmithKline

DESCRIPTION
Simplirix is a recombinant vaccine being developed for genital herpes prophylaxis. Simplirix consists of a recombinant glycoprotein from herpes simplex virus 2 (HSV-2), in combination with an adjuvant "derivative endotoxin." Results of two large, placebo-controlled, randomized international trials were presented at the 40th annual Interscience Conference on Antimicrobials and Chemotherapy in 2000. Both were "discordant partner studies," in which one of the partners had genital herpes and the other did not. The first trial included 847 subjects who tested negative for HSV-1 and HSV-2 at baseline, and the second trial involved 1,867 subjects who were negative for HSV-2. The vaccine had no effect in the men in either group; however, a notable effect was observed in the women. In the first study, the vaccine efficacy in women was 73%. Similarly, among the seronegative women in the second study, the vaccine efficacy was 74%. The vaccine was not protective in the women who were HSV-1-positive and HSV-2-negative.

INDICATION(S) AND RESEARCH PHASE
Genital Herpes – Phase II
Vaccines – Phase II

vaccine, genital herpes
unknown

MANUFACTURER
Corixa Montana

DESCRIPTION
This immunostimulant vaccine uses monophosphoryl lipid A (MPL) adjuvant for prevention and treatment of herpes simplex virus types 1 and 2 that cause genital herpes. The vaccine is in phase III trials.

INDICATION(S) AND RESEARCH PHASE
Genital Herpes – Phase III
Herpes Simplex Infections – Phase III

Genital Warts

HspE7
unknown

MANUFACTURER
StressGen

DESCRIPTION
HspE7 is a recombinant fusion product composed of the heat shock protein 65 (Hsp65) from *M. bovis* BCG and the protein E7. The E7 protein is derived from the human papillomavirus (HPV) and is involved in the malignant transformation of anal and cervical epithelial cells. E7 is a tumor-specific antigen and represents a precise target for immune system attack on abnormal cells.

StressGen has initiated a phase III trial to investigate HspE7 as a novel immunotherapeutic for anal dysplasia (AIN) caused by HPV. Phase II trials in women with HPV-related cervical dysplasia and cervical cancer are under way. In January 2001, a phase II trial was initiated to test HspE7 on 52 subjects suffering from genital warts caused by HPV.

Genital Warts

INDICATION(S) AND RESEARCH PHASE
Cervical Dysplasia/Cancer – Phase II
Anal dysplasia caused by HPV – Phase III
Genital Warts – Phase II

---

interferon (IFN) alfa-n3
Alferon N Gel

MANUFACTURER
Interferon Sciences

DESCRIPTION
Alferon N Gel is a human leukocyte-derived natural interferon (IFN) treatment being tested for vaginal infections in phase II trials. Interferons are naturally produced chemicals that modulate and boost the immune system. These trials are testing the drug in a topical gel formulation.

Already on the market, interferon alfa-n3 (human leukocyte-derived) is an injectable formulation of natural alpha interferon, approved by the FDA in 1989 for the intralesional treatment of refractory or recurring external condylomata acuminata in subjects 18 years of age or older.

INDICATION(S) AND RESEARCH PHASE
Genital Warts – Phase II
Vaginal Infection – Phase II
Viral Infection – Phase II

PEN203
unknown

MANUFACTURER
CoPharma

DESCRIPTION
PEN203 represents a novel class of small molecule pharmaceuticals with broad spectrum antiviral activity. These anti-proliferative compounds are designed to act through a natural antiviral pathway induced by interferon. Like interferon, they are believed to work by enhancing the body's natural mechanism for protection against viruses. Unlike injectable interferon or ablative topical therapies, however, PEN203 can be topically applied and is designed to be well tolerated by patients.

PEN203 is currently in phase IIb trials for treatment of basal cell carcinoma, psoriasis, and genital warts.

INDICATION(S) AND RESEARCH PHASE
Genital Warts – Phase IIb
Psoriasis and Psoriatic Disorders – Phase IIb
Basal Cell Carcinoma – Phase IIb

TA-GW pharmaccine
unknown

MANUFACTURER
Cantab Pharmaceuticals plc

DESCRIPTION
TA-GW pharmaccine is a novel therapeutic vaccine for genital warts. The compound, in an intravenous formulation, combines an HPV (human papillomavirus) protein with an adjuvant to produce an immune reaction directed against the virus. SmithKline Beecham (now GlaxoSmithKline), who have been responsible for funding development, have decided to discontinue investment in TA-GW. This decision was based on results of a phase II trial, which showed that at six months there was no significant difference in the wart recurrence rate between subjects who received TA-GW and those in the control group.

INDICATION(S) AND RESEARCH PHASE
Genital Warts – Phase II discontinued

---

unknown
Polyphenon E

MANUFACTURER
MediGene AG

DESCRIPTION
Polyphenon E consists of polyphenols, which inhibit viruses causing genital warts. In addition, polyphenols have anti-tumor and anti-inflammatory properties. Polyphenon E is in a phase III trial to treat genital warts caused by human papillomaviruses and will enroll 260 subjects, 50% male and 50% female, in 30 sites throughout Germany and Russia. The trial will be randomized, double-blinded, and placebo-controlled.

INDICATION(S) AND RESEARCH PHASE
Genital Warts – Phase III

Hepatitis

ACH-126,443
unknown

MANUFACTURER
Achillion Pharmaceuticals

DESCRIPTION
ACH-126,443 is an orally administered antiviral agent with potent activity against the hepatitis B virus and the human immunodeficiency virus (HIV). The drug is currently in phase I development. MediChem Life Sciences, a drug discovery technology and services company, conducted chemical route development that provided the scaleable synthetic pathway used to manufacture kilogram quantities of this drug candidate. Kilogram-scale synthesis was then performed to supply large quantities of ACH-126,443 for the clinical trials.

INDICATION(S) AND RESEARCH PHASE
Hepatitis – Phase I
HIV Infection – Phase I

---

adefovir dipivoxil, GS-840
unknown

MANUFACTURER
Gilead Sciences

DESCRIPTION
Adefovir dipivoxil is a prodrug of PMEA, a nucleotide that inhibits hepatitis B virus DHA polymerase, an enzyme essential to viral replication. Currently, it is being tested in a phase III trial for hepatitis B. This two year trial is recruiting about 500 subjects and is evaluating dosages of 10 and 30 mg/day orally.

INDICATION(S) AND RESEARCH PHASE
Hepatitis – Phase III

---

anti-hepatitis B

unknown

MANUFACTURER
Cangene Corporation

DESCRIPTION
Anti-hepatitis B is part of the company's hyperimmune products, which are highly purified antibodies made from human plasma obtained from people with high antibody titers to the hepatitis B virus. A phase III trial for use in the treatment of chronic hepatitis B virus infection was completed in Europe at the end of 2000 and results suggested that the product was efficacious. The company anticipates filing an NDS in Canada.

INDICATION(S) AND RESEARCH PHASE
Hepatitis – Phase III completed

anti-hepatitis C
unknown

MANUFACTURER
Cangene Corporation

DESCRIPTION
Anti-hepatitis C is part of the company's hyperimmune products, which are highly purified antibodies made from specialty human plasma used for therapeutic purposes. It is being tested in a phase II trial in liver transplantation recipients infected with the hepatitis C virus. The phase II trial will evaluate the effects of the antibodies to prevent re-infection of the transplanted liver. The trial is being conducted at multiple sites throughout Canada.

INDICATION(S) AND RESEARCH PHASE
Hepatitis – Phase II

BMS-200475
Entecavir

MANUFACTURER
Bristol-Myers Squibb

DESCRIPTION
Viruses such as hepatitis B need to be able to replicate their viral genetic material in order to reproduce themselves. Bristol-Myers Squibb is developing a treatment for chronic hepatitis B infection, a common and serious liver condition, which works by disrupting the viral replication process.

Genetic material is made up of proteins called nucleic acids. By using a synthesized protein (2'-deoxyguanosine carbocyclic analogue) that mimics one of the building blocks of nucleic acids, scientists hope to stop the production of viral genetic information, and thus prevent viruses from creating the genetic machinery they require to keep reproducing.

Studies are under way in phase II trials to understand if this novel drug will improve the symptoms and prognosis of chronic hepatitis B infection.

INDICATION(S) AND RESEARCH PHASE
Hepatitis – Phase II
Viral Infection – Phase II

cidofovir
Vistide

MANUFACTURER
Gilead Sciences

DESCRIPTION
Vistide is being tested as an injectable formulation for treatment of central nervous system infections and hepatitis B virus respiratory tumors, and tumors or disorders of the larynx. The drug is in phase I/II trials for HBV respiratory tumors, laryngeal papillomatosis, and progressive multifocal leukoencephalopathy.

INDICATION(S) AND RESEARCH PHASE
Hepatitis – Phase I/II
Laryngeal Tumors/Disorders – Phase I/II
Viral Infection – Phase I/II
Brain Cancer – Phase I/II

clevudine
unknown

MANUFACTURER
Triangle Pharmaceuticals

DESCRIPTION
Clevudine (formerly L-FMAU) is a pyrimidine nucleoside analogue that has shown inhibitory activity against hepatitis B virus (HBV) replication invitro. The drug is currently in phase I development for the treatment of HBV.

INDICATION(S) AND RESEARCH PHASE
Hepatitis – Phase I

EHT899
unknown

MANUFACTURER
Enzo Biochem

DESCRIPTION
EHT899 is currently in phase II development for the treatment of hepatitis B (HBV). Hepatitis B virus can cause a chronic infection in the liver of infected people. Liver damage is the result of direct viral effects and the person's immune system response to the infection. In preclinical work, it was shown that the immune response against the virus could be altered by oral administration of certain viral proteins developed by Enzo.

Eighty percent of subjects in a phase I trial of EHT899 responded favorably as measured by a decrease in viral load, decrease in liver inflammation, or reduction of elevated levels of liver enzymes. Nine of the 15 subjects experienced significant decreases in viral load, while ten subjects showed complete normalization of liver enzymes. The trial was conducted in Jerusalem.

INDICATION(S) AND RESEARCH PHASE
Hepatitis – Phase II

emtricitabine
Coviracil

MANUFACTURER
Triangle Pharmaceuticals

DESCRIPTION
Coviracil, a nucleoside reverse transcript inhibitor (NRTI), has been shown to be a potent inhibitor of hepatitis B virus (HBV)

replication. In October 2000, results of a phase I/II trial of Coviracil involving subjects chronically infected with HBV indicated that a daily dose of 200 mg was most effective. As a result, the 200 mg/day dosage was selected for a phase III trial, which was initiated in October 2000. Coviracil is also in phase II and III trials for the treatment of HIV infection.

INDICATION(S) AND RESEARCH PHASE
HIV Infection – Phase III
Hepatitis – Phase III
Pediatric, AIDS/HIV – Phase III

HCI-436
unknown

MANUFACTURER
Wyeth-Ayerst

DESCRIPTION
HCI-436 is a novel drug being developed for the treatment of hepatitis C virus. It works by inhibiting viral activities essential to the replication of the virus. The drug is being jointly developed with ViroPharma and is in phase II trials.

INDICATION(S) AND RESEARCH PHASE
Hepatitis – Phase II

hepatitis A
Nothav

MANUFACTURER
Chiron Corporation

DESCRIPTION
Nothav is a second-generation vaccine for hepatitis A. It is currently in phase III trials for adults in Europe. The company plans to develop a formulation for pediatric subjects as well.

INDICATION(S) AND RESEARCH PHASE
Hepatitis – Phase III

hepatitis B immune globulin
HBVIg

MANUFACTURER
Nabi

DESCRIPTION
HBVIg is a human hepatitis B immune globulin in development for the treatment of acute exposure to blood containing hepatitis B virus surface antigen. It is also being developed in an intravenous formulation to prevent hepatitis B virus re-infection of transplanted livers in subjects with hepatitis B. A biologics license application has been submitted for the first indication, and the drug is in phase III trials regarding liver transplants.

An NDA has been submitted for the prevention of perinatal transmission of hepatitis B.

INDICATION(S) AND RESEARCH PHASE
Hepatitis – NDA submitted
Liver Transplant – Phase III
Pediatric – NDA submitted

hepatitis B immunotherapy, HBV/MF59
unknown

MANUFACTURER
Chiron Corporation

DESCRIPTION
HBV/MF59 is an immunotherapy combining the company's hepatitis B vaccine and a novel proprietary adjuvant, MF59. The adjuvant is needed to enhance the response to the vaccine. Even with a complete series of three injections, approximately 20% of people receiving the licensed HBV vaccine do not respond. It is currently in phase II trials for chronic hepatitis B.

INDICATION(S) AND RESEARCH PHASE
Hepatitis – Phase II

hepatitis C protein
unknown

MANUFACTURER
Enzo Biochem

DESCRIPTION
A new broad-spectrum immune regulatory compound is in a phase I trial for treatment of hepatitis C virus infection (HCV) or its associated hepatocellular carcinoma secondary to HCV infection. The trial will treat each subject for 30 weeks and will be followed for another 20 weeks. The trial is taking place in Israel.

INDICATION(S) AND RESEARCH PHASE
Hepatitis – Phase I

IDN-6556
unknown

MANUFACTURER
IDUN Pharmaceuticals

DESCRIPTION
IDN-6556 is a caspase inhibitor, resulting in the inhibition of apoptosis. The compound is in a phase I trial for the treatment of acute alcoholic hepatitis, a condition that is characterized by increased apoptosis of hepatocytes.

INDICATION(S) AND RESEARCH PHASE
Hepatitis – Phase I

immune globulin
Nabi Civacir

MANUFACTURER
Nabi

DESCRIPTION
Nabi Civacir is a human antibody product containing antibodies that neutralize hepatitis C virus (HCV). It is being developed to prevent liver transplant subjects with hepatitis C from experiencing liver re-infection. It is also being developed for the treatment of chronic hepatitis C virus infections. Nabi Civacir is currently in phase I trials.

INDICATION(S) AND RESEARCH PHASE
Hepatitis – Phase I

immune globulin intravenous
Venoglobulin-S

MANUFACTURER
Alpha Therapeutic

DESCRIPTION
Venoglobulin-S is a solution of antibodies that are being tested for use in two indications. The first one is a phase III clinical trial to prevent infection (prophylaxis) from the hepatitis A virus and the second use is for prevention of acute graft versus host disease (GVHD) in subjects needing a bone marrow transplant. Sometimes drug therapy is helpful to prevent the body from rejecting a transplanted organ, or in the opposite case of the organ rejecting its new host.

This immune globulin product may replace missing antibodies, especially in subjects that have a compromised immune system or primary immunodeficiencies, which may be present at birth. This biological product is given to a subject by intramuscular injection.

INDICATION(S) AND RESEARCH PHASE
Bone Marrow Transplant – Phase III
Hepatitis – Phase III

immunostimulatory sequences (ISS) candidate
unknown

MANUFACTURER
Triangle Pharmaceuticals

DESCRIPTION
Immunostimulatory sequences (ISS) are short strands of DNA believed to elicit immune responses. Triangle Pharmaceuticals currently has an ISS candidate in phase I development for the treatment of hepatitis B.

INDICATION(S) AND RESEARCH PHASE
Hepatitis – Phase I

immunotherapeutic, AML
Ceplene

MANUFACTURER
Maxim Pharmaceuticals

DESCRIPTION
Ceplene (formally Maxamine) is a histamine-2 (H_2) receptor stimulator (agonist) that is being co-administered with immunotherapies, including cytokines and interleukin-2 (IL-2). Clinical testing includes treatment of acute myelogenous leukemia (AML), chronic hepatitis C, malignant melanoma, multiple myeloma, and renal cell carcinoma.

Results from a phase III 300 subject trial of Ceplene (histamine dihydrochloride) in stage IV malignant melanoma indicated that Ceplene used in combination with a lower dose of IL-2 improved survival rates for stage IV malignant melanoma subjects compared with those treated with the same doses of IL-2 alone. Treatment with Ceplene and IL-2 improved overall survival, increased survival rates at 12, 18, and 24 months, and improved time-to-disease progression over treatment with IL-2 alone. Twenty-five percent of subjects treated with Ceplene and lower-dose IL-2 survived for a 24-month period. Overall response was achieved in 38% of the subjects treated with Ceplene and lower-dose IL-2. The company received an NDA non-approvable letter in January 2001 because the FDA stated that the phase III trial forming the basis of the NDA would not be adequate as a single study to support approval.

INDICATION(S) AND RESEARCH PHASE
Hepatitis – Phase II
Leukemia – Phase III completed
Malignant Melanoma – NDA denied
Multiple Myeloma – Phase II
Renal Cell Carcinoma – Phase II

interferon (IFN) alfa-n3
Alferon N Injection

MANUFACTURER
Interferon Sciences

DESCRIPTION
Alferon N is a human leukocyte-derived natural interferon (IFN) treatment being tested for chronic hepatitis C in subjects previously untreated with IFN.

Alferon N is given by injection and has completed a phase III trial. The company reported that the FDA rejected the drug application and advised for the conduct of another phase III study with an improved endpoint design before approval may be granted. At the present time, the company does not have the resources necessary to continue development.

INDICATION(S) AND RESEARCH PHASE
Hepatitis – NDA denied
HIV Infection – Phase II

interferon alfa-2b
PEG-Intron

MANUFACTURER
Schering-Plough Corporation

DESCRIPTION
PEG-Intron is a long-acting antiviral/biological response modifier. Clinical trials include testing for the treatment of chronic myelogenous leukemia, solid tumors, and malignant melanoma.

PEG-Intron was developed by Enzon for Schering-Plough who owns the exclusive rights. The drug was approved by the FDA for the treatment of hepatitis C in January 2001.

INDICATION(S) AND RESEARCH PHASE
Cancer/Tumors (Unspecified) – Phase II
Hepatitis – FDA approved
Leukemia – Phase III
Malignant Melanoma – Phase III

interferon alfa-2b/ribavirin
PEG-Intron/Rebetol

MANUFACTURER
Enzon

DESCRIPTION
PEG-Intron + Rebetol is a combination therapy of biosynthetic interferon and ribavirin for the treatment of hepatitis C virus infection. Rebetol is an oral formulation of ribavirin, a synthetic nucleoside analog with broad-spectrum antiviral activity. Intron A is a recombinant version of naturally occurring alpha interferon, which has been shown to exert both antiviral and immunomodulatory effects. Intron A must be given three

times a week. PEG-Intron is a longer-acting form of Intron A that uses proprietary PEG technology developed by Enzon, and can be given once weekly.

Results of a phase III trial indicated that combination therapy with once-weekly PEG-Intron injection plus daily Rebetol capsules achieved a 54% rate of sustained virologic response overall in previously untreated adult subjects with chronic hepatitis C. Sustained virologic response (SVR) is defined as sustained loss of detectable hepatitis C virus.

INDICATION(S) AND RESEARCH PHASE
Hepatitis – Phase III

---

interleukin-10
Tenovil

MANUFACTURER
Schering-Plough

DESCRIPTION
Tenovil is an immunomodulator being developed in an injectable formulation. It is currently being evaluated for the treatment of ischemia reperfusion injury, hepatic fibrosis, hepatitis C, and psoriasis.

INDICATION(S) AND RESEARCH PHASE
Liver Disease – Phase II
Hepatitis – Phase I
Ischemia Reperfusion Injury – Phase I
Psoriasis and Psoriatic Disorders – Phase II

---

interleukin-12 (IL-12)
unknown

MANUFACTURER
Genetics Institute

DESCRIPTION
Interleukin-12 (IL-12) is a novel genetically engineered, human immune modulator being tested in phase II trials for the treatment of hepatitis C, chronic liver disease due to hepatitis infection, and AIDS. There is an additional indication for renal carcinoma, which may have an orphan drug status.

INDICATION(S) AND RESEARCH PHASE
Acquired Immune Deficiency Syndrome (AIDS) and AIDS-Related Infections – Phase II
Hepatitis – Phase II
Renal Cell Carcinoma – Phase II

IP501
unknown

MANUFACTURER
Interneuron Pharmaceuticals

DESCRIPTION
IP501 is a purified phospholipid, which helps to repair damaged cells. It is indicated for the treatment and prevention of alcohol-induced cirrhosis of the liver and hepatitis C. IP501 is currently in phase III trials. The drug is in tablet form.

INDICATION(S) AND RESEARCH PHASE
Alcohol Dependence – Phase III
Hepatitis – Phase III
Liver Disease – Phase III

ISIS-14803
unknown

MANUFACTURER
Isis Pharmaceuticals

DESCRIPTION
ISIS 14803 is a novel antisense drug designed specifically to inhibit the replication of the virus. Its preclinical trials in mice and cell cultures showed marked reduction of the HCV RNA expression. It consists of a 20-base phosphorothioate oligonucleotide that is administered using a microfusion pump called Medipad. The Elan Corporation of Ireland has developed the pump and is the co-developer of the drug.

INDICATION(S) AND RESEARCH PHASE
Hepatitis – Phase I/II

LY466700
Heptazyme

MANUFACTURER
Ribozyme Pharmaceuticals

DESCRIPTION
Heptazyme is an anti-hepatitis C virus ribozyme. It works by cleaving the hepatitis C (HCV) genetic material in a region of the HCV gene that is highly conserved. Heptazyme has been designed to target a specific region necessary for the viral life cycle; when this region is cut, the virus is unable to replicate. Phase II trials testing Heptazyme are planned for first quarter 2001.

Two phase I results demonstrated that Heptazyme was well tolerated at all doses given, in contrast to the significant side effects associated with currently available HCV treatments. Further, 12 HCV positive subjects with elevations in serum ALT were treated at doses ranging from 10 to 90 mg/subject in the multi-dose trials. Three of these subjects had transient decreases in serum HCV RNA of approximately 1 log10. Ribozyme is preparing for upcoming phase II trials.

INDICATION(S) AND RESEARCH PHASE
Hepatitis – Phase II

MIV-210
unknown

MANUFACTURER
Medivir

DESCRIPTION
MIV-210 is a nucleoside analogue in a phase I trial for treatment of hepatitis B virus infection. The initial phase I trials are being conducted in the United Kingdom and are expected to be completed during the third quarter of 2001. In animal tests, MIV-210 shows good efficacy against the hepatitis B virus.

INDICATION(S) AND RESEARCH PHASE
Hepatitis – Phase I

OST 577
Ostavir

MANUFACTURER

Protein Design Labs

DESCRIPTION
Ostavir is a humanized monoclonal antibody (Mab) in ongoing phase II trials for the treatment of chronic hepatitis B, either combined with interferon or as a sole agent. Additional indications may include infectious diseases and viral diseases.

INDICATION(S) AND RESEARCH PHASE
Hepatitis – Phase II
Viral Infection – Phase II

peginterferon alfa-2a
Pegasys

MANUFACTURER
Hoffmann-La Roche

DESCRIPTION
Pegasys is a longer-lasting form of interferon, which is a naturally produced immune boosting substance. This drug is given in an injectable formulation that is being tested in phase III trials for the treatment of complications of hepatitis C.

INDICATION(S) AND RESEARCH PHASE
Hepatitis – Phase III
Malignant Melanoma – Phase II
Renal Cell Carcinoma – Phase II
Leukemia – Phase III

PeNta-HepB-IPV, vaccine
Infanrix

MANUFACTURER
GlaxoSmithKline

DESCRIPTION
This recombinant vaccine has been developed to address several indications. It has been approved by the European Union for diphtheria, tetanus, pertussis, hepatitis B, and polio. An NDA has also been submitted for these indications.

INDICATION(S) AND RESEARCH PHASE
Pediatric, Diphtheria, Tetanus, Pertussis, and Polio – NDA submitted
Hepatitis – NDA submitted

recombinant human interferon beta-1a
Rebif

MANUFACTURER
Serono Laboratories

DESCRIPTION
Rebif is an interferon beta-1a product being developed for a variety of indications. These include non-small cell lung cancer, chronic hepatitis C, Crohn's disease, ulcerative colitis, Guillain-Barré syndrome, as an early treatment of multiple sclerosis (phase III) and as a treatment for secondary progressive multiple sclerosis (filed) and rheumatoid arthritis. Rebif has been approved in several countries for the treatment of relapsing-remitting multiple sclerosis.

INDICATION(S) AND RESEARCH PHASE
Multiple Sclerosis – Phase III
Lung Cancer – Phase II
Hepatitis – Phase II
Crohn's Disease – Phase II
Inflammatory Bowel Disease – Phase II
Guillain-Barré Syndrome – Phase II
Rheumatoid Arthritis – Phase II

SB M00026
unknown

MANUFACTURER
GlaxoSmithKline

DESCRIPTION
SB M00026 is a recombinant compound being developed for the treatment of chronic infection with hepatitis B virus. It is currently in phase II development.

INDICATION(S) AND RESEARCH PHASE
Hepatitis – Phase II

thymalfasin
Zadaxin

MANUFACTURER
SciClone Pharmaceuticals

DESCRIPTION
Zadaxin is a twenty-eight amino acid peptide originally isolated from the thymus gland now produced synthetically. The compound has been shown to promote the maturation of T-cells, which are involved in the control of various immune responses. Zadaxin has been administered to over 3,000 subjects in over 70 clinical trials without serious drug-related side effects.

Zadaxin is presently in phase II trials in the United States in combination with lamivudine for the treatment of hepatitis B. SciClone plans to initiate additional U.S. phase II Zadaxin clinical programs in liver cancer and malignant melanoma. Pivotal phase III hepatitis B studies are currently ongoing in Japan. SciClone plans to start a pivotal phase III hepatitis C trial in the United States, which will be complemented by a pivotal phase III hepatitis C trial in Europe to be conducted by Sigma-Tau S.p.A., SciClone's European partner.

INDICATION(S) AND RESEARCH PHASE
Hepatitis – Phase II
Hepatitis – Phase III
Viral Infection – Phase III
Liver Cancer – Phase II
Malignant Melanoma – Phase II

unknown
Omniferon

MANUFACTURER
Viragen

DESCRIPTION
Omniferon is a multi-subtype alpha interferon derived from human white blood cells. This specific interferon is being studied in the treatment of hepatitis C virus infection. Favorable interim dose escalation results from the first phase II trial have been reported. None of the subjects had to undergo dose reduction or discontinue treatment because of side effects at any of the three dosing levels. There was a significant decrease in hepatitis C virus concentrations in the blood with some evidence that this reduction was more rapid than that observed with other drug regimens used to treat this infection.

INDICATION(S) AND RESEARCH PHASE
Hepatitis – Phase II

unknown
Albuferon

MANUFACTURER
Human Genome Sciences

DESCRIPTION
Albuferon is a new protein created by fusing the gene for interferon alpha to the gene of another human protein, albumin. The fused gene produces a protein with characteristics of both interferon alpha and albumin. Based on preclinical studies, Albuferon should provide a longer acting therapeutic activity and an improved side-effect profile when compared to the current first line therapy for hepatitis C virus infection, recombinant human interferon alpha. In October 2000, Human Genome Sciences submitted an IND application with the FDA in order to initiate phase I trials.

INDICATION(S) AND RESEARCH PHASE
Hepatitis – Phase I

ursodiol
Urso

MANUFACTURER
Axcan Pharma

DESCRIPTION
Urso is an oral tablet composed of a bile acid (ursodeoxycholic acid) found in small amounts in normal human bile and in larger quantities in the bile of certain bears. This drug has been marketed in the United States for the treatment of primary biliary cirrhosis (PBC) since 1998. It is also approved in Canada for the treatment of cholestatic liver diseases such as PBC and the dissolution of gallstones. Additionally, Urso is being tested in trials for at least five other indications: hypercholesterolemia, treatment with chemoprevention of colorectal polyps, treatment of colorectal cancer, treatment of non-alcoholic steatohepatitis, and treatment of viral hepatitis. The drug is licensed by Sanofi-Synthelabo to Axcan Pharma in a joint venture with Schwarz Pharma.

INDICATION(S) AND RESEARCH PHASE
Cholesterol, High Levels – Phase II
Colon Polyps – Phase II
Colorectal Cancer – Phase II
Gallbladder Disorders – Phase III/IV
Hepatitis – Phase II

vaccine, hepatitis E
unknown

MANUFACTURER
GlaxoSmithKline

DESCRIPTION
GlaxoSmithKline is developing a recombinant vaccine for hepatitis E prophylaxis. It is currently in phase I development.

INDICATION(S) AND RESEARCH PHASE
Hepatitis – Phase I

vaccine, HCV/MF59, hepatitis C
unknown

MANUFACTURER
Chiron Corporation

DESCRIPTION
HCV/MF59 is a prophylactic vaccine for the prevention of hepatitis C. It is currently in phase II trials.

INDICATION(S) AND RESEARCH PHASE
Hepatitis – Phase II

vaccine, hepatitis
Twinrix-three doses

MANUFACTURER
GlaxoSmithKline

DESCRIPTION
Twinrix is a recombinant vaccine that immunizes recipients against both hepatitis A and hepatitis B. Benefits of this vaccine may include greater convenience and protection for subjects, since immunization against two diseases can be achieved with one injection. An NDA has been submitted for Twinrix (three doses) for combined hepatitis A and B prophylaxis in adults.

INDICATION(S) AND RESEARCH PHASE
Hepatitis – NDA submitted
Vaccines – NDA submitted

vaccine, hepatitis B
unknown

MANUFACTURER
GlaxoSmithKline

DESCRIPTION
GlaxoSmithKline is developing a recombinant vaccine for extra strength hepatitis B prophylaxis (poor/non-responders). It is currently in phase III trials.

INDICATION(S) AND RESEARCH PHASE
Hepatitis – Phase III

vaccine, hepatitis B
Hepagene

MANUFACTURER
Celltech Chiroscience plc

DESCRIPTION
Hepagene is a novel third generation recombinant vaccine for the prevention of hepatitis B virus infection. Hepagene mimics the surface of the hepatitis B virus, which elicits an immune response. The success of this vaccine is significantly improved because it incorporates all three surface antigens: pre-S1, pre-S2, and S of the virus. Current vaccines contain only one or two of these surface antigens, providing for a much weaker immune stimulus. An MAA has been filed in Europe.

INDICATION(S) AND RESEARCH PHASE
Hepatitis – MAA filed

vaccine, hepatitis B DNA
unknown

MANUFACTURER
PowderJect Vaccines

DESCRIPTION

This DNA vaccine, which uses PowderJect delivery technology, is being developed for the treatment of hepatitis B. The ability of DNA vaccines to induce a cellular response is believed to be critical in eliminating chronic viral infections such as hepatitis B. An earlier clinical trial demonstrated that PowderJect's preventive hepatitis B DNA vaccine induced cellular immune responses in all evaluable subjects. This trial also indicated the vaccine elicited protective levels of antibodies in all volunteers.

The needle-free PowderJect system delivers vaccines, drugs, and diagnostics in a dry powder formulation of microscopic solid particles. These particles are accelerated to high velocity in a jet of gas generated from a helium microcylinder contained inside the hand-held PowderJect device. The medicine is propelled down a specially designed nozzle into the outer layers of the skin. The vaccine is being developed as part of a multi-product strategic alliance with GlaxoSmithKline.

INDICATION(S) AND RESEARCH PHASE
Hepatitis – Phase I

vaccine, viral hepatitis (HBV)
GENEVAX-HBV

MANUFACTURER
Wyeth-Lederle Vaccines

DESCRIPTION
Genevax is a novel DNA-based immunotherapeutic vaccine being developed against the hepatitis B virus (HBV).

INDICATION(S) AND RESEARCH PHASE
Hepatitis – Phase II

VML 600, R-848
unknown

MANUFACTURER
Vernalis

DESCRIPTION
VML 600 is a novel immune response modifier (IRM) that stimulates the production of cytokines and boosts cell-mediated immunity. It is being developed for the treatment of hepatitis C virus infections and herpes virus infections. Vernalis completed phase IIa studies in Europe and the United States in 2000 and is planning to conduct a larger phase II trial in 2001.

INDICATION(S) AND RESEARCH PHASE
Hepatitis – Phase II

VP 50406
unknown

MANUFACTURER
ViroPharma

DESCRIPTION
VP 50406 is an orally administered small molecule being developed for the treatment of hepatitis C virus infection. The drug has demonstrated an ability to inhibit RNA replication of hepatitis C virus invitro. VP 50406 is currently in phase II trials.

INDICATION(S) AND RESEARCH PHASE
Hepatitis – Phase II

VX-497
unknown

MANUFACTURER
Vertex Pharmaceuticals

DESCRIPTION
This oral drug contains a novel inhibitor of inosine monophosphate dehydrogenase (IMPDH), an enzyme responsible for stimulating production of lymphocytes. VX-497 has the potential to exert direct antiviral activity, as well as affect the immune response by affecting lymphocyte migration and proliferation. Consequently, VX-497 may be an effective treatment for hepatitis C virus (HCV) infection as the disease involves both viral proliferation and liver inflammation.

Vertex plans to initiate a pivotal trial of VX-497 plus pegylated interferon in subjects with HCV in 2001.

INDICATION(S) AND RESEARCH PHASE
Hepatitis – Phase II

XTL-001
unknown

MANUFACTURER
XTL Biopharmaceuticals

DESCRIPTION
XTL-001, a combination of two high affinity human monoclonal antibodies (Mabs), is directed against two different epitopes of hepatitis B surface antigen HbsAg of the hepatitis B virus (HBV) and binds to all major HBV subtypes. Phase I trial results indicated that XTL-001 produced a rapid and consistent decrease in HBV-DNA and HBsAg levels in subjects with chronic HBV. Twelve subjects received multiple infusions of XTL-001 in doses ranging from 10 mg to 80 mg per week for four consecutive weeks followed by four weeks of observation. HBV-DNA levels decreased by as much as 100,000-fold (5 logs), while lowered HbsAg levels were sustained for a short period of time in several subjects receiving the two highest doses of XTL-001 (40 mg/week and 80 mg/week). XTL Biopharmaceuticals plans to initiate a phase II trial of XTL-001 combined with currently available antivirals in 2001.

INDICATION(S) AND RESEARCH PHASE
Hepatitis – Phase I completed

Herpes Labialis Infections (Cold Sores)

ME-609
unknown

MANUFACTURER
Medivir

DESCRIPTION
ME-609 is a cream currently in development for the treatment of oral herpes simplex infections. In December 2000, preliminary results of a phase II trial demonstrated that the cream reduced the healing time of cold sores by 15% compared to placebo.

The double-blind, placebo-controlled, randomized trial was carried out by university clinics in North America. Subjects with a history of sun-induced herpes simplex virus infections around the mouth were irradiated with UV light. Treatment began after 48 hours; half of the subjects were treated with ME-609 and half with an inactive placebo cream. Medivir has conducted phase I and II trials in collaboration with AstraZeneca; however, this partnership will not be continued for the remainder of development.

INDICATION(S) AND RESEARCH PHASE
Herpes Labialis Infections (Cold Sores) – Phase II completed

Herpes Simplex Infections

AG-701
unknown

MANUFACTURER
Antigenics

DESCRIPTION
AG-701 is a recombinant human HSP complexed to a synthetic peptide derived from HSV-2 being tested in a phase I trial in subjects diagnosed with herpes simplex virus type 2 (HSV-2).

INDICATION(S) AND RESEARCH PHASE
Herpes Simplex Infections – Phase I

vaccine, genital herpes
unknown

MANUFACTURER
Corixa Montana

DESCRIPTION
This immunostimulant vaccine uses monophosphoryl lipid A (MPL) adjuvant for prevention and treatment of herpes simplex virus types1 and 2 that cause genital herpes. The vaccine is in phase III trials.

INDICATION(S) AND RESEARCH PHASE
Genital Herpes – Phase III
Herpes Simplex Infections – Phase III

valaciclovir
Valtrex, Zelitrex

MANUFACTURER
GlaxoSmithKline

DESCRIPTION
Valtrex (valaciclovir) is a nucleoside analogue in phase III development. It is being tested for three new indications: the prevention of herpes simplex virus (HSV) transmission, HSV suppression in immunocompromised subjects, and cold sores. Valtrex is also marketed under the trade name Zelitrex.

INDICATION(S) AND RESEARCH PHASE
Herpes Simplex Infections – Phase III
Cold Sores – Phase III

Herpes Zoster Infections

ADL2-1294
unknown

MANUFACTURER
Adolor

DESCRIPTION
ADL2-1294 is a peripheral opiate (synthetic narcotic) being tested for the treatment of pain and itching associated with burns, abrasions, eczema, and dermatitis. The drug, in a topical formulation, is in phase II trials for atopic dermatitis, burns and burn infections, herpes zoster infections, psoriasis and psoriatic disorders, as well as for eye disorders and infections.

INDICATION(S) AND RESEARCH PHASE
Atopic Dermatitis – Phase II
Burns and Burn Infections – Phase II
Herpes Zoster Infections – Phase II
Psoriasis and Psoriatic Disorders – Phase II
Eye Disorders/Infections – Phase II
Skin Infections/Disorders – Phase II

HIV Infection

abacavir
Ziagen

MANUFACTURER
GlaxoSmithKline

DESCRIPTION
Ziagen is a nucleoside reverse transcriptase inhibitor (NRTI) approved by the FDA for the treatment of HIV-1 infection in adults and children (ages three months and above). It is also in phase II trials in combination with the reverse transcriptase inhibitor Epivir for the treatment of HIV infection.

INDICATION(S) AND RESEARCH PHASE
HIV Infection – Phase II
Pediatric, HIV Infection – FDA approved

ACH-126,443
unknown

MANUFACTURER
Achillion Pharmaceuticals

DESCRIPTION
ACH-126,443 is an orally administered antiviral agent with potent activity against the hepatitis B virus and the human immunodeficiency virus (HIV). The drug is currently in phase I development. MediChem Life Sciences, a drug discovery technology and services company, conducted chemical route development that provided the scaleable synthetic pathway used to manufacture kilogram quantities of this drug candidate. Kilogram-scale synthesis was then performed to supply large quantities of ACH-126,443 for the clinical trials.

INDICATION(S) AND RESEARCH PHASE
Hepatitis – Phase I
HIV infection – Phase I

AIDS gene therapy
unknown

MANUFACTURER
Aventis

DESCRIPTION

This gene therapy for AIDS involves genetically engineered T-cells that may target and eliminate residual virus in HIV-infected cells. The AIDS virus can remain dormant as reservoirs for future infection even after treatment with the best available antiviral drugs. This therapy is being tested in phase II trials for the treatment of AIDS. Future therapeutic studies may include cancer.

INDICATION(S) AND RESEARCH PHASE

Acquired Immune Deficiency Syndrome (AIDS) and AIDS-Related Infections – Phase II
HIV Infection – Phase II

aldesleukin, interleukin-2 (IL-2)
Proleukin

MANUFACTURER
Chiron Corporation

DESCRIPTION

Proleukin is a genetically engineered (recombinant) form of interleukin-2, which is a naturally occurring immune modulator. Proleukin is being evaluated for the treatment of leukemia, non-Hodgkin's lymphoma, and HIV infection. Additionally, Proleukin was approved in July 2000 for advanced-stage kidney cancer and melanoma.

INDICATION(S) AND RESEARCH PHASE

HIV Infection – Phase III
Leukemia – Phase III
Lymphoma, Non-Hodgkin's – Phase III
Renal Cell Carcinoma – FDA approved
Melanoma – FDA approved

ALVAC-HIV 1
unknown

MANUFACTURER
Aventis Pasteur

DESCRIPTION

ALVAC-HIV 1 is a vaccine that uses live canary poxvirus, which does not infect human beings. The poxvirus is acting as a carrier or vector to deliver a preparation of genetically engineered HIV surface glycoproteins (gp 160). This complex was developed to stimulate the body's production of HIV-neutralizing antibodies to protect against AIDS. This vaccine is being tested in phase II trials.

INDICATION(S) AND RESEARCH PHASE

Acquired Immune Deficiency Syndrome (AIDS) and AIDS-Related Infections – Phase II
HIV Infection – Phase II

AMD-3100
unknown

MANUFACTURER
AnorMED

DESCRIPTION

AMD-3100, a fusion inhibitor for the treatment of human immunodeficiency virus (HIV), acts by blocking the binding of the virus's CXCR4 receptor with a human host cell. The drug is being tested in phase II trials in an intravenous infusion formulation.

INDICATION(S) AND RESEARCH PHASE

Acquired Immune Deficiency Syndrome (AIDS) and AIDS-Related Infections – Phase II
HIV Infection – Phase II

BCX-34
unknown

MANUFACTURER
BioCryst Pharmaceuticals

DESCRIPTION

BCX-34 is an inhibitor of the enzyme called purine nucleoside phosphorylase (PNP), which may be essential for T-cells to replicate. T-cells are part of the body's immune system that normally attack invading bacteria and viruses. When T-cells multiply abnormally or attack healthy body tissue, then these disorders are considered proliferative diseases, such as cutaneous T-cell lymphoma (CTCL) and T-cell leukemia.

The company plans to test high dose BCX-34 in phase II trials for both CTCL and HIV-infected subjects for AIDS disease. Future clinical trials may include investigation for other T-cell diseases such as rheumatoid arthritis, Crohn's disease, atopic dermatitis, and multiple sclerosis.

INDICATION(S) AND RESEARCH PHASE

HIV Infection – Phase I/II
Leukemia – Trial discontinued
Lymphomas – Phase I/II

BMS-232632
unknown

MANUFACTURER
Bristol-Myers Squibb

DESCRIPTION

BMS-232632 is a new protease inhibitor that may enable HIV subjects to take their medication once a day, rather than taking multiple pills several times a day. Protease inhibitors act against the HIV virus by inhibiting the action of the protease enzyme that the virus needs in order to reproduce. When this enzyme is blocked, HIV makes copies of itself that cannot infect new cells. Because these drugs reduce HIV production, they help to decrease the total amount of virus in a subject's system.

Among the many challenges that face subjects with HIV is the necessity of having to take up to eighty pills throughout the day. In preclinical studies, BMS-232632 has been shown to be effective against the HIV virus when administered only once a day. This frequency of dosing represents a more convenient way for subjects to take their antiviral medication, and it could enhance subject compliance and therefore, improve the effective outcome. Early research has demonstrated that the reason BMS-232632 is effective in once daily administration is because it is one of the more potent protease inhibitors. Further study is necessary to confirm preliminary animal findings. BMS-232632 is currently being tested in phase II clinical trials.

INDICATION(S) AND RESEARCH PHASE

Acquired Immune Deficiency Syndrome (AIDS) and AIDS-Related Infections – Phase II

HIV Infection – Phase II

capravirine
unknown

MANUFACTURER
Pfizer

DESCRIPTION
The compound capravirine is a member of an important class of anti-HIV agents called non-nucleoside reverse transcriptase inhibitors (NNRTIs). In January 2001, Pfizer announced that it has restricted use of capravirine for some subjects in clinical trials based on results of a 12-month animal toxicology study, which demonstrated an unexpected finding of vasculitis in animals that received very high doses of capravirine. The drug is presently the subject of phase II and III trials to determine its safety and efficacy in people living with HIV. The FDA is permitting treatment-experienced subjects who previously have failed NNRTIs, but are responding well to capravirine, to continue their current capravirine drug regimens. The remaining subjects will discontinue use of capravirine but will remain on study protocols.

INDICATION(S) AND RESEARCH PHASE
Acquired Immune Deficiency Syndrome (AIDS) and AIDS-Related Infections – Phase III
HIV Infection – Phase III

DAPD
unknown

MANUFACTURER
Triangle Pharmaceuticals

DESCRIPTION
DAPD is a novel dioxolane guanosine reverse transcriptase inhibitor for the treatment of HIV. DXG is a metabolite of DAPD and a potent inhibitor of HIV reverse transcriptase.

Results of a phase I/II trial of DAPD showed that after 15 days of therapy, the maximum median reduction in HIV viral load ranged from 0.5 to 1.1 log units. The 20 treatment-experienced subjects had previously failed an average of seven antiretroviral drugs and had been treated for an average of four years.

INDICATION(S) AND RESEARCH PHASE
HIV Infection – Phase I/II completed

difluoromethylornithine (DFMO)
unknown

MANUFACTURER
Aventis

DESCRIPTION
Difluoromethylornithine (DFMO) is a potent, irreversible inhibitor of ornithine decarboxylase (OCD), an enzyme that is elevated in most tumors and pre-malignant lesions.

Difluoromethylornithine is currently in a phase III clinical trial to determine the effectiveness of the drug in treating subjects who have newly-diagnosed or recurrent bladder cancer. The drug is administered orally in tablet form.

DFMO is also in trials for the prevention and treatment of HIV infections and skin, breast, prostate, and cervical dysplasia/cancer.

INDICATION(S) AND RESEARCH PHASE
Bladder Cancer – Phase III
Breast Cancer – Phase II/III
Cervical Dysplasia/Cancer – Phase II
HIV Infection – Phase II
Prostate Cancer – Phase II
Skin Cancer – Phase III

DMP-450
unknown

MANUFACTURER
Du Pont

DESCRIPTION
DMP-450, a second-generation protease inhibitor, belongs to a class of chemicals that are novel for the treatment of HIV infections: the cyclic ureas. The company completed a phase I study and plans phase I/II studies outside the United States. The initiation of potential efficacy studies in the United States awaits the outcome of further discussions with the FDA who have placed the DMP-450 program on partial clinical hold.

INDICATION(S) AND RESEARCH PHASE
Acquired Immune Deficiency Syndrome (AIDS) and AIDS-Related Infections – Phase I/II
HIV Infection – Phase I/II

emivirine
Coactinon

MANUFACTURER
Triangle Pharmaceuticals

DESCRIPTION
Coactinon is a nucleoside analogue derivative that functions as a non-nucleoside reverse transcriptase inhibitor (NNRTI). In August 2000, the company announced its intention to continue developing Coactinon for the treatment of HIV infection, following notification in 1999 that additional phase III trials may be necessary to prove that regimens containing Coactinon are equivalent or superior to current first-line therapies. MKC-401 is currently ongoing and has been amended to enroll an additional 280 subjects.

INDICATION(S) AND RESEARCH PHASE
Acquired Immune Deficiency Syndrome (AIDS) and AIDS-Related Infections – Phase III
HIV Infection – Phase III
Pediatric, AIDS/HIV – Phase III

emtricitabine
Coviracil

MANUFACTURER
Triangle Pharmaceuticals

DESCRIPTION
Coviracil, a nucleoside reverse transcript inhibitor (NRTI), has been shown to be a potent inhibitor of hepatitis B virus (HBV) replication. Results of a phase I/II trial of Coviracil involving subjects chronically

infected with HBV indicated that a daily dose of 200 mg was most effective. As a result, the 200 mg/day dosage was selected for a phase III trial, which was initiated in October 2000. Coviracil is also in phase II and III trials for the treatment of HIV infection.

INDICATION(S) AND RESEARCH PHASE
HIV Infection – Phase III
Hepatitis – Phase III
Pediatric, AIDS/HIV – Phase III

EWBH treatment
unknown

MANUFACTURER
First Circle Medical

DESCRIPTION
Extracorporeal whole body hyperthermia (EWBH) is being developed to treat HIV and AIDS subjects who have not responded to standard therapies. EWBH is a technique in which the core body temperature is raised by removing blood from the subject, heating it, and then returning it to the subject. Special equipment designed by First Circle Medical is being developed to carry out this process.

Ever since the ancient Greeks, the concept of elevating body temperature to fight disease has been present in medicine. Raising the temperature of the body actually simulates the body's own fever response as part of its immune reaction to disease. The artificial "fever" state created by EWBH may increase the rate of viral killing in subjects with HIV and AIDS.

Results of a phase I study demonstrated lower levels of the HIV virus in subjects' blood after EWBH, as well as improvement in overall functioning. Using the blood, in effect, to warm the body from the inside out may result in greater control of desired temperatures, higher uniformity of heat distribution throughout the body, and fewer side effects, since the process is carried out at a slow, monitored rate. If results from further studies confirm safety and effectiveness findings, hyperthermia centers would be set up where subjects could receive this therapy outside of the hospital.

INDICATION(S) AND RESEARCH PHASE
Acquired Immune Deficiency Syndrome (AIDS) and AIDS-Related Infections – Phase II
HIV Infection – Phase II

GEM-92
unknown

MANUFACTURER
Hybridon

DESCRIPTION
GEM-92 is not being actively developed for the treatment of HIV/AIDS at this time. Further development is pending the availability of a partner to contribute to the expenses of further trials. A pilot study has been completed, while phase I has been initiated but not completed.

INDICATION(S) AND RESEARCH PHASE
Acquired Immune Deficiency Syndrome (AIDS) and AIDS-Related Infections – Phase I
HIV Infection – Phase I

Gallium maltolate
unknown

MANUFACTURER
Titan Pharmaceuticals

DESCRIPTION
Gallium is a semi-metallic element that has shown some therapeutic activity in metabolic bone disease, hypercalcemia of malignancy, and cancer. Gallium maltolate can displace divalent iron from the iron transporting protein, transferrin; thus gallium maltolate causes interference with iron metabolism with inhibition of enzymes requiring divalent iron. The most important of these in the cancer setting appears to be ribonucleotide reductase (RNR). In addition, gallium appears to form salts with calcium and phosphate and get incorporated into bone. The bone that is created with gallium incorporated appears to be at least as strong as normal bone; however, it appears to be more resistant to degradation by osteoclasts and tumor cells.

INDICATION(S) AND RESEARCH PHASE
Prostate Cancer – Phase I/II
Lymphomas – Phase I/II
Myeloma – Phase I/II
Bladder Cancer – Phase I/II
HIV Infection – Phase I/II

GW 433908
unknown

MANUFACTURER
GlaxoSmithKline

DESCRIPTION
GW 433908 is a protease inhibitor and a prodrug of Agenerase (amprenavir). Protease inhibitors act against the HIV virus by inhibiting the action of the protease enzyme, which is essential for viral replication. GW 433908 is in phase III trials for the treatment of HIV infection.

INDICATION(S) AND RESEARCH PHASE
HIV Infection – Phase III

HE2000
unknown

DESCRIPTION
HE2000 inhibits HIV replication by manipulating host cellular factors. In vitro studies showed that HE2000 significantly inhibited various strains of HIV including wild type, reverse transcriptase inhibitor resistant and multiple drug resistant isolates. These in vitro studies showed no toxicity at up to 100 times the expected human dose.

HE2000 is being evaluated in a phase I/II and II trials for HIV/AIDS in both the United States and South Africa in intramuscular, subcutaneous, and buccal formulations. Buccal administartion involves delivering the compound through the mucosal layer in the mouth with a specially formulated tablet designed for rapid absorption. The company believes that HE2000 may be acting through a unique mechanism of action on the host cell rather than on the virus itself. As a result, an extensive set of analytical measurements on a number of different virologic and immunologic markers of therapeutic activity are being evaluated. In the phase I/II trial all the patients will be monitored during dosing and up to three months after completion of treatment.

Since HE2000 does not target specific viral proteins, the company believes it may be a more durable treatment and less prone to viral mutations and the resulting resistance to drug therapy.

Hollis-Eden also is planning future trials for the drug for treatment of malaria and hepatitis.

INDICATION(S) AND RESEARCH PHASE
HIV Infection – Phase I/II
HIV Infection – Phase II

HGP-30W
unknown

MANUFACTURER
CEL-SCI Corporation

DESCRIPTION
HGP-30W is a vaccine designed to induce cellular (e.g., T-cell) and humoral (antibody) immune responses against the predominant subtype of HIV-1. The hope is that the vaccine will target multiple HIV subtypes and be more effective than other HIV vaccines in preventing infection. It is currently in phase II trials for HIV.

INDICATION(S) AND RESEARCH PHASE
HIV Infection – Phase II
Vaccines – Phase II

HGTV-43
unknown

MANUFACTURER
Enzo Biochem

DESCRIPTION
HGTV-43 is a gene medicine product developed to protect human immune cells from infection by HIV-1, including its mutational variants. This is accomplished by the insertion of an "antisense molecule" into blood cells in order to block the virus. HGTV-43 also utilizes a novel vector designed to deliver the antisense molecule to the cell; in this manner newly inserted genes can become integrated into the chromosome of the cell.

In January 2001, positive results were reported from a phase I trial of HGTV43. All five HIV-1 infected subjects enrolled in the trial tolerated the procedure well, and in each case stem cells infected with anti-HIV antisense genes engrafted, propagated and were producing differentiated CD4+ cells. Antisense RNA has been detected in circulating immune cells for as long as one year after the initial infusion of the engineered stem cells. Additionally, the anti HIV-1 antisense RNA was found in the bone marrow of four of the five subjects; while the fifth subject had antisense RNA in both his circulating immune cells and CD4+ cells, his bone marrow produced an insufficient number of stem cells for a valid assay. The company plans to extend the trial to two additional sites and has begun the transition to phase II.

INDICATION(S) AND RESEARCH PHASE
HIV Infection – Phase I completed

HIV-1 immunogen
Remune

MANUFACTURER
Immune Response Corporation

DESCRIPTION
Remune (HIV-1 immunogen) is designed to stimulate an individual's immune system to attack HIV-infected cells and slow the progression of the disease. Trial results have indicated the drug produces a favorable impact on important indicators of HIV disease progression including CD4 cell levels, viral burden, weight gain, and the stimulation of cell-mediated immune responses to HIV.

Immune Response is also conducting a phase I trial, in collaboration with the National Institutes of Health, in up to 32 HIV-infected children. The trial is designed to demonstrate the safety and immunogenicity of the product in a pediatric population.

Remune is co-developed by the Immune Response Corporation and Agouron Pharmaceuticals.

INDICATION(S) AND RESEARCH PHASE
HIV Infection – Phase III
Pediatric, HIV Infection – Phase I

HMR-4004
unknown

MANUFACTURER
Aventis

DESCRIPTION
CD4 cells are specific types of immune cells that the HIV virus targets and destroys. Hoechst Marion Roussel was developing a genetically resistant variety of CD4 cells that cannot be infected by the HIV virus. CD4 cells, once stimulated by foreign material, signal the production of other immune cells to attack the incoming pathogen. Therefore, with a decreased number of these cells, a person's immune system is severely compromised.

There is a protein found on the outer surface of the HIV molecule (gp 120) that binds to CD4 cells. This specialized binding site allows the virus to infiltrate these CD4 cells and destroy them. This systematic decimation of a person's CD4 immune cells may lead to the serious symptoms of AIDS since the body cannot protect itself from infection. It is thought that if HIV or AIDS subjects could be supplied with these cells, the severity of the disease could potentially be mitigated and subjects' lifespan may be prolonged.

Scientists were modifying a CD4 cell gene in order to make it more resistant to HIV infection. This modification could make it more difficult for the HIV virus to bind to the CD4 cell or prevent its replication once the virus gains access to the interior of the cell. According to the company phase II trials using HMR-4004 have stopped and all further development has been discontinued.

INDICATION(S) AND RESEARCH PHASE
Acquired Immune Deficiency Syndrome (AIDS) and AIDS-Related Infections – Phase II discontinued
HIV Infection – Phase II discontinued

interferon (IFN) alfa-n3

Alferon N Injection

MANUFACTURER
Interferon Sciences

DESCRIPTION
Alferon N is a human leukocyte-derived natural interferon (IFN) treatment being tested for chronic hepatitis C in subjects previously untreated with IFN.

Alferon N is given by injection and has completed a phase III trial. The company reported that the FDA rejected the drug application and advised for the conduct of another phase III study with an improved endpoint design before approval may be granted. At the present time, the company does not have the resources necessary to continue development.

INDICATION(S) AND RESEARCH PHASE
Hepatitis – Phase III
HIV Infection – Phase II

interferon (IFN) alfa-n3
Alferon LDO

MANUFACTURER
Interferon Sciences

DESCRIPTION
Alferon LDO is a human leukocyte-derived natural interferon (IFN) treatment being developed for ARC, AIDS, and HIV infections. The drug is given in a low-dose liquid oral formulation. Alferon completed a phase III trial.

INDICATION(S) AND RESEARCH PHASE
HIV Infection – Phase III completed

interleukin (IL)
Multikine

MANUFACTURER
CEL-SCI Corporation

DESCRIPTION
Multikine is a multiple combination therapy made from a natural, cytokine cocktail (which includes IL-2, IL-β, TNF-α, Gm-CSF, and an IFN-γ/immunomodulator). It is being tested for the treatment of advanced head and neck cancer subjects who have previously failed standard therapy, and head and neck cancer subjects prior to surgery.

Multikine has completed two phase II trials for head and neck cancer. The first trial consisted of 16 subjects and tested four different doses of Multikine in four subjects each. The treatment regimen involved five injections of Multikine per week over a period of two weeks every month for a minimum of two months. To qualify for the trial, the subjects must have had a recurrence of the cancer and failed conventional therapy.

MultiKine is also in trials for the treatment of prostate cancer, HIV, and head and neck cancer.

INDICATION(S) AND RESEARCH PHASE
Head and Neck Cancer – Phase II completed
HIV Infection – Phase I
Breast Cancer – Phase Preclinical
Prostate Cancer – Phase I/II

lamivudine
Epivir

MANUFACTURER
GlaxoSmithKline

DESCRIPTION
Epivir (lamivudine) is a reverse transcriptase inhibitor that has been approved by the FDA for the treatment of HIV infection. Epivir is currently approved for twice-daily administration in combination with other antiretroviral agents. Aa MAA has been submited for a once-daily formulation of the drug for the treatment of HIV infection.

INDICATION(S) AND RESEARCH PHASE
HIV Infection – MAA submitted

MIV-150
unknown

MANUFACTURER
Chiron Corporation

DESCRIPTION
MIV-150 is a new compound being developed in collaboration with Medivir AB for the treatment of HIV infection. It is currently in phase I studies.

INDICATION(S) AND RESEARCH PHASE
HIV Infection – Phase I

mozenavir dimesylate
unknown

MANUFACTURER
Triangle Pharmaceuticals

DESCRIPTION
Mozenavir dimesylate is a protease inhibitor that belongs to a novel chemical class called cyclic ureas. The drug is currently being developed for the treatment of HIV infection. In an ongoing phase I/II trial conducted outside the United States, mozenavir dimesylate was found to suppress the viral load of the majority of subjects in all groups to undetectable levels. Antiretroviral drug naïve subjects were randomized to receive mozenavir dimesylate or indinavir in combination with stavudine and lamivudine. Preliminary data indicate that mozenavir dimesylate is generally well tolerated and no significant laboratory toxicities have been observed. The initiation of efficacy trials in the United States hinges on further discussions with the FDA.

INDICATION(S) AND RESEARCH PHASE
HIV Infection – Phase I/II

pentafuside, T-20
unknown

MANUFACTURER
Trimeris

DESCRIPTION
Pentafuside (T-20) belongs to a new class of investigational anti-HIV treatments called fusion inhibitors. Unlike existing anti-retroviral drugs that work in the cell to target enzymes involved in viral replication, T-20 inhibits fusion of HIV with host cells before the virus can begin replicating and infecting

other cells. T-20 is co-developed by Trimeris and Hoffmann-La Roche.

Results of an open-label, randomized phase II trial of T-20 in combination with oral antiretrovirals suggested that the addition of T-20 to a standard antiretroviral regimen was well tolerated and provided additional decreases in viral load compared to the antiretroviral control regimen alone in HIV subjects.

Also in January 2001, preliminary results of a phase I/II trial suggested that short-term (up to 12 weeks) subcutaneous dosing with T-20 was well tolerated by children with HIV. Additionally, in the highest dose group (60 mg/m^2), T-20 caused rapid suppression of HIV RNA of approximately 10-fold average reduction from baseline levels in seven days. The trial evaluated 12 treatment-experienced or treatment-naïve children ages three to 12. It was conducted in collaboration with the Pediatric AIDS Clinical Trials Group (PACTG) of the National Institute of Allergy and Infectious Diseases.

INDICATION(S) AND RESEARCH PHASE
HIV Infection – Phase II
Pediatric, HIV Infection – Phase II

poly I:poly C-12-U
Ampligen

MANUFACTURER
Hemispherx Biopharma

DESCRIPTION
Ampligen is a novel therapeutic treatment composed of genetic building blocks (polyribonucleotide and synthetic nucleic acid) for the treatment of metastatic renal carcinoma, as an orphan indication. This intravenous drug is being evaluated in trials for renal carcinoma, malignant melanoma, chronic fatigue syndrome, and HIV.

INDICATION(S) AND RESEARCH PHASE
Renal Cell Carcinoma – Phase II/III
Malignant Melanoma – Phase I/II
Chronic Fatigue Syndrome – Phase III
HIV Infection – Phase III

PRO 140
unknown

MANUFACTURER
Progenics Pharmaceuticals

DESCRIPTION
PRO 140 is a monoclonal antibody against CCR5, a protein that is expressed on the surface of different cell types. This receptor is utilized by HIV to enter the cells. PRO 140 is one of a new category of anti-HIV drugs broadly known as "entry inhibitors" that blocks HIV infection at concentrations that do not affect CCR5's normal function, which involves activation of certain immune system cells. HIV-infected individuals who possess a defective CCR5 gene experience a milder, slower course of disease, providing clinical proof-of-concept for CCR5-directed therapies. Progenics has a collaboration with Protein Design Labs to develop a humanized PRO 140 antibody. PRO 140 is in a phase I/II trial for the treatment of HIV.

INDICATION(S) AND RESEARCH PHASE
HIV Infection – Phase I/II

PRO 2000 Gel
unknown

MANUFACTURER
Procept

DESCRIPTION
PRO 2000 gel is a synthetic naphthalene sulfonate polymer of approximately 5,000 molecular weight. Its high solubility and lack of color and odor make it well suited for topical use. Thus, PRO 2000 gel, a topical microbicide, can be used for the prevention of human immunodeficiency virus (HIV) infection and sexually transmitted diseases (STDs).

Results from preclinical studies showed PRO 2000 gel reduced the infection rate in female rhesus macaques exposed to a high dose of an HIV-like virus, protected mice completely from vaginal HSV-2 infection, as well as being a contraceptive in rabbits.

Phase I/II trials in the United States and South Africa are testing the safety and acceptability of PRO 2000 gel in healthy, sexually active women and in sexually abstinent, asymptomatic and HIV-seropositive women were completed. Phase II/III trials will begin in Africa and India in late 2001.

INDICATION(S) AND RESEARCH PHASE
HIV Infection – Phase I/II completed
Contraception – Phase I/II completed

PRO 367
unknown

MANUFACTURER
Progenics Pharmaceuticals

DESCRIPTION
PRO 367, a fusion protein, binds to gp120 (a glycoprotein receptor on the surface of HIV-infected cells) via an engineered molecule linked to a therapeutic radioisotope. This targeted complex releases a low but lethal dose of radiation, killing the cell and halting the spread of viral infection. This proprietary technology models the fusion of HIV cells in a way that makes the use of a live virus unnecessary.

INDICATION(S) AND RESEARCH PHASE
Acquired Immune Deficiency Syndrome (AIDS) and AIDS-Related Infections – Phase I/II
HIV Infection – Phase I/II

PRO 542
unknown

MANUFACTURER
Progenics Pharmaceuticals

DESCRIPTION
PRO 542, a novel fusion protein, incorporates the HIV-binding region of the human cell surface receptor (CD4) into a human antibody molecule. This complex binds to the HIV surface glycoprotein (gp120) and blocks the virus from attaching itself to human host cells. This mechanism of action is unique among antiretrovirals that are either approved or in late stage clinical development.

Additionally, PRO 542 is being evaluated in a multi-dose phase II pediatric trial sponsored by the AIDS Clinical Trials Group of the National Institutes of Health. Engineered to provide a different strategy for treating and preventing HIV infection, subjects have been able to tolerate PRO 542 in early clinical testing.

Results from a phase I trial demonstrated PRO 542 had strong antiviral effects and was considered safe and effective in subjects who were infected with HIV. The subjects received a single injection of PRO 542 at one of four dose levels. Subjects receiving high doses of PRO 542 showed a statistically significant acute reduction in plasma HIV RNA or viral load, which is considered an accepted clinical endpoint for antiretroviral therapies. Phase II testing is under way.

INDICATION(S) AND RESEARCH PHASE
Acquired Immune Deficiency Syndrome (AIDS) and AIDS-Related Infections – Phase II
HIV Infection – Phase II
Pediatric, HIV Infection – Phase II

procaine HCl
Anticort

MANUFACTURER
Steroidogenesis Inhibitors International

DESCRIPTION
Cortisol is the primary steroid hormone involved in carbohydrate metabolism and the body's response to stress. It is known that high cortisol levels play a major role in destroying the immune system in such diseases as AIDS and cancer. Anticort is an anti-cortisol, steroidogenesis inhibitor drug being tested for the treatment of immune deficiency in AIDS/HIV infection and other diseases. Procaine (the active ingredient of Anticort) has been used clinically for more than 40 years, primarily as the injectable local anesthetic Novocaine.

INDICATION(S) AND RESEARCH PHASE
Acquired Immune Deficiency Syndrome (AIDS) and AIDS-Related Infections – Phase I/II
HIV Infection – Phase I/II

Proleukin Interleukin-2 and standard anti-HIV therapy
unknown

MANUFACTURER
Chiron Corporation

DESCRIPTION
Proleukin is a genetically engineered (recombinant) form of interleukin-2, which is a naturally occurring immune modulator. The use of Proleukin may represent a new approach to treat HIV because this drug is designed to bolster and help rebuild the compromised immune system rather than target the virus specifically like other treatments. This combination therapy has produced increases in CD4+ counts and an improvement in other immune function parameters that appear to be sustained over the course of one year.

An international phase III study is evaluating the safety and effectiveness of Proleukin (aldesleukin) Interleukin-2 in combination with standard anti-HIV therapy in 1,400 subjects living with HIV with low CD4+ T-cell counts. The objective of this study is to determine if intermittent cycles of Proleukin delay the progression of HIV disease compared to what is observed with anti-HIV therapy alone in people with advanced HIV infection.

INDICATION(S) AND RESEARCH PHASE
Acquired Immune Deficiency Syndrome (AIDS) and AIDS-Related Infections – Phase III
HIV Infection – Phase III

ribozyme gene therapy
unknown

MANUFACTURER
Ribozyme Pharmaceuticals

DESCRIPTION
Gene therapies represent a promising direction for treatment of retroviral and other diseases. This therapeutic construct, based on the ability of ribozymes to alter RNA molecules, began its proof-of-principle phase II study in AIDS/lymphoma subjects. The trial was designed to test the viability of the gene therapy approach, that is, to measure the extent to which ribozyme-containing "stem cells" are re-engrafted into the bone marrow as part of a bone marrow transplant procedure.

Ribozymes are RNA enzymes that perform numerous functions, including the cleavage of ribonucleic acid (RNA) molecules. Ribozymes can be designed to selectively recognize, bind and cleave any mRNA sequence. As human therapeutics, ribozymes can be chemically synthesized to selectively inhibit disease-causing proteins through the specific cleavage of the disease-causing mRNA. The company has made proprietary chemical modifications to ribozymes that allow them to be stable and active in human serum for several days, thus broadening their potential therapeutic applications.

INDICATION(S) AND RESEARCH PHASE
Acquired Immune Deficiency Syndrome (AIDS) and AIDS-Related Infections – Phase II
HIV Infection – Phase II
Lymphoma, Non-Hodgkin's – Phase II

T-1249
unknown

MANUFACTURER
Trimeris

DESCRIPTION
T-1249 is a rationally designed proprietary peptide, which blocks fusion of HIV with host cells. T-1249 has demonstrated potent HIV suppression in animal models and is highly active against a wide range of HIV strains in culture.

In January 2001, results of a phase I/II dose escalation trial of the second-generation fusion inhibitor, T-1249, indicated that the drug was well tolerated over 14 days, had pharmacokinetic characteristics that support once-daily dosing and conferred dose-related suppression of plasma HIV RNA. The trial assessed 72 HIV positive, treatment-experienced adults with no concomitant antiretroviral therapy. Based on the favorable tolerability and activity observed with T-1249, Trimeris and Roche will continue to explore higher doses in subsequent cohorts of this trial.

INDICATION(S) AND RESEARCH PHASE
HIV Infection – Phase I/II completed
Acquired Immune Deficiency Syndrome (AIDS) and AIDS-Related Infections – Phase I/II completed

tenofovir disoproxil fumarate
Tenofovir DF

MANUFACTURER
Gilead Sciences

DESCRIPTION
Tenofovir disoproxil fumarate (tenofovir DF) is a nucleotide analogue formulated as an oral pill taken once daily as part of combination antiretroviral regimens. It is being tested in a phase III study for HIV that plans to enroll a total of 600 subjects at nearly 70 sites in the United States, Europe, and Australia.

The phase III trial is a 48-week randomized, double-blind combination antiretroviral regimen in treatment-experienced subjects. The trial is testing subjects who have HIV RNA levels greater than or equal to 10,000 copies/mL, and who have maintained a stable antiretroviral regimen for at least eight weeks prior to enrollment. Based on results from the phase II study, subjects will be randomized to receive a dose of tenofovir DF 300 mg or placebo in addition to their antiretroviral regimen for 24 weeks of blinded dosing. After 24 weeks, subjects receiving tenofovir DF 300 mg may make changes in their background antiretroviral therapy, and subjects assigned to receive placebo will cross over to open label active tenofovir DF for the remainder of the 48 week study period.

INDICATION(S) AND RESEARCH PHASE
Acquired Immune Deficiency Syndrome (AIDS) and AIDS-Related Infections – Phase III
HIV Infection – Phase III

unknown
unknown

MANUFACTURER
BioChem Pharma

DESCRIPTION
dOTC is a novel nucleoside substitute (analogue) that inhibits the AIDS virus from multiplying. It works by slowing down or inhibiting the enzyme, reverse transcriptase, from copying the genetic code of the virus. This drug is being tested on HIV strains that have developed resistance to AZT and 3TC and to certain protease inhibitors.

INDICATION(S) AND RESEARCH PHASE
Acquired Immune Deficiency Syndrome (AIDS) and AIDS-Related Infections – Phase II
HIV Infection – Phase II

unknown
VIR201

MANUFACTURER
Virax

DESCRIPTION
VIR201 is a live viral vector vaccine based on the company's platform technology, Co-X-Gene with FPV, a method for delivering vaccines. VIR201 uses a FPV to carry genes from HIV and a human cytokine to cells in the human body to trigger a directed immune response. VIR201 is in a phase I/IIa trial in Australia for treatment of HIV infection.

INDICATION(S) AND RESEARCH PHASE
HIV Infection – Phase I/IIa

vaccine, HIV
Aidsvax

MANUFACTURER
VaxGen

DESCRIPTION
Aidsvax is a genetically engineered, aluminum-adjuvanted subunit vaccine cloned from a protein (gp120) found on the surface of the HIV virus. Because it is a subunit vaccine it does not contain viral DNA, and therefore, no participant in the trial can become infected by HIV due to the vaccination.

Aidsvax is currently being tested in phase III trials. The subjects are between the ages of 18 and 60 and do not have HIV-1 infection, but they are at risk of acquiring HIV-1 infection through sexual contact.

INDICATION(S) AND RESEARCH PHASE
Acquired Immune Deficiency Syndrome (AIDS) and AIDS-Related Infections – Phase III
HIV Infection – Phase III
Vaccines – Phase III

vaccine, HIV
GeneVax-HIV-Px

MANUFACTURER
Wyeth-Lederle Vaccines

DESCRIPTION
GeneVax-HIV-Px is a novel prophylactic DNA vaccine for the treatment of HIV infection. It is an injectable therapeutic that uses the proprietary GeneVax delivery technology. The drug is in phase II trials.

INDICATION(S) AND RESEARCH PHASE
Acquired Immune Deficiency Syndrome (AIDS) and AIDS-Related Infections – Phase II
HIV Infection – Phase II

vaccine, HIV
unknown

MANUFACTURER
GlaxoSmithKline

DESCRIPTION
This is a recombinant vaccine for HIV prophylaxis in phase I development.

INDICATION(S) AND RESEARCH PHASE
HIV Infection – Phase I
Vaccines – Phase I

vaccine, HIV-1 gp-120

prime-boost
unknown

MANUFACTURER
Chiron Corporation

DESCRIPTION
Chiron Corporation is developing a vaccine for AIDS that works in two ways. There is a protein found on the outer surface of the HIV molecule (gp 120) that binds to important human immune cells (CD4). This specialized binding site allows the virus to infiltrate these CD4 cells and destroy them. This systematic decimation of a person's CD4 immune cells leads to the serious symptoms of AIDS since the body cannot adequately compensate for the loss in immune protection.

This new vaccine is composed of synthetically made proteins that closely resemble the gp 120 proteins of the AIDS virus. Scientists believe that, upon immunization, the body makes antibodies to these synthetic proteins, and these antibodies will act against the real HIV molecule as well. This vaccine also contains another protein that enhances the immune response. This protein (MF59) is known as an adjuvant because it causes the body to produce a stronger and longer lasting immune reaction than would occur with the vaccine alone. These two mechanisms may potentially immunize people against this pervasive and serious disease. Phase II trials are currently taking place using this intravenous vaccination.

INDICATION(S) AND RESEARCH PHASE
Acquired Immune Deficiency Syndrome (AIDS) and AIDS-Related Infections – Phase II
HIV Infection – Phase II
Vaccines – Phase II

VX-175
unknown

MANUFACTURER
Vertex Pharmaceuticals

DESCRIPTION
VX-175 (also known as GW433908) is a prodrug of the HIV protease inhibitor amprenavir. It has been formulated to allow a dosing regimen of three pills, twice a day. VX-175 is being tested in two phase III trials. The first trial will enroll 210 subjects at 30 sites in the United States and will compare three tablets of VX-175 dosed twice daily with the protease inhibitor nelfinavir dosed twice daily in subjects who have not previously received antiretroviral therapy. In addition, all subjects will also receive the reverse transcriptase inhibitors abacavir and 3TC twice daily. The second phase III trial will enroll more than 600 subjects who have not previously received antiretroviral therapy at 50 sites. Subjects will be randomized to receive either a combination of three tablets of VX-175 + ritonavir once daily, or 1,250 mg nelfinavir twice daily. In addition, all subjects will receive 3TC twice daily as well.

VX-175 was discovered by Vertex Pharmaceuticals and is licensed by Glaxo Wellcome.

INDICATION(S) AND RESEARCH PHASE
HIV Infection – Phase III

WF10
unknown

MANUFACTURER
OXO Chemie

DESCRIPTION
WF10 is an immune therapeutic that targets macrophage function. The active ingredient in WF10 is a chemically stabilized chlorite matrix called tetrachlorodecaoxygen (TDCO). WF10 has completed phase III trials for HIV.

Results from phase II trials showed WF10 lowered frequency of infections, required fewer hospitalizations, and increased survival rates for subjects who had AIDS.

Additionally, WF10 is in phase III trials for the treatment of chronic inflammatory diseases.

INDICATION(S) AND RESEARCH PHASE
Acquired Immune Deficiency Syndrome (AIDS) and AIDS-Related Infections – Phase III completed
HIV Infection – Phase III completed

Immunosuppressive

AI-502
unknown

MANUFACTURER
AutoImmune

DESCRIPTION
Donor organ rejection is a major, and sometimes fatal, problem in organ transplantation. AI-502, a tolerizing peptide, acts by permitting the recipient's immune system to tolerate the foreign tissue instead of attacking it. The company is conducting phase I/II trials of an oral formulation of the drug for prevention of chronic organ transplant rejection.

INDICATION(S) AND RESEARCH PHASE
Immunosuppressive – Phase I/II

anti B-7 humanized antibodies
unknown

MANUFACTURER
Wyeth-Ayerst

DESCRIPTION
Anti B-7 humanized antibodies are being developed for the prevention of graft versus host disease (GVHD) following haploidentical bone marrow transplant and preventing kidney rejection. Clinical trials are currently in phase I/II development.

INDICATION(S) AND RESEARCH PHASE
Immunosuppressive – Phase I/II
Kidney Transplant Surgery – Phase I/II
Bone Marrow Transplant – Phase I/II

Anti-LFA-1, odulimomab
unknown

MANUFACTURER
SangStat Medical

DESCRIPTION
Odulimomab is a monoclonal antibody designed to help prevent renal rejection

after a kidney transplant and reduce the delay in graft functioning. The drug, in an intravenous formulation, is in phase III trials for kidney transplant rejection as an immunosuppressant.

INDICATION(S) AND RESEARCH PHASE
Immunosuppressive – Phase III
Kidney Transplant Surgery – Phase III

BTI-322, MEDI-507
unknown

MANUFACTURER
BioTransplant

DESCRIPTION
MEDI-507 is a novel, humanized monoclonal antibody which binds specifically to the CD2 surface antigen receptor found on T-cells and natural killer (NK) cells. MEDI-507 was engineered from BTI-322, a murine antibody, in order to reduce potential immunogenicity and allow for long-term administration. Laboratory studies have suggested that MEDI-507 and BTI-322 primarily inhibit the response of specific activated T-cells while subsequently allowing other immune cells to respond normally. Therefore, these drugs may be able to prevent the host rejection of a transplanted organ without compromising the entire immune system. MEDI-507 may prove to induce long-term functional transplantation tolerance in humans, increase the therapeutic benefit of bone marrow transplants, and reduce or eliminate the need for lifelong immunosuppressive therapy.

The drug is currently in multiple phase II clinical trials for treatment of graft versus host disease, a frequent and often fatal outcome of bone marrow transplantation, caused when donor white blood cells in a bone marrow transplant attack the tissue of the recipient. Clinical manifestations include skin rash, severe diarrhea, liver abnormalities, and jaundice.

Phase II trials are also in progress for kidney transplant rejection and treatment of psoriasis as a proof of concept for its use in autoimmune diseases.

INDICATION(S) AND RESEARCH PHASE
Immunosuppressive – Phase II
Kidney Transplant Surgery – Phase II
Psoriasis and Psoriatic Disorders – Phase II
Liver Transplant Rejection – Phase II
Graft Versus Host Disease (GVHD) – Phase II

everolimus
Certican

MANUFACTURER
Novartis

DESCRIPTION
Certican is a novel oral proliferation signal inhibitor (PSI) designed to protect transplant recipients from acute and chronic rejection and from the toxicities of conventional agents. It is being developed for combination therapy with cyclosporine, and it is currently in phase III trials.

INDICATION(S) AND RESEARCH PHASE
Immunosuppressive – Phase III

FTY 720
unknown

MANUFACTURER
Novartis

DESCRIPTION
FTY 720 is an orally administered immunosuppressant being developed for the prevention of rejection following organ transplantation. FTY 720 has been shown to reduce the number of circulating peripheral blood lymphocytes. It may induce the sequestration of circulating mature lymphocytes within lymph nodes and Peyer's patches through the acceleration of lymphocyte homing. FTY 720 is currently in phase II development.

INDICATION(S) AND RESEARCH PHASE
Immunosuppressive – Phase II

ISAtx247
Unknown

MANUFACTURER
Isotechnika

DESCRIPTION
ISAtx247 is a novel immunosuppressant for prevention of organ rejection after transplantation and for treatment of autoimmune diseases such as rheumatoid arthritis and psoriasis.

INDICATION(S) AND RESEARCH PHASE
Psoriasis and Psoriatic Disorders – Phase I
Rheumatoid Arthritis – Phase I
Immunosuppressant – Phase I

monoclonal antibody, ABX-CBL
unknown

MANUFACTURER
Abgenix

DESCRIPTION
ABX-CBL is an antibody designed to help subjects with steroid-resistant graft versus host disease (GVHD). The transplant or graft is intended to restore normal circulating blood cells and immune cells in subjects who cannot mount a sufficient immune response because their own bone marrow and immune system have been suppressed by radiation and/or chemotherapy. GVHD results when a portion of the graft recognizes the subject's own genetically different (allogeneic) cells as foreign, becomes activated, and attacks them.

ABX-CBL acts by seeking out and destroying these activated immune cells, including T-cells, B-cells, and monocytes. Because ABX-CBL can distinguish between activated and resting immune cells, it can destroy subsets of immune cells without causing general immune suppression. The drug is delivered in an intravenous formulation.

The phase III trial is expected to enroll 92 subjects and to be completed in 18 to 24 months.

INDICATION(S) AND RESEARCH PHASE
Immunosuppressive – Phase III

organ transplantation system
AlloMune

MANUFACTURER
BioTransplant

DESCRIPTION
AlloMune is an organ transplantation system for the creation of specific immune tolerance in solid organ transplants from human donor organs using a novel anti-CD2 antibody/immunosuppressive monoclonal antibody (MAb). The drug is designed to re-educate the recipient's immune system to recognize the foreign tissue as "self." The AlloMune™ System for cancer applications is designed to attack tumor cells more aggressively than the subject's own immune defenses. Phase I/II trials are being conducted for kidney transplant surgery and use as an immunosuppressant. Additional indications include refractory lymphoma, hematological disorders, and other types of cancers.

INDICATION(S) AND RESEARCH PHASE
Immunosuppressive – Phase I/II
Kidney Transplant Surgery – Phase I/II
Lymphomas – Phase I/II

---

pentostatin
Nipent

MANUFACTURER
SuperGen

DESCRIPTION
Nipent (pentostatin) belongs to a group of drugs called antimetabolites. Pentostatin inhibits the enzyme adenosine deaminase, which leads to cytotoxicity and cell death. This drug is in phase II trials for rheumatoid arthritis and non-Hodgkin's lymphoma. Nipent is also being tested in phase III trials for chronic lymphocytic leukemia.

In December 2000, results of a phase II trial of Nipent indicated the drug has significant activity (75% overall response rate) in the treatment of graft versus host disease (GVHD). Twelve subjects with steroid refractory GVHD received Nipent as "salvage therapy" because each had previously failed all other treatments. SuperGen plans to initiate a phase III trial in early 2001.

INDICATION(S) AND RESEARCH PHASE
Leukemia – Phase III
Lymphoma, Non-Hodgkin's – Phase II
Rheumatoid Arthritis – Phase II
Immunosuppressive – Phase III
CTCL/ PTCL – Phase II

SDZ RAD
unknown

MANUFACTURER
Novartis

DESCRIPTION
SDZ RAD is a potent immunosuppressive that inhibits growth factor-driven cell proliferation. It is currently in development for kidney, liver, and lung transplantation, including a pediatric phase II/III trial in children ages two through 16 years.

INDICATION(S) AND RESEARCH PHASE
Immunosuppressive – Phase II/III
Pediatric, Transplantation – Phase II/III

SMART anti-CD3
Nuvion

MANUFACTURER
Protein Design Labs

DESCRIPTION
Nuvion is an IgG2 monoclonal antibody that targets the CD3 antigen present on all T-cells. Nuvion is an immunosuppressive drug in phase I/II trials for the treatment of psoriasis and phase I trials for graft vs. host disease and t-cell malignancies.

INDICATION(S) AND RESEARCH PHASE
Psoriasis and Psoriatic Disorders – Phase I/II
Immunosuppressant – Phase I

SR-31747
unknown

MANUFACTURER
Sanofi-Synthelabo Pharmaceuticals

DESCRIPTION
SR-31747 is being tested to treat autoimmune diseases and prevent transplant rejection. It is currently in Phase II clinical trials and is to be given in intravenous formulation. Autoimmune diseases occur when the body's immune cells see the body's own tissues as foreign material that needs to be attacked and eradicated. For example, when these immune cells attack joint tissue, the disease rheumatoid arthritis results. This process can also result in transplant organ rejection, as the immune cells attack the transplanted organ, seeing it as a foreign invader instead of a needed transplant.

There are many types of cells that constitute the attack mechanism in immune reactions. SR-31747 inhibits the action of several cells. It acts against a couple different types of immune signaling cells, called interleukins, that when stimulated, spur the production of immunogenic white blood cells (T-cells). In this way, SR-31747 results in decreased T-cell production, and thus a decreased immune response. In addition, SR-31747 acts directly to inhibit a certain type of T-cell (Th1 lymphocytes) by attaching itself to a sigma receptor on the cell's surface. Further studies are under way.

INDICATION(S) AND RESEARCH PHASE
Immunosuppressive – Phase II

---

thalidomide
Thalomid

MANUFACTURER
Celgene Corporation

DESCRIPTION
Thalomid is an oral formulation of the immunomodulatory agent thalidomide. Thalidomide has a notorious history of having caused birth defects when the medical profession unsuspectingly prescribed it for pregnant women as a treatment for nausea and insomnia. Celgene is investigating new applications for the drug, while being particularly mindful of the potential risks of thalidomide treatment. Thalomid is currently being tested for numerous indications in the areas of oncology and immunology.

INDICATION(S) AND RESEARCH PHASE
Multiple Myeloma – Phase II

Myelodysplastic Syndrome – Phase II
Leukemia – Phase II
Brain Cancer – Phase II
Liver Cancer – Phase II
Kidney Cancer – Phase II
Prostate Cancer – Phase II
Kaposi's Sarcoma – Phase II
Cachexia – Phase II
Recurrent Aphthous Stomatitis – Phase III
Crohn's Disease – Phase II
Inflammatory Bowel Disease – Phase II
Sarcoidosis – Phase II
Scleroderma – Phase II

VAS981
unknown

MANUFACTURER
Vasogen

DESCRIPTION
VAS 981 is Vasogen's proprietary cell-processing technology being developed for the prevention of graft versus host disease (GVHD). Results of preclinical studies suggested that the clinical utility of the VAS981 cell-processing technology may extend to transplant situations where there are no appropriately matched bone marrow donors and the risk of the subject developing life-threatening GvHD is extremely high—thus offering a potential therapeutic option for subjects for whom none currently exists.

INDICATION(S) AND RESEARCH PHASE
Immunosuppressive – Phase II

Influenza

adjuvanted influenza
Fluad

MANUFACTURER
Chiron Corporation

DESCRIPTION
Fluad is a vaccine for the prevention of influenza that incorporates the company's proprietary adjuvant MF59. Filing has already taken place in Italy.

INDICATION(S) AND RESEARCH PHASE
Influenza – MAA submitted

RWJ 241947
unknown

MANUFACTURER
R. W. Johnson Pharmaceutical Research Institute

DESCRIPTION
RWJ 241947 is in phase III trials for influenza.

INDICATION(S) AND RESEARCH PHASE
Influenza – Phase II

RWJ 270201
unknown

MANUFACTURER
R. W. Johnson Pharmaceutical Research Institute

DESCRIPTION
RWJ 270201 is in phase III trials for influenza.

INDICATION(S) AND RESEARCH PHASE
Influenza – Phase III

unknown
FluMist

MANUFACTURER
Wyeth-Ayerst

DESCRIPTION
FluMist is an investigational cold-adapted intranasal influenza vaccine. It is designed to be effective in children by inducing immunity via the nasal mucosa. In October 2000, Aviron and American Home Products Corporation announced that a Biologics License Application for FluMist has been submitted to the FDA. Wyeth-Ayerst is the pharmaceutical division of American Home Products.

INDICATION(S) AND RESEARCH PHASE
Influenza – Phase III
Pediatric, Influenza – Phase III
Vaccines – Phase III

vaccine, DPT/ Haemophilus influenzae type B
unknown

MANUFACTURER
Chiron Corporation

DESCRIPTION
Chiron Corporation has formulated a combination vaccine that might effectively immunize children against four serious diseases: *Haemophilus influenzae* type B, diphtheria, pertussis, and tetanus—with a single injection. This vaccine has the potential to simplify pediatric vaccination schedules, thereby lowering costs, increasing convenience, and improving compliance. The vaccine is composed of inactive molecules of diphtheria toxin, pertussis toxin, and tetanus toxin. Toxins are the destructive molecules that cause most of the pathology seen in these diseases. The vaccine also contains inactivated *H. influenzae* proteins.

INDICATION(S) AND RESEARCH PHASE
Bacterial Infection – Phase III
Pediatric, Influenza – Phase III
Pediatric, Vaccines – Phase III
Viral Infection – Phase III

vaccine, influenza
unknown

MANUFACTURER
BioChem Pharma

DESCRIPTION
Influenza is one of the most pervasive illnesses known. The best weapon against the influenza virus is annual vaccination. However, since the influenza vaccine is administered as an injection, many needle-shy people avoid being vaccinated. The decision not to be immunized due to discomfort from intramuscular injection results in much unnecessary and preventable illness each year.

In order to improve vaccination rates, BioChem Pharma is developing an influenza vaccine that can be taken as a nasal spray. This method of vaccination might not only create a helpful systemic immune response (in the blood and throughout the body), but also stimulate a local immune response in the mucosal lining of the nose, mouth, and throat, which would create an additional barrier to influenza infection and increase efficacy.

INDICATION(S) AND RESEARCH PHASE
Influenza – Phase I
Vaccines – Phase I

vaccine, influenza
unknown

MANUFACTURER
GlaxoSmithKline

DESCRIPTION
This subunit vaccine is being developed for influenza prophylaxis. It is currently in phase I development.

INDICATION(S) AND RESEARCH PHASE
Influenza – Phase I
Vaccines – Phase I

vaccine, nasal proteosome influenza
unknown

MANUFACTURER
Intellivax International

DESCRIPTION
Nasal proteosome influenza vaccine is a nasally administered vaccine that may provide mucosal as well as systemic immunity, which could offer people more effective protection against the influenza virus than standard injectable flu vaccine. The phase I trial will compare the novel Intellivax product to the standard injectable vaccine. Preclinical studies demonstrated the nasal proteosome flu vaccine has induced high levels of antibodies in serum as well as in lung and nasal mucosal secretions and has protected animals in experimental models of influenza disease.

INDICATION(S) AND RESEARCH PHASE
Influenza – Phase I

vaccine, parainfluenza
unknown

MANUFACTURER
Wyeth-Lederle Vaccines

DESCRIPTION
This is a novel vaccine for prevention of parainfluenza virus (PIV)-mediated serious respiratory illness in children. The vaccine is made from live attenuated (cold-adapted) influenza A virus administered as a nasal spray. These live attenuated vaccines stimulate local antibody production more efficiently than conventional inactivated vaccines. The drug is in phase II testing in adults and a phase I/II in infants and toddlers.

INDICATION(S) AND RESEARCH PHASE
Influenza – Phase II
Pediatric, Influenza – Phase I/II

vaccine, Pseudomonas infection
Pseudostat

MANUFACTURER
Provalis

DESCRIPTION
Pseudostat is an oral (mucosal) therapeutic vaccine against *Pseudomonas aeruginosa* infections in cystic fibrosis subjects and subjects with chronic bronchitis, bronchiectasis, and influenza. The company intended to re-enter phase II trials in Australia, and, if successful, plans to initiate phase II trials in the United States, where it has been in discussion with the National Institute of Health and the Cystic Fibrosis Foundation. In addition, the developer has filed for Orphan Drug Designation in the United States.

INDICATION(S) AND RESEARCH PHASE
Bronchitis – Phase I/II
Bacterial Infection – Phase I/II
Cystic Fibrosis – Phase I/II
Influenza – Phase I/II
Vaccines – Phase I/II

Pediatric, Influenza – FDA approved

zanamavir
Relenza

MANUFACTURER
GlaxoSmithKline

DESCRIPTION
Relenza (zanamivir) is an anti-viral drug for the treatment of influenza. The proposed mechanism of action of zanamivir is via inhibition of influenza virus neuraminidase with the possibility of alteration of virus particle aggregation and release. The FDA has approved Relenza for persons ages seven years and older for the treatment of uncomplicated influenza virus. This product is approved to treat types A and B influenza, the two types most responsible for flu epidemics. It is also in phase III trials for two additional indications: influenza prophylaxis and influenza treatment in subjects with asthma/COPD (label update).

INDICATION(S) AND RESEARCH PHASE
Influenza – Phase III

Kaposi's Sarcoma

Col-3
Metastat

MANUFACTURER
CollaGenex Pharmaceuticals

DESCRIPTION
Metastat is an anti-angiogenesis compound used to treat subjects with HIV-related Kaposi's sarcoma. It is an anti-tumor agent that reduces the amount of inflammatory cytokines that are involved in metastasis and cell proliferation. The compound has been well tolerated in phase I clinical trials.

INDICATION(S) AND RESEARCH PHASE
Kaposi's Sarcoma – Phase I

IM862
unknown

MANUFACTURER
Cytran

DESCRIPTION
IM862 is a small peptide comprised of two amino acids that may inhibit new blood vessel formation (angiogenesis). When there is excessive growth of new blood vessels, a number of pathological conditions result, including malignant tumors, age-related macular degeneration, and vascular diseases. Limiting the growth of new blood vessels in tumors deprives them of nourishment and can ultimately kill these cancers. This drug is being developed in phase III trials for Kaposi's sarcoma and phase I/II trials for ovarian cancer.

INDICATION(S) AND RESEARCH PHASE
Kaposi's Sarcoma – Phase III
Ovarian Cancer – Phase I/II
Malignant Melanoma – Phase Preclinical
Prostate Cancer – Phase Preclinical

Malaria

tafenoquine, SB 252263
unknown

MANUFACTURER
GlaxoSmithKline

DESCRIPTION
Tafenoquine is an analogue of primaquine being developed for malaria prophylaxis in adults. It is currently in phase III development.

INDICATION(S) AND RESEARCH PHASE
Malaria – Phase III

vaccine, malaria
unknown

MANUFACTURER
Aventis Pasteur

DESCRIPTION
This malaria vaccine uses DNA malaria molecules to stimulate an immune response in the human body. Using DNA molecules represents a new strategy in the formulation of vaccines. Production of a certain kind of immune cells (T-cells) is generated by the DNA vaccine, and these T-cells are capable of attacking and destroying the malaria organism.

Preliminary studies demonstrated the majority of the subjects developed potent "killer" T-cells, which can destroy malaria organisms and defend the body against the disease. The development of an effective new malaria vaccine is important since the standard therapies, mefloquine or doxycycline, are not always effective since some strains of malaria have become drug resistant. The goal of the scientists developing this vaccine is to design a long lasting, effective, safe vaccine that can be administered to people before they enter malarial geographic zones. This vaccine is given by intramuscular injection and it is being tested in phase II trials. It is being developed in conjunction with Vical.

INDICATION(S) AND RESEARCH PHASE
Malaria – Phase II
Vaccines – Phase II

vaccine, malaria
unknown

MANUFACTURER
GlaxoSmithKline

DESCRIPTION
GlaxoSmithKline Beecham is developing a new malaria vaccine that they believe might offer stronger protection and greater efficacy against the disease. Malaria is an infection by microscopic organisms known as protozoans and is transmitted to humans by mosquitoes. There are four types of malarial diseases, all causing symptoms of different quality and severity. Malaria infection can present as fevers, seizures, disturbances in mental functioning, coma, and ultimately, result in death.

The new malaria vaccine under development is a combination of the standard malaria vaccine together with two separate proteins that are designed to enhance and strengthen the body's immune response to the vaccine. These "helper vaccine" proteins are known as adjuvants, and they may enhance the duration and overall effectiveness of the vaccine. This formulation contains two different adjuvants, known as Ribi adjuvants, one of which is called a monophosphoryl lipid A (MPL) formulation. Ribi adjuvants are natural and synthetic derivatives of immunomodulatory bacterial components that mimic the beneficial properties of those parent compounds.

This malaria vaccine is currently being tested in phase II trials, under development collaboration among Ribi ImmunoChem Research, GlaxoSmithKline, Walter Reed Army of Research, and the Medical Research Council.

INDICATION(S) AND RESEARCH PHASE
Malaria – Phase II
Vaccines – Phase II

Meningitis

cytarabine liposome injection
DepoCyt

MANUFACTURER
Skye Pharma

DESCRIPTION
DepoCyt is an injectable sustained-release formulation that gradually releases cytarabine into the cerebral spinal fluid (CSF). Cytarabine is a cell cycle phase-specific drug that stops or slows the maturation and spread of tumor cells, affecting cells only during the S-phase of cell division. DepoCyt was approved by the FDA in 1999 for the treatment of lymphomatous meningitis. It is currently in phase I pediatric trials for newborns to children 18 years old.

DepoCyt is being co-developed by DepoTech Corporation (a wholly owned subsidiary of SkyPharma) and Chiron for the U.S. market; Pharmacia & Upjohn will market the product internationally.

INDICATION(S) AND RESEARCH PHASE
Meningitis – FDA approved
Pediatric, Meningitis – Phase I

nystatin, AR-121
Nyotran

MANUFACTURER
Aronex Pharmaceuticals

DESCRIPTION
Nyotran is an intravenous liposomal formulation of nystatin being developed for the treatment of serious systemic, opportunistic fungal infections. Phase III trials have been completed for systemic fungal infections and confirmed cryptococcal meningitis. Additionally, phase II trials have been completed for candidiasis and aspergillosis.

Nyotran is under agreement with Abbott Laboratories for worldwide commercialization. Abbott will fund clinical development and will submit marketing registration outside the United States.

INDICATION(S) AND RESEARCH PHASE
Aspergillosis – Phase II completed
Candidiasis – Phase II completed
Systemic Fungal Infections – Phase III completed
Meningitis – Phase III completed

opebecan, rBPI-21, recombinant human bactericidal/permeability-increasing protein
Neuprex

MANUFACTURER
XOMA Corporation

DESCRIPTION
Neuprex is a systemic formulation of recombinant bactericidal/permeability-increasing protein, rBPI-21, for the treatment of severe meningococcemia, a rare systemic gram-negative bacterial infection that primarily affects children. The active molecule in Neuprex, rBPI-21, binds to endotoxin molecules (LOS and LPS, lipopolysaccharide) in living bacteria, disrupting their cell walls, killing the bacteria or making them more susceptible to antibiotics. Phase III data were released in September 2000 for both pediatric and adult trials.

XOMA is pursuing various indications for Neuprex: One indication is severe meningococcemia in children who become infected with these harmful bacteria that attack their brain and spinal cord's protective sheathing after entering the bloodstream. The gram-negative bacteria, called *Neisseria meningitidis*, cause meningococcemia and produce spiking high fever and a classic rigid stiff neck. Shock and death may occur in just a few hours after infection. Additionally, Neuprex is being tested in trials for the treatment of serious lung complications (pneumonia and acute respiratory distress Syndrome (ARDS)), in combination with other antibiotics and subjects who had their liver removed during surgery.

INDICATION(S) AND RESEARCH PHASE
Bacterial Infection – Phase III
Pediatric, Meningococcemia – Phase III completed
Meningitis – Phase III
Acute Respiratory Distress Syndrome (ARDS) – Phase III
Pneumonia – Phase III
Liver Disease – Phase II
Intra-abdominal Infection – Phase I/II

vaccine, meningococcal C conjugate
Meningitec

MANUFACTURER
Wyeth-Ayerst

DESCRIPTION
Meningitec is a conjugate vaccine for the prevention of meningococcal Group C disease. In October 1999, the vaccine was approved for use in the United Kingdom. Meningitec is being evaluated in phase III clinical trials in the United States.

INDICATION(S) AND RESEARCH PHASE
Meningitis – Phase III
Pediatric, Meningococcal Group C Meningitis – Phase III
Vaccines – Phase III

vaccine, meningococcus C
unknown

MANUFACTURER
Chiron Corporation

DESCRIPTION
Chiron Corporation is working on a new vaccine for meningococcal bacterial infections. The bacteria known as *Neisseria meningitidis* produce these infections. This organism can cause a variety of diseases ranging from benign upper respiratory infections to serious blood infections, which can lead to rashes, muscle and joint aches, and meningitis. Meningococcal meningitis begins when the organism crosses the meninges, which are the membranes surrounding the brain and spinal cord. This bacterial invasion into the central nervous system can result in fever, neck stiffness, headache, and coma. In a third of affected subjects, overwhelming infection causes the body to go into shock with associated blood clotting problems, lung and heart infections, and death. If subjects survive, they could experience residual problems such as deafness, paralysis, and mental retardation. Approximately half of all cases of meningococcal meningitis occur in children under the age of 15 years, with most cases of meningitis occurring among infants three to eight months of age.

INDICATION(S) AND RESEARCH PHASE
Meningitis – Phase III
Vaccines – Phase III
Pediatric, Meningitis – Phase III
Pediatric, Vaccines – Phase II

vaccine, Streptococcus pneumoniae
unknown

MANUFACTURER
GlaxoSmithKline

DESCRIPTION
This conjugated pediatric vaccine is currently in phase III trials for Streptococcus pneumoniae disease prophylaxis. The vaccine contains antigens for prevention of pneumonia, middle ear infections, and meningitis in pediatric patients.

INDICATION(S) AND RESEARCH PHASE

Pediatric, Bacterial Infection—Phase III
Pediatric, Ear Infections —Phase III
Pediatric, Meningitis —Phase III
Pediatric, Pneumonia— Phase III

Parasites and Protozoa

nitazoxanide (NTZ)
unknown

MANUFACTURER
BioChem Pharma

DESCRIPTION
Nitazoxanide (NTZ) is a medication that is being developed to treat diarrhea caused by cryptosporidial parasites in immunocompromised people, such as AIDS subjects. Currently this drug is in phase III trials and it is to be given orally. Cryptosporidiosis is an infection of the intestinal lining with the parasite *Cryptosporidium parvum* that can be found in contaminated food and water. Forty-five million people each year may be exposed to this parasite through municipal water systems. This parasite is found in up to 20% of people with AIDS.

Symptoms of this infection include watery diarrhea, with up to twenty bowel movements each day. NTZ is a molecule (thiazolide derivative) that acts not only against parasites such as protozoa and helminths (worms), but against bacteria as well. This drug is already available in developing countries where parasitic infections are common. People who are immunocompromised due to AIDS, steroid treatment, or cancer treatment are the most susceptible to infection by the *Cryptosporidium* organism and these subjects may potentially derive the greatest benefit from this new therapy.

INDICATION(S) AND RESEARCH PHASE
Diarrhea – Phase III
Parasites and Protozoa – Phase III
Acquired Immune Deficiency Syndrome (AIDS) and AIDS-Related Infections – Phase III

roxithromycine, RU-28,965
unknown

MANUFACTURER
Aventis

DESCRIPTION
Roxithromycine is a new antibiotic similar in action and composition to existing antibiotics such as erythromycin and clarithromycin. It is being developed to treat a wide array of bacterial infections including those of the lungs, genitals, urinary tract, skin, and soft tissues. It also may have potent action against parasitic infections from parasites such as cryptosporidium, *Pneumocystis carinii* (PCP), and *Toxoplasma gondii*. Many of these parasites infect people with compromised immune systems, such as AIDS subjects. Roxithromycine, if proved effective, may help improve quality of life and decrease mortality in these subjects.

Development has been discontinued.

INDICATION(S) AND RESEARCH PHASE
Bacterial Infection – Phase discontinued
Parasites & Protozoa – Phase discontinued

vaccine, malaria
Quilimmune-M

MANUFACTURER
Aquila Biopharmaceuticals

DESCRIPTION
Quilimmune-M, a genetically engineered sporozoite malaria vaccine, combines an immune system modulator isolated from the *Quillaja saponaria* tree and highly purified as an adjuvant with the peptide antigen SPF-66. The company uses genetic engineering technologies to identify biological molecules that are strongly associated with a target pathogen. These molecules can then be used to stimulate disease-specific immune responses.

Aquila Biopharmaceuticals in cooperation with the World Health Organization and Dr. Manuel Patarroyo of the Instituto de Immunologia in Bogota, Colombia, are conducting phase III trials in Colombia, South America.

INDICATION(S) AND RESEARCH PHASE
Parasites and Protozoa – Phase II
Vaccines – Phase II

Rhinitis

AG7088, anti-rhinoviral agent
unknown

MANUFACTURER
Agouron Pharmaceuticals

DESCRIPTION
AG7088 is a small synthetic molecule designed to inhibit the rhinovirus 3C protease and presents a broad spectrum of potent anti-rhinoviral activity in preclinical testing.

Results showed that AG7088 was well tolerated and it significantly reduced total cold symptoms and respiratory symptoms. Based on these results the company plans to initiate a larger phase II/III trial in more than 50 sites throughout the United States.

INDICATION(S) AND RESEARCH PHASE
Rhinitis – Phase II/III
Sinus Infections – Phase II/III

desloratadine, descarboethoxyloratadine
unknown

MANUFACTURER
Sepracor

DESCRIPTION
Desloratadine is an active metabolite of Claritin, a non-sedating antihistamine, for the treatment of seasonal allergic rhinitis. The drug selectively blocks histamine-1 receptors in the bloodstream, and thereby prevents the release of histamine by inflammatory cells. Desloratadine is being developed under an agreement between Sepracor and Schering-Plough Corporation.

INDICATION(S) AND RESEARCH PHASE
Allergy – NDA submitted
Rhinitis – NDA submitted

DNK 333
unknown

MANUFACTURER
Novartis

DESCRIPTION
DNK 333 is a dual NK_1/NK_2 antagonist being developed in an oral formulation. It is in phase II development for rhinitis, asthma, and chronic obstructive pulmonary disease.

INDICATION(S) AND RESEARCH PHASE
Asthma – Phase II
Rhinitis – Phase II
Chronic Obstructive Pulmonary Disease (COPD) – Phase II

fluticasone/salmeterol
unknown

MANUFACTURER
GlaxoSmithKline

DESCRIPTION
This combination product includes a beta-2 adrenergic agonist (salmeterol) and an inhaled corticosteroid (fluticasone) to be administered by intranasal inhalation. It is currently in phase I development for the treatment of rhinitis.

INDICATION(S) AND RESEARCH PHASE
Rhinitis – Phase I

loratadine/montelukast sodium
Claritin/Singulair

MANUFACTURER
Schering-Plough Corporation

DESCRIPTION
Schering-Plough and Merck are collaborating for the development of a once-daily fixed-combination tablet containing Claritin (loratadine) and Singulair (montelukast sodium). Claritin is a once-daily nonsedating antihistamine indicated for the treatment of seasonal allergic rhinitis, while Singulair is a once-daily leukotriene receptor antagonist for the treatment of asthma. The combination drug is currently being developed for the treatment of seasonal allergic rhinitis.

INDICATION(S) AND RESEARCH PHASE
Rhinitis – Phase III

norastemizole
unknown

MANUFACTURER
Sepracor

DESCRIPTION
Norastemizole, a noncardiotoxic metabolite of astemizole (Hismanal), is in phase III trials for the treatment of seasonal and perennial allergic rhinitis in a once-daily formulation. The company claims that the drug is nonsedating and has no harmful effects on the heart, which are improvements over previous generations of antihistamines.

INDICATION(S) AND RESEARCH PHASE
Allergy – Phase III
Rhinitis – Phase III

omalizumab
Xolair

MANUFACTURER
Genentech

DESCRIPTION
Xolair is a recombinant humanized monoclonal antibody to immunoglobulin (Ig) E. It is being developed for the treatment of asthma and the prevention of seasonal allergic rhinitis. A BLA has been submitted for the two above indications and pediatric subjects ages six to 12. This drug is being developed in partnership with Novartis and Tanox. It is currently awaiting FDA approval.

INDICATION(S) AND RESEARCH PHASE
Asthma – NDA submitted
Rhinitis – NDA submitted
Pediatric – NDA submitted

rofleponide palmitate
unknown

MANUFACTURER
AstraZeneca

DESCRIPTION
Rofleponide palmitate is an intranasal steroid indicated for the treatment of rhinitis. It is currently in phase II trials.

INDICATION(S) AND RESEARCH PHASE
Rhinitis – Phase II

Sepsis and Septicemia

anti-tumor necrosis factor-alpha
CytoTAb

MANUFACTURER
Protherics

DESCRIPTION
Whenever there are large amounts of bacteria in the blood, this condition is known as blood poisoning or sepsis. Sepsis is a life-threatening condition in which there can be severe infections and compromise of crucial organs such as the heart and lungs. In a septic state, the body can become so overwhelmed by the bacteria that it can go into shock, with a sharp drop in blood pressure that can result in multi-organ failure and subsequent death.

When the body is invaded by infectious organisms, it usually releases molecules that produce inflammatory responses in order to fight off the infection. One of these inflammatory molecules is called tumor necrosis factor-alpha (TNF-α). Ironically, the action of these molecules themselves, because of the strong chemicals they release in their attempt to destroy bacteria, may result in serious or life-threatening effects. CytoTAb is designed to neutralize the destructive effects of TNF-α on the body.

Initial clinical trials have demonstrated that CytoTAb may potentially block the effects of TNF-α to the degree that it might contribute to significant clinical improvement in disease states ranging from sepsis to inflammatory bowel disease. Further study is necessary to delineate its potential benefits, indications, and possible side effects. CytoTAb, an intravenous formulation, is being evaluated in phase II trials.

INDICATION(S) AND RESEARCH PHASE

Sepsis and Septicemia – Phase II

antithrombin III
unknown

MANUFACTURER
Aventis

DESCRIPTION
Whenever there are large amounts of bacteria in the blood, blood poisoning (sepsis) can result. Sepsis is a life-threatening condition in which there can be severe infections and compromise of crucial organs such as the heart and lungs. In a septic state, the body can become so overwhelmed by the bacteria that it can go into shock, with a sharp drop in blood pressure that can result in multi-organ failure and subsequent death.

When the body is invaded by infectious organisms, it usually releases molecules that produce inflammatory responses in order to fight off the infection. Ironically, these inflammatory molecules themselves, because of the strong chemicals they release in their attempt to destroy bacteria, may result in serious or life-threatening effects. One of these potentially serious effects is that in sepsis, the blood becomes more viscous, increasing the risk of clots in the blood vessels and strokes arising from those clots.

Rhone-Poulenc Rorer is developing a molecule called antithrombin III that could correct this blood disorder. In fact, antithrombin III is normally found in the body, but when a septic state occurs, the body may not have adequate amounts of the molecule to prevent clots. By giving subjects more antithrombin, along with other therapies such as antibiotics, scientists hope to limit the severity of sepsis and prevent strokes that could result in permanent disability. This antithrombin III drug is delivered in an intravenous solution. Development of this drug has been discontinued by Aventis. It was formerly being evaluated in phase III clinical trials for the treatment of sepsis.

INDICATION(S) AND RESEARCH PHASE
Sepsis and Septicemia – Phase III discontinued

atelimomab
Segard

MANUFACTURER
Knoll Pharmaceutical

DESCRIPTION
When the body is invaded by infectious organisms, it usually releases molecules that produce inflammatory responses in order to fight off bacterial infection. One of these inflammatory molecules is called tumor necrosis factor-alpha (TNF-α). Ironically, the action of these molecules themselves, because of the strong chemicals they release in their attempt to destroy bacteria, may result in serious or life-threatening effects. Atelimomab is a protein that can block the activity of these TNF-α molecules.

Atelimomab is a protein known as a monoclonal antibody. Monoclonal antibodies are formulated to target certain proteins, and attach themselves to special receptors (antigens) on the cell surfaces of these proteins. By attaching themselves to the proteins, in this case TNF-α molecules, these antibodies can shut down their activity. These antibodies could contribute to significant clinical improvement in disease states ranging from sepsis to inflammatory bowel disease. Further study is necessary to delineate atelimomab's potential benefits, indications, and possible side effects. This monoclonal antibody is formulated in an intravenous solution, which is undergoing testing in phase III clinical trials.

INDICATION(S) AND RESEARCH PHASE
Sepsis and Septicemia – Phase III

drotrecogin alfa
Zovant

MANUFACTURER
Eli Lilly

DESCRIPTION
Zovant is a recombinant version of naturally occurring activated protein C. The compound may help ameliorate many of the chemical processes that occur during sepsis, including inflammation and clotting in the blood vessels.

In February 2001, results of a phase III trial indicated that Zovant reduced the relative risk of death from sepsis with associated acute organ dysfunction by 19.4%. The double-blind, placebo-controlled PROWESS (Recombinant Human Activated Protein C Worldwide Evaluation in Severe Sepsis) trial included 1,690 subjects from 11 countries. Eli Lilly has applied for regulatory approval in the United States, European Union, and Australia.

INDICATION(S) AND RESEARCH PHASE
Sepsis and Septicemia – NDA submitted
Sepsis and Septicemia – MAA submitted

E5531
unknown

MANUFACTURER
Eisai

DESCRIPTION
When the body is invaded by infectious organisms like bacteria such as *E. coli*, chemicals (endotoxins) that are part of the bacteria's outer membrane are released into the bloodstream. These endotoxins are responsible for many of the destructive effects that bacterial infections can cause in the human body. When enough endotoxins are present in the blood, shock can occur. E5531 works by blocking the noxious action of bacterial-released endotoxins in the body. It occupies receptor sites in human tissues to which the endotoxin molecule would ordinarily bind, resulting in blockage of the effects of the endotoxins.

Further research is necessary to determine how strongly E5531 can inactivate endotoxin molecules, and if this drug is at all effective in a clinical setting. E5531 is being tested in phase II trials in an intravenous formulation.

INDICATION(S) AND RESEARCH PHASE
Sepsis and Septicemia – Phase II

GW 270773
unknown

MANUFACTURER
GlaxoSmithKline

DESCRIPTION
GW 270773 is a phospholipid anti-endotoxin emulsion being developed for the treatment of sepsis. It is currently in phase II trials.

INDICATION(S) AND RESEARCH PHASE
Sepsis and Septicemia – Phase II

IC14
unknown

MANUFACTURER
ICOS Corporation

DESCRIPTION
IC14 is an antibody that targets the CD14 cell surface receptor found on white blood cells. By blocking the CD14 receptor, IC14 may block a damaging cascade of immune system responses that can be initiated by localized bacterial infection. IC14 is in phase I development for the treatment of sepsis.

INDICATION(S) AND RESEARCH PHASE
Sepsis and Septicemia – Phase I

pyridoxalated hemoglobin polyoxyethylene (PHP)
unknown

MANUFACTURER
Apex Bioscience

DESCRIPTION
Apex Bioscience has manufactured a human red blood cell substitute called pyridoxalated hemoglobin polyoxyethylene (PHP). The primary indication is for nitric oxide (NO)-induced shock subjects, which may lead to therapy in the treatment of surgical septic shock. Other indications may include anemia and as a helpful aid to cancer chemotherapy.

INDICATION(S) AND RESEARCH PHASE
Anemia – Phase II/III
Effects of Chemotherapy – Phase II/III
Sepsis and Septicemia – Phase II/III

recombinant human activated protein C (rhAPC)
unknown

MANUFACTURER
Eli Lilly

DESCRIPTION
Recombinant human activated protein C (rhAPC) is a genetically engineered biological drug. Clinical trials are in phase III testing for the treatment of severe sepsis.

INDICATION(S) AND RESEARCH PHASE
Sepsis and Septicemia – Phase III
Pediatric, Sepsis – Phase III

SB 249417
unknown

MANUFACTURER
GlaxoSmithKline

DESCRIPTION
SB 249417 is an anti-factor IX monoclonal antibody being developed for the treatment of severe sepsis, septic shock, and stroke. It is currently in phase I development.

INDICATION(S) AND RESEARCH PHASE
Sepsis and Septicemia – Phase I
Strokes – Phase I

tifacogin
unknown

MANUFACTURER
Chiron Corporation

DESCRIPTION
Tifacogin, a recombinant form of tissue factor pathway inhibitor (TFPI), is believed to block a critical event in sepsis, namely tissue-factor mediated clotting in small blood vessels, which potentially leads to organ failure and death. Phase III trials are under way testing tifacogin to delineate its potential risks and benefits in treating sepsis. Tifacogin is being developed under an agreement with Pharmacia.

INDICATION(S) AND RESEARCH PHASE
Sepsis and Septicemia – Phase III

unknown
Pafase

MANUFACTURER
ICOS Corporation

DESCRIPTION
Pafase is a genetically engineered enzyme formerly called rPAF-AH. The body normally manufactures and releases rapidly acting molecules that amplify the inflammatory response. These amplification signals may become harmful to normal cells if they remain for a prolonged period of time. One of these inflammatory precursor compounds is the platelet-activating factor (PAF). ICOS has cloned the gene that produces acetylhydrolase, a naturally occurring human enzyme that breaks down PAF and inhibits its actions.

A phase III trial for the treatment of sepsis is expected to enroll subjects in the first quarter of 2001. Pafase is part of a joint venture between ICOS and Suntory.

INDICATION(S) AND RESEARCH PHASE
Sepsis and Septicemia – Phase III

Staph Bacterial Infections

hyperimmune globulin
Nabi-Altastaph

MANUFACTURER
Nabi

DESCRIPTION
Nabi-Altastaph is an antibody-based product that contains high levels of antibodies against *Staphylococcus aureus*. It is currently in development for the prevention of *Staphylococcus aureus* infections in subjects who are unable to respond to a vaccine, or who are at immediate risk of infection (i.e., trauma subjects, low birth weight newborns). Nabi Altastaph is currently in phase II trials in neonates, and Nabi also plans to evaluate the product

as a therapeutic drug for the treatment of diagnosed *Staphylococcus aureus* infections.

INDICATION(S) AND RESEARCH PHASE
Staph Bacterial Infections – Phase II Pediatric, Staph Bacterial Infections – Phase II

SA-IGIV
unknown

MANUFACTURER
Inhibitex

DESCRIPTION
SA-IGIV (*S. aureus* immune globulin intravenous human) is a purified immunoglobulin G product derived from pooled adult human plasma selected for elevated levels of antibodies specific for *S. aureus*. According to the company, the selection of donors is based on the company's proprietary MSCRAMM (microbial surface components recognizing adhesive matrix molecules) technology platform. MSCRAMM are a family of naturally occurring proteins on the cell surface of pathogenic microorganisms. These proteins mediate the adherence of bacteria to human tissues—the critical first step in the initiation of most infections.

Inhibitex has begun subject enrollment for a phase II trial of SA-IGIV. The multisite trial is designed to demonstrate that treatment with SA-IGIV can reduce the duration of *S. aureus* bacteremia in subjects with infectious endocarditis.

INDICATION(S) AND RESEARCH PHASE
Staph Bacterial Infections – Phase II

unknown
Ramoplanin Oral

MANUFACTURER
IntraBiotics Pharmaceuticals

DESCRIPTION
The presence of multi-drug resistant bacteria in hospital settings has become a major health problem. One such bacterium is vancomycin-resistant *Enterococcus faecium* (VRE). It is one of the major multi-drug resistant pathogens that cause life-threatening hospital-acquired infections. The prevalence of VRE in hospitalized subjects has increased dramatically since its first occurrence in 1989. VRE infections are particularly problematic in very sick or immunocompromised subjects, many of which are present in hospital ICUs and transplant units. The pathogen is carried in the intestine from where it may be inadvertently transferred through fecal contamination to wound sites, or enter the bloodstream via catheter entry sites or damaged intestinal lining.

Ramoplanin Oral antibiotic acts against multi-drug resistant, gram-positive bacteria such as vancomycin-resistant *Enterococcus faecium* and methicillin-resistant *Staphylococcus aureus*.

Ramoplanin's advantages derive from its potency against these key pathogens, its speed of bacterial killing, and its novel mechanism of action. In multiple comparative studies, Ramoplanin has been shown to be more potent than many other antibiotics, and it has not demonstrated cross-resistance with other antibiotics. Results of a company-sponsored phase II trial showed that administration of Ramoplanin suppressed VRE below detectable levels from 90% of the subjects who carried VRE prior to the study.

INDICATION(S) AND RESEARCH PHASE
Vancomycin Resistant Enterococci (VRE) – Phase III
Staph Bacterial Infections – Phase II

unknown
MBI 853NL

MANUFACTURER
Micrologix

DESCRIPTION
MBI 853NL, a novel drug candidate for preventing hospital-acquired infections caused by *Staphylococcus aureus* (*S. aureus*), including methicillin-resistant *S. aureus*. (MRSA), is in a phase Ib trial. The phase Ib trial is anticipated to be completed in the second quarter of 2001 in the United States.

INDICATION(S) AND RESEARCH PHASE
Staph Bacterial Infections – Phase Ib

vaccine, Staphylococcus aureus
Nabi StaphVAX

MANUFACTURER
Nabi

DESCRIPTION
Nabi StaphVAX is a proprietary, capsular polysaccharide vaccine designed to provide protection against infection caused by *Staphylococcus aureus*. Nabi StaphVAX works by activating specific antibodies in vaccinated individuals that bind to and help kill the invading bacteria. The company claims that phase II trials indicated the vaccine induces high levels of functional antibody in both normal subjects and hemodialysis subjects, with antibody titers persisting through one year or more of follow-up. The injectable vaccine is in phase III testing.

INDICATION(S) AND RESEARCH PHASE
Staph Bacterial Infections – Phase III
Vaccines – Phase III

Tuberculosis

CDC 801
SelCID

MANUFACTURER
Celgene Corporation

DESCRIPTION
SelCIDs (selective cytokine inhibitory drugs) are oral immunotherapeutic agents that treat various inflammatory diseases by inhibiting phosphodiesterase type-4 enzyme (PDE-4). The inhibition of PDE-4 decreases production of tumor necrosis factor-alpha (TNF-α), a protein manufactured by cells of the immune system. This inhibition reduces the level of circulating TNF-α and, therefore, its ability to cause inflammation in cells. At normal levels, the protein is essential for effective immune function. However, overproduction of TNF as a result of age,

genetic, and other influences contributes to the pathology of numerous diseases.

SelCIDs are in phase II trials for the following indications: inflammatory bowel disease, rheumatoid arthritis, multiple sclerosis, asthma, tuberculosis, autoimmune diseases, and mycobacteriosis such as leprosy.

INDICATION(S) AND RESEARCH PHASE
Inflammatory Bowel Disease – Phase II
Rheumatoid Arthritis – Phase II
Multiple Sclerosis – Phase II
Asthma – Phase discontinued
Tuberculosis – Phase II
Autoimmune Diseases – Phase II
Bacterial Infection – Phase II
Multiple Myeloma – Phase II

Vaccines

A streptococcus vaccine
StreptAvax

MANUFACTURER
ID Biomedical

DESCRIPTION
StreptAvax is a multivalent recombinant vaccine developed to cover 26 serotypes of group A streptococcus. A phase I/II trial was initiated in January 2001 in a small group of adults. With positive results, a phase II trial will be initiated in children of two different age groups; adolescents, ages 10 to 14 years old and the target group, pre-school children ages three to six years old.

Results from the phase I trial demonstrated StreptAvax was safe and well tolerated at the 50 ug dose. All subjects in the study developed antibody responses to the vaccine. The FDA has determined that StreptAvax may proceed in human testing at a higher dose.

INDICATION(S) AND RESEARCH PHASE
Vaccines – Phase I/II

BLP-25
unknown

MANUFACTURER
Biomira

DESCRIPTION
BLP-25 is a vaccine designed to induce an immune response to cancer cells. This vaccine incorporates a 25-amino acid sequence of the MUC-1 cancer mucin, encapsulated in a liposomal delivery system that enhances recognition by the immune system and provides better delivery to the tumor.

The company has initiated a phase IIb trial for advanced non-small cell lung cancer at the Cross Cancer Institute in Edmonton, Alberta, which involves seven to ten subjects. The purpose of this trial is to determine whether a higher dose and more frequent administration of the vaccine will enhance its effect. A randomized and comparative phase IIb trial is currently under way.

The company reported that the results of the phase I trial showed the product was well tolerated and excited a cytotoxic T-lymphocyte (CTL) immune response against cancer cells. In addition, BLP-25 has shown an early subjective indication of improved quality of life compared to that seen in chemotherapy subjects in previous trials for non-small cell lung cancer.

INDICATION(S) AND RESEARCH PHASE
Lung Cancer – Phase IIb
Vaccines – Phase IIb

C. difficile vaccine, CdVax
unknown

MANUFACTURER
Acambis

DESCRIPTION
CdVax is a vaccine being developed for the prevention of antibiotic-associated colitis caused by *Clostridium difficile* (*C. difficile*). The *C. difficile* bacteria produce A and B toxins that cause intestinal inflammation and fluid secretion. CdVax contains chemically inactivated A and B toxins, which could potentially stimulate high-level anti-toxin antibodies in plasma donors. These plasma donations could then be used to prepare an immune globulin product (IVIG) for use in the short-term prophylaxis and therapy of *C. difficile* infection.

INDICATION(S) AND RESEARCH PHASE
Bacterial Infection – Phase I/II completed
Vaccines – Phase I/II completed
Gastrointestinal Diseases and Disorders, miscellaneous – Phase I/II completed

Epstein-Barr virus vaccine
unknown

MANUFACTURER
GlaxoSmithKline

DESCRIPTION
This is a recombinant vaccine to prevent infection with Epstein-Barr virus. It is currently in phase II development.

INDICATION(S) AND RESEARCH PHASE
Vaccines – Phase II
Viral Infection – Phase II

ETEC vaccine
unknown

MANUFACTURER
Acambis

DESCRIPTION
This is an oral live attenuated vaccine being developed for the prevention of traveler's diarrhea. The vaccine is designed to be orally administered and to induce mucosal immune responses against the predominant disease-causing strains of ETEC. The vaccine is currently in phase I testing.

INDICATION(S) AND RESEARCH PHASE
Diarrhea – Phase I
Vaccines – Phase I
Bacterial Infection – Phase I

gene therapy, IL-2 and superantigen gene (SEB)
unknown

MANUFACTURER
Valentis

DESCRIPTION

The treatment of malignant melanoma using a combination of cytokine gene (IL-2) and superantigen gene is in phase II trials. The vaccine is injected directly into the tumor, producing an immune response to kill it.

INDICATION(S) AND RESEARCH PHASE
Malignant Melanoma – Phase II
Vaccines – Phase II

H. pylori vaccine
unknown

MANUFACTURER
Acambis

DESCRIPTION
Acambis is developing vaccines designed to prevent and treat peptic ulcers and chronic gastritis caused by *H. pylori*. The vaccines would be used to treat *H. pylori* infection, to prevent reinfection in previously infected persons and to stimulate immunity in uninfected persons. The vaccines are being developed under a joint venture with Aventis Pasteur.

INDICATION(S) AND RESEARCH PHASE
Vaccines – Phase II
Bacterial Infection – Phase II
Gastrointestinal Diseases and Disorders, miscellaneous – Phase II

hepatitis vaccine
Twinrix-2 doses

MANUFACTURER
GlaxoSmithKline

DESCRIPTION
Twinrix (2 doses) is a recombinant vaccine that immunizes recipients against both hepatitis A and hepatitis B. Benefits of this vaccine may include greater convenience and protection for subjects, since immunization against two diseases can be achieved with one injection. Twinrix (two doses) is in phase III trials for combined hepatitis A and B prophylaxis in children and adolescents.

INDICATION(S) AND RESEARCH PHASE
Pediatric, Hepatitis – Phase III
Vaccines – Phase III

HER-2/neu dendritic cell vaccine
unknown

MANUFACTURER
Corixa Corporation

DESCRIPTION
The HER-2/*neu* dendritic cell vaccine is currently undergoing phase I trials for breast and ovarian cancer.

INDICATION(S) AND RESEARCH PHASE
Breast Cancer – Phase I
Ovarian Cancer – Phase I
Vaccines – Phase I

HGP-30W
unknown

MANUFACTURER
CEL-SCI Corporation

DESCRIPTION
HGP-30W is a vaccine designed to induce cellular (e.g., T-cell) and humoral (antibody) immune responses against the predominant subtype of HIV-1. The hope is that the vaccine will target multiple HIV subtypes and be more effective than other HIV vaccines in preventing infection. It is currently in phase II trials for HIV.

INDICATION(S) AND RESEARCH PHASE
HIV Infection – Phase II
Vaccines – Phase II

IR208
NeuroVax

MANUFACTURER
Immune Response Corporation

DESCRIPTION
IR208 is a synthetic T-cell receptor (TCR) vaccine being developed for the treatment of multiple sclerosis. Clinical testing for the IR208 vaccine is in phase I/II.

INDICATION(S) AND RESEARCH PHASE
Multiple Sclerosis – Phase I/II
Vaccines – Phase I/II

IR501
Ravax

MANUFACTURER
Immune Response Corporation

DESCRIPTION
IR501 is a therapeutic vaccine being evaluated for the treatment of rheumatoid arthritis in individuals with stage II or III disease. This T-cell receptor (TCR) vaccine consists of three synthetic peptides (VB3, VB14, and VB17) combined with a potent immune system stimulant known as incomplete Freund's adjuvant (IFA). The vaccine is designed to cause the immune system to inhibit T-cells attacking the joints and causing abnormal cellular damage.

IR501 recently completed a phase II trial for rheumatoid arthritis. Results showed the drug to be safe and well tolerated in 99 subjects; additionally, the drug demonstrated clinically meaningful improvement in subjects after 24 weeks of treatment. However, the results also showed that IR501 may be more effective in subjects with early-stage disease, and that continued monthly injections of the vaccine may be required in order to maintain a positive clinical response.

INDICATION(S) AND RESEARCH PHASE
Rheumatoid Arthritis – Phase II/III
Vaccines – Phase II/III

IR502
Zorcell

MANUFACTURER
Immune Response Corporation

DESCRIPTION
IR502 is a therapeutic vaccine consisting of synthetic peptides combined with a potent immune system stimulant called incomplete Freund's adjuvant (IFA). This T-cell receptor (TCR) vaccine is designed to cause the immune system to shut down activated T-

cells attacking the joints and causing tissue damage. It is being tested for the treatment of moderate to severe psoriasis.

INDICATION(S) AND RESEARCH PHASE
Psoriasis and Psoriatic Disorders – Phase II
Vaccines – Phase II

N. meningitidis A/C
unknown

MANUFACTURER
GlaxoSmithKline

DESCRIPTION
N. meningitidis A/C is a conjugated vaccine in phase II trials for meningitis prophylaxis in children.

INDICATION(S) AND RESEARCH PHASE
Pediatric, Meningitis – Phase II
Vaccines – Phase II

PeNta-HepB-IPV, vaccine
Infanrix

MANUFACTURER
GlaxoSmithKline

DESCRIPTION
This recombinant vaccine has been developed to address several indications. It has been approved by the European Union for diphtheria, tetanus, pertussis, hepatitis B, and polio. An NDA has also been submitted for these indications.

INDICATION(S) AND RESEARCH PHASE
Pediatric, Vaccines – NDA submitted
Hepatitis – NDA submitted

Peru-15
unknown

MANUFACTURER
AVANT Immunotherapeutics

DESCRIPTION
Peru-15 is a cholera vaccine formulation currently in phase IIb development at the Children's Hospital in Cincinnati. Avant Immunotherapeutics announced initiation of the placebo-controlled, double-blind trial in October 2000. The trial will test the safety, immunogenicity, and protective capacity of the vaccine against a challenge with live bacteria that cause cholera.

Results from two previous trials conducted at the U.S. Army Medical Research Institute of Infectious Diseases (USAMRIID) and the John's Hopkins University showed Peru-15 was safe, immunogenic, and protective against a cholera challenge.

INDICATION(S) AND RESEARCH PHASE
Vaccines – Phase II

QS-21
unknown

MANUFACTURER
Aquila Biopharmaceuticals

DESCRIPTION
QS-21 is a potent immunological adjuvant flu vaccine in a phase I clinical trial. This NIAID/DMID-sponsored trial will evaluate the effect of QS-21 on improving the magnitude and the pattern of the immune responses that are found when immunizing with a flu vaccine. The trial will enroll 30 subjects ages 18-40. The eventual goal is the development of an optimized flu vaccine for testing in the elderly.

INDICATION(S) AND RESEARCH PHASE
Vaccines – Phase I

raltitrexed, ZD-1694
Tomudex

MANUFACTURER
AstraZeneca

DESCRIPTION
Tomudex is a cytotoxic enzyme inhibitor of thymidylate synthase, which is being developed for the treatment of solid tumors and advanced colorectal cancer, and adjuvant therapy for colorectal cancer. The drug is administered as a single-agent infusion. Tomudex is in trials for the treatment of colorectal cancer, other unspecified tumors, and as a cancer vaccine.

INDICATION(S) AND RESEARCH PHASE
Colorectal Cancer – Phase II
Cancer/Tumors (Unspecified) – Phase II/III
Vaccines – Phase III

rotavirus vaccine
Rotarix

MANUFACTURER
GlaxoSmithKline

DESCRIPTION
Rotarix is an oral pediatric live attenuated vaccine derived from a naturally occurring isolate of rotavirus found in children. Roatrix is currently in phase II development for rotavirus prophylaxis.

INDICATION(S) AND RESEARCH PHASE
Pediatric, Rotavirus Prophylaxis – Phase II
Vaccines – Phase II

T-cell peptide vaccines
unknown

MANUFACTURER
Immune Response Corporation

DESCRIPTION
T-cell receptor (TCR) peptide vaccines are composed of TCR peptides (BV5S2, BV6S5 and BV13S1) in incomplete Freund's adjuvant (IFA). The rationale for the vaccines is to elicit an antibody response to the T-cell receptor and thereby decrease T-cell activity. This would have anti-inflammatory effects. The IFA should enhance the immunogenicity of peptides. A phase I/II trial will evaluate T-cell receptor (TCR) peptide vaccines for safety, the ability to increase anti-inflammatory immune responses and changes in neurologic evaluations including MRI (magnetic resonance imaging) in multiple sclerosis.

INDICATION(S) AND RESEARCH PHASE
Multiple Sclerosis – Phase I/II
Vaccines – Phase I/II

Td-IPV
unknown

MANUFACTURER
Chiron Corporation

DESCRIPTION
Td-IPV is a new vaccine derived to protect against tetanus, diphtheria, and polio. It contains inactivated polio vaccine in addition to tetanus toxoid and inactivated diphtheria toxin. An application has been filed in Germany.

INDICATION(S) AND RESEARCH PHASE
Vaccines – Filed

tetanus/diphtheria booster
unknown

MANUFACTURER
Celltech Chiroscience plc

DESCRIPTION
This tetanus/diphtheria vaccine is for prevention of tetanus and diphtheria in adults. It is currently in phase III trials.

INDICATION(S) AND RESEARCH PHASE
Vaccines – Phase III

typhoid vaccine
unknown

MANUFACTURER
Acambis

DESCRIPTION
This is an oral live vaccine for the prevention of typhoid that consists of attenuated S. typhi bacteria. The vaccine contains bacteria that have been weakened enough to not cause the disease, but they are still capable of inducing an immune response. A phase II trial was successfully completed. The company is currently seeking a partner for the remainder of development.

INDICATION(S) AND RESEARCH PHASE
Vaccines – Phase II completed
Bacterial Infection – Phase II completed

unknown
ChimeriVax JE

MANUFACTURER
Acambis

DESCRIPTION
ChimeriVax JE is a live, attenuated, injectable vaccine being developed for the prevention of Japanese encephalitis viral infections.

INDICATION(S) AND RESEARCH PHASE
Vaccines – Phase I
Viral Infection – Phase I

unknown
Detox

MANUFACTURER
Corixa Corporation

DESCRIPTION
Detox is a novel vaccine adjuvant contained in Melacine and Biomira's Theratope vaccines. It is currently in phase III trials for breast cancer.

INDICATION(S) AND RESEARCH PHASE
Breast Cancer – Phase III
Vaccines – Phase III

unknown
MPL vaccine adjuvant

MANUFACTURER
Corixa Corporation

DESCRIPTION
MPL, a vaccine adjuvant, is currently undergoing phase II and III trials in Europe for use in allergy vaccines marketed by Allergy Therapeutics.

INDICATION(S) AND RESEARCH PHASE
Allergy – Phase III
Vaccines – Phase III

unknown
FluMist

MANUFACTURER
Wyeth-Ayerst

DESCRIPTION
FluMist is an investigational cold-adapted intranasal influenza vaccine. It is designed to be effective in children by inducing immunity via the nasal mucosa. In October 2000, Aviron and American Home Products Corporation announced that a Biologics License Application for FluMist has been submitted to the FDA. Wyeth-Ayerst is the pharmaceutical division of American Home Products.

INDICATION(S) AND RESEARCH PHASE
Influenza – Phase III
Vaccines – Phase III
Pediatric, Influenza – Phase III

vaccine
Onyvax P

MANUFACTURER
Onyvax

DESCRIPTION
Onyvax P is an allogenic whole-cell vaccine being developed for the treatment of prostate cancer. Phase I/II trials have been completed, and the vaccine is scheduled to enter phase II development in the first quarter of 2001. The phase I/II trial involved 60 subjects with advanced disease. Results showed the vaccine to be safe and capable of generating cancer-specific immune responses.

INDICATION(S) AND RESEARCH PHASE
Prostate Cancer – Phase I/II completed
Vaccines – Phase I/II completed

vaccine
Onyvax CR

MANUFACTURER
Onyvax

DESCRIPTION
Onyvax CR is an allogeneic whole-cell colorectal cancer vaccine. It is currently in a phase I/II trial in subjects with

advanced metastatic disease, which was initiated in 2000. The trial is being conducted at St. George's Hospital in London and is designed to principally examine the safety and immunogenicity of the vaccine. The vaccine is initially administered every two weeks for six weeks, and then monthly for up to a year.

INDICATION(S) AND RESEARCH PHASE
Colorectal Cancer – Phase I/II
Vaccines – Phase I/II

vaccine, 105AD7
Onyvax 105

MANUFACTURER
Onyvax

DESCRIPTION
Onyvax 105 is a human monoclonal antibody being developed for the treatment of colorectal cancer. The drug works by inducing immune responses against the widespread tumor antigen CD55. CD55 is overexpressed in numerous cancers, including those of the prostate, colon, and pancreas. Onyvax 105 will bind to cancer cells overexpressing CD55. This direct attack on the tumor may subsequently produce a therapeutic response. Onyvax 105 is currently in phase I/II trials.

INDICATION(S) AND RESEARCH PHASE
Colorectal Cancer – Phase I/II
Vaccines – Phase I/II

vaccine, adjuvant
AdjuVax-100a

MANUFACTURER
Jenner BioTherapies

DESCRIPTION
AdjuVax-100a is a proprietary emulsion formulation being tested with OncoVax-P prostate cancer vaccine. The combination therapy is in phase II trials.

INDICATION(S) AND RESEARCH PHASE
Prostate Cancer – Phase II
Vaccines – Phase II

vaccines, allergy
unknown

MANUFACTURER
Corixa Montana

DESCRIPTION
MPL is a supplemental molecule (adjuvant) that could make allergy injections stronger and more effective. Phase II studies have shown that it may potentially reduce the total number of injections necessary for desensitization to foreign material (allergens). MPL is formulated from a protein found in a certain species of bacterium. These bacteria and the proteins that compose them provoke a strong immune reaction in humans. By adding this protein to an allergy vaccine, MDL stimulates the body to react more strongly than it would have to the vaccine components alone.

If clinical studies demonstrate the effectiveness of the MDL adjuvant molecule, a chemical that signals the immune system to further boost its response to foreign material, this technology may be useful not only with allergy vaccines, but with cancer and infectious disease therapies as well. Testing of this vaccine is currently in phase III.

INDICATION(S) AND RESEARCH PHASE
Allergy – Phase III
Vaccines – Phase III

vaccine, allogeneic and autologous neuroblastoma cells
unknown

MANUFACTURER
St. Jude Children's Research Hospital

DESCRIPTION
Currently, phase II/III clinical trials are evaluating gene-modified cancer vaccines using autologous and allogeneic tumor cells from interleukin-2 (IL-2) secreting neuroblastomas after autologous bone marrow transplant in first remission. According to the researchers, they are conducting parallel clinical trials in children with recurrent neuroblastoma who are receiving either allogenic or autologous tumor cells that are gene-modified to secrete small amounts of IL-2.

In the autologous trial, one subject had a complete tumor response, one had a partial response, and three had stable disease following the tumor immunogen alone. Four of the five subjects with tumor responses had co-existing neuroblastoma-specific cytotoxic T-lymphocyte activity, as opposed to only one of the subjects with non-responsive disease. These results show a promising correlation between immune response and clinical outcome with autologous vaccines.

In the allogenic group, one child had a very good partial response, five had stable disease and four had progressive disease. Although immunization with autologous vaccine produces superior immune responses, these results offer encouragement for the continued pursuit of allogeneic vaccine strategies in human cancer.

INDICATION(S) AND RESEARCH PHASE
Pediatric, Neuroblastoma – Phase II/III
Pediatric, Vaccines – Phase II/III

vaccine, cancer
Gvax

MANUFACTURER
Cell Genesys

DESCRIPTION
Gvax is an allogeneic compound involving genetic modification of prostate cancer cell lines. These cancer cells have been irradiated and modified to secrete granulocyte-macrophage colony stimulating factor (GM-CSF), a hormone which plays a key role in stimulating the body's immune response to vaccines. The compound is in trials for prostate cancer, pancreatic cancer, lung cancer, leukemia, and malignant melanoma.

The Gvax prostate cancer vaccine demonstrated anti-tumor activity in an initial phase II trial in subjects with advanced metastatic prostate cancer who have not responded to hormone therapy. Prior to initiating a phase III trial, Cell Genesys plans to initiate further trials of Gvax prostate cancer vaccine in 2001, which will employ a higher potency version of the same product.

In addition, the product may be tested in combination with chemotherapy since future phase III trials in hormone refractory prostate cancer subjects may compare Gvax vaccine in combination with chemotherapy to chemotherapy alone.

INDICATION(S) AND RESEARCH PHASE
Prostate Cancer – Phase II
Lung Cancer – Phase I/II completed
Malignant Melanoma – Phase I/II
Vaccines – Phase I/II
Pancreatic Cancer – Phase II
Leukemia – Phase I/II

vaccine, cancer, (pSa)
GeneVax

MANUFACTURER
Centocor

DESCRIPTION
Apollon's cancer vaccine in development uses their patented GeneVax delivery system to deliver genetic material to colorectal cancer cells. This medication, which is administered intravenously, is currently being evaluated in phase II clinical trials. Apollon's GeneVax delivery system is being tested for a variety of different conditions, such as HIV, cervical cancer, herpes infection, hepatitis B, and tuberculosis. But their most active application of this vaccine technology has been in colon cancer. Certain types of colorectal cancers have a strong genetic component that could potentially be targeted by gene therapy. For this type of cancer, Apollon has formulated a DNA vaccine that inserts DNA material into affected cancer cells, so as to arrest the progression and proliferation of cancer growth.

In order to achieve this DNA insertion, Apollon has developed a GeneVax vaccine delivery system that combines DNA molecules with a substance called bupivacaine that facilitates uptake of the DNA by colorectal cells. By potentially improving delivery of the DNA to the affected cancer cells, Apollon is trying to establish clinical efficacy such that cancer growth will be slowed or stopped altogether. The development of new delivery systems for gene therapy is important since one of the major disappointments of gene therapy as it has been administered thus far has been the failure of cells to adequately take up the DNA gene therapy molecules. Further studies will demonstrate whether the GeneVax delivery system will be an improvement compared to established delivery systems.

INDICATION(S) AND RESEARCH PHASE
Vaccines – Phase II
Breast Cancer – Phase I
Prostate Cancer – Phase I

vaccine, DPT/ Haemophilus influenzae type B
unknown

MANUFACTURER
Chiron Corporation

DESCRIPTION
Chiron Corporation has formulated a combination vaccine that might effectively immunize children against four serious diseases: *Haemophilus influenzae* type B, diphtheria, pertussis, and tetanus—with a single injection. This vaccine has the potential to simplify pediatric vaccination schedules, thereby lowering costs, increasing convenience, and improving compliance. The vaccine is composed of inactive molecules of diphtheria toxin, pertussis toxin, and tetanus toxin. Toxins are the destructive molecules that cause most of the pathology seen in these diseases. The vaccine also contains inactivated *H. influenza* proteins.

INDICATION(S) AND RESEARCH PHASE
Bacterial Infection – Phase III
Influenza – Phase III
Pediatric, Influenza – Phase III
Vaccines – Phase III
Viral Infection – Phase III

vaccine, Epstein-Barr virus
unknown

MANUFACTURER
Aviron

DESCRIPTION
The vaccine against EBV/infectious mononucleosis is based on the single surface protein antigen responsible for most of the neutralizing antibodies stimulated by EBV infection, and it combines Aviron's antigen with SmithKline's proprietary adjuvant technology.

Results from a phase I clinical trial showed the vaccine tested was safe and well tolerated, whether or not subjects had been exposed to EBV prior to the study. The trial was a randomized, double-blind study to evaluate safety and immunogenicity of two formulations of intramuscularly injected vaccines in healthy young adults.

INDICATION(S) AND RESEARCH PHASE
Vaccines – Phase II
Viral Infection – Phase I/II

vaccine, genital herpes
Simplirix

MANUFACTURER
GlaxoSmithKline

DESCRIPTION
Simplirix is a recombinant vaccine being developed for genital herpes prophylaxis. Simplirix consists of a recombinant glycoprotein from herpes simplex virus 2 (HSV-2), in combination with an adjuvant "derivative endotoxin." Results of two large, placebo-controlled, randomized international trials were presented at the 40th annual Interscience Conference on Antimicrobials and Chemotherapy in 2000. Both were "discordant partner studies," in which one of the partners had genital herpes and the other did not. The first trial included 847 subjects who tested negative for HSV-1 and HSV-2 at baseline, and the second trial involved 1867 subjects who were negative for HSV-2. The vaccine had no effect in the men in either group; however, a notable effect was observed in the women. In the first study, the vaccine efficacy in women was 73%. Similarly, among the seronegative women in the second study, the vaccine efficacy was 74%. The vaccine was not protective in the women who were HSV-1 positive and HSV-2 negative.

INDICATION(S) AND RESEARCH PHASE

Genital Herpes – Phase II
Vaccines – Phase II

vaccine, GMK
unknown

MANUFACTURER
Progenics Pharmaceuticals

DESCRIPTION
GMK is a vaccine composed of the ganglioside antigen GM2, conjugated to the immunogenic carrier protein KLH and combined with an adjuvant that is the immunological stimulator, QS-21. GMK stimulates the production of antibodies, which has been shown invitro to recognize and destroy cancer cells.

GMK is an injectable vaccine treatment being tested in a phase III trial for melanoma in subjects who are at risk of relapse after surgery. In order for subjects to qualify for the trial they must have had either a deep primary melanoma (4 mm or thicker), or disease that has spread to regional lymph nodes and who are free of disease after surgery. This vaccine is administered on an outpatient basis and it is being tested at hundreds of sites throughout the United States.

INDICATION(S) AND RESEARCH PHASE
Malignant Melanoma – Phase III
Vaccines – Phase III

vaccine, hepatitis
Twinrix-three doses

MANUFACTURER
GlaxoSmithKline

DESCRIPTION
Twinrix is a recombinant vaccine that immunizes recipients against both hepatitis A and hepatitis B. Benefits of this vaccine may include greater convenience and protection for subjects, since immunization against two diseases can be achieved with one injection. An NDA has been submitted for Twinrix (three doses) for combined hepatitis A and B prophylaxis in adults.

INDICATION(S) AND RESEARCH PHASE
Hepatitis – NDA submitted
Vaccines – NDA submitted

vaccine, HIV
Aidsvax

MANUFACTURER
VaxGen

DESCRIPTION
Aidsvax is a genetically engineered, aluminum-adjuvanted subunit vaccine cloned from a protein (gp120) found on the surface of the HIV virus. Because it is a subunit vaccine it does not contain viral DNA, and therefore, no participant in the trial can become infected by HIV due to the vaccination.

Aidsvax is currently being tested in phase III trials. The subjects are between the ages of 18 and 60 and do not have HIV-1 infection, but they are at risk of acquiring HIV-1 infection through sexual contact.

INDICATION(S) AND RESEARCH PHASE
Acquired Immune Deficiency Syndrome (AIDS) and AIDS-Related Infections – Phase III
HIV Infection – Phase III
Vaccines – Phase III

vaccine, HIV
unknown

MANUFACTURER
GlaxoSmithKline

DESCRIPTION
This is a recombinant vaccine for HIV prophylaxis in phase I development.

INDICATION(S) AND RESEARCH PHASE
HIV Infection – Phase I
Vaccines – Phase I

vaccine, HIV-1 gp-120 prime-boost
unknown

MANUFACTURER
Chiron Corporation

DESCRIPTION
Chiron Corporation is developing a vaccine for AIDS that works in two ways. There is a protein found on the outer surface of the HIV molecule (gp 120) that binds to important human immune cells (CD4). This specialized binding site allows the virus to infiltrate these CD4 cells and destroy them. This systematic decimation of a person's CD4 immune cells leads to the serious symptoms of AIDS since the body cannot adequately compensate for the loss in immune protection.

This new vaccine is composed of synthetically made proteins that closely resemble the gp 120 proteins of the AIDS virus. Scientists believe that, upon immunization, the body makes antibodies to these synthetic proteins, and these antibodies will act against the real HIV molecule as well. This vaccine also contains another protein that enhances the immune response. This protein (MF59) is known as an adjuvant because it causes the body to produce a stronger and longer lasting immune reaction than would occur with the vaccine alone. These two mechanisms may potentially immunize people against this pervasive and serious disease. Phase II trials are currently taking place using this intravenous vaccination.

INDICATION(S) AND RESEARCH PHASE
Acquired Immune Deficiency Syndrome (AIDS) and AIDS-Related Infections – Phase II
HIV Infection – Phase II
Vaccines – Phase II

vaccine, HPV
unknown

MANUFACTURER
GlaxoSmithKline

DESCRIPTION
This recombinant vaccine is being developed for the prevention of human papillomavirus (HPV). This vaccine is currently being tested in phase II trials.

INDICATION(S) AND RESEARCH PHASE

vaccine, HPV-16 VLP
unknown

MANUFACTURER
Novavax

DESCRIPTION
HPV-16 VLP, or recombinant human papilloma virus type 16 (HPV-16) virus-like particle (VLP) vaccine, is in development for the prevention of papillomavirus-induced infection and associated diseases, including cervical cancer. Phase I and II trial results indicated that the HPV-16 L1 VLP vaccines elicited virus-specific neutralizing antibodies in immunized human volunteers. In animal models, these antibodies have been shown to prevent virus infection. No serious adverse effects attributable to the vaccine were observed. In October 2000, the National Cancer Institute awarded a contract to Novavax's Biomedical Services Division to manufacture HPV-16 VLP vaccine for a pivotal large-scale clinical efficacy trial to be initiated in 2001.

INDICATION(S) AND RESEARCH PHASE
Viral Infection – Phase II completed
Vaccines – Phase II completed

vaccine, human papilloma virus
unknown

MANUFACTURER
Merck & Co.

DESCRIPTION
This quadrivalent vaccine acts against four of the many herpes viruses: human papilloma virus (HPV) types 6, 11, 16, and 18, and cervical cancer. Papillomas are benign tumors arising from the epithelium in various parts of the body. Phase II trials are under way.

INDICATION(S) AND RESEARCH PHASE
Vaccines – Phase II
Viral Infection – Phase II

vaccine, influenza
unknown

MANUFACTURER
GlaxoSmithKline

DESCRIPTION
This subunit vaccine is being developed for influenza prophylaxis (new delivery). It is currently in phase I development.

INDICATION(S) AND RESEARCH PHASE
Influenza – Phase I
Vaccines – Phase I

vaccine, influenza
unknown

MANUFACTURER
BioChem Pharma

DESCRIPTION
The best weapon against the influenza virus is annual vaccination. However, since the influenza vaccine is administered as an injection, many needle-shy people avoid being vaccinated. The decision not to be immunized due to discomfort from intramuscular injection results in much unnecessary and preventable illness each year.

In order to improve vaccination rates, BioChem Pharma is developing an influenza vaccine that can be taken as a nasal spray. This method of vaccination might not only create a helpful systemic immune response (in the blood and throughout the body), but also stimulate a local immune response in the mucosal lining of the nose, mouth, and throat, which would create an additional barrier to influenza infection and increase efficacy. Phase I results demonstrated comparable immunization responses to that of the injectable vaccine. Clinical testing is in phase III for this nasal inhalation vaccination against the influenza virus.

INDICATION(S) AND RESEARCH PHASE
Influenza – Phase III
Vaccines – Phase III
Pediatric, Influenza – Phase III
Pediatric, Vaccines – Phase III

vaccine, malaria
unknown

MANUFACTURER
GlaxoSmithKline

DESCRIPTION
GlaxoSmithKline is developing a new malaria vaccine that they believe might offer stronger protection and greater efficacy against the disease. Malaria is an infection by microscopic organisms known as protozoans and is transmitted to humans by mosquitoes. There are four types of malarial diseases, all causing symptoms of different quality and severity.

The new malaria vaccine is a combination of the standard malaria vaccine together with two separate proteins that are designed to enhance and strengthen the body's immune response to the vaccine. These "helper vaccine" proteins are known as adjuvants, and they may enhance the duration and overall effectiveness of the vaccine. This formulation contains two different adjuvants, known as Ribi adjuvants, one of which is called a monophosphoryl lipid A (MPL) formulation. Ribi adjuvants are natural and synthetic derivatives of immunomodulatory bacterial components that mimic the beneficial properties of those parent compounds.

This malaria vaccine is currently being tested in phase II trials, under development collaboration among Ribi ImmunoChem Research, GlaxoSmithKline, Walter Reed Army of Research, and the Medical Research Council.

INDICATION(S) AND RESEARCH PHASE
Malaria – Phase II
Vaccines – Phase II

vaccine, malaria
unknown

MANUFACTURER
Aventis Pasteur

DESCRIPTION
This malaria vaccine uses DNA malaria molecules to stimulate an immune response

in the human body. Using DNA molecules represents a new strategy in the formulation of vaccines. Production of a certain kind of immune cells (T-cells) is generated by the DNA vaccine, and these T-cells are capable of attacking and destroying the malaria organism.

Preliminary studies demonstrated the majority of the subjects developed potent "killer" T-cells, which can destroy malaria organisms and defend the body against the disease. The development of an effective new malaria vaccine is important since the standard therapies, mefloquine or doxycycline, are not always effective since some strains of malaria have become drug resistant. The goal of the scientists developing this vaccine is to design a long-lasting, effective, safe vaccine that can be administered to people before they enter malarial geographic zones. This vaccine is given by intramuscular injection and it is being tested in phase II trials. It is being developed in conjunction with Vical.

INDICATION(S) AND RESEARCH PHASE
Malaria – Phase II
Vaccines – Phase II

vaccine, malaria
Quilimmune-M

MANUFACTURER
Aquila Biopharmaceuticals

DESCRIPTION
Quilimmune-M, a genetically engineered sporozoite malaria vaccine, combines an immune system modulator isolated from the *Quillaja saponaria* tree and highly purified as an adjuvant with the peptide antigen SPF-66. The company uses genetic engineering technologies to identify biological molecules that are strongly associated with a target pathogen. These molecules can then be used to stimulate disease-specific immune responses.

Quilimmune-M is being co-developed with Aquila Biopharmaceuticals in cooperation with the World Health Organization and Dr. Manuel Patarroyo of the Instituto de Immunologia in Bogota, Colombia. A Phase I clinical study conducted in Colombia, South America, showed very compelling immunological results.

INDICATION(S) AND RESEARCH PHASE
Parasites and Protozoa – Phase II
Vaccines – Phase II

vaccine, melanoma
Melacine

MANUFACTURER
Schering-Plough Corporation

DESCRIPTION
Melacine is a melanoma vaccine in phase III trials for treatment of late-stage (III and IV) melanoma. The company reported that previous phase III trials demonstrated the vaccine provided a survival rate equal to the standard four-drug chemotherapy.

Melacine consists of lysed cells from two human melanoma cell lines combined with the company's proprietary Detox adjuvant. Detox adjuvant includes MPL immunostimulant (monophosphoryl lipid A) and mycobacterial cell wall skeleton, both of which have a powerful effect on activating the human immune system.

Melacine is being developed under a collaborative agreement between Schering-Plough and Corixa.

INDICATION(S) AND RESEARCH PHASE
Malignant Melanoma – Phase III
Vaccines – Phase III

vaccine, meningitis B
unknown

MANUFACTURER
GlaxoSmithKline

DESCRIPTION
This subunit vaccine has been designed for prevention of *Neisseria meningitides* type B meningitis in children. It is in phase II development.

INDICATION(S) AND RESEARCH PHASE
Pediatric, Meningitis – Phase II
Pediatric, Vaccines – Phase II

vaccine, meningococcal C conjugate
Meningitec

MANUFACTURER
Wyeth-Ayerst

DESCRIPTION
Meningitec is a conjugate vaccine for the prevention of meningococcal Group C disease. In October 1999, the vaccine was approved for use in the United Kingdom.

INDICATION(S) AND RESEARCH PHASE
Meningitis – Phase III
Pediatric, Meningococcal Group C
  Meningitis – Phase III
Vaccines – Phase III

vaccine, meningococcus C
unknown

MANUFACTURER
Chiron Corporation

DESCRIPTION
Chiron Corporation is working on a new vaccine for meningococcal bacterial infections. The bacteria known as *Neisseria meningitidis* produce these infections. This organism can cause a variety of diseases ranging from benign upper respiratory infections to serious blood infections, which can lead to rashes, muscle and joint aches, and meningitis.

Chiron Corporation has developed a synthetic vaccine to immunize against one important subtype of this bacteria (*N. meningitidis* serotype C). This new vaccine is composed of synthetically created proteins that resemble meningococcal proteins. Preliminary studies demonstrated these designed proteins stimulated a stronger immunization response than achieved if the subject had been vaccinated with the normal meningococcal proteins. This new vaccine may be especially helpful in young children whose immune systems are not fully mature and might not respond adequately to the standard vaccine. This intramuscular vaccination is being tested in phase III trials as a treatment against meningococcal infection for children older than twelve months of age, adults with immune deficiencies, complement deficiencies, asplenia, and HIV infection. A phase II trial is also under way for infants.

INDICATION(S) AND RESEARCH PHASE
Meningitis – Phase III
Vaccines – Phase III
Pediatric, Meningitis – Phase III
Pediatric – Phase II

vaccine, MMR-varicella
unknown

MANUFACTURER
GlaxoSmithKline

DESCRIPTION
This is a live attenuated vaccine for the prevention of measles, mumps, rubella, and varicella. It is currently in phase III trials.

INDICATION(S) AND RESEARCH PHASE
Vaccines – Phase III
Pediatric, Measles, Mumps, Rubella, and Varicella Prophylaxis – Phase III

vaccine, pneumococcal infections
Quilimmune-P

MANUFACTURER
Aquila Biopharmaceuticals

DESCRIPTION
Quilimmune-P is designed to enhance the immune response to *Streptococcus pneumoniae*, a prominent bacterial pathogen, and to provide improved protection in the elderly against diseases such as pneumonia, bacteremia, and meningitis. *S. pneumoniae* is a leading cause of morbidity and mortality in the United States and in the world, especially among the very young and the elderly.

A phase IIb trial involves 30 elderly subjects who have received a single immunization of Quilimmune-P in the original phase IIa trial. The subjects will receive a second immunization of Quilimmune-P approximately 12 months after the first one. The primary endpoint of the study is safety. The secondary objectives are to evaluate the immune response to two immunizations given one year apart, and the persistence of the immune response at 12 months following the first immunization.

INDICATION(S) AND RESEARCH PHASE
Pneumonia – Phase II
Vaccines – Phase II

vaccine, prostate cancer (rV-psa)
Prostvac

MANUFACTURER
Therion Biologics

DESCRIPTION
Prostvac is a genetically engineered vaccine that is derived from the poxvirus. This immunotherapeutic is being tested in phase II trials for the treatment of prostate cancer.

INDICATION(S) AND RESEARCH PHASE
Prostate Cancer – Phase II
Vaccines – Phase II

vaccine, Pseudomonas infection
Pseudostat

MANUFACTURER
Provalis

DESCRIPTION
Pseudostat is an oral (mucosal) therapeutic vaccine against *Pseudomonas aeruginosa* infections in cystic fibrosis subjects and subjects with chronic bronchitis, bronchiectasis and influenza. The company intends to re-enter phase II trials in Australia and plans to initiate phase II trials in the United States, where it has been in discussion with the National Institute of Health and the Cystic Fibrosis Foundation. In addition, the developer has filed for Orphan Drug Designation in the United States.

INDICATION(S) AND RESEARCH PHASE
Bronchitis – Phase I/II
Bacterial Infection – Phase I/II
Cystic Fibrosis – Phase I/II
Influenza – Phase I/II
Vaccines – Phase I/II

vaccine, respiratory syncytial virus
unknown

MANUFACTURER
Aventis Pasteur

DESCRIPTION
Respiratory syncytial virus (RSV), a common cause of winter outbreaks of acute respiratory disease, may cause an estimated 90,000 hospitalizations and 4,500 deaths each year from lower respiratory tract disease in both infants and young children. RSV is a common, but preventable cause of hospital-acquired (nosocomial) infection. The source of this virus transmission may include other infected subjects, staff, and visitors.

Most severe manifestations of infection with RSV (e.g., pneumonia and bronchiolitis) occur in infants aged two to six months; however, children of any age with underlying cardiac or pulmonary disease or who are immunocompromised are at risk for serious complications from this infection. Because natural infection with RSV provides limited protective immunity, RSV causes repeated symptomatic infections throughout life. In adults, RSV usually causes upper respiratory tract manifestations but may cause lower respiratory tract disease, especially in the elderly and in immunocompromised persons.

The company has an RSV-mediated lower respiratory disease vaccination for at-risk children and the elderly being tested in phase I/II trials.

INDICATION(S) AND RESEARCH PHASE
Bronchitis – Phase I/II
Lung Disease – Phase I/II
Pediatric, Respiratory Syncytial Virus – Phase I/II
Pneumonia – Phase I/II
Vaccines – Phase I/II
Viral Infection – Phase I/II

vaccine, Shigella flexneri and sonneii
unknown

MANUFACTURER
Intellivax International

DESCRIPTION
This novel vaccine, in a nasal spray formulation, in phase II trials.

INDICATION(S) AND RESEARCH PHASE
Bacterial Infection – Phase II
Diarrhea – Phase II
Vaccines – Phase II

vaccine, Staphylococcus aureus
Nabi StaphVAX

MANUFACTURER
Nabi

DESCRIPTION
Nabi StaphVAX is a proprietary, capsular polysaccharide vaccine designed to provide protection against infection caused by *Staphylococcus aureus*. Nabi StaphVAX works by activating specific antibodies in vaccinated individuals that bind to and help kill the invading bacteria. The company claims that phase II trials indicated the vaccine induces high levels of functional antibody in both normal subjects and hemodialysis subjects, with antibody titers persisting through one year or more of follow-up. The injectable vaccine is in phase III testing.

INDICATION(S) AND RESEARCH PHASE
Staph Bacterial Infections – Phase III
Vaccines – Phase III

vaccine, Streptococcus pneumoniae
unknown

MANUFACTURER
GlaxoSmithKline

DESCRIPTION
This conjugated pediatric vaccine is currently in phase III trials for Streptococcus pneumoniae disease prophylaxis. The vaccine contains antigens for prevention of pneumonia, middle ear infections, and meningitis in pediatric patients.

INDICATION(S) AND RESEARCH PHASE
Pediatric, Bacterial Infection—Phase III
Pediatric, Ear Infections —Phase III
Pediatric, Meningitis —Phase III
Pediatric, Pneumonia— Phase III

yellow fever vaccine
Arilvax

MANUFACTURER
Acambis

DESCRIPTION
Arilvax is a live attenuated vaccine being developed for the prevention of yellow fever. The vaccine is based on a live attenuated yellow fever virus (17D strain). In June 2000, positive results were obtained from a U.S. phase III trial of Arilvax. The multicenter, double-blind, randomized trial compared the safety and immunogenicity of Arilvax with a control yellow fever vaccine, YF-VAX. Celltech Medeva is responsible for manufacturing Arilvax.

INDICATION(S) AND RESEARCH PHASE
Vaccines – Phase III completed
Viral Infection – Phase III completed

Vancomycin Resistant Enterococci (VRE)

unknown
Ramoplanin Oral

MANUFACTURER
IntraBiotics Pharmaceuticals

DESCRIPTION
The presence of multi-drug resistant bacteria in hospital settings has become a major health problem. One such bacterium is vancomycin-resistant *Enterococcus faecium* (VRE). It is one of the major multi-drug resistant pathogens that cause life-threatening hospital-acquired infections. The prevalence of VRE in hospitalized subjects has increased dramatically since its first occurrence in 1989. VRE infections are particularly problematic in very sick or immunocompromised subjects, many of which are present in hospital ICUs and transplant units. The pathogen is carried in the intestine from where it may be inadvertently transferred through fecal contamination to wound sites, or enter the bloodstream via catheter entry sites or damaged intestinal lining.

Ramoplanin Oral antibiotic acts against multi-drug resistant, gram-positive bacteria such as vancomycin-resistant *Enterococcus faecium* and methicillin-resistant *Staphylococcus aureus*.

Ramoplanin's advantages derive from its potency against these key pathogens, its speed of bacterial killing, and its novel mechanism of action. In multiple comparative studies, Ramoplanin has been shown to be more potent than many other antibiotics, and it has not demonstrated cross-resistance with other antibiotics. Results of a company-sponsored phase II trial showed that administration of Ramoplanin suppressed VRE below detectable levels from 90% all of the subjects who carried VRE prior to the study. Based upon these positive results, phase III clinical trials were initiated.

INDICATION(S) AND RESEARCH PHASE
Vancomycin Resistant Enterococci (VRE) – Phase III
Staph Bacterial Infections – Phase II

Viral Infection

BMS-200475
Entecavir

MANUFACTURER
Bristol-Myers Squibb

DESCRIPTION
Viruses such as hepatitis B need to be able to replicate their viral genetic material in order to reproduce themselves. Bristol-Myers Squibb is developing a treatment for chronic hepatitis B infection, a common and serious liver condition, which works by disrupting the viral replication process.

Genetic material is made up of proteins called nucleic acids. By using a synthesized protein (2'-deoxyguanosine carbocyclic analogue) that mimics one of the building blocks of nucleic acids, scientists hope to stop the production of viral genetic information, and thus prevent viruses from creating the genetic machinery they require to keep reproducing.

Studies are under way in phase II trials to understand if this novel drug will improve the symptoms and prognosis of chronic hepatitis B infection.

INDICATION(S) AND RESEARCH PHASE
Hepatitis – Phase II
Viral Infection – Phase II

cidofovir
Vistide

MANUFACTURER
Gilead Sciences

DESCRIPTION
Vistide is being tested as an injectable formulation for treatment of central nervous system infections and hepatitis B virus respiratory tumors, and tumors or disorders of the larynx. The drug is in phase I/II trials for HBV respiratory tumors, laryngeal papillomatosis, and progressive multifocal leukoencephalopathy.

INDICATION(S) AND RESEARCH PHASE
Hepatitis – Phase I/II
Laryngeal Tumors/Disorders – Phase I/II
Viral Infection – Phase I/II
Brain Cancer – Phase I/II

cidofovir
unknown

MANUFACTURER
Gilead Sciences

DESCRIPTION
Cidofovir is a broad-spectrum antiviral for the treatment of a variety of ophthalmic viruses, including adenovirus and viral keratoconjunctivitis. The drug, which is made in a topical ophthalmic formulation, is in phase II trials.

INDICATION(S) AND RESEARCH PHASE
Eye Disorders/Infections – Phase II
Viral Infection – Phase II

cidofovir
Vistide

MANUFACTURER
Gilead Sciences

DESCRIPTION
Vistide is being tested as an injectable formulation for treatment of central nervous system infections and hepatitis B virus respiratory tumors, and tumors or disorders of the larynx. The drug is in phase I/II trials for HBV respiratory tumors, laryngeal papillomatosis, and progressive multifocal leukoencephalopathy.

INDICATION(S) AND RESEARCH PHASE
Hepatitis – Phase I/II
Laryngeal Tumors/Disorders – Phase I/II
Viral Infection – Phase I/II
Brain Cancer – Phase I/II

Epstein-Barr virus vaccine
unknown

MANUFACTURER
GlaxoSmithKline

DESCRIPTION
This is a recombinant vaccine to prevent infection with Epstein-Barr virus. It is currently in phase II development.

INDICATION(S) AND RESEARCH PHASE
Vaccines – Phase II
Viral Infection – Phase II

interferon (IFN) alfa-n3
Alferon N Gel

MANUFACTURER
Interferon Sciences

DESCRIPTION
Alferon N Gel is a human leukocyte-derived natural interferon (IFN) treatment being tested for vaginal infections in phase II trials. Interferons are naturally produced chemicals that modulate and boost the immune system. These trials are testing the drug in a topical gel formulation.

Already on the market, interferon alfa-n3 (human leukocyte derived) is an injectable formulation of natural alpha interferon, approved by the FDA in 1989 for the intralesional treatment of refractory or recurring external condylomata acuminata in subjects 18 years of age or older.

INDICATION(S) AND RESEARCH PHASE
Genital Warts – Phase II
Vaginal Infection – Phase II
Viral Infection – Phase II

MEDI-517
unknown

MANUFACTURER
MedImmune

DESCRIPTION
MEDI-517 is a virus-like particle vaccine designed to elicit an immune response against the human papilloma virus (HPV). HPVs have been implicated in the development of genital warts and cervical cancer, with specific types of HPVs associated with each condition. HPV-6 and HPV-11 cause the majority of genital warts, while HPV-16 and HPV-18 cause the majority of cervical cancers. MEDI-517 is currently in phase II trials for the prevention of cervical cancer.

INDICATION(S) AND RESEARCH PHASE
Viral Infection – Phase II
Cervical Dysplasia/Cancer – Phase II

OST 577
Ostavir

MANUFACTURER
Protein Design Labs

DESCRIPTION
Ostavir is a humanized monoclonal antibody (Mab) in ongoing phase II trials for the treatment of chronic hepatitis B, either combined with interferon or as a sole agent. Additional indications may include infectious diseases and viral diseases.

INDICATION(S) AND RESEARCH PHASE
Hepatitis – Phase II
Viral Infection – Phase II

---

pleconaril
unknown

MANUFACTURER
ViroPharma

DESCRIPTION
Pleconaril is an orally active broad-spectrum anti-viral agent that possesses anti-picornaviral activity. Pleconaril belongs to a class of compounds that inhibits capsid function of picornaviruses, which is essential for viral infection. The agent is currently being tested in two phase III trials in adult subjects with viral respiratory infection (VRI).

INDICATION(S) AND RESEARCH PHASE
Viral Infection – Phase III

---

psoralen, S-59
unknown

MANUFACTURER
Cerus Corporation

DESCRIPTION
Psoralen uses ultraviolet-A light to initiate a platelet pathogen inactivation system. This invitro process works on blood temporarily drawn outside of the body for sterilization of viruses, bacteria, and other pathogens that may be present. Psoralen is being tested in phase III trials with blood components (platelets, fresh frozen plasma (FFP), and red blood cells) used in transfusions. The purpose is to enhance the safety of blood transfusions by inactivating pathogens in the blood components.

Additionally, psoralen may help inactivate white blood cells, which are responsible for a variety of adverse transfusion reactions. This therapy may be useful for treatment of thrombocytopenia and red and white blood cell disorders.

Cerus Corporation is developing psoralen in collaboration with Baxter Healthcare.

INDICATION(S) AND RESEARCH PHASE
Bacterial Infection – Phase III
Red Blood Cell Disorders – Phase III
Thrombocytopenia – Phase III
Viral Infection – Phase III

---

ribavirin
Virazole

MANUFACTURER
ICN Pharmaceuticals

DESCRIPTION
Virazole is a brand name for ribavirin, a synthetic nucleoside analog with broad-spectrum antiviral activity, currently marketed by ICN in a variety of dosage forms for at least one of 10 indications in 44 countries.

The drug is in phase II trials against human papilloma virus and phase III trials against respiratory syncytial virus (RSV-BMT). In cell cultures the inhibitory activity of ribavirin for respiratory syncytial virus is selective. The mechanism of action is unknown. Reversal of the invitro antiviral activity by guanosine or xanthosine suggests ribavirin may act as an analogue of these cellular metabolites.

INDICATION(S) AND RESEARCH PHASE
Lung Disease – Phase III
Viral Infection – Phase II
Viral Infection – Phase III

T611
unknown

MANUFACTURER
Tularik

DESCRIPTION
T611 is an orally administered anti-cytomegalovirus drug. Cytomegalovirus (CMV) belongs to the family of herpes viruses and can produce a serious infection in subjects with compromised immune systems. T611 interferes with CMV replication. Phase I trials were initiated in August 2000.

INDICATION(S) AND RESEARCH PHASE
Viral Infection – Phase I

---

thymalfasin
Zadaxin

MANUFACTURER
SciClone Pharmaceuticals

DESCRIPTION
Zadaxin is a twenty-eight amino acid peptide originally isolated from the thymus gland and now produced synthetically. The compound has been shown to promote the maturation of T-cells, which are involved in the control of various immune responses.

The company has conducted phase II/III trials of Zadaxin in combination with lamivudine and famciclovir for the treatment of chronic hepatitis B and hepatitis C.

Zadaxin is also in trials for the treatment of malignant melanoma, hepatitis C, hepatitis B (Japan), and hepatitis C (Europe). Zadaxin was FDA approved in March 2000 for liver cancer.

INDICATION(S) AND RESEARCH PHASE
Hepatitis – Phase II/III
Viral Infection – Phase II/III
Liver Cancer – FDA approved
Malignant Melanoma – Phase II
Lung Cancer – Phase Preclinical

---

unknown
ChimeriVax JE

MANUFACTURER
Acambis

DESCRIPTION
ChimeriVax JE is a live attenuated injectable vaccine being developed for the prevention of Japanese encephalitis viral infections. In September 2000, Acambis began a phase I safety and immunogenicity trial.

INDICATION(S) AND RESEARCH PHASE
Vaccines – Phase I
Viral Infection – Phase I

---

vaccine, DPT/ Haemophilus influenzae type B
unknown

MANUFACTURER
Chiron Corporation

DESCRIPTION
Chiron Corporation has formulated a combination vaccine that might effectively immunize children against four serious diseases: *Haemophilus influenzae* type B, diphtheria, pertussis, and tetanus—with a single injection. This vaccine has the potential to simplify pediatric vaccination schedules, thereby lowering costs, increasing convenience and improving compliance. The vaccine is composed of inactive molecules of diphtheria toxin, pertussis toxin, and tetanus toxin. Toxins are the destructive molecules that cause most of the pathology seen in these diseases. The vaccine also contains inactivated *H. influenzae* proteins.

Diphtheria is an infection that can cause upper respiratory symptoms, heart problems, or nerve damage. Five to ten percent of cases are fatal. Tetanus causes nerve and muscle destruction as a result of the toxin that the bacterium *Clostridium tetani* releases. Affected subjects can experience muscular rigidity and spasms, and if untreated, have difficulty breathing and subsequent death. Pertussis (whooping cough) affects the respiratory tract and can progress to cause pneumonia, seizures, and brain damage. *Haemophilus influenzae* type B is a bacterium that is responsible for a significant percentage of bacterial sepsis in infants under four months of age. It can also cause upper airway, lung, skin, and joint infections. The combination vaccine given as an intramuscular injection is currently in phase III trials.

INDICATION(S) AND RESEARCH PHASE
Bacterial Infection – Phase III
Influenza – Phase III
Pediatric – Phase III
Vaccines – Phase III
Viral Infection – Phase III

vaccine, Epstein-Barr virus
unknown

MANUFACTURER
Aviron

DESCRIPTION
The vaccine against EBV/infectious mononucleosis is based on the single surface protein antigen responsible for most of the neutralizing antibodies stimulated by EBV infection, and it combines Aviron's antigen with SmithKline's proprietary adjuvant technology.

A phase I clinical trial demonstrated the vaccine tested was safe and well tolerated, whether or not subjects had been exposed to EBV prior to the study. The trial was a randomized, double-blind study to evaluate safety and immunogenicity of two formulations of intramuscularly injected vaccines in healthy young adults.

INDICATION(S) AND RESEARCH PHASE
Vaccines – Phase II
Viral Infection – Phase I/II

vaccine, HPV
unknown

MANUFACTURER
GlaxoSmithKline

DESCRIPTION
This recombinant vaccine is being developed for the prevention of human papillomavirus (HPV). This vaccine is currently being tested in phase II trials.

INDICATION(S) AND RESEARCH PHASE
Vaccines – Phase II
Viral Infection – Phase II

vaccine, HPV-16 VLP
unknown

MANUFACTURER
Novavax

DESCRIPTION
HPV-16 VLP, or recombinant human papilloma virus type 16 (HPV-16) virus-like particle (VLP) vaccine, is in development for the prevention of papillomavirus-induced infection and associated diseases, including cervical cancer. Phase I and II trial results indicated that the HPV-16 L1 VLP vaccines elicited virus-specific neutralizing antibodies in immunized human volunteers. In animal models, these antibodies have been shown to prevent virus infection. No serious adverse effects attributable to the vaccine were observed. In October 2000, the National Cancer Institute awarded a contract to Novavax's Biomedical Services Division to manufacture HPV-16 VLP vaccine for a pivotal large-scale clinical efficacy trial to be initiated in 2001.

INDICATION(S) AND RESEARCH PHASE
Viral Infection – Phase II completed
Vaccines – Phase II completed

vaccine, human papilloma virus
unknown

MANUFACTURER
Merck & Co.

DESCRIPTION
This quadrivalent vaccine acts against four of the many herpes viruses: human papilloma virus (HPV) types 6, 11, 16, and 18, and cervical cancer. Papillomas are benign tumors arising from the epithelium in various parts of the body. Phase II trials were under way for these indications.

INDICATION(S) AND RESEARCH PHASE
Vaccines – Phase II
Viral Infection – Phase II

vaccine, respiratory syncytial virus
unknown

MANUFACTURER
Aventis Pasteur

DESCRIPTION
Respiratory syncytial virus (RSV), a common cause of winter outbreaks of acute respiratory disease, may cause an estimated 90,000 hospitalizations and 4,500 deaths each year from lower respiratory tract disease in both infants and young children. RSV is a common, but preventable cause of hospital-acquired (nosocomial) infection. The source of this virus transmission may include other infected subjects, staff, and

visitors.

Most severe manifestations of infection with RSV (e.g., pneumonia and bronchiolitis) occur in infants aged two to six months; however, children of any age with underlying cardiac or pulmonary disease or who are immunocompromised are at risk for serious complications from this infection. Because natural infection with RSV provides limited protective immunity, RSV causes repeated symptomatic infections throughout life. In adults, RSV usually causes upper respiratory tract manifestations but may cause lower respiratory tract disease, especially in the elderly and in immunocompromised persons.

The company has an RSV-mediated lower respiratory disease vaccination for at-risk children and the elderly being tested in phase I/II trials.

INDICATION(S) AND RESEARCH PHASE
Bronchitis – Phase I/II
Lung Disease – Phase I/II
Pediatric, Respiratory Syncytial Virus – Phase I/II
Pneumonia – Phase I/II
Vaccines – Phase I/II
Viral Infection – Phase I/II

vaccine, rotavirus
unknown

MANUFACTURER
Merck & Co.

DESCRIPTION
Rotavirus vaccine is in a phase III for the prevention of of diarrhea and dehydration due to rotavirus.

INDICATION(S) AND RESEARCH PHASE
Viral Infection – Phase III

votumumab
HumaSPECT/Infectious Diseases

MANUFACTURER
INTRACEL Corporation

DESCRIPTION
HumaSPECT is the trade name for votumumab, which is being tested in different formulations for a variety of indications. HumaSPECT/Infectious Diseases is an imaging agent using tumor specific, human monoclonal antibodies (MAbs). This intravenous formulation is in phase II trials against viral infections.

INDICATION(S) AND RESEARCH PHASE
Viral Infection – Phase II

VP 14637
unknown

MANUFACTURER
ViroPharma

DESCRIPTION
VP 14637 is a small molecule that has been shown to inhibit respiratory syncytial virus (RSV) replication invitro. It is currently being evaluated in phase I trials for the treatment of diseases caused by RSV.

INDICATION(S) AND RESEARCH PHASE
Viral Infection – Phase I

VX-148
unknown

MANUFACTURER
Vertex Pharmaceuticals

DESCRIPTION
VX-148 is an inhibitor of inosine monophosphate dehydrogenase (IMPDH), a cellular enzyme essential for production of guanine nucleotides, one of the building blocks of RNA and DNA. Inhibiting IMPDH may be an effective strategy for blocking the growth of lymphocytes and the replication of viruses, since both depend on nucleotide synthesis for replication. Vertex's IMPDH inhibitors have the potential to treat viral infections, autoimmune diseases, and psoriasis. These three indications are currently being tested in phase I trials.

INDICATION(S) AND RESEARCH PHASE
Viral Infection – Phase I
Autoimmune Diseases – Phase I
Psoriasis and Psoriatic Disorders – Phase I

yellow fever vaccine
Arilvax

MANUFACTURER
Acambis

DESCRIPTION
Arilvax is a live attenuated vaccine being developed for the prevention of yellow fever. The vaccine is based on a live attenuated yellow fever virus (17D strain). In June 2000, positive results were obtained from a U.S. phase III trial of Arilvax. The multicenter, double-blind, randomized trial compared the safety and immunogenicity of Arilvax with a control yellow fever vaccine, YF-VAX. Celltech Medeva is responsible for manufacturing Arilvax.

INDICATION(S) AND RESEARCH PHASE
Vaccines – Phase III completed
Viral Infection – Phase III completed

7 | Pulmonary and Respiratory

Population with illnesses in this category	150 million[1]
Drugs in the development pipeline	331[2]
Number of drugs in preclinical testing	176
Number of drugs in clinical testing	140

Source: 1. World Health Organization, worldwide figures 2. Parexel

Pulmonary and respiratory diseases affect millions of individuals, and the therapeutic area includes conditions such as chronic obstructive pulmonary disease (COPD), asthma, respiratory distress syndrome and cystic fibrosis. COPD includes emphysema and chronic bronchitis—diseases that are characterized by airflow obstruction and loss of the normal elasticity of the lungs. Both the prevalence of and mortality from COPD is increasing, even in industrialized countries. According to the World Health Organization, COPD will be the third most common cause of death worldwide by 2020. CenterWatch research indicates that there are 15 to 20 drugs in trials for COPD at a cost of approximately $75 million to 95 million.

Chronic bronchitis is characterized by inflammation and eventual scarring of the bronchial epithelium. Symptoms include chronic cough, increased mucus production, and shortness of breath. Emphysema is a degenerative disease that usually develops from long-term exposure to cigarette smoke or other toxins. Symptoms of emphysema include cough, shortness of breath, especially with exertion, and limited exercise tolerance.

The quality of life for a person suffering from COPD diminishes as the disease progresses. Eventually the person may require supplemental oxygen and may have to rely on mechanical respiratory assistance. Current treatment is tailored to the severity of the disease and may include bronchodilators and exercise to strengthen muscles. Antibiotics are sometimes used to treat superimposed infection. Investigational drugs that hold promise for the treatment of COPD include AstraZeneca's Viozan, a novel dual D2 dopamine receptor and beta-2-adrenoceptor agonist, and GlaxoSmithKline's Ariflo, a novel oral phosphodiesterase (PDE)-IV inhibitor.

Asthma, a chronic inflammatory lung disease, affects as many as 17 million Americans and is responsible for 5,000 deaths annually. According to CenterWatch research, 30 to 40 drugs are currently in trials for the treatment of asthma, costing approximately $170 million to $196 million. Children account for approximately one-third of the diagnosed cases, and asthma is the second most common cause of school absenteeism, after the common cold. The condition is characterized by shortness of breath, wheezing, tightness in the chest, and cough. Since asthma is a chronic condition, the goal of treatment is management rather than cure.

In addition to the many compounds moving through the pipeline, researchers are also examining new methods for delivering asthma treatment. Incorrect use of inhalers has been implicated as a cause of failed treatment, with patients experiencing difficulties such as the mistiming of inhalation. Delivery systems that react to patient inhalation, in addition to other delivery methods, have been developed to address this problem. The use of spacers has been another solution. A spacer attaches to a metered dose inhaler, and consists of a chamber that traps medicine for the individual to inhale in one or two breaths rather than the mandatory one breath of many currently used inhalers.

Recent FDA approvals that address incorrect inhalation include Novartis' Foradil Aerolizer (formoterol fumarate inhalation powder), a selective beta-2-agonist for the maintenance treatment of asthma and prevention of bronchospasm. Foradil capsules are administered via a new device called the Aerolizer Inhaler, a delivery system that allows patients to "see, hear, feel" that they have correctly taken their medication. In contrast to traditional metered-dose inhalers, patients can visually inspect the Aerolizer Inhaler to confirm they have received the full dose. The Aerolizer Inhaler also produces a whirring noise, which signals that the drug is being dispensed.

Cystic fibrosis (CF) is a genetic disease affecting approximately 55,000 children and adults in the United States and Europe. CenterWatch estimates that there are nine to 15 drugs in trials for cystic fibrosis at a cost of approximately $50 million to $70 million. In individuals with the disease, the defective CFTR gene results in the production of an abnormally thick, sticky mucus, due to the faulty transport of sodium and chloride in epithelial cells of the lungs and pancreas. Abnormal mucus in the gastrointestinal tract results in pancreatic duct obstruction. These thick secretions predispose the body to infections that damage organ tissue and ultimately lead to death. The median survival age of patients with CF today is approximately 30 years. There is no cure for cystic fibrosis and the standard treatments, including antibiotics and mucus thinning therapies, are often less than optimal.

Until 1989 when researchers discovered the defective gene, only CF symptoms could be treated. The standard treatments then and now depend on the disease stage and organs involved. These include chest physical therapy to dislodge secretions from the lungs, antibiotics to treat lung infections, and enriched diets and replacement vitamins and enzymes. The discovery that gene therapy may potentially correct defective CF cells opened the door to a new area of research. Research is underway to evaluate methods of delivering the normal CF gene, such as via synthetic vectors, modified viruses or liposomes.

Acute Respiratory Distress Syndrome (ARDS)

lucinactant
Surfaxin

MANUFACTURER
Discovery Laboratories

DESCRIPTION
Surfaxin, has been granted a fast track designation by the FDA for development as a treatment for meconium aspiration syndrome (MAS), acute respiratory distress syndrome (ARDS), and acute lung injury (ALI). The drug is currently in late stage phase III trials in premature babies.

A surfactant is a surface-active agent secreted by alveolar type II cells that decreases the surface tension of pulmonary fluids and increases elasticity of lung tissue, thus helping the lungs to breathe easier. Surfaxin is a novel surfactant, containing a peptide mimic of the human protein B. It cleanses the lung and restores surfactant inactivated by MAS. An injectable formulation of the drug is in phase III trials.

INDICATION(S) AND RESEARCH PHASE
Acute Respiratory Distress Syndrome (ARDS) – Phase III
Respiratory Failure – Phase III
Pediatric, Meconium Aspiration Syndrome – Phase III

opebecan, rBPI-21, recombinant human bactericidal/permeability-increasing protein
Neuprex

MANUFACTURER
XOMA Corporation

DESCRIPTION
Neuprex is a systemic formulation of recombinant bactericidal/permeability-increasing protein rBPI-21, being developed for the treatment of severe meningococcemia, a rare systemic gram-negative bacterial infection that primarily affects children. After entering the bloodstream, the harmful bacteria attack the brain and spinal cord's protective sheathing. The gram-negative bacteria, called *Neisseria meningitidis*, cause meningococcemia and produce spiking high fever and a classic rigid stiff neck. Shock and death may occur in just a few hours after infection.

The active molecule in Neuprex, rBPI-21, binds to the endotoxin molecules LOS and LPS, lipopolysaccharides in living bacteria, disrupting their cell walls, killing the bacteria, or making them more susceptible to antibiotics. Phase III data were released in September 2000 from both pediatric and adult trials.

A 1,650 subject phase III trauma trial evaluating whether Neuprex can prevent pneumonia and acute respiratory distress syndrome (ARDS) is under way. Subjects are enrolled after experiencing a severe accident, in which they have lost at least two units of blood. More than 800 subjects are currently enrolled. Supporting this study was a previous 401 subject phase II trial, with the results published in the *Journal of Trauma* in April 1999.

Acute intra-abdominal infection is another potential use for Neuprex, in combination with other antibiotics. The drug is currently in phase I/II trials for this indication.

A phase II trial is currently enrolling subjects who have had part of their liver removed during surgery. Neuprex may prevent post-surgical infection and complications.

INDICATION(S) AND RESEARCH PHASE
Bacterial Infection – Phase III completed
Pediatric, Bacterial Infection - Meningococcemia – Phase III completed
Meningitis – Phase III
Acute Respiratory Distress Syndrome (ARDS) – Phase III
Pneumonia – Phase III
Liver Disease – Phase II
Intra-abdominal Infection – Phase I/II

perflubron
LiquiVent

MANUFACTURER
Alliance Pharmaceutical

DESCRIPTION
LiquiVent (perfluorooctylbromide) is an intrapulmonary liquid oxygen-carrying drug for treatment of acute lung injury (ALI) and acute respiratory distress syndrome (ARDS). The drug is administered directly into the lungs of subjects on a mechanical ventilator, via a proprietary partial liquid ventilation technique that opens collapsed or debris-filled alveoli and assists in respiratory gas exchange. The FDA has granted this drug a fast track status. LiquiVent is being tested in phase III trials for pulmonary complications.

INDICATION(S) AND RESEARCH PHASE
Acute Respiratory Distress Syndrome (ARDS) – Phase II/III
Respiratory Failure – Phase II/III

TP10
unknown

MANUFACTURER
AVANT Immunotherapeutics

DESCRIPTION
TP10 is a genetically engineered (recombinant) soluble complement receptor-1 (sCR1). Complement-1 is a naturally occurring substance that binds to antibodies as part of the immune response to infection or foreign bodies. Clinical trials are testing TP10 in an intravenous formulation for a variety of disorders including the treatment of acute respiratory distress syndrome (ARDS), reperfusion injury, heart attack, cardiac surgery, organ reperfusion, xenotransplantation, allotransplantation, and post-surgical complications in infants.

A phase IIb trial was initiated in January 2001 in approximately 30 infants undergoing high risk cardiac surgery utilizing cardiopulmonary bypass. The trial will be conducted at seven sites in the United States.

INDICATION(S) AND RESEARCH PHASE
Acute Respiratory Distress Syndrome (ARDS) – Phase II/III
Cardiac Ischemia – Phase I/II
Cardiac Surgery – Phase IIb
Myocardial Infarction – Phase I/II
Pediatric, Post-surgical complications –

Phase I/II
Pediatric, Cardiac Surgery – Phase IIb

ZD-8321
unknown

MANUFACTURER
AstraZeneca

DESCRIPTION
ZD-8321 is a new drug under development for treatment of chronic obstructive pulmonary disease (COPD) and acute respiratory distress syndrome (ARDS).

The lungs are composed of thousands of tiny air sacs, called alveoli, that function to oxygenate the blood from inspired air. In COPD and ARDS, the delicate walls of these alveoli are eroded away, resulting in less functional lung tissue. Because of fewer working alveoli, oxygen taken in cannot be transferred to the blood vessels, making the lungs more susceptible to infection and therefore requiring bronchodilators and oxygen for support.

In COPD and ARDS, the enzyme elastase is hyperstimulated by the toxins involved, from smoking in COPD and infection or trauma in ARDS. This enzyme destroys elastin and collagen, two proteins that are important structural components of lung tissue. Scientists believe that ZD-8321, which blocks the action of the elastase enzyme, may slow down or stop completely the destruction of lung tissue characteristic of both these conditions. ZD-8321 is an orally formulated drug that was being evaluated in phase II clinical trials for the treatment of ARDS and COPD. As of December 2000, the trials have been discontinued until further notice.

INDICATION(S) AND RESEARCH PHASE
Acute Respiratory Distress Syndrome (ARDS) – Phase III discontinued
Chronic Obstructive Pulmonary Disease (COPD) – Phase III discontinued

Aspergillosis

FK463, echinocandin
unknown

MANUFACTURER
Fujisawa Healthcare

DESCRIPTION
Echinocandin is a novel antifungal agent for the treatment of systemic fungal infections. The drug is used as prophylaxis, empirical therapy, and second line treatment for candidiasis and aspergillosis. Echinocandin is in phase II/III trials for these indications and other fungal infections.

INDICATION(S) AND RESEARCH PHASE
Aspergillosis – Phase II/III
Candidiasis – Phase II/III
Fungal Infections – Phase II/III

nystatin, AR-121
Nyotran

MANUFACTURER
Aronex Pharmaceuticals

DESCRIPTION
Nyotran is an intravenous liposomal formulation of nystatin being developed for the treatment of serious systemic, opportunistic fungal infections. Phase III trials have been completed for systemic fungal infections and confirmed cryptococcal meningitis. Additionally, phase II trials have been completed for candidiasis and aspergillosis.

Nyotran is under agreement with Abbott Laboratories for worldwide commercialization. Abbott will fund clinical development and will submit marketing registration outside the United States.

INDICATION(S) AND RESEARCH PHASE
Aspergillosis – Phase II completed
Candidiasis – Phase II completed
Systemic Fungal Infections – Phase III completed
Meningitis – Phase III completed

Asthma

(R,R)-formoterol
unknown

MANUFACTURER
Sepracor

DESCRIPTION
(R,R)-formoterol is a single-isomer bronchdilator with a rapid onset of action. This drug is currently in phase II b trials in subjects with asthma and emphysema.

INDICATION(S) AND RESEARCH PHASE
Asthma – Phase II b
Emphysema – Phase IIb

albuterol
Ventolin

MANUFACTURER
GlaxoSmithKline

DESCRIPTION
Ventolin, a beta-2 agonist, is currently on the market in several formulations for the treatments of asthma and chronic obstructive pulmonary disease (COPD). The drug acts by relaxing the bronchial smooth muscle and inhibiting the release of immediate hypersensitivity mediators. Ventolin has received European Union (EU) approval for both indications in a formulation that uses non-CFC propellant (GR106642) in a metered dose inhaler. An approvable letter was received from the FDA in January 2001. Ventolin has also received EU approval for the same indications via delivery by Diskus/Accuhaler, a dry powder inhaler. An FDA approvable letter was received in July 2000.

INDICATION(S) AND RESEARCH PHASE
Asthma – FDA recommend approval letter
Chronic Obstructive Pulmonary Disease (COPD) – FDA recommend approval letter

anti-interleukin-5 MAb (Anti-IL-5)
unknown

MANUFACTURER
Schering-Plough Corporation

DESCRIPTION
Anti-interleukin-5 MAb (Anti-IL-5) is a

monoclonal antibody to interleukin-5 being developed in an injectable formulation. It is currently in phase II trials for the treatment of asthma.

INDICATION(S) AND RESEARCH PHASE
Asthma – Phase II

CDC 801
SelCIDs

MANUFACTURER
Celgene Corporation

DESCRIPTION
SelCIDs, selective cytokine inhibitory drugs, are oral immunotherapeutic agents that treat various inflammatory diseases by inhibiting phosphodiesterase type-4 enzyme (PDE-4). The inhibition of PDE-4 decreases production of tumor necrosis factor-alpha (TNF-α), a protein manufactured by cells of the immune system. This inhibition reduces the level of circulating TNF-α and, therefore, its ability to cause inflammation in cells. At normal levels, the protein is essential for effective immune function. However, overproduction of TNF as a result of age, genetic, and other influences contributes to the pathology of numerous diseases.

SelCIDs are in phase II trials for the following indications: inflammatory bowel disease, rheumatoid arthritis, multiple sclerosis, tuberculosis, autoimmune diseases, multiple myeloma, and mycobacterial infections such as leprosy.

INDICATION(S) AND RESEARCH PHASE
Inflammatory Bowel Disease – Phase II
Rheumatoid Arthritis – Phase II
Multiple Sclerosis – Phase II
Asthma – Phase discontinued
Tuberculosis – Phase II
Autoimmune Diseases – Phase II
Bacterial Infection – Phase II
Multiple Myeloma – Phase II

CpG compound
unknown

MANUFACTURER
Coley Pharmaceutical

DESCRIPTION
CpG compound is a novel immune modulator designed to redirect hypersensitivity allergic and asthmatic reactions into more normal responses, thereby eliminating or reducing the appearance of symptoms. CpG molecules simultaneously suppress allergic immune responses that result in airway inflammation and bronchial spasm, and induce normal immune responses that promote antibody and cellular responses. In October 2000, Coley initiated a phase II trial in the United Kingdom for the treatment of allergic asthma.

INDICATION(S) AND RESEARCH PHASE
Asthma – Phase II
Allergy – Phase I

cromolyn sodium
Intal HFA-227

MANUFACTURER
Aventis

DESCRIPTION
Intal, in its original formulation, is currently on the market for the treatment of asthma. The active ingredient, cromolyn sodium, inhibits both the immediate and non-immediate bronchoconstrictive reactions to inhaled antigen. Cromolyn sodium also decreases bronchospasm caused by exercise, toluene diisocyanate, aspirin, cold air, sulfur dioxide, and environmental pollutants. Although the exact mechanism of action of cromolyn sodium is unknown, its effects are mediated through the secondary messenger, cyclic-AMP. The drug has no intrinsic bronchodilator or antihistamine activity. This new non-CFC formulation, Intal HFA-227, is in phase III trials for the treatment of asthma in both adults and children.

INDICATION(S) AND RESEARCH PHASE
Asthma – Phase III
Pediatric, Asthma – Phase III

DNK 333
unknown

MANUFACTURER
Novartis

DESCRIPTION
DNK 333 is a dual NK_1/NK_2 antagonist being developed in an oral formulation. It is in phase II development for rhinitis, asthma and chronic obstructive pulmonary disease (COPD).

INDICATION(S) AND RESEARCH PHASE
Asthma – Phase II
Rhinitis – Phase II
Chronic Obstructive Pulmonary Disease (COPD) – Phase II

EPI-2010
unknown

MANUFACTURER
EpiGenesis Pharmaceuticals

DESCRIPTION
EPI-2010 is an antisense oligonucleotide that targets the adenosine A1 receptor, which is produced in excess in virtually all asthma subjects. In animal models the drug was effective for nearly seven days, and appeared to be metabolized within the lung, causing no systemic toxicity. Phase I trials of EPI-2010 in inhalation formulation are under way.

INDICATION(S) AND RESEARCH PHASE
Asthma – Phase I

flunisolide
Aerobid

MANUFACTURER
Forest Laboratories

DESCRIPTION
Aerobid, a steroid inhaler containing flunisolide may be more effective than currently prescribed steroid inhalers and may also produce fewer side effects. In preliminary trials, Aerobid has been shown to have strong anti-inflammatory and anti-allergic action on airways. In addition, after Aerobid is absorbed into the body, it is quickly converted into a conjugate that has little or no effect on other organs in the body. Aerobid

is in phase III trials for the treatment of asthma in both children and adults.

INDICATION(S) AND RESEARCH PHASE
Asthma – Phase III
Pediatric, Asthma – Phase III

fluticasone propionate
Flixotide, Flovent

MANUFACTURER
GlaxoSmithKline

DESCRIPTION
Flovent is an inhaled glucocorticoid being developed for the treatment of asthma. While the precise mechanism of action of glucocorticoid is unknown, these steroids demonstrate anti-inflammatory influences on multiple cell types and mediator production or secretion involved in the asthmatic response.

This drug is being developed in the United States as Flovent and internationally as Flixotide. It is in phase III trials in the United States for the treatment of asthma, in a once-daily dosing formulation. The drug received European Union (EU) approval for the treatment of chronic obstructive pulmonary disease (COPD) in September 1999, for both asthma and COPD in a formulation that uses non-CFC propellant (GR 106642) in a metered dose inhaler. Flovent has been FDA approved for use in inhaled corticosteroid, CFC propellant, and Diskus/Accuhaler (dry powder) formulations.

INDICATION(S) AND RESEARCH PHASE
Asthma – Phase III
Chronic Obstructive Pulmonary Disease (COPD) – Phase EU approved
Asthma – Phase EU approved
Asthma – FDA approved

formoterol
Budoxis, Oxis

MANUFACTURER
AstraZeneca

DESCRIPTION
Otis combines a long-acting beta-2 agonist, formoterol, with budesonide, an inhaled glucocorticoid. Formoterol has been approved by the FDA for use in the Oxis Turbuhaler, which administers the drug through a multi-dose dry powder inhalation device. Clinical documentation of the Oxis Turbuhaler demonstrated the combination of a rapid onset of symptom relief and long-lasting bronchodilation.

The Oxis Turbuhaler is currently in three phase III trials for treatment of asthma, both in children and adults, and for chronic obstructive pulmonary disease (COPD).

INDICATION(S) AND RESEARCH PHASE
Asthma – Phase III
Chronic Obstructive Pulmonary Disease (COPD) – Phase III
Pediatric, asthma – Phase III

formoterol
Foradil

MANUFACTURER
Novartis

DESCRIPTION
Foradil (formoterol), a long-acting beta2-agonist, is a bronchodilator for the treatment of asthma and chronic obstructive pulmonary disease. It is currently being tested in phase II trials in a multi-dose dry powder inhaler. It has been approved for twice-daily use via the Aerolizer inhaler (a single-dose powder inhalation device) for use in adults and children ages five and older.

The multi-dose dry powder formulation is being tested in phase II trials for the treatment of asthma. In February 2001, Foradil Aerolizer was approved by the FDA for long-term, twice daily administration in the maintenance treatment of asthma and in the prevention of bronchospasm in adults and children five years of age and older with reversible obstructive airways disease.

INDICATION(S) AND RESEARCH PHASE
Asthma – Phase II
Asthma – FDA approved
Reversible Obstructive Airways Disease – FDA approved
Pediatric, Asthma – FDA approved

GW 328267
unknown

MANUFACTURER
GlaxoSmithKline

DESCRIPTION
GW 328267 is an adenosine A2 agonist. It is currently in phase I development for the treatment of asthma and chronic obstructive pulmonary disease (COPD).

INDICATION(S) AND RESEARCH PHASE
Asthma – Phase I
Chronic Obstructive Pulmonary Disease (COPD) – Phase I

IDEC-152
unknown

MANUFACTURER
IDEC Pharmaceuticals

DESCRIPTION
IDEC-152 is an anti-CD23 monoclonal antibody that targets the CD23 receptor on immune cells. The anti-CD23 antibody is part of IDEC's primatized antibody technology that may be useful in treating allergic conditions such as allergic asthma, allergic rhinitus, and atopic conditions. This antibody enables the treatment of specific allergy conditions by combining with the CD23 factor to regulate the production of the allergy-triggering immuno-globulin (IgE), while generating no further IgE production. In February 2000, IDEC initiated a phase I trial for allergic asthma. IDEC-152 is being developed by IDEC Pharmaceuticals and Seikagaku Corporation of Japan.

INDICATION(S) AND RESEARCH PHASE
Asthma – Phase I
Allergy – Phase I

interleukin-4 (IL-4)
Nuvance

MANUFACTURER

Immunex Corporation

DESCRIPTION
Interleukin-4 (IL-4) is an immune system protein commonly associated with asthma and respiratory allergies. IL-4 binds to an IL-4 receptor (IL-4R) on the surface of certain cells, triggering a cascade of events leading to clinical symptoms. When IL-4 binds to soluble IL-4R instead of cell-surface IL-4R, its effects may be blocked.

Nuvance is a novel, genetically engineered IL-4R protein being evaluated for the symptomatic treatment of allergic asthma. The drug is administered in an inhalation formulation. It is currently in phase II trials with asthma subjects not receiving corticosteroid treatment.

INDICATION(S) AND RESEARCH PHASE
Asthma – Phase II

IPL 576,092
unknown

MANUFACTURER
Inflazyme Pharmaceuticals

DESCRIPTION
Canadian scientists originally derived this orally administered anti-inflammatory drug from the molecules of a sea sponge. The drug appears to have a strong effect on the mediators in inflammation and is the most promising candidate from the company's IPL 576 series of anti-inflammatory compounds. Its chief advantage is that it appears to have similar results to the inhalation of glucocorticoids without the side effects. It is currently being developed for asthma and related respiratory conditions.

Phase II trials are expected to be completed in 2001, at which point, partner company Aventis will have the option to continue trials and will also be responsible for marketing the product after a royalty payment to Inflazyme.

In phase I trials, IPL 576,092 demonstrated a strong effect on the mediators of inflammation invitro, and in its oral and inhalation formulations invivo. It compared quite favorably to a control in reducing bronchoconstriction in animal testing.

INDICATION(S) AND RESEARCH PHASE
Asthma – Phase II

LDP-977
unknown

MANUFACTURER
LeukoSite

DESCRIPTION
LDP-977 is an orally active, small molecule compound that has demonstrated the ability to selectively inhibit the production of leukotrienes, a class of molecules that play an important role in triggering bronchial asthma. Leukotrienes are produced by activated, inflammatory white blood cells or leukocytes (eosinophils, basophils, and mast cells), which are present in elevated numbers in the airways of subjects with asthma. LeukoSite is evaluating LDP-977 in phase II trials for the treatment of asthma.

INDICATION(S) AND RESEARCH PHASE
Asthma – Phase II

mepolizumab, SB 240563
unknown

MANUFACTURER
GlaxoSmithKline

DESCRIPTION
SB 240563 is a steroid sparing anti-interleukin (IL-5) monoclonal antibody in phase II trials for the treatment of asthma. Similar to other drugs used for the treatment of asthma, SB 240563 works by shutting down the inflammatory process that causes the symptoms of asthma.

Interleukins are immune proteins that modulate the inflammatory response by stimulating the growth and function of white blood cells. Research is needed to determine whether administration of this anti-IL-5 antibody will neutralize the interleukin molecules, and thus halt the inflammatory process.

INDICATION(S) AND RESEARCH PHASE
Asthma – Phase II

mometasone furoate
Asmanex

MANUFACTURER
Schering-Plough Corporation

DESCRIPTION
Asmanex is an orally inhaled steroid that works by stabilizing cell membranes, and thereby suppressing the inflammatory process frequently seen in asthma subjects. Asmanex is being tested both as a metered-dose inhaler that regulates the quantity of the drug delivered with each puff and as a dry powder inhaler. The metered-dose inhaler is currently in phase III trials. An NDA is currently under review for the dry-powder inhaler.

INDICATION(S) AND RESEARCH PHASE
Asthma, metered-dose inhaler – Phase III
Asthma, dry powder inhaler – NDA submitted

omalizumab
Xolair

MANUFACTURER
Genentech

DESCRIPTION
Xolair is a recombinant humanized monoclonal antibody to immunoglobulin (IgE). It is being developed for the treatment of asthma and the prevention of seasonal allergic rhinitis. An NDA has been submitted for the two above indications and for treatment in pediatric asthma subjects ages six to 12. This drug is being developed in partnership with Novartis and Tanox. It is currently awaiting FDA approval.

INDICATION(S) AND RESEARCH PHASE
Asthma – NDA submitted
Rhinitis – NDA submitted
Pediatric, Asthma – NDA submitted

PDE4i, SCH351591
unknown

MANUFACTURER

Celltech Chiroscience plc

DESCRIPTION
PDE4i are a series of PDE4 inhibitors that Celltech is developing in conjunction with Schering-Plough. The PDE4 enzyme regulates activities in cells that lead to inflammation in the lungs and increased sensitivity to allergens. Inhibitors of this enzyme may reduce the symptoms of asthma and decrease sensitivity to allergens. PDE4 inhibitors have generally been associated with negative side effects. This PDE4 inhibitor preferentially binds to the catalytic site of PDE4, which should result in an anti-inflammatory effect with fewer side effects. This therapy is currently in phase I development for treatment of asthma.

INDICATION(S) AND RESEARCH PHASE
Asthma – Phase I

pumactant
unknown

MANUFACTURER
Britannia Pharmaceuticals Limited

DESCRIPTION
Pumactant is a sterile mixture of the two phospholipids palmitoyl-phosphatidylcholine and phosphatidylglycerol. It is in phase III development in the United Kingdom and Australia for surgical adhesions and phase II development in the United Kingdom for asthma.

INDICATION(S) AND RESEARCH PHASE
Asthma – Phase II
Surgical Adhesions – Phase III

salbutamol
Ultrahaler

MANUFACTURER
Aventis

DESCRIPTION
Salbutamol, a short-acting beta-2 agonist for symptomatic relief of bronchial asthma, relieves the most serious symptom of asthma, the constriction of the smooth muscle lining the bronchi of the lungs. The drug is widely manufactured in various formulations.

Ultrahaler is a dry powder inhalation formulation that was formerly being tested in phase III trials. Development for this device has been discontinued.

INDICATION(S) AND RESEARCH PHASE
Asthma – Phase III discontinued

salmeterol xinafoate
Serevent

MANUFACTURER
GlaxoSmithKline

DESCRIPTION
Serevent is a beta-2 agonist for the treatment of asthma and chronic obstructive pulmonary disease (COPD). The drug is thought to stimulate intracellular adenyl cyclase, the enzyme that catalyzes the conversion of adenosine triphosphate (ATP) to cyclic C-3',5'-adenosine monophosphate (cyclic AMP). Increased cyclic AMP levels cause relaxation of bronchial smooth muscle and inhibit release of mediators of immediate hypersensitivity from cells.

The drug is in phase III trials for the treatment of asthma and COPD in a formulation that uses non-CFC propellant (GR106642) in a metered dose inhaler. Additionally, Serevent is in phase III trials for COPD with delivery via Diskus/Accuhaler, a dry powder inhaler.

INDICATION(S) AND RESEARCH PHASE
Asthma – Phase III
Chronic Obstructive Pulmonary Disease (COPD) – Phase III

salmeterol/fluticasone propionate
Seretide, Advair

MANUFACTURER
GlaxoSmithKline

DESCRIPTION
Seretide is a combination therapy consisting of a beta-2 agonist and a synthetic glucocorticoid with potent anti-inflammatory activity. The beta-2 agonist is thought to stimulate intracellular adenyl cyclase, the enzyme that catalyzes the conversion of adenosine triphosphate (ATP) to cyclic C-3',5'-adenosine monophosphate (cyclic AMP). Increased cyclic AMP causes relaxation of bronchial smooth muscle and inhibits the release of mediators of immediate hypersensitivity.

While the precise mechanism of glucocorticoid action in asthma is unknown, they have been shown to inhibit many types of cells and mediator production, or secretion, involved in the asthmatic response. These anti-inflammatory actions may contribute to the efficacy of glucocorticoids in asthma.

Seretide has received European Union (EU) approval for the treatment of pediatric asthma using the Diskus/Accuhaler dry powder inhaler. An NDA has been submitted for the CFC-free formulation for the treatment of adult asthma. Seretide is also in phase III trials for the treatment of COPD and as a first-line therapy for asthma via delivery by the Diskus/Accuhaler inhaler. Seretide is being developed under the trade name Advair in the United States.

INDICATION(S) AND RESEARCH PHASE
Pediatric, Asthma – Phase EU approved
Chronic Obstructive Pulmonary Disease (COPD) – Phase III
Asthma – NDA submitted

SB 207499
Ariflo

MANUFACTURER
GlaxoSmithKline

DESCRIPTION
Ariflo, a novel oral phosphodiesterase (PDE)-IV inhibitor, is being developed for the treatment of chronic obstructive pulmonary disease (COPD) and asthma. The company claims that clinical trials thus far suggest that Ariflo significantly improved lung function in subjects with moderate-to-severe COPD. It also improved exercise tolerance, which enhances the ability to perform activities of daily living. The drug is in phase II trials for the treatment of asthma and phase III trials for COPD.

INDICATION(S) AND RESEARCH PHASE
Chronic Obstructive Pulmonary Disease (COPD) – Phase III
Asthma – Phase II

SB 683698, TR 14035
unknown

MANUFACTURER
GlaxoSmithKline

DESCRIPTION
SB 683698 is a dual alpha4 integrin antagonist (VLA4). It is currently in phase II trials for the treatment of asthma and rheumatoid arthritis.

INDICATION(S) AND RESEARCH PHASE
Asthma – Phase II
Rheumatoid Arthritis – Phase II

SCH55700
unknown

MANUFACTURER
Celltech Chiroscience plc

DESCRIPTION
SCH5570 is a humanized antibody to interleukin-5 (IL-5), a key factor in the maturation of eosinophils. Eosinophil activity in the lungs is a major component of asthmatic disease. SCH5570 neutralizes IL-5, preventing eosinophil accumulation and activity in the lung, thereby possibly reducing the symptoms of asthma.

The drug is being developed in collaboration with Schering-Plough and is currently in phase II studies around the world.

INDICATION(S) AND RESEARCH PHASE
Asthma – Phase II

SR-140333
unknown

MANUFACTURER
Sanofi-Synthelabo Pharmaceuticals

DESCRIPTION
SR-140333 is a new drug that blocks the action of substances that can cause airway inflammation in asthmatics. SR-140333 is currently in phase II trials in an inhaled suspension formulation.

Many substances have a role in producing the inflammatory process that results in the symptoms of asthma. Asthmatics may be more sensitive to these irritating substances than non-asthmatic individuals. One of these, Substance P, is a molecule known as a tachykinin that acts on the NK_1 receptor to cause airway contraction, mucus secretion, and the accumulation of white blood cells in the lungs.

SR-140333 blocks the receptor to which Substance P attaches, thus preventing the negative effects of its action. It will most likely have the strongest action in blocking the production of mucus and the aggregation of white blood cells, both of which obstruct lung passageways. In preclinical studies, SR-140333 was shown to have efficacy in blocking the bronchoconstricting effects of Substance P.

INDICATION(S) AND RESEARCH PHASE
Asthma – Phase II

T3
unknown

MANUFACTURER
AstraZeneca

DESCRIPTION
T3 is a dry powder inhaler, non-reservoir currently in phase I trials for the treatment of asthma.

INDICATION(S) AND RESEARCH PHASE
Asthma – Phase I

TBC-1269
unknown

MANUFACTURER
Texas Biotechnology

DESCRIPTION
Texas Biotechnology is developing a new drug that may prevent some of the inflammation that causes the main symptoms of asthma. TBC-1269 inhibits the action of selectins, small molecules that play an important role in the inflammatory process. They help white blood cells, which release substances that directly cause inflammation, to adhere to blood vessels near the area of sensitization. By blocking one link in the chain of events leading to an inflammatory reaction, this adhesion of white blood cells may prevent allergic asthmatic attacks.

TBC-1269 appears to have inhibitory action against all of the principal selectin types—E selectin, L selectin, and P selectin. In preclinical research, TBC-1269 has been shown to reduce the incidence of asthma attacks in study subjects. In addition, since this medication is not a steroid, it does not result in the side effects commonly experienced by chronic steroid use. This orally formulated drug is currently being tested in phase II trials for the treatment of asthma.

INDICATION(S) AND RESEARCH PHASE
Asthma – Phase II

theophylline
Theolan

MANUFACTURER
Elan Pharmaceutical Research

DESCRIPTION
Theolan is one of many formulations of theophylline used in the treatment of asthma. It causes the relaxation of bronchial smooth muscles and modulation of mediator release by inhibiting cyclic-AMP degradation by the enzyme phosphodiesterase. The drug is in phase III trials in a pediatric liquid suspension formulation, using twice-daily proprietary PharmaZome oral delivery technology.

INDICATION(S) AND RESEARCH PHASE
Asthma – Phase III
Pediatric, Asthma – Phase III

unknown
Symbicort Turbuhaler

MANUFACTURER
AstraZeneca

DESCRIPTION
Symbicort Turbuhaler is an inhaled steroid indicated for the treatment of asthma and chronic obstructive pulmonary disease (COPD). The drug is a long-acting formulation of a beta-2 agonist and is currently in phase III trials.

INDICATION(S) AND RESEARCH PHASE
Asthma – Phase III
Chronic Obstructive Pulmonary Disease (COPD) – Phase III

unknown
Albuterol

MANUFACTURER
Alkermes

DESCRIPTION
Alkermes is developing a long-acting inhalable formulation of the asthma drug albuterol. This new formulation is based on Alkermes' AIR pulmonary drug delivery technology and is designed to provide several hours of therapeutic benefit from a single administration.

In November 2000, Alkermes announced a phase II of the drug, designed to test the efficacy of a range of doses in subjects with mild to moderate asthma. It will enroll 48 subjects and is expected to be completed in 2001.

INDICATION(S) AND RESEARCH PHASE
Asthma – Phase II

unknown
MSI-Albuterol

MANUFACTURER
Zambon S.p.A.

DESCRIPTION
The metered solution inhaler (MSI) system is a small, portable hand-held nebulizer designed to combine the therapeutic benefits of nebulization with the convenience of pressurized metered dose inhalers (MDIs).

In June 2000, Zambon Group and Sheffield Pharmaceuticals announced the successful completion and preliminary results of the second phase II trial evaluating the MSI-Albuterol system. The randomized, cross over, cumulative dose trial demonstrated that it was comparable to the market-leading albuterol product delivered through an MDI. Both the MSI-Albuterol and MDI-Albuterol were given as cumulative doses in 24 adult subjects with moderate, persistent asthma. A phase I trial in pediatric subjects is currently in progress.

INDICATION(S) AND RESEARCH PHASE
Asthma – Phase II completed
Pediatric, Asthma – Phase I

unknown
Symbicort pMDI

MANUFACTURER
AstraZeneca

DESCRIPTION
Symbicort pMDI is an inhaled steroid indicated for the treatment of asthma and chronic obstructive pulmonary disease (COPD). The drug is a long-acting formulation of a beta-2 agonist. It is currently in development in phase I trials.

INDICATION(S) AND RESEARCH PHASE
Asthma – Phase I
Chronic Obstructive Pulmonary Disease (COPD) – Phase I

very late antigen-4 inhibitor (VLA-4)
unknown

MANUFACTURER
Biogen

DESCRIPTION
Very late antigen-4 (VLA-4) is a receptor on most white blood cells. The binding of VLA-4 to VCAM-1, a protein found on certain endothelial cells, facilitates the migration of white blood cells into tissue as part of an inflammatory response. This response can be very damaging, when it abnormally acts against the body's own tissue in chronic inflammatory diseases like asthma. VLA-4 blocks the inflammation process in a highly specific manner.

By blocking the VLA-4/VCAM-pathway and the subsequent movement of white blood cells into tissues, it may be possible to prevent injury and damage.

Biogen and Merck are collaborating to develop small molecule VLA-4 inhibitors in oral and aerosolized formulations in phase II trials for treatment of asthma.

INDICATION(S) AND RESEARCH PHASE
Asthma – Phase II

Bronchitis

HP-3
unknown

MANUFACTURER
Milkhaus Laboratory

DESCRIPTION
HP-3 is a nucleic acid medication in an oral formulation. It is a novel therapeutic agent being tested in phase II and III trials for the treatment of chronic bronchitis (CB), chronic obstructive pulmonary disease (COPD), and cystic fibrosis (CF). HP-3 is also being tested in pediatric subjects, ages six to 21 years old.

Results from a phase II trial for CF showed significant improvement in pulmonary function and an increase in sputum clearance.

Results for all three indications showed that HP-3 increased sputum expectoration and significantly improved pulmonary function. The company believes that the drug evokes such responses through a mechanism common to all three diseases. Consequently, HP-3 may have a broad potential utility in relieving the debilitating symptoms of respiratory distress, which afflict more than 15 million subjects.

INDICATION(S) AND RESEARCH PHASE
Bronchitis – Phase III
Chronic Obstructive Pulmonary Disease (COPD) – Phase II completed
Cystic Fibrosis – Phase II completed
Pediatric, Cystic Fibrosis – Phase II completed

INS365
unknown

MANUFACTURER
Inspire Pharmaceuticals

DESCRIPTION
INS365 is a novel P2Y2-receptor stimulator, stabilized uridine nucleotide analogue, being developed for the treatment of acute and chronic lung diseases, such as chronic bronchitis (CB) and cystic fibrosis (CF). The drug hydrates and clears mucus from a subject's airways, principally by acting on the P2Y2 receptor.

A phase III trial for dry eye was initiated in January 2001 in approximately 1,000 subjects at 60 ophthalmology centers.

CB, caused primarily by smoking and pollution, involves excessive retention of mucus as well as inflamed airways leading to impaired mucociliary clearance and causing subjects to experience frequent respiratory infections. INS365 is in phase I/II trials for CB treatment.

CF is a disorder in which a genetic mutation in airway cells causes dehydrated secretions and production of thickened mucus and impaired mucociliary clearance. This plugging effect leads to frequent pulmonary infections and severely impaired quality of life. INS365 is in phase III trials for treatment of CF.

INDICATION(S) AND RESEARCH PHASE
Bronchitis – Phase I/II
Cystic Fibrosis – Phase II
Eye Disorders, Infections – Phase III

moxifloxacin
Avelox

MANUFACTURER
Bayer Corporation

DESCRIPTION
At the end of 1999, the FDA approved Bayer's respiratory antibiotic Avelox (moxifloxacin) for the treatment of acute exacerbations of chronic bronchitis, community-acquired pneumonias and acute sinusitis. The company is evaluating the drug in phase III trials for additional indications of respiratory tract infections and lung disease.

INDICATION(S) AND RESEARCH PHASE
Bacterial Infection – Phase III
Lung Disease – Phase III
Bronchitis – FDA approved
Pneumonia – FDA approved
Sinus Infection – FDA approved

vaccine, Pseudomonas infection
Pseudostat

MANUFACTURER
Provalis

DESCRIPTION
Pseudostat is an oral therapeutic vaccine against *Pseudomonas aeruginosa* infections in cystic fibrosis subjects and subjects with chronic bronchitis, bronchiectasis, and influenza. Phase II trials are being run in Australia. Pending their success, Provalis plans to initiate phase II trials in the United States, where it has been in discussion with the National Institutes of Health and the Cystic Fibrosis Foundation. In addition, the developer has filed for orphan drug designation in the United States.

INDICATION(S) AND RESEARCH PHASE
Bronchitis – Phase II
Bacterial Infection – Phase II
Cystic Fibrosis – Phase II
Influenza – Phase II
Vaccines – Phase II

vaccine, respiratory syncytial virus
unknown

MANUFACTURER
Aventis Pasteur

DESCRIPTION
Respiratory syncytial virus (RSV) is a common cause of winter outbreaks of acute respiratory disease. RSV is a common, but preventable cause of hospital-acquired infection. The source of this virus transmission may include other infected subjects, staff, and visitors.

Most severe manifestations of RSV infection, including pneumonia and bronchiolitis, occur in infants aged two to six months. However, children of any age with underlying cardiac or pulmonary disease, or who are immunocompromised, are at risk for serious complications from this infection. Because natural infection with RSV provides limited protective immunity, RSV causes repeated symptomatic infections. In adults, RSV usually causes upper respiratory tract manifestations, but may cause lower respiratory tract disease, especially in the elderly and in immunocompromised persons.

Aventis Pasteur has an RSV-mediated lower respiratory disease vaccination for at-risk children and the elderly being developed in phase I/II trials.

INDICATION(S) AND RESEARCH PHASE
Bronchitis – Phase I/II
Lung Disease – Phase I/II
Pediatric, Respiratory Syncytial Virus – Phase I/II
Pneumonia – Phase I/II
Vaccines – Phase I/II
Viral Infection – Phase I/II

Chronic Obstructive Pulmonary Disease (COPD)

albuterol
Ventolin

MANUFACTURER
GlaxoSmithKline

DESCRIPTION
Ventolin, a beta-2 agonist, is currently on the market in several formulations for the treatments of asthma and chronic obstructive pulmonary disease (COPD). The drug acts by relaxing the bronchial smooth muscle and inhibiting the release of immediate hypersensitivity mediators. Ventolin has received European Union (EU) approval for both indications in a formulation that uses non-CFC propellant (GR106642) in a metered dose inhaler. An approvable letter was received from the FDA in January 2001.

Ventolin has also received EU approval for the same indications via delivery by Diskus/Accuhaler, a dry powder inhaler. An FDA approvable letter was received in July 2000.

INDICATION(S) AND RESEARCH PHASE
Asthma – FDA recommend approval letter
Chronic Obstructive Pulmonary Disease (COPD) – FDA recommend approval letter

AR-C68397AA
Viozan

MANUFACTURER
AstraZeneca

DESCRIPTION
Viozan is a novel dual D_2 dopamine receptor, beta-2-adrenoceptor agonist, which stimulates dopamine receptors on afferent nerves in the lung, leading to the suppression of sensory nerve activity. This reduces reflex-induced symptoms such as coughing, sputum, and shortness of breath. Phase II trials showed statistically significant improvement in relief of symptoms in subjects with chronic obstructive pulmonary disease (COPD). Viozan is currently in phase III trials in both the United States and Europe.

INDICATION(S) AND RESEARCH PHASE
Chronic Obstructive Pulmonary Disease (COPD) – Phase III

AR-C89855
unknown

MANUFACTURER
AstraZeneca

DESCRIPTION
AR-C89855 is a dual dopamine beta-2 agonist indicated for the treatment of chronic obstructive pulmonary disease (COPD). It is currently in phase I trials.

INDICATION(S) AND RESEARCH PHASE
Chronic Obstructive Pulmonary Disease (COPD) – Phase I

DNK 333
unknown

MANUFACTURER
Novartis

DESCRIPTION
DNK 333 is a dual NK_1/NK_2 antagonist being developed in an oral formulation. It is in phase II development for rhinitis, asthma, and chronic obstructive pulmonary disease.

INDICATION(S) AND RESEARCH PHASE
Asthma – Phase II
Rhinitis – Phase II
Chronic Obstructive Pulmonary Disease (COPD) – Phase II

fluticasone propionate
Flixotide, Flovent

MANUFACTURER
GlaxoSmithKline

DESCRIPTION
Flovent is an inhaled glucocorticoid being developed for the treatment of asthma. While the precise mechanism of action of glucocorticoid is unknown, these steroids demonstrate anti-inflammatory influences on multiple cell types and mediator production or secretion involved in the asthmatic response.

This drug is being developed in the United States as Flovent and internationally as Flixotide. It is in phase III trials in the United States for the treatment of asthma, in a once-daily dosing formulation. The drug received European Union (EU) approval for the treatment of chronic obstructive pulmonary disease (COPD) in September 1999, as well as for both asthma and COPD in a formulation that uses non-CFC propellant (GR 106642) in a metered dose inhaler. Flovent has been FDA approved for use in inhaled corticosteroid, CFC propellant, and Diskus/Accuhaler (dry powder) formulations.

INDICATION(S) AND RESEARCH PHASE
Asthma – Phase III
Chronic Obstructive Pulmonary Disease (COPD) – Phase EU approved
Asthma – Phase EU approved
Asthma – FDA approved
Pediatric – Phase

formoterol
Budoxis, Oxis

MANUFACTURER
AstraZeneca

DESCRIPTION
Otis combines a long-acting beta-2 agonist, formoterol, with budesonide, an inhaled glucocorticoid. Formoterol has been approved by the FDA for use in the Oxis Turbuhaler, which administers the drug through a multi-dose dry powder inhalation device. Clinical documentation of the Oxis Turbuhaler demonstrated the combination of a rapid onset of symptom relief and long-lasting bronchodilation.

The Oxis Turbuhaler is currently in three phase III trials for treatment of asthma, both in children and adults, and for chronic obstructive pulmonary disease (COPD).

INDICATION(S) AND RESEARCH PHASE
Asthma – Phase III
Chronic Obstructive Pulmonary Disease (COPD) – Phase III
Pediatric, asthma – Phase III

GW 328267
unknown

MANUFACTURER
GlaxoSmithKline

DESCRIPTION
GW 328267 is an adenosine A2 agonist. It is currently in phase I development for the treatment of asthma and chronic obstructive pulmonary disease (COPD).

INDICATION(S) AND RESEARCH PHASE
Asthma – Phase I
Chronic Obstructive Pulmonary Disease (COPD) – Phase I

HP-3
unknown

MANUFACTURER
Milkhaus Laboratory

DESCRIPTION
HP-3 is a nucleic acid medication in an oral formulation. It is a novel therapeutic agent being tested in phase II and III trials for the treatment of chronic bronchitis (CB), chronic obstructive pulmonary disease (COPD), and cystic fibrosis (CF). HP-3 is also being tested in pediatric subjects, ages six to 21 years old.

Results from a phase II trial for CF showed significant improvement in pulmonary function and an increase in sputum clearance.

Results for all three indications showed that HP-3 increased sputum expectoration and significantly improved pulmonary function. The company believes that the drug evokes such responses through a mechanism common to all three diseases. Consequently, HP-3 may have a broad potential utility in relieving the debilitating symptoms of respiratory distress, which afflict more than 15 million subjects.

INDICATION(S) AND RESEARCH PHASE
Bronchitis – Phase III
Chronic Obstructive Pulmonary Disease (COPD) – Phase II
Cystic Fibrosis – Phase II completed
Pediatric, Cystic Fibrosis – Phase II completed

LTB 019
unknown

MANUFACTURER
Novartis

DESCRIPTION
LTB 019 is a leukotriene B4 antagonist being developed in an oral formulation. It is in phase II trials for the treatment of chronic obstructive pulmonary disease.

INDICATION(S) AND RESEARCH PHASE
Chronic Obstructive Pulmonary Disease (COPD) – Phase II

oxandrolone, CO221
unknown

MANUFACTURER
Bio-Technology General

DESCRIPTION
CO221 is an anabolic steroid for treatment of chronic obstructive pulmonary disease (COPD) and pressure ulcers. The drug, in oral tablet formulation, is being developed in phase II trials.

INDICATION(S) AND RESEARCH PHASE
Chronic Obstructive Pulmonary Disease (COPD) – Phase II
Pressure Ulcers – Phase II

salmeterol xinafoate
Serevent

MANUFACTURER
GlaxoSmithKline

DESCRIPTION
Serevent is a beta-2 agonist for the treatment of asthma and chronic obstructive pulmonary disease (COPD). The drug is thought to stimulate intracellular adenyl cyclase, the enzyme that catalyzes the conversion of adenosine triphosphate (ATP) to cyclic C-3',5'-adenosine monophosphate (cyclic AMP). Increased cyclic AMP levels cause relaxation of bronchial smooth muscle and inhibit release of mediators of immediate hypersensitivity from cells.

The drug is in phase III trials for the treatment of asthma and COPD in a formulation that uses non-CFC propellant (GR106642) in a metered dose inhaler. Additionally, Serevent is in phase III trials for COPD with delivery via Diskus/Accuhaler, a dry powder inhaler.

INDICATION(S) AND RESEARCH PHASE
Asthma – Phase III
Chronic Obstructive Pulmonary Disease (COPD) – Phase III

salmeterol/fluticasone propionate
Seretide, Advair

MANUFACTURER
GlaxoSmithKline

DESCRIPTION
Seretide is a combination therapy consisting of a beta-2 agonist and a synthetic glucocorticoid with potent anti-inflammatory activity. The beta-2 agonist is thought to stimulate intracellular adenyl cyclase, the enzyme that catalyzes the conversion of adenosine triphosphate (ATP) to cyclic C-3',5'-adenosine monophosphate (cyclic AMP). Increased cyclic AMP causes relaxation of bronchial smooth muscle and inhibits the release of mediators of immediate hypersensitivity.

While the precise mechanism of glucocorticoid action in asthma is unknown, they have been shown to inhibit many types of cells and mediator production, or secretion, involved in the asthmatic response. These anti-inflammatory actions may contribute to the efficacy of glucocorticoids in asthma.

Seretide has received European Union (EU) approval for the treatment of pediatric asthma using the Diskus/Accuhaler dry powder inhaler. An NDA has been submitted for the CFC-free formulation for the treatment of adult asthma. Seretide is also in phase III trials for the treatment of COPD and as a first-line therapy for asthma via delivery by the Diskus/Accuhaler inhaler. Seretide is being developed under the trade name Advair in the United States.

INDICATION(S) AND RESEARCH PHASE
Pediatric, Asthma – Phase EU approved
Chronic Obstructive Pulmonary Disease (COPD) – Phase III
Asthma – NDA submitted

SB 207499
Ariflo

MANUFACTURER
GlaxoSmithKline

DESCRIPTION

DESCRIPTION

Ariflo, a novel oral phosphodiesterase (PDE)-IV inhibitor, is being developed for the treatment of chronic obstructive pulmonary disease (COPD) and asthma. The company claims that clinical trials thus far suggest that Ariflo significantly improved lung function in subjects with moderate-to-severe COPD. It also improved exercise tolerance, which enhances the ability to perform activities of daily living. The drug is in phase II trials for the treatment of asthma and phase III trials for COPD.

INDICATION(S) AND RESEARCH PHASE
Chronic Obstructive Pulmonary Disease (COPD) – Phase III
Asthma – Phase II

SB 223412
unknown

MANUFACTURER
GlaxoSmithKline

DESCRIPTION
SB 223412 is a tachykinin (NK$_3$) receptor antagonist. It is currently in phase I development for the treatment of urinary incontinence and chronic obstructive pulmonary disease (COPD).

INDICATION(S) AND RESEARCH PHASE
Urinary Incontinence – Phase I
Chronic Obstructive Pulmonary Disease (COPD) – Phase I

TBC-11251
unknown

MANUFACTURER
Texas Biotechnology

DESCRIPTION
TBC-11251 is a small molecule that blocks the endothelin-A receptor. This drug is being evaluated in a phase II trial for the treatment of congestive heart failure and pulmonary hypertension associated with chronic obstructive pulmonary disease (COPD) or primary pulmonary hypertension. It is in an oral formulation.

INDICATION(S) AND RESEARCH PHASE
Congestive Heart Failure – Phase II
Chronic Obstructive Pulmonary Disease (COPD) – Phase II
Lung Disease – Phase II

ThGRF 1-44
unknown

MANUFACTURER
Theratechnologies

DESCRIPTION
ThGRF 1-44 is a growth hormone releasing factor analogue indicated for the treatment of chronic obstructive pulmonary disease (COPD) and sleep impairment. The drug is currently being developed in phase II trials.

INDICATION(S) AND RESEARCH PHASE
Chronic Obstructive Pulmonary Disease (COPD) – Phase II
Sleep Disorders – Phase II

unknown
Symbicort Turbuhaler

MANUFACTURER
AstraZeneca

DESCRIPTION
Symbicort Turbuhaler is an inhaled steroid indicated for the treatment of asthma and chronic obstructive pulmonary disease (COPD). The drug is a long-acting formulation of a beta-2 agonist and is currently in phase III trials.

INDICATION(S) AND RESEARCH PHASE
Asthma – Phase III
Chronic Obstructive Pulmonary Disease (COPD) – Phase III

unknown
Symbicort pMDI

MANUFACTURER
AstraZeneca

DESCRIPTION
Symbicort pMDI is an inhaled steroid indicated for the treatment of asthma and chronic obstructive pulmonary disease (COPD). The drug is a long-acting formulation of a beta-2 agonist. It is currently in development in phase I trials.

INDICATION(S) AND RESEARCH PHASE
Asthma – Phase I
Chronic Obstructive Pulmonary Disease (COPD) – Phase I

ZD-8321
unknown

MANUFACTURER
AstraZeneca

DESCRIPTION
ZD-8321 is a new drug under development for treatment of chronic obstructive pulmonary disease (COPD) and acute respiratory distress syndrome (ARDS).

The lungs are composed of thousands of tiny air sacs, called alveoli, that function to oxygenate the blood from inspired air. In COPD and ARDS, the delicate walls of these alveoli are eroded away, resulting in less functional lung tissue. Because of fewer working alveoli, oxygen taken in cannot be transferred to the blood vessels, making the lungs more susceptible to infection and therefore requiring bronchodilators and oxygen for support.

In COPD and ARDS, the enzyme elastase is hyperstimulated by the toxins involved, from smoking in COPD and infection or trauma in ARDS. This enzyme destroys elastin and collagen, two proteins that are important structural components of lung tissue. Scientists believe that ZD-8321, which blocks the action of the elastase enzyme, may slow down or stop completely the destruction of lung tissue characteristic of both these conditions. ZD-8321 is an orally formulated drug that was being evaluated in phase II clinical trials for the treatment of ARDS and COPD. As of December 2000, the trials have been discontinued until further notice.

INDICATION(S) AND RESEARCH PHASE
Acute Respiratory Distress Syndrome (ARDS) – Phase III discontinued

Chronic Obstructive Pulmonary Disease (COPD) – Phase III discontinued

ZD4407
unknown

MANUFACTURER
AstraZeneca

DESCRIPTION
ZD4407 is a 5-lipoxygenase inhibitor indicated for the treatment of chronic obstructive pulmonary disease (COPD). It is currently in phase I trials.

INDICATION(S) AND RESEARCH PHASE
Chronic Obstructive Pulmonary Disease (COPD) – Phase I

Cystic Fibrosis

8-cyclopentyl 1,3-dipropylxanthine, CPX
unknown

MANUFACTURER
SciClone Pharmaceuticals

DESCRIPTION
CPX (8-cyclopentyl 1,3-dipropylxanthine) is an oral drug being tested in a phase II trial for cystic fibrosis (CF). The trial will enroll 50 subjects with mild to moderately severe CF at four centers. Subjects will receive an oral dose of CPX or placebo up to four times daily for one week. Trial results will be evaluated by the changes in the sweat chloride content and changes in nasal epithelial transmembrane potential difference (NEPD). The measurement of sweat chloride content is currently the standard diagnostic test for CF.

INDICATION(S) AND RESEARCH PHASE
Cystic Fibrosis – Phase II

alfa inhalation solution
unknown

MANUFACTURER
Aradigm Corporation

DESCRIPTION
Dornase alfa is a recombinant human protein that received its first marketing approval by the FDA in December 1993 for the management of cystic fibrosis (CF), to improve lung function. Currently, phase IIa trials for alfa inhalation solution are studying the effects of dornase alfa administration using Aradigm's patented AERx Pulmonary Drug Delivery System, a broadly applicable technology platform that converts molecules into fine particle aerosols and deposits them deep into the lungs. It is expected that delivery of dornase alfa with the AERx System will provide similar clinical benefits to subjects with CF as with those documented using dornase alfa delivered via a nebulizer, but in significantly less time.

INDICATION(S) AND RESEARCH PHASE
Cystic Fibrosis – Phase IIa

alpha-1 antitrypsin (AAT)
unknown

MANUFACTURER
PPL Therapeutics plc

DESCRIPTION
Alpha-1-antitrypsin (AAT), an alpha-1-protease inhibitor, is a human blood protein whose prime physiological target is neutrophil elastase. AAT is in phase II trials for cystic fibrosis.

Many respiratory diseases, including cystic fibrosis, create an imbalance of AAT elastase in the lung. An abundance of elastase is thought to contribute to damage of the pulmonary epithelium. AAT supplements may eliminate some of the surplus.

INDICATION(S) AND RESEARCH PHASE
Cystic Fibrosis – Phase II

CFTR, GR-213487B
unknown

MANUFACTURER
Valentis

DESCRIPTION
CFTR, a gene therapy for the treatment of cystic fibrosis, uses an aerosol-based delivery system as a carrier for the CFTR gene. This therapy is in a partnership between Valentis and GlaxoWellcome. The companies claim that results from a phase I/II clinical trial show the product to be safe and non-inflammatory. The decision to proceed to phase III trials is pending.

INDICATION(S) AND RESEARCH PHASE
Cystic Fibrosis – Phase I/II completed

gamma interferon
unknown

MANUFACTURER
InterMune Pharmaceuticals

DESCRIPTION
Gamma interferon is an immune system modulator formulated to help cystic fibrosis (CF) patients avoid progressive lung damage that can lead to respiratory failure. This novel inhaled therapy is being tested in a phase II trial in 60 CF patients at eight medical centers around the country. This trial is the first attempt to prevent lung damage by controlling the patients' immune response to infection. Researchers hope that gamma interferon will block the destructive cycle of infection and inflammation in the lungs of CF patients by simultaneously stimulating the infection-fighting properties of lung macrophages and suppressing the activity of neutrophils that cause airway inflammation and destruction.

INDICATION(S) AND RESEARCH PHASE
Cystic Fibrosis Phase II

HP-3
unknown

MANUFACTURER
Milkhaus Laboratory

DESCRIPTION
HP-3 is a nucleic acid medication in an oral formulation. It is a novel therapeutic agent being tested in phase II and III trials for the

treatment of chronic bronchitis (CB), chronic obstructive pulmonary disease (COPD), and cystic fibrosis (CF). HP-3 is also being tested in pediatric subjects, ages six to 21 years old.

Results from a phase II trial for CF showed significant improvement in pulmonary function and an increase in sputum clearance.

Results for all three indications showed that HP-3 increased sputum expectoration and significantly improved pulmonary function. The company believes that the drug evokes such responses through a mechanism common to all three diseases. Consequently, HP-3 may have a broad potential utility in relieving the debilitating symptoms of respiratory distress, which afflict more than 15 million subjects.

INDICATION(S) AND RESEARCH PHASE
Bronchitis – Phase III
Chronic Obstructive Pulmonary Disease (COPD) – Phase II
Cystic Fibrosis – Phase II completed
Pediatric, Cystic Fibrosis – Phase II completed

INS365
unknown

MANUFACTURER
Inspire Pharmaceuticals

DESCRIPTION
INS365 is a novel P2Y2-receptor stimulator, stabilized uridine nucleotide analogue, being developed for the treatment of acute and chronic lung diseases, such as chronic bronchitis (CB) and cystic fibrosis (CF). The drug hydrates and clears mucus from a subject's airways, principally by acting on the P2Y2 receptor.

A phase III trial for dry eye was initiated in January 2001 in approximately 1,000 subjects at 60 ophthalmology centers.

CB, caused primarily by smoking and pollution, involves excessive retention of mucus as well as inflamed airways leading to impaired mucociliary clearance and causing subjects to experience frequent respiratory infections. INS365 is in phase I/II trials for CB treatment.

CF is a disorder in which a genetic mutation in airway cells causes dehydrated secretions and production of thickened mucus and impaired mucociliary clearance. This plugging effect leads to frequent pulmonary infections and severely impaired quality of life. INS365 is in phase III trials for treatment of CF.

INDICATION(S) AND RESEARCH PHASE
Bronchitis – Phase I/II
Cystic Fibrosis – Phase II
Eye Disorders, Infections – Phase III

INS37217 respiratory
unknown

MANUFACTURER
Inspire Pharmaceuticals

DESCRIPTION
INS37217 respiratory is a second-generation P2Y(2) agonist being tested in a phase I clinical trial for cystic fibrosis (CF) in an inhalation formulation. INS37217 is designed to enhance the lung's innate mucosal hydration and mucociliary clearance mechanisms, which are seriously impaired in CF subjects due to genetic defect. Pre-clinical results demonstrated INS37217 respiratory has extended duration of action. Inspire Pharmaceuticals is co-developing the drug with Genentech.

In addition, a phase II/III trial is under way for testing INS37217 for the treatment of retinal detachment and retinal edema.

INDICATION(S) AND RESEARCH PHASE
Cystic Fibrosis – Phase I
Eye Disorders/Infections – Phase II/III

protegrin IB-367, aerosol
unknown

MANUFACTURER
IntraBiotics Pharmaceuticals

DESCRIPTION
Protegrin IB-367 is a synthetic antimicrobial peptide molecule that belongs to a new class of agents called protegrins. Studies suggest that protegrin IB-367 kills bacteria by integrating with and disrupting the integrity of bacterial cell membranes. This aerosol formulation is being tested in cystic fibrosis subjects with chronic respiratory infections. A phase I trial has been completed.

INDICATION(S) AND RESEARCH PHASE
Cystic Fibrosis – Phase I completed

tgAAV-CF
unknown

MANUFACTURER
Targeted Genetics

DESCRIPTION
tgAAV-CF is a gene therapy compound administered in an aerosol formulation. It is thought to decrease the amount of IL-8, an inflammatory cytokine, present in the lungs of cystic fibrosis (CF) subjects. A phase I trial was completed at the Stanford University Medical Center in collaboration with the Cystic Fibrosis Foundation's Therapeutics Development Network. The drug was well tolerated, with a greater distribution area than other formulations. A phase IIa trial was initiated November 2000 for adults. In addition, a phase II trial is testing tgAAV-CF in CF subjects 15 years and older. tgAAV-CF is being co-developed with Celltech Chiroscience plc.

INDICATION(S) AND RESEARCH PHASE
Cystic Fibrosis – Phase II a
Pediatric, Cystic Fibrosis – Phase II

tyloxapol
SuperVent

MANUFACTURER
Discovery Laboratories

DESCRIPTION
SuperVent Aerosol Solution is a potent antioxidant that has anti-inflammatory activity through the inhibition of NF-(Kappa)B. This drug reduces the viscosity of sputum. A phase IIa clinical trial will evaluate this triple mechanism of action in cystic fibrosis subjects and examine the benefits of SuperVent Aerosol Solution on pulmonary

function. In addition, a phase II trial is being run in pediatric subjects.

According to the company, SuperVent Aerosol Solution was shown to be safe and well tolerated at concentrations up to 1.25% in a phase I study with 20 subjects. The phase II trials are being conducted at the Intermountain Cystic Fibrosis Center at the University of Utah in Salt Lake City.

INDICATION(S) AND RESEARCH PHASE
Cystic Fibrosis – Phase IIa
Pediatric, Cystic Fibrosis – Phase II

Unknown
Merrem

MANUFACTURER
AstraZeneca

DESCRIPTION
Merrem is a carbepenem antibiotic currently involved in numerous phase III line extension studies. The indications being tested include hospital- and community-acquired pneumonia, cystic fibrosis, skin and soft tissue infections, abdominal infections, and for use in neutropenics.

INDICATION(S) AND RESEARCH PHASE
Skin Infections/Disorders – Phase III
Cystic Fibrosis – Phase III
Pneumonia – Phase III
Neutropenics – Phase III
Abdominal Infections – Phase III

vaccine, Pseudomonas infection
Pseudostat

MANUFACTURER
Provalis

DESCRIPTION
Pseudostat is an oral therapeutic vaccine against *Pseudomonas aeruginosa* infections in cystic fibrosis subjects and subjects with chronic bronchitis, bronchiectasis, and influenza. Phase II trials are being run in Australia. Pending their success, Provalis plans to initiate phase II trials in the United States, where it has been in discussion with the National Institutes of Health and the Cystic Fibrosis Foundation. In addition, the developer has filed for orphan drug designation in the United States.

INDICATION(S) AND RESEARCH PHASE
Bronchitis – Phase II
Bacterial Infection – Phase II
Cystic Fibrosis – Phase II
Influenza – Phase II
Vaccines – Phase II

Emphysema

(R,R)-formoterol
unknown

MANUFACTURER
Sepracor

DESCRIPTION
(R,R)-formoterol is a single-isomer bronchdilator with a rapid onset of action. This drug is currently in phase IIb trials in subjects with asthma and emphysema.

INDICATION(S) AND RESEARCH PHASE
Asthma – Phase IIb
Emphysema – Phase IIb

alpha-1 proteinase inhibitor
unknown

MANUFACTURER
Alpha Therapeutic

DESCRIPTION
Alpha-1 proteinase inhibitor is a protein produced naturally in the body, primarily by liver cells but also by some white blood cells. It protects the lungs by blocking the effects of powerful enzymes called elastases. Elastase is normally carried in white blood cells and protects the delicate tissue of the lung by killing bacteria and neutralizing tiny particles inhaled into the lung. Once the protective work of this enzyme is finished, the alpha-1-proteinase inhibitor blocks further action by this enzyme. Without alpha-1-proteinase inhibitor, elastase can destroy the air sacs of the lung.

Some people inherit a certain combination of genes that are not able to produce adequate amounts of alpha-1-proteinase inhibitor. This may lead to damage to the lungs and liver, resulting in emphysema in the lungs, and cirrhosis in the liver. Phase III trials evaluating the effect of administering alpha-1-proteinase to subjects with hereditary emphysema who have inherited this gene deficiency are being conducted.

INDICATION(S) AND RESEARCH PHASE
Emphysema – Phase III
Liver Disease – Phase III

alpha-1-proteinase inhibitor
unknown

MANUFACTURER
Aventis

DESCRIPTION
Alpha-1-proteinase inhibitor is a gene therapy being developed for the treatment of alpha-1 antitrypsin deficiency, a rare condition that can cause hereditary emphysema. This condition occurs when an individual is unable to neutralize the leukocytic proteolytic enzymes that are associated with inflammation of lung tissue. The drug, in an intravenous formulation, was in phase III trials for the treatment of emphysema. Development has been discontinued.

INDICATION(S) AND RESEARCH PHASE
Emphysema – Phase III discontinued

Hyponatremia

YM-087, conivaptan
unknown

MANUFACTURER
Yamanouchi Pharmaceutical

DESCRIPTION
YM-087 is a receptor antagonist to the peptide hormone vasopressin, which is released by the hypothalamus to regulate water balance in the body. The drug is currently in phase III trials for the treatment of hyponatremia, and phase II trials for the treatment

of heart failure. It is being developed in both Europe and the United States. The drug is also part of Yamanouchi's domestic pipeline; YM-087 is in phase II trials for both hyponatremia and heart failure. YM-087 is manufactured in oral and injectable formulations.

INDICATION(S) AND RESEARCH PHASE
Congestive Heart Failure (United States and Japan) – Phase II
Hyponatremia (United States) – Phase III
Hyponatremia (Japan) – Phase II

Influenza

adjuvanted influenza
Fluad

MANUFACTURER
Chiron Corporation

DESCRIPTION
Fluad is a vaccine for the prevention of influenza that incorporates Chiron's proprietary adjuvant MF59. Filing has already taken place in Italy.

INDICATION(S) AND RESEARCH PHASE
Influenza – NDA submitted (Italy)

RWJ 241947
unknown

MANUFACTURER
R.W. Johnson Pharmaceutical Research Institute

DESCRIPTION
RWJ 241947 is in phase III clinical trials for the treatment of influenza.

INDICATION(S) AND RESEARCH PHASE
Influenza – Phase II

RWJ 270201
unknown

MANUFACTURER
R.W. Johnson Pharmaceutical Research Institute

DESCRIPTION
RWJ 270201 is in phase III trials for the treatment of influenza.

INDICATION(S) AND RESEARCH PHASE
Influenza – Phase III

unknown
FluMist

MANUFACTURER
Wyeth-Ayerst

DESCRIPTION
FluMist is an investigational cold-adapted intranasal influenza vaccine. It is designed to induce immunity via the nasal mucosa in pediatric subjects. In October 2000, Aviron and American Home Products Corporation announced that a Biologics License Application for FluMist has been submitted to the FDA. Wyeth-Ayerst is the pharmaceutical division of American Home Products.

INDICATION(S) AND RESEARCH PHASE
Influenza – Phase III
Vaccines – Phase III
Pediatric, Influenza – Phase III

vaccine, DPT/ Haemophilus influenzae type B
unknown

MANUFACTURER
Chiron Corporation

DESCRIPTION
Chiron Corporation has formulated a combination vaccine to immunize children against *Haemophilus influenzae* type B, diphtheria, pertussis, and tetanus in a single injection formulation. This vaccine has the potential to simplify pediatric vaccination schedules, thereby lowering costs, increasing convenience and improving compliance. The vaccine is composed of inactive molecules of diphtheria toxin, pertussis toxin, and tetanus toxin. Toxins are the destructive molecules that cause most of the pathology seen in these diseases. The vaccine also contains inactivated *H. influenzae* proteins.

This combination vaccine, given as an intramuscular injection, is currently in phase III trials.

INDICATION(S) AND RESEARCH PHASE
Pediatric, Bacterial Infection – Phase III
Pediatric, Influenza – Phase III
Pediatric, Bacterial Infection, Influenza, Viral Infection – Phase III
Pediatric, Vaccines – Phase III
Pediatric, Viral Infection – Phase III

vaccine, influenza
unknown

MANUFACTURER
GlaxoSmithKline

DESCRIPTION
This new delivery, subunit vaccine is being developed for influenza prophylaxis. It is currently in phase I development.

INDICATION(S) AND RESEARCH PHASE
Influenza – Phase I
Vaccines – Phase I

vaccine, influenza
unknown

MANUFACTURER
BioChem Pharma

DESCRIPTION
Currently, the best weapon against the influenza virus is an annual vaccination. However, since the vaccine is administered as an injection, many needle-shy people avoid being vaccinated. The decision not to be immunized due to discomfort from intramuscular injection results in much unnecessary and preventable illness each year.

In order to improve vaccination rates, BioChem Pharma is developing an influenza vaccine to be taken as a nasal spray. This method of vaccination may create a helpful systemic immune response in the blood and throughout the body, and may stimulate a local immune response in the mucosal lining of the nose, mouth, and throat, which would create an additional barrier to influenza infection and increase efficacy. Phase I results have shown comparable immunization responses to that of the injectable vaccine. Clinical testing is in phase II for the influenza virus in both children and adults.

INDICATION(S) AND RESEARCH PHASE
Influenza – Phase II
Vaccines – Phase II
Pediatric, Influenza – Phase II

vaccine, nasal proteosome influenza
unknown

MANUFACTURER
Intellivax International

DESCRIPTION
Nasal proteosome influenza vaccine is a nasally administered vaccine that may provide mucosal as well as systemic immunity to the influenza virus. This could offer people more effective protection against the virus than the standard injectable flu vaccine. A phase I trial is comparing this novel nasal vaccine to the standard injectable vaccine. Preclinical studies demonstrated the nasal proteosome flu vaccine to induce high levels of antibodies in serum and lung and nasal mucosal secretions. It has also protected animals in experimental models of influenza disease.

INDICATION(S) AND RESEARCH PHASE
Influenza – Phase I
Vaccine – Phase I

vaccine, parainfluenza
unknown

MANUFACTURER
Wyeth-Lederle Vaccines

DESCRIPTION
This product is a novel vaccine for prevention of parainfluenza virus (PIV), a mediated serious respiratory illness in children. The vaccine is made from live attenuated influenza A virus and is administered as a nasal spray. These live attenuated vaccines stimulate local antibody production more efficiently than conventional inactivated vaccines. The drug is in phase II testing in adults and phase I/II in infants and toddlers.

INDICATION(S) AND RESEARCH PHASE
Influenza – Phase II
Pediatric, Influenza – Phase I/II

vaccine, Pseudomonas infection
Pseudostat

MANUFACTURER
Provalis

DESCRIPTION
Pseudostat is an oral therapeutic vaccine against *Pseudomonas aeruginosa* infections in cystic fibrosis subjects and subjects with chronic bronchitis, bronchiectasis, and influenza. Phase II trials are being run in Australia. Pending their success, Provalis plans to initiate phase II trials in the United States, where it has been in discussion with the National Institutes of Health and the Cystic Fibrosis Foundation. In addition, the developer has filed for orphan drug designation in the United States.

INDICATION(S) AND RESEARCH PHASE
Bronchitis – Phase II
Bacterial Infection – Phase II
Cystic Fibrosis – Phase II
Influenza – Phase II
Vaccines – Phase II

zanamivir
Relenza

MANUFACTURER
GlaxoSmithKline

DESCRIPTION
Relenza (zanamivir) is an anti-viral drug for the treatment of influenza. The proposed mechanism of action of Relenza is via inhibition of influenza virus neuraminidase with the possibility of alteration of virus particle aggregation and release. The FDA has approved Relenza for persons ages seven years and older for the treatment of uncomplicated influenza virus. This product is approved to treat type A and B influenza, the two types most responsible for flu epidemics. It is also in phase III trials for the additional indications of influenza prophylaxis and influenza treatment in subjects with asthma and chronic obstructive pulmonary disease.

INDICATION(S) AND RESEARCH PHASE
Influenza – Phase III
Influenza – FDA approved

Lung Disease

moxifloxacin
Avelox

MANUFACTURER
Bayer Corporation

DESCRIPTION
At the end of 1999, the FDA approved Bayer's respiratory antibiotic Avelox (moxifloxacin) for the treatment of acute exacerbations of chronic bronchitis, community-acquired pneumonia, and acute sinusitis. The company is evaluating the drug in phase III trials for additional indications of respiratory tract infections and lung disease.

INDICATION(S) AND RESEARCH PHASE
Bacterial Infection – Phase III
Lung Disease – Phase III
Bronchitis – FDA approved
Pneumonia – FDA approved
Sinus Infection – FDA approved

poloxamer 188 N.F., CRL-5861
Flocor

MANUFACTURER
CytRx Corporation

DESCRIPTION
Flocor is an injectable drug that may improve blood flow. It is a type of surfactant, a purified form of poloxamer 188, non-ionic copolymer, which is a surface-active agent, like soap, that helps reduce sur-

face tension on blood cells to keep fluids flowing.

Flocor is in a phase I/II study in subjects with acute lung injury. This clinical trial is being conducted at Vanderbilt University Medical Center in Nashville, Tennessee. In acute lung injury, arterial and venous microvascular obstructions contribute to the severity of pulmonary dysfunction. Flocor is being evaluated for the prevention of secondary platelet aggregation and stasis-related capillary obstruction, and the development and propagation of dynamic blood clots, or thrombi.

Flocor is also being evaluated in a pivotal phase III study for the treatment of the acute painful crisis in sickle cell subjects ages ten and over, and a phase I study in sickle cell subjects with acute chest syndrome.

INDICATION(S) AND RESEARCH PHASE
Anemia – Phase III
Anemia – Phase I
Lung Disease – Phase I/II
Sickle Cell Disease – Phase I
Thrombosis – Phase I/II
Pediatric, Sickle Cell Disease – Phase III

ribavirin
Virazole

MANUFACTURER
ICN Pharmaceuticals

DESCRIPTION
Virazole (ribavirin) is a synthetic nucleoside analog with broad-spectrum antiviral activity. It is currently marketed by ICN in a variety of dosage forms for up to ten indications in 44 countries.

Virazole is in phase II trials for treatment of human papilloma virus and phase III trials for respiratory syncytial virus (RSV-BMT). In cell cultures, the inhibitory activity of ribavirin for respiratory syncytial virus is selective. The mechanism of action is unknown. Reversal of the invitro antiviral activity by guanosine or xanthosine suggests that ribavirin may act as an analogue of these cellular metabolites.

INDICATION(S) AND RESEARCH PHASE
Lung Disease – Phase III
Viral Infection, Human Papilloma Virus – Phase II
Viral Infection, Respiratory Syncytial Virus – Phase III

TBC-11251
unknown

MANUFACTURER
Texas Biotechnology

DESCRIPTION
TBC-11251 is a small molecule that blocks the endothelin-A receptor. This drug is being evaluated in a phase II trial for the treatment of congestive heart failure and pulmonary hypertension associated with chronic obstructive pulmonary disease (COPD) or primary pulmonary hypertension. It is in an oral formulation.

INDICATION(S) AND RESEARCH PHASE
Congestive Heart Failure – Phase II
Chronic Obstructive Pulmonary Disease (COPD) – Phase II
Lung Disease – Phase II

vaccine, respiratory syncytial virus
unknown

MANUFACTURER
Aventis Pasteur

DESCRIPTION
Respiratory syncytial virus (RSV) is a common cause of winter outbreaks of acute respiratory disease. RSV is a common, but preventable cause of hospital-acquired infection. The source of this virus transmission may include other infected subjects, staff, and visitors.

Most severe manifestations of RSV infection, including pneumonia and bronchiolitis, occur in infants aged two to six months. However, children of any age with underlying cardiac or pulmonary disease, or who are immunocompromised, are at risk for serious complications from this infection. Because natural infection with RSV provides limited protective immunity, RSV causes repeated symptomatic infections. In adults, RSV usually causes upper respiratory tract manifestations, but may cause lower respiratory tract disease, especially in the elderly and in immunocompromised persons.

Aventis Pasteur has a RSV-mediated lower respiratory disease vaccination for at-risk children and the elderly being developed in phase I/II trials.

INDICATION(S) AND RESEARCH PHASE
Bronchitis – Phase I/II
Lung Disease – Phase I/II
Pediatric, respiratory syncytial virus – Phase I/II
Pneumonia – Phase I/II
Vaccines – Phase I/II
Viral Infection – Phase I/II

Pneumonia

amikacin
Mikasome

MANUFACTURER
Gilead Sciences

DESCRIPTION
Mikasome, an aminoglycoside antibiotic, is in phase II trials for treatment of serious bacterial and mycobacterial infections including nosocomial *Pseudomonas* pneumonia, complicated urinary tract infections, and *Pseudomonas*-colonized subjects with cystic fibrosis. The drug is delivered in a liposomal formulation.

INDICATION(S) AND RESEARCH PHASE
Bacterial Infection – Phase II
Pneumonia – Phase II
Urinary Tract Infections – Phase II

cefditoren pivoxil
unknown

MANUFACTURER
Abbott Laboratories

DESCRIPTION
Cefditoren pivoxil is an advanced genera-

tion oral cephalosporin that has a broad spectrum of activity against gram-positive and gram-negative pathogens. It is being tested in phase III trials as a first-line agent for pneumonia in adults and children.

INDICATION(S) AND RESEARCH PHASE
Pneumonia – Phase III
Pediatric, Pneumonia – Phase III

DB-289
unknown

MANUFACTURER
Immtech International/NextEra Therapeutics

DESCRIPTION
DB-289 is currently in development for the treatment of *Pneumocystis carinii* pneumonia (PCP) and trypanosomiasis. DB-289 is effective due to neutralized positive charges that enable it to cross the digestive membranes. Once DB-289 enters the circulatory system, naturally occurring enzymes remove the patented masking or neutralizing charges, to expose the active drug. The drug is in a phase I trial in Germany, consisting of 54 subjects who will be given a single dose of DB-289. In the second part of the trial, which will be the last four weeks, subjects will receive multiple doses. The company has hired Parexel International to manage the study in Berlin.

INDICATION(S) AND RESEARCH PHASE
Pneumonia – Phase I/II
Trypanosomiasis – Phase I/II

HMR-3647, RU-64,004
unknown

MANUFACTURER
Aventis

DESCRIPTION
HMR-3647 is an anti-infective drug that was being tested against a broad range of bacteria, including drug-resistant, susceptible strains of *Streptococcus pneumoniae* and other common pathogens. The company reported that development on this antibiotic was discontinued.

INDICATION(S) AND RESEARCH PHASE
Bacterial Infection – Phase discontinued
Pneumonia – Phase discontinued

MK-826, carbepenem
unknown

MANUFACTURER
Merck & Co.

DESCRIPTION
MK-826 is a broad-spectrum antibiotic being developed in phase III trials for the treatment of bacterial infections including pneumonia, intra-abdominal infections, skin and skin structure infections, urinary tract infection, and obstetric and gynecologic infections.

INDICATION(S) AND RESEARCH PHASE
Pneumonia – Phase III
Skin Infections/Disorders – Phase III
Urinary Tract Infections – Phase III
Gynecologic Infections – Phase III
Bacterial Infection – Phase III
Gastrointestinal Diseases and Disorders, miscellaneous – Phase III

moxifloxacin
Avelox

MANUFACTURER
Bayer Corporation

DESCRIPTION
At the end of 1999, the FDA approved Bayer's respiratory antibiotic Avelox (moxifloxacin) for the treatment of acute exacerbations of chronic bronchitis, community-acquired pneumonia, and acute sinusitis. The company is evaluating the drug in phase III trials for additional indications of respiratory tract infections and lung disease.

INDICATION(S) AND RESEARCH PHASE
Bacterial Infection – Phase III
Lung Disease – Phase III
Bronchitis – FDA approved
Pneumonia – FDA approved
Sinus Infection – FDA approved

opebecan, rBPI-21, recombinant human bactericidal/permeability-increasing protein
Neuprex

MANUFACTURER
XOMA Corporation

DESCRIPTION
Neuprex is a systemic formulation of recombinant bactericidal/permeability-increasing protein rBPI-21, being developed for the treatment of severe meningococcemia, a rare systemic gram-negative bacterial infection that primarily affects children. After entering the bloodstream, the harmful bacteria attack the brain and spinal cord's protective sheathing. The gram-negative bacteria, called *Neisseria meningitidis*, cause meningococcemia and produce spiking high fever and a classic rigid stiff neck. Shock and death may occur in just a few hours after infection.

The active molecule in Neuprex, rBPI-21, binds to the endotoxin molecules LOS and LPS, lipopolysaccharides in living bacteria, disrupting their cell walls, killing the bacteria, or making them more susceptible to antibiotics. Phase III data were released in September 2000 from both pediatric and adult trials.

A 1650 subject phase III trauma trial evaluating whether Neuprex can prevent pneumonia and acute respiratory distress syndrome (ARDS) is under way. Subjects are enrolled after experiencing a severe accident, in which they have lost at least two units of blood. More than 800 subjects are currently enrolled. Supporting this study was a previous 401 subject phase II trial, with the results published in the *Journal of Trauma* in April 1999.

Acute intra-abdominal infection is another potential use for Neuprex, in combination with other antibiotics. The drug is currently in phase I/II trials for this indication.

A phase II trial is currently enrolling subjects who have had part of their liver removed during surgery. Neuprex may prevent post-surgical infection and complications.

INDICATION(S) AND RESEARCH PHASE

Bacterial Infection – Phase III completed
Pediatric, Bacterial Infection -
 Meningococcemia – Phase III completed
Meningitis – Phase III
Acute Respiratory Distress Syndrome
 (ARDS) – Phase III
Pneumonia – Phase III
Liver Disease – Phase II
Intra-abdominal Infection – Phase I/II

protegrin IB-367, rinse, gel
unknown

MANUFACTURER
IntraBiotics Pharmaceuticals

DESCRIPTION
Protegrin IB-367 is a synthetic antimicrobial peptide molecule that belongs to a new class of agents, called protegrins. Studies suggest that Protegrin IB-367 kills bacteria by integrating with and disrupting the integrity of bacterial cell membranes. The antibiotic has a broad spectrum of microbicidal activity against gram-positive and gram-negative bacteria that are frequent pathogens in ventilator-associated pneumonia.

Results of a single-dose phase I trial indicate that protegrin IB-367 safely reduces bacterial levels in the mouths of subjects at risk of experiencing ventilator-associated pneumonia. A rinse and gel formulation of protegrin IB-367 was topically applied to the mouth to reduce the number of oral and oropharyngeal bacteria in intubated subjects. A single administration of 9 mg of the rinse formulation more safely and rapidly reduced the total bacteria in orally intubated subjects compared to placebo. The magnitude and duration of effect after a single 9 mg dose of Protegrin IB-367 rinse similar to the response measured after a single 30 mg dose. In November 2000, IntraBiotics began subject enrollment for a phase IIa trial.

The rinse formulation of Protegrin IB-367 is also undergoing evaluation in two phase III trials for the prevention of oral mucositis. As of February 2001, one trial had completed enrollment of subjects receiving high-dose chemotherapy, while the other continues to enroll subjects receiving radiotherapy.

INDICATION(S) AND RESEARCH PHASE
Effects of Chemotherapy – Phase III
Bacterial Infection – Phase IIa
Pneumonia – Phase IIa

quinupristin/dalfopristin
Synercid

MANUFACTURER
Aventis

DESCRIPTION
Synercid is a combination therapy of two semi-synthetic antibacterial agents, quinupristin and dalfopristin. The antibiotic blocks bacterial protein synthesis.

Synercid has been FDA approved for the treatment of bloodstream infections due to vancomycin-resistant *Enterococcus faecium* (VREF) and skin and skin structure infections (SSTI) caused by methicillin-susceptible *Staphylococcus aureus* or *Streptococcus pyogenes*. Synercid is in intravenous formulation. It is currently in pediatric trials for pneumonia.

INDICATION(S) AND RESEARCH PHASE
Bacterial Infection – FDA approved
Skin Infections/Disorders – FDA approved
Pediatric, Pneumonia – Phase III
Pneumonia – Phase III

unknown
Merrem

MANUFACTURER
AstraZeneca

DESCRIPTION
Merrem is a carbepenem antibiotic currently involved in numerous phase III line extension studies. The indications being tested include hospital and community acquired pneumonia, cystic fibrosis, skin and soft tissue infections, abdominal infections, and for use in neutropenics.

INDICATION(S) AND RESEARCH PHASE
Skin Infections/Disorders – Phase III
Cystic Fibrosis – Phase III
Pneumonia – Phase III
Neutropenics – Phase III
Abdominal Infections – Phase III

vaccine, pneumococcal infections
Quilimmune-P

MANUFACTURER
Aquila Biopharmaceuticals

DESCRIPTION
Quilimmune-P is designed to enhance the immune response to *Streptococcus pneumoniae*, a prominent bacterial pathogen, and to provide improved protection in the elderly against diseases such as pneumonia, bacteremia, and meningitis.

A phase IIb study involves 30 elderly subjects who have received a single immunization of Quilimmune-P in the previous phase IIa trial. The subjects will receive a second immunization of Quilimmune-P approximately 12 months after the first to evaluate the persistence of the immune response.

INDICATION(S) AND RESEARCH PHASE
Pneumonia – Phase IIb
Vaccines – Phase IIb

vaccine, respiratory syncytial virus
unknown

MANUFACTURER
Aventis Pasteur

DESCRIPTION
Respiratory syncytial virus (RSV) is a common cause of winter outbreaks of acute respiratory disease. RSV is a common, but preventable cause of hospital-acquired infection. The source of this virus transmission may include other infected subjects, staff, and visitors.

Most severe manifestations of RSV infection with RSV, including pneumonia and bronchiolitis, occur in infants aged two to six months. However, children of any age with underlying cardiac or pulmonary disease, or who are immunocompromised, are at risk for serious complications from this infection. Because natural infection with RSV provides limited protective immunity,

RSV causes repeated symptomatic infections. In adults, RSV usually causes upper respiratory tract manifestations, but may cause lower respiratory tract disease, especially in the elderly and in immunocompromised persons.

Aventis Pasteur has an RSV-mediated lower respiratory disease vaccination for at-risk children and the elderly being developed in phase I/II trials.

INDICATION(S) AND RESEARCH PHASE
Bronchitis – Phase I/II
Lung Disease – Phase I/II
Pediatric, Respiratory Syncytial Virus – Phase I/II
Pneumonia – Phase I/II
Vaccines – Phase I/II
Viral Infection – Phase I/II

Pulmonary Fibrosis

interferon, beta-1a
Avonex

MANUFACTURER
Biogen

DESCRIPTION
Interferons are proteins naturally produced by the body to help fight viral infections and regulate the immune system. Avonex is a biosynthetic compound that contains the same arrangement of amino acids as the interferon beta-1a produced by the body. It is believed that Avonex regulates the body's immune response to decrease an attack against myelin, a possible mechanism for the nervous system destruction caused by multiple sclerosis (MS).

Approved by the FDA for the treatment of relapsing forms of MS, Avonex is currently in phase II trials for the treatment of brain cancer and idiopathic pulmonary fibrosis (IPF). For IPF, treatment is aimed at minimizing the disease progression from inflammation to fibrosis.

In January 2001, results of a phase III trial of Avonex for the treatment of secondary progressive MS demonstrated that the drug reduced the progression of disability by 27% versus treatment with placebo.

IMPACT (International Multiple Sclerosis Secondary Progressive Avonex Controlled Trial) was a randomized, double-blind, placebo-controlled trial involving 436 subjects at 42 sites in the United States, Canada, and Europe.

INDICATION(S) AND RESEARCH PHASE
Pulmonary Fibrosis – Phase II
Brain Cancer – Phase II
Multiple Sclerosis, Secondary Progressive – Phase III
Multiple Sclerosis – FDA approved

pirfenidone
Deskar

MANUFACTURER
Marnac

DESCRIPTION
Deskar is a broad-spectrum anti-fibrotic drug being tested in clinical trials for treatment of fibrotic conditions. These diseases include pulmonary fibrosis, uterine fibroids, peritoneal sclerosis, and scleroderma. The drug is also a tumor necrosis factor (TNF) alpha agent, which is effective in multiple sclerosis (MS). The phase II trials for pulmonary fibrosis and MS use a capsule formulation of Deskar.

INDICATION(S) AND RESEARCH PHASE
Pulmonary Fibrosis – Phase II
Multiple Sclerosis – Phase II

Respiratory Failure

lucinactant
Surfaxin

MANUFACTURER
Discovery Laboratories

DESCRIPTION
A surfactant is a surface-active agent secreted by alveolar type II cells that decreases the surface tension of pulmonary fluids and increases elasticity of lung tissue, thus helping the lungs to breathe easier. Surfaxin is a novel surfactant, containing a peptide mimic of the human protein B. It cleanses the lung and restores surfactant inactivated by MAS. An injectable formulation of the drug is in phase II/III trials.

Additionally, Surfaxin, has been granted a fast track designation by the FDA for development as a treatment for meconium aspiration syndrome (MAS), acute respiratory distress syndrome (ARDS), and acute lung injury (ALI). The drug is currently in late stage phase III trials in premature babies.

INDICATION(S) AND RESEARCH PHASE
Acute Respiratory Distress Syndrome (ARDS) – Phase III
Respiratory Failure – Phase III
Pediatric, Meconium Aspiration Syndrome – Phase III

perflubron
LiquiVent

MANUFACTURER
Alliance Pharmaceutical

DESCRIPTION
LiquiVent (perfluorooctylbromide) is an intrapulmonary liquid oxygen-carrying drug for treatment of acute lung injury (ALI) and acute respiratory distress syndrome (ARDS). The drug is administered directly into the lungs of subjects on a mechanical ventilator, via a proprietary partial liquid ventilation technique that opens collapsed or debris-filled alveoli and assists in respiratory gas exchange. The FDA has granted this drug a fast track status. LiquiVent has completed phase II/III trials for pulmonary complications.

INDICATION(S) AND RESEARCH PHASE
Acute Respiratory Distress Syndrome (ARDS) – Phase II/III completed
Respiratory Failure – Phase II/III completed

Reversible Obstructive Airways Disease

formoterol
Foradil

MANUFACTURER
Novartis

DESCRIPTION
Foradil (formoterol), a long-acting beta2-agonist, is a bronchodilator for the treatment of asthma and chronic obstructive pulmonary disease. It is currently being tested in phase II trials in a multi-dose dry powder inhaler. It has been approved for twice-daily use via the Aerolizer inhaler (a single-dose powder inhalation device) for use in adults and children ages five and older.

The multi-dose dry powder formulation is being tested in phase II trials for the treatment of asthma. In February 2001, Foradil Aerolizer was approved by the FDA for long-term, twice daily administration in the maintenance treatment of asthma and in the prevention of bronchospasm in adults and children five years of age and older with reversible obstructive airways disease.

INDICATION(S) AND RESEARCH PHASE
Asthma – Phase II
Asthma – FDA approved
Reversible Obstructive Airways Disease – FDA approved
Pediatric, Asthma – FDA approved
Pediatric, Reversible Obstructive Airways Disease – FDA approved

Sinus Infections

AG7088, anti-rhinoviral agent
unknown

MANUFACTURER
Agouron Pharmaceuticals

DESCRIPTION
AG7088 is a small, synthetic molecule designed to inhibit the rhinovirus 3C protease. The drug presented a broad spectrum of potent antirhinoviral activity in preclinical testing.

In a phase II trial, subjects were administered multiple daily intranasal doses of AG7088 starting 24 hours after exposure to human rhinovirus. Results showed that AG7088 was well tolerated and that it significantly reduced total cold symptoms and respiratory symptoms. Based on these results, Agouron is initiating a larger phase II/III trial at more than 50 sites throughout the United States.

INDICATION(S) AND RESEARCH PHASE
Rhinitis – Phase II/III
Sinus Infections – Phase II/III

moxifloxacin
Avelox

MANUFACTURER
Bayer Corporation

DESCRIPTION
At the end of 1999, the FDA approved Bayer's respiratory antibiotic Avelox (moxifloxacin) for the treatment of acute exacerbations of chronic bronchitis, community-acquired pneumonia, and acute sinusitis. The company is evaluating the drug in phase III trials for additional indications of respiratory tract infections and lung disease.

INDICATION(S) AND RESEARCH PHASE
Bacterial Infection – Phase III
Lung Disease – Phase III
Bronchitis – FDA approved
Pneumonia – FDA approved
Sinus Infection – FDA approved

mupirocin
Bactroban

MANUFACTURER
GlaxoSmithKline

DESCRIPTION
Bactroban is an antibiotic currently marketed in a topical cream formulation for the treatment of secondarily infected traumatic skin lesions due to susceptible strains of *Staphylococcus aureus* and *Streptococcus pyogenes*. Bactroban is also being developed in phase II trials for the prevention of recurrent sinusitis.

INDICATION(S) AND RESEARCH PHASE
Sinus Infections – Phase II
Skin Infections, Disorders – FDA approved

SB 275833
unknown

MANUFACTURER
GlaxoSmithKline

DESCRIPTION
SB 275833 is a bacterial protein synthesis inhibitor being developed for the prevention of recurrent sinusitis. It is currently in phase I development.

INDICATION(S) AND RESEARCH PHASE
Sinus Infections – Phase I

Smoking Cessation

CP-526,555
unknown

MANUFACTURER
Pfizer

DESCRIPTION
CP-526,555 is an oral treatment for smoking cessation. As a partial agonist, CP-526,555 partially stimulates the nicotine receptor in the brain to satisfy a smoker's nicotine craving while, at the same time, blocking the nicotine receptor from the reinforcing value of nicotine in smoke. Phase II trials are currently under way.

INDICATION(S) AND RESEARCH PHASE
Smoking Cessation – Phase II

GW 468816
unknown

MANUFACTURER
GlaxoSmithKline

DESCRIPTION
GW 468816 is a glycine receptor antagonist currently in phase I development for migraine prophylaxis and for smoking cessation.

INDICATION(S) AND RESEARCH PHASE
Migraine and Cluster Headaches – Phase I

Smoking Cessation – Phase I

LY-354740
unknown

MANUFACTURER
Eli Lilly

DESCRIPTION
LY-354740 is a glutamate receptor agonist used as a smoking cessation aid and in the treatment of anxiety. This drug is currently in phase II trials.

INDICATION(S) AND RESEARCH PHASE
Smoking Cessation – Phase II
Anxiety Disorders – Phase II

nicotine addiction product
unknown

MANUFACTURER
Algos Pharmaceutical

DESCRIPTION
This novel nicotine addiction product is being tested in a phase II trial for smoking cessation. It is made in an oral capsule formulation.

INDICATION(S) AND RESEARCH PHASE
Smoking Cessation – Phase II

SR-141716
unknown

MANUFACTURER
Sanofi-Synthelabo Pharmaceuticals

DESCRIPTION
SR-141716 is a medication that may provide for the treatment of schizophrenia, obesity, and smoking addiction. It is in an oral formulation and is currently being tested in phase IIa clinical trials. Marijuana activates cannabinoid (CB1) receptors. The human body itself makes a substance, anandamide, which also activates these receptors. It has long been observed that marijuana use increases appetite, probably through activation of these cannabinoid receptors. Scientists hope that by blocking these receptors with SR-141716, appetite will be reduced, leading to weight loss.

In addition, cannabinoid receptors may play a role in drug and alcohol abuse, possibly by affecting the activity of brain reward systems. By lowering the pleasant sensation that the brain experiences from smoking, drinking, or using mood altering drugs, blockage of these receptors may help control such addictive behaviors.

The cannabinoid receptor also may contribute to schizophrenic behavior. Preliminary studies have shown that when these receptors were blocked with SR-141716, the hyperactive, psychotic behavior associated with schizophrenia was decreased. Overactivity or overproduction of cannabinoid receptors in the body may contribute to an imbalance in dopamine, the neurotransmitter most commonly associated with schizophrenia.

INDICATION(S) AND RESEARCH PHASE
Schizophrenia and Schizoaffective Disorders – Phase IIa
Obesity – Phase IIa
Smoking Cessation – Phase IIa

Tuberculosis

CDC 801
SelCID

MANUFACTURER
Celgene Corporation

DESCRIPTION
SelCIDs, selective cytokine inhibitory drugs, are oral immunotherapeutic agents that treat various inflammatory diseases by inhibiting phosphodiesterase type-4 enzyme (PDE-4). The inhibition of PDE-4 decreases production of tumor necrosis factor-alpha (TNF-α), a protein manufactured by cells of the immune system. This inhibition reduces the level of circulating TNF-α and, therefore, its ability to cause inflammation in cells. At normal levels, the protein is essential for effective immune function. However, overproduction of TNF as a result of age, genetic, and other influences contributes to the pathology of numerous diseases.

SelCIDs are in phase II trials for the following indications: inflammatory bowel disease, rheumatoid arthritis, multiple sclerosis, tuberculosis, autoimmune diseases, multiple myeloma, and mycobacterial infections such as leprosy.

INDICATION(S) AND RESEARCH PHASE
Inflammatory Bowel Disease – Phase II
Rheumatoid Arthritis – Phase II
Multiple Sclerosis – Phase II
Asthma – Phase discontinued
Tuberculosis – Phase II
Autoimmune Diseases – Phase II
Bacterial Infection – Phase II
Multiple Myeloma – Phase II

8 | Endocrine and Metabolism

Drugs in the development pipeline	481*
Number of drugs in preclinical testing	231
Number of drugs in clinical testing	205

Source: Parexel

Two major targets of investigation in the endocrine and metabolic therapeutic area are diabetes and hormone replacement therapy. Growth hormone deficiencies, obesity and thyroid disorders are additional diseases that fall into this therapeutic category.

The World Health Organization estimates there are 125 million people worldwide with diabetes. This number has increased 15% in the last ten years and is expected to double by 2005. According to the American Diabetes Association, there are 15.7 million people who have diabetes, or 5.9 percent of the population, in the United States. Diabetes is also a costly and deadly disease; each year in the United States it is estimated to account for nearly $100 billion in direct and indirect health care costs, and 193,000 deaths. According to CenterWatch research, there are approximately 40 to 50 drugs in development for the treatment of diabetes and associated complications, at a cost of approximately $190 million to $240 million dollars.

Diabetes is a chronic disease characterized by the body's inability to produce or properly use insulin, a hormone that is needed to metabolize sugars, starches and other food into the energy needed for daily life. There are three types of diabetes mellitus. Type 1 diabetes, also referred to as insulin-dependent diabetes mellitus or juvenile-onset diabetes, occurs when the body's white blood cells attack insulin-producing cells in the pancreas. The second type, gestational diabetes, usually develops during pregnancy but then disappears once the pregnancy is over. The most common form is type 2 diabetes, formerly known as non-insulin dependent diabetes mellitus. Unlike the insulin-dependent type of diabetes, people with non-insulin-dependent diabetes produce some insulin. However, either their bodies do not produce enough insulin or their cells are resistant to the action of insulin.

Whereas type 1 diabetes is often diagnosed in children, type 2 diabetes has typically been associated with an older, middle-aged population. However, in recent years diabetes experts have seen a dramatic increase in the number of children and young adults with type 2 diabetes. According to a panel report from an American Diabetes Association sponsored conference, anywhere from 8% to 45% of all cases of diabetes in children may be type 2. Possible explanations for this increase include decreased physical activity and widespread obesity among the younger population.

A lack of knowledge concerning this rise presents a problem for both the diagnosis and treatment of younger patients. Because type 2 diabetes has been associated with older patients, physicians may not be accustomed to considering it as a diagnosis. Additionally, many diabetes drugs have not yet been tested in pediatric populations, leaving physicians without age-appropriate information. Currently, the FDA has approved injected insulin and Bristol-Myers Squibb's Glucophage (metformin HCl) for the treatment of type 2 diabetes in pediatric patients, with other companies planning to initiate pediatric testing.

Scientists have yet to find a cure for diabetes. In the meantime, the goal of diabetes management is to keep blood glucose levels as close to the normal, non-diabetic range as safely possible. Diet, exercise and blood testing for glucose are the basis for management of type 2 diabetes. While type 1 diabetics must have daily injections of insulin, some people with type 2 diabetes also take insulin or oral drugs to lower their blood glucose levels.

Researchers have long searched for an alternative to administering insulin by injection in the hopes of increasing patient compliance, which is a critical factor for minimizing the long-term effects of diabetes. However, this has proven a daunting task over past decades. Insulin is a large protein, and therefore has been unable to pass the barrier of digestive acids in an oral formulation. In terms of inhaled insulin, particle size may also be a challenge—if the particle is too large or small it may be exhaled or otherwise misdirected.

Despite these and other challenges, alternative delivery methods for insulin are being actively pursued by pharmaceutical companies. This includes an inhaled insulin product being co-developed by Aventis and Pfizer, with additional support from Inhale Therapeutic Systems. A device aerosolizes a powder formulation of insulin, which is absorbed into the alveoli of the lungs. The hormone then passes from the lung tissue into the blood. Other companies are also testing inhaled insulin products, such as Dura Pharmaceuticals and Aradigm, but Pfizer's is the most advanced product, with a New Drug Application (NDA) and Marketing Authorization Application (MAA) filing expected in late 2001.

While inhaled insulin appears close to approval and may produce a sizeable market impact, it is not the only new delivery method in development. Eli Lilly and Generex are testing an oral form of insulin that is absorbed through the inner cheek walls, and in contrast to injected insulin, does not require refrigeration. Additional products with promise include an insulin pump, manufactured by MiniMed, which can be implanted under the skin - an improvement in administration compared to current insulin pumps, which are worn outside the body.

Another endocrine category receiving much attention is hormone replacement therapy. According to CenterWatch research, approximately five to nine drugs are in the pipeline for this indication. Hormone replacement therapy (HRT) for post-menopausal women has long been the subjects of debate. After menopause, the body makes less of the female hormones, estrogen and progesterone. Symptoms during the years around menopause include hot flashes, sleep problems, or vaginal dryness. Estrogen loss also increases the risk for more serious health problems, including heart disease, stroke, and osteoporosis.

Hormone replacement therapies have proven useful in relieving post-menopausal symptoms; however, research suggests these therapies may carry risks. Estrogen supplements, particularly in high doses, can lead to endometrial cancer, a cancer of the lining of the uterus. As a result, lower doses of estrogen are prescribed in combination with progestin (a form of progesterone) for women who still have a uterus. Women who have had their uterus, including the cervix, removed can use estrogen alone (estrogen replacement therapy or ERT).

In the Journal of the American Medical Association, scientists from the American Cancer Society reported that women who use estrogen after menopause for 10 years or more have a substantially increased risk of death from ovarian cancer. In a new analysis of the Society's large prospective United States cohort study, Cancer Prevention Study II (CPSII), researchers followed the health status of 211,581 post-menopausal women from enrollment in 1982 to 1996. According to the authors, one possible mechanism to account for these findings may be that post-menopausal estrogen therapy raises levels of serum estradiol and estrogen, the forms of estrogen found circulating in the body. These substances have a direct effect on cells in the ovary. Increased exposure to estrogen is known to increase proliferation of ovarian cells, and some women with ovarian cancer experience a beneficial effect when treated with the drug tamoxifen, a powerful anti-estrogen. Further research is necessary to confirm these results, and it is also noteworthy that the study did not evaluate hormone therapy that combines estrogen and progesterone.

Acromegaly

pegvisomant
Somavert

MANUFACTURER
Sensus Drug Development

DESCRIPTION
Somavert (pegvisomant), a genetically modified form of human growth hormone, is being tested for the treatment of acromegaly. The drug is designed to block the effects of excessive growth hormone production by a pituitary tumor. Eighty-nine percent of subjects experienced normalized serum insulin-like growth factor one (IGF-I) at 12 weeks, compared to 10% receiving placebo. At least 75% of the IGF-I reduction occurred within two weeks of initiating treatment. The Somavert-treated group also experienced decreases in soft-tissue swelling, excessive perspiration, and fatigue.

INDICATION(S) AND RESEARCH PHASE
Acromegaly – Phase III completed

Alopecia

GI 198745
unknown

MANUFACTURER
GlaxoSmithKline

DESCRIPTION
GI 198745 is a dual inhibitor of 5-alpha-reductase type 1 and 2 isozymes. GlaxoSmithKline has developed the drug for the treatment of benign prostatic hyperplasia (BPH). An NDA was submitted for this indication in December 2000. Additionally, GI 198745 is in phase II trials for the treatment of alopecia.

INDICATION(S) AND RESEARCH PHASE
Alopecia – Phase II
Benign Prostatic Hyperplasia – NDA submitted

Diabetes Mellitus Types 1 and 2

AC2993
unknown

MANUFACTURER
Amylin Pharmaceuticals

DESCRIPTION
AC2993 (synthetic exendin-4) is a 39 amino acid peptide that exhibits prolonged and anti-diabetic actions. AC2993 completed phase II trials for type 2 diabetes and related metabolic disorders in June 2000. A second phase II trial was initiated in November 2000 in 100 subjects for type 2 diabetes who are not achieving adequate blood glucose target levels with their current oral agent therapies.

Phase II results of AC2993 (synthetic exendin-4) showed that AC2993 administered at different frequencies lowered blood glucose in subjects with type 2 diabetes. In the double-blind, placebo-controlled crossover study, 12 subjects with type 2 diabetes were given a daily dose of AC2993 totaling 0.2 μg/kg, with injection frequencies of one, two, and four times a day. All three injection frequencies resulted in lower 24-hour mean plasma glucose concentrations compared to placebo. Amylin Pharmaceuticals plans to submit the results of this study for presentation to international diabetes conferences.

INDICATION(S) AND RESEARCH PHASE
Diabetes Mellitus Types 1 and 2 – Phase II

AC2993 LAR
unknown

MANUFACTURER
Amylin Pharmaceuticals

DESCRIPTION
AC2993 is a 39-amino acid peptide that exhibits several of the anti-diabetic actions of the mammalian hormone glucagon-like peptide (GLP-1). Amylin and Alkermes are developing an injectable long-acting formulation of AC2993, known as AC2993 LAR, utilizing Alkermes' Medisorb injectable sustained release drug delivery technology. Based upon results obtained to date from initial feasibility studies, the goal of the Alkermes-Amylin agreement is a formulation that would allow once a month administration of AC2993 for the treatment of type 2 diabetes.

INDICATION(S) AND RESEARCH PHASE
Diabetes Mellitus Types 1 and 2 – Phase I

AERx diabetes management system
unknown

MANUFACTURER
Aradigm Corporation

DESCRIPTION
AERx diabetes management system is a drug delivery device for insulin that is being tested for the treatment of diabetes, types 1 and 2. This device produces a fine aerosol mist of insulin that is inhaled into the lungs for absorption into the bloodstream. This system uses a hand-held electronic inhaler that may direct a more consistent dose of insulin for each use.

Results of the first phase II U.S. trial, which stated that insulin inhaled through the AERx diabetes management system immediately before a meal controlled blood glucose comparable to regular insulin injected 30 minutes prior to mealtime. This trial enrolled 20 adult, insulin-dependent (type 1) diabetes subjects. It was suggested that the inhaled system was as effective and more convenient than needle injected insulin, especially since dosing can be timed with a meal instead of waiting for 30 minutes after injection. A phase IIb trial was initiated November 2000.

INDICATION(S) AND RESEARCH PHASE
Diabetes Mellitus Types 1 and 2 – Phase IIb

AI-401
unknown

MANUFACTURER
AutoImmune

DESCRIPTION
AI-401 is genetically engineered (recombinant) human insulin. It is being evaluated for either delaying or preventing the onset of insulin-dependent diabetes mellitus (IDDM or type 1). AI-401 is manufactured in an oral crystalline capsule formulation.

INDICATION(S) AND RESEARCH PHASE
Diabetes Mellitus Types 1 and 2 – Phase II/III

AJ-9677, TAK-677
unknown

MANUFACTURER
Dainippon Pharmaceutical

DESCRIPTION
AJ-9677, TAK-677 is a beta-3-adrenergic receptor agonist, which improves both lipid and glycemic metabolism by reducing insulin resistance and is accordingly expected to be a new class of anti-diabetic agent for type 2 diabetes. Since this compound promotes energy consumption, it also has a potential to be developed as an anti-obesity drug. Clinical trials are taking place in the United States and Japan. Takeda will receive the development and marketing rights in the world except Japan, China, Taiwan, and South Korea.

INDICATION(S) AND RESEARCH PHASE
Diabetes Mellitus Types 1 and 2 – Phase II

AR-H049020
unknown

MANUFACTURER
AstraZeneca

DESCRIPTION
AR-H049020 is a PPAR agonist indicated for the treatment of diabetes and insulin resistance. It is in phase I trials.

INDICATION(S) AND RESEARCH PHASE
Diabetes Mellitus Types 1 and 2 – Phase I

AZ 242 (AR-H039242)
unknown

MANUFACTURER
AstraZeneca

DESCRIPTION
AZ 242 is a PPAR agonist indicated for the treatment of diabetes and insulin resistance. It is currently in phase II trials.

INDICATION(S) AND RESEARCH PHASE
Diabetes Mellitus Types 1 and 2 – Phase II

BetaRx
unknown

MANUFACTURER
VivoRx

DESCRIPTION
BetaRx is being tested for the treatment of insulin-dependent diabetes mellitus (IDDM), especially in subjects on immunosuppressive therapy. This drug delivery system is made up of an encapsulated pancreatic islet cell implant. Since the pancreas is the organ responsible for making insulin in the the islets of Langerhans, a device surgically implanted in the body that delivers insulin made from these types of pancreatic cells may demonstrate usefulness for diabetic subjects. This program is considered as an orphan indication and may receive a faster regulatory review.

INDICATION(S) AND RESEARCH PHASE
Diabetes Mellitus Types 1 and 2 – Phase I/II

candesartan cilexetil
Blopress

MANUFACTURER
Takeda Chemical Industries

DESCRIPTION
Blopress is an angiotensin II receptor antagonist being developed in Japan for the treatment of congestive heart failure and for diabetic nephropathy.

INDICATION(S) AND RESEARCH PHASE
Congestive Heart Failure – Phase III
Diabetes Mellitus Types 1 and 2 – Phase II

CLX-0901
unknown

MANUFACTURER
Calyx Therapeutics

DESCRIPTION
CLX-0901 is an orally active small molecule that had, in previous animal trials, lowered blood glucose levels and concentrations of serum triglycerides, free fatty acids, and cholesterol associated with type 2 diabetes.

The results of a phase Ib trial showed that CLX-0901 was well tolerated at each of several ascending multiple doses in healthy volunteers and in subjects with type 2 diabetes. The trial was a randomized, double-blind, placebo-controlled study involving 18 subjects in the Netherlands.

INDICATION(S) AND RESEARCH PHASE
Diabetes Mellitus Types 1 and 2 – Phase II

DPC-444
unknown

MANUFACTURER
Du Pont

DESCRIPTION
DPC-444 is a pharmaceutical agent that is radioactively labeled with Tc-99m. This radiopharmaceutical is being tested for blood clot (thrombosis) imaging and diabetes.

INDICATION(S) AND RESEARCH PHASE
Thrombosis – Phase III
Diabetes Mellitus Types 1 and 2 – Phase III completed

DPP 728/LAF 237
unknown

MANUFACTURER
Novartis

DESCRIPTION
DPP 728/ LAF 237 belong to a new class of

orally active antidiabetic drugs (DPP-IV inhibitors) that appear to have multiple functional benefits beyond simple blood-glucose control. One of these is the potential ability to restore beta cell function and thereby enhance endogenous insulin secretion.

INDICATION(S) AND RESEARCH PHASE
Diabetes Mellitus Types 1 and 2 – Phase II

---

exendin
Exendin-4

MANUFACTURER
Amylin Pharmaceuticals

DESCRIPTION
Exendin is a synthetic version of exendin-4 and a naturally occurring peptide that has certain GLP-1-like activities for treatment of type 2 or noninsulin-dependent diabetes mellitus (NIDDM). In animal studies, exendin-4 treatment resulted in near normalization of glucose control in type 2 diabetes.

Positive results were reported from a phase I trial of the safety and tolerability of a single subcutaneous dose of exendin-4 in healthy volunteers. Significant stimulation of insulin secretion was observed at the lowest tested dose (0.01 ug/kg), and doses above (0.5 ug/kg) caused a significant reduction of plasma glucose.

INDICATION(S) AND RESEARCH PHASE
Diabetes Mellitus Type 2 – Phase II

GI 262570
unknown

MANUFACTURER
GlaxoSmithKline

DESCRIPTION
GI 262570 is a peroxisome proliferator activated receptor (PPAR) gamma agonist being developed for the treatment of type 2 diabetes. Data from a double-blind, placebo-controlled phase III trial in 376 subjects with type 2 diabetes showed a dose-dependent improvement of baseline fasting HbA1c and plasma glucose levels with all GI-262570 doses over 0.25 mg. A significant metabolic improvement in fasting triglyceride and HDL cholesterol levels was also seen in 2, 5, and 10 mg treatment groups relative to placebo, with the maximum reduction in triglycerides achieved after 4 weeks and maintained for 12 weeks. GI 262570 is in phase III trials.

INDICATION(S) AND RESEARCH PHASE
Diabetes Mellitus Types 1 and 2 – Phase III

GW 427353
unknown

MANUFACTURER
GlaxoSmithKline

DESCRIPTION
GW 427353 is a beta-3-adrenergic receptor agonist. It is currently in phase I trials for the treatment of type 2 diabetes and obesity.

INDICATION(S) AND RESEARCH PHASE
Diabetes Mellitus Types 1 and 2 – Phase I
Obesity – Phase I

---

inhaled insulin
unknown

MANUFACTURER
Pfizer

DESCRIPTION
Pfizer is currently developing inhaled insulin, a new route of administration for the treatment of diabetes, in collaboration with Aventis and Inhale Therapeutic Systems. This may help minimize the need for injections. The inhaled insulin system has been as effective as subcutaneous injections of short-acting insulin in the treatment of insulin-dependent or type 1 diabetes, in preliminary studies. Inhaled insulin is currently being tested in phase III trials; the NDA and MAA will be filed in late 2001.

INDICATION(S) AND RESEARCH PHASE
Pediatric – Phase III
Diabetes Mellitus Types 1 and 2 – Phase III

---

insulin
Oralgen

MANUFACTURER
Generex Biotechnology

DESCRIPTION
Oralgen is a oral liquid form of insulin that is being evaluated for treatment of type 1 and type 2 diabetes. Phase II/III trials will test this insulin form in an oral metered-dose dispenser.

INDICATION(S) AND RESEARCH PHASE
Diabetes Mellitus Types 1 and 2 – Phase II/III

KRP-297
unknown

MANUFACTURER
Merck & Co.

DESCRIPTION
KRP-297 is a peroxisome proliferator-activated receptor (PPAR) agonist in a phase II trial for the treatment of diabetes.

INDICATION(S) AND RESEARCH PHASE
Diabetes Mellitus Types 1 and 2 – Phase II

---

leptin
unknown

MANUFACTURER
Amgen

DESCRIPTION
Leptin is a genetically engineered (recombinant) form of a protein that is naturally made by the human body. This gene therapy is being evaluated in phase II trials for the treatment of obesity and type 2 diabetes. Leptin is made in a subcutaneous injectable formulation.

INDICATION(S) AND RESEARCH PHASE
Diabetes Mellitus Types 1 and 2 – Phase II
Obesity – Phase II

MBX-102
unknown

MANUFACTURER
Metabolex

DESCRIPTION
MBX-102 is the active isomer of a compound that was studied extensively in the 1970's as a potential lipid lowering agent. Metabolex has re-analyzed the patent compound and discovered that this active isomer displays good characteristics as a potential treatment for diabetes. MBX-102 lowers glucose by reducing insulin resistance as well as lowering LDL cholesterol. MBX-102, an isomer, is in a phase I trial for diabetes.

INDICATION(S) AND RESEARCH PHASE
Diabetes Mellitus Types 1 and 2 – Phase I

metformin hydrochloride, ADX-155
Metformin XT

MANUFACTURER
Andrx

DESCRIPTION
Metformin XT is being tested for the treatment of diabetes mellitus. Phase II results demonstrated that this once-a-day drug has a safety and efficacy profile comparable to multiple-daily doses of Glucophage (metformin hydrochloride) in diabetic subjects.

INDICATION(S) AND RESEARCH PHASE
Diabetes Mellitus Types 1 and 2 – Phase III

metformin/sulfonylureas
unknown

MANUFACTURER
Merck KgaA

DESCRIPTION
This combination therapy is made of metformin and sulfonylureas. It is being tested in a phase III study for the treatment of noninsulin-dependent diabetes (type 2).

INDICATION(S) AND RESEARCH PHASE
Diabetes Mellitus Types 1 and 2 – Phase III

NBI-6024
unknown

MANUFACTURER
Neurocrine Biosciences

DESCRIPTION
NBI-6024 is an altered peptide ligand that is designed to induce an immune response capable of regulating autoreactive T-cells that are involved in the destruction of (beta)-islet cells of the pancreas of type 1 diabetes. A phase I/II trial is currently taking place at six centers. The company plans to commence a phase II trial in the third quarter of 2001 in 600 subjects.

INDICATION(S) AND RESEARCH PHASE
Diabetes Mellitus Types 1 and 2 – Phase I/II

NN 1215
unknown

MANUFACTURER
Novo Nordisk

DESCRIPTION
NN 1215 is a long-acting insulin formulation to be administered by injection. The drug is in phase I trials for types 1 and 2 diabetes.

INDICATION(S) AND RESEARCH PHASE
Diabetes Mellitus Types 1 and 2 – Phase I

NN 1998, Insulin (r-human)
unknown

MANUFACTURER
Novo Nordisk

DESCRIPTION
NN 1998 is a pulmonary delivery system designed to administer insulin by inhalation. NN 1998 is in phase IIa trials for the treatment of types 1 and 2 diabetes, and is being developed in collaboration with Aradigm Corporation.

INDICATION(S) AND RESEARCH PHASE
Diabetes Mellitus Types 1 and 2 – Phase IIa

NN 2344, DRF-2593
unknown

MANUFACTURER
Novo Nordisk

DESCRIPTION
NN 2344 is an insulin sensitizer that increases glucose uptake in peripheral tissue, thereby lowering blood concentrations of glucose. It in phase II trials for the treatment of type 2 diabetes.

INDICATION(S) AND RESEARCH PHASE
Diabetes Mellitus Types 1 and 2 – Phase II

NN 304, insulin detemir
unknown

MANUFACTURER
Novo Nordisk

DESCRIPTION
NN 304 is a long-acting insulin-like drug. This insulin analog contains human recombinant insulin attached to a fatty acid (acylated with a 14-C fatty acid chain). It is in a phase III trial for types 1 and 2 diabetes.

INDICATION(S) AND RESEARCH PHASE
Diabetes Mellitus Types 1 and 2 – Phase III

NN 414
unknown

MANUFACTURER
Novo Nordisk

DESCRIPTION
NN 414 is a potassium channel opener that works directly on beta cells, which are located in the islets of Langerhans in the pancreas. Beta cells produce insulin, a hormone that controls the level of glucose in the blood. In type 2 diabetes this production may be decreased, causing an increase in blood glucose. NN 414 is in phase I development for type 2 diabetes.

INDICATION(S) AND RESEARCH PHASE
Diabetes Mellitus Type 2 – Phase I

NN 4201, NNC-42-1001
unknown

MANUFACTURER
Novo Nordisk

DESCRIPTION
NN 4201 is a glycogen phosphorylase inhibitor that reduces glucose output from the liver. It is in phase I trials for the treatment of type 2 diabetes.

INDICATION(S) AND RESEARCH PHASE
Diabetes Mellitus Type 2 – Phase I

NN 622, DRF-2725
unknown

MANUFACTURER
Novo Nordisk

DESCRIPTION
NN 622 is an anti-diabetic molecule discovered by Dr. Reddy's Research Foundation and licensed to Novo Nordisk. It is an insulin sensitizer that lowers blood glucose and produces favorable effects on lipid profile. NN 622 is in phase II trials for type 2 diabetes.

INDICATION(S) AND RESEARCH PHASE
Diabetes Mellitus Types 1 and 2 – Phase II

NNC-90-1170, NN 2211
unknown

MANUFACTURER
Novo Nordisk

DESCRIPTION
NNC-90-1170 is a glucagon-like peptide-1 (GLP-1) derivative that decreases the level of glucagon, a hormone that raises the amount of glucose in the blood. Therefore, NNC-90-1170 results in lower glucose levels. The drug is in phase I trials for type 2 diabetes.
  NN 2211 is being developed under an agreement between Novo Nordisk and Scios.

INDICATION(S) AND RESEARCH PHASE
Diabetes Mellitus Type 2 – Phase I

orlistat
Xenical

MANUFACTURER
Hoffmann-La Roche

DESCRIPTION
Xenical (orlistat) is a lipase inhibitor that inhibits the absorption of dietary fats. It is currently being marketed by Hoffmann-La Roche in the United States for the treatment of obesity. It is in phase III trials for children 12 to 16 years of age for obesity and phase III trials for diabetes.

INDICATION(S) AND RESEARCH PHASE
Obesity – FDA approved
Pediatric, Obesity – Phase III
Diabetes Mellitus Type 2 – Phase III

pimagedine HCl
unknown

MANUFACTURER
Alteon

DESCRIPTION
Pimagedine is a compound (aminoguanidine inhibitor) designed to slow down or stop the progression of kidney disease in type 1 (insulin-dependent) diabetic subjects. A common problem for diabetics is that too much protein may be lost in the urine, a condition known as proteinuria. Alteon claims that a phase II/III trial showed a significant and clinically meaningful reduction of urinary protein excretion.

INDICATION(S) AND RESEARCH PHASE
Diabetes Mellitus Types 1 and 2 – Phase II/III completed
Kidney Disease – Phase II/III completed

pioglitazone HCl
Actos

MANUFACTURER
Takeda Chemical Industries

DESCRIPTION
Actos (pioglitazone hydrochloride) is an orally administered antidiabetic agent that acts primarily by decreasing insulin resistance. Actos improves sensitivity to insulin in muscle and adipose tissue and inhibits hepatic gluconeogenesis. The drug has been approved by the FDA for the improvement of glycemic control in subjects with type 2 diabetes. Actos is currently in phase III trials in Japan.

INDICATION(S) AND RESEARCH PHASE
Diabetes Mellitus Types 1 and 2 – Phase III

pramlintide
Symlin

MANUFACTURER
Amylin Pharmaceuticals

DESCRIPTION
Symlin is a synthetic reproduction (analog) of human amylin for treatment of type 1 and type 2 noninsulin-dependent diabetes mellitus (NIDDM). Results have indicated that Symlin produced a statistically significant lowering of the primary glucose control endpoint in a one-year study in people with type 2 diabetes who use insulin. Additionally, study participants who received Symlin experienced a statistically significant reduction in body weight.
  Amylin Pharmaceuticals has completed its phase III trials for Symlin which included 4,400 participants in the trials. The design of the study was the following: People with type 2 diabetes who use diabetes treatment regimens comprised of insulin with or without oral hypoglycemic agents were enrolled in over 75 research centers in the United States. At least 90% of those enrolled in the study were using multiple injections of insulin each day. Participants continued their usual diabetes treatment regimes and were randomized to receive Symlin 120 μg twice a day (BID), Symlin 90 μg BID, or placebo. HbA1C, an accepted clinical standard, was measured to assess glucose control during the one-year study. The primary

evaluation criteria (endpoint) was change in HbA1C from baseline to 6 months for the Symlin groups compared with the control group. A predefined secondary endpoint was HbA1C change from baseline study participants who were identified as glycemic responders by having achieved at least a 0.5% HbA1 reduction four weeks after the initiation of study drug. No safety issues of concern were identified during the study, and the data indicated that all dosages were well tolerated. There was no difference in the annual event rate for severe hypoglycemia between the Symlin and control groups.

The company submitted an NDA with a submission for regulatory approval in Europe to follow.

INDICATION(S) AND RESEARCH PHASE
Diabetes Mellitus Types 1 and 2 – NDA submitted

pulmonary insulin
unknown

MANUFACTURER
Alkermes

DESCRIPTION
Short-acting (mealtime) and long-acting (once to twice a day) formulations of inhaled insulin are administered from small, simple inhalers to provide diabetic subjects with an alternative to frequent injections. Alkermes' inhaled insulin formulations utilize the company's AIR pulmonary drug delivery technology. A phase I trial has been successfully completed.

INDICATION(S) AND RESEARCH PHASE
Diabetes Mellitus Types 1 and 2 – Phase I completed

pyrazinoylguanidine (PZG)
unknown

MANUFACTURER
SuperGen

DESCRIPTION
A ring-unsubstiuted derivative of a 2-pyrazionic acid possesses several pharmacological activities that may be useful in the treatment of noninsulin-dependent (type 2) diabetes. Pyrazinoylguanidine is currently in a phase I trial.

INDICATION(S) AND RESEARCH PHASE
Diabetes Mellitus Types 1 and 2 – Phase I

repaglinide
NovoNorm

MANUFACTURER
Novo Nordisk

DESCRIPTION
NovoNorm is a prandial glucose regulator. This drug rapidly stimulates insulin secretion, which makes it well suited for dosing at mealtime. Because NovoNorm stops stimulating insulin secretion within a very short time, the risk of hypoglycemia is less than with longer-acting oral antidiabetic drugs.

In January 2001, results of a multinational trial showed that Novo Nordisk's NovoNorm tablets, in a flexible mealtime regimen, improved glycemic control without significantly increasing body weight in subjects with type 2 diabetes. In the double-blind, placebo-controlled trial, a total of 408 type 2 diabetes subjects were randomly assigned to take either NovoNorm (0.5–1.0 mg) or placebo immediately prior to main meals. Those taking NovoNorm showed a significant improvement in glycemic control. These improvements were achieved without a significant increase in body weight irrespective of the subjects' meal patterns.

NovoNorm is known as Prandin in the United States. The drug is marketed in Europe and the United States and is in phase III trials in Japan.

INDICATION(S) AND RESEARCH PHASE
Diabetes Mellitus Types 1 and 2 – FDA approved
Diabetes Mellitus Types 1 and 2 – Phase III

RF-1051
unknown

MANUFACTURER
SuperGen

DESCRIPTION
RF-1051 is a human hormonal replica (analogue) that appears to cause cells to burn more fat to produce the same amount of energy. This agent is being tested in phase II trials for the treatment of obesity and diabetes. RF-1051 is made in an oral capsule formulation.

INDICATION(S) AND RESEARCH PHASE
Diabetes Mellitus Types 1 and 2 – Phase II
Obesity – Phase II
Metabolic Disease – Phase II

rosiglitazone
Avandia

MANUFACTURER
GlaxoSmithKline

DESCRIPTION
Avandia enhances the action of insulin in the body to reduce blood-sugar levels in subjects with type 2 diabetes. It also improves beta cell function in the pancreas, resulting in the release of more insulin. Avandia has been approved by the FDA as an adjunct to diet and exercise to improve glycemic control in subjects with type 2 diabetes mellitus. It is indicated as a monotherapy and for use in combination with a sulfonylurea or metformin when diet, exercise and a single agent do not result in adequate glycemic control. An NDA and a Marketing Authorization Application (MAA) were submitted in February 2000 for the use of Avandia in combination with insulin.

INDICATION(S) AND RESEARCH PHASE
Diabetes Mellitus Types 1 and 2 – NDA submitted
Diabetes Mellitus Types 1 and 2 – MAA submitted

SB 418790
unknown

MANUFACTURER
GlaxoSmithKline

DESCRIPTION
SB 418790 is a beta-3-adrenergic receptor agonist being tested in phase I trials for the treatment of type 2 diabetes and obesity.

INDICATION(S) AND RESEARCH PHASE
Diabetes Mellitus Types 1 and 2 – Phase I
Obesity – Phase I

unknown
Diamyd

MANUFACTURER
Diamyd Medical

DESCRIPTION
Diamyd is a type 1 diabetes vaccine. Diamyd is the proprietary name for recombinant human glutamic acid decarboxylase (GAD65). Results of a phase II trial showed there were no adverse clinical effects, a dose of 0.5 mg/person was well tolerated, and autoantibodies to GAD65, insulin, or IA-2 were not induced. A phase II trial was initiated in Sweden in August 2000.

INDICATION(S) AND RESEARCH PHASE
Diabetes Mellitus Types 1 and 2 – Phase II

voglibose
Basen

MANUFACTURER
Takeda Chemical Industries

DESCRIPTION
Basen is a disaccharidase inhibitor that was approved in Japan in 1994 for the treatment of subjects with diabetes. It is currently in phase II trials in Japan for the indication of impaired glucose tolerance.

INDICATION(S) AND RESEARCH PHASE
Impaired Glucose Tolerance – Phase II

Diabetes Prevention

acetyl-L-carnitine
Alcar

MANUFACTURER
Sigma-Tau Pharmaceuticals

DESCRIPTION
Alcar, an orally formulated drug, is being evaluated in phase III studies for early onset Alzheimer's disease and diabetic peripheral neuropathy. Alcar causes the growth and repair of neurons through the stimulation of nerve growth factor, which should lessen the cognitive deterioration resulting from Alzheimer's disease.

INDICATION(S) AND RESEARCH PHASE
Alzheimer's Disease – Phase III
Diabetes Prevention – Phase III

Diabetic Foot Ulcers

becaplermin
Regranex

MANUFACTURER
Chiron Corporation

DESCRIPTION
Regranex is a wound healing therapeutic for pressure ulcers. These skin ulcers may develop in weight-bearing areas due to many different disease conditions, especially diabetes. The drug is currently being tested in phase III trials. Chiron Corporation has a licensing agreement with R.W. Johnson Pharmaceutical Research Institute for developing Regranex.

INDICATION(S) AND RESEARCH PHASE
Diabetic Foot Ulcers (Pressure Ulcers) – Phase III
Skin Wounds – Phase III

therapeutic, wound healing
unknown

MANUFACTURER
Mylan

DESCRIPTION
This drug is an unspecified therapeutic being tested in phase III trials for both wound healing and diabetic foot ulcers.

INDICATION(S) AND RESEARCH PHASE
Diabetic Foot Ulcers – Phase III
Wounds – Phase III

transforming growth factor beta-2 (TGF-b2)
unknown

MANUFACTURER
Genzyme Tissue Repair

DESCRIPTION
This synthetic drug is known as transforming growth factor beta-2 (TGF-β2). It is normally made in the body to help stimulate the formation of granulation tissue for treating chronic skin ulcers. Results of a phase II double blind, randomized trial were collected over a three year period with testing at 15 study centers with diabetic foot ulcer subjects. Both safety and dose ranging efficacy were evaluated. The two important criteria used to study TGF-β2 were the frequency of complete wound closure and time to wound closure.

The study subjects were randomly assigned to one of five groups. The first group of 24 subjects received standard care only, which consisted of surgical debridement, compression dressing, and off-loading of weight from the wound site. The remainder of the subjects was enrolled in the blinded part of the trial. One group of 22 subjects received placebo sponges and standardized care. The remaining 131 subjects were evenly divided among three doses in addition to standardized care. All the subjects were treated twice a week for 20 weeks or until their ulcer healed.

Results from the phase II trial suggested that TGF-β2 was safe and effective at all dose levels tested. The subject group which received the highest dosage of TGF-β2 (5 μg /cm^2) demonstrated statistically significant improvement compared to placebo in both the efficacy endpoints, frequency of complete closure and time to closure. Subjects in the groups which received the middle or low doses of TGF-β2 also showed improvements in both endpoints but did not consistently achieve statistical significance.

The company, Genzyme Tissue Repair is actively seeking a partner to work with them in the final stages of development and commercialization for the TGF-β2 drug.

INDICATION(S) AND RESEARCH PHASE
Diabetic Foot Ulcers – Phase II completed
Skin Infections/Disorders – Phase II

VM-301, OAS 1000
unknown

MANUFACTURER
Nexell Therapeutics

DESCRIPTION
VM-301 is a topical wound healing agent that is being tested in phase II trials. Indications include treatment of skin graft donor sites of both partial and full thickness wounds, including burns, surgical wounds, diabetic skin ulcers and decubitus ulcers.

INDICATION(S) AND RESEARCH PHASE
Burns and Burn Infections – Phase II
Decubitus Ulcers (Bed Sores) – Phase II
Diabetic Foot Ulcers – Phase II
Wounds – Phase II

Diabetic Kidney Disease

EXO-226
unknown

MANUFACTURER
Exocell

DESCRIPTION
EXO-226 inhibits the formation of glycated albumin, which results from the attachment of a sugar unit to a protein. Reducing the concentration of glycated albumin, which is elevated in diabetes, can prevent kidney pathology and abnormal kidney function. The company believes that the benefits of reduced glycated albumin may be observed even though blood sugar concentrations remained elevated. EXO-226 is in a phase III trial for diabetic kidney disease. The trial will enroll approximately 350 subjects in 15 centers in the United States.

INDICATION(S) AND RESEARCH PHASE
Diabetic Kidney Disease – Phase III

Female Hormonal Deficiencies/ Abnormalities

estrogens/methyltestosterone
Estratest

MANUFACTURER
Solvay Pharmaceuticals

DESCRIPTION
Estratest is a hormone replacement therapy that consists of esterified estrogens and methyltestosterone administered as an oral tablet. It is already approved by the FDA for moderate to severe vasomotor symptoms associated with menopause. Estratest is currently being evaluated in phase III trials for the treatment of sexual dysfunction in women.

INDICATION(S) AND RESEARCH PHASE
Sexual Dysfunction – Phase III
Female Hormonal
  Deficiencies/Abnormalities – Phase III

Growth Hormone Deficiencies/ Abnormalities

growth hormone releasing factor (GRF)
unknown

MANUFACTURER
ICN Pharmaceuticals

DESCRIPTION
This drug is known as growth hormone releasing factor (GRF) and is being evaluated in phase II/III trials for the treatment of growth retardation. GRF is a precursor chemical naturally made by the body to stimulate the release of growth hormone. This hormone is essential for proper maturation and body development in infants and children. Lack of growth hormone may cause diseases such as dwarfism, whereas too much release of the hormone may cause gigantism. ICN Pharmaceuticals has a licensing agreement with Fujisawa for the development and marketing GRF.

INDICATION(S) AND RESEARCH PHASE
Growth Hormone
  Deficiencies/Abnormalities – Phase II/III

NN 703, NNC 26-0703, r-Somatropin
unknown

MANUFACTURER
Novo Nordisk

DESCRIPTION
NN 703 is a growth hormone releasing peptide being tested in phase II trials for the treatment of growth hormone deficiency and insufficiency. Dwarfism and other maturational diseases may be treated by this growth hormone stimulant. The drug is available in an oral formulation.

INDICATION(S) AND RESEARCH PHASE
Growth Hormone
  Deficiencies/Abnormalities – Phase II

pralmorelin
unknown

MANUFACTURER
Fujisawa Healthcare

DESCRIPTION
Pralmorelin is a growth hormone releasing factor that is being developed for treatment of growth retardation. The releasing factor may activate the anterior lobe of the pituitary gland to secrete growth hormone into the bloodstream. Pralmorelin is being tested in phase II/III clinical trials. Fujisawa Healthcare has a licensing agreement with ICN Pharmaceuticals for this drug product.

INDICATION(S) AND RESEARCH PHASE
Pediatric, Growth Hormone
  Deficiencies/Abnormalities – Phase II/III

somatropin

Nutropin Depot

MANUFACTURER
Genentech

DESCRIPTION
Nutropin Depot is a long-acting dosage formulation of Genetech's human growth hormone, which employs Alkermes' ProLease injectable extended-release drug delivery system. The drug is indicated for the long-term treatment of growth failure in pediatric subjects due to a lack of adequate endogenous growth hormone secretion. Nutropin Depot, somatropin (rDNA) for injectable suspension, entered a phase II/III trial in January 2001 for treatment of adults with growth hormone deficiencies. Nutropin Depot was approved for marketing by the FDA in December 1999. Genentech is co-developing Nutropin Depot with Alkermes.

INDICATION(S) AND RESEARCH PHASE
Growth Hormone Deficiencies/
  Abnormalities – Phase II/III
Hormone Deficiencies – Phase II
Pediatric, Hormone Deficiencies – FDA
  approved

Hormone Deficiencies

somatropin, r-hGH
Serostim

MANUFACTURER
Serono Laboratories

DESCRIPTION
Serostim is a recombinant human growth hormone in trials for several indications. The drug is currently marketed for the treatment of AIDS wasting (cachexia), and is in development for growth hormone deficiency in adults, short bowel syndrome, lipodystrophy, and congestive heart failure.

INDICATION(S) AND RESEARCH PHASE
Acquired Immune Deficiency Syndrome
  (AIDS) and AIDS-Related Infections –
  FDA approved
Hormone Deficiencies – Phase III
Gastrointestinal Diseases and Disorders,
  Miscellaneous – Phase III
Lipodystrophy – Phase II
Congestive Heart Failure – Phase II

Hormone Replacement Therapy/Menopause

17-beta estradiol/trimegestone
unknown

MANUFACTURER
Wyeth-Ayerst

DESCRIPTION
17-beta estradiol/trimegestone is being evaluated in late clinical trials for the treatment of menopausal symptoms and osteoporosis.

INDICATION(S) AND RESEARCH PHASE
Menopause – Phase III
Hormone Replacement
  Therapy/Menopause – Phase III
Osteoporosis – Phase III

conjugated estrogen tablets
Premarin/Trimegesterone

MANUFACTURER
Wyeth-Ayerst

DESCRIPTION
Premarin/Trimegesterone is being evaluated in phase III trials for relieving menopausal symptoms as well as decreasing the incidence of endometrial hyperplasia seen with estrogen-alone therapy. Premarin for oral administration contains a mixture of estrogens obtained exclusively from natural sources. Trimegesterone is a progestational molecule originated by Aventis for hormone replacement therapy.

INDICATION(S) AND RESEARCH PHASE
Menopause – Phase III
Hormone Replacement
  Therapy/Menopause – Phase III

estradiol
Estrasorb

MANUFACTURER
Novavax

DESCRIPTION
Estrasorb is an estrogen replacement therapy developed for symptomatic menopausal women. It is applied as a typical cosmetic lotion, and is designed to deliver 17-beta-etradiol through the skin.

Results of a randomized, placebo-controlled, dose ranging study in 117 subjects showed that Estrasorb successfully delivered therapeutic doses of estradiol transdermally. No skin irritation was found and no significant fluctuations in blood hormone levels were observed.

INDICATION(S) AND RESEARCH PHASE
Hormone Replacement
  Therapy/Menopause – Phase III completed

estradiol, 17-beta
Estrogel

MANUFACTURER
Solvay Pharmaceuticals

DESCRIPTION
Estrogel is a topical gel steroid (17-beta estradiol) developed for use as an estrogen hormone replacement therapy. The estradiol accumulates in the skin and forms a reservoir, providing a steady release of the drug. Estrogel is under FDA review as a transdermal treatment for vasomotor symptoms of menopause, including hot flashes and night sweats. An NDA was submitted by Unimed Pharmaceuticals, which is a subsidiary of Solvay Pharmaceuticals.

INDICATION(S) AND RESEARCH PHASE
Hormone Replacement
  Therapy/Menopause – NDA submitted

estradiol/progestin
unknown

MANUFACTURER
Watson Pharmaceuticals

DESCRIPTION

Watson Laboratories has conducted phase III trials for a combination estradiol/progestin hormone replacement therapy (HRT) patch using their transdermal (patch) delivery system. The patch administers a continuous dose of both estrogen and progestin through the patch's adhesive into the skin for body absorption. The company received a non-approvable letter in November 2000 because of lack of sufficient evidence to support the safety and efficacy of the estradiol/progestin for the prevention of hyperplasia and required that an additional endometrial protection trial be submitted. The company anticipates filing an amendment.

INDICATION(S) AND RESEARCH PHASE
Hormone Replacement
  Therapy/Menopause – FDA denied
Osteoporosis – Phase III

testosterone
unknown

MANUFACTURER
Watson Pharmaceuticals

DESCRIPTION
Testosterone is a naturally produced hormone, which is responsible for proper development of male secondary sex characteristics. This hormone, which has been formulated in the MTX transdermal patch, is being tested in phase II trials for several indications, which include the treatment of sexual dysfunction in surgically menopausal subjects, menopause associated hormone replacement therapy, and osteoporosis. Additionally, this drug is in phase III clinical trials for male hormonal deficiencies and abnormalities.

This hormone regime is also being evaluated in phase II trials for treatment of female AIDS wasting. Testosterone is an anabolic steroid that may help build up muscle mass in subjects suffering from AIDS.

INDICATION(S) AND RESEARCH PHASE
Acquired Immune Deficiency Syndrome
  (AIDS) and AIDS-Related Infections –
  Phase II
Hormone Replacement
  Therapy/Menopause – Phase II
Male Hormonal Deficiencies/Abnormalities
  – Phase III
Osteoporosis – Phase II
Sexual Dysfunction – Phase II completed

transdermal testosterone gel
Tostrelle

MANUFACTURER
Cellegy Pharmaceuticals

DESCRIPTION
Tostrelle (transdermal testosterone gel) is indicated for the treatment of low levels of testosterone in menopausal women. Testosterone deficiency in women is a frequent cause of diminished libido or low sex drive.

INDICATION(S) AND RESEARCH PHASE
Menopause – Phase I/II
Hormone Replacement
  Therapy/Menopause – Phase II
Sexual Dysfunction – Phase I/II

Hyponatremia

YM-087, conivaptan
unknown

MANUFACTURER
Yamanouchi Pharmaceutical

DESCRIPTION
YM-087 is a receptor antagonist to the peptide hormone vasopressin, which is released by the hypothalamus to regulate water balance in the body. The drug is currently in phase III trials for the treatment of hyponatremia, and phase II trials for the treatment of heart failure. It is being developed in both Europe and the United States. The drug is also part of Yamanouchi's domestic pipeline; YM-087 is in phase II trials for both hyponatremia and heart failure. YM-087 is manufactured in oral and injectable formulations.

INDICATION(S) AND RESEARCH PHASE
Congestive Heart Failure – Phase II
Hyponatremia (Europe) – Phase III
Hyponatremia (United States) – Phase II

Limb Preservation and Amputation

AS-013
Circulase

MANUFACTURER
Alpha Therapeutic

DESCRIPTION
Circulase is being tested in a phase II/III study for the prevention of limb amputation in subjects with decreased tissue blood flow. Circulase may help blood flow in the arms and legs.

INDICATION(S) AND RESEARCH PHASE
Limb Preservation and Amputation – Phase II/III

Male Hormonal Deficiencies/ Abnormalities

dihydrotestosterone
Andractim

MANUFACTURER
Unimed Pharmaceuticals

DESCRIPTION
Andractim is a hormone replacement therapy for the treatment of male testosterone deficiency. It is a clear, odorless, non-irritating, topical gel that delivers dihydrotestosterone transdermally to the bloodstream. Dihydrotestosterone is a natural male hormone that can assist in building muscle mass. It is being tested in phase III trials for geriatric hypogonadism, a condition characterized by abnormally decreased sexual function of the testes in elderly males.

The anabolic steroid is also being tested in phase II trials for the treatment of weight loss associated with HIV wasting in AIDS subjects.

Unimed Pharmaceuticals has a collaborative agreement with BioChem Pharma to develop Andractim, which is licensed from Laboratoires Besins Iscovesco S.A., France.

INDICATION(S) AND RESEARCH PHASE
Acquired Immune Deficiency Syndrome (AIDS) and AIDS-Related Infections – Phase II
Male Hormonal Deficiencies/Abnormalities – Phase III

testosterone
Androsorb

MANUFACTURER
Novavax

DESCRIPTION
Androsorb is a cream for testosterone replacement therapy in phase II clinical trials for testosterone deficient men and phase I trials for post-menopausal women. A phase I trial will test 21 postmenopausal women at two sites. Androsorb is being developed using Novavax's proprietary micellar nanoparticle technology, a microemulsion drug delivery platform.

INDICATION(S) AND RESEARCH PHASE
Male Hormonal Deficiencies/Abnormalities – Phase II
Menopause – Phase I

testosterone
unknown

MANUFACTURER
Watson Pharmaceuticals

DESCRIPTION
Testosterone is a naturally produced hormone, which is responsible for proper development of male secondary sex characteristics. This hormone, which has been formulated in the MTX transdermal patch, is being tested for several indications, which include the treatment of sexual dysfunction in surgically menopausal subjects, menopause associated hormone replacement therapy, osteoporosis, male hormonal deficiencies, and abnormalities. This hormone regime is also being evaluated for treatment of female AIDS wasting. Testosterone is an anabolic steroid that may help build up muscle mass in subjects suffering from AIDS.

INDICATION(S) AND RESEARCH PHASE
Acquired Immune Deficiency Syndrome (AIDS) and AIDS-Related Infections – Phase II
Hormone Replacement Therapy/Menopause – Phase II
Male Hormonal Deficiencies/Abnormalities – Phase III
Osteoporosis – Phase II
Sexual Dysfunction – Phase II completed

Transdermal testosterone gel
Tostrex

MANUFACTURER
Cellegy Pharmaceuticals

DESCRIPTION
This transdermal testosterone gel is currently in phase III trials for the treatment of male hormone hypogonadism, a disorder frequently characterized by diminished libido and reduced muscle mass. This hormonal gel is a more convenient treatment than injections and a less irritating alternative to the current patch products. Additionally, it is in trials for the treatment of impotence.

INDICATION(S) AND RESEARCH PHASE
Male Hormonal Deficiencies/Abnormalities – Phase III
Impotence – Phase II/III

Menopause

17-beta estradiol/trimegestone
unknown

MANUFACTURER
Wyeth-Ayerst

DESCRIPTION
17-beta estradiol/trimegestone is being evaluated in late clinical trials for the treatment of menopausal symptoms and osteoporosis.

INDICATION(S) AND RESEARCH PHASE
Menopause – Phase III
Hormone Replacement Therapy/Menopause – Phase III
Osteoporosis – Phase III

conjugated estrogen tablets
Premarin/Trimegesterone

MANUFACTURER
Wyeth-Ayerst

DESCRIPTION
Premarin/Trimegesterone is being evaluated in phase III trials for relieving menopausal symptoms as well as decreasing the incidence of endometrial hyperplasia seen with estrogen-alone therapy. Premarin for oral administration contains a mixture of estrogens obtained exclusively from natural sources. Trimegesterone is a progestational molecule originated by Aventis for hormone replacement therapy.

INDICATION(S) AND RESEARCH PHASE
Menopause – Phase III
Hormone Replacement Therapy/Menopause – Phase III

estrogen
Vivelle-Dot

MANUFACTURER
Noven Pharmaceuticals

DESCRIPTION
Vivelle-Dot is an estrogen transdermal system designed to be exceptionally small and provide hormone replacement therapy for the treatment of menopausal symptoms. Vivelle-Dot utilizes dot matrix adhesive technology to deliver 17-beta-estradiol through the skin and into the bloodstream. It is FDA approved for the treatment of menopausal symptoms, and is also in clinical development for the treatment of osteoporosis.

INDICATION(S) AND RESEARCH PHASE
Menopause – FDA approved

Osteoporosis – NDA submitted

estrogen
Vivelle/Menorest

MANUFACTURER
Noven Pharmaceuticals

DESCRIPTION
Vivelle/Menorest is an estradiol transdermal system to be used as hormone replacement therapy (HRT) for the treatment of menopausal symptoms and the prevention of osteoporosis. The product delivers 17-beta estradiol, the primary estrogen produced by the ovaries, through a patch that is applied twice weekly. It has been approved by the FDA for menopausal symptoms, and an application has been filed and results are pending for the osteoporosis indication.

Marketing rights have been licensed to Novogyne in the United States, to Novartis in Canada, and to Aventis in all other territories. The product is being sold as Menorest in 19 foreign countries, including France, Germany, and the United Kingdom, while being marketed as Vivelle in the United States and Canada.

INDICATION(S) AND RESEARCH PHASE
Osteoporosis – NDA submitted
Menopause – FDA approved

transdermal testosterone gel
Tostrelle

MANUFACTURER
Cellegy Pharmaceuticals

DESCRIPTION
Tostrelle (transdermal testosterone gel) is indicated for the treatment of low levels of testosterone in menopausal women. Testosterone deficiency in women is a frequent cause of diminished libido or low sex drive.

INDICATION(S) AND RESEARCH PHASE
Menopause – Phase I/II
Hormone Replacement
   Therapy/Menopause – Phase II
Sexual Dysfunction – Phase I/II

Neuropathy, Diabetic

BMS-186295, SR-47436 (irbesartan)
Avapro

MANUFACTURER
Bristol-Myers Squibb

DESCRIPTION
Avapro is a very selective, long-acting angiotensin-II receptor antagonist. By inhibiting the potent vasoconstrictor, angiotensin-II, Avapro works to lower blood pressure.

Avapro (irbesartan) is an approved drug (September 1997) in the United States and indicated for the treatment of hypertension. Additionally, the company is trying to extend the product line by conducting a phase III trial for the indication of diabetic neuropathy. Avapro alters the renin-angiotensin-aldosterone system, which are hormones involved with kidney function. A phase IV trial for heart failure is planned for 2001.

INDICATION(S) AND RESEARCH PHASE
Neuropathy, Diabetic – Phase III
Congestive Heart Failure – Phase III completed

LY-333531
unknown

MANUFACTURER
Eli Lilly

DESCRIPTION
LY-333531 is an enzyme inhibitor (of PKC). It is being tested in diabetes subjects in a phase II trial for the treatment of neuropathy and eye disease (macular edema), which are pathological diabetic complications.

INDICATION(S) AND RESEARCH PHASE
Neuropathy, Diabetic – Phase II
Eye Disorders/Infections – Phase II

memantine
unknown

MANUFACTURER
Neurobiological Technologies

DESCRIPTION
Memantine is an orally available compound that appears to restore the function of damaged nerve cells and reduce abnormal excitatory signals. This is accomplished by the modulation of N-methyl-D-aspartate (NMDA) receptor activity.

Memantine is in trials for diabetic neuropathy (phase II completed), AIDS-related dementia and neurological function (phase II), and moderate to severe dementia and Alzheimer's disease (phase III). Forest Laboratories intends to prepare an NDA for submission around the end of 2001 for the treatment of Alzheimer's disease, but will also begin additional phase III trials in both mild to moderate and moderately severe to severe Alzheimer's disease.

Forest Laboratories has entered into an agreement with Merz & Co. (collaborator of Neurobiological Technologies) for the development and marketing of memantine in the United States.

INDICATION(S) AND RESEARCH PHASE
Alzheimer's Disease – Phase III
Acquired Immune Deficiency Syndrome
   (AIDS) and AIDS-Related Infections –
   Phase II
Neuropathy, Diabetic – Phase II completed

timcodar dimesylate
Timcodar

MANUFACTURER
Vertex Pharmaceuticals

DESCRIPTION
Timcodar dimesylate is an orally bioavailable neuroprotective agent being evaluated in a phase II trial for reversal of neural dysfunction in subjects with diabetic neuropathy. This neurophilin compound is made up of small molecules that may promote nerve growth and recovery of nerve function.

In 1998, Vertex began collaborating with Schering AG on the discovery, development and commercialization of neurophilin ligands for the treatment of neurological disease. Vertex and Schering AG are working to clarify the development track for Timcodar.

INDICATION(S) AND RESEARCH PHASE
Neuropathy, Diabetic – Phase II

zenarestat
unknown

MANUFACTURER
Pfizer

DESCRIPTION
Pfizer announced in October 2000 that it is suspending development of its aldose reductase inhibitor research candidate, zenarestat, for the treatment of diabetic neuropathy. The company based its decision on an evaluation of safety data from two large phase III trials. In a small number of subjects, zenarestat was noted to have potential renal toxicity, which appears to be dose dependent with the majority of cases at the highest dose (1200 mg/day). However with regard to efficacy, zenarestat was shown in phase II development to have a beneficial effect on nerve conduction velocity, which was confirmed in an interim efficacy analysis of one of the phase III trials.

INDICATION(S) AND RESEARCH PHASE
Neuropathy, Diabetic – Phase III discontinued

Obesity

bromocriptine, ER-230
Ergoset

MANUFACTURER
Ergo Science

DESCRIPTION
Ergoset stimulates dopamine (D_2) receptors and is being tested in phase II trials for the treatment of obesity. This drug was made in a low-dose oral tablet formulation.

INDICATION(S) AND RESEARCH PHASE
Obesity – Phase II

ecopipam
unknown

MANUFACTURER
Schering-Plough Corporation

DESCRIPTION
Ecopipam is a D_1/D_5 dopamine receptor antagonist being developed in an oral formulation. It is in phase II trials for the management of obesity.

INDICATION(S) AND RESEARCH PHASE
Obesity – Phase II

GI 181771
unknown

MANUFACTURER
GlaxoSmithKline

DESCRIPTION
GI 181771 is a cholecystokinin (CCK)-A receptor agonist being tested in phase I trials for the treatment of obesity and gallstone prophylaxis.

INDICATION(S) AND RESEARCH PHASE
Gallbladder Disorders – Phase I
Obesity – Phase I

GW 427353
unknown

MANUFACTURER
GlaxoSmithKline

DESCRIPTION
GW 427353 is a beta-3-adrenergic receptor agonist. It is currently in phase I trials for the treatment of type 2 diabetes and obesity.

INDICATION(S) AND RESEARCH PHASE
Diabetes Mellitus Types 1 and 2 – Phase I
Obesity – Phase I

leptin
unknown

MANUFACTURER
Amgen

DESCRIPTION
Leptin is a genetically engineered (recombinant) form of a protein that is naturally made by the human body. This gene therapy is being evaluated in phase II trials for the treatment of obesity and type 2 diabetes. Leptin is made in a subcutaneous injectable formulation.

INDICATION(S) AND RESEARCH PHASE
Diabetes Mellitus Types 1 and 2 – Phase II
Obesity – Phase II

orlistat
Xenical

MANUFACTURER
Hoffmann-La Roche

DESCRIPTION
Xenical (orlistat) is a lipase inhibitor that inhibits the absorption of dietary fats. It is currently being marketed by Hoffmann-La Roche in the United States for the treatment of obesity. It is also in phase III trials for children 12 to 16 years of age.

INDICATION(S) AND RESEARCH PHASE
Obesity – FDA approved
Pediatric, Obesity – Phase III
Diabetes Mellitus Types 1 and 2 – Phase III

RF-1051
unknown

MANUFACTURER
SuperGen

DESCRIPTION
RF-1051 is a human hormonal replica (analogue) that appears to cause cells to burn more fat to produce the same amount of energy. This agent is being tested in phase II trials for the treatment of obesity and diabetes. RF-1051 is made in an oral capsule formulation.

INDICATION(S) AND RESEARCH PHASE
Diabetes Mellitus Types 1 and 2 – Phase II

Obesity – Phase II
Metabolic Disease – Phase II

SB 418790
unknown

MANUFACTURER
GlaxoSmithKline

DESCRIPTION
SB 418790 is a beta-3-adrenergic receptor agonist being tested in phase I trials for the treatment of type 2 diabetes and obesity.

INDICATION(S) AND RESEARCH PHASE
Diabetes Mellitus Types 1 and 2 – Phase I
Obesity – Phase I

SR-141716
unknown

MANUFACTURER
Sanofi-Synthelabo Pharmaceuticals

DESCRIPTION
SR-141716 is a medication that may provide for the treatment of schizophrenia, obesity, and smoking addiction. It is in an oral formulation and is currently being tested in phase IIa clinical trials. Marijuana activates receptors in the body called cannabinoid (CB1) receptors. The human body itself makes a substance, anandamide, which also activates these receptors. It has long been observed that marijuana use increases appetite, probably through activation of these cannabinoid receptors. Scientists hope that by blocking these receptors with SR-141716, appetite will be reduced, leading to weight loss. Currently, this drug is being evaluated as a new weight loss therapy.

These cannabinoid receptors also may play a role in drug and alcohol abuse, possibly by affecting the activity of brain reward systems. By lowering the "reward" (the pleasant sensation) that the brain experiences from smoking, drinking, or using mood altering drugs, blockage of these receptors may help control addictive behaviors.

Additionally, the cannabinoid receptor may contribute to schizophrenic behavior. The company reported that preliminary studies have shown that when these receptors were blocked with SR-141716, the hyperactive, psychotic behavior associated with schizophrenia was decreased. Overactivity or overproduction of cannabinoid receptors in the body may contribute to an imbalance in dopamine, the neurotransmitter most commonly associated with schizophrenia. Current clinical trials for all these indications are under way.

INDICATION(S) AND RESEARCH PHASE
Schizophrenia and Schizoaffective Disorders – Phase IIa
Obesity – Phase II
Smoking Cessation – Phase II

unknown
Axokine

MANUFACTURER
Regeneron Pharmaceuticals

DESCRIPTION
Axokine is a genetically engineered version of a naturally occurring human protein known as ciliary neurotrophic factor (CNTF).

In November 2000, results of a double-blind, placebo-controlled phase II trial indicated that Axokine produced statistically significant weight loss in a dose-dependent manner. Enrolled subjects were morbidly obese, with an average baseline weight of 240 pounds and a body mass index between 35 and 50 kg/square meter. Subjects who received the optimal dose of Axokine averaged 10 pounds greater weight loss than subjects on placebo, and continued to lose weight over the 12-week treatment period. Regeneron Pharmaceuticals plans to initiate phase III testing in 2001.

INDICATION(S) AND RESEARCH PHASE
Obesity – Phase II completed

Pancreatic Cancer

CEP-701
unknown

MANUFACTURER
Cephalon

DESCRIPTION
CEP-701 is an orally active inhibitor of the enzyme, tyrosine kinase that works as a signal transduction modulator for the treatment of various cancers. It is being evaluated in phase II studies for prostate cancer and pancreatic ductal adenocarcinoma.

INDICATION(S) AND RESEARCH PHASE
Pancreatic Cancer – Phase II
Prostate Cancer – Phase II

CI-1042, ONYX-015
unknown

MANUFACTURER
Onyx Pharmaceuticals

DESCRIPTION
CI-1042 (ONYX-015) is a tumor-selective, modified adenovirus that has been genetically engineered to replicate in and kill cancer cells that possess a mutated oncogene called p53, while sparing normal cells with functioning p53. p53 Is a tumor suppressor gene that is mutated in approximately 50% of all human cancers. CI-1042 is in development for several indications, including pancreatic cancer, liver metastases of colorectal cancer, and lung cancer.

Results of a phase II trial demonstrated that CI-1042 administered as a single-agent replicates and causes tumor regression in refractory head and neck cancer. CI-1042 was shown to selectively target cancer cells containing a mutant p53 gene, while sparing normal cells with a functioning p53 gene. Of the 19 subjects who received the standard dosing regimen, four (21%) had an objective response, including two complete responses and two partial responses. CI-1042 is being co-developed with Pfizer.

INDICATION(S) AND RESEARCH PHASE
Colorectal Cancer – Phase II
Pancreatic Cancer – Phase II
Head and Neck Cancer – Phase III
Cervical Dysplasia/Cancer – Phase I completed
Lung Cancer – Phase II

Bladder Cancer – Phase I completed
Brain Cancer – Phase I completed

CTP-37
Avicine

MANUFACTURER
AVI BioPharma

DESCRIPTION
Avicine is a hormone vaccine derived from human chorionic gonadotropin peptide that is being tested for prevention of colorectal, pancreatic and prostate cancer. AVI BioPharma is partnering with the company SuperGen and under the terms of the agreement, SuperGen will be responsible for U.S. marketing and sales of Avicine, and AVI will be responsible for product manufacturing.

INDICATION(S) AND RESEARCH PHASE
Colorectal Cancer – Phase III
Pancreatic Cancer – Phase III
Prostate Cancer – Phase II

diethylnorspermine
DENSPM

MANUFACTURER
GelTex Pharmaceuticals

DESCRIPTION
DENSPM (diethylnorspermine) is similar to a naturally produced polyamine, except that it may interrupt the rapid growth of tumor cells that need polyamines for growth. The drug is in phase II trials for renal cell carcinoma, pancreatic cancer, malignant melanoma, and non-small cell lung cancer. Additional indications may include ovarian and colon cancers.

INDICATION(S) AND RESEARCH PHASE
Renal Cell Carcinoma – Phase II
Pancreatic Cancer – Phase II
Malignant Melanoma – Phase II
Lung Cancer – Phase II

GBC-590
unknown

MANUFACTURER
Safe Sciences

DESCRIPTION
GBC-590 is a designed carbohydrate representing a new class of drugs, lectin inhibitors that specifically interfere with cellular interactions. GBC-590 competitively binds to unique lectins (special protein cell-surface receptors) on cancer cells and disrupts the metastatic process. GBC-590's affinity for cancer lectins is the core reason for its' significant biological activity and specificity.

GBC-590 is being tested in phase II studies for pancreatic and colorectal cancer and plans to be tested in phase II trials for prostate cancer.

INDICATION(S) AND RESEARCH PHASE
Colorectal Cancer – Phase II
Pancreatic Cancer – Phase II
Prostate Cancer – Phase I/II

gemcitabine HCl
Gemzar

MANUFACTURER
Eli Lilly

DESCRIPTION
Gemzar, a nucleoside analogue, mimics a natural building block of DNA. Gemzar disrupts the process of cell replication and thereby slows or stops progression of the disease. The drug is administered intravenously. Gemzar is being tested for the treatment of breast cancer and ovarian cancer.

Gemzar is approved as first-line treatment of locally advanced or metastatic pancreatic cancer and, in combination with cisplatin, for locally advanced or metastatic non-small cell lung cancer.

INDICATION(S) AND RESEARCH PHASE
Breast Cancer – Phase III
Lung Cancer – FDA approved
Ovarian Cancer – Phase III
Pancreatic Cancer – FDA approved

HSPPC-96
Oncophage

MANUFACTURER
Antigenics

DESCRIPTION
Oncophage cancer vaccine is an injectable protein that contains the unique profile ("antigenic fingerprint") of each subject's cancer. The antigens activate the immune system to elicit an anti-tumor response. Oncophage is in clinical trials for several indications, including renal cell carcinoma (phase III), melanoma (phase II), colorectal cancer (phase II), gastric cancer (phase I/II), pancreatic cancer (phase I/II completed), and non-Hodgkin's lymphoma (phase II).

A phase II trial of Oncophage is being conducted in subjects who have been diagnosed with sarcoma, also known as soft tissue cancer. The study is expected to initially enroll 20 subjects diagnosed with recurrent metastatic or unresectable soft tissue sarcoma and may be expanded to include an additional 15 subjects depending on preliminary results.

INDICATION(S) AND RESEARCH PHASE
Renal Cell Carcinoma – Phase III
Malignant Melanoma – Phase I/II
Colorectal Cancer – Phase II
Gastric Cancer – Phase I/II
Pancreatic Cancer – Phase I/II completed
Lymphoma, non-Hodgkin's – Phase II
Sarcoma – Phase II

HuC242-DM1/SB-408075
unknown

MANUFACTURER
ImmunoGen

DESCRIPTION
HuC242-DM1/SB-408075 is a tumor-activated prodrug (TAP) designed for the treatment of colorectal, pancreatic, and certain non-small cell lung cancers. Tumor-activated prodrugs consist of chemically linked monoclonal antibodies and potent, cell-killing chemicals. HuC242-DM1 in particular is created by joining the cytotoxic maytansinoid drug DM1 with the humanized monoclonal antibody C242.

The attached chemical remains inactive until the monoclonal antibody reaches its targeted tumor cell and the TAP is drawn inside. Once inside, DM1 is able to kill the tumor cell without affecting surrounding healthy cells. HuC242-DM1 is currently in phase I/II trials.

INDICATION(S) AND RESEARCH PHASE
Colorectal Cancer – Phase I/II
Pancreatic Cancer – Phase I/II
Lung Cancer – Phase I/II

IMC-C225, CPT-11
unknown

MANUFACTURER
ImClone Systems

DESCRIPTION
C225 is a chimerized (part mouse, part human) monoclonal antibody that may help fight cancer cells when used in conjunction with radiation therapy or other chemotherapy agents. This antibody selectively blocks a receptor, the epidermal growth factor receptor (EGFr), which may be present in greater amounts on actively growing tumor cells. Since many cancers use specific growth factors to stimulate tumor cell growth, blocking this receptor may inhibit the cancer from increasing in size and spreading throughout the body. This biological drug is given by intravenous infusion using an initial (loading) dose of 400 mg/m² followed by weekly maintenance doses of 250 mg/m².

Two phase III clinical trials of its lead cancer therapeutic, C225, are being conducted; the first trial is in combination with radiation in subjects with advanced squamous cell cancer of the head and neck and the second is testing the effect of C225 in combination with cisplatin (a chemotherapy drug) in approximately 114 subjects with advanced squamous cell cancer of the head and neck. Subjects will be treated with cisplatin alone or cisplatin plus weekly infusions of C225 per the protocol. The primary endpoint of the trial will be response and time to disease progression.

Additionally, two phase II clinical trials are being conducted for newly diagnosed cases of renal cell carcinoma or metastatic disease. Subjects will be treated with C225 in combination with interleukin-2 or interferon, to determine the response rate to therapy and safety profiles. Lastly, a dose-ranging phase Ib/IIa clinical trial for subjects with metastatic breast cancer is open to enrollment. This study is testing of the safety and efficacy of C225 in combination with Taxol (a chemotherapy agent).

Other clinical trial indications testing C225 include small cell lung cancer using combination therapy with cisplatin, and prostate cancer using C225 combined with doxorubicin. C225 is licensed from Rhone-Poulenc Rorer.

INDICATION(S) AND RESEARCH PHASE
Breast Cancer – Phase I/II
Head and Neck Cancer – Phase II/III
Lung Cancer – Phase III
Prostate Cancer – Phase I/II
Renal Cell Carcinoma – Phase II
Pancreatic Cancer – Phase II
Colorectal Cancer – Phase II

IMMU-MN14, anti-CEA
CEA-Cide

MANUFACTURER
Immunomedics

DESCRIPTION
Carcinoembryonic antigen (CEA) is a protein-polysaccharide complex released in the bloodstream by certain cancers, especially colon carcinoma. This antigenic substance may provide early diagnosis when used as a therapeutic marker in immunologic tests. The CEA complex may also be targeted by specialized monoclonal antibodies in the design of a biologic therapeutic.

CEA-Cide is a novel monoclonal antibody that is designed for radioimmunotherapy (with 90 Y-labeled humanized MN-14). This drug is being tested in phase II trials for the treatment of subjects with advanced metastatic, CEA-producing cancers, particularly colorectal cancer. Other indications may include breast cancer, female reproductive system cancer, ovarian cancer, lung cancer, and pancreatic cancer.

INDICATION(S) AND RESEARCH PHASE
Breast Cancer – Phase II
Cancer/Tumors (Unspecified) – Phase II
Colorectal Cancer – Phase II
Lung Cancer – Phase II
Ovarian Cancer – Phase II
Pancreatic Cancer – Phase II

ISIS-2503
unknown

MANUFACTURER
Isis Pharmaceuticals

DESCRIPTION
ISIS 2503 is a potent, selective antisense inhibitor of H-ras gene expression. Antisense drugs inhibit the production of disease-causing proteins by altering the genetic information, which messenger RNA uses to produce new protein. H-ras is one of a family of ras genes that are involved in the process by which cells receive and send signals that affect their behavior. The company claims that substantial evidence exists to support a direct role for the ras gene products in the development and maintenance of human cancers.

In phase II trials of ISIS 2503, the compound is being evaluated as a single-agent in subjects with colon, breast, pancreatic and non-small cell lung cancers. These trials will provide preliminary data on the antitumor activity of ISIS 2503 against these common tumor types. Approximately ten sites in the United States and Europe will enroll 15–30 subjects per tumor type in these trials. The company plans future trials of ISIS 2503 in combination with approved cancer therapies.

INDICATION(S) AND RESEARCH PHASE
Breast Cancer – Phase II
Colon Malignancies – Phase II
Lung Cancer – Phase II
Pancreatic Cancer – Phase II

ISIS-5132, CGP-69846A
unknown

MANUFACTURER
Isis Pharmaceuticals

DESCRIPTION

ISIS-5132 is a potent antisense inhibitor of the enzyme, c-Raf-1 kinase. Antisense drugs inhibit the production of disease-causing proteins by altering the genetic information, which messenger RNA uses to produce new protein. c-Raf kinase plays a role in signal processes that regulate cell growth and proliferation. It is one of a family of raf genes thought to play an important role in the development of some solid tumors. The company reports that activated-Raf has also been detected in a substantial variety of human cancers including small cell lung carcinoma and breast cancer. For example, it has been reported that 60% of all lung carcinoma cells express unusually high levels of normal c-Raf mRNA and protein.

Results from phase I studies, which examined subjects with a wide variety of solid tumors, demonstrated that the drug was well tolerated and that several subjects experienced disease stabilization. The developing companies plan additional phase I safety studies involving the drug in combination with currently approved chemotherapies. Phase II clinical trials examining ISIS-5132 as a single agent therapy for the treatment of breast, lung, colon, pancreatic and prostate cancers are under way.

INDICATION(S) AND RESEARCH PHASE
Breast Cancer – Phase II
Cancer/Tumors (Unspecified) – Phase II
Colon Malignancies – Phase II
Lung Cancer – Phase II
Pancreatic Cancer – Phase II
Prostate Cancer – Phase II

marimastat, BB-2516
unknown

MANUFACTURER
British Biotech plc

DESCRIPTION

Marimastat is an inhibitor of matrix metalloproteinase (MMP), a family of naturally occurring enzymes that are over-produced in a number of disease states, especially in cancer, where MMPs are involved in the spread and local growth of tumors. Both angiogenesis and metastasis require MMPs during tumor invasion. Anti-angiogenic strategies, unlike other therapeutic approaches, do not aim to directly destroy or "kill" the tumor or cause tumor regression. Rather, they are designed to prevent the further growth of tumors by limiting their blood supply. Because peripheral tumor cells could theoretically survive on a diffusion-dependent basis, anti-angiogenic drugs may prove most effective when given in combination with other standard cytotoxic regimens. Marimastat is in phase III development for the treatment of cancer.

British Biotech and Schering-Plough Corporation signed an agreement to develop and commercialize British Biotech's metalloproteinase inhibitors, including marimastat.

INDICATION(S) AND RESEARCH PHASE
Pancreatic Cancer – Phase III
Lung Cancer – Phase III
Breast Cancer – Phase III
Brain Cancer – Phase III completed
Ovarian Cancer – Phase III

MDX-210
unknown

MANUFACTURER
Medarex

DESCRIPTION

MDX-210 is a bispecific (target-trigger) monoclonal antibody (MAb)-based treatment being developed for prostate cancer and other cancers with specific markers (HER-2/*neu* positive), including renal cell, non-small cell lung, pancreatic, prostate, and kidney cancers. Phase II trials have been completed for kidney, prostate, and ovarian cancers. The additional indications were in phase II trials. Phase III trials have been commenced in Europe under a partnership with Immuno-Designed Molecules.

INDICATION(S) AND RESEARCH PHASE
Prostate Cancer – Phase II
Renal Cell Carcinoma – Phase II
Colon Malignancies – Phase II
Breast Cancer – Phase II
Renal Cell Carcinoma – Phase II
Gastric Cancer – Phase II
Pancreatic Cancer – Phase II
Lung Cancer – Phase II
Ovarian Cancer (Europe) – Phase III

MDX-220
unknown

MANUFACTURER
Medarex

DESCRIPTION

MDX-220 is a bispecific (target-trigger) monoclonal antibody (MAb) that targets Tag-72 in the treatment of a variety of cancers, including lung, colon, prostate, ovarian, endometrial, pancreatic, and gastric cancer. These indications are in phase I/II trials.

INDICATION(S) AND RESEARCH PHASE
Endometrial Cancer – Phase I/II
Gastric Cancer – Phase I/II
Lung Cancer – Phase I/II
Ovarian Cancer – Phase I/II
Pancreatic Cancer – Phase I/II
Prostate Cancer – Phase II
Colorectal Cancer – Phase II

MGI-114, hydroxymethylacylfulvene, HMAF
Irofulven

MANUFACTURER
MGI Pharma

DESCRIPTION

Irofulven (MGI-114) is the first product candidate being developed by MGI Pharma from its family of anti-cancer compounds called acylfulvenes. Early trials demonstrated that Irofulven is absorbed rapidly by tumor cells, and once inside binds to DNA and protein targets. The binding interferes with DNA replication and cell division, leading to tumor-specific cell death. The drug is being tested in a series of phase I and II trials for a variety of cancers.

Results from a phase II trial of Irofulven indicated that the drug produced anti-tumor activity in subjects with advanced pancreatic cancer who were refractory to gemcitabine (Gemzar). Ten of the 53 subjects enrolled achieved six-month survival and two subjects demonstrated objective responses: one subject experienced tumor shrinkage of 100% and another subject experienced an 84% decrease in tumor mass. A phase III trial was initiated in February 2001.

INDICATION(S) AND RESEARCH PHASE
Breast Cancer – Phase II
Colon Malignancies – Phase II
Renal Cell Carcinoma – Phase II
Cervical Dysplasia/Cancer – Phase II
Lung Cancer – Phase II
Ovarian Cancer – Phase I/II
Colorectal Cancer – Phase II
Prostate Cancer – Phase I/II
Cancer/Tumors (Unspecified) – Phase I/II
Pancreatic Cancer – Phase III
Liver Cancer – Phase II

RFS-2000
Rubitecan

MANUFACTURER
SuperGen

DESCRIPTION
Rubitecan is a novel drug that works by inhibiting an enzyme called topoisomerase-I. This drug is made in an oral form that is an advantage for outpatient treatment compared to intravenous type cancer drugs that may require a visit to a hospital setting.

Rubitecan is being evaluated in treating advanced pancreatic cancer and a variety of solid tumors, such as in breast, colorectal, lung, ovarian, and prostate cancers, as well as metastatic melanoma and advanced gastric carcinoma. Also, phase II trials in the United States and Europe are testing Rubitecan in blood cancers such as chronic myelomonocytic leukemia (CMML/myelodysplastic syndrome).

Some expected side effects reported are blood toxicities, bladder irritation (cystitis), and some gastrointestinal disorders.

INDICATION(S) AND RESEARCH PHASE
Pancreatic Cancer – Phase III
Breast Cancer – Phase II
Colorectal Cancer – Phase II
Gastric Cancer – Phase II
Leukemia – Phase II
Malignant Melanoma – Phase II
Ovarian Cancer – Phase II
Myelodysplastic Syndrome – Phase III

SR-27897B
unknown

MANUFACTURER
Sanofi-Synthelabo Pharmaceuticals

DESCRIPTION
CCK-A (cholecystokinin-A) is a molecule that is secreted from the lining of the small intestine, and is also present in the central nervous system. It is a substance that causes many different actions throughout the body, including gallbladder contraction, release of pancreatic digestive enzymes, and promotion of the feeling of digestive fullness or satiety. CCK also promotes cell growth and division, especially in the pancreas. It also has a regulating effect on the amount of the neurotransmitters dopamine and serotonin present in the body.

SR-27897 is a potent substance that blocks the receptors to which CCK would ordinarily bind, thus blocking CCK's effects on the body. By negating the action of CCK, people may lose their sense of satiety, potentially making SR-27897 a good therapy for anorexia. In addition, CCK's probable role in the pathogenesis of pancreatic cancer (since it can cause abnormal pancreatic cell division) may also be reduced with the use of SR-27897. Potential applications for this drug may also include treatment for autism, although no clinical trials for this indication are under way as of yet.

INDICATION(S) AND RESEARCH PHASE
Pancreatic Cancer – Phase II
Anorexia – Phase II

troxacitabine, BCH-4556
Troxatyl

MANUFACTURER
BioChem Pharma

DESCRIPTION
Troxatyl is a dioxolane nucleoside analog being investigated as an anticancer agent. The drug is a complete DNA chain terminator and DNA polymerase inhibitor. It acts by incorporating itself into the growing DNA chain of cancer cells, interfering with their ability to replicate further. Currently, Troxatyl is being evaluated as a single agent or in combination therapy in a number of ongoing single and multicenter trials in hematologic malignancies, including acute myeloid leukemia, chronic myeloid leukemia—blastic phase, and in lymphoproliferative disorders such as lymphoma, chronic lymphocytic leukemia, and myeloma. It is also being evaluated as a single agent in pancreatic cancer and in combination therapy in a number of solid tumors. Troxatyl is currently in phase II development.

INDICATION(S) AND RESEARCH PHASE
Cancer/Tumors (Unspecified) – Phase II
Colorectal Cancer – Phase II
Head and Neck Cancer – Phase II
Leukemia – Phase II
Lung Cancer – Phase II
Malignant Melanoma – Phase II
Ovarian Cancer – Phase II
Pancreatic Cancer – Phase II
Prostate Cancer – Phase II
Renal Cell Carcinoma – Phase II

vaccine, anti-gastrin
Gastrimmune

MANUFACTURER
Aphton Corporation

DESCRIPTION
Gastrimmune is a therapeutic vaccine that neutralizes specific hormones (G17 & Gly-extended G17). The drug is in phase III trials for the treatment of cancers of the gastrointestinal tract, including gastric cancer, colorectal cancer, liver cancer, esophageal cancer and two phase III trials for advanced pancreatic cancer—one in the the United States and one in Europe.

INDICATION(S) AND RESEARCH PHASE
Colorectal Cancer – Phase III
Esophageal Cancer – Phase III
Gastric Cancer – Phase III
Liver Cancer – Phase II/III

Pancreatic Cancer – Phase III

vaccine, cancer
Gvax

MANUFACTURER
Cell Genesys

DESCRIPTION
Gvax is an allogeneic compound involving genetic modification of prostate cancer cell lines. These cancer cells have been irradiated and modified to secrete granulocyte-macrophage colony stimulating factor (GM-CSF), a hormone that plays a key role in stimulating the body's immune response to vaccines. The compound is in phase II trials for prostate and pancreatic cancer, and phase I/II trials for lung cancer, leukemia, and malignant melanoma.

The Gvax prostate cancer vaccine demonstrated anti-tumor activity in an initial phase II trial in subjects with advanced metastatic prostate cancer who have not responded to hormone therapy. Prior to initiating a phase III trial, Cell Genesys plans to initiate further trials of Gvax prostate cancer vaccine in 2001, which will employ a higher potency version of the same product. In addition, the product may be tested in combination with chemotherapy since future phase III trials in hormone refractory prostate cancer subjects may compare Gvax vaccine in combination with chemotherapy to chemotherapy alone.

INDICATION(S) AND RESEARCH PHASE
Prostate Cancer – Phase II
Lung Cancer – Phase I/II completed
Malignant Melanoma – Phase I/II
Vaccines – Phase I/II
Pancreatic Cancer – Phase II
Leukemia – Phase I/II

pancrelipase
Viokase

MANUFACTURER
Axcan Pharma

DESCRIPTION
Viokase is a pancreatic enzyme preparation containing standardized lipase, protease, and amylase in fixed proportions. It is indicated for the treatment of subjects with exocrine pancreatic enzyme deficiency as is often associated with cystic fibrosis, chronic pancreatitis, and post-pancreatectomy. It has been prescribed for years to assist in the digestion and absorption of food. Axcan is currently conducting phase II trials of Viokase at elevated dosages (8,000 units/day) to alleviate pain often associated with pancreatic disorders.

INDICATION(S) AND RESEARCH PHASE
Pain, Acute or Chronic – Phase II
Pancreatic Disorders – Phase II

Parathyroid Disease

calcimimetics
unknown

MANUFACTURER
Amgen

DESCRIPTION
Calcimimetics are small molecules that activate calcium receptors and suppress the secretion of excessive amounts of parathyroid hormone. These compounds are orally-active and are beneficial in treating hyperthyroidism. The drug is currently in phase II trials for treatment of dialysis study volunteers with secondary HTP.

The body has four small parathyroid glands which are located on the back of the thyroid gland in the neck. The parathyroid gland secretes a hormone called parathyroid hormone (PTH) which breaks down the bones to increase calcium and decrease phosphorus levels in the blood. Excessive amounts of PTH may weaken muscles, fracture bones, and cause rare seizures.

In primary hyperparathyroidism some problem exists within the gland itself to cause oversecretion of PTH. Secondary hyperparathyroidism is an adaptive response to conditions that cause low calcium, like intestinal malabsorption syndromes or kidney failure. Calcimimetics may be helpful to dialysis subjects who frequently experience kidney failure.

The calcimimetic compounds are licensed for development from NPS Pharmaceuticals to Amgen who is conducting two phase II trials in the United States. The first study is testing subjects with primary HPT; and, the other trial is evaluating dialysis subjects with secondary HPT.

INDICATION(S) AND RESEARCH PHASE
Parathyroid Disease – Phase II

AMG 073
unknown

MANUFACTURER
NPS Allelix Corp

DESCRIPTION
AMG 073 is NPS's lead calcimimetic, a group of orally active compounds being developed for the treatment of hyperparathyroidism (HPT). They act on calcium receptors located on parathyroid cells to restore normal levels of parathyroid hormone (PTH) and calcium in the bloodstream.

Preliminary phase II results demonstrated that administration of single doses of AMG 073 produced dose-dependent decreases in PTH in subjects with secondary HPT. Further results indicated that daily doses of AMG 073 administered over 8 days were associated with decreases in PTH and calcium values. A larger phase II study is currently being conducted in subjects with secondary HPT to confirm and build upon these preliminary results.

INDICATION(S) AND RESEARCH PHASE
Parathyroid Disorders – Phase II

Thyroid Cancer

arcitumomab
CEA-Scan

MANUFACTURER
Immunomedics

DESCRIPTION
CEA-Scan is a monoclonal antibody

attached to carcinoembryonic (CEA) antigen that is radioactively labeled with technetium (Tc99m). CEA is an important cell surface marker expressed by certain tumor cells. This imaging agent can detect various cancer cells associated with CEA expressed tumors. CEA-Scan utilizes the proprietary technetium (RAID) technology.

Currently, CEA-Scan is being tested in three trials: A phase II/III trial for breast cancer that is using CEA-scan to evaluate subjects with suspicious mammograms and palpable and non-palpable lesions. A phase II trial for thyroid cancer. CEA-Scan is used for the diagnosis and localization of primary, residual, recurrent, and metastatic medullary thyroid carcinoma. Lastly, a phase III for lung cancer, in which CEA-scan determines the presence, location, and the extent of the metastatic disease in primary and recurrent lung cancer.

INDICATION(S) AND RESEARCH PHASE
Breast Cancer – Phase II/III
Lung Cancer – Phase III
Thyroid Cancer – Phase II

Turner's Syndrome

human growth hormone
unknown

MANUFACTURER
Cangene Corporation

DESCRIPTION
Natural human growth hormone is a protein produced by the pituitary gland that acts on the long bones of the body until the onset of puberty and promotes growth to normal stature. A deficiency of this hormone during childhood results in abnormally small stature. This drug is being tested in a phase III European trial for the treatment of Turner's syndrome in girls as well as to combat short stature in children with growth hormone deficiency.

INDICATION(S) AND RESEARCH PHASE
Pediatric, Turner's Syndrome – Phase III

9 | Gastroenterology

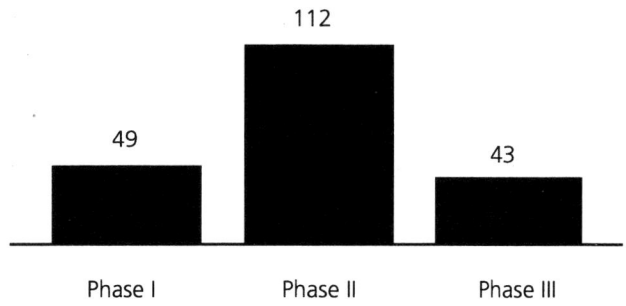

Drugs in the development pipeline

Phase I: 49
Phase II: 112
Phase III: 43

Source: CenterWatch, 2001

Digestive system disorders affect a large portion of the population, causing conditions that range from discomfort to life-threatening illnesses. Major diseases in this therapeutic area include peptic ulcer disease, hepatitis, colorectal cancer, gastroesophageal reflux disease, inflammatory bowel disease and irritable bowel syndrome.

According to the Crohn's & Colitis Foundation of America, it is estimated that there may be up to one million Americans with inflammatory bowel disease (IBD). IBD refers to both ulcerative colitis and Crohn's disease. Symptoms of Crohn's disease include abdominal pain, fever and gastrointestinal bleeding, and flare-ups can be mild to severe. Ulcerative colitis is characterized by an inflammation of the mucosal lining and sub-mucosal tissues of the colon, and symptoms include diarrhea with or without rectal bleeding and abdominal pain. CenterWatch estimates that there are 20 to 25 drugs in development for IBD, at a cost of approximately $105 million to $125 million annually in investigator grants.

IBD treatment options include aminosalicylic acid (5-ASA), immunosuppressive agents, steroids and anti-tumor necrosis factor-alpha (TNF-α)—all of which are designed to reduce intestinal inflammation. Colazal, a 5-ASA product, was the first new chemical entity approved in ten years and the first new therapy approved in seven years by the FDA for the treatment of mildly to moderately active ulcerative colitis. To avoid the side effects associated with sulfapyridine, 5-ASA is linked to a less toxic carrier molecule in Colazal.

Anti-TNF agents, in particular, have surfaced as a promising new approach to IBD. Remicade, the first biologic agent approved for the treatment of Crohn's disease, is made from a combination of human and mouse antibodies. Additional anti-TNF drugs containing less mouse and more human antibody are now in development. Researchers are also investigating other biological products such as LDP-02 (an antibody to alpha4-beta7), in addition to probiotics, growth hormone therapy, and compounds such as thalidomide as treatment options.

According to the International Foundation for Functional Gastrointestinal Disorders, as many as 35 million American adults experience irritable bowel syndrome (IBS) symptoms. IBS is characterized by multiple symptoms, including chronic or recurrent abdominal pain and discomfort and irregular bowel function, characterized by diarrhea and/or constipation. Female patients outnumber male patients by a ratio of three to one. Therapy may include first-line options such as over-the-counter fiber supplements or laxatives, along with regulated low-fat diets. Current drugs used in the treatment of IBS include antidepressants, anticholinergics, and antidiarrheal agents.

The area of IBS drug development experienced a recent setback with the withdrawal of GlaxoSmithKline's Lotronex (alosetron) from the market due to reports of serious complications. An antagonist of the serotonin 5-HT$_3$ receptor type, Lotronex was originally approved for the treatment of female patients with diarrhea-predominant IBS. However, other investigational compounds may reestablish the usefulness of 5-HT modulators. This includes Novartis' Zelmac, a 5-HT$_4$ agonist for which an NDA has been submitted. Additional compounds being developed for IBS include gastroprokinetic agents and cholecystokinin antagonists.

One of the most common gastrointestinal disorders in gastroesophageal reflux disease (GERD), which affects more than 60 million Americans. GERD is a chronic, severe form of heartburn with the potential to erode the esophageal epitherlium. The condition is characterized by reflux of acid from the stomach into the esophagus. According to CenterWatch, there are approximately seven to 12 drugs in trials for the treatment of GERD, costing approximately $30 million to $40 million in investigator grants.

Once GERD is diagnosed, there are several ways to treat it effectively. The first intervention usually involves lifestyle and diet changes; if this is not successful, individuals may be prescribed medication such as promotility agents, H2-blockers or proton pump inhibitors. In addition to approved formulations, these three drug types are also well represented in the developmental pipeline for GERD. Preclinical testing includes the development of isomers of currently approved proton pump inhibitors. Based on previous studies, these drugs may provide more consistent dosing and greater efficacy. At the other end of the spectrum, the first intravenous formulation of a proton pump inhibitor was recently approved, which will compete in the hospital market with intravenous H2-antagonists. Other avenues of GERD research include the development of vaccines, such as Aphton's anti-gastrin vaccine, or the use of 5-hydroxytryptamine (5-HT) modulators.

Anal Fissures

nitroglycerin ointment
Anogesic

MANUFACTURER
Cellegy Pharmaceuticals

DESCRIPTION
Anogesic is a nitroglycerin-based ointment applied topically for the treatment of anal fissures and hemorrhoids. Although used for more than a century for the treatment of certain cardiovascular diseases, nitroglycerin has only recently been tested in this proprietary formulation for anal fissures and hemorrhoids.

Anogesic works because the active ingredient, nitroglycerin, relaxes the muscles surrounding the blood vessels supplying the anal tissue. Studies demonstrated that the use of nitroglycerin ointment promotes healing of chronic anal fissures, offers significant pain reduction, and eliminates the need for surgery in many cases.

Phase III results showed that Anogesic produced a statistically significant reduction in pain associated with chronic anal fissures. Subjects with chronic anal fissures were randomly assigned to one of eight treatment regimens utilizing several concentrations of nitroglycerin or placebo for up to eight weeks. Statistical significance was not achieved with the primary endpoint, but treatment with 0.4% nitroglycerin ointment resulted in a highly significant decrease in pain intensity compared with placebo. In a second study, 34 hemorrhoidectomy subjects were randomly assigned to 0.2% nitroglycerin ointment or placebo applied three times daily following surgery. It was found that use of an oral narcotic drug was higher in the placebo group than the nitroglycerin group, indicating that the ointment promoted pain relief.

INDICATION(S) AND RESEARCH PHASE
Anal Fissures – Phase III completed
Hemorrhoids – Phase II

Colon Malignancies

APC8024
unknown

MANUFACTURER
Dendreon Corporation

DESCRIPTION
APC8024 is a vaccine designed to elicit an antibody response to a protein antigen called HER-2/*neu*. HER-2/*neu* is overexpressed in approximately 25% of metastatic breast cancers, ovarian, pancreatic, and colon cancers. APC8024 is being tested in phase I trials.

INDICATION(S) AND RESEARCH PHASE
Breast Cancer – Phase I
Ovarian Cancer – Phase I
Colon Malignancies – Phase I

GL-331
unknown

MANUFACTURER
Genelabs Technologies

DESCRIPTION
GL-331 is an inhibitor of topoisomerase II. It is a semi-synthetic derivative of podophyllotoxin, which is a chemotherapeutic agent designed to overcome multidrug resistant (MDR) cancers. At this time, trials have been discontinued.

INDICATION(S) AND RESEARCH PHASE
Colon Malignancies – Trial discontinued
Leukemia – Trial discontinued
Lung Cancer – Trial discontinued
Renal Cell Carcinoma – Trial discontinued

ISIS-2503
unknown

MANUFACTURER
Isis Pharmaceuticals

DESCRIPTION
ISIS-2503 is a potent, selective antisense inhibitor of H-Ras gene expression. Antisense drugs are designed to target particular genes and selectively block them. These drugs provide an exact complementary sequence to a unique part of the target gene, so that the drug will bind to and affect only that gene.

H-Ras is one of a family of ras genes that are involved in the process by which cells receive and send signals that affect their behavior. According to the company, evidence supports a direct role for ras gene products in the development and maintenance of human cancers.

In phase II trials, the compound is being evaluated as a single-agent in subjects with colon, breast, pancreatic, and non-small cell lung cancers. These trials will provide preliminary data on the anti-tumor activity of ISIS-2503 against these common tumor types. Approximately ten sites in the United States and Europe will enroll 15–30 subjects per tumor type. The company may initiate future trials of ISIS-2503 in combination with approved cancer therapies.

INDICATION(S) AND RESEARCH PHASE
Breast Cancer – Phase II
Colon Malignancies – Phase II
Lung Cancer – Phase II
Pancreatic Cancer – Phase II

ISIS-5132, CGP-69846A
unknown

MANUFACTURER
Isis Pharmaceuticals

DESCRIPTION
ISIS-5132 is a potent antisense inhibitor of the enzyme c-Raf-1 kinase. Antisense drugs are designed to target particular genes and selectively block them. These drugs provide an exact complementary sequence to a unique part of the target gene, so that the drug will bind to and affect only that gene.

c-Raf kinase plays a role in signal processes that regulate cell growth and proliferation. It is one of a family of Raf genes thought to play an important role in the development of various solid tumors. The company reported that activated Raf has also been detected in a substantial variety of cancers including small cell lung carcinoma and breast cancer. It has been reported that 60% of all lung carcinoma cells express unusually high levels of normal c-Raf mRNA and protein.

The sponsor companies reported that results from phase I studies, which examined subjects with a wide variety of solid tumors, demonstrated that the drug was well tolerated and that several subjects experienced disease stabilization. The companies are planning additional phase I safety studies involving the drug in combination with currently approved chemotherapies. Phase II clinical trials examining ISIS-5132 as a single agent therapy in subjects with breast, lung, colon, pancreatic, and prostate cancers are under way.

INDICATION(S) AND RESEARCH PHASE
Breast Cancer – Phase II
Cancer/Tumors (Unspecified) – Phase II
Colon Malignancies – Phase II
Lung Cancer – Phase II
Pancreatic Cancer – Phase II
Prostate Cancer – Phase II

MDX-210
unknown

MANUFACTURER
Medarex

DESCRIPTION
MDX-210 is a bispecific (target-trigger) monoclonal antibody-based treatment being developed for the treatment of cancers with specific markers (HER-2/*neu* positive), including renal cell, non-small cell lung, pancreatic, and kidney cancers. Phase II trials have been completed for kidney, prostate, and ovarian cancer. Phase III development for ovarian cancer has commenced in Europe.

INDICATION(S) AND RESEARCH PHASE
Prostate Cancer – Phase II completed
Renal Cell Carcinoma – Phase II completed
Colon Malignancies – Phase II
Breast Cancer – Phase II
Gastric Cancer – Phase II
Pancreatic Cancer – Phase II
Lung Cancer – Phase II
Ovarian Cancer – Phase III

MGI-114, hydroxymethylacylfulvene, HMAF
Irofulven

MANUFACTURER
MGI Pharma

DESCRIPTION
Irofulven (MGI-114) is the first product candidate being developed by MGI Pharma from its family of anti-cancer compounds called acylfulvenes. Early trials demonstrated that Irofulven is absorbed rapidly by tumor cells, and once inside binds to DNA and protein targets. The binding interferes with DNA replication and cell division, leading to tumor-specific cell death.

Results from a phase II trial of Irofulven indicated that the drug produced anti-tumor activity in subjects with advanced pancreatic cancer who were refractory to gemcitabine (Gemzar). Ten of the 53 subjects enrolled achieved six-month survival and two subjects demonstrated objective responses: one subject experienced tumor shrinkage of 100% and another subject experienced an 84% decrease in tumor mass. A phase III trial was initiated in February 2001.

INDICATION(S) AND RESEARCH PHASE
Breast Cancer – Phase II
Colon Malignancies – Phase II
Renal Cell Carcinoma – Phase II
Cervical Dysplasia/Cancer – Phase II
Lung Cancer – Phase II
Ovarian Cancer – Phase I/II
Colorectal Cancer – Phase II
Prostate Cancer – Phase I/II
Cancer/Tumors (Unspecified) – Phase I/II
Pancreatic Cancer – Phase III
Liver Cancer – Phase II

SGN-15/Taxotere
unknown

MANUFACTURER
Seattle Genetics

DESCRIPTION
SGN-15 is an antibody drug conjugate composed of the chimeric monoclonal antibody (mAb) BR96 chemically linked to the drug doxorubicin. SGN-15 works by binding to a cell surface Ley-related antigen expressed on many tumor types, rapidly internalizing, and then releasing its payload of drug at the low pH present within the cell through acid catalyzed hydrolysis in the endosome.

This mechanism of targeted drug delivery allows for relative sparing of tissues normally affected by non-specific chemotherapy, and represents an attractive strategy for the treatment of tumors expressing the BR96 antigen.

SGN-15 is being tested as a combination therapy with Aventis' Taxotere in a phase I/II trial in subjects with breast or colon cancer. This trial is being co-funded by Aventis. In addition, a phase II trial is testing SGN-15/Taxotere in hormone refractory prostate cancer.

INDICATION(S) AND RESEARCH PHASE
Breast Cancer – Phase I/II
Prostate Cancer – Phase II
Colon Malignancies – Phase I/II

SR-48692
unknown

MANUFACTURER
Sanofi-Synthelabo Pharmaceuticals

DESCRIPTION
SR-48692 is a neurotensin antagonist. This orally formulated drug is in phase II trials for colon cancer, prostate cancer, and depression. It is also in phase IIa development for the treatment of psychosis and schizophrenia.

INDICATION(S) AND RESEARCH PHASE
Colon Malignancies – Phase II
Prostate Cancer – Phase II
Schizophrenia and Schizoaffective Disorders – Phase IIa
Psychosis – Phase IIa
Depression – Phase II

TLK286
Unknown

MANUFACTURER

Telik

DESCRIPTION
TLK286 is a tumor activated drug candidate for the treatment of major cancers that are resistant to standard treatments. The small molecule drug candidate was developed through the application of Telik's proprietary TRAP chemogenomics technology. According to the company, its mechanism of activation in tumor cells suggests a potentially safer, more effective and directed cancer drug, especially against resistant cancers.

In March 2001, Telik announced that a phase II trial has begun to evaluate TLK286 for the treatment of refractory colon cancer. This multicenter, single-arm, open-label trial is designed to enroll up to 75 subjects who had relapsed or failed to respond to standard treatments for colon cancer.

INDICATION(S) AND RESEARCH PHASE
Colon Malignancies – Phase II

Colon Polyps

exisulind
Aptosyn

MANUFACTURER
Cell Pathways

DESCRIPTION
Aptosyn (exisulind) belongs to a novel class of compounds called selective apoptotic anti-neoplastic drugs (SAANDs). SAANDs inhibit a form of cyclic GMP phosphodiesterase and selectively induce apoptosis in abnormally growing precancerous and cancerous cells. Aptosyn is being tested for several indications and is in five different trials for adenomatous polyposis coli (APC) and familial adenomatous polyposis coli; two of these trials are specifically for pediatric subjects.

The company received a non-approvable letter from the FDA in September 2000 for one of the trials for the treatment of familial adenomatous polyposis. The company intends to amend the NDA and request a meeting with the FDA to address the deficiencies and the possible requirement for additional clinical data.

INDICATION(S) AND RESEARCH PHASE
Adenomatous polyposis coli – Non-approvable letter
Pediatric, Familial Adenomatous Polyposis coli – Phase II
Adenomatous polyposis coli – Phase I/II
Barrett's Esophagus Disease – Phase II
Prostate Cancer – Phase II/III
Breast Cancer – Phase II/III
Lung Cancer – Phase Ib
Colon Polyps – Phase II/III

ursodiol
Urso

MANUFACTURER
Axcan Pharma

DESCRIPTION
Urso is an oral tablet composed of a bile acid (ursodeoxycholic acid) found in small amounts in normal human bile and in larger quantities in the bile of certain bears. This drug has been marketed in the United States for the treatment of primary biliary cirrhosis (PBC) since 1998. It is also approved in Canada for the treatment of cholestatic liver diseases such as PBC and the dissolution of gallstones.

Urso is being tested in trials for at least five other indications: the treatment of hypercholesterolemia, treatment with chemo-prevention of colorectal polyps, treatment of colorectal cancer, treatment of non-alcoholic steatohepatitis, and treatment of viral hepatitis. The drug was licensed by Sanofi-Synthelabo to Axcan Pharma in a joint venture with Schwarz Pharma.

INDICATION(S) AND RESEARCH PHASE
Cholesterol (High Levels) – Phase II
Colon Polyps – Phase II
Colorectal Cancer – Phase II
Gallbladder Disorders – Phase III/IV
Hepatitis – Phase II

Colorectal Cancer

capecitabine
Xeloda

MANUFACTURER
Hoffmann-La Roche

DESCRIPTION
Xeloda is an anticancer agent and the prodrug of 5-fluorouracil (5-FU). 5-Fluorouracil is a pyrimidine analog that works by interfering with the synthesis of DNA and RNA. An NDA has been submitted for the treatment of colorectal cancer.

INDICATION(S) AND RESEARCH PHASE
Colorectal Cancer – NDA submitted

CI-1042, ONYX-015
unknown

MANUFACTURER
Onyx Pharmaceuticals

DESCRIPTION
CI-1042 (ONYX-015) is a tumor-selective, modified adenovirus (similar to the common cold virus) that has been genetically engineered to replicate in and kill cancer cells that possess a mutated oncogene called p53, while sparing normal cells with functioning p53. p53 Is a tumor suppressor gene that is mutated in approximately 50% of all human cancers.

CI-1042 is in development for several indications, including pancreatic cancer, liver metastases of colorectal cancer, and lung cancer. Results of a phase II trial demonstrated that CI-1042 administered as a single-agent replicates and causes tumor regression in refractory head and neck cancer. CI-1042 was shown to selectively target cancer cells containing a mutant p53 gene, while sparing normal cells with a functioning p53 gene. Of the 19 subjects who received the standard dosing regimen, four (21%) had an objective response, including two complete responses and two partial responses. CI-1042 is being co-developed with Pfizer.

INDICATION(S) AND RESEARCH PHASE
Colorectal Cancer – Phase II

Pancreatic Cancer – Phase II
Head and Neck Cancer – Phase III
Cervical Dysplasia/Cancer – Phase I completed
Lung Cancer – Phase II
Bladder Cancer – Phase I completed
Brain Cancer – Phase I completed

cisplatin/epinephrine
IntraDose

MANUFACTURER
Matrix Pharmaceutical

DESCRIPTION
IntraDose is a biodegradable collagen carrier matrix combined with a vasoconstrictor. The gel is injected directly into tumors where it localizes high concentrations of cisplatin, a widely used anticancer drug. IntraDose is currently being tested for several indications, including head and neck, breast, malignant melanoma, esophageal, and primary hepatocellular cancer.

A phase II trail of IntraDose Injectable Gel produced durable responses in subjects with colorectal cancer that has metastasized to the liver. Nine of 31 subjects who received IntraDose responded to therapy. Six subjects experienced a complete response (100% reduction in viable tumor volume of treated tumors) while the other three subjects demonstrated a partial response (at least a 50% reduction of viable tumor volume). Eight of the nine treatment responders have had durable responses with no relapse at the site of treatment.

INDICATION(S) AND RESEARCH PHASE
Breast Cancer – Phase II
Cancer/Tumors (Unspecified) – Phase II
Colorectal Cancer – Phase II completed
Esophageal Cancer – Phase II
Liver Cancer – Phase II
Malignant Melanoma – Phase II
Head and Neck Cancer – NDA submitted

CTP-37
Avicine

MANUFACTURER
AVI BioPharma

DESCRIPTION
Avicine is a hormone vaccine derived from human chorionic gonadotropin peptide. It is being developed for the prevention of colorectal, pancreatic, and prostate cancer. The pharmaceutical company SuperGen will be responsible for U.S. marketing and sales of Avicine, while AVI BioPharma will be responsible for product manufacturing.

INDICATION(S) AND RESEARCH PHASE
Colorectal Cancer – Phase III
Pancreatic Cancer – Phase III
Prostate Cancer – Phase II

declopramide
unknown

MANUFACTURER
OXiGENE

DESCRIPTION
Declopramide is a DNA repair inhibitor being developed for the treatment of various cancers. DNA repair inhibitors may increase the effectiveness of standard treatment by inhibiting the ability of tumor cells to repair damaged DNA, leading to apoptosis.

Two phase I trials demonstrated that declopramide increases the vulnerability of cancer cells to conventional forms of chemotherapy and radiation. The two trials took place at the Ireland Cancer Center in Cleveland, Ohio, and at St. John's Mercy Medical Center in St. Louis, Missouri. Subjects were given declopramide with either 5-fluorouracil or cisplatin. Results determined the recommended combination dose for the phase II trial that was initiated in January 2001 for colon cancer.

INDICATION(S) AND RESEARCH PHASE
Colorectal Cancer – Phase II

FMdC
unknown

MANUFACTURER
Matrix Pharmaceutical

DESCRIPTION
FMdC is a nucleoside analogue being evaluated as a possible treatment for cancer. Nucleoside analogues are a class of drugs that affect DNA synthesis, and they have long been used to treat hematologic cancers such as leukemia. The early members of this drug class were minimally effective against solid tumors.

DNA synthesis occurs during cell division and is critical to successful replication. FMdC enters cells and is metabolized into two active forms: FMdC diphosphate and FMdC triphosphate. These two active metabolites of FMdC interrupt the process of DNA synthesis, which leads to cell death. FMdC is being evaluated in phase II studies for the treatment of non-small cell lung, colorectal, and ovarian cancer.

INDICATION(S) AND RESEARCH PHASE
Colorectal Cancer – Phase II
Lung Cancer – Phase II
Ovarian Cancer – Phase II

G3139/irinotecan
Genasense/irinotecan

MANUFACTURER
Genta

DESCRIPTION
Genasense (G3139) is designed to reduce levels of bcl-2, a protein that contributes to the resistance of cancer cells to current forms of cancer treatment. Treatment with Genasense may markedly improve the effectiveness of standard anticancer therapies. Genasense in combination with irinotecan is in phase II trials for the treatment of colorectal cancer.

INDICATION(S) AND RESEARCH PHASE
Colorectal Cancer – Phase II

G3139/mitoxantrone
Genasense/mitoxantrone

MANUFACTURER
Genta

DESCRIPTION
Genasense (G3139) is designed to reduce

levels of bcl-2, a protein that contributes to the resistance of cancer cells to current forms of cancer treatment. Treatment with Genasense may markedly improve the effectiveness of standard anticancer therapies. G-3139 in combination with mitoxantrone is in trials for the treatment of prostate and colorectal cancers.

INDICATION(S) AND RESEARCH PHASE
Colorectal Cancer – Phase II
Prostate Cancer – Phase I/II

GBC-590
unknown

MANUFACTURER
Safe Sciences

DESCRIPTION
GBC-590 belongs to a new class of drugs called lectin inhibitors that specifically interfere with cellular interactions. GBC-590 competitively binds to unique lectins on cancer cells and disrupts the metastatic process. GBC-590's affinity for cancer lectins is the core reason for its significant biological activity and specificity.

GBC-590 is being tested in phase II trials for pancreatic and colorectal cancer, and the company plans to test it in phase II trials for prostate cancer.

INDICATION(S) AND RESEARCH PHASE
Colorectal Cancer – Phase II
Pancreatic Cancer – Phase II
Prostate Cancer – Phase I/II

HSPPC-96
Oncophage

MANUFACTURER
Antigenics

DESCRIPTION
Oncophage cancer vaccine is an injectable protein that contains the unique profile ("antigenic fingerprint") of each subject's cancer. The antigens activate the immune system to elicit an anti-tumor response.

Antigenics has initiated a phase II trial of Oncophage in subjects who have been diagnosed with sarcoma, also known as soft tissue cancer. The study is expected to initially enroll 20 subjects diagnosed with recurrent metastatic or unresectable soft tissue sarcoma and may be expanded to include an additional 15 subjects depending on preliminary results.

Oncophage is also in clinical trials for several other indications, including renal cell carcinoma (phase III), melanoma (phase II), colorectal cancer (phase II), gastric cancer (phase I/II), pancreatic cancer (phase I/II completed), and non-Hodgkin's lymphoma (phase II).

INDICATION(S) AND RESEARCH PHASE
Renal Cell Carcinoma – Phase III
Malignant Melanoma – Phase II
Colorectal Cancer – Phase II
Gastric Cancer – Phase I/II
Pancreatic Cancer – Phase I/II completed
Lymphoma, Non-Hodgkin's – Phase II
Sarcoma – Phase II

HuC242-DM1/SB-408075
unknown

MANUFACTURER
ImmunoGen

DESCRIPTION
HuC242-DM1/SB-408075 is a tumor-activated prodrug (TAP) designed for the treatment of colorectal, pancreatic, and certain non-small cell lung cancers. Tumor-activated prodrugs consist of chemically linked monoclonal antibodies and potent, cell-killing chemicals. HuC242-DM1, in particular, is created by joining the cytotoxic maytansinoid drug DM1 with the humanized monoclonal antibody C242. The attached chemical remains inactive until the monoclonal antibody reaches its targeted tumor cell and the TAP is drawn inside. Once inside, DM1 is able to kill the tumor cell without affecting surrounding healthy cells. HuC242-DM1 is currently in phase I/II trials.

INDICATION(S) AND RESEARCH PHASE
Colorectal Cancer – Phase I/II
Pancreatic Cancer – Phase I/II
Lung Cancer – Phase I/II

IMC-1C11
unknown

MANUFACTURER
ImClone Systems

DESCRIPTION
IMC-1C11 is a chimerized monoclonal antibody that inhibits the KDR report, also known as vascular endothelial growth factor receptor (VEGFr), on vascular endothelial cells by blocking the binding of VEGF to the receptor. In animal models, IMC-1C11 demonstrated that it inhibited new blood vessel formation, and by doing so deprived tumors of required nutrients. IMC-1C11 is currently being tested in a phase I trial for the treatment of metastatic colorectal cancer.

INDICATION(S) AND RESEARCH PHASE
Colorectal Cancer – Phase I

IMC-C225, CPT-11
unknown

MANUFACTURER
ImClone Systems

DESCRIPTION
IMC-C225 is a chimerized (part mouse, part human) monoclonal antibody that may help fight cancer cells when used in conjunction with radiation therapy or chemotherapy agents. This antibody selectively blocks the epidermal growth factor receptor (EGFr), which may be present in greater amounts on actively growing tumor cells. Since many cancers use specific growth factors to stimulate tumor cell growth, blocking this receptor may inhibit the cancer from increasing in size and spreading throughout the body.

The company is conducting phase III trials evaluating IMC-C225 in combination with radiotherapy and with chemotherapy in subjects with advanced squamous cell head and neck carcinoma. IMC-C225 is in trials for several other indications in combination with various anti-cancer agents.

INDICATION(S) AND RESEARCH PHASE

408 / Colorectal Cancer

Breast Cancer – Phase I/II
Head and Neck Cancer – Phase III
Lung Cancer – Phase III
Prostate Cancer – Phase I/II
Renal Cell Carcinoma – Phase II
Pancreatic Cancer – Phase II
Colorectal Cancer – Phase II

IMMU-MN14, anti-CEA
CEA-Cide

MANUFACTURER
Immunomedics

DESCRIPTION
Carcinoembryonic antigen (CEA) is a protein-polysaccharide complex released into the bloodstream by certain cancers, particularly colon carcinoma. This antigenic substance may provide early diagnosis when used as a therapeutic marker in immunologic tests. The CEA complex may also be targeted by specialized monoclonal antibodies in the design of a biologic therapeutic.

CEA-Cide is a novel monoclonal antibody directed against carcinoembryonic antigen and designed for radioimmunotherapy (with 90 Y-labeled humanized MN-14). This drug is being tested in phase II trials for the treatment of subjects with advanced metastatic CEA-producing cancers.

INDICATION(S) AND RESEARCH PHASE
Breast Cancer – Phase II
Cancer/Tumors (Unspecified) – Phase II
Colorectal Cancer – Phase II
Lung Cancer – Phase II
Ovarian Cancer – Phase II
Pancreatic Cancer – Phase II

MDX-220
unknown

MANUFACTURER
Medarex

DESCRIPTION
MDX-220 is a bispecific (target-trigger) monoclonal antibody that targets Tag-72 in the treatment of a variety of cancers, including lung, colon, prostate, and gastric cancer.

INDICATION(S) AND RESEARCH PHASE
Endometrial Cancer – Phase I/II
Gastric Cancer – Phase I/II
Lung Cancer – Phase I/II
Ovarian Cancer – Phase I/II
Pancreatic Cancer – Phase I/II
Prostate Cancer – Phase II
Colorectal Cancer – Phase II

MGI-114, hydroxymethylacylfulvene, HMAF
Irofulven

MANUFACTURER
MGI Pharma

DESCRIPTION
Irofulven (MGI-114) is the first product candidate being developed by MGI Pharma from its family of anti-cancer compounds called acylfulvenes. Early trials demonstrated that Irofulven is absorbed rapidly by tumor cells, and once inside binds to DNA and protein targets. The binding interferes with DNA replication and cell division, leading to tumor-specific cell death.

Results from a phase II trial of Irofulven indicated that the drug produced anti-tumor activity in subjects with advanced pancreatic cancer who were refractory to gemcitabine (Gemzar). Ten of the 53 subjects enrolled achieved six-month survival and two subjects demonstrated objective responses: one subject experienced tumor shrinkage of 100% and another subject experienced an 84% decrease in tumor mass. A phase III trial was initiated in February 2001.

INDICATION(S) AND RESEARCH PHASE
Breast Cancer – Phase II
Colon Malignancies – Phase II
Renal Cell Carcinoma – Phase II
Cervical Dysplasia/Cancer – Phase II
Lung Cancer – Phase II
Ovarian Cancer – Phase I/II
Colorectal Cancer – Phase II
Prostate Cancer – Phase I/II
Cancer/Tumors (Unspecified) – Phase I/II
Pancreatic Cancer – Phase III
Liver Cancer – Phase II

raltitrexed, ZD-1694
Tomudex

MANUFACTURER
AstraZeneca

DESCRIPTION
Tomudex is a cytotoxic enzyme inhibitor of thymidylate synthase. It is administered as a single agent via infusion. Tomudex is in trials for colorectal cancer, other unspecified tumors, and as a cancer vaccine.

INDICATION(S) AND RESEARCH PHASE
Colorectal Cancer – Phase II
Cancer/Tumors (Unspecified) – Phase II/III
Vaccines – Phase III

RFS-2000
Rubitecan

MANUFACTURER
SuperGen

DESCRIPTION
Rubitecan is a novel drug that inhibits an enzyme called topoisomerase I. The drug is made in an oral formulation, which may prove to be an advantage for outpatient treatment in comparison to intravenous type drugs that require a visit to a hospital setting.

Rubitecan is being tested as a potential treatment for a variety of solid tumors, as well as for metastatic melanoma, advanced pancreatic cancer, and advanced gastric carcinoma. Additionally, phase II trials in the United States and Europe are testing Rubitecan for blood cancers such as chronic myelomonocytic leukemia (CMML).

SuperGen has announced positive preliminary results from an ongoing study on the efficacy of rubitecan in CMML, chronic myeloid leukemia (CML) and myelodysplastic syndrome (MDS). Of the 54 subjects treated, 43% experienced a complete response, partial response, or hematologic improvement.

INDICATION(S) AND RESEARCH PHASE
Pancreatic Cancer – Phase III
Breast Cancer – Phase II

Colorectal Cancer – Phase II
Gastric Cancer – Phase II
Leukemia – Phase II
Malignant Melanoma – Phase II
Ovarian Cancer – Phase II
Myelodysplastic Syndrome – Phase III

SB 408075
unknown

MANUFACTURER
GlaxoSmithKline

DESCRIPTION
SB 408075 is a tumor activated pro-drug (maytansine-antibody conjugate) in phase I trials. It is being tested as a second-line therapy for the treatment of colorectal cancer.

INDICATION(S) AND RESEARCH PHASE
Colorectal Cancer – Phase I

T67
unknown

MANUFACTURER
Tularik

DESCRIPTION
T67 is an anti-cancer compound that binds irreversibly to tubulin and inhibits the growth of multi-drug resistant tumors. Tubulin is a protein that polymerizes into chains to form microtubules. Microtubules are essential for cell division, and by disrupting their function, T67 produces cell death and potentially causes tumor shrinkage.

The drug is currently in phase II trials in subjects with non-small cell lung cancer, glioma, colorectal cancer, and breast cancer. It is also in a phase I/II trial for the treatment of hepatocellular carcinoma. These trials are being conducted in the United States, the United Kingdom, Hong Kong, and Taiwan.

INDICATION(S) AND RESEARCH PHASE
Lung Cancer – Phase II
Brain Cancer – Phase II
Colorectal Cancer – Phase II
Breast Cancer – Phase II
Hepatocellular Carcinoma – Phase I/II

TBA-CEA
unknown

MANUFACTURER
Therion Biologics

DESCRIPTION
TBA-CEA is being developed for the treatment of colorectal cancer. This biological drug targets carcinoembryonic antigen, which is a marker of colorectal cancer. Clinical trials are in phase II development.

INDICATION(S) AND RESEARCH PHASE
Colorectal Cancer – Phase II

topotecan HCl
Hycamtin

MANUFACTURER
GlaxoSmithKline

DESCRIPTION
Hycamtin (topotecan HCl) is a topoisomerase I inhibitor administered by injection. It is currently indicated for the treatment of metastatic carcinoma of the ovary after failure of initial or subsequent chemotherapy. Hycamtin is also indicated for the treatment of small cell lung cancer sensitive disease after failure of first-line chemotherapy.

Hycamtin is being evaluated in a variety of phase II and III trials. It is being tested as a second-line therapy for the treatment of colorectal cancer (phase II), as first-line therapy for small cell and non-small cell lung cancer (phase II), as oral second-line therapy for small cell lung cancer (phase III), and as first-line therapy for ovarian cancer (phase III). Lastly, Hycamtin is in phase III trials for the treatment of myelodysplastic syndrome.

INDICATION(S) AND RESEARCH PHASE
Colorectal Cancer – Phase II
Lung Cancer – Phase II
Lung Cancer – Phase III
Ovarian Cancer – Phase III
Myelodysplastic Syndrome – Phase III

trimetrexate glucuronate/ leucovorin
NeuTrexin/leucovorin

MANUFACTURER
MedImmune

DESCRIPTION
NeuTrexin, a product already approved in 13 countries for the management of moderate-to-severe *Pneumocystis carinii* pneumonia (PCP), one of the most serious complications of HIV infection, may have potential oncologic applications. NeuTrexin works by disrupting DNA, RNA, and protein synthesis, causing cell death. It is being tested in combination with leucovorin for the treatment of colorectal cancer.

INDICATION(S) AND RESEARCH PHASE
Colorectal Cancer – Phase III

troxacitabine, BCH-4556
Troxatyl

MANUFACTURER
BioChem Pharma

DESCRIPTION
Troxatyl is a dioxolane nucleoside analog being investigated as an anticancer agent. The drug is a complete DNA chain terminator and DNA polymerase inhibitor. It acts by incorporating itself into the DNA chain of cancer cells, interfering with their ability to further replicate.

Troxatyl is being evaluated as a single agent or in combination therapy in a number of ongoing trials in hematologic malignancies, including acute myeloid leukemia and chronic myeloid leukemia (blastic phase), and in lymphoproliferative disorders such as lymphoma, chronic lymphocytic leukemia, and myeloma. It is also being evaluated as a single agent in pancreatic cancer and in combination therapy in a number of solid tumors. Troxatyl is currently in phase II development.

INDICATION(S) AND RESEARCH PHASE
Cancer/Tumors (Unspecified) – Phase II
Colorectal Cancer – Phase II

410/Colorectal Cancer

Head and Neck Cancer – Phase II
Leukemia – Phase II
Lung Cancer – Phase II
Malignant Melanoma – Phase II
Ovarian Cancer – Phase II
Pancreatic Cancer – Phase II
Prostate Cancer – Phase II
Renal Cell Carcinoma – Phase II

UFT/leucovorin calcium
unknown

MANUFACTURER
Bristol-Myers Squibb

DESCRIPTION
UFT capsules, in combination with leucovorin calcium tablets, have been developed as a treatment for advanced colorectal cancer. UFT plus leucovorin could potentially provide patients with an oral chemotherapy option, removing the need for invasive intravenous chemotherapy. Oral chemotherapy also offers patients the convenience of administering their chemotherapy at home.

UFT's clinical development program included two large phase III trials in metastatic colorectal cancer, comparing the oral regimen of UFT and leucovorin with a standard intravenous regimen of 5-fluorouracil and leucovorin. However, the FDA has decided that the NDA submission did not meet its standards for approval, and the company received a "not approvable" letter in March 2001.

INDICATION(S) AND RESEARCH PHASE
Colorectal Cancer – FDA denied

unknown
CEA-Tricom

MANUFACTURER
Therion Biologics

DESCRIPTION
CEA-Tricom is a recombinant pox virus-based vaccine that targets carcinoembryonic antigen (CEA), a protein found on the surface of colorectal, pancreatic, breast, and lung cancer cells. CEA-Tricom is administered using two pox virus vectors, rV-CEA-Tricom and rF-CEA-Tricom. The Tricom component of the vaccine consists of three co-stimulatory molecules known to elicit strong cellular immune responses necessary for complete tumor destruction. A phase I trial testing CEA-Tricom will treat 42 subjects who have advanced metastatic colorectal cancer. This trial is being co-sponsored by NCI.

INDICATION(S) AND RESEARCH PHASE
Colorectal Cancer – Phase I

ursodiol
Urso

MANUFACTURER
Axcan Pharma

DESCRIPTION
Urso is an oral tablet composed of a bile acid (ursodeoxycholic acid) found in small amounts in normal human bile and in larger quantities in the bile of certain bears. This drug has been marketed in the United States for the treatment of primary biliary cirrhosis (PBC) since 1998. It is also approved in Canada for the treatment of cholestatic liver diseases such as PBC and the dissolution of gallstones.

Urso is being tested in trials for at least five other indications: the treatment of hypercholesterolemia, treatment with chemo-prevention of colorectal polyps, treatment of colorectal cancer, treatment of non-alcoholic steatohepatitis, and treatment of viral hepatitis. The drug is licensed by Sanofi-Synthelabo to Axcan Pharma in a joint venture with Schwarz Pharma.

INDICATION(S) AND RESEARCH PHASE
Cholesterol (High Levels) – Phase II
Colon Polyps – Phase II
Colorectal Cancer – Phase II
Gallbladder Disorders – Phase III/IV
Hepatitis – Phase II

vaccine
Onyvax CR

MANUFACTURER
Onyvax

DESCRIPTION
Onyvax CR is an allogeneic whole-cell colorectal cancer vaccine. It is currently in a phase I/II trial in subjects with advanced metastatic disease. The trial is being conducted at St. George's Hospital in London, and it is designed to principally examine the safety and immunogenicity of the vaccine. The vaccine is initially administered every two weeks for six weeks, and then monthly for up to a year.

INDICATION(S) AND RESEARCH PHASE
Colorectal Cancer – Phase I/II
Vaccines – Phase I/II

vaccine, anti-cancer
CEAVac

MANUFACTURER
Titan Pharmaceuticals

DESCRIPTION
CEAVac is an anti-cancer monoclonal antibody based product designed to help the subject's immune system recognize and kill tumor cells. Early phase I/II results of CEAVac in subjects with colorectal cancer suggested a positive clinical effect, with nine of 15 subjects continuing without disease. Phase III trials are under way.

INDICATION(S) AND RESEARCH PHASE
Colorectal Cancer – Phase III

vaccine, anti-cancer
CEAVac/TriAb

MANUFACTURER
Titan Pharmaceuticals

DESCRIPTION
Both CEAVac and TriAb are anti-cancer monoclonal antibody based products designed to help the subject's immune system recognize and kill tumor cells. They are being tested in a combined therapy for the treatment of non-small cell lung cancer and colorectal cancer.

INDICATION(S) AND RESEARCH PHASE
Lung Cancer – Phase II
Colorectal Cancer – Phase II

vaccine, anti-gastrin
Gastrimmune

MANUFACTURER
Aphton Corporation

DESCRIPTION
Gastrimmune is a therapeutic vaccine that neutralizes specific hormones (G17 & Gly-extended G17). The drug is in phase III trials for the treatment of cancers of the gastrointestinal tract, including gastric cancer and colorectal cancer. It is also in trials for liver cancer, esophageal cancer and two phase III trials in subjects with advanced pancreatic cancer—one in the United States and one in Europe.

INDICATION(S) AND RESEARCH PHASE
Colorectal Cancer – Phase III
Esophageal Cancer – Phase III
Gastric Cancer – Phase III
Liver Cancer – Phase II/III
Pancreatic Cancer – Phase III

vaccine, 105AD7
Onyvax 105

MANUFACTURER
Onyvax

DESCRIPTION
Onyvax 105 is a human monoclonal antibody being developed for the treatment of colorectal cancer. The drug works by inducing immune responses against the widespread tumor antigen CD55. CD55 is overexpressed in numerous cancers, including those of the prostate, colon and pancreas. Onyvax 105 is currently in phase I/II trials.

INDICATION(S) AND RESEARCH PHASE
Colorectal Cancer – Phase I/II
Vaccines – Phase I/II

VNP 40101M
unknown

MANUFACTURER
Vion Pharmaceuticals

DESCRIPTION
Sulfonyl hydrazine prodrugs (SHPs) are a series of unique, small molecule anti-tumor alkylating agents that prevent cell division upon interaction with DNA. VNP 40101M has been identified as the lead candidate of these compounds for clinical development. The drug has demonstrated broad anti-tumor activity in animal models including tumors resistant to standard alkylating agents. A phase I trial was initiated in February 2001 for the treatment of colorectal cancer in 42 subjects.

INDICATION(S) AND RESEARCH PHASE
Colorectal Cancer – Phase I

YMB-6H9
unknown

MANUFACTURER
YM Biosciences

DESCRIPTION
YMB-6H9 is an anti-CEA super high affinity monoclonal antibody (SHMAs). Phase I/II development is planned for 2001 for the treatment of colorectal cancer.

INDICATION(S) AND RESEARCH PHASE
Colorectal Cancer – Phase I

ZD-0473/AMD 473
unknown

MANUFACTURER
AstraZeneca

DESCRIPTION
ZD-0473 is a new platinum-based anti-cancer agent designed to deliver an extended spectrum of activity and overcome resistance to currently approved platinum drugs, such as cisplatin and carboplatin. It is being evaluated for the treatment of a range of solid-tumor cancers, including colorectal, non-small cell lung, and bladder cancer, which are resistant to carboplatin. ZD-0473 is being tested in both intravenous (IV) and oral formulations. The IV formulation is in phase II trials and the oral formulation is in preclinical development. AnorMED has a licensing agreement with AstraZeneca, who is conducting the phase II development of ZD-0473.

INDICATION(S) AND RESEARCH PHASE
Bladder Cancer – Phase II
Cancer/Tumors (Unspecified) – Phase II
Colorectal Cancer – Phase II
Lung Cancer – Phase II
Ovarian Cancer – Phase II
Prostate Cancer – Phase II
Breast Cancer – Phase II
Cervical Dysplasia/Cancer – Phase II

ZD-1839
Iressa

MANUFACTURER
AstraZeneca

DESCRIPTION
Iressa binds to the epidermal growth factor receptor (EGFR) and inhibits tyrosine kinase, thereby blocking signals for cancer growth and survival. The company reported encouraging results from phase I trials in a variety of tumors, but particularly in non-small cell lung cancer (NSCLC).

Iressa is being investigated both as a monotherapy and in combination with other anti-tumor drugs in NSCLC, gastric, colorectal, and hormone-resistant prostate cancers. The drug is currently in phase III studies for solid tumors.

INDICATION(S) AND RESEARCH PHASE
Cancer/Tumors (Unspecified) – Phase III
Colorectal Cancer – Phase III
Gastric Cancer – Phase III
Lung Cancer – Phase III
Prostate Cancer – Phase III

Constipation

neurotrophin-3, NT-3
unknown

MANUFACTURER

Regeneron Pharmaceuticals

DESCRIPTION
This drug is an injectable formulation of neurotrophin-3, a naturally occurring human protein. It acts on the neurons of the intestinal tract and is being tested for severe constipation and various constipating conditions caused by spinal cord injuries, narcotic analgesics, and Parkinson's disease. NT-3 is currently in phase II development.

INDICATION(S) AND RESEARCH PHASE
Constipation – Phase II
Spinal Cord Injuries – Phase II
Parkinson's Disease – Phase II
Pain, Acute or Chronic – Phase II

prucalopride
Resolor

MANUFACTURER
Janssen Pharmaceutica

DESCRIPTION
Resolor is a colonic motility agent for the treatment of chronic constipation. The drug is administered in an oral capsule formulation, and it is currently in phase III trials. Resolor is also being tested in an injectable subcutaneous formulation in phase I/II trials for post-operative ileus. Pediatric trials for this drug have been discontinued.

INDICATION(S) AND RESEARCH PHASE
Constipation – Phase III
Ileus – Phase I/II
Pediatric – Trial discontinued

tegaserod
Zelmac

MANUFACTURER
Novartis

DESCRIPTION
Zelmac selectively targets $5HT_4$ receptors present throughout the gastrointestinal (GI) tract. It is being developed for the treatment of functional dyspepsia (phase II), gastroesophageal reflux disease (phase II) and chronic constipation (phase III). Additionally, an NDA has been submitted for the treatment of irritable bowel syndrome.

INDICATION(S) AND RESEARCH PHASE
Irritable Bowel Syndrome (IBS) – NDA submitted
Gastrointestinal Diseases and Disorders, miscellaneous – Phase II
Gastroesophageal Reflux Disease (GERD) – Phase II
Constipation – Phase III

Crohn's Disease

5D12
unknown

MANUFACTURER
Tanox

DESCRIPTION
5D12 is an anti-CD40 antibody that blocks the activation of lymphocytes by binding to the CD40 molecule. According to the company, this antibody may prove useful for the treatment of several autoimmune diseases. 5D12 is currently being tested in a phase I/II trial for the treatment of Crohn's disease. The antibody is being developed by Tanox's European subsidiary, Tanox Pharma.

INDICATION(S) AND RESEARCH PHASE
Crohn's Disease – Phase I/II

budesonide
Entocort

MANUFACTURER
AstraZeneca

DESCRIPTION
Entocort contains the compound budesonide, which is a synthetic corticosteroid. AstraZeneca has submitted an NDA for Entocort modified-release capsules for the treatment of mild to moderate, active Crohn's disease. The application, which was submitted to the FDA in January 2001, has been granted priority review status.

INDICATION(S) AND RESEARCH PHASE
Crohn's Disease – NDA submitted

CBP-1011
Colirest

MANUFACTURER
Inkine Pharmaceutical Company

DESCRIPTION
Colirest is an oral steroid-like drug in development for the treatment of idiopathic thrombocytopenic purpura (ITP) and other conditions. ITP is a disorder in which the immune system attacks its own platelets, targeting them with antibodies and then destroying the resulting immune complexed platelets. Preliminary studies have indicated Colirest may help increase platelet counts. Additionally, CPB-1011 is being tested for the treatment of Crohn's disease and ulcerative colitis.

In December 2000, positive results were announced from a multicenter, open-label phase II trial of Colirest in subjects with mild or moderate active ulcerative colitis. Nine of 11 evaluable subjects completed eight weeks of Colirest treatment. Seven of the nine (78%) subjects responded to Colirest treatment in the disease activity index (DAI) and investigator global assessment (IGA) evaluations. Inkine Pharmaceutical Company plans to move Colirest into later stage pivotal trials.

INDICATION(S) AND RESEARCH PHASE
Thrombocytopenia – Phase III
Crohn's Disease – Phase II completed
Inflammatory Bowel Disease – Phase II completed

CDC-801
SelCID

MANUFACTURER
Celgene Corporation

DESCRIPTION
SelCIDs (selective cytokine inhibitory drugs) are a group of novel, orally available small molecules that are anti-angiogenic and potent modulators of tumor necrosis

factor-alpha (TNF-α). They selectively inhibit type-4 phosphodiesterase (PDE-4), a key class of cell-signaling enzymes that are linked to the overproduction of TNF-α.

Previously, Celgene reported that a phase I human safety trial evaluating CDC-801 (the most advanced SelCID) was completed and data showed that the compound had no serious adverse effects and no gastrointestinal toxicity. Currently, a phase II trial under Celgene's sponsorship is evaluating CDC-801 in Crohn's disease. Additional trials for CDC-801 are being planned by Celgene for a variety of oncology and immunomodulatory indications such as ulcerative colitis, hematological malignancies, dermatology, rheumatoid arthritis, and respiratory disorders.

INDICATION(S) AND RESEARCH PHASE
Crohn's Disease – Phase II

CDP-571, BAY 10-356
Humicade

MANUFACTURER
Celltech Chiroscience plc

DESCRIPTION
CDP-571 is a recombinant humanized IgG4 antibody that blocks the activity of tumor necrosis factor-alpha (TNF-α). Tumor necrosis factor, a cytokine naturally produced by the body, is an important mediator of inflammation.

CDP-571 is being tested in phase IIb trials for the treatment of various inflammatory conditions, including Crohn's disease, ulcerative colitis, rheumatoid arthritis, and inflammatory bowel disease. The drug is administered by intravenous infusion.

INDICATION(S) AND RESEARCH PHASE
Crohn's Disease – Phase IIb
Inflammatory Bowel Disease – Phase IIb
Rheumatoid Arthritis – Phase IIb

ISIS-2302
unknown

MANUFACTURER
Isis Pharmaceuticals

DESCRIPTION
ISIS-2302 is an inhibitor of antisense intracellular adhesion molecule-1 (ICAM-1), which is a chemical that plays a central role in inflammation. Antisense drugs work at the genetic level to interrupt the process by which disease-causing proteins are produced. Proteins play a central role in virtually every aspect of human metabolism. Many human diseases are the result of inappropriate protein production (or disordered protein performance). This is true of both host diseases (such as cancer) and infectious diseases (such as AIDS).

Traditional drugs are designed to interact with protein molecules throughout the body that support or cause diseases. Antisense drugs are designed to inhibit the production of disease-causing proteins. They can be designed to treat a wide range of diseases including infectious, inflammatory, and cardiovascular diseases, as well as cancer.

ISIS-2302 is being tested in a phase II trial using an enema formulation to treat subjects with ulcerative colitis. This method of administration allows potentially therapeutic amounts of the drug to be absorbed by the lining of the intestine, which is inflamed in subjects with ulcerative colitis.

In addition, ISIS-2302 is in trials for kidney transplant surgery, psoriasis and Crohn's disease.

INDICATION(S) AND RESEARCH PHASE
Crohn's Disease – Phase III
Psoriasis and Psoriatic Disorders – Phase II
Inflammatory Bowel Disease – Phase II
Kidney Transplant Surgery – Phase II

LDP-02
unknown

MANUFACTURER
Millennium Pharmaceuticals

DESCRIPTION
LDP-02 is an investigational humanized monoclonal antibody for the treatment of inflammatory bowel disease (IBD), which includes Crohn's disease and ulcerative colitis. LDP-02 targets a protein called alpha-4-beta-7, an integrin on inflammatory cells that causes these cells to adhere to the gastrointestinal tract.

In preclinical models, LDP-02 eliminated or reduced diarrhea, chronic inflammation, and tissue damage associated with IBD. The drug is currently in trials for ulcerative colitis and Crohn's disease. It is being developed by Millennium Pharmaceuticals in collaboration with Genentech.

INDICATION(S) AND RESEARCH PHASE
Crohn's Disease – Phase II
Inflammatory Bowel Disease – Phase II

natalizumab
Antegren

MANUFACTURER
Elan Pharmaceutical Research

DESCRIPTION
Antegren is a humanized monoclonal antibody that belongs to a new class of potential therapeutics known as alpha-4 integrin inhibitors. It is designed to block immune cell adhesion to blood vessel walls and subsequent migration of lymphocytes into tissue. Antegren binds to cell surface receptors known as alpha-4-beta-1 (VLA-4) and alpha-4-beta-7.

In January 2001, positive results were announced from preliminary analyses of two large phase II trials of Antegren in subjects with multiple sclerosis (MS) and Crohn's disease. The first double-blind, placebo-controlled trial included 213 MS subjects and was conducted at 26 sites in the United States, Canada, and the United Kingdom. The primary endpoint of a reduction in new gadolinium enhancing lesions compared to placebo over the six-month treatment period was achieved with a high degree of statistical significance. The second trial included 240 subjects with moderate to severe Crohn's disease and was conducted at 38 sites in eight European countries. Statistically significant positive results were obtained for multiple endpoints, including induction of remission as measured by the Crohn's disease activity index.

Elan Corporation and Biogen plan to initiate phase III trials in 2001 for both MS and Crohn's disease. Additionally, Antegren is being studied in a phase II trial for inflammatory bowel disease.

INDICATION(S) AND RESEARCH PHASE
Multiple Sclerosis – Phase II completed
Inflammatory Bowel Disease – Phase II
Crohn's Disease – Phase II completed

r-hTBP-1
unknown

MANUFACTURER
Serono Laboratories

DESCRIPTION
This drug is a recombinant human tumor necrosis factor-binding protein (r-hTBP-1). It is currently in phase II development for rheumatoid arthritis, Crohn's disease, and cardiac reperfusion injury.

INDICATION(S) AND RESEARCH PHASE
Rheumatoid Arthritis – Phase II
Crohn's Disease – Phase II
Cardiac Reperfusion Injury – Phase II

recombinant human interferon beta-1a
Rebif

MANUFACTURER
Serono Laboratories

DESCRIPTION
Rebif is an interferon beta-1a product being developed for a variety of indications. These include non-small cell lung cancer, chronic hepatitis C, Crohn's disease, ulcerative colitis, Guillain-Barré syndrome, and rheumatoid arthritis. Rebif has been approved in several countries for the treatment of relapsing-remitting multiple sclerosis. It is currently being evaluated as an early treatment of multiple sclerosis (phase III) and as a treatment for secondary progressive multiple sclerosis (filed).

INDICATION(S) AND RESEARCH PHASE
Multiple Sclerosis – Phase III
Lung Cancer – Phase II
Hepatitis – Phase II
Crohn's Disease – Phase II
Inflammatory Bowel Disease – Phase II
Guillain-Barré Syndrome – Phase II
Rheumatoid Arthritis – Phase II

rhIL-11
unknown

MANUFACTURER
Wyeth-Ayerst

DESCRIPTION
Recombinant human interleukin-11 (rhIL-11) is a pleiotropic cytokine that affects multiple cell types. IL-11 is currently marketed in the United States as Neumega—a thrombopoietic growth factor for preventing severe thrombocytopenia and the corresponding need for platelet transfusions following chemotherapy. rhIL-11 is currently in trials for mucositis and Crohn's disease.

INDICATION(S) AND RESEARCH PHASE
Effects of Chemotherapy – Phase II/III
Crohn's Disease – Phase II/III

SMART Anti-Gamma Interferon Antibody
unknown

MANUFACTURER
Protein Design Labs

DESCRIPTION
SMART Anti-Gamma Interferon Antibody is a humanized monoclonal antibody directed against Interferon-gamma. It was recently evaluated in healthy subjects in a dose-escalating phase I trial. Results suggested that the drug can be administered in a range of doses and may be useful in the treatment of various autoimmune conditions. A phase I/II trial in subjects with Crohn's disease is under way.

INDICATION(S) AND RESEARCH PHASE
Crohn's Disease – Phase I/II

tazofelone
unknown

MANUFACTURER
Roberts Pharmaceutical

DESCRIPTION
Crohn's disease and ulcerative colitis are both inflammatory bowel diseases. In both, it is thought that the body essentially reacts against its own colon tissue. This reaction can result in recurrent abdominal pain, fever, nausea, vomiting, weight loss, bloody and non-bloody diarrhea, and in severe cases, intestinal perforation.

The inflammatory process actually consists of many small molecules signaling cytokines to abnormally attack tissue that the body now considers foreign. Tazofelone, formulated at Roberts Pharmaceutical, acts against one of these inflammatory signal molecules known as cyclo-oxygenase. Tazofelone combines with the cyclo-oxygenase molecule and disables it, preventing it from activating other molecules responsible for the inflammation process. By blocking this particular route that the body uses to promote the cascade of inflammation, tazofelone may decrease the symptoms and tissue destruction typical of Crohn's disease and ulcerative colitis.

INDICATION(S) AND RESEARCH PHASE
Crohn's Disease – Phase II
Inflammatory Bowel Disease – Phase II

thalidomide
Thalomid

MANUFACTURER
Celgene Corporation

DESCRIPTION
Thalomid is an oral formulation of the immunomodulatory agent thalidomide. Thalidomide has a notorious history of having caused birth defects when the medical profession unsuspectingly prescribed it for pregnant women as a treatment for nausea and insomnia. Celgene is investigating new applications for the drug, while being particularly mindful of the potential risks of thalidomide treatment. Thalomid is currently being tested for numerous indications in the areas of oncology and immunology.

INDICATION(S) AND RESEARCH PHASE
Multiple Myeloma – Phase II
Myelodysplastic Syndrome – Phase II
Leukemia – Phase II
Brain Cancer – Phase II
Liver Cancer – Phase II
Kidney Cancer – Phase II
Prostate Cancer – Phase II
Kaposi's Sarcoma – Phase II
Cachexia – Phase II
Recurrent Aphthous Stomatitis – Phase III
Crohn's Disease – Phase II
Inflammatory Bowel Disease – Phase II
Sarcoidosis – Phase II
Scleroderma – Phase II

Diarrhea

DB-075
unknown

MANUFACTURER
Immtech International/NextEra Therapeutics

DESCRIPTION
DB-075 is in a phase I trial for the treatment of diarrhea caused by two common parasites found in water, *Cryptosoporidum parvum* and *Giardia lamblia*. Results from invivo tests conducted by the Scientific consortium at Tufts University showed DB-075 to be safe and less toxic then current treatments. Furthermore, results demonstrated that DB-075 stays in the digestive tract where the parasite is found, and less than 2% of the drug moves into the circulation, which greatly reduces its toxicity. Tufts is currently performing more advanced dosing tests on DB-075 for treatment of *Giardia*. Immtech intends to seek fast-track FDA approval for the drug.

INDICATION(S) AND RESEARCH PHASE
Diarrhea – Phase I

ETEC vaccine
unknown

MANUFACTURER
Acambis

DESCRIPTION
This is an oral, live attenuated vaccine being developed for the prevention of traveler's diarrhea. The vaccine is designed to induce mucosal immune responses against the predominant disease-causing strains of ETEC. The vaccine is currently in phase I testing.

INDICATION(S) AND RESEARCH PHASE
Diarrhea – Phase I
Vaccines – Phase I
Bacterial Infection – Phase I

immune globulin (IgG)
DiffGAM

MANUFACTURER
ImmuCell Corporation

DESCRIPTION
DiffGAM is a hyperimmune bovine antibody that uses cow's milk-derived passive antibody technology as an alternative to antibiotics in the treatment and/or prevention of *Clostridium difficile*-associated diarrhea and other bacterial infections. The development of this drug is currently on hold until the company can find a development partner.

INDICATION(S) AND RESEARCH PHASE
Bacterial Infection – Phase I/II
Diarrhea – Phase I/II

nitazoxanide (NTZ)
unknown

MANUFACTURER
BioChem Pharma

DESCRIPTION
Nitazoxanide (NTZ) is being developed to treat diarrhea caused by cryptosporidial parasites in immunocompromised individuals, such as those with AIDS. Cryptosporidiosis is an infection of the intestinal lining caused by the parasite *Cryptosporidium parvum*, which can be found in contaminated food and water.

Symptoms of this infection include watery diarrhea, with up to twenty bowel movements each day. NTZ is a molecule (thiazolide derivative) that acts not only against parasites such as protozoa and helminths (worms), but against bacteria as well. This drug is already available in developing countries where parasitic infections are common. People who areimmuno-compromised due to AIDS, steroid treatment, or cancer treatment are the most susceptible to infection by the *Cryptosporidium* organism—these subjects may potentially derive the greatest benefit from this new therapy.

INDICATION(S) AND RESEARCH PHASE
Diarrhea – Phase III
Parasites & Protozoa – Phase III
Acquired Immune Deficiency Syndrome (AIDS) and AIDS-Related Infections – Phase III

OPHE001
unknown

MANUFACTURER
Ophidian Pharmaceuticals

DESCRIPTION
OPHE001 is an antitoxin made to neutralize the bacterium Clostridium difficile, which may cause debilitating diarrhea.

INDICATION(S) AND RESEARCH PHASE
Diarrhea – Phase II

saccharomyces boulardii
unknown

MANUFACTURER
Biocodex

DESCRIPTION
Saccharomyces boulardii is a yeast that appears to have an inhibitory effect against a type of bacteria (*Clostridium difficile*) that causes severe diarrhea in a variety of subjects. Sixty-one percent of neonates are colonized with this bacteria, and in a study at the Children's Hospital in Philadelphia, one-third of the children tested were found to have toxins made by *C. difficile* bacteria in their stools.

Scientists are not certain how exactly this

yeast exerts its destructive effect against bacterial infection, but it might produce an enzyme that destroys one of the toxins produced by the bacteria. It also may prevent invading bacteria from binding to the intestinal walls, or it might stimulate the production of immune cells that helps attack the invading bacteria. One French study showed that subjects who were producing four to eight liters of diarrhea a day had normal stools after an eight-day course of *Saccharomyces boulardii*.

People taking antibiotics for infections are susceptible to *C. difficile* infection, since antibiotics strip the intestinal walls of normal bacteria that protect against infection. In a study of people taking antibiotics, the group receiving *Saccharomyces boulardii* experienced a lower incidence of *C. difficile* diarrhea than those receiving other anti-diarrheal therapies. Further study is under way to determine exactly how effective this yeast may be in treating infection and what subjects might receive the most benefit from it.

INDICATION(S) AND RESEARCH PHASE
Bacterial Infection – Phase II
Diarrhea – Phase II
Pediatric, Clostridium difficile Diarrhea-colitis – Phase II

SP-303
Provir

MANUFACTURER
Shaman Pharmaceuticals

DESCRIPTION
Provir is a naturally occurring compound derived from the red, viscous latex of the Croton tree (Croton lechlerli), which grows in the Amazonian jungles of South America. Provir is an oral drug that acts as a specific inhibitor of fluid loss via an antisecretory mechanism. Provir has entered phase III trials for the treatment of AIDS-associated diarrhea, and for the treatment of acute watery and traveler's diarrhea.

INDICATION(S) AND RESEARCH PHASE
Acquired Immune Deficiency Syndrome (AIDS) and AIDS-Related Infections – Phase III
Diarrhea – Phase III

vaccine, campylobacter
Campyvax

MANUFACTURER
Antex Biologics

DESCRIPTION
This orally administered vaccine, developed under a Cooperative Research and Development Agreement (CRADA) with the U.S. Navy and Army, is designed to prevent gastroenteritis and traveler's diarrhea caused by *Campylobacter jejuni*. A novel proprietary technology combines the vaccine, consisting of inactivated whole cells, with an adjuvant. While vaccines typically provide protection after bacteria enter the body, this new genetic engineering technology provides the platform for vaccines that prevent bacterial infection.

According to the companies involved, phase II trials showed encouraging results for continued development of the vaccine.

INDICATION(S) AND RESEARCH PHASE
Bacterial Infection – Phase II completed
Diarrhea – Phase II completed
Gastroenteritis – Phase II completed
Pediatric, Campylobacter Infection – Phase II completed

vaccine, Shigella flexneri and sonneii
unknown

MANUFACTURER
Intellivax International

DESCRIPTION
Shigella infections cause 200 million cases of dysentery and diarrhea worldwide every year. Shigellosis, infectious dysentery caused by bacteria of the genus *Shigella*, is marked by intestinal pain, tenesmus, diarrhea with mucus and blood in the stools, and toxemia. This novel vaccine is being developed in a nasal spray formulation.

INDICATION(S) AND RESEARCH PHASE
Bacterial Infection – Phase II
Diarrhea – Phase II
Vaccines – Phase II

Diet and Nutrition

L-glutathione
Cachexon

MANUFACTURER
Telluride Pharmaceutical

DESCRIPTION
Cachexon is an oral capsule formulation of glutathione, an antioxidant produced naturally by the body. Cancer and AIDS subjects have lowered levels of glutathione. This capsule is designed as a replacement therapy for glutathione in order to provide direct protection to intestinal epithelial cells (enterocytes) against oxidative stress. Oxidative stress leads to activation of HIV replication, resulting in damage to enterocytes, malabsorption, and cachexia.

INDICATION(S) AND RESEARCH PHASE
Acquired Immune Deficiency Syndrome (AIDS) and AIDS-Related Infections – Phase III
Cancer/Tumors (Unspecified) – Phase III
Diet and Nutrition – Phase III

Esophageal Cancer

cisplatin/epinephrine
IntraDose

MANUFACTURER
Matrix Pharmaceutical

DESCRIPTION
IntraDose is a biodegradable collagen carrier matrix combined with a vasoconstrictor. The gel is injected directly into tumors where it localizes high concentrations of cisplatin, a widely used anticancer drug. It is currently being tested for several indications, including head and neck, breast, malignant melanoma, esophageal, and primary hepatocellular cancer.

A phase II trial of IntraDose Injectable Gel produced durable responses in subjects with colorectal cancer that had metastasized to the liver. Nine of 31 subjects who received IntraDose responded to therapy. Six subjects experienced a complete response (100% reduction in viable tumor volume of treated tumors) while the other three subjects demonstrated a partial response (at least a 50% reduction of viable tumor volume). Eight of the nine treatment responders have had durable responses with no relapse at the site of treatment. IntraDose was well tolerated by subjects.

INDICATION(S) AND RESEARCH PHASE
Breast Cancer – Phase II
Cancer/Tumors (Unspecified) – Phase II
Colorectal Cancer – Phase II completed
Esophageal Cancer – Phase II
Liver Cancer – Phase II
Malignant Melanoma – Phase II
Head and Neck Cancer – NDA submitted

flavopiridol, HMR-1275
unknown

MANUFACTURER
Aventis

DESCRIPTION
Flavopiridol belongs to a new class of drugs for cancer therapy known as cyclin-dependent kinase (CDK) inhibitors. It is being tested in phase II trials as a treatment for chronic lymphatic leukemia, esophageal cancer, and non-small cell lung cancer.

INDICATION(S) AND RESEARCH PHASE
Esophageal Cancer – Phase II
Leukemia – Phase II
Lung Cancer – Phase II

vaccine, anti-gastrin
Gastrimmune

MANUFACTURER
Aphton Corporation

DESCRIPTION
Gastrimmune is a therapeutic vaccine that neutralizes specific hormones (G17 & Gly-extended G17). The drug is in phase III trials for the treatment of cancers of the gastrointestinal tract, including gastric cancer and colorectal cancer. It is also in trials for liver cancer, esophageal cancer and two phase III trials in subjects with advanced pancreatic cancer—one in the United States and one in Europe.

INDICATION(S) AND RESEARCH PHASE
Colorectal Cancer – Phase III
Esophageal Cancer – Phase III
Gastric Cancer – Phase III
Liver Cancer – Phase II/III
Pancreatic Cancer – Phase III

Esophageal Disorders

exisulind
Aptosyn

MANUFACTURER
Cell Pathways

DESCRIPTION
Aptosyn (exisulind) belongs to a novel class of compounds called selective apoptotic anti-neoplastic drugs (SAANDs). SAANDs inhibit a form of cyclic GMP phosphodiesterase and selectively induce apoptosis in abnormally growing precancerous and cancerous cells. Aptosyn is being tested for several indications and is in five different trials for adenomatous polyposis coli (APC) and familial adenomatous polyposis coli; two of these trials are specifically for pediatric subjects.

The company received a non-approvable letter from the FDA in September 2000 for one of the trials for familial adenomatous polyposis. The company intends to amend the NDA and request a meeting with the FDA to address the deficiencies and the possible requirement for additional clinical data.

INDICATION(S) AND RESEARCH PHASE
Adenomatous polyposis coli – Non-approvable letter
Pediatric, Familial Adenomatous Polyposis coli – Phase II
Adenomatous Polyposis coli – Phase I/II
Barrett's Esophagus Disease – Phase II
Prostate Cancer – Phase II/III
Breast Cancer – Phase II/III
Lung Cancer – Phase Ib
Colon Polyps – Phase II/III

V-Echinocandin
unknown

MANUFACTURER
Versicor

DESCRIPTION
V-Echinocandin is a novel intravenous drug being developed for the treatment of fungal infections. The drug selectively inhibits an enzyme in fungi involved in cell wall synthesis. V-Echinocandin has shown invitro activity against various fungi, including *Candida* and *Aspergillus*.

V-Echinocandin has been well tolerated in five trials involving over 100 subjects. In one phase II trial of subjects with esophagitis, over 80% of evaluable subjects were cured or improved (as defined by endoscopy) by the end of the treatment. Twenty-nine evaluable subjects were treated with daily intravenous infusions of V-Echinocandin for up to 21 days. Phase III trials in subjects with esophageal candidiasis are currently under way. In these trials, an increased dose of V-Echinocandin will be compared to fluconazole.

INDICATION(S) AND RESEARCH PHASE
Fungal Infections – Phase II completed
Esophageal Disorders – Phase III

Gallbladder Disorders

GI 181771
unknown

MANUFACTURER
GlaxoSmithKline

DESCRIPTION
GI 181771 is a cholecystokinin (CCK)-A receptor agonist being tested in phase I trials for the treatment of obesity and gallstone prophylaxis.

INDICATION(S) AND RESEARCH PHASE
Gallbladder Disorders – Phase I
Obesity – Phase I

ursodiol
Urso

MANUFACTURER
Axcan Pharma

DESCRIPTION
Urso is an oral tablet composed of a bile acid (ursodeoxycholic acid) found in small amounts in normal human bile and in larger quantities in the bile of certain bears. This drug has been marketed in the United States for the treatment of primary biliary cirrhosis (PBC) since 1998. It is also approved in Canada for the treatment of cholestatic liver diseases such as PBC and the dissolution of gallstones.

Urso is being tested in trials for at least five other indications: the treatment of hypercholesterolemia, treatment with chemo-prevention of colorectal polyps, treatment of colorectal cancer, treatment of non-alcoholic steatohepatitis, and treatment of viral hepatitis. The drug was licensed by Sanofi-Synthelabo to Axcan Pharma in a joint venture with Schwarz Pharma.

INDICATION(S) AND RESEARCH PHASE
Cholesterol (High Levels) – Phase II
Colon Polyps – Phase II
Colorectal Cancer – Phase II
Gallbladder Disorders – Phase III/IV
Hepatitis – Phase II

Gastric Cancer

docetaxel hydrate
Taxotere

MANUFACTURER
Aventis

DESCRIPTION
Drugs for the treatment of cancer and other diseases often originate in plants, many of them highly poisonous. Taxotere (docetaxel hydrate), an agent that inhibits the formation of new protoplasm, is derived from the renewable evergreen needles of the genus Taxus (Yew). Taxotere acts by disrupting the microtubular network in cells, which is essential for cell division and other cellular functions.

Taxotere is approved for use in the United States for treatment of refractory breast cancer, refractory non-small cell lung cancer (NSCLC), and locally advanced or metastatic breast cancer. New phase II/III trials are under way in head and neck, gastric, and ovarian cancers. Taxotere is also being tested either alone or in combination with other chemotherapy agents in the earlier stages of breast cancer, NSCLC, and others tumors.

Phase I extension studies are under way for brain metastasis and lung cancer.

INDICATION(S) AND RESEARCH PHASE
Gastric Cancer – Phase II/III
Head and Neck Cancer – Phase II/III
Lung Cancer – Phase II/III
Ovarian Cancer – Phase II/III
Breast Cancer – Phase III/IV
Brain Cancer – Phase I
Lung Cancer – Phase I

fluoropyrimidine, S-1
unknown

MANUFACTURER
Bristol-Myers Squibb

DESCRIPTION
Fluoropyrimidine is a combination medication that is being tested in subjects with solid tumors. One of the active components in fluoropyrimidine is tegafur, which is a type of a chemotherapeutic drug known as 5-fluorouracil (5-FU). 5-FU prevents the metabolic activities of cancer cells, thus limiting their ability to grow and replicate. In clinical use for over forty years, 5-FU has been used to treat gastrointestinal, breast, head and neck, and bladder cancers. Problems associated with 5-FU use include subject tolerance to its anti-cancer effects, serious side effects, and toxicity to the digestive tract when taken orally.

Fluoropyrimidine may be an improvement over 5-FU alone because it also contains the molecule otastat potassium, which protects the GI tract from toxic effects, and the substance gimestat, which increases the action of 5-FU by inhibiting the enzyme in the body that breaks it down. Studies will demonstrate whether these two molecules will allow the drug to be given orally, producing fewer resultant adverse effects. This may mean that subjects will be able to tolerate the drug for longer periods of time, thus increasing subject compliance and potentially the effectiveness of the drug. It also may reduce the variability of clinical response to the drug among subjects, allowing doctors to better predict the effect its administration will have on their subjects' condition and what doses would be optimal for them.

Preliminary studies have shown that fluoropyrimidine produces greater efficacy and less toxicity than conventional chemotherapeutic agents. The drug is given orally at 80 mg twice a day, and it is currently being tested in phase II clinical trials.

INDICATION(S) AND RESEARCH PHASE
Cancer/Tumors (Unspecified) – Phase II
Gastric Cancer – Phase II

HSPPC-96
Oncophage

MANUFACTURER
Antigenics

DESCRIPTION
Oncophage cancer vaccine is an injectable protein that contains the unique profile ("antigenic fingerprint") of each subject's cancer. The antigens activate the immune system to elicit an anti-tumor response.

In October 2000, Antigenics announced that it had initiated a phase II trial of Oncophage in subjects who have been diagnosed with sarcoma, also known as soft tissue cancer. The study is expected to initially enroll 20 subjects diagnosed with recurrent metastatic or unresectable soft tissue sarcoma and may be expanded to include an additional 15 subjects depending on preliminary results.

INDICATION(S) AND RESEARCH PHASE
Renal Cell Carcinoma – Phase III

Malignant Melanoma – Phase II
Colorectal Cancer – Phase II
Gastric Cancer – Phase I/II
Pancreatic Cancer – Phase I/II completed
Lymphoma, Non-Hodgkin's – Phase II
Sarcoma – Phase II

Liposomal Encapsulated Paclitaxel
unknown

MANUFACTURER
Pharmacia

DESCRIPTION
Liposomal Encapsulated Paclitaxel (LEP) is being developed for the treatment of cancer. LEP was licensed to Pharmacia for worldwide development and commercialization in February 1999. It is currently in phase II/III clinical trials in a number of countries worldwide.

INDICATION(S) AND RESEARCH PHASE
Gastric Cancer – Phase II/III
Esophageal Cancer – Phase II/III

MDX-210
unknown

MANUFACTURER
Medarex

DESCRIPTION
MDX-210 is a bispecific (target-trigger) monoclonal antibody (MAb)-based treatment being developed for cancers with specific markers (HER-2/*neu* positive), including renal cell, non-small cell lung, pancreatic, and kidney cancers. Phase II trials have been completed for kidney, prostate, and ovarian cancer. Phase III development for ovarian cancer has commenced in Europe.

INDICATION(S) AND RESEARCH PHASE
Prostate Cancer – Phase II completed
Renal Cell Carcinoma – Phase II completed
Colon Malignancies – Phase II
Breast Cancer – Phase II
Gastric Cancer – Phase II
Pancreatic Cancer – Phase II
Lung Cancer – Phase II
Ovarian Cancer – Phase III

MDX-220
unknown

MANUFACTURER
Medarex

DESCRIPTION
MDX-220 is a bispecific (target-trigger) monoclonal antibody that targets Tag-72. It is being developed for the treatment of a variety of cancers, including lung, colon, prostate, ovarian, endometrial, pancreatic, and gastric cancer.

INDICATION(S) AND RESEARCH PHASE
Endometrial Cancer – Phase I/II
Gastric Cancer – Phase I/II
Lung Cancer – Phase I/II
Ovarian Cancer – Phase I/II
Pancreatic Cancer – Phase I/II
Prostate Cancer – Phase II
Colorectal Cancer – Phase II

murine monoclonal antibody
Theragyn

MANUFACTURER
Antisoma plc

DESCRIPTION
Theragyn is composed of a mouse monoclonal antibody (HMFG1) linked to a radioactive isotope. It is thought that small numbers of residual tumor cells remaining in the abdomen after surgery and chemotherapy are one of the main causes of relapse. These residual tumor cells are the targets of Theragyn. Theragyn uses the natural targeting ability of antibodies to selectively deliver radioactivity to tumor cells.

Theragyn is being tested as an adjuvant treatment in trials for gastric cancer and ovarian cancer.

INDICATION(S) AND RESEARCH PHASE
Gastric Cancer – Phase II
Ovarian Cancer – Phase III

RFS-2000
Rubitecan

MANUFACTURER
SuperGen

DESCRIPTION
Rubitecan is a novel drug that inhibits an enzyme called topoisomerase I. The drug is made in an oral formulation, which may prove to be an advantage for outpatient treatment in comparison to intravenous type drugs that require a visit to a hospital setting.

Rubitecan is being tested as a potential treatment for a variety of solid tumors, as well as for metastatic melanoma, advanced pancreatic cancer and advanced gastric carcinoma. Additionally, phase II trials in the United States and Europe are testing Rubitecan for blood cancers such as chronic myelomonocytic leukemia (CMML).

SuperGen has announced positive preliminary results from an ongoing study on the efficacy of rubitecan in CMML, chronic myeloid leukemia (CML), and myelodysplastic syndrome (MDS). Of the 54 subjects treated, 43% experienced a complete response, partial response, or hematologic improvement.

INDICATION(S) AND RESEARCH PHASE
Pancreatic Cancer – Phase III
Breast Cancer – Phase II
Colorectal Cancer – Phase II
Gastric Cancer – Phase II
Leukemia – Phase II
Malignant Melanoma – Phase II
Ovarian Cancer – Phase II
Myelodysplastic Syndrome – Phase III

vaccine, anti-gastrin
Gastrimmune

MANUFACTURER
Aphton Corporation

DESCRIPTION
Gastrimmune is a therapeutic vaccine that neutralizes specific hormones (G17 & Gly-extended G17). The drug is in phase III trials for the treatment of cancers of the gas-

trointestinal tract, including gastric cancer and colorectal cancer. It is also in trials for liver cancer, esophageal cancer and two phase III trials in subjects with advanced pancreatic cancer—one in the United States and one in Europe.

INDICATION(S) AND RESEARCH PHASE
Colorectal Cancer – Phase III
Esophageal Cancer – Phase III
Gastric Cancer – Phase III
Liver Cancer – Phase II/III
Pancreatic Cancer – Phase III

ZD-1839
Iressa

MANUFACTURER
AstraZeneca

DESCRIPTION
Iressa binds to the epidermal growth factor receptor (EGFR) and inhibits tyrosine kinase, thereby blocking signals for cancer growth and survival. The company reported encouraging results from phase I trials in a variety of tumors, but particularly in non-small cell lung cancer (NSCLC). Iressa is being investigated both as a monotherapy and in combination with other anti-tumor drugs in NSCLC, gastric, colorectal, and hormone-resistant prostate cancers. In 1999, the FDA gave Iressa fast track status.

INDICATION(S) AND RESEARCH PHASE
Cancer/Tumors (Unspecified) – Phase III
Colorectal Cancer – Phase III
Gastric Cancer – Phase III
Lung Cancer – Phase III
Prostate Cancer – Phase III

Gastric Ulcers

AG-1749, lansoprazole
unknown

MANUFACTURER
Takeda Chemical Industries

DESCRIPTION
Lansoprazole, marketed in Japan as Takepron, is a proton pump inhibitor being developed for use in several countries. For the indication of non-steroidal anti-inflammatory drug (NSAID) induced ulcers, an NDA has been filed in the United States and the product has been launched in the United Kingdom, France, and Italy. Additionally, an NDA has also been filed for the treatment of non-ulcer dyspepsia.

INDICATION(S) AND RESEARCH PHASE
Gastric Ulcers – NDA submitted
Gastrointestinal Diseases and Disorders, miscellaneous – NDA submitted

Gastroenteritis

ibuprofen
Elangesic

MANUFACTURER
Elan Pharmaceutical Research

DESCRIPTION
Non-steroidal anti-inflammatory drugs (NSAIDs), such as ibuprofen, are very effective agents for the relief of pain and inflammation. But many individuals cannot use these drugs due to adverse effects, such as irritation of the lining of the stomach. NSAIDs may cause gastritis and ulcers, or exacerbate these conditions when already present.

Elan Pharmaceuticals has developed a new product called Elangesic that may potentially increase the tolerability of NSAIDs. Elangesic works by formulating drugs into high density, controlled-release beads. Each bead contains a core of the desired drug, and an outer coating which discharges the drug in a time-release fashion. Clinical testing is in phase II trials using this once- and twice-daily intestinal protective drug absorption system (IPDAS).

INDICATION(S) AND RESEARCH PHASE
Gastroenteritis – Phase II
Inflammatory Bowel Disease – Phase II
Ulcers – Phase II

vaccine, campylobacter
Campyvax

MANUFACTURER
Antex Biologics

DESCRIPTION
This orally administered vaccine, developed under a Cooperative Research and Development Agreement (CRADA) with the United States Navy and Army, is designed to prevent gastroenteritis and traveler's diarrhea caused by *Campylobacter jejuni*. A novel proprietary technology combines the vaccine, consisting of inactivated whole cells, with an adjuvant. While vaccines typically provide protection after bacteria enter the body, this new genetic engineering technology provides the platform for vaccines that prevent bacterial infection.

According to the companies involved, phase II trials showed encouraging results for continued development of the vaccine.

INDICATION(S) AND RESEARCH PHASE
Bacterial Infection – Phase II completed
Diarrhea – Phase II completed
Gastroenteritis – Phase II completed
Pediatric, Campylobacter Infection – Phase II completed

Gastroesophageal Reflux Disease (GERD)

(+)-norcisapride
unknown

MANUFACTURER
Janssen Pharmaceutica

DESCRIPTION
(+)-norcisapride is an active metabolite of Propulsid (cisapride), a product marketed by Johnson & Johnson. Propulsid is indicated for the treatment of nocturnal heartburn associated with gastroesophageal reflux disease (GERD); however, it has been associated with cardiac toxicity and is only available in a limited access program. (+)-norcisapride offers the possibility of treating GERD and other indications without the risk of cardiac toxicity.

Sepracor has licensed its norcisapride

rights to Janssen Pharmaceutical, a wholly owned subsidiary of Johnson & Johnson. The drug is currently in phase II clinical development.

INDICATION(S) AND RESEARCH PHASE
Gastroesophageal Reflux Disease (GERD) – Phase II

AR-H047108
unknown

MANUFACTURER
AstraZeneca

DESCRIPTION
AR-H047108 is a reversible acid pump inhibitor for the treatment of acid related gastrointestinal disease. It is currently in phase I/II trials.

INDICATION(S) AND RESEARCH PHASE
Gastrointestinal Diseases and Disorders, miscellaneous – Phase I/II
Gastroesophageal Reflux Disease (GERD) – Phase I/II

KC-11458
unknown

MANUFACTURER
Solvay Pharmaceuticals

DESCRIPTION
KC-11458 is a non-peptidergic motilin agonist with a 12-ring macrolide structure. It is currently in phase I/IIa trials for the treatment of gastroesophageal reflux disease (GERD).

INDICATION(S) AND RESEARCH PHASE
Gastroesophageal Reflux Disease (GERD) – Phase I/II

---

lansoprazole
Takepron

MANUFACTURER
Takeda Chemical Industries

DESCRIPTION
Takepron suppresses gastric acid secretion by specific inhibition of (H+, K+)-ATPase. The drug is currently under application in Japan for the treatment of reflux esophagitis and phase II trials for gastritis.

INDICATION(S) AND RESEARCH PHASE
Gastroesophageal Reflux Disease (GERD) – Under Application in Japan
Gastrointestinal Diseases and Disorders, miscellaneous – Phase II

R 149524
unknown

MANUFACTURER
Janssen Pharmaceutica

DESCRIPTION
R 149524 is the major metabolite of cisapride. It is currently in phase II development for the treatment of gastroesophageal reflux disease (GERD).

INDICATION(S) AND RESEARCH PHASE
Gastroesophageal Reflux Disease (GERD) – Phase II

---

reflux inhibitor
unknown

MANUFACTURER
AstraZeneca

DESCRIPTION
AstraZeneca's reflux inhibitor is an inhibitor of transient lower esophageal sphincter relaxations (TLESR). It is currently in phase I/II trials for the treatment of gastroesophageal reflux disease (GERD).

INDICATION(S) AND RESEARCH PHASE
Gastroesophageal Reflux Disease (GERD) – Phase I/II

SLV 305
unknown

MANUFACTURER
Solvay Pharmaceuticals

DESCRIPTION
SLV 305 is a motilin agonist in phase I development for the treatment of gastrointestinal motility disorders.

INDICATION(S) AND RESEARCH PHASE
Gastrointestinal Diseases and Disorders, miscellaneous – Phase I
Gastroesophageal Reflux Disease (GERD) – Phase I

SLV 311
unknown

MANUFACTURER
Solvay Pharmaceuticals

DESCRIPTION
SLV 311 is a motilin agonist being developed for the treatment of gastrointestinal motility disorders. It is currently in phase I trials.

INDICATION(S) AND RESEARCH PHASE
Gastrointestinal Diseases and Disorders, miscellaneous – Phase I
Gastroesophageal Reflux Disease (GERD) – Phase I

---

tegaserod
Zelmac

MANUFACTURER
Novartis

DESCRIPTION
Zelmac selectively targets $5HT_4$ receptors present throughout the gastrointestinal (GI) tract. It is being developed for the treatment of functional dyspepsia (phase II), gastroesophageal reflux disease (phase II) and chronic constipation (phase III). Additionally, an NDA has been submitted for the treatment of irritable bowel syndrome.

INDICATION(S) AND RESEARCH PHASE
Irritable Bowel Syndrome (IBS) – NDA submitted
Gastrointestinal Diseases and Disorders, miscellaneous – Phase II
Gastroesophageal Reflux Disease (GERD) –

Phase II
Constipation – Phase III

vaccine, anti-gastrin II
unknown

MANUFACTURER
Aphton Corporation

DESCRIPTION
Aphton's anti-gastrin II vaccine induces antibodies in subjects that neutralize gastrin-17. The drug is currently being developed for the treatment of gastroesophageal reflux disease (GERD).

INDICATION(S) AND RESEARCH PHASE
Gastroesophageal Reflux Disease (GERD) – Phase III

YH-1885, SB 641257
unknown

MANUFACTURER
GlaxoSmithKline

DESCRIPTION
YH-1885 is a reversible proton pump inhibitor. It is currently in phase I trials in Korea for the treatment of gastroesophageal reflux disease.

INDICATION(S) AND RESEARCH PHASE
Gastroesophageal Reflux Disease (GERD) – Phase I

Gastrointestinal Diseases and Disorders, Miscellaneous

ADL 8-2698
unknown

MANUFACTURER
Adolor

DESCRIPTION
ADL 8-2698 is a gastrointestinal tract-restricted opioid narcotic antagonist that treats or prevents the gastrointestinal side effects of opioid analgesics such as morphine and codeine. These side effects include nausea, vomiting, and constipation (in subjects who take opioid analgesics for a longer duration for chronic pain).

Results of two phase II trials of ADL 8-2698 indicated that the compound mitigates severe opioid-induced bowel dysfunction in subjects taking narcotics without interfering with their analgesic effects. In the first trial, 26 subjects with chronic opioid-induced constipation received increasing doses of ADL 8-2698 or placebo for four consecutive days. An effective dose as measured by stimulating a bowel movement within 24 hours of dose administration was identified in all subjects receiving ADL 8-2698 with a statistically significant difference obtained versus placebo.

The second trial was a double-blind, placebo-controlled single dose trial in which 75 subjects received either a placebo or one of three doses of ADL 8-2698. Subjects receiving ADL 8-2698 were substantially more likely to have a bowel movement within twelve hours after treatment compared to subjects receiving placebo. The company plans to advance ADL 8-2698 into phase III development for opioid induced bowel dysfunction in early 2001.

INDICATION(S) AND RESEARCH PHASE
Gastrointestinal Diseases and Disorders, miscellaneous – Phase II/III

AG-1749, lansoprazole
unknown

MANUFACTURER
Takeda Chemical Industries

DESCRIPTION
Lansoprazole, marketed in Japan as Takepron, is a proton pump inhibitor being developed for use in several countries. For the indication of non-steroidal anti-inflammatory drug (NSAID) induced ulcers, an NDA has been filed in the United States and the product has been launched in the United Kingdom, France, and Italy. Additionally, an NDA has also been filed for the treatment of non-ulcer dyspepsia.

INDICATION(S) AND RESEARCH PHASE
Gastric Ulcers – NDA submitted
Gastrointestinal Diseases and Disorders, miscellaneous – NDA submitted

ALX-0600
unknown

MANUFACTURER
NPS Allelix Corp

DESCRIPTION
ALX-0600 is a subcutaneously administered therapy for the treatment of several gastrointestinal disorders, including short bowel syndrome (SBS). The drug is a proprietary analogue of the naturally occurring gastrointestinal peptide, glucagon-like peptide-2 (GLP-2). GLP-2 acts as a potent stimulator of cell growth in the lining of the small bowel.

INDICATION(S) AND RESEARCH PHASE
Gastrointestinal Diseases and Disorders, miscellaneous – Phase II

AR-H047108
unknown

MANUFACTURER
AstraZeneca

DESCRIPTION
AR-H047108 is a reversible acid pump inhibitor for the treatment of acid related gastrointestinal disease. It is currently in phase I/II trials.

INDICATION(S) AND RESEARCH PHASE
Gastrointestinal Diseases and Disorders, miscellaneous – Phase I/II
Gastroesophageal Reflux Disease (GERD) – Phase I/II

C. difficile vaccine, CdVax
unknown

MANUFACTURER
Acambis

DESCRIPTION

CdVax is a vaccine being developed for the prevention of antibiotic-associated colitis caused by *Clostridium difficile* (*C. difficile*). The *C. difficile* bacteria produce A and B toxins that cause intestinal inflammation and fluid secretion. CdVax contains chemically inactivated A and B toxins, which could potentially stimulate high-level antitoxin antibodies in plasma donors. These plasma donations could then be used to prepare an immune globulin product (IVIG) for use in the short-term prophylaxis and therapy of *C. difficile* infection.

INDICATION(S) AND RESEARCH PHASE
Bacterial Infection – Phase I/II completed
Vaccines – Phase I/II completed
Gastrointestinal Diseases and Disorders, miscellaneous – Phase I/II completed

H. pylori vaccine
unknown

MANUFACTURER
Acambis

DESCRIPTION
Acambis is developing vaccines designed to prevent and treat peptic ulcers and chronic gastritis caused by *H. pylori*. The vaccines would be used to treat *H. pylori* infection, prevent reinfection in previously infected persons, and stimulate immunity in uninfected individuals. The vaccines are being developed under a joint venture with Aventis Pasteur.

INDICATION(S) AND RESEARCH PHASE
Vaccines – Phase II
Bacterial Infection – Phase II
Gastrointestinal Diseases and Disorders, miscellaneous – Phase II

intranasal metoclopramide
Emitasol, Pramidin

MANUFACTURER
Questcor

DESCRIPTION
Metoclopramide is a prokinetic agent that interferes with dopamine receptors in the brain. Emitasol is an intranasal formulation of metoclopramide being developed for the treatment of chemotherapy-induced nausea and vomiting, as well as diabetic gastroparesis.

A phase II trial for diabetic gastroparesis has been completed and results were presented in October 2000. Both 10 mg and 20 mg Emitasol dosages showed faster absorption than an already FDA approved metoclopramide oral tablet. At the end of the trial, subjects taking both doses of Emitasol reported a greater reduction in symptoms of gastroparesis than those taking the oral form. Questcor plans to initiate a pivotal phase III trial for gastroparesis in 2001.

Emitasol is marketed in Italy as Pramidin, and an application has been submitted for approval in six Eastern European countries. Questcor has partnered with Roberts Pharmaceutical, a subsidiary of Shire Pharmaceuticals, to co-develop the patented product for North America.

INDICATION(S) AND RESEARCH PHASE
Gastrointestinal Diseases and Disorders, miscellaneous – Phase II completed
Gastroparesis – Phase II completed

keratinocyte growth factor (KGF)
unknown

MANUFACTURER
Amgen

DESCRIPTION
Keratinocyte growth factor (KGF) is a recombinant form of a naturally occurring epithelial tissue growth factor that stimulates the growth of cells comprising the surface lining (epithelium) of the gastrointestinal tract. Phase II trials are ongoing to determine whether KGF can reduce the incidence, severity, and duration of oral and gastrointestinal mucositis in cancer subjects receiving forms of chemotherapy and radiation therapy. KGF is administered by intravenous injection.

INDICATION(S) AND RESEARCH PHASE
Effects of Chemotherapy – Phase II
Gastrointestinal Diseases and Disorders, miscellaneous – Phase II

lansoprazole
Takepron

MANUFACTURER
Takeda Chemical Industries

DESCRIPTION
Takepron suppresses gastric acid secretion by specific inhibition of (H+, K+)-ATPase. The drug is currently under application in Japan for the treatment of reflux esophagitis and in phase II trials for gastritis.

INDICATION(S) AND RESEARCH PHASE
Gastroesophageal Reflux Disease (GERD) – Under application in Japan
Gastrointestinal Diseases and Disorders, miscellaneous – Phase II

MB-U820
Oralex

MANUFACTURER
Molecular Biosystems

DESCRIPTION
Oralex is a novel agent for the enhancement of ultrasound contrast imaging of the pancreas and gastrointestinal tract. The drug is delivered in an oral formulation, and it is being tested for use in gastrointestinal diseases and disorders. Phase II trials are complete in the United States, and phase III development is awaiting a corporate partnership.

INDICATION(S) AND RESEARCH PHASE
Gastrointestinal Diseases and Disorders, miscellaneous – Phase II complete

MK-826, carbapenem
unknown

MANUFACTURER
Merck & Co.

DESCRIPTION
Carbapenem is a broad-spectrum antibiotic being developed for the treatment of bacterial infections including pneumonia, intra-abdominal infections, skin and skin

structure infections, urinary tract infection and obstetric and gynecologic infections.

INDICATION(S) AND RESEARCH PHASE
Pneumonia – Phase III
Skin Infections/Disorders – Phase III
Urinary Tract Infections – Phase III
Gynecological Infections – Phase III
Bacterial Infection – Phase III
Gastrointestinal Diseases and Disorders, miscellaneous – Phase III

radiolabeled monoclonal antibody
LeuTech

MANUFACTURER
Palatin Technologies

DESCRIPTION
LeuTech is a monoclonal antibody labeled with a radioactive isotope (technetium 99). When injected into the body, LeuTech attaches itself to neutrophils, which naturally accumulate in areas of infection or inflammation. When imaged using a standard gamma camera, the accumulated LeuTech appears as a bright spot, indicating an area of infection.

Researchers participating in a phase III clinical trial of LeuTech concluded that the drug is safe and effective in diagnosing cases of equivocal appendicitis. LeuTech also demonstrated a significant positive impact on the management of these subjects. The trial included 200 subjects at ten sites across the United States. The FDA recommended approval of LeuTech in July 2000.

In addition, LeuTech is in multiple phase II trials for other types of infection, such as osteomyelitis and ulcerative colitis.

INDICATION(S) AND RESEARCH PHASE
Gastrointestinal Diseases and Disorders, miscellaneous – FDA approval letter
Inflammatory Bowel Disease – Phase II
Osteomyelitis – Phase II

rifaximin
unknown

MANUFACTURER
Salix Pharmaceuticals

DESCRIPTION
Rifaximin is a broad-spectrum, gastrointestinal-targeted antibiotic licensed from Alfa Wassermann, S.p.A. Research indicates that rifaximin may exert its antimicrobial action by inhibiting bacterial RNA synthesis and that it may be active against numerous Gram-positive and Gram-negative bacteria. Rifaximin is currently in phase III development for the potential treatment of infections of the gastrointestinal tract.

INDICATION(S) AND RESEARCH PHASE
Bacterial Infection – Phase III
Gastrointestinal Diseases and Disorders, miscellaneous – Phase III

scopolamine
unknown

MANUFACTURER
Elan Transdermal Technologies

DESCRIPTION
Scopolamine acts as a central nervous system depressant. It is an alkaloid derived from plants of the Solanaceae family (Deadly Nightshade), particularly Datura metel and Scopolia carniolica. The drug is in phase II trials for the prevention of motion sickness and for the treatment of gastrointestinal disorders, central and peripheral nervous system disorders, and vertigo. It is administered in a transdermal patch formulation.

INDICATION(S) AND RESEARCH PHASE
Gastrointestinal Diseases and Disorders, miscellaneous – Phase II
Vestibular Hypofunction – Phase II

SLV 305
unknown

MANUFACTURER
Solvay Pharmaceuticals

DESCRIPTION
SLV 305 is a motilin agonist in phase I development for the treatment of gastrointestinal motility disorders.

INDICATION(S) AND RESEARCH PHASE
Gastrointestinal Diseases and Disorders, miscellaneous – Phase I
Gastroesophageal Reflux Disease (GERD) – Phase I

SLV 311
unknown

MANUFACTURER
Solvay Pharmaceuticals

DESCRIPTION
SLV 311 is a motilin agonist being developed for the treatment of gastrointestinal motility disorders. It is currently in phase I trials.

INDICATION(S) AND RESEARCH PHASE
Gastrointestinal Diseases and Disorders, miscellaneous – Phase I
Gastroesophageal Reflux Disease (GERD) – Phase I

somatropin, r-hGH
Serostim

MANUFACTURER
Serono Laboratories

DESCRIPTION
Serostim is a recombinant human growth hormone in trials for several indications. The drug is currently marketed for the treatment of AIDS wasting (cachexia), and it is in development for growth hormone deficiency in adults, short bowel syndrome, lipodystrophy, and congestive heart failure.

INDICATION(S) AND RESEARCH PHASE
Acquired Immune Deficiency Syndrome (AIDS) and AIDS-Related Infections – FDA approved
Hormone Deficiencies – Phase III
Gastrointestinal Diseases and Disorders, miscellaneous – Phase III
Lipodystrophy – Phase II
Congestive Heart Failure – Phase II

tarazepide
unknown

MANUFACTURER
Solvay Pharmaceuticals

DESCRIPTION
Tarazepide is an orally administered medication developed for the treatment of motility disorders of the digestive tract. The drug is designed to have a regulatory effect on the gastrointestinal organs by acting on the nerves and muscles of the digestive tract. At this time, development of tarazepide has been discontinued.

INDICATION(S) AND RESEARCH PHASE
Gastrointestinal Diseases and Disorders, miscellaneous – Trial discontinued

---

tegaserod
Zelmac

MANUFACTURER
Novartis

DESCRIPTION
Zelmac selectively targets and acts on $5HT_4$ receptors present throughout the gastrointestinal (GI) tract. It is being developed for the treatment of functional dyspepsia (phase II), gastroesophageal reflux disease (phase II), and chronic constipation (phase III). An NDA has been submitted for the indication of irritable bowel syndrome.

INDICATION(S) AND RESEARCH PHASE
Irritable Bowel Syndrome (IBS) – NDA submitted
Gastrointestinal Diseases and Disorders, miscellaneous – Phase II
Gastroesophageal Reflux Disease (GERD) – Phase II
Constipation – Phase III

Gastroparesis

intranasal metoclopramide
Emitasol, Pramidin

MANUFACTURER
Questcor

DESCRIPTION
Metoclopramide is a prokinetic agent that interferes with dopamine receptors in the brain. Emitasol is an intranasal formulation of metoclopramide being developed for the treatment of chemotherapy-induced nausea and vomiting, as well as diabetic gastroparesis.

A phase II trial for diabetic gastroparesis has been completed and results were presented in October 2000. Both 10 mg and 20 mg Emitasol dosages showed faster absorption than an already FDA approved metoclopramide oral tablet. At the end of the trial, subjects taking both doses of Emitasol reported a greater reduction in symptoms of gastroparesis than those taking the oral form. Questcor plans to initiate a pivotal phase III trial for gastroparesis in 2001.

Emitasol is marketed in Italy as Pramidin, and an application has been submitted for approval in six Eastern European countries. Questcor has partnered with Roberts Pharmaceutical, a subsidiary of Shire Pharmaceuticals, to co-develop the patented product for North America.

INDICATION(S) AND RESEARCH PHASE
Gastrointestinal Diseases and Disorders, miscellaneous – Phase II completed
Gastroparesis – Phase II completed

Helicobacter Pylori

bismuth subcitrate/ metronidazole/tetracycline
Helicide

MANUFACTURER
Axcan Pharma

DESCRIPTION
Helicide is a single capsule containing colloidal bismuth subcitrate, metronidazole, and tetracycline (a bismuth compound and two antibiotics) for the treatment of *Helicobacter pylori*, the main cause of gastric and duodenal ulcers. This capsule formulation simplifies the problem of taking multiple drugs at different times of the day.

Results of a phase III North American trial of Helicide confirmed that it has potential to be used as a first-line therapy for *Helicobacter pylori*. The trial was conducted in 62 centers in the United States and Canada, and involved 282 subjects with a history of duodenal ulcer. Helicide's 10-day treatment was shown to be at least as efficacious as OAC—a combination of omeprazole, clarithromycin, and amoxicillin. The trial also confirmed that unlike OAC, which does not work in subjects infected with clarithromycin resistant *H. pylori*, Helicide overcomes metronidazole resistance.

Axcan Pharma intends to file an NDA application with the FDA in the beginning of 2001.

INDICATION(S) AND RESEARCH PHASE
Helicobacter Pylori – Phase III completed

NE-0080
unknown

MANUFACTURER
Neose Technologies

DESCRIPTION
NE-0080 is a naturally occurring human gastrointestinal oligosaccharide and antibacterial agent for the treatment and prevention of gastritis and ulcers due to the bacterium, *Helicobacter pylori*. According to Neose Technologies, development of the product is not being actively pursued at this time.

INDICATION(S) AND RESEARCH PHASE
Helicobacter Pylori – Trial discontinued

---

vaccine, Helicobacter pylori
Helivax

MANUFACTURER
Antex Biologics

DESCRIPTION
This vaccine/adjuvant combination is designed for the prevention and treatment of peptic ulcers and gastrointestinal disorders caused by the bacterium, *Helicobacter*

pylori. The vaccine is given in an oral liquid formulation.

INDICATION(S) AND RESEARCH PHASE
Helicobacter Pylori – Phase II
Pediatric, Helicobacter pylori infection – Phase I/II

Hemorrhoids

nitroglycerin ointment
Anogesic

MANUFACTURER
Cellegy Pharmaceuticals

DESCRIPTION
Anogesic is a nitroglycerin-based ointment applied topically for the treatment of anal fissures and hemorrhoids. Although used for more than a century for the treatment of certain cardiovascular diseases, nitroglycerin has only recently been tested in this proprietary formulation for anal fissures and hemorrhoids.

Anogesic works because the active ingredient, nitroglycerin, relaxes the muscles surrounding the blood vessels supplying the anal tissue. Studies demonstrated that the use of nitroglycerin ointment promotes healing of chronic anal fissures, offers significant pain reduction, and eliminates the need for surgery in many cases.

Phase III results showed that Anogesic produced a statistically significant reduction in pain associated with chronic anal fissures. Subjects with chronic anal fissures were randomly assigned to one of eight treatment regimens utilizing several concentrations of nitroglycerin or placebo for up to eight weeks. Statistical significance was not achieved with the primary endpoint, but treatment with 0.4% nitroglycerin ointment resulted in a highly significant decrease in pain intensity compared with placebo. In a second study, 34 hemorrhoidectomy subjects were randomly assigned to 0.2% nitroglycerin ointment or placebo applied three times daily following surgery. It was found that use of an oral narcotic drug was higher in the placebo group than the nitroglycerin group, indicating that the ointment promoted pain relief.

INDICATION(S) AND RESEARCH PHASE
Anal Fissures – Phase III completed
Hemorrhoids – Phase II

Hepatic Encephalopathy

ABT-594, epibatidine
unknown

MANUFACTURER
Abbott Laboratories

DESCRIPTION
In 1976, scientists with the National Institutes of Health (NIH) isolated a compound from the skin of Epipedobates tricolor, an Ecuadorian frog. Named epibatidine, this alkaloid was found to block pain 200 times more effectively than morphine, without morphine's addictive and harmful side effects. A potent antinociceptive agent for acute and persistent pain, this compound works predominately by targeting central neuronal acetylcholine receptors (nAChRs).

After successfully eliminating the paralyzing effects of the poison, epibatidine is now being tested for hepatic encephalopathy in subjects with advanced liver disease. Most analgesics modulate the feeling of pain by binding to opiate receptors. Epibatidine has a very low affinity for the nicotine receptors in the neuromuscular junction that cause the paralysis effect, but it has a high affinity for the nicotine receptors in the central nervous system that regulate pain perception.

INDICATION(S) AND RESEARCH PHASE
Hepatic Encephalopathy – Phase II
Pain, Acute or Chronic – Phase II

Hepatitis

ACH-126,443
unknown

MANUFACTURER
Achillion Pharmaceuticals

DESCRIPTION
ACH-126,443 is an orally administered antiviral agent with potent activity against the hepatitis B virus and the human immunodeficiency virus (HIV). The drug is currently in phase I development. MediChem Life Sciences, a drug discovery technology and services company, conducted chemical route development that provided the scaleable synthetic pathway used to manufacture kilogram quantities of this drug candidate. Kilogram-scale synthesis was then performed to supply large quantities of ACH-126,443 for the clinical trials.

INDICATION(S) AND RESEARCH PHASE
Hepatitis – Phase I
HIV infection – Phase I

adefovir dipivoxil, GS-840
unknown

MANUFACTURER
Gilead Sciences

DESCRIPTION
Adefovir dipivoxil is a prodrug of PMEA, a nucleotide that inhibits hepatitis B virus DHA polymerase, an enzyme essential to viral replication. Currently, it is being tested in a phase III trial for hepatitis B. This two-year trial is recruiting about 500 subjects and is evaluating dosages of 10 and 30 mg/day orally.

INDICATION(S) AND RESEARCH PHASE
Hepatitis – Phase III

anti-hepatitis B
unknown

MANUFACTURER
Cangene Corporation

DESCRIPTION
Anti-hepatitis B is part of the company's hyperimmune products, which are highly purified antibodies made from human plasma obtained from people with high antibody titers to the hepatitis B virus. A phase III trial of the compound for use in the treatment of people with chronic hepatitis B

virus infection was completed in Europe at the end of 2000 and results suggested that the product was efficacious. The company anticipates filing an NDS in Canada.

INDICATION(S) AND RESEARCH PHASE
Hepatitis – Phase III completed

anti-hepatitis C
unknown

MANUFACTURER
Cangene Corporation

DESCRIPTION
Anti-hepatitis C is part of the company's hyperimmune products, which are highly purified antibodies made from specialty human plasma used for therapeutic purposes. It is being tested in a phase II trial in liver transplantation recipients infected with hepatitis C virus. The phase II trial will evaluate the effects of the antibodies to prevent re-infection of the transplanted liver. The trial is being conducted at multiple sites throughout Canada.

INDICATION(S) AND RESEARCH PHASE
Hepatitis – Phase II

BMS-200475
Entecavir

MANUFACTURER
Bristol-Myers Squibb

DESCRIPTION
Viruses such as hepatitis B need to be able to replicate their viral genetic material in order to reproduce themselves. Bristol-Myers Squibb is developing a treatment for chronic hepatitis B infection, a common and serious liver condition, which works by disrupting the viral replication process.

Genetic material is made up of proteins called nucleic acids. By using a synthesized protein (2'-deoxyguanosine carbocyclic analogue) that mimics one of the building blocks of nucleic acids, scientists hope to stop the production of viral genetic information, and thus prevent viruses from creating the genetic machinery they require to keep reproducing.

Studies are under way in phase II trials to understand if this novel drug will improve the symptoms and prognosis of chronic hepatitis B infection.

INDICATION(S) AND RESEARCH PHASE
Hepatitis – Phase II
Viral Infection – Phase II

cidofovir
Vistide

MANUFACTURER
Gilead Sciences

DESCRIPTION
Vistide is being tested as an injectable formulation for treatment of central nervous system infections and hepatitis B virus respiratory tumors, and tumors or disorders of the larynx. The drug is in phase I/II trials for HBV respiratory tumors, laryngeal papillomatosis, and progressive multifocal leukoencephalopathy.

INDICATION(S) AND RESEARCH PHASE
Hepatitis – Phase I/II
Laryngeal Tumors/Disorders – Phase I/II
Viral Infection – Phase I/II
Brain Cancer – Phase I/II

clevudine
unknown

MANUFACTURER
Triangle Pharmaceuticals

DESCRIPTION
Clevudine (formerly L-FMAU) is a pyrimidine nucleoside analogue that has shown inhibitory activity against hepatitis B virus (HBV) replication invitro. The drug is currently in phase I development for the treatment of HBV.

INDICATION(S) AND RESEARCH PHASE
Hepatitis – Phase I

EHT899
unknown

MANUFACTURER
Enzo Biochem

DESCRIPTION
EHT899 is currently in phase II development for the treatment of hepatitis B (HBV). Hepatitis B virus can cause a chronic infection in the liver of infected people. Liver damage is the result of direct viral effects and the person's immune system response to the infection. In preclinical work, it was shown that the immune response against the virus could be altered by oral administration of certain viral proteins developed by Enzo.

Eighty percent of subjects in a phase I trial of EHT899 responded favorably as measured by a decrease in viral load, decrease in liver inflammation, or reduction of elevated levels of liver enzymes. Nine of the 15 subjects experienced significant decreases in viral load, while ten subjects showed complete normalization of liver enzymes. The trial was conducted in Jerusalem.

INDICATION(S) AND RESEARCH PHASE
Hepatitis – Phase II

emtricitabine
Coviracil

MANUFACTURER
Triangle Pharmaceuticals

DESCRIPTION
Coviracil, a nucleoside reverse transcript inhibitor (NRTI), has been shown to be a potent inhibitor of hepatitis B virus (HBV) replication. In October 2000, results of a phase I/II trial of Coviracil involving subjects chronically infected with HBV indicated that a daily dose of 200 mg was most effective. As a result, the 200 mg/day dosage was selected for a phase III trial, which was initiated in October 2000. Coviracil is also in phase II and III trials for the treatment of HIV infection.

INDICATION(S) AND RESEARCH PHASE
HIV Infection – Phase III
Hepatitis – Phase III
Pediatric, AIDS/HIV – Phase III

HCI-436
unknown

MANUFACTURER
Wyeth-Ayerst

DESCRIPTION
HCI-436 is a novel drug being developed for the treatment of hepatitis C virus. It works by inhibiting viral activities essential to the replication of the virus. The drug is being jointly developed with ViroPharma and is in phase II trials.

INDICATION(S) AND RESEARCH PHASE
Hepatitis – Phase II

HE2000
unknown

MANUFACTURER
Hollis-Eden Pharmaceuticals

DESCRIPTION
HE2000 inhibits HIV replication by manipulating host cellular factors. Invitro studies showed that HE2000 significantly inhibited various strains of HIV including wild type, reverse transcriptase inhibitor resistant and multiple drug resistant isolates. These invitro studies showed no toxicity at up to 100 times the expected human dose.

HE2000 is being evaluated in a phase I/II trial for HIV/AIDS in both the United States and South Africa. The company believes that HE2000 may be acting through a unique mechanism of action on the host cell rather than on the virus itself. As a result, an extensive set of analytical measurements on a number of different virologic and immunologic markers of therapeutic activity are being evaluated. In the phase I/II trial all the subjects will be monitored during dosing and up to three months after completion of treatment.

Since HE2000 does not target specific viral proteins, the company believes it may be a more durable treatment and less prone to viral mutations and the resulting resistance to drug therapy.

Additionally, HE2000 is being tested in early-stage trials for malaria and hepatitis.

INDICATION(S) AND RESEARCH PHASE
Acquired Immune Deficiency Syndrome (AIDS) and AIDS-Related Infections – Phase I/II
HIV Infection – Phase I/II
Hepatitis – Phase I
Malaria – Phase I/II

hepatitis A
Nothav

MANUFACTURER
Chiron Corporation

DESCRIPTION
Nothav is a second-generation vaccine for hepatitis A. It is currently in phase III trials for adults in Europe. The company plans to develop a formulation for pediatric subjects as well.

INDICATION(S) AND RESEARCH PHASE
Hepatitis – Phase III

hepatitis B immune globulin
HBVIg

MANUFACTURER
Nabi

DESCRIPTION
HBVIg is a human hepatitis B immune globulin in development for the treatment of acute exposure to blood containing hepatitis B virus surface antigen. It is also being developed in an intravenous formulation to prevent hepatitis B virus re-infection of transplanted livers in subjects with hepatitis B. A Biologics License Application has been submitted for the first indication, and the drug is in phase III trials regarding liver transplants.

An NDA has been submitted for the prevention of perinatal transmission of hepatitis B.

INDICATION(S) AND RESEARCH PHASE
Hepatitis – Phase III

hepatitis B immunotherapy, HBV/MF59
unknown

MANUFACTURER
Chiron Corporation

DESCRIPTION
HBV/MF59 is an immunotherapy combining the company's hepatitis B vaccine and a novel proprietary adjuvant, MF59. The adjuvant is needed to enhance the response to the vaccine. Even with a complete series of three injections, approximately 20% of people receiving the licensed HBV vaccine, do not respond. It is currently in phase II trials for chronic hepatitis B.

INDICATION(S) AND RESEARCH PHASE
Hepatitis – Phase II

hepatitis C protein
unknown

MANUFACTURER
Enzo Biochem

DESCRIPTION
A new broad-spectrum immune regulatory compound is in a phase I trial for treatment of hepatitis C virus infection (HCV) or its associated hepatocellular carcinoma secondary to HCV infection. The trial will treat each subject for 30 weeks and will be followed for another 20 weeks. The trial is taking place in Israel.

INDICATION(S) AND RESEARCH PHASE
Hepatitis – Phase I

IDN-6556
unknown

MANUFACTURER
IDUN Pharmaceuticals

DESCRIPTION
IDN-6556 is a caspase inhibitor, resulting in the inhibition of apoptosis. The compound is in a phase I trial for the treatment of acute alcoholic hepatitis, a condition that is characterized by increased apoptosis of hepatocytes.

INDICATION(S) AND RESEARCH PHASE
Hepatitis – Phase I

immune globulin
Nabi Civacir

MANUFACTURER
Nabi

DESCRIPTION
Nabi Civacir is a human antibody product containing antibodies that neutralize hepatitis C virus (HCV). It is being developed to prevent liver transplant subjects with hepatitis C from experiencing liver re-infection. It is also being developed for the treatment of chronic hepatitis C virus infections. Nabi Civacir is currently in phase I trials.

INDICATION(S) AND RESEARCH PHASE
Hepatitis – Phase I

immune globulin intravenous
Venoglobulin-S

MANUFACTURER
Alpha Therapeutic

DESCRIPTION
Venoglobulin-S is a solution of antibodies that are being tested for use in two indications. The first one is a phase III clinical trial to prevent infection (prophylaxis) from the hepatitis A virus; and the second use is for prevention of acute graft versus host disease (GVHD) in subjects needing a bone marrow transplant. Sometimes drug therapy is helpful to prevent the body from rejecting a transplanted organ, or in the opposite case of the organ rejecting its new host.

This immune globulin product may replace missing antibodies, especially in subjects that have a compromised immune system or primary immunodeficiencies, which may be present at birth. This biological product is given to a subject by intramuscular injection.

INDICATION(S) AND RESEARCH PHASE
Bone Marrow Transplant – Phase III
Hepatitis – Phase III

immunostimulatory sequences (ISS) candidate
unknown

MANUFACTURER
Triangle Pharmaceuticals

DESCRIPTION
Immunostimulatory sequences (ISS) are short strands of DNA believed to elicit immune responses. Triangle Pharmaceuticals currently has an ISS candidate in phase I development for the treatment of hepatitis B.

INDICATION(S) AND RESEARCH PHASE
Hepatitis – Phase I

immunotherapeutic, AML
Ceplene

MANUFACTURER
Maxim Pharmaceuticals

DESCRIPTION
Ceplene (formally Maxamine) is a histamine-2 (H_2) receptor stimulator (agonist) that is being co-administered with immunotherapies, including cytokines and interleukin-2 (IL-2). Clinical testing includes treatment of acute myelogenous leukemia (AML), chronic hepatitis C, malignant melanoma, multiple myeloma, and renal cell carcinoma.

Results from a phase III 300 subject trial of Ceplene (histamine dihydrochloride) in stage-IV malignant melanoma indicated that Ceplene used in combination with a lower dose of interleukin-2 (IL-2) improved survival rates for stage IV malignant melanoma subjects compared with those treated with the same doses of IL-2 alone. Treatment with Ceplene and IL-2 improved overall survival, increased survival rates at 12, 18, and 24 months, and improved time-to-disease progression over treatment with IL-2 alone. Twenty-five percent of subjects treated with Ceplene and lower-dose IL-2 survived for a 24-month period. Overall response was achieved in 38% of the subjects treated with Ceplene and lower-dose IL-2. The company received an NDA non-approvable letter in January 2001 because the FDA stated that the phase III trial forming the basis of the NDA would not be adequate as a single study to support approval.

INDICATION(S) AND RESEARCH PHASE
Hepatitis – Phase II
Leukemia – Phase III completed
Malignant Melanoma – NDA denied
Multiple Myeloma – Phase II
Renal Cell Carcinoma – Phase II

interferon (IFN), alfa-n3
Alferon N Injection

MANUFACTURER
Interferon Sciences

DESCRIPTION
Alferon N is a human leukocyte-derived natural interferon (IFN) treatment being tested for chronic hepatitis C in subjects previously untreated with IFN.

Alferon N is given by injection and has completed a phase III trial. The company reported that the FDA rejected the drug application and advised for the conduct of another phase III study with an improved endpoint design before approval may be granted. At the present time, the company does not have the resources necessary to continue development.

INDICATION(S) AND RESEARCH PHASE
Hepatitis – NDA denied
HIV Infection – Phase II

interferon alfa-2b
PEG-Intron

MANUFACTURER
Schering-Plough Corporation

DESCRIPTION
PEG-Intron is a long-acting antiviral/biological response modifier. Clinical trials include testing for the treatment of chronic myelogenous leukemia, solid tumors, and malignant melanoma.

PEG-Intron was developed by Enzon for Schering-Plough who owns the exclusive rights. The drug was approved by the FDA for the treatment of hepatitis C in January 2001.

INDICATION(S) AND RESEARCH PHASE
Cancer/Tumors (Unspecified) – Phase II
Hepatitis – FDA approved
Leukemia – Phase III
Malignant Melanoma – Phase III

interferon alfa-2b/ribavirin
PEG-Intron/Rebetol

MANUFACTURER
Enzon

DESCRIPTION
PEG-Intron + Rebetol is a combination therapy of biosynthetic interferon and ribavirin for the treatment of hepatitis C virus infection. Rebetol is an oral formulation of ribavirin, a synthetic nucleoside analog with broad-spectrum antiviral. Intron A is a recombinant version of naturally occurring alpha interferon, which has been shown to exert both antiviral and immunomodulatory effects. Intron A must be given three times a week. PEG-Intron is a longer-acting form of Intron A that uses proprietary PEG technology developed by Enzon, and can be given once weekly.

Results of a phase III trial indicated that combination therapy with once-weekly PEG-Intron injection plus daily Rebetol capsules achieved a 54% rate of sustained virologic response overall in previously untreated adult subjects with chronic hepatitis C. Sustained virologic response (SVR) is defined as sustained loss of detectable hepatitis C virus.

INDICATION(S) AND RESEARCH PHASE
Hepatitis – Phase III

interleukin-10 (IL-10)
Tenovil

MANUFACTURER
Schering-Plough Corporation

DESCRIPTION
Tenovil is an immunomodulator being developed in an injectable formulation. It is currently being evaluated for the treatment of ischemia reperfusion injury, hepatic fibrosis, and hepatitis C.

INDICATION(S) AND RESEARCH PHASE
Liver Disease – Phase II
Hepatitis – Phase I
Ischemia Reperfusion Injury – Phase I

interleukin-12 (IL-12)
unknown

MANUFACTURER
Genetics Institute

DESCRIPTION
Interleukin-12 (IL-12) is a novel, genetically engineered, human immune modulator being tested in phase II trials for the treatment of hepatitis C, chronic liver disease due to hepatitis infection, and AIDS. There is an additional indication for renal carcinoma, which may have an orphan drug status.

INDICATION(S) AND RESEARCH PHASE
Acquired Immune Deficiency Syndrome (AIDS) and AIDS-Related Infections – Phase II
Hepatitis – Phase II
Renal Cell Carcinoma – Phase II

IP501
unknown

MANUFACTURER
Interneuron Pharmaceuticals

DESCRIPTION
IP501 is a purified phospholipid, which helps to repair damaged cells. It is indicated for the treatment and prevention of alcohol-induced cirrhosis of the liver and hepatitis C. IP501 is currently in phase III trials. The drug is in tablet form.

INDICATION(S) AND RESEARCH PHASE
Alcohol Dependence – Phase III
Hepatitis – Phase III
Liver Disease – Phase III

ISIS-14803
unknown

MANUFACTURER
Isis Pharmaceuticals

DESCRIPTION
ISIS 14803 is a novel antisense drug designed specifically to inhibit the replication of the virus. Its preclinical trials in mice and cell cultures showed marked reduction of the HCV RNA expression. It consists of a 20-base phosphorothioate oligonucleotide that is administered using a microfusion pump called Medipad. The Elan Corporation of Ireland has developed the pump and is the co-developer of the drug.

INDICATION(S) AND RESEARCH PHASE
Hepatitis – Phase I/II

LY466700
Heptazyme

MANUFACTURER
Ribozyme Pharmaceuticals

DESCRIPTION
Heptazyme is an anti-hepatitis C virus ribozyme. It works by cleaving the hepatitis C (HCV) genetic material in a region of the HCV gene that is highly conserved. Heptazyme has been designed to target a specific region necessary for the viral life cycle; when this region is cut, the virus is unable to replicate. Phase II trials testing Heptazyme is planned for first quarter 2001.

Two phase I results demonstrated that Heptazyme was well tolerated at all doses given, in contrast to the significant side effects associated with currently available HCV treatments. Further, 12 HCV positive subjects with elevations in serum ALT were treated at doses ranging from 10 to 90 mg/subject in the multi-dose trials. Three of these subjects had transient decreases in serum HCV RNA of approximately 1 log10. Ribozyme is preparing for upcoming phase II trials.

INDICATION(S) AND RESEARCH PHASE
Hepatitis – Phase II

MIV-210
unknown

MANUFACTURER
Medivir

DESCRIPTION
MIV-210 is a nuceloside analogue in a phase I trial for treatment of hepatitis B virus infection. The initial phase I trials are being conducted in the United Kingdom and are expected to be completed during the third quarter of 2001. In animal tests, MIV-210 shows good efficacy against the hepatitis B virus.

INDICATION(S) AND RESEARCH PHASE
Hepatitis – Phase I

OST 577
Ostavir

MANUFACTURER
Protein Design Labs

DESCRIPTION
Ostavir is a humanized monoclonal antibody (Mab) in ongoing phase II trials for the treatment of chronic hepatitis B, either combined with interferon or as a sole agent. Additional indications may include infectious diseases and viral diseases.

INDICATION(S) AND RESEARCH PHASE
Hepatitis – Phase II
Viral Infection – Phase II

peginterferon alfa-2a
Pegasys

MANUFACTURER
Hoffmann-La Roche

DESCRIPTION
Pegasys is a longer-lasting form of interferon, which is a naturally produced immune boosting substance. This drug is given in an injectable formulation that is being tested in phase III trials for the treatment of complications of hepatitis C.

INDICATION(S) AND RESEARCH PHASE
Hepatitis B & C – Phase III
Malignant Melanoma – Phase II
Renal Cell Carcinoma – Phase II
Leukemia – Phase III

PeNta-HepB-IPV, vaccine
Infanrix

MANUFACTURER
GlaxoSmithKline

DESCRIPTION
This recombinant vaccine has been developed to address several indications. It has been approved by the European Union for diphtheria, tetanus, pertussis, hepatitis B, and polio. An NDA has also been submitted for these indications.

INDICATION(S) AND RESEARCH PHASE
Pediatric, Vaccines – NDA submitted
Hepatitis – NDA submitted

recombinant human interferon beta-1a
Rebif

MANUFACTURER
Serono Laboratories

DESCRIPTION
Rebif is an interferon beta-1a product being developed for a variety of indications. These include non-small cell lung cancer, chronic hepatitis C, Crohn's disease, ulcerative colitis, Guillain-Barré syndrome, as an early treatment of multiple sclerosis (phase III) and as a treatment for secondary progressive multiple sclerosis (filed) and rheumatoid arthritis. Rebif has been approved in several countries for the treatment of relapsing-remitting multiple sclerosis.

INDICATION(S) AND RESEARCH PHASE
Multiple Sclerosis – Phase III
Lung Cancer – Phase II
Hepatitis – Phase II
Crohn's Disease – Phase II
Inflammatory Bowel Disease – Phase II
Neurologic Disorders, Guillain-Barré Syndrome – Phase II
Rheumatoid Arthritis – Phase II

ritonavir
Norvir/ABT-378

MANUFACTURER
Abbott Laboratories

DESCRIPTION
Norvir is a peptide-imitating protease inhibitor currently used by itself or with other antiretroviral agents for the treatment of HIV infection. The drug acts by making the enzyme incapable of processing a gag-pol polyprotein precursor, which leads to production of a non-infectious immature HIV particles. ABT-378, another protease inhibitor is itself in phase III trials for HIV infections, has been combined with Norvir in capsule form for use against HIV infections and hepatitis. Abbott Laboratories has submitted an NDA for this combination therapy to treat HIV and AIDS.

INDICATION(S) AND RESEARCH PHASE
HIV Infection – NDA submitted
Hepatitis – Phase III
Pediatric – FDA approved

SB M00026
unknown

MANUFACTURER
GlaxoSmithKline

DESCRIPTION
SB M00026 is a recombinant compound being developed for the treatment of chronic infection with hepatitis B virus. It is currently in phase II development.

INDICATION(S) AND RESEARCH PHASE
Hepatitis – Phase II

thymalfasin
Zadaxin

MANUFACTURER
SciClone Pharmaceuticals

DESCRIPTION

Zadaxin is a twenty-eight amino acid peptide originally isolated from the thymus gland and now produced synthetically. The compound has been shown to promote the maturation of T-cells, which are involved in the control of various immune responses. The company has conducted phase II/III trials of Zadaxin in combination with lamivudine and famciclovir for the treatment of chronic hepatitis B and hepatitis C. Additionally, a phase III study for hepatitis B is currently ongoing in Japan. Sigma-Tau S.p.A. is conducting a phase III trial in Europe for hepatitis C. Zadaxin was FDA approved in March 2000 for liver cancer.

INDICATION(S) AND RESEARCH PHASE
Hepatitis – Phase II/III
Viral Infection – Phase II/III
Liver Cancer – FDA approved
Malignant Melanoma – Phase II
Lung Cancer – Phase Preclinical

unknown
Omniferon

MANUFACTURER
Viragen

DESCRIPTION
Omniferon is a multi-subtype alpha interferon derived from human white blood cells. This specific interferon is being studied in the treatment of hepatitis C virus infection. Favorable interim dose escalation results from the first phase II trial have been reported. None of the subjects had to undergo dose reduction or discontinue treatment because of side effects at any of the three dosing levels. There was a significant decrease in hepatitis C virus concentrations in the blood with some evidence that this reduction was more rapid than that observed with other drug regimens used to treat this infection.

INDICATION(S) AND RESEARCH PHASE
Hepatitis – Phase II

unknown
Albuferon

MANUFACTURER
Human Genome Sciences

DESCRIPTION
Albuferon is a new protein created by fusing the gene for interferon alpha to the gene of another human protein, albumin. The fused gene produces a protein with characteristics of both interferon alpha and albumin. Based on preclinical studies, Albuferon should provide a longer acting therapeutic activity and an improved side-effect profile when compared to the current first line therapy for hepatitis C virus infection, recombinant human interferon alpha. In October 2000, Human Genome Sciences submitted an IND application with the FDA in order to initiate phase I trials.

INDICATION(S) AND RESEARCH PHASE
Hepatitis – Phase I

ursodiol
Urso

MANUFACTURER
Axcan Pharma

DESCRIPTION
Urso is an oral tablet composed of a bile acid (ursodeoxycholic acid) found in small amounts in normal human bile and in larger quantities in the bile of certain bears. This drug has been marketed in the United States for the treatment of primary biliary cirrhosis (PBC) since 1998. It is also approved in Canada for the treatment of cholestatic liver diseases such as PBC and the dissolution of gallstones. Additionally, Urso is being tested in trials for at least five other indications: the treatment of hypercholesterolemia, treatment with chemo-prevention of colorectal polyps, treatment of colorectal cancer, treatment of non-alcoholic steatohepatitis, and treatment of viral hepatitis. The drug is licensed by Sanofi-Synthelabo to Axcan Pharma in a joint venture with Schwarz Pharma.

INDICATION(S) AND RESEARCH PHASE
Cholesterol (High Levels) – Phase II
Colon Polyps – Phase II
Colorectal Cancer – Phase II
Gallbladder Disorders – Phase III/IV
Hepatitis – Phase II

vaccine, hepatitis E
unknown

MANUFACTURER
GlaxoSmithKline

DESCRIPTION
GlaxoSmithKline is developing a recombinant vaccine for hepatitis E prophylaxis. It is currently in phase I development.

INDICATION(S) AND RESEARCH PHASE
Hepatitis – Phase I

vaccine, HCV/MF59, hepatitis C
unknown

MANUFACTURER
Chiron Corporation

DESCRIPTION
HCV/MF59 is a prophylactic vaccine for the prevention of hepatitis C. It is currently in phase II trials.

INDICATION(S) AND RESEARCH PHASE
Hepatitis – Phase II

vaccine, hepatitis
Twinrix-three doses

MANUFACTURER
GlaxoSmithKline

DESCRIPTION
Twinrix is a recombinant vaccine that immunizes recipients against both hepatitis A and hepatitis B. Benefits of this vaccine may include greater convenience and protection for subjects, since immunization against two diseases can be achieved with one injection. An NDA has been submitted for Twinrix (three doses) for combined hepatitis A and B prophylaxis in adults.

INDICATION(S) AND RESEARCH PHASE
Hepatitis – NDA submitted
Vaccines – NDA submitted

vaccine, hepatitis B
unknown

MANUFACTURER
GlaxoSmithKline

DESCRIPTION
GlaxoSmithKline is developing a recombinant vaccine for extra strength hepatitis B prophylaxis (poor/non-responders). It is currently in phase III trials.

INDICATION(S) AND RESEARCH PHASE
Hepatitis – Phase III

---

vaccine, hepatitis B
Hepagene

MANUFACTURER
Celltech Chiroscience plc

DESCRIPTION
Hepagene is a novel third generation recombinant vaccine for the prevention of hepatitis B virus infection. Hepagene mimics the surface of the hepatitis B virus, which elicits an immune response. The success of this vaccine is significantly improved because it incorporates all three surface antigens: pre-S1, pre-S2, and S of the virus. Current vaccines only contain one or two of these surface antigens, providing for a much weaker immune stimulus. An MAA has been filed in Europe.

INDICATION(S) AND RESEARCH PHASE
Hepatitis – MAA submitted

---

vaccine, hepatitis B DNA
unknown

MANUFACTURER
PowderJect Vaccines

DESCRIPTION
This DNA vaccine, which uses PowderJect delivery technology, is being developed for the treatment of hepatitis B. The ability of DNA vaccines to induce a cellular response is believed to be critical in eliminating chronic viral infections such as hepatitis B.

An earlier clinical trial demonstrated that PowderJect's preventive hepatitis B DNA vaccine induced cellular immune responses in all evaluable subjects. This trial also indicated the vaccine elicited protective levels of antibodies in all volunteers.

The needle-free PowderJect system delivers vaccines, drugs, and diagnostics in a dry powder formulation of microscopic solid particles. These particles are accelerated to high velocity in a jet of gas generated from a helium microcylinder contained inside the hand-held PowderJect device. The medicine is propelled down a specially designed nozzle into the outer layers of the skin. The vaccine is being developed as part of a multiproduct strategic alliance with GlaxoSmithKline.

INDICATION(S) AND RESEARCH PHASE
Hepatitis – Phase I

---

vaccine, viral hepatitis (HBV)
GENEVAX—HBV

MANUFACTURER
Wyeth-Lederle Vaccines

DESCRIPTION
Genevax is a novel DNA-based immunotherapeutic vaccine being developed against the hepatitis B virus (HBV).

INDICATION(S) AND RESEARCH PHASE
Hepatitis – Phase II

VML 600, R-848
unknown

MANUFACTURER
Vernalis

DESCRIPTION
VML 600 is a novel immune response modifier (IRM) that stimulates the production of cytokines and boosts cell-mediated immunity. It is being developed for the treatment of hepatitis C virus infections and herpes virus infections. Vernalis completed phase IIa studies in Europe and the United States in 2000 and is planning to conduct a larger phase II trial in 2001.

INDICATION(S) AND RESEARCH PHASE
Hepatitis – Phase II

VP 50406
unknown

MANUFACTURER
ViroPharma

DESCRIPTION
VP 50406 is an orally administered small molecule being developed for the treatment of hepatitis C virus infection. The drug has demonstrated an ability to inhibit RNA replication of hepatitis C virus invitro. VP 50406 is currently in phase II trials.

INDICATION(S) AND RESEARCH PHASE
Hepatitis – Phase II

VX-497
unknown

MANUFACTURER
Vertex Pharmaceuticals

DESCRIPTION
This oral drug contains a novel inhibitor of inosine monophosphate dehydrogenase (IMPDH), an enzyme responsible for stimulating production of lymphocytes. VX-497 has the potential to exert direct antiviral activity, as well as affect the immune response by effecting on lymphocyte migration and proliferation. Consequently, VX-497 may be an effective treatment for hepatitis C virus (HCV) infection as the disease involves both viral proliferation and liver inflammation.

Vertex plans to initiate a pivotal trial of VX-497 plus pegylated interferon in subjects with HCV in 2001.

INDICATION(S) AND RESEARCH PHASE
Hepatitis – Phase II

XTL-001
unknown

MANUFACTURER
XTL Biopharmaceuticals

Hepatitis

DESCRIPTION

XTL-001, a combination of two high affinity human monoclonal antibodies (Mabs), is directed against two different epitopes of hepatitis B surface antigen HbsAg of the hepatitis B virus (HBV) and binds to all major HBV subtypes. Phase I trial results indicated that XTL-001 produced a rapid and consistent decrease in HBV-DNA and HBsAg levels in subjects with chronic HBV. Twelve subjects received multiple infusions of XTL-001 in doses ranging from 10 mg to 80 mg per week for four consecutive weeks followed by four weeks of observation. HBV-DNA levels decreased by as much as 100,000 fold (5 logs), while lowered HbsAg levels were sustained for a short period of time in several subjects receiving the two highest doses of XTL-001 (40 mg/week and 80 mg/week). XTL Biopharmaceuticals plan to initiate a phase II trial of XTL-001 combined with currently available antivirals in 2001.

INDICATION(S) AND RESEARCH PHASE
Hepatitis – Phase I completed

Ileus

prucalopride
Resolor

MANUFACTURER
Janssen Pharmaceutica

DESCRIPTION

Resolor is a colonic motility agent for the treatment of chronic constipation. The drug is administered in an oral capsule formulation, and it is currently in phase III trials. Resolor is also being tested in an injectable subcutaneous formulation in phase I/II trials for post-operative ileus. Pediatric trials for this drug have been discontinued.

INDICATION(S) AND RESEARCH PHASE
Constipation – Phase III
Ileus – Phase I/II
Pediatric – Trial discontinued

Inflammatory Bowel Disease

APC 2059
unknown

MANUFACTURER
Axys Pharmaceuticals

DESCRIPTION

APC 2059 is an inhibitior of tryptase, an enzyme found in mast cells. Research suggests that tryptase functions pathologically as a potent mediator of mast cell-related allergic inflammatory conditions. In the gastrointestinal tract, mast cell infiltration and tryptase activity have been associated with several pathologies, including inflammatory bowel disease, caliginous colitis, and gastrointestinal allergy. Significantly elevated tryptase secretion and enzyme activity have been measured relative to controls for ulcerative colitis. Taken together, these observations have suggested that ulcerative colitis may be a mast cell and tryptase-mediated disease.

Results of an open-label phase II trial of APC 2059 for the treatment of moderate to severe flares of ulcerative colitis demonstrated that 58% of evaluable subjects achieved "clinically significant benefit" as measured by the Investigators' Global Assessment. APC 2059 was delivered by subcutaneous injection twice a day, and by the end of the trial there were 53 evaluable subjects out of 56 enrolled. Axys Pharmaceuticals plans to initiate placebo-controlled phase IIb/III trials for ulcerative colitis based on the phase II results.

INDICATION(S) AND RESEARCH PHASE
Inflammatory Bowel Disease – Phase II completed

budesonide
Entocort CR

MANUFACTURER
AstraZeneca

DESCRIPTION

One of the mainstays of treatment for Crohn's disease has been steroids. Unfortunately, side effects of corticosteroids often are severe and can include swelling of the face, arms, and legs, "buffalo" hump of the upper back, easy bruisability, increased body hair, and acne. These adverse effects are caused by the strong effect of steroids on parts of the body other than the colon.

Entocort, inserted rectally, may have a lower side effect profile. Currently in phase III trials, it has been designed to have a strong effect on tissues where it is topically applied (such as the colon) because of its high affinity for surface steroid receptors. But soon after Entocort is absorbed through the colon into the bloodstream, it passes through the liver where it is rapidly metabolized into relatively inactive molecules that have little effect on the rest of the body. The susceptibility of the drug to the liver's metabolizing action limits distribution of Entocort in the body, thus limiting side effects.

INDICATION(S) AND RESEARCH PHASE
Crohn's Disease – Phase III
Inflammatory Bowel Disease – Phase III

Carn 1000
Aliminase

MANUFACTURER
Carrington Laboratories

DESCRIPTION

Aliminase is derived from the gel of the plant Aloe barbadense Miller (aloe vera L.). It is an off-white powder comprised of a mixture of naturally occurring substances, principally complex carbohydrates. Results of phase III trials revealed that Aliminase showed little therapeutic effect in subjects with ulcerative colitis. As a result, the company is discontinuing testing of Aliminase for the treatment of ulcerative colitis.

INDICATION(S) AND RESEARCH PHASE
Inflammatory Bowel Disease – Phase discontinued

CBP-1011

Colirest

MANUFACTURER
Inkine Pharmaceutical Company

DESCRIPTION
Colirest is an oral steroid-like drug in development for the treatment of idiopathic thrombocytopenic purpura (ITP) and other conditions. ITP is a disorder in which the immune system attacks its own platelets, targeting them with antibodies and then destroying the resulting immune complexed platelets. Preliminary studies have indicated Colirest may help increase platelet counts. Additionally, CPB-1011 is being tested for the treatment of Crohn's disease and ulcerative colitis.

In December 2000, positive results were announced from a multicenter, open-label phase II trial of Colirest in subjects with mild or moderate active ulcerative colitis. Nine of 11 evaluable subjects completed eight weeks of Colirest treatment. Seven of the nine (78%) subjects responded to Colirest treatment in the disease activity index (DAI) and investigator global assessment (IGA) evaluations. Inkine Pharmaceutical Company plans to move Colirest into later stage pivotal trials.

INDICATION(S) AND RESEARCH PHASE
Thrombocytopenia – Phase III
Crohn's Disease – Phase II completed
Inflammatory Bowel Disease – Phase II completed

CDP-571, BAY 10-356
Humicade

MANUFACTURER
Celltech Chiroscience plc

DESCRIPTION
CDP-571 is a recombinant humanized IgG4 antibody that blocks the activity of tumor necrosis factor-alpha (TNF-α), an important mediator of inflammation. This biological drug is being tested in phase IIb trials for the treatment of various inflammatory conditions, including Crohn's disease, ulcerative colitis, rheumatoid arthritis, and inflammatory bowel disease. The drug is administered by intravenous infusion.

INDICATION(S) AND RESEARCH PHASE
Crohn's Disease – Phase IIb
Inflammatory Bowel Disease – Phase IIb
Rheumatoid Arthritis – Phase IIb

ibuprofen
Elangesic

MANUFACTURER
Elan Pharmaceutical Research

DESCRIPTION
Non-steroidal anti-inflammatory drugs (NSAIDs), such as ibuprofen, are very effective agents for the relief of pain and inflammation. But many individuals cannot use these drugs due to adverse effects, such as irritation of the lining of the stomach. NSAIDs may cause gastritis and ulcers, or exacerbate these conditions when already present.

Elan Pharmaceuticals has developed a new product called Elangesic that may potentially increase the tolerability of NSAIDs. Elangesic works by formulating drugs into high density, controlled-release beads. Each bead contains a core of the desired drug, and an outer coating which discharges the drug in a time-release fashion. Clinical testing is in phase II trials using this once- and twice-daily Intestinal Protective Drug Absorption System (IPDAS).

INDICATION(S) AND RESEARCH PHASE
Gastroenteritis – Phase II
Inflammatory Bowel Disease – Phase II
Ulcers – Phase II

ISIS-2302
unknown

MANUFACTURER
Isis Pharmaceuticals

DESCRIPTION
ISIS-2302 is an inhibitor of antisense intracellular adhesion molecule-1 (ICAM-1), which is a chemical that plays a central role in inflammation. Antisense drugs work at the genetic level to interrupt the process by which disease-causing proteins are produced. Proteins play a central role in virtually every aspect of human metabolism. Many human diseases are the result of inappropriate protein production or disordered protein performance. This is true of both host diseases (such as cancer) and infectious diseases (such as AIDS).

ISIS-2302 is being tested in a phase II trial using an enema formulation to treat subjects with ulcerative colitis. This method of administration allows potentially therapeutic amounts of the drug to be absorbed by the lining of the intestine, which is inflamed in subjects with ulcerative colitis.

In addition, ISIS-2302 is in trials for kidney transplant surgery, psoriasis and Crohn's Disease.

INDICATION(S) AND RESEARCH PHASE
Crohn's Disease – Phase III
Psoriasis and Psoriatic Disorders – Phase II
Inflammatory Bowel Disease – Phase II
Kidney Transplant Surgery – Phase II

keratinocyte growth factor-2 (KGF-2)
Repifermin

MANUFACTURER
Human Genome Sciences

DESCRIPTION
Repifermin is a genomics-derived therapeutic protein drug, also known as keratinocyte growth factor-2 (KGF-2). KGF-2 stimulates the growth of keratinocyte cells, which make up 95% of the epidermal cells. Together, keratinocyte and melanocyte cells form the epidermis of the body.

According to the company, KGF-2 has demonstrated beneficial effects on both the dermal and epidermal tissues of the skin, healing full-thickness wounds in a short period of time. In subjects with mucositis, Repifermin may stimulate the creation of new mucosal tissue.

Additionally, results of phase I clinical trials showed that systemically administered Repifermin is safe and well tolerated in healthy human subjects at doses proposed for subsequent clinical studies. None of the subjects withdrew from the study or required dose modification because of adverse effects.

Repifermin is in a phase II trial for the treatment of mucositis associated with bone marrow transplantation for the treatment of cancer. This randomized, double-blind, placebo-controlled, dose-escalation trial is being conducted at several sites in the United States. In addition, Repifermin is in a phase IIb trial for topical wound healing treatment of venous ulcers and a phase II trial for inflammatory bowel disease (IBD).

INDICATION(S) AND RESEARCH PHASE
Bone Marrow Transplant – Phase II
Effects of Chemotherapy – Phase II
Oral Medicine – Phase II
Skin Wounds – Phase IIb
Inflammatory Bowel Disease – Phase II

LDP-02
unknown

MANUFACTURER
Millennium Pharmaceuticals

DESCRIPTION
LDP-02 is an investigational humanized monoclonal antibody for the treatment of inflammatory bowel disease (IBD), which includes Crohn's disease and ulcerative colitis. LDP-02 targets a protein called alpha-4-beta-7, an integrin on inflammatory cells that causes these cells to adhere to the gastrointestinal tract.

In preclinical models, LDP-02 eliminated or reduced diarrhea, chronic inflammation, and tissue damage associated with IBD. The drug is currently in trials for ulcerative colitis and Crohn's disease. It is being developed by Millennium Pharmaceuticals in collaboration with Genentech.

INDICATION(S) AND RESEARCH PHASE
Crohn's Disease – Phase II
Inflammatory Bowel Disease – Phase II

mesalamine
Pentasa

MANUFACTURER
Shire Pharmaceuticals

DESCRIPTION
Pentasa (mesalamine) is an anti-inflammatory drug that acts on the gastrointestinal endothelium to reduce inflammation. Phase II trials have been completed with this 500 mg tablet formulation for the treatment of ulcerative colitis.

INDICATION(S) AND RESEARCH PHASE
Inflammatory Bowel Disease – Phase II completed

natalizumab
Antegren

MANUFACTURER
Elan Pharmaceutical Research

DESCRIPTION
Antegren is a humanized monoclonal antibody that belongs to a new class of potential therapeutics known as alpha-4 integrin inhibitors. It is designed to block immune cell adhesion to blood vessel walls and subsequent migration of lymphocytes into tissue. Antegren binds to the cell surface receptors known as alpha-4-beta-1 (VLA-4) and alpha-4-beta-7.

Positive results were announced from preliminary analyses of two large phase II trials of Antegren in subjects with multiple sclerosis (MS) and Crohn's disease. The first double-blind, placebo-controlled trial included 213 MS subjects and was conducted at 26 sites in the United States, Canada, and the United Kingdom. The primary endpoint of a reduction in new gadolinium enhancing lesions compared to placebo over the six-month treatment period was achieved with a high degree of statistical significance. The second trial included 240 subjects with moderate to severe Crohn's disease and was conducted at 38 sites in eight European countries. Statistically significant positive results were obtained for multiple endpoints, including induction of remission as measured by the Crohn's disease activity index.

Elan Corporation and Biogen plan to initiate phase III trials in 2001 for both MS and Crohn's disease. Additionally, Antegren is being studied in a phase II trial for inflammatory bowel disease. Biogen and Elan have announced a worldwide, exclusive collaboration to develop, manufacture and commercialize Antegren.

INDICATION(S) AND RESEARCH PHASE
Multiple Sclerosis – Phase II completed
Inflammatory Bowel Disease – Phase II
Crohn's Disease – Phase II completed

NCX 1015
unknown

MANUFACTURER
NicOx SA

DESCRIPTION
NCX 1015 is a nitric oxide-releasing derivative of prednisolone being developed for the treatment of acute episodes of inflammatory bowel disease. Currently under way, a randomized, double-blind, placebo-controlled, parallel-group, single dose escalation phase I trial is testing an enema formulation. Four single escalating dose levels will be evaluated.

INDICATION(S) AND RESEARCH PHASE
Inflammatory Bowel Disease – Phase I

radiolabeled monoclonal antibody
LeuTech

MANUFACTURER
Palatin Technologies

DESCRIPTION
LeuTech is a monoclonal antibody labeled with a radioactive isotope (technetium 99). When injected into the body, LeuTech attaches itself to neutrophils, which naturally accumulate in areas of infection or inflammation. When imaged using a standard gamma camera, the accumulated LeuTech appears as a bright spot, indicating an area of infection.

Researchers participating in a phase III clinical trial of LeuTech concluded that the drug is safe and effective in diagnosing cases of equivocal appendicitis. LeuTech also demonstrated a significant positive impact on the management of these subjects. The trial included 200 subjects at ten sites across the United States. The FDA recommended approval of LeuTech in July 2000.

In addition, LeuTech is in multiple phase II trials for other types of infection, such as osteomyelitis and ulcerative colitis.

INDICATION(S) AND RESEARCH PHASE
Gastrointestinal Diseases and Disorders, miscellaneous – FDA approval letter
Inflammatory Bowel Disease – Phase II
Osteomyelitis – Phase II

recombinant human interferon beta-1a
Rebif

MANUFACTURER
Serono Laboratories

DESCRIPTION
Rebif is an interferon beta-1a product being developed for a variety of indications. These include non-small cell lung cancer, chronic hepatitis C, Crohn's disease, ulcerative colitis, Guillain-Barré syndrome, and rheumatoid arthritis. Rebif has been approved in several countries for the treatment of relapsing-remitting multiple sclerosis. It is currently being evaluated as an early treatment of multiple sclerosis (phase III) and as a treatment for secondary progressive multiple sclerosis (filed).

INDICATION(S) AND RESEARCH PHASE
Multiple Sclerosis – Phase III
Lung Cancer – Phase II
Hepatitis – Phase II
Crohn's Disease – Phase II
Inflammatory Bowel Disease – Phase II
Guillain-Barré Syndrome – Phase II
Rheumatoid Arthritis – Phase II

rofleponide
unknown

MANUFACTURER
AstraZeneca

DESCRIPTION
Rofleponide is a topical steroid in phase I trials for the treatment of inflammatory bowel disease.

INDICATION(S) AND RESEARCH PHASE
Inflammatory Bowel Disease – Phase I

tazofelone
unknown

MANUFACTURER
Roberts Pharmaceutical

DESCRIPTION
Crohn's disease and ulcerative colitis are both inflammatory bowel diseases. In both, it is thought that the body essentially reacts against its own colon tissue. This reaction can result in recurrent abdominal pain, fever, nausea, vomiting, weight loss, bloody and non-bloody diarrhea, and in severe cases, intestinal perforation.

The inflammatory process actually consists of many small molecules signaling cytokines to abnormally attack tissue that the body now considers foreign. Tazofelone, formulated at Roberts Pharmaceutical, acts against one of these inflammatory signal molecules known as cyclo-oxygenase. Tazofelone combines with the cyclo-oxygenase molecule and disables it, preventing it from activating other molecules responsible for the inflammation process. By blocking this particular route that the body uses to promote the cascade of inflammation, tazofelone may decrease the symptoms and tissue destruction typical of Crohn's disease and ulcerative colitis.

INDICATION(S) AND RESEARCH PHASE
Crohn's Disease – Phase II
Inflammatory Bowel Disease – Phase II

unknown
Balsalazide

MANUFACTURER
Shire Pharmaceuticals

DESCRIPTION
Balsalazide is a prodrug of 5-ASA (mesalamine, mesalazine) being developed for the treatment of ulcerative colitis in certain European markets. Available data on the drug are being evaluated to determine if additional testing is necessary prior to submitting an application for marketing approval. According to the company, the drug can be considered post-phase II.

INDICATION(S) AND RESEARCH PHASE
Inflammatory Bowel Disease – Phase II completed

Irritable Bowel Syndrome (IBS)

cilansetron
unknown

MANUFACTURER
Solvay Pharmaceuticals

DESCRIPTION
Cilansetron is an orally formulated medication that blocks the action of 5-hydroxy-tryptamine 3 ($5HT_3$) receptors. The drug was developed for the treatment of symptoms associated with irritable bowel syndrome. It is designed to potentiate the effects of other drugs used for this condition, such as duspatalin and dicetel. Solvay Pharmaceuticals has temporarily suspended phase III trials.

INDICATION(S) AND RESEARCH PHASE
Irritable Bowel Syndrome (IBS) – Phase III on hold

NK-2 antagonist
Saredutant

MANUFACTURER
Sanofi-Synthelabo Pharmaceuticals

DESCRIPTION
Saredutant is a new medication that may be useful in the treatment of irritable bowel syndrome. It is currently in phase II clinical trials and will be administered in an oral formulation.

Several substances found in the body may make the intestines more motile and hyperactive than normal, resulting in cramping and diarrhea. One of these potentially causative substances is neurokinin A, which overstimulates muscle by activating the NK_2 receptor. Saredutant blocks NK_2 receptors and prevents them from being stimulated. By reducing the effect of neurokinin A on intestinal tissue, hypermotility of the bowel may be decreased with this medication. Further studies are under way to determine the efficacy of Saredutant.

INDICATION(S) AND RESEARCH PHASE
Irritable Bowel Syndrome (IBS) – Phase II

TAK-637
unknown

MANUFACTURER
Takeda Chemical Industries

DESCRIPTION
TAK-637 is an NK_1 receptor antagonist being developed for the treatment of various indications. It is currently in phase I trials in Japan for urinary incontinence. Additionally, TAK-637 is in phase II trials in Europe and the United States for urinary incontinence, depression, and irritable bowel syndrome.

INDICATION(S) AND RESEARCH PHASE
Urinary Incontinence – Phase I
Urinary Incontinence – Phase II
Depression – Phase II
Irritable Bowel Syndrome (IBS) – Phase II

tegaserod
Zelmac

MANUFACTURER
Novartis

DESCRIPTION
Zelmac selectively targets and acts on $5HT_4$ receptors present throughout the gastrointestinal tract. It is being developed for the treatment of functional dyspepsia (phase II), gastroesophageal reflux disease (phase II), and chronic constipation (phase III). An NDA has been submitted for the indication of irritable bowel syndrome.

INDICATION(S) AND RESEARCH PHASE
Irritable Bowel Syndrome (IBS) – NDA submitted
Gastrointestinal Diseases and Disorders, miscellaneous – Phase II
Gastroesophageal Reflux Disease (GERD) – Phase II
Constipation – Phase III

unknown
Dexloxiglumide

MANUFACTURER
Forest Laboratories

DESCRIPTION
Dexloxiglumide is a selective cholecystokinin type A (CCKA) receptor antagonist. CCKA antagonists target receptors in the gastrointestinal system to increase gastric emptying, increase intestinal motility, and modulate intestinal sensitivity to distension. Forest Laboratories has entered into an agreement with Rotta Research Laboratorium S.p.A. of Monza, Italy, for the development and marketing of dexloxiglumide in the United States. The drug is being developed for the treatment of irritable bowel syndrome and is scheduled to begin phase III trials in 2001.

INDICATION(S) AND RESEARCH PHASE
Irritable Bowel Syndrome (IBS) – Phase II completed

Liver Disease

human liver cells
unknown

MANUFACTURER
Diacrin

DESCRIPTION
Human liver cells can be injected into the spleen or into a liver diseased and damaged by cirrhosis. If these healthy cells survive after the transplantation, they can maintain healthy liver function and drastically reduce the effects of the disease. A phase I study is testing whether or not this transplantation therapy can significantly increase the quality of life of subjects waiting for a liver transplant or eliminate the need for transplantation altogether.

INDICATION(S) AND RESEARCH PHASE
Liver Disease – Phase I
Liver Transplant Surgery – Phase I

interleukin-10 (IL-10)
Tenovil

MANUFACTURER
Schering-Plough Corporation

DESCRIPTION
Tenovil is an immunomodulator being developed in an injectable formulation. It is currently being evaluated for the treatment of ischemia reperfusion injury, hepatic fibrosis, and hepatitis C.

INDICATION(S) AND RESEARCH PHASE
Liver Disease – Phase II
Hepatitis – Phase I
Ischemia Reperfusion Injury – Phase I

IP501
unknown

MANUFACTURER
Interneuron Pharmaceuticals

DESCRIPTION
IP501 is a purified phospholipid that helps to repair damaged cells. It is being developed for the treatment and prevention of alcohol-induced cirrhosis of the liver and hepatitis C. The drug is manufactured in a tablet formulation.

INDICATION(S) AND RESEARCH PHASE
Alcohol Dependence – Phase III
Hepatitis – Phase III
Liver Disease – Phase III

r-FVIIa
NovoSeven

MANUFACTURER
Novo Nordisk

DESCRIPTION

The coagulant NovoSeven is a recombinant Factor VIIa developed for the treatment of hemophilia in subjects with inhibitors to Factor VIIa. This recombinant protein induces hemostasis at the site of injury independent of the presence of Factor VIII or Factor IX by forming complexes with exposed tissue factor (TF). In the United States, NovoSeven has been approved for the treatment of bleeding episodes in hemophilia A or B subjects with inhibitors to Factor VIII or Factor IX.

NovoSeven is also in phase III trials for the prevention and treatment of bleeding episodes in subjects with coagulopathy associated with liver disease.

INDICATION(S) AND RESEARCH PHASE

Hemophilia – FDA approved
Liver Disease – Phase III

Liver Transplant Surgery

human liver cells
unknown

MANUFACTURER
Diacrin

DESCRIPTION

Human liver cells can be injected into the spleen, or into a liver diseased and damaged by cirrhosis. If these healthy cells survive after the transplantation, they can maintain healthy liver function and drastically reduce the effects of the disease. A phase I study is testing whether or not this transplantation therapy can significantly increase the quality of life of subjects waiting for a liver transplant or eliminate the need for transplantation altogether.

INDICATION(S) AND RESEARCH PHASE

Liver Disease – Phase I
Liver Transplant Surgery – Phase I

Pancreatic Cancer

CEP-701
unknown

MANUFACTURER
Cephalon

DESCRIPTION

CEP-701 is an orally active inhibitor of the enzyme tyrosine kinase. It works as a signal transduction modulator for the treatment of various cancers. CEP-701 is being evaluated in phase II studies for prostate cancer and pancreatic ductal adenocarcinoma.

INDICATION(S) AND RESEARCH PHASE

Pancreatic Cancer – Phase II
Prostate Cancer – Phase II

CI-1042, ONYX-015
unknown

MANUFACTURER
Onyx Pharmaceuticals

DESCRIPTION

CI-1042 (ONYX-015) is a tumor-selective, modified adenovirus (similar to the common cold virus) that has been genetically engineered to replicate in and kill cancer cells that possess a mutated oncogene called p53, while sparing normal cells with functioning p53. p53 Is a tumor suppressor gene that is mutated in approximately 50% of all human cancers.

CI-1042 is in development for several indications, including pancreatic cancer, liver metastases of colorectal cancer, and lung cancer. Results of a phase II trial demonstrated that CI-1042 administered as a single-agent replicates and causes tumor regression in refractory head and neck cancer. CI-1042 was shown to selectively target cancer cells containing a mutant p53 gene, while sparing normal cells with a functioning p53 gene. Of the 19 subjects who received the standard dosing regimen, four (21%) had an objective response, including two complete responses and two partial responses. CI-1042 is being co-developed with Pfizer.

INDICATION(S) AND RESEARCH PHASE

Colorectal Cancer – Phase II
Pancreatic Cancer – Phase II
Head and Neck Cancer – Phase III
Cervical Dysplasia/Cancer – Phase I completed
Lung Cancer – Phase II
Bladder Cancer – Phase I completed
Brain Cancer – Phase I completed

CTP-37
Avicine

MANUFACTURER
AVI BioPharma

DESCRIPTION

Avicine is a hormone vaccine derived from human chorionic gonadotropin peptide that is being tested for the prevention of colorectal, pancreatic, and prostate cancer. The drug is in phase II trials for prostate cancer, and phase III trials for colorectal and pancreatic cancer. The pharmaceutical company SuperGen will be responsible for U.S. marketing and sales of Avicine, while AVI BioPharma will be responsible for product manufacturing.

INDICATION(S) AND RESEARCH PHASE

Colorectal Cancer – Phase III
Pancreatic Cancer – Phase III
Prostate Cancer – Phase II

diethylnorspermine
DENSPM

MANUFACTURER
GelTex Pharmaceuticals

DESCRIPTION

DENSPM (diethylnorspermine) is similar to a naturally produced polyamine, except that it may interrupt the rapid growth of tumor cells that need polyamines for growth. The drug is in phase II trials for renal cell carcinoma, pancreatic cancer, malignant melanoma, and non-small cell lung cancer. Additional indications may include ovarian and colon cancers.

INDICATION(S) AND RESEARCH PHASE

Renal Cell Carcinoma – Phase II
Pancreatic Cancer – Phase II
Malignant Melanoma – Phase II

Lung Cancer – Phase II

GBC-590
unknown

MANUFACTURER
Safe Sciences

DESCRIPTION
GBC-590 belongs to a new class of drugs called lectin inhibitors that specifically interfere with cellular interactions. GBC-590 competitively binds to unique lectins on cancer cells and disrupts the metastatic process. GBC-590's affinity for cancer lectins is the core reason for its significant biological activity and specificity.

GBC-590 is being tested in phase II trials for pancreatic and colorectal cancer, and the company plans to test the drug in phase II trials for prostate cancer.

INDICATION(S) AND RESEARCH PHASE
Colorectal Cancer – Phase II
Pancreatic Cancer – Phase II
Prostate Cancer – Phase I/II

gemcitabine HCl
Gemzar

MANUFACTURER
Eli Lilly

DESCRIPTION
Gemzar is under review as a combination therapy for use with cisplatin for the treatment of locally advanced or metastatic transitional cell carcinoma (advanced bladder cancer). The drug is a nucleoside analogue. It is a novel chemotherapeutic agent that mimics a natural building block of DNA. Gemzar disrupts the process of cell replication and thereby slows or stops progression of the disease. The drug is administered intravenously.

Gemzar is also indicated as first-line treatment of locally advanced or metastatic pancreatic cancer and, in combination with cisplatin, for locally advanced or metastatic non-small cell lung cancer.

Additionally, Gemzar is in trials for the treatment of breast, ovarian, and pancreatic cancers.

INDICATION(S) AND RESEARCH PHASE
Breast Cancer – Phase III
Bladder Cancer – Phase III
Lung Cancer – FDA approved
Ovarian Cancer – Phase III
Pancreatic Cancer – Phase II completed

HSPPC-96
Oncophage

MANUFACTURER
Antigenics

DESCRIPTION
Oncophage cancer vaccine is an injectable protein that contains the unique profile ("antigenic fingerprint") of each subject's cancer. The antigens activate the immune system to elicit an anti-tumor response.

In October 2000, Antigenics announced that it had initiated a phase II trial of Oncophage in subjects who have been diagnosed with sarcoma, also known as soft tissue cancer. The study is expected to initially enroll 20 subjects diagnosed with recurrent metastatic or unresectable soft tissue sarcoma and may be expanded to include an additional 15 subjects depending on preliminary results.

INDICATION(S) AND RESEARCH PHASE
Renal Cell Carcinoma – Phase III
Malignant Melanoma – Phase II
Colorectal Cancer – Phase II
Gastric Cancer – Phase I/II
Pancreatic Cancer – Phase I/II completed
Lymphoma, Non-Hodgkin's – Phase II
Sarcoma – Phase II

HuC242-DM1/SB-408075
unknown

MANUFACTURER
ImmunoGen

DESCRIPTION
HuC242-DM1/SB-408075 is a tumor-activated prodrug (TAP) designed for the treatment of colorectal, pancreatic, and certain non-small cell lung cancers. Tumor-activated prodrugs consist of chemically linked monoclonal antibodies and potent, cell-killing chemicals. HuC242-DM1, in particular, is created by joining the cytotoxic maytansinoid drug DM1 with the humanized monoclonal antibody C242. The attached chemical remains inactive until the monoclonal antibody reaches its targeted tumor cell and the TAP is drawn inside. Once inside, DM1 is able to kill the tumor cell without affecting surrounding healthy cells. HuC242-DM1 is currently in phase I/II trials.

INDICATION(S) AND RESEARCH PHASE
Colorectal Cancer – Phase I/II
Pancreatic Cancer – Phase I/II
Lung Cancer – Phase I/II

IMC-C225, CPT-11
unknown

MANUFACTURER
ImClone Systems

DESCRIPTION
IMC-C225 is a chimerized (part mouse, part human) monoclonal antibody that may help fight cancer cells when used in conjunction with radiation therapy or other chemotherapy agents. This antibody selectively blocks the epidermal growth factor receptor (EGFr), which may be present in greater amounts on actively growing tumor cells. Since many cancers use specific growth factors to stimulate tumor cell growth, blocking this receptor may inhibit the cancer from increasing in size and spreading throughout the body.

The company is conducting phase III clinical trials evaluating IMC-C225 in combination with radiotherapy and with chemotherapy in subjects with advanced squamous cell head and neck carcinoma. IMC-C225 is in trials for several other indications in combination with various anti-cancer agents.

INDICATION(S) AND RESEARCH PHASE
Breast Cancer – Phase I/II
Head and Neck Cancer – Phase III
Lung Cancer – Phase III
Prostate Cancer – Phase I/II

Renal Cell Carcinoma – Phase II
Pancreatic Cancer – Phase II
Colorectal Cancer – Phase II

IMMU-MN14, anti-CEA
CEA-Cide

MANUFACTURER
Immunomedics

DESCRIPTION
Carcinoembryonic antigen (CEA) is a protein-polysaccharide complex released in the bloodstream by certain cancers, especially colon carcinoma. This antigenic substance may provide early diagnosis when used as a therapeutic marker in immunologic tests. The CEA complex may also be targeted by specialized monoclonal antibodies in the design of a biologic therapeutic.

CEA-Cide is a novel monoclonal antibody that is designed for radioimmunotherapy (with 90 Y-labeled humanized MN-14). This drug is being tested in phase II trials for the treatment of subjects with advanced metastatic, CEA-producing cancers.

INDICATION(S) AND RESEARCH PHASE
Breast Cancer – Phase II
Cancer/Tumors (Unspecified) – Phase II
Colorectal Cancer – Phase II
Lung Cancer – Phase II
Ovarian Cancer – Phase II
Pancreatic Cancer – Phase II

ISIS-2503
unknown

MANUFACTURER
Isis Pharmaceuticals

DESCRIPTION
ISIS-2503 is a potent, selective antisense inhibitor of H-Ras gene expression. Antisense drugs are designed to target particular genes and selectively block them. These drugs provide an exact complementary sequence to a unique part of the target gene, so that the drug will bind to and affect only that gene.

H-Ras is one of a family of ras genes that are involved in the process by which cells receive and send signals that affect their behavior. According to the company, evidence supports a direct role for ras gene products in the development and maintenance of human cancers.

In phase II trials, the compound is being evaluated as a single-agent in subjects with colon, breast, pancreatic, and non-small cell lung cancers. These trials will provide preliminary data on the anti-tumor activity of ISIS 2503 against these common tumor types. Approximately ten sites in the United States and Europe will enroll 15–30 subjects per tumor type. The company may initiate future trials of ISIS 2503 in combination with approved cancer therapies.

INDICATION(S) AND RESEARCH PHASE
Breast Cancer – Phase II
Colon Malignancies – Phase II
Lung Cancer – Phase II
Pancreatic Cancer – Phase II

ISIS-5132, CGP-69846A
unknown

MANUFACTURER
Isis Pharmaceuticals

DESCRIPTION
ISIS-5132 is a potent antisense inhibitor of the enzyme c-Raf-1 kinase. Antisense drugs are designed to target particular genes and selectively block them. These drugs provide an exact complementary sequence to a unique part of the target gene, so that the drug will bind to and affect only that gene.

c-Raf kinase plays a role in signal processes that regulate cell growth and proliferation. It is one of a family of Raf genes thought to play an important role in the development of various solid tumors. The company reported that activated Raf has also been detected in a substantial variety of cancers including small cell lung carcinoma and breast cancer. It has been reported that 60% of all lung carcinoma cells express unusually high levels of normal c-Raf mRNA and protein.

The sponsor companies reported that results from phase I studies, which examined subjects with a wide variety of solid tumors, demonstrated that the drug was well tolerated and that several subjects experienced disease stabilization. The companies are planning additional phase I safety studies involving the drug in combination with currently approved chemotherapies. Phase II clinical trials examining ISIS-5132 as a single agent therapy in subjects with breast, lung, colon, pancreatic, and prostate cancers are under way.

INDICATION(S) AND RESEARCH PHASE
Breast Cancer – Phase II
Cancer/Tumors (Unspecified) – Phase II
Colon Malignancies – Phase II
Lung Cancer – Phase II
Pancreatic Cancer – Phase II
Prostate Cancer – Phase II

marimastat, BB-2516
unknown

MANUFACTURER
British Biotech plc

DESCRIPTION
Marimastat is an anti-angiogenic inhibitor of matrix metalloproteinase (MMP), a family of naturally occurring enzymes that are over-produced in a number of diseases. This is especially true of cancer, where MMPs are involved in the spread and local growth of tumors.

Anti-angiogenic strategies, unlike other therapeutic approaches, do not aim to directly destroy or "kill" the tumor or cause tumor regression. Rather, they are designed to prevent the further growth of tumors by limiting their blood supply. Because peripheral tumor cells could theoretically survive on a diffusion-dependent basis, anti-angiogenic drugs may prove most effective when given in combination with other standard cytotoxic regimens.

Marimastat is in phase III development for the treatment of cancer. In 1999, British Biotech and Schering-Plough Corporation signed an agreement to develop and commercialize British Biotech's metalloproteinase inhibitors, including marimastat.

INDICATION(S) AND RESEARCH PHASE
Pancreatic Cancer – Phase III
Lung Cancer – Phase III

Breast Cancer – Phase III
Brain Cancer – Phase III completed
Ovarian Cancer – Phase III

MDX-210
unknown

MANUFACTURER
Medarex

DESCRIPTION
MDX-210 is a bispecific (target-trigger) monoclonal antibody-based treatment being developed for cancers with specific markers (HER-2/*neu* positive), including renal cell, non-small cell lung, pancreatic and kidney cancers. Phase II trials have been completed for kidney, prostate, and ovarian cancer. Phase III development for ovarian cancer has commenced in Europe.

INDICATION(S) AND RESEARCH PHASE
Prostate Cancer – Phase II completed
Renal Cell Carcinoma – Phase II completed
Colon Malignancies – Phase II
Breast Cancer – Phase II
Gastric Cancer – Phase II
Pancreatic Cancer – Phase II
Lung Cancer – Phase II
Ovarian Cancer – Phase III

MDX-220
unknown

MANUFACTURER
Medarex

DESCRIPTION
MDX-220 is a bispecific (target-trigger) monoclonal antibody that targets Tag-72. It is being developed for the treatment of a variety of cancers, including lung, colon, prostate, ovarian, endometrial, pancreatic, and gastric cancer.
Endometrial Cancer – Phase I/II
Gastric Cancer – Phase I/II
Lung Cancer – Phase I/II
Ovarian Cancer – Phase I/II
Pancreatic Cancer – Phase I/II
Prostate Cancer – Phase II
Colorectal Cancer – Phase II

MGI-114, hydroxymethylacylfulvene, HMAF
Irofulven

MANUFACTURER
MGI Pharma

DESCRIPTION
Irofulven (MGI-114) is the first product candidate being developed by MGI Pharma from its family of anti-cancer compounds called acylfulvenes. Early trials demonstrated that Irofulven is absorbed rapidly by tumor cells, and once inside binds to DNA and protein targets. The binding interferes with DNA replication and cell division, leading to tumor-specific cell death.

Results from a phase II trial of Irofulven indicated that the drug produced anti-tumor activity in subjects with advanced pancreatic cancer who were refractory to gemcitabine (Gemzar). Ten of the 53 subjects enrolled achieved six-month survival and two subjects demonstrated objective responses: one subject experienced tumor shrinkage of 100% and another subject experienced an 84% decrease in tumor mass. A phase III trial was initiated in February 2001.

INDICATION(S) AND RESEARCH PHASE
Breast Cancer – Phase II
Colon Malignancies – Phase II
Renal Cell Carcinoma – Phase II
Cervical Dysplasia/Cancer – Phase II
Lung Cancer – Phase II
Ovarian Cancer – Phase I/II
Colorectal Cancer – Phase II
Prostate Cancer – Phase I/II
Cancer/Tumors (Unspecified) – Phase I/II
Pancreatic Cancer – Phase III
Liver Cancer – Phase II

RFS-2000
Rubitecan

MANUFACTURER
SuperGen

DESCRIPTION
Rubitecan is a novel drug that inhibits an enzyme called topoisomerase I. The drug is made in an oral formulation, which may prove to be an advantage for outpatient treatment in comparison to intravenous type drugs that require a visit to a hospital setting.

Rubitecan is being tested as a potential treatment for a variety of solid tumors, as well as for metastatic melanoma, advanced pancreatic cancer, and advanced gastric carcinoma. Additionally, phase II trials in the United States and Europe are testing Rubitecan for blood cancers such as chronic myelomonocytic leukemia (CMML).

SuperGen has announced positive preliminary results from an ongoing study on the efficacy of rubitecan in CMML, chronic myeloid leukemia (CML), and myelodysplastic syndrome (MDS). Of the 54 subjects treated, 43% experienced a complete response, partial response, or hematologic improvement.

INDICATION(S) AND RESEARCH PHASE
Pancreatic Cancer – Phase III
Breast Cancer – Phase II
Colorectal Cancer – Phase II
Gastric Cancer – Phase II
Leukemia – Phase II
Malignant Melanoma – Phase II
Ovarian Cancer – Phase II
Myelodysplastic Syndrome – Phase III

SR-27897B
unknown

MANUFACTURER
Sanofi-Synthelabo Pharmaceuticals

DESCRIPTION
CCKa (cholecystokinin a) is a molecule that is present in the central nervous system and also secreted from the lining of the small intestine. It causes many different actions throughout the body, including gallbladder contraction, release of pancreatic digestive enzymes, and promotion of the feeling of digestive fullness. CCK also promotes cell growth and division, especially in the pancreas, and it has a regulating effect on the amount of dopamine and serotonin present in the body.

SR-27897 is a potent substance that blocks the receptors to which CCK would ordinarily bind, thus blocking CCK's effects on the body. By negating the action of CCK, people may lose their sense of satiety, making SR-27897 a potential therapy for anorexia. In addition, CCK's probable role in the pathogenesis of pancreatic cancer (because it can cause abnormal pancreatic cell division) may also be reduced with the use of SR-27897.

INDICATION(S) AND RESEARCH PHASE
Pancreatic Cancer – Phase II
Anorexia – Phase II

troxacitabine, BCH-4556
Troxatyl

MANUFACTURER
BioChem Pharma

DESCRIPTION
Troxatyl is a dioxolane nucleoside analog being investigated as an anticancer agent. The drug is a complete DNA chain terminator and DNA polymerase inhibitor. It acts by incorporating itself into the growing DNA chain of cancer cells, interfering with their ability to replicate further.

Troxatyl is being evaluated as a single agent or in combination therapy in a number of ongoing trials for hematologic malignancies, including acute myeloid leukemia and chronic myeloid leukemia (blastic phase), and in lymphoproliferative disorders such as lymphoma, chronic lymphocytic leukemia, and myeloma. It is also being evaluated as a single agent in pancreatic cancer and in combination therapy in a number of solid tumors. Troxatyl is currently in phase II development.

INDICATION(S) AND RESEARCH PHASE
Cancer/Tumors (Unspecified) – Phase II
Colorectal Cancer – Phase II
Head and Neck Cancer – Phase II
Leukemia – Phase II
Lung Cancer – Phase II
Malignant Melanoma – Phase II
Ovarian Cancer – Phase II
Pancreatic Cancer – Phase II
Prostate Cancer – Phase II
Renal Cell Carcinoma – Phase II

vaccine, anti-gastrin
Gastrimmune

MANUFACTURER
Aphton Corporation

DESCRIPTION
Gastrimmune is a therapeutic vaccine that neutralizes specific hormones (G17 & Gly-extended G17). The drug is in phase III trials for the treatment of cancers of the gastrointestinal tract, including gastric cancer and colorectal cancer. It is also in trials for liver cancer, esophageal cancer and two phase III trials in subjects with advanced pancreatic cancer—one in the United States and one in Europe.

INDICATION(S) AND RESEARCH PHASE
Colorectal Cancer – Phase III
Esophageal Cancer – Phase III
Gastric Cancer – Phase III
Liver Cancer – Phase II/III
Pancreatic Cancer – Phase III

vaccine, cancer
Gvax

MANUFACTURER
Cell Genesys

DESCRIPTION
Gvax is an allogeneic compound that involves the genetic modification of prostate cancer cell lines. These cancer cells have been irradiated and modified to secrete granulocyte-macrophage colony stimulating factor (GM-CSF), a hormone which plays a key role in stimulating the body's immune response to vaccines.

The Gvax prostate cancer vaccine demonstrated anti-tumor activity in an initial phase II trial in subjects with advanced metastatic prostate cancer who have not responded to hormone therapy. Prior to initiating a phase III trial, Cell Genesys plans to initiate further trials of Gvax prostate cancer vaccine in 2001 that will employ a higher potency version of the same product. In addition, future phase III trials in hormone refractory prostate cancer subjects may compare Gvax vaccine in combination with chemotherapy to chemotherapy alone.

INDICATION(S) AND RESEARCH PHASE
Prostate Cancer – Phase II
Lung Cancer – Phase I/II completed
Malignant Melanoma – Phase I/II
Vaccines – Phase I/II
Pancreatic Cancer – Phase II
Leukemia – Phase I/II

virulizin
unknown

MANUFACTURER
Lorus Therapeutics

DESCRIPTION
Virulizin, which is isolated from bovine bile, is a potent activator of monocytes and macrophages. The compound has demonstrated significant antitumor activity against several tumor types including pancreatic cancer, melanoma, and AIDS related lymphoma.

In a phase I/II study, 26 patients with advanced pancreatic cancer who previously failed standard therapies were enrolled. A total of 19 evaluable patients were treated with different doses of Virulizin (1.5, 3.0, 6.0 ml, 3 times per week and 3.0 ml, 5 times per week) for at least 4 weeks. The maximum dose level was well-tolerated. Seven patients (37%) achieved stable disease and one patient in the last cohort achieved a complete response. The patients treated with Virulizin had a median survival of 6.7 months with a 6-month survival rate of 58% and showed a significant improvement in quality of life. The company initiated phase III trials for pancreatic cancer in early 2001.

INDICATION(S) AND RESEARCH PHASE
Pancreatic cancer – Phase III

Pancreatic Disorders

pancrelipase
Viokase

MANUFACTURER
Axcan Pharma

DESCRIPTION
Viokase is a pancreatic enzyme preparation containing standardized lipase, protease, and amylase in fixed proportions. It is indicated for the treatment of subjects with exocrine pancreatic enzyme deficiency, which is often associated with cystic fibrosis, chronic pancreatitis, and post-pancreatectomy. It has been prescribed for years to assist the digestion and absorption of food. Axcan is currently conducting phase II trials of Viokase at elevated dosages (8,000 units/day) to alleviate pain often associated with pancreatic disorders.

INDICATION(S) AND RESEARCH PHASE
Pain, Acute or Chronic – Phase II
Pancreatic Disorders – Phase II

Ulcers

ibuprofen
Elangesic

MANUFACTURER
Elan Pharmaceutical Research

DESCRIPTION
Non-steroidal anti-inflammatory drugs (NSAIDs), such as ibuprofen, are very effective agents for the relief of pain and inflammation. But many individuals cannot use these drugs due to adverse effects, such as irritation of the lining of the stomach. NSAIDs may cause gastritis and ulcers, or exacerbate these conditions when already present.

Elan Pharmaceuticals has developed a new product called Elangesic that may potentially increase the tolerability of NSAIDs. Elangesic works by formulating drugs into high density, controlled-release beads. Each bead contains a core of the desired drug, and an outer coating which discharges the drug in a time-release fashion. Clinical testing is in phase II trials using this once- and twice-daily intestinal protective drug absorption system (IPDAS).

INDICATION(S) AND RESEARCH PHASE
Gastroenteritis – Phase II
Inflammatory Bowel Disease – Phase II
Ulcers – Phase II

nisin
Ambicin

MANUFACTURER
AstraZeneca

DESCRIPTION
Ambicin is an anti-microbial peptide administered as a dietary supplement to help maintain or restore a healthy microbial balance in the intestine and colon. The company is deciding whether or not they will conduct further studies with Ambicin.

INDICATION(S) AND RESEARCH PHASE
Ulcers – Phase I/II

10 | Urology

Population with illnesses in this category	37 million[1]
Drugs in the development pipeline	87[2]
Number of drugs in preclinical testing	31
Number of drugs in clinical testing	51

Source: 1. World Health Organization, worldwide figures 2. Parexel

According to the National Kidney Foundation, kidney and urologic diseases affect approximately 20 million Americans. This therapeutic area covers diseases associated with the urinary tract and reproductive organs, including renal cell carcinoma, prostate cancer, benign prostatic hyperplasia (BPH), impotence, end-stage renal disease, and urinary incontinence, among other indications.

Kidney cancer and its most common form, renal cell carcinoma, are a major target of research and clinical drug development. The National Cancer Institute has reported that carcinoma of the kidney affects approximately 27,000 Americans each year. CenterWatch estimates there are between 20 and 25 drugs in development for the treatment of renal cell carcinoma, costing approximately $100 million to $120 million per year in investigator grants.

Surgery is the initial and primary treatment approach for patients diagnosed with kidney cancer. Surgical options include a radical or partial nephrectomy, depending on the extent of the tumor, as well as laparoscopic techniques designed to remove the malignancy. While radiation therapy is another possible treatment option, kidney cancer has unfortunately proven highly resistant to chemotherapy. However, unlike other solid tumors, kidney cancer appears to be susceptible to immunotherapy. As a result, cytokines, such as interleukin-2 and interferon-alpha have been of value to some patients, although they are not an effective therapy for all individuals.

Because immune-mediated anticancer effects have been observed against cancers such as leukemia and lymphoma following conventional allogeneic stem cell transplantation, some researchers have investigated whether similar anticancer effects can be produced in patients with treatment resistant kidney cancer. Researchers at the National Institutes of Health have reported positive results from transplants utilizing blood stem cells from healthy sibling donors. Patients are given immunosuppressive drugs to allow for the transplanted donor cells to repopulate the bone marrow and grow. The differentiated transplanted cells can then attack the tumor cells and hopefully lead to tumor regression. Although substantial regression was observed in initial studies, this stem cell transplant therapy was shown to result in severe complications such as graft vs. host disease and bacterial infections.

Other treatments in development for kidney cancer include antiangiogenic compounds, gene therapies, and vaccines. A vaccine consisting of fused dendritic and cancer cells is being evaluated. The hypothesis is these chimeric cells will result in immune system activation to cancer cell antigens and the resultant immune response will help to eradicate the patient's tumor cells. Antiangiogenic compounds such Aeterna's Neovastat are in late-stage phase III development.

More than 13 million Americans experience incontinence, according to the National Kidney and Urologic Diseases Information Clearinghouse. Women represent a large portion of this population, with approximately 11 million suffering from the disease. The World Health Organization has reported that urinary incontinence costs may surpass approximately $16 billion per year. CenterWatch has identified approximately 12 to 16 drugs in the pipeline for urinary incontinence at an annual cost of $70 million to $80 million.

Urinary incontinence can be generally defined as the involuntary leakage of urine. Major types include stress incontinence, where leakage occurs as a result of a sneeze, laugh, cough or other pressure-producing event, and urge incontinence, where the individual experiences a strong urge to urinate but is unable to maintain control until a facility can be reached. A third type, overflow incontinence, occurs when the bladder is continually full, leading to frequent, small volume leakage of urine. This type of incontinence is most common in men suffering from benign prostatic hypertrophy (BPH). Current treatment varies significantly depending on the type of incontinence and the individual patient, and can involve surgery, devices, pelvic muscle exercises, and collagen injections, as well as estrogen replacement therapy for post-menopausal women.

Pharmaceutical companies are showing an increased interest in the field of urinary incontinence, and many are searching for drug options that will provide efficacy without the side effects associated with current therapies. The major drugs used in the treatment of urinary incontinence include oxybutynin chloride and tolterodine tartrate. Unfortunately, these drugs cause dry mouth, which often discourages patients from continuing with treatment.

Alza has developed an extended-release form of oxybutynin chloride (Ditropan XL) that reportedly reduces this side effect. Ditropan XL was involved in a head-to-head phase IV trial known as OBJECT, designed to compare the two leading medications for the treatment of urinary incontinence: Ditropan XL(oxybutynin chloride) and Pharmacia's Detrol (tolterodine tartrate). Results from this study indicated that Ditropan XL might be the more effective treatment, while significantly reducing the incidence of severe dry mouth.
However, Pharmacia recently obtained marketing approval for a daily extended-release formulation of Detrol, called Detrol LA, which may offer similar results. There are also several drugs in the pipeline that may provide benefit to patients, including a single-isomer version of Ditropan, the selective muscarinic antagonist darifenacin, and a transdermal delivery system for oxybutynin.

Benign Prostatic Hyperplasia

alfuzosin
Xatral

MANUFACTURER
Sanofi-Synthelabo Pharmaceuticals

DESCRIPTION
Xatral is a new medication being developed in phase III trials to treat benign prostatic hypertrophy (BPH).

Treatments for BPH include surgical removal of part of the enlarged prostate gland, drugs that lower the active hormone (DHT) that is causing excessive prostate growth, and alpha receptor blockers which prevent abnormal prostate muscular contraction. By relaxing prostate tissue, alpha receptor blockers open up urine passageways. Alpha receptors are located throughout the body, and have many actions, including cardiac and respiratory effects. Because of their widespread activity, current alpha blocker medications can produce serious cardiac and respiratory side effects. Xatral works on blocking a specific type of alpha receptor that is primarily located in the urinary tract and prostate gland, allowing the drug to act only where it is needed. This specificity of action may lead to fewer side effects than seen with drugs that block alpha receptors throughout the body.

INDICATION(S) AND RESEARCH PHASE
Benign Prostatic Hyperplasia – NDA submitted

GI 198745
unknown

MANUFACTURER
GlaxoSmithKline

DESCRIPTION
GI 198745 is a dual inhibitor of 5-alpha-reductase type 1 and 2 isozymes. GlaxoSmithKline has developed the drug for the treatment of benign prostatic hyperplasia (BPH). An NDA was submitted in December 2000. Additionally, GI 198745 is in phase II trials for the treatment of alopecia.

INDICATION(S) AND RESEARCH PHASE
Alopecia – Phase II
Benign Prostatic Hyperplasia – NDA submitted

S-doxazosin
unknown

MANUFACTURER
Sepracor

DESCRIPTION
S-doxazosin is the single-isomer version of Cardura, developed and marketed by Pfizer. S-doxazosin has the potential to significantly reduce orthostatic hypotension with a greater potency than Cardura. This drug could reduce the cost of treatment by reducing the number of doctor visits required for dosage titration. S-doxazosin is currently in phase I study for benign prostatic hyperplasia (BPH).

INDICATION(S) AND RESEARCH PHASE
Benign Prostatic Hyperplasia – Phase I

Bladder Cancer

arsenic trioxide (ATO)
Trisenox

MANUFACTURER
Cell Therapeutics

DESCRIPTION
Trisenox is believed to kill cancer cells through apoptosis, or programmed cell death. The mechanism of action of Trisenox is not fully understood, but the drug appears to induce apoptosis in a different manner than other anti-cancer agents such as retinoids.

Trisenox is FDA approved to treat acute promyelocytic leukemia (APL), and it is also in numerous trials in the United States for indications including other types of leukemia, prostate cancer, multiple myeloma, renal cell cancer, cervical cancer, and bladder cancer.

INDICATION(S) AND RESEARCH PHASE
Leukemia – Phase I
Lymphoma, Non-Hodgkin's – Phase II
Leukemia – Phase II
Multiple Myeloma – Phase II
Prostate Cancer – Phase II
Renal Cell Carcinoma – Phase II
Cervical Dysplasia/Cancer – Phase II
Bladder Cancer – Phase II

CI-1042, ONYX-015
unknown

MANUFACTURER
Onyx Pharmaceuticals

DESCRIPTION
CI-1042 (ONYX-015) is a tumor-selective, modified adenovirus (similar to the common cold virus) that has been genetically engineered to replicate in and kill cancer cells that possess a mutated oncogene called p53, while sparing normal cells with functioning p53. p53 Is a tumor suppressor gene that is mutated in approximately 50% of all human cancers. CI-1042 is in development for several indications, including pancreatic cancer, liver metastases of colorectal cancer, and lung cancer.

In November 2000, results of a phase II trial demonstrated that CI-1042 administered as a single agent replicates and causes tumor regression in refractory head and neck cancer. CI-1042 was shown to selectively target cancer cells containing a mutant p53 gene, while sparing normal cells with a functioning p53 gene. Of the 19 subjects who received the standard dosing regimen, four (21%) had an objective response, including two complete responses and two partial responses. CI-1042 is being co-developed with Pfizer.

INDICATION(S) AND RESEARCH PHASE
Colorectal Cancer – Phase II
Pancreatic Cancer – Phase II
Head and Neck Cancer – Phase III
Cervical Dysplasia/Cancer – Phase I completed
Lung Cancer – Phase II

Bladder Cancer – Phase I completed
Brain Cancer – Phase I completed

cytostatics
unknown

MANUFACTURER
Bioenvision

DESCRIPTION
Cytostatics are a group of compounds that inhibit retinoic acid metabolizing enzyme, leading to an accumulation of retinoic acid. Retinoic acid is important in maintaining differentiation of cells and has been shown to have an anti-proliferative effect on malignant cells. There are three potential products being developed in this group. One product, still unnamed, is currently being developed for the treatment of bladder cancer. A phase I trial for this indication is planned for 2001.

INDICATION(S) AND RESEARCH PHASE
Bladder Cancer – Phase I

eflornithine, DFMO (difluoromethylornydil)
Unknown

MANUFACTURER
Aventis

DESCRIPTION
Eflornithine is a potent, irreversible inhibitor of ornithine decarboxylase (OCD), an enzyme that is elevated in most tumors and pre-malignant lesions. Eflornithine is currently in a phase III clinical trial to determine the effectiveness of the drug in treating subjects who have newly diagnosed or recurrent bladder cancer. The drug is administered orally in tablet form.

Eflornithine is also in trials for the prevention and treatment of HIV infections, skin cancer, breast cancer, prostate cancer, and cervical dysplasia/cancer.

INDICATION(S) AND RESEARCH PHASE
Bladder Cancer – Phase III
Breast Cancer – Phase II/III
Cervical Dysplasia/Cancer – Phase II
HIV Infection – Phase II
Prostate Cancer – Phase II
Skin Cancer – Phase III

EMD 82633
unknown

MANUFACTURER
Merck KgaA

DESCRIPTION
EMD 82633 is a humanized and bispecific monoclonal antibody derived from mice. These antibodies are altered in such a way that they no longer appear different from human antibodies. This genetic modification prevents immune reactions against foreign substances of animal origin used in humans. In this bispecific drug, one component binds to tumor cells, while the other activates the body's own CD8 "killer cells" to attack cancer cells.

This new drug is being given as an adjuvant therapy to subjects who have not been adequately helped by conventional forms of treatment, such as chemotherapy. EMD 82633 is being tested in trials for the treatment of renal cancer, head and neck cancer, breast cancer, bladder cancer, and ovarian cancer.

INDICATION(S) AND RESEARCH PHASE
Bladder Cancer – Phase II
Breast Cancer – Phase II
Cancer/Tumors (Unspecified) – Phase II
Head and Neck Cancer – Phase II
Ovarian Cancer – Phase II
Renal Cell Carcinoma – Phase II

gemcitabine HCl
Gemzar

MANUFACTURER
Eli Lilly

DESCRIPTION
Gemzar is under review as a combination therapy for use with cisplatin for the treatment of locally advanced or metastatic transitional cell carcinoma. The drug is a novel chemotherapeutic agent that mimics a natural building block of DNA. Gemzar disrupts the process of cell replication and thereby slows or stops progression of the disease. The drug is administered intravenously.

Gemzar is also indicated as first-line treatment of locally advanced or metastatic pancreatic cancer and, in combination with cisplatin, for locally advanced or metastatic non-small cell lung cancer.

INDICATION(S) AND RESEARCH PHASE
Bladder Cancer – Phase III
Lung Cancer – FDA approved
Pancreatic Cancer – Phase II completed

gallium maltolate
unknown

MANUFACTURER
Titan Pharmaceuticals

DESCRIPTION
Gallium is a semi-metallic element that has shown some therapeutic activity in metabolic bone disease, hypercalcemia of malignancy, and cancer. Gallium maltolate can displace divalent iron from the iron transporting protein, transferrin; thus gallium maltolate causes interference with iron metabolism with inhibition of enzymes requiring divalent iron. The most important of these in the cancer setting appears to be ribonucleotide reductase (RNR). In addition, gallium appears to form salts with calcium and phosphate and become incorporated into bone. The bone that is created with incorporated gallium appears to be at least as strong as normal bone, and it appears to be more resistant to degradation by osteoclasts and tumor cells.

INDICATION(S) AND RESEARCH PHASE
Prostate Cancer – Phase I/II
Lymphomas – Phase I/II
Myeloma – Phase I/II
Bladder Cancer – Phase I/II
HIV Infection – Phase I/II

INGN-201, adenoviral p53
Unknown

MANUFACTURER
Introgen Therapeutics

DESCRIPTION

INGN-201 is a p53 gene therapy cancer product. It has been tested as a treatment for a variety of solid tumor cancers with administration via intratumoral injection. The drug was well tolerated according to the company, and additional trials are under way using an intravenous infusion in order to reach more types of cancers. The tumor-suppressing p53 gene encodes a protein that responds to damage involving cellular DNA by terminating cell division. Normal p53 genes are delivered into cancer cells of the subject through an adenoviral vector.

The developers of INGN-201 have signed a Cooperative Research and Development Agreement (CRADA) with the National Cancer Institute to evaluate the potential effectiveness and superiority of the drug over other treatments against breast, ovarian, bladder, prostate, and brain cancers in phase I and phase II trials. A phase III trial in head and neck cancer was initiated in March 2000.

INDICATION(S) AND RESEARCH PHASE

Head and Neck Cancer – Phase III
Bladder Cancer – Phase I
Brain Cancer – Phase I
Breast Cancer – Phase I
Bronchoalveolar Cancer – Phase I
Ovarian Cancer – Phase I
Prostate Cancer – Phase I
Lung Cancer – Phase II
Cancer/Tumors (Unspecified) – Phase I

MCC
unknown

MANUFACTURER
Bioniche Life Sciences

DESCRIPTION

MCC is a cell wall complex prepared from the non-pathogenic bacterium *Mycobacterium phlei* (*M. phlei*) that inhibits cancer cell division, induces apoptosis and stimulates a profound immune response in a wide range of human cancer cells. Based on extensive preclinical research, the company believes these therapeutic activities are not affected by the presence of multi-drug resistance in cancer cells. MCC is in a phase I/II trial for bladder cancer in Canada and Australia.

INDICATION(S) AND RESEARCH PHASE
Bladder Cancer – Phase I/II

MDX-447, H-447
unknown

MANUFACTURER
Medarex

DESCRIPTION

MDX-477 is a novel biological drug designed to stimulate an immune response against cancer cells. Certain cancer cells contain and express large amounts of unique proteins (such as epidermal growth factor receptors), which MDX-477 is directed to recognize. MDX-477 attaches itself both to these cancer proteins and to macrophages that specialize in killing foreign material.

The binding together of the cancer and the immune cells by MDX-477 signals the body to destroy the tumor. MDX-477 may offer a new therapeutic alternative to cancer subjects who have been unresponsive to conventional therapies. This agent is unique since it has two receptors on its surface, one that can attract the cancer cell, and the other that can attract a killer immune cell. This dual nature of the drug is why it is known as a "bispecific antibody."

This type of drug is designed to be more efficient than current anti-cancer therapies, and may have effects that last longer. This technology may also be useful in the development of an "anti-cancer vaccine" in the future. MDX-477 is currently being tested as an intravenous solution in phase II trials for multiple tumor indications, which include brain, bladder, breast, head and neck, and lung cancer.

INDICATION(S) AND RESEARCH PHASE
Brain Cancer – Phase II
Bladder Cancer – Phase II
Breast Cancer – Phase II
Head and Neck Cancer – Phase II
Lung Cancer – Phase II

unknown
BCI-Immune Activator

MANUFACTURER
INTRACEL Corporation

DESCRIPTION

BCI-Immune Activator is a non-specific immunotherapy for bladder cancer. The drug acts by inducing a non-specific inflammatory response in the bladder. In turn, this response stimulates macrophages and other immune cells to attack the site of the inflammation, thereby killing the tumor. BCI-Immune Activator is formulated as a liquid and delivered to the subject in two steps. First, a small amount of the drug is injected subcutaneously to stimulate or sensitize the immune system. Then, it is injected directly into the tumor.

Based on positive results from a phase I/II study of the effects of increasing doses, a phase III clinical trial has begun to test the efficacy of BCI-Immune Activator for treatment of refractory bladder cancer.

INDICATION(S) AND RESEARCH PHASE
Bladder Cancer – Phase III

valrubicin
Valstar

MANUFACTURER
Anthra Pharmaceuticals

DESCRIPTION

Valstar Intravesical Solution is a lipophilic anthracycline-like chemotherapeutic agent. The drug acts by penetrating cells where it affects a variety of biological functions, most of which involve nucleic acid metabolism.

Previously approved for treatment of subjects with BCG-refractory carcinoma-in-situ (CIS) for whom surgical removal of the bladder would present unacceptable risks of morbidity or mortality, Valstar is in phase III trials for treatment of papillary bladder cancer.

Valstar is also in phase III trials for treatment of refractory ovarian cancer. For this indication, the drug is administered through the abdomen (intraperitoneal).

INDICATION(S) AND RESEARCH PHASE
Bladder Cancer – Phase III
Ovarian Cancer – Phase III

ZD-0473/AMD 473
unknown

MANUFACTURER
AstraZeneca

DESCRIPTION
ZD-0473 is a new platinum-based anti-cancer agent designed to deliver an extended spectrum of activity and overcome resistance to currently approved platinum drugs, such as cisplatin and carboplatin. It is being evaluated for the treatment of a range of solid-tumor cancers, including colorectal, non-small cell lung, and bladder cancer, which are resistant to carboplatin. ZD-0473 is formulated in both intravenous and oral forms. The intravenous formulation is in phase II trials and the oral form is in preclinical development.

INDICATION(S) AND RESEARCH PHASE
Bladder Cancer – Phase II
Cancer/Tumors (Unspecified) – Phase II
Colorectal Cancer – Phase II
Lung Cancer – Phase II
Ovarian Cancer – Phase II
Prostate Cancer – Phase II
Breast Cancer – Phase II
Cervical Dysplasia/Cancer – Phase II

ZD0473
unknown

MANUFACTURER
AstraZeneca

DESCRIPTION
ZD0473 is a third generation platinum compound for the treatment of cisplatin- and carboplatin-resistant tumors, including non-small cell lung cancer, ovarian, colorectal, and bladder cancers. ZD0473 is a new generation platinum agent designed to deliver an extended spectrum of anti-cancer activity and overcome platinum resistance.

AnorMED has a licensing agreement with AstraZeneca, who is conducting the phase II study development of ZD0473.

INDICATION(S) AND RESEARCH PHASE
Bladder Cancer – Phase II
Colorectal Cancer – Phase II
Head and Neck Cancer – Phase II
Lung Cancer – Phase II
Ovarian Cancer – Phase II

Erectile Dysfunction

alprostadil
Topiglan

MANUFACTURER
MacroChem Corporation

DESCRIPTION
Topiglan is a topical gel that is being evaluated in phase II and phase III studies for the treatment of male erectile dysfunction. Topiglan is a naturally occurring compound that may relax disease-constricted penile blood vessels in impotent men. This drug is a specific type of biochemical called prostaglandin E-1 (PGE-1), which increases blood flow and may help males to produce an erection.

Topiglan is formulated with a special drug delivery technology, known as SEPA (soft enhancement of percutaneous absorption), that increases absorption across the skin. Previous administrations of Topiglan included injection into the penis with a hypodermic syringe, or insertion into the urethra as a suppository.

Macrochem Corporation reported a preliminary review for a phase IIB double-blind study in which half of the subjects received placebo, and the other half received either the active drug plus the SEPA-formulated gel, or only the SEPA-gel without the drug. The test article was applied topically to the head of the penis in sixty subjects with known erectile dysfunction. Many of the subjects were reported to have previously failed to respond to available therapies, including Viagra, MUSE, and surgical revascularization.

According to the company, the results indicated that Topiglan application was associated with a statistically greater penile rigidity and swelling (tumescence) as compared to placebo, as assessed by physicians. Subject's assessment also rated Topiglan results as better. Six times more subjects stated that the erection produced by using Topiglan was sufficient for vaginal intercourse compared to placebo treated subjects. Treatment was associated with transient, minor to mild symptoms of localized warmth, occasionally mild burning or tingling in some subjects, with no difference observed between the drug and placebo treatments.

A pivotal phase III trial was initiated in July 2000 for impotence and will be conducted at 20 sites and will include 400 subjects. In addition, a phase III trial was initiated in January 2001 for the treatment of male erectile dysfunction.

INDICATION(S) AND RESEARCH PHASE
Impotence – Phase III
Sexual Dysfunction – Phase III
Erectile Dysfuction – Phase III

alprostadil
Alprox-TD, Befar

MANUFACTURER
NexMed

DESCRIPTION
Alprox-TD is a topical treatment that contains alprostadil, which has been used for the treatment of erectile dysfunction (ED). Alprostadil is a vasodilator that relaxes blood vessels and increases blood flow. NexMed's Alprox-TD combines alprostadil with the NexACT transdermal penetration enhancing technology. According to NexMed, NexACT contains skin penetration-enhancing molecules that allow a drug to be quickly absorbed to a localized disease site.

Results of a phase II trial of Alprox-TD indicated that three different dose levels of the drug were more effective than placebo in the treatment of mild to moderate ED. The randomized, double-blind, placebo-controlled trial was conducted at 12 clinical sites in the United States. The response to the Global Assessment Questionnaire, which measures improvement in erectile function, indicated an effectiveness rate of 73% in the highest dose group compared to 23% in the placebo group.

Additionally, phase III trials have been completed in China, where Alprox-TD will be marketed as Befar. The company has a New Drug Application for marketing approval pending with the State Drug Administration of China.

INDICATION(S) AND RESEARCH PHASE
Erectile Dysfunction – Phase II completed
Erectile Dysfunction – Application submitted (China)

alprostadil/prazosin hydrochloride
Alibra

MANUFACTURER
Vivus

DESCRIPTION
Alibra is a urethral microsuppository of alprostadil and prazosin hydrochloride and is indicated for the treatment of male erectile dysfunction. An NDA was withdrawn in October 2000 because additional information is needed by the FDA.

INDICATION(S) AND RESEARCH PHASE
Erectile Dysfunction – NDA withdrawn

apomorphine HCl
Uprima

MANUFACTURER
Abbott Laboratories

DESCRIPTION
Uprima is a dopamine receptor agonist being developed in a novel sublingual formulation. This formulation allows for the specific stimulation of parts of the brain involved in the erectile process, thereby replicating the way the body naturally produces an erection.

Uprima has had a somewhat troubled history in terms of safety concerns; however, in January 2001 Abbott Laboratories reported that the European Union's Committee for Proprietary Medicinal Products (CPMP) has adopted a positive opinion on Uprima for the treatment of erectile dysfunction. The CPMP opinion will be considered by the European Commission, which will make a final decision regarding the issue of marketing authorization.

Abbott Laboratories holds non-exclusive rights to Uprima in markets outside the United States and Canada. Abbott licensed the drug from TAP Pharmaceuticals.

INDICATION(S) AND RESEARCH PHASE
Erectile Dysfunction – Phase III

BMS-193884
unknown

MANUFACTURER
Bristol-Myers Squibb

DESCRIPTION
BMS-193884 is an endothelin-A receptor stimulator for both congestive heart failure and male erectile dysfunction. It is made in an oral formulation. Clinical testing is in phase II.

INDICATION(S) AND RESEARCH PHASE
Congestive Heart Failure – Phase II
Erectile Dysfunction – Phase II

BMS-223131
unknown

MANUFACTURER
Bristol-Myers Squibb

DESCRIPTION
BMS-223131 is being developed for the treatment of erectile dysfunction. It is currently in phase I/II development.

INDICATION(S) AND RESEARCH PHASE
Erectile Dysfunction – Phase I/II

IC351
Cialis

MANUFACTURER
Eli Lilly

DESCRIPTION
Cialis (IC351) is an orally administered phosphodiesterase type 5 (PDE5) inhibitor that has been tested in more than 20 phase I and II trials. Cialis targets PDE5, which is an enzyme involved in controlling blood flow to the penis. When PDE5 is inhibited, natural sexual stimuli produce a more pronounced effect, facilitating the ability of men with erectile dysfunction (ED) to attain and maintain an erection.

In November 2000, results of a phase II trial indicated that up to 88% of men taking Cialis reported improved erections relative to placebo. Subjects with mild-to-severe ED were randomized to receive either placebo or Cialis at doses up to 25 mg over an eight-week period. Data obtained from sexual encounter profile diaries showed increased reports from both men and their partners of successful intercourse attempts.

Lilly ICOS has initiated a global phase III trial for ED, and Cialis is also in phase II trials for female sexual dysfunction (FSD).

INDICATION(S) AND RESEARCH PHASE
Erectile Dysfunction – Phase III
Sexual Dysfunction – Phase II

phentolamine mesylate
Vasomax

MANUFACTURER
Zonagen

DESCRIPTION
Vasomax is an oral drug being developed for the treatment of male erectile dysfunction. This drug works by blocking alpha-receptors, which are located on the interior of blood vessels. An NDA has been submitted for Vasomax, which has been approved in Mexico under the name Z-Max. The drug has been developed under and agreement between Schering-Plough and Zonagen.

INDICATION(S) AND RESEARCH PHASE
Erectile Dysfunction – NDA submitted

PT-141

unknown

MANUFACTURER
Palatin Technologies

DESCRIPTION
PT-141 is a synthetic modification of PT-14, which is an analogue of a naturally occurring peptide hormone called alpha MSH. A phase I trial was initiated in January 2001 testing PT-141 as a nasal spray for erectile dysfunction. Results from a small pilot study found PT-141 was approximately 80% effective in treating men with erectile dysfunction.

INDICATION(S) AND RESEARCH PHASE
Erectile Dysfunction – Phase I

(S)-sibutramine
unknown

MANUFACTURER
Sepracor

DESCRIPTION
According to in vitro studies, (S)-sibutramine is a potent inhibitor of both dopamine and norepinephrine. This dual pharmacology may improve both erectile and ejaculatory dysfunction, and a preclinical model has shown that the (S)-sibutramine metabolite facilitates sexual performance. Sepracor is developing (S)-sibutramine as a treatment for both sexual dysfunction and stress urinary incontinence.

INDICATION(S) AND RESEARCH PHASE
Erectile Dysfunction – Phase I
Urinary Incontinence – Phase I

TA-1790
unknown

MANUFACTURER
Vivus

DESCRIPTION
TA-1790 is a highly selective phosphodiesterase type 5 (PDE5) inhibitor. The compound is being developed for the treatment of male and female sexual dysfunction. Vivus has a licensing agreement with Tanabe Seiyaku regarding this product.

INDICATION(S) AND RESEARCH PHASE
Sexual Dysfunction – Phase I
Erectile Dysfunction – Phase I

TAK-251, apomorphine
unknown

MANUFACTURER
Takeda Chemical Industries

DESCRIPTION
TAK-251 is a dopamine receptor agonist in testing for the treatment of erectile dysfunction. The drug is in phase I trials in Japan, phase III trials in the United States and an application has been filed in Europe.

INDICATION(S) AND RESEARCH PHASE
Erectile Dysfunction (Japan) – Phase I
Erectile Dysfunction – Phase III
Erectile Dysfunction – MAA submitted

testosterone
unknown

MANUFACTURER
MacroChem Corporation

DESCRIPTION
This drug product is a SEPA enhanced formulation of testosterone that is being developed for the treatment of male erectile dysfunction. The phase II trial is completed, and the phase III study is pending protocol design modifications.

INDICATION(S) AND RESEARCH PHASE
Erectile Dysfunction – Phase II completed

Transdermal testosterone gel
Tostrex

MANUFACTURER
Cellegy Pharmaceuticals

DESCRIPTION
This transdermal testosterone gel is currently in phase III trials for the treatment of male hormone hypogonadism, a disorder frequently characterized by diminished libido and reduced muscle mass. This hormonal gel is a more convenient treatment than injections and a less irritating alternative to the current patch products.

INDICATION(S) AND RESEARCH PHASE
Male Hormonal Deficiencies/Abnormalities – Phase III
Erectile Dysfunction – Phase II/III

unknown
Daproxetine

MANUFACTURER
PPD Genupro

DESCRIPTION
Daproxetine is a selective serotonin reuptake inhibitor for the treatment of premature ejaculation. Daproxetine has recently completed a phase II trial in thirteen centers throughout the United States. The double-blind, placebo-controlled, three way crossover study enrolled 155 subjects. It evaluated two different dose levels of the oral drug and placebo. In each period of the study, each subject took the medication 1-3 hours prior to intercourse, and the subject's partner recorded ejaculatory latency in a diary. Each period included four attempts over four weeks. Results showed that daproxetine therapy resulted in a significant prolongation of ejaculatory latency compared to placebo.

INDICATION(S) AND RESEARCH PHASE
Erectile Dysfunction – Phase II
Sexual Dysfunction – Phase II

unknown
Invicorp

MANUFACTURER
Senetek PLC

DESCRIPTION
Invicorp is a combination of vasoactive intestinal peptide (VIP) and 1 to 2 mg of phentolamine mesylate (PMS). The drug is administrated using a novel drug delivery

system that makes the self-injection process pain free.

In phase III trials in the United Kingdom, Denmark, Ireland and Australia, an efficacy of 83% was achieved without serious side effects. The most frequent side effect was transient facial flushing which resolved minutes after using Invicorp.

Invicorp has received approval for the treatment of erectile dysfunction in the United Kingdom, Denmark and New Zealand. In the United States, the FDA has upgraded the status of the Invicorp IND to a partial clinical hold.

INDICATION(S) AND RESEARCH PHASE
Erectile Dysfunction – Phase III

vardenafil
unknown

MANUFACTURER
Bayer Corporation

DESCRIPTION
Vardenafil is a phosphodiesterase type 5 (PDE5) inhibitor being developed for the treatment of erectile dysfunction (ED). Phase II results indicated that men with ED reported a significant increase in their ability to achieve erection and complete intercourse with ejaculation after vardenafil treatment. The drug is currently in phase III trials.

INDICATION(S) AND RESEARCH PHASE
Erectile Dysfunction – Phase III

Hypertension

BMS-186716, omapatrilat
Vanlev

MANUFACTURER
Bristol-Myers Squibb

DESCRIPTION
BMS-186716 is a combination medicine made of two enzyme inhibitors for angiotensin converting enzyme (ACE) and neural endopeptidase (NEP). This dual drug is being evaluated in phase II trials for the treatment of heart failure and phase III trials for hypertension.

In April 2000 Bristol-Myers Squibb volunatarily withdrew its current NDA for Vanlev treating hypertension because of questions regarding the side effect angioedema. Angioedema is a localized swelling that generally affects the face, throat, lips, or tongue that can be triggered by food and commonly used drugs such as ACE-inhibitors, nonsteroidal anti-inflammatory agents, and some antibotics. The company plans to continue with further controlled trials and identify additional data to answer the FDA's questions.

INDICATION(S) AND RESEARCH PHASE
Congestive Heart Failure – Phase II
Hypertension – NDA withdrawn

bosentan
Tracleer

MANUFACTURER
Actelion Pharmaceuticals

DESCRIPTION
Tracleer is an orally active dual endothelin receptor agonist, blocking the action of endothelin at two different receptors, ETA and ETB. Endothelin is a potent vasoconstrictor that appears to play a fundamental mechanistic role in the development of pulmonary hypertension (PHT). Results of a double-blind, placebo-controlled phase III trial of Tracleer showed that subjects receiving the drug experienced significant improvements in terms of exercise ability and hemodynamics. At 12 weeks, subjects who received Tracleer demonstrated a 20% increase in exercise ability compared to the placebo group, in the standardized six minute walk test.

INDICATION(S) AND RESEARCH PHASE
Hypertension – Phase III completed

candesartan cilexetil
Atacand

MANUFACTURER
AstraZeneca

DESCRIPTION
Atacand (candesartan cilexetil) is an angiotensin II receptor blocker (ARB) being tested for the treatment of hypertension. Results of two multicenter, double-blind, randomized studies in more than 1,200 hypertensive subjects demonstrated Atacand to be significantly more effective in lowering both diastolic and systolic blood pressure than the most prescribed ARB Cozaar (losartan). During the double-blind treatment period, subjects were randomized to receive either 16 mg of Atacand or 50 mg of losartan. At week two, all subjects were titrated to double their current dose to 32 mg of Atacand or 100 mg of losartan. Duration of treatment was eight weeks unless a subject discontinued due to an adverse event, had an insufficient therapeutic response, or withdrew consent. The incidence of discontinuation was only 2.7% for Atacand and 1.8% for losartan. The most commonly reported adverse events for both medications were headache, dizziness, sinusitis, and respiratory infection.

The drug is currently being tested in phase III trials for hypertension outcomes (SCOPE study), congestive heart failure outcomes (CHARM study), and diabetic retinopathy. Pediatric phase III trials for hypertension are ongoing. Atacand Plus, a diuretic formula, is FDA approved for hypertension in adults.

INDICATION(S) AND RESEARCH PHASE
Hypertension – Phase III
Pediatric, Hypertension – Phase III
Congestive Heart Failure – Phase III
Diabetic Retinopathy – Phase III

captopril
Captelan

MANUFACTURER
Elan Pharmaceutical Research

DESCRIPTION
Captelan is a once-daily oral product made available by a technology that improves oral drug delivery. Captelan is a specific competitive inhibitor of the angiotensin I convert-

ing enzyme (ACE), the enzyme responsible for converting angiotensin I to angiotensin II. As an ACE inhibitor, Captelan has the potential to lower blood pressure and to indirectly reduce the workload on the heart. Clinical testing is in phase II for hypertension and congestive heart failure.

INDICATION(S) AND RESEARCH PHASE
Congestive Heart Failure – Phase II
Hypertension – Phase II

CS-866
unknown

MANUFACTURER
Sankyo

DESCRIPTION
CS-866 is an anti-hypertensive drug that works by blocking the receptor on angiotensin-2, a very potent natural agent that raises blood pressure. CS-866 is made in an oral formulation and is currently in a phase III trial for the treatment of hypertension. Sankyo is collaborating development of this product with Recordati Industria Chimica e Farmaceutica S.p.A.

INDICATION(S) AND RESEARCH PHASE
Hypertension – Phase III

diltiazem HCl
Verzem

MANUFACTURER
Verex Laboratories

DESCRIPTION
Verzem is an oral tablet formulation of diltiazem hydrochloride, a calcium channel blocker. This drug works by inhibiting the influx of calcium ions during the normal electrical discharge, or membrane depolarization, of cardiac and vascular smooth muscle. As a treatment for hypertension, Verzem is thought to relax blood vessel muscles, which decreases peripheral vascular resistance. In angina subjects, it may reduce oxygen demand in heart muscle. Verzem is currently in a phase II trial for hypertension.

INDICATION(S) AND RESEARCH PHASE
Hypertension – Phase II

GW 660511
unknown

MANUFACTURER
GlaxoSmithKline

DESCRIPTION
GW 660511 is an angiotensin-converting enzyme (ACE)/neutral-endopeptidase enzyme (NEP) inhibitor being developed for the treatment of hypertension. It is currently in phase I trials.

INDICATION(S) AND RESEARCH PHASE
Hypertension – Phase I

isradipine
unknown

MANUFACTURER
Elan Pharmaceutical Research

DESCRIPTION
Isradipine is a calcium channel blocker being evaluated in a once-daily formulation, using the insoluble drug absorption system (INDAS) manufactured by Elan Pharmaceutical Research. Clinical testing is in a phase II trial for treatment of hypertension.

INDICATION(S) AND RESEARCH PHASE
Hypertension – Phase II

lercanidipine
unknown

MANUFACTURER
Forest Laboratories

DESCRIPTION
Lercanidipine belongs to the dihydropyridine calcium channel blocker class of antihypertensives. The drug is currently marketed in nineteen countries, and clinical experience has shown that it has comparable efficacy to other drugs in its class. Forest Laboratories has entered into an agreement with Recordati of Milan, Italy, for the marketing of lercanidipine in the United States. It is expected that an NDA will be filed for approval in the United States mid-2001.

INDICATION(S) AND RESEARCH PHASE
Hypertension – Phase III

sitaxsentan
unknown

MANUFACTURER
ICOS Corporation

DESCRIPTION
Sitaxsentan is an endothelin receptor antagonist with a long duration of action and high specificity for type A endothelin (ETA) receptors. Blocking ETA may reverse the vasoconstrictive effects of endothelin-1 (ET-1) on the pulmonary vasculature, while maintaining the vasodilator functions of the type B (ETB) receptor.

Sitaxsentan is being developed by ICOS and Texas Biotechnology for the treatment of pulmonary hypertension. It is currently enrolling subjects in a phase II/III trial.

INDICATION(S) AND RESEARCH PHASE
Hypertension – Phase II/III

SLV 306
unknown

MANUFACTURER
Solvay Pharmaceuticals

DESCRIPTION
SLV 306 is an anti-hypertensive drug being tested in phase II trials for the treatments of both hypertension and congestive heart failure.

INDICATION(S) AND RESEARCH PHASE
Congestive Heart Failure – Phase II
Hypertension – Phase II

SPP 100
unknown

MANUFACTURER

Speedel Pharma

DESCRIPTION
SPP 100 is an oral renin inhibitor being developed in a phase II fast track program. The ongoing multicenter trial, treating 300 hypertensive subjects, will establish the dose-response of the blood pressure lowering effect. SPP 100 was outlicensed to Speedel from Novartis.

INDICATION(S) AND RESEARCH PHASE
Hypertension – Phase II

TBC-3711
unknown

MANUFACTURER
Texas Biotechnology

DESCRIPTION
TBC-3711 is an oral endothelin A receptor antagonist (ETA). Endothelin is a potent vasoconstrictor that exerts its effects through the activation of endothelin A and B receptors. The endothelin A receptor is believed to contribute to increased pulmonary and systemic artery pressures. Thus in blocking the endothelin A receptor, vasoconstriction may be prevented or reserved. The company plans to initiate a phase II trial for either congestive heart failure or essential hypertension by the second half of 2001. TBC-3711 is being co-developed with ICOS Corporation and is currently in phase I development for congestive heart failure and essential hypertension.

INDICATION(S) AND RESEARCH PHASE
Congestive Heart Failure – Phase I
Hypertension – Phase I

TCV-116C
unknown

MANUFACTURER
Takeda Chemical Industries

DESCRIPTION
TCV-116C is a combination of TCV-116, an angiotensin II receptor antagonist, and a diuretic. The drug is in phase II trials in Japan for the treatment of hypertension.

INDICATION(S) AND RESEARCH PHASE
Hypertension – Phase II

telmisartan
unknown

MANUFACTURER
GlaxoSmithKline

DESCRIPTION
Telmisartan is an angiotensin II receptor antagonist. Binding sites for angiotensin II are found in many tissues. Blockade of these binding sites inhibits vasoconstriction and facilitates blood flow, thereby reducing blood pressure.

Telmisartan is currently in phase III trials in combination with hydrochlorothiazide (HCTZ) for the treatment of hypertension. HCTZ is a diuretic commonly prescribed in combination with other anti-hypertensives. It flushes excess water and sodium from the body by increasing urine formation. This decreases the amount of fluid in the blood vessels, thereby increasing blood flow and reducing blood pressure.

INDICATION(S) AND RESEARCH PHASE
Hypertension – Phase III

unknown
Beraprost

MANUFACTURER
United Therapeutics

DESCRIPTION
Beraprost is a chemically stable oral form of prostacyclin that dilates blood vessels, prevents platelet aggregation and prevents proliferation of smooth muscle cells surrounding blood vessels. It is in phase III trials for both early-stage peripheral vascular disease and early-stage pulmonary hypertension, in an immediate-release oral formulation.

INDICATION(S) AND RESEARCH PHASE
Peripheral Vascular Disease – Phase III
Hypertension – Phase III

UT-15
unknown

MANUFACTURER
United Therapeutics

DESCRIPTION
UT-15 is a formulation of prostacyclin that is delivered continuously through the MiniMed subcutaneous system. UT-15 is a particularly long-lived and stable version of prostacyclin, and because the MiniMed system operates by subcutaneous infusion rather than intravenous injection, there is less risk of infection. The product is in phase II development for the treatment of late-stage peripheral vascular disease and has also been developed for treatment of pulmonary hypertension.

In November 2000, United Therapeutics announced that the NDA submitted for treatment of pulmonary hypertension was accepted by the FDA. The company anticipates a six-month priority review status.

INDICATION(S) AND RESEARCH PHASE
Hypertension – NDA submitted
Peripheral Vascular Disease – Phase II

valsartan
Diovan

MANUFACTURER
Novartis

DESCRIPTION
Diovan is an oral angiotensin II receptor antagonist in phase III development for the treatment of post- and pre-myocardial infarction and congestive heart failure. Diovan blocks the action of angiotensin II (AT-II), a hormone formed when a precursor (angiotensin I) is cleaved by an enzyme in the lungs and blood vessels. In this manner, Diovan blocks the vasoconstriction of blood vessels and the aldosterone-secreting effects of AT-II.

Diovan has been FDA approved for the treatment of hypertension in elderly subjects. It is currently being marketed by Novartis with this indication.

INDICATION(S) AND RESEARCH PHASE
Congestive Heart Failure – Phase III
Myocardial Infarction – Phase III
Hypertension – FDA approved

Hyponatremia

YM-087, conivaptan
unknown

MANUFACTURER
Yamanouchi Pharmaceutical

DESCRIPTION
YM-087 is a receptor antagonist to the peptide hormone vasopressin, which is released by the hypothalamus to regulate water balance in the body. The drug is currently in phase III trials for the treatment of hyponatremia, and phase II trials for the treatment of heart failure. It is being developed in both Europe and the United States. The drug is also part of Yamanouchi's domestic pipeline; YM-087 is in phase II trials for both hyponatremia and heart failure. YM-087 is manufactured in oral and injectable formulations.

INDICATION(S) AND RESEARCH PHASE
Congestive Heart Failure (United States and Japan) – Phase II
Hyponatremia (United States) – Phase III
Hyponatremia (Japan) – Phase II

Kidney Disease

5G1.1
unknown

MANUFACTURER
Alexion

DESCRIPTION
5G1.1 is a monoclonal antibody that inhibits C5, a major protein in the complement system, important in inflammation. This antibody will result in an anti-inflammatory response. In February 2001, positive interim results were announced for a double-blind, randomized, placebo-controlled phase II trial of 5G1.1 in subjects with rheumatoid arthritis. Additionally, 5G1.1 is in a phase II trial for the treatment of membranous nephritis and in phase Ib pilot studies for the treatment of psoriasis, dermatomyositis, and pemphigoid.

INDICATION(S) AND RESEARCH PHASE
Rheumatoid Arthritis – Phase II
Kidney Disease – Phase II
Skin Infections/Disorders – Phase Ib

CVT-124
Adentri

MANUFACTURER
Biogen

DESCRIPTION
Adentri is believed to act by blocking the selective adenosine A-1 receptor that is present in several locations within the kidney. The selectivity of this compound offers the potential to promote excretion of excess fluid without causing side effects such as renal failure, diuretic resistance, or potassium loss.

This drug was shown to be active in a placebo-controlled, phase II trial evaluating various doses of Adentri in comparison to and in combination with furosemide for congestive heart failure. Biogen plans to move ahead with phase III studies. Adentri has also been evaluated in 70 subjects and it was shown that the glomerular filtration rate (GFR), a measure of kidney function, is preserved, while causing useful increases in sodium and urine excretion. Other useful indications may include acute renal failure following kidney transplantation, and high risk surgical procedures.

INDICATION(S) AND RESEARCH PHASE
Kidney Disease – Phase II
Congestive Heart Failure – Phase II

darbepoetin alfa
Aranesp

MANUFACTURER
Amgen

DESCRIPTION
Aranesp (darbepoetin alfa) is a sustained release form of Epogen (epoetin alfa), a drug developed by Amgen for the treatment of anemia in subjects with kidney disease and other conditions. Chronic kidney disease is characterized by decreased levels of erythropoietin, a hormone that stimulates the production of red blood cells. Aranesp is a novel erythropoiesis stimulating protein developed to treat anemia with less frequent administration than recombinant epoetin alfa.

In December 2000, trial results for Aranesp indicated that the drug was effective when given once every three weeks to anemic cancer subjects with solid tumors. In a double-blind, placebo-controlled, dose-finding phase I/II trial of 163 subjects, a dose response was seen between four different doses of Aranesp as demonstrated by increases in hemoglobin as well as a decrease in transfusions. Amgen has completed NDA filing for Aranesp as a treatment for anemia in subjects with kidney disease. Development for Aranesp as a treatment for anemia in cancer subjects is currently in phase II.

INDICATION(S) AND RESEARCH PHASE
Kidney Disease – NDA submitted
Cancer/Tumors (Unspecified) – Phase II

doxercalciferol
Hectorol Capsules

MANUFACTURER
Bone Care International

DESCRIPTION
Hectorol Capsules provide vitamin D-hormone replacement, which reduces elevated parathyroid hormone levels in subjects with end stage renal disease (ESRD) and secondary hyperparathyroidism. Doxercalciferol undergoes metabolic activation to form a naturally occurring, biologically active form of vitamin D2. The active vitamin D metabolites act directly on bone cells, called osteoblasts, to stimulate skeletal growth, and on the parathyroid glands to suppress parathyroid hormone synthesis and secretion.

Positive results were reported for the first of two phase III trials of Hectorol Capsules in 30 subjects with ESRD who were not yet receiving dialysis. Treatment for 24 weeks reduced abnormally elevated parathyroid hormone by approximately 60%, and did not adversely influence renal function or produce significant adverse side effects. Hectorol Capsules are currently approved by the FDA for the treatment of secondary hyperparathyroidism in subjects with end-stage renal disease currently on dialysis. Bone Care intends to file a supplemental NDA in early 2001 for the new indication of ESRD in subjects not yet receiving dialysis.

INDICATION(S) AND RESEARCH PHASE
Kidney Disease – Phase III

fenoldopam mesylate, SK&F-82526
Corlopam

MANUFACTURER
Elan Pharmaceutical Research

DESCRIPTION
Corlopam is a dopamine-1 receptor facilitator that acts as a systemic vasodilator, opening up blood vessels throughout the body. This drug is being tested in phase II trials for the treatment of congestive heart failure and acute renal failure.

INDICATION(S) AND RESEARCH PHASE
Congestive Heart Failure – Phase II
Kidney Disease – Phase II

icodextrin, Extraneal
Icodial

MANUFACTURER
ML Laboratories plc

DESCRIPTION
Icodial is a peritoneal dialysis solution for treatment of end stage renal disease, which is an orphan indication. The active ingredient of the solution, icodextrin, is a unique polymer of glucose. The company states that Icodial is the only dialysis solution to exhibit a prolonged duration of action. The drug is in phase III trials.

INDICATION(S) AND RESEARCH PHASE
Kidney Disease – Phase III

lanthanum carbonate
Lambda

MANUFACTURER
Shire Pharmaceuticals

DESCRIPTION
Lambda is being developed to reduce the amount of phosphate in the blood of subjects with chronic kidney failure. These subjects generally experience hyperphosphatemia because their kidneys are unable to filter out the excess phosphate acquired by food intake.

Lambda is being evaluated as a phosphate binder to be given with food. Lanthanum phosphate, the compound resulting from this binding reaction, is insoluble and will pass through the gut and into the stools, preventing the phosphate from entering the bloodstream.

Lambda is in phase III development in Europe and the United States, and is in phase I development in Japan.

INDICATION(S) AND RESEARCH PHASE
Kidney Disease – Phase III

LJP-394
unknown

MANUFACTURER
La Jolla Pharmaceutical

DESCRIPTION
LJP-394 is a novel compound derived from La Jolla's proprietary tolerance technology. The mechanism of action of LJP-394 is thought to involve inhibition of B cell antibody production. Antibodies are thought to be important in the pathogenesis of systemic lupus erythematosus (SLE). In a phase II/III trial, LPJ-394 reduced renal flares in lupus subjects with poor renal function. In subjects with high-affinity antibodies to LJP 394, time to renal flare, the primary endpoint of the trial, was significantly increased in the drug treated population as compared to the placebo treated group. In the high-affinity group, there were one-third as many renal flares in LJP 394 treated subjects compared to placebo treated subjects. A phase III trial for LJP 394 is currently in progress.

INDICATION(S) AND RESEARCH PHASE
Kidney Disease – Phase III
Systemic Lupus Erythematosus – Phase III

midodrine HCl
ProAmatine

MANUFACTURER
Shire Pharmaceuticals

DESCRIPTION
ProAmatine is being tested in clinical trials for the relief of urinary incontinence, a serious problem that causes disability and erosion of quality of life for many people. Incontinence occurs when there is weakening of the bladder muscle, the urethral muscle, or the muscle of the urinary sphincter. Especially in the case of the sphincter, a tight circle of muscle that regulates passage of urine from the bladder to the urethra when voiding, any decrease in muscle strength can cause urine leakage when exercising, coughing, sneezing, laughing, or putting any pressure on the body.

ProAmatine acts to stimulate alpha-1 adrenergic receptors in the sphincter and bladder that increase muscle tone. This action strengthens the tone of the bladder sphincter and delays bladder emptying, giving people more control over urination. Since this medication cannot cross from the bloodstream into the brain or nervous system, it is thought that ProAmatine may cause fewer side effects compared to other drugs used for urinary incontinence.

In addition to urinary incontinence, other indications undergoing phase II clinical testing include ejaculation disorders and hypotension caused by kidney dialysis, infection, or drugs. Roberts Pharmaceutical has licensed ProAmantine from Nycomed Pharma.

INDICATION(S) AND RESEARCH PHASE

458/Kidney Disease

Kidney Disease – Phase II
Urinary Incontinence – Phase II
Sexual Dysfunction – Phase II

novel erythropoiesis stimulating protein (NESP)
unknown

MANUFACTURER
Amgen

DESCRIPTION
Novel erythropoiesis stimulating protein (NESP) is a compound that stimulates bone marrow to produce more red blood cells. NESP is currently in phase III trials to treat anemia associated with chronic renal failure, especially for pre-dialysis subjects.

INDICATION(S) AND RESEARCH PHASE
Anemia – Phase III
Kidney Disease – Phase III

pimagedine HCl
unknown

MANUFACTURER
Alteon

DESCRIPTION
Pimagedine HCl is an aminoguanidine inhibitor compound designed to slow down or stop the progression of kidney disease in type 1, insulin dependent, diabetic subjects. A common problem for diabetics is that too much protein may be lost in the urine, a condition known as proteinuria. Alteon reports that a large phase III trial of pigagedine HCl showed a significant and clinically meaningful reduction of urinary protein excretion.

INDICATION(S) AND RESEARCH PHASE
Diabetes Mellitus Types 1 and 2 – Phase III completed
Kidney Disease – Phase III completed

triacetyl uridine
unknown

MANUFACTURER
Repligen Corporation

DESCRIPTION
Uridine is one of the four main riboside components of ribonucleic acid. Results of a phase I trial indicated that therapy with uridine, or a prodrug of uridine (triacetyl uridine (TAU)), was well-tolerated in children with severe to moderate mitochondrial disease. Data were also presented on four subjects with a form of kidney disease called renal tubular acidosis, a condition that can lead to severe acidosis, susceptibility to infections, malnutrition and failure to thrive. All four subjects showed a rapid improvement or correction of kidney function with TAU treatment.

Repligen plans to initiate a double-blind, placebo-controlled phase II trial evaluating the potential of TAU to correct kidney disease in subjects with mitochondrial disease and renal tubular acidosis.

INDICATION(S) AND RESEARCH PHASE
Kidney Disease – Phase II

unknown
NOX-100

MANUFACTURER
Medinox

DESCRIPTION
NOX-100 is a nitric oxide neutralizer currently being tested in a phase I/II trial for intradialytic hypotension in subjects with end-stage renal disease currently on hemodialysis. Dialysis can activate the immune system and cause overproduction of nitric oxide, a vasodilator resulting in low blood pressure. NOX-100 is given as an intravenous bolus during dialysis and is intended to bind only excessively produced nitric oxide and not remove the low levels of nitric oxide required to perform important necessary functions in the body.

The phase I/II trial is being conducted at The University of California-San Diego Medical Center in La Jolla, California with 28 subjects.

INDICATION(S) AND RESEARCH PHASE
Kidney Disease – Phase I/II

Kidney Transplant Surgery

5c8 (Anti CD-40 ligand antibody)
Antova

MANUFACTURER
Biogen

DESCRIPTION
Biogen has engineered 5c8 (Anti CD-40 ligand antibody), a humanized monoclonal antibody for the potential treatment of a number of autoimmune disorders. These include idiopathic thrombocytopenic purpura (ITP), systemic lupus erythematosus, kidney transplantation, and Factor VIII antibody inhibition.

In the aforementioned autoimmune diseases, it is thought that activated white blood cells, called T cell lymphocytes, bind to other tissue cells through a cell surface receptor, the CD-40 ligand. Abnormal antibodies are produced that will then recognize healthy body tissues as foreign, and thereby cause an inflammatory response. The 5c8 antibody may stop this abnormal immune cycle by binding to the CD-40 ligand and inhibiting its ability to bind with its receptor on a variety of other normal cells.

INDICATION(S) AND RESEARCH PHASE
Thrombocytopenia – Phase II discontinued
Systemic Lupus Erythematosus – Phase II discontinued
Kidney Transplant Surgery – Phase II discontinued
Factor VIII Antibody Inhibition – Phase II discontinued

anti B-7 humanized antibodies
unknown

MANUFACTURER
Wyeth-Ayerst

DESCRIPTION
Anti B-7 humanized antibodies are being developed for the prevention of graft-versus-host disease (GvHD) following haploidentical bone marrow transplant and

for preventing kidney rejection. Clinical trials are currently in phase I/II development.

INDICATION(S) AND RESEARCH PHASE
Immunosuppressive – Phase I/II
Kidney Transplant Surgery – Phase I/II
Bone Marrow Transplant – Phase I/II

---

anti-CD11a, hu1124
unknown

MANUFACTURER
XOMA Corporation

DESCRIPTION
This drug is a monoclonal antibody made from the fusion of an antibody producing cell and a myeloma cell, developed for the treatment of moderate to severe plaque psoriasis. It works by inhibiting T cells, a type of white blood cell, and targeting a specific cell marker, CD11a, on the T cell surface. Anti-CD11a then potentially turns off the abnormal autoimmune response in psoriasis subjects. The drug is given intravenously.

These T cell lymphocytes play a large role in the immune system, helping the body fight off infection and recognize foreign materials. Sometimes the immune system becomes short-circuited and the body starts attacking itself. This widely diverse group of problems is called autoimmune diseases. Psoriasis is one such type, in which the immune system sends lymphocytes to attack parts of the skin around the hands, elbows, and other areas. The skin becomes chronically inflamed and then red, scaly plaques form. Drugs that suppress this abnormal immune response may provide new therapies for autoimmmune diseases.

A phase II placebo-controlled clinical trial conducted in Canada tested the anti-CD11a antibody in 145 moderate to severe psoriasis subjects who received an eight week course of therapy with either the antibody or placebo. XOMA claims that preliminary analysis of the data demonstrated a clinical response of 75% or better improvement over baseline, as measured by physician's global assessment, in 25% of the subjects treated with the drug versus two percent of the subjects in the placebo group. Side effects included a temporary hearing loss in one subject that may or may not be related to the drug. The more common adverse effects were mild headaches and low body temperature increases, usually after the first dose. The drug is currently in phase III testing for treatment of psoriasis and in phase II development in kidney transplant subjects.

INDICATION(S) AND RESEARCH PHASE
Psoriasis and Psoriatic Disorders – Phase III
Kidney Transplant Surgery – Phase II

Anti-LFA-1, odulimomab
unknown

MANUFACTURER
SangStat Medical

DESCRIPTION
Odulimomab is a monoclonal antibody designed to help prevent renal rejection after a kidney transplant and reduce the delay in graft functioning. The drug, in an intravenous formulation, is in phase III trials for kidney transplant rejection, acting as an immunosuppressant.

INDICATION(S) AND RESEARCH PHASE
Immunosuppressive – Phase III
Kidney Transplant Surgery – Phase III

BTI-322, MEDI-507
unknown

MANUFACTURER
BioTransplant

DESCRIPTION
MEDI-507 is a novel, humanized monoclonal antibody which binds specifically to the CD2 surface antigen receptor found on T cells and natural killer (NK) cells. MEDI-507 was engineered from BTI-322, a murine antibody, in order to reduce potential immunogenicity and allow for long-term administration. Laboratory studies have suggested that MEDI-507 and BTI-322 primarily inhibit the response of specific activated T cells, while subsequently allowing other immune cells to respond normally. Therefore, these drugs may be able to prevent the host rejection of a transplanted organ without compromising the entire immune system. MEDI-501 may prove to induce long-term functional transplantation tolerance in humans, increase the therapeutic benefit of bone marrow transplants, and reduce or eliminate the need for lifelong immunosuppressive therapy.

The drug is currently in multiple phase II clinical trials for treatment of graft versus host disease and for kidney transplant rejection. MEDI-507 is also being evaluated for treatment of psoriasis, as a proof of concept for its use in autoimmune diseases.

INDICATION(S) AND RESEARCH PHASE
Immunosuppressive – Phase II
Kidney Transplant Surgery – Phase II
Psoriasis and Psoriatic Disorders – Phase II

ISIS-2302
unknown

MANUFACTURER
Isis Pharmaceuticals

DESCRIPTION
ISIS-2302 is an inhibitor of antisense intracellular adhesion molecule-1 (ICAM-1), a chemical that plays a central role in inflammation. Antisense drugs work at the genetic level to interrupt the process by which disease-causing proteins are produced. Proteins play a central role in virtually every aspect of human metabolism. Many human diseases are the result of inappropriate protein production or disordered protein performance. This is true of both host diseases, such as cancer, and infectious diseases, such as AIDS.

Traditional drugs are designed to interact with protein molecules throughout the body that support or cause diseases. Antisense drugs are designed to inhibit the production of disease-causing proteins. They can be designed to treat a wide range of diseases including infectious, inflammatory, and cardiovascular diseases, as well as cancer.

ISIS-2302 is being tested in a phase II trial using an enema formulation to treat subjects with ulcerative colitis. This method of administration allows potentially therapeutic amounts of the drug to be absorbed by the lining of the intestine, which is inflamed in subjects with ulcerative colitis.

ISIS-2302 is in additional phase II trials for kidney transplant and psoriasis, and is in a phase III trial for treatment of Crohn's disease.

INDICATION(S) AND RESEARCH PHASE
Crohn's Disease – Phase III
Psoriasis and Psoriatic Disorders – Phase II
Inflammatory Bowel Disease – Phase II
Kidney Transplant Surgery – Phase II

organ transplantion system
AlloMune

MANUFACTURER
BioTransplant

DESCRIPTION
AlloMune is an organ transplantation system for the creation of specific immune tolerance in solid organ transplants from human donor organs, using a novel anti-CD2 antibody/immunosuppressive monoclonal antibody (MAb). The drug is designed to re-educate the recipient's immune system to recognize the foreign tissue as "self." The AlloMune system for cancer applications is designed to attack tumor cells more aggressively than the subject's own immune defenses. Phase I/II trials are being conducted for therapy refractory lymphoma, kidney transplant surgery, and for use as an immunosuppressant.

INDICATION(S) AND RESEARCH PHASE
Immunosuppressive – Phase I/II
Kidney Transplant Surgery – Phase I/II
Lymphomas – Phase I/II

SMART Anti-CD3
unknown

MANUFACTURER
Protein Design Labs

DESCRIPTION
The SMART humanized anti-CD3 monoclonal antibody (Mab) combines, through genetic engineering, the binding site of a mouse antibody, the small part of the antibody that attaches to its target, with approximately 90% of a human antibody for treatment of autoimmune diseases and transplant rejection. Using such a small part of the mouse antibody avoids the human anti-mouse antibody (HAMA) response in which the human body produces an immune reaction against the foreign antibodies of the mouse.

This Mab is in phase I/II trials for the treatment of kidney transplant rejection, and the treatment of psoriasis and psoriatic disorders.

INDICATION(S) AND RESEARCH PHASE
Kidney Transplant Surgery – Phase I/II
Psoriasis and Psoriatic Disorders – Phase I/II

Peyronie's Disease

collagenase for injection
Cordase

MANUFACTURER
Biospecifics Technologies

DESCRIPTION
Cordase is an injectable formulation of purified collagenase, an enzyme that induces changes in collagen, causing it to degrade within the connective tissue. This drug is currently in phase II testing for treatment of Peyronie's disease and Dupuytren's disease, a contracture deformity that may cause the fingers to become stuck in a flexed position. These trials also include evaluation for treatment of adhesive capsulitis, or frozen shoulder. Cordase is considered an orphan drug since there are limited therapies for these uncommon conditions. Research is under development by Advance Biofactures, a subsidiary of Biospecifics Technologies.

INDICATION(S) AND RESEARCH PHASE
Dupuytren's Disease – Phase II
Peyronie's Disease – Phase II
Adhesive Capsulitis – Phase II

Prostate Cancer

abarelix depot, PPI-149
unknown

MANUFACTURER
Praecis Pharmaceuticals

DESCRIPTION
Approximately 85% of newly diagnosed prostate cancers are hormone-dependent tumors that require the male hormone testosterone for their continued growth. Lowering the body's normal production of testosterone, therefore, is the primary goal of hormonal treatment. However, available hormonal therapies may cause an initial surge or increase in the level of testosterone before the desired effect of lowering testosterone occurs. Abarelix depot is designed to rapidly block the production of testosterone and avoid the initial testosterone level surge. An NDA was submitted in December 2000.

Additionally, a multisite, blinded phase II/III trial of abarelix depot for the treatment of endometriosis is under way. Subject enrollment in this study is complete, with 365 subjects enrolled. Praecis is developing abarelix depot under an agreement with Amgen and Sanofi-Synthelabo.

INDICATION(S) AND RESEARCH PHASE
Prostate Cancer – NDA submitted
Endometriosis – Phase II/III

abiraterone acetate
unknown

MANUFACTURER
BTG International

DESCRIPTION
Abiraterone acetate, an approved drug in the United Kingdom, inhibits both testicular and adrenal androgen production by selective inhibition of 17 alpha-hydroxylase/C17-20 lyase, the key enzyme in the androgen biosynthetic pathway. Due to abiraterone acetate's high inhibitory potency, a phase I trial for the treatment of prostate cancer was conducted. The trial examined the effects of single or multiple doses of abiraterone acetate in chemically castrated or untreated subjects. Results indicated that the drug is a

potent inhibitor of testosterone production and can itself reduce testosterone to sub-castrate levels.

INDICATION(S) AND RESEARCH PHASE
Prostate Cancer – Phase I completed

ABT-627
unknown

MANUFACTURER
Abbott Laboratories

DESCRIPTION
ABT-627 is a drug that is being developed to halt the progression of late-stage, metastatic prostate cancer. Cancer requires the growth of blood vessels that will nourish the cancer cells as they grow and divide. If there is a limited blood supply, the cancer cells will die and the growth of the tumor will be slowed. ABT-627 acts to restrict the blood supply to newly forming cancer cells.

ABT-627 blocks the action of a potent substance in the body (endothelin-A). This substance is a strong constrictor of blood vessels that also stimulates cell proliferation. By preventing the action of endothelin-A, it is thought that blood vessel and cancer cell growth will be slowed or halted altogether. In initial trials, ABT-627 decreased the amount of a prostate protein (PSA) that is used to monitor the progression of prostate cancer therapy. Additionally, the drug decreased pain resulting from cancerous spread to the bone, and it enabled subjects to decrease their narcotic use.

This new medication has shown that it can stabilize the progression of prostate cancer for up to fifteen months and improve the quality of life of prostate cancer subjects. Phase II studies are currently under way.

INDICATION(S) AND RESEARCH PHASE
Prostate Cancer – Phase II

APC8015
Provenge

MANUFACTURER
Dendreon Corporation

DESCRIPTION
Provenge is a dendritic exvivo cell therapy being tested for the treatment of advanced prostate cancer. The aim of the therapy is to heighten the immunologic response to cancer cells by removing dendritic cells from a subject, pulsing them with a prostate cancer antigen, and reinjecting them into the subject. The dendritic cells help the immune system by attaching pieces of the tumor proteins to their own surface and presenting them to lymphocytes, which then learn to recognize the antigens as foreign matter and attack them.

Phase II trial results published in December 2000 indicated that Provenge was safe, well tolerated, and stimulated an immune response in subjects with prostate cancer. Phase III trials are under way throughout the United States.

INDICATION(S) AND RESEARCH PHASE
Prostate Cancer – Phase III

arsenic trioxide (ATO)
Trisenox

MANUFACTURER
Cell Therapeutics

DESCRIPTION
Trisenox is believed to kill cancer cells through apoptosis. The mechanism of action of Trisenox is not fully understood, but the drug appears to induce apoptosis in a different manner than other anti-cancer agents such as retinoids.

Trisenox is FDA approved to treat acute promyelocytic leukemia (APL), and it is also in numerous trials in the United States for indications including other types of leukemia, prostate cancer, multiple myeloma, renal cell cancer, cervical cancer, and bladder cancer.

INDICATION(S) AND RESEARCH PHASE
Leukemia – Phase I
Lymphoma, Non-Hodgkin's – Phase II
Leukemia – Phase II
Multiple Myeloma – Phase II
Prostate Cancer – Phase II
Renal Cell Carcinoma – Phase II
Cervical Dysplasia/Cancer – Phase II
Bladder Cancer – Phase II

bicalutimide
Casodex

MANUFACTURER
AstraZeneca

DESCRIPTION
Casodex is a non-steroidal anti-androgen for the treatment of advanced prostate cancer. Prostate cancer is known to be sensitive to androgen—it responds to treatment that counteracts the effects of androgen and/or removes the source of androgen. Data suggest that this oral hormonal medication shows no statistical difference in overall survival or time-to-progression when compared to castration in subjects with non-metastatic, locally advanced prostate cancer. The company has submitted a supplemental NDA for this indication. Casodex is given in an oral tablet form.

INDICATION(S) AND RESEARCH PHASE
Prostate Cancer – Phase sNDA submitted

CEP-2563
unknown

MANUFACTURER
Cephalon

DESCRIPTION
CEP-2563 is an orally active inhibitor of tyrosine kinase. It is currently in phase I development for the treatment of prostate cancer. Cephalon has CEP-2563 development agreements with TAP Pharmaceuticals and Abbott Laboratories.

INDICATION(S) AND RESEARCH PHASE
Prostate Cancer – Phase I

CEP-701
unknown

MANUFACTURER
Cephalon

DESCRIPTION

CEP-701 is an orally active inhibitor of the enzyme tyrosine kinase. It is being evaluated in phase II studies for prostate cancer and pancreatic ductal adenocarcinoma.

INDICATION(S) AND RESEARCH PHASE
Pancreatic Cancer – Phase II
Prostate Cancer – Phase II

CT-2584
Apra

MANUFACTURER
Cell Therapeutics

DESCRIPTION
Apra is a novel synthetic inhibitor of phosphatidic acid metabolism in tumor cells. This antineoplastic agent kills cancer cells without having to depend on cell division to exert its effect. Additionally, Apra may also help inhibit multi-drug resistance of certain cancers. The drug is in trials for the treatment of prostate cancer and sarcomas. Additional indications may include cancers of the colon, breast, and female reproductive system including the ovaries.

INDICATION(S) AND RESEARCH PHASE
Prostate Cancer – Phase II
Sarcoma – Phase II

CTP-37
Avicine

MANUFACTURER
AVI BioPharma

DESCRIPTION
Avicine is a hormone vaccine derived from human chorionic gonadotropin peptide that is being tested for prevention of colorectal, pancreatic, and prostate cancer. The drug is in phase II trials for prostate cancer, and phase III trials for colorectal and pancreatic cancer. AVI BioPharma has partnered with SuperGen and under the terms of the agreement, SuperGen will be responsible for U.S. marketing and sales of Avicine, and AVI will be responsible for product manufacturing.

INDICATION(S) AND RESEARCH PHASE
Colorectal Cancer – Phase III
Pancreatic Cancer – Phase III
Prostate Cancer – Phase II

CV706
unknown

MANUFACTURER
Calydon

DESCRIPTION
CV706 is an oncolytic virus that is able to replicate in and kill targeted cancer cells, leaving non-cancer cells unharmed. It is currently in development for the treatment of prostate cancer. In October 2000, phase I/II trial results indicated that CV706 displayed anti-tumor activity and that the drug was well tolerated. Subjects showing the greatest anti-tumor response were treated at one of the top two doses evaluated; four of these 11 subjects exhibited a prostate specific antigen (PSA) partial response, defined as a 50% or greater reduction in serum PSA for at least four weeks. In three of the subjects, their partial response lasted at least nine months. PSA levels decreased from baseline in nine of the 11 subjects (80%) treated in the top two dose groups. A study of post-treatment biopsy samples demonstrated that adenoviral replication—the mechanism upon which CV706 has been designed to both target and kill prostate cancer cells—had occurred in subjects.

INDICATION(S) AND RESEARCH PHASE
Prostate Cancer – Phase I/II completed

CV787
unknown

MANUFACTURER
Calydon

DESCRIPTION
CV787 is a genetically engineered adenovirus type-5 that is cytolytic to cells expressing prostate specific antigen (PSA). It is being evaluated in a phase I/II trial in subjects with locally recurrent prostate cancer following definitive radiotherapy and/or brachytherapy. The phase I/II trial is an open-label, dose finding study designed to determine the safety and tolerance of an injection of CV787 directly into the prostate. The trial is being conducted at six hospitals in the United States.

INDICATION(S) AND RESEARCH PHASE
Prostate Cancer – Phase I/II

cVax-Pr
unknown

MANUFACTURER
Jenner BioTherapies

DESCRIPTION
cVax-Pr is a vaccine designed from DNA pieces from a protein (prostate-specific antigen, PSA) found in both healthy and cancerous prostate cancer cells. Scientists add molecules to this DNA that stimulate the body's immune system. In this manner, the body is manipulated into recognizing PSA-DNA as foreign material. Consequently, this immune response attacks both normal and cancerous prostate cells.

In preliminary studies, administration of cVax-Pr stimulated antibody and white blood cell production. cVax-Pr is being tested in phase II trials.

INDICATION(S) AND RESEARCH PHASE
Prostate Cancer – Phase II

doxorubicin HCl
Doxil, Caelyx

MANUFACTURER
Alza (Sequus Pharmaceuticals)

DESCRIPTION
Doxil is a liposomal formulation of doxorubicin hydrochloride, an intravenous chemotherapy agent. This anthracycline anti-tumor agent is currently on the market for the treatment of Kaposi's sarcoma. The drug uses a novel, targeted delivery system to help evade recognition and uptake by the immune system so that the liposomes can circulate in the body longer. A long circulation time increases the likelihood that the liposomes and their pharmaceutical con-

tents will reach their targeted tumor site. Doxil may act through its ability to bind DNA and inhibit nucleic acid synthesis.

Doxil is being tested in trials for the treatment of breast, liver, lung, and prostate cancers, as well as for unspecified cancers and tumors.

Alza markets this product in the United States under the tradename Doxil; however, it is marketed under the name Caelyx in other areas. Schering-Plough has exclusive international marketing rights to Caelyx, excluding Japan and Israel, through a distribution agreement with Alza.

INDICATION(S) AND RESEARCH PHASE
Breast Cancer – Phase II/III
Liver Cancer – Phase II/III
Lung Cancer – Phase II/III
Prostate Cancer – Phase II/III
Cancer/Tumors (Unspecified) – Phase II

DPPE
unknown

MANUFACTURER
Bristol-Myers Squibb

DESCRIPTION
DPPE is being developed to potentiate the effects of chemotherapy in subjects with late-stage prostate cancer. There are many substances in the body that play a role in the regulation of cell growth. When there is an imbalance or problem with one of these regulatory substances, uncontrolled cell growth or cancer may result.

An example of one such substance is histamine, which acts as a growth factor in both normal and cancer cells. It spurs cell growth by stimulating growth receptors located within the cell.

DPPE is a drug designed to block these receptors for histamine. By blocking the effects of histamine, it is proposed that unregulated cell growth will decrease. When given with standard chemotherapy agents, DPPE may help these agents better destroy cancer cells.

INDICATION(S) AND RESEARCH PHASE
Prostate Cancer – Phase II

eflornithine, DFMO (difluoromethylornydil)
unknown

MANUFACTURER
Aventis

DESCRIPTION
Eflornithine is a potent, irreversible inhibitor of ornithine decarboxylase (OCD), an enzyme that is elevated in most tumors and pre-malignant lesions. Eflornithine is currently in a phase III clinical trial to determine the effectiveness of the drug in treating subjects who have newly diagnosed or recurrent bladder cancer. The drug is administered orally in tablet form.

Eflornithine is also in trials for the prevention and treatment of HIV infections, skin cancer, breast cancer, prostate cancer, and cervical dysplasia/cancer.

INDICATION(S) AND RESEARCH PHASE
Bladder Cancer – Phase III
Breast Cancer – Phase II/III
Cervical Dysplasia/Cancer – Phase II
HIV Infection – Phase II
Prostate Cancer – Phase II
Skin Cancer – Phase III

exisulind
Aptosyn/LHRH agonist

MANUFACTURER
Cell Pathways

DESCRIPTION
Aptosyn (exisulind) belongs to a novel class of compounds called selective apoptotic anti-neoplastic drugs (SAANDs). SAANDs inhibit a form of cyclic GMP phosphodiesterase and selectively induce apoptosis in abnormally growing precancerous and cancerous cells. Aptosyn is being tested with LHRH agonist hormone therapy for the treatment of prostate cancer. The objective of this study is to determine the preliminary efficacy of Aptosyn in subjects who are receiving LHRH agonist hormone therapy and have rising prostate specific antigen (PSA) levels. This open-label, 12-month phase II trial will include 15 subjects.

INDICATION(S) AND RESEARCH PHASE
Prostate Cancer – Phase II

exisulind
Aptosyn

MANUFACTURER
Cell Pathways

DESCRIPTION
Aptosyn (exisulind) belongs to a novel class of compounds called selective apoptotic anti-neoplastic drugs (SAANDs). SAANDs inhibit a form of cyclic GMP phosphodiesterase and selectively induce apoptosis in abnormally growing precancerous and cancerous cells. Aptosyn is being tested for several indications and is in five different trials for adenomatous polyposis coli (APC) and familial adenomatous polyposis coli; two of these trials are specifically for pediatric subjects.

The company received a non-approvable letter from the FDA in September 2000 for one of the trials for familial adenomatous polyposis. The company intends to amend the NDA and request a meeting to address the deficiencies and the possible requirement for additional clinical data.

Additionally, Aptosyn is being tested in trials for the treatment of prostate cancer, lung cancer, breast cancer, sporadic colonic polyps, and Barrett's esophagus disease.

INDICATION(S) AND RESEARCH PHASE
Adenomatous Polyposis Coli – Phase Non-approvable letter
Pediatric, Familial Adenomatous Polyposis Coli – Phase II
Adenomatous Polyposis Coli – Phase I/II
Barrett's Esophagus Disease – Phase II
Prostate Cancer – Phase II/III
Breast Cancer – Phase II/III
Lung Cancer – Phase Ib
Colon Polyps – Phase II/III

exisulind/docetaxel
Aposyn/Taxotere

MANUFACTURER
Cell Pathways

DESCRIPTION

Aptosyn (exisulind) belongs to a novel class of compounds called selective apoptotic anti-neoplastic drugs (SAANDs). SAANDs inhibit a form of cyclic GMP phosphodiesterase and selectively induce apoptosis in abnormally growing precancerous and cancerous cells. Because SAANDs do not induce apoptosis in normal cells, they do not produce the serious side effects normally associated with traditional chemotherapeutic agents. They also do not inhibit cyclooxygenase (COX I or COX II) and have not exhibited the gastric and renal toxicities associated with non-steroidal anti-inflammatory drugs (NSAIDs), including the COX II inhibitors.

Aptosyn is being tested with Rhone-Poulenc Rorer's Taxotere for the treatment of prostate, lung, and breast cancer as well as for solid tumors. Both companies will jointly share the cost of the trials and will retain all marketing rights to its respective products.

INDICATION(S) AND RESEARCH PHASE
Prostate Cancer – Phase I/II
Breast Cancer – Phase I/II
Lung Cancer – Phase I/II
Lung Cancer – Phase III
Cancer/Tumors (Unspecified) – Phase I

FK-317
unknown

MANUFACTURER
Fujisawa Healthcare

DESCRIPTION
Fujisawa has developed a new anti-cancer medication, FK-317, that originally was developed as an antibiotic. The molecule, known as a dihydrobenzoxazine, underwent preliminary testing in thirty-one subjects with solid tumors that were refractory to other chemotherapeutic treatments. The company reported that tumor reduction was observed in four subjects, two of whom achieved complete remission. Side effects and other toxicities such as leukopenia (decreased white blood cells) and neutropenia were modest in comparison to other established treatments.

It is unclear how exactly this compound works to limit the growth of cancer, but it seems to influence the process by which cells reproduce themselves. Currently, FK-317 is given at a dose of 24 mg/day intravenously and it is being evaluated in phase II trials. Scientists are testing it in a variety of solid tumors such as prostate, breast, and skin cancer.

INDICATION(S) AND RESEARCH PHASE
Breast Cancer – Phase II
Cancer/Tumors (Unspecified) – Phase II
Prostate Cancer – Phase II
Skin Cancer – Phase II

G3139/mitoxantrone
Genasense/mitoxantrone

MANUFACTURER
Genta

DESCRIPTION
Genasense (G3139) is designed to reduce levels of Bcl-2, a protein that contributes to the resistance of cancer cells to current forms of cancer treatment. Treatment with Genasense may markedly improve the effectiveness of standard anticancer therapies; it is being tested in combination with mitoxantrone for treatment of prostate and colorectal cancers.

INDICATION(S) AND RESEARCH PHASE
Colorectal Cancer – Phase II
Prostate Cancer – Phase I/II

G3139/docetaxel
Genasense/Taxotere

MANUFACTURER
Genta

DESCRIPTION
Genasense (G3139) attacks Bcl-2, a protein that is over-expressed in many forms of cancer. Bcl-2 appears to contribute to the resistance of these diseases to standard treatment. Genta is using its proprietary antisense approach to first decrease the expression of Bcl-2, and then to administer state-of-the-art anticancer therapy in an effort to improve subject outcome. Genasense in combination with docetaxel is in trials for treatment of breast and prostate cancer.

INDICATION(S) AND RESEARCH PHASE
Breast Cancer – Phase I/II
Prostate Cancer – Phase II

G3139/androgen blockade
Genasense/androgen blockade

MANUFACTURER
Genta

DESCRIPTION
Genasense (G3139) is designed to reduce levels of Bcl-2, a protein that contributes to the resistance of cancer cells to current forms of cancer treatment. Genasense in combination with androgen blockade is in phase I/II trials for the treatment of androgen-insensitive metastatic prostate cancer.

INDICATION(S) AND RESEARCH PHASE
Prostate Cancer – Phase I/II

GBC-590
unknown

MANUFACTURER
Safe Sciences

DESCRIPTION
GBC-590 belongs to a new class of drugs called lectin inhibitors that specifically interfere with cellular interactions. GBC-590 competitively binds to unique lectins (special protein cell-surface receptors) on cancer cells and disrupts the metastatic process. GBC-590's affinity for cancer lectins is the core reason for its significant biological activity and specificity.

GBC-590 is being tested in phase II studies for pancreatic and colorectal cancer, and the company plans to test it in phase II trials for prostate cancer.

INDICATION(S) AND RESEARCH PHASE
Colorectal Cancer – Phase II
Pancreatic Cancer – Phase II
Prostate Cancer – Phase I/II

gallium maltolate
unknown

MANUFACTURER
Titan Pharmaceuticals

DESCRIPTION
Gallium is a semi-metallic element that has shown some therapeutic activity in metabolic bone disease, hypercalcemia of malignancy, and cancer. Gallium maltolate can displace divalent iron from the iron transporting protein, transferrin; thus gallium maltolate causes interference with iron metabolism with inhibition of enzymes requiring divalent iron. The most important of these in the cancer setting appears to be ribonucleotide reductase (RNR). Additionally, gallium appears to form salts with calcium and phosphate and become incorporated into bone. The bone that is created with incorporated gallium appears to be at least as strong as normal bone, and it appears to be more resistant to degradation by osteoclasts and tumor cells.

INDICATION(S) AND RESEARCH PHASE
Prostate Cancer – Phase I/II
Lymphomas – Phase I/II
Myeloma – Phase I/II
Bladder Cancer – Phase I/II
HIV Infection – Phase I/II

IM862
unknown

MANUFACTURER
Cytran

DESCRIPTION
IM862 is a small peptide comprised of two amino acids that may inhibit new blood vessel formation (angiogenesis). When there is excessive growth of new blood vessels, a number of pathological conditions result, including malignant tumors, age-related macular degeneration, and vascular diseases. Limiting the growth of new blood vessels in tumors deprives them of nourishment and can ultimately kill these cancers. This drug is being developed in phase III trials for Kaposi's sarcoma and phase I/II trials for ovarian cancer.

INDICATION(S) AND RESEARCH PHASE
Kaposi's Sarcoma – Phase III
Ovarian Cancer – Phase I/II
Malignant Melanoma – Preclinical
Prostate Cancer – Preclinical

IMC-C225, CPT-11
unknown

MANUFACTURER
ImClone Systems

DESCRIPTION
IMC-C225 is a chimerized (part mouse, part human) monoclonal antibody that may help fight cancer cells when used in conjunction with radiation therapy or other chemotherapy agents. This antibody selectively blocks the epidermal growth factor receptor (EGFr), which may be present in greater amounts on actively growing tumor cells. Since many cancers use specific growth factors to stimulate tumor cell growth, blocking this receptor may inhibit the cancer from increasing in size and spreading throughout the body.

The company is conducting phase III clinical trials evaluating IMC-C225 in combination with radiotherapy and with chemotherapy in subjects with advanced squamous cell head and neck carcinoma. IMC-C225 is in trials for several other indications in combination with various anticancer agents.

INDICATION(S) AND RESEARCH PHASE
Breast Cancer – Phase I/II
Head and Neck Cancer – Phase III
Lung Cancer – Phase III
Prostate Cancer – Phase I/II
Renal Cell Carcinoma – Phase II
Pancreatic Cancer – Phase II
Colorectal Cancer – Phase II

INGN-201, adenoviral p53
unknown

MANUFACTURER
Introgen Therapeutics

DESCRIPTION
INGN-201 is a p53 gene therapy product. It has been tested as a treatment for a variety of solid tumor cancers with administration via intratumoral injection. The drug was well tolerated according to the company, and additional trials are under way using an intravenous infusion in order to reach more types of cancers. The tumor-suppressing p53 gene encodes a protein that responds to damage involving cellular DNA by terminating cell division. Normal p53 genes are delivered into cancer cells of the subject through an adenoviral vector.

The developers of INGN-201 have signed a Cooperative Research and Development Agreement (CRADA) with the National Cancer Institute to evaluate the potential effectiveness and superiority of the drug over other treatments against breast, ovarian, bladder, prostate, and brain cancers in phase I and phase II trials. A phase III trial in head and neck cancer was initiated in March 2000.

INDICATION(S) AND RESEARCH PHASE
Head and Neck Cancer – Phase III
Bladder Cancer – Phase I
Brain Cancer – Phase I
Breast Cancer – Phase I
Bronchoalveolar Cancer – Phase I
Ovarian Cancer – Phase I
Prostate Cancer – Phase I
Lung Cancer – Phase II
Cancer/Tumors (Unspecified) – Phase I

interleukin (IL)
MultiKine

MANUFACTURER
CEL-SCI Corporation

DESCRIPTION
MultiKine is a multiple combination therapy made from a natural, cytokine cocktail (which includes interleukin-2 (IL-2), IL-β, TNF-α, Gm-CSF and an IFN-γ/immunomodulator). It is being tested for the treatment of advanced head and neck cancer in subjects who have previously failed standard therapy, and for head and neck cancer treatment prior to surgery.

MultiKine has just completed two phase II

trials for head and neck cancer. The first trial consisted of 16 subjects and tested four different doses of MultiKine in four subjects each. To qualify for the trial, the subjects must have had a recurrence of the cancer and failed conventional therapy.

The company reported that in an earlier and still ongoing study conducted in newly diagnosed head and neck cancer subjects, 10 subjects had tumor reductions prior to surgery within a short time period. Three of ten subjects had tumor reductions exceeding 50%, and one additional subject with a tumor that was nearly three inches in diameter had a complete clinical response. Lastly, two subjects refused surgery because they were satisfied with their condition after treatment with MultiKine.

INDICATION(S) AND RESEARCH PHASE
Head and Neck Cancer – Phase II
HIV Infection – Phase II
Breast Cancer – Phase I
Prostate Cancer – Phase I/II

ISIS-5132, CGP-69846A
unknown

MANUFACTURER
Isis Pharmaceuticals

DESCRIPTION
ISIS-5132 is a potent antisense inhibitor of the enzyme cRaf-1 kinase. Antisense drugs inhibit the production of disease-causing proteins by altering the genetic information that messenger RNA uses to produce new protein. cRaf kinase plays a role in signal processes that regulate cell growth and proliferation. It is one of a family of Raf genes thought to play an important role in the development of some solid tumors. The company reports that activated-Raf has also been detected in a substantial variety of human cancers including small cell lung carcinoma and breast cancer. For example, it has been reported that 60% of all lung carcinoma cells express unusually high levels of normal cRaf mRNA and protein.

The sponsor companies reported that results from phase I studies, which examined subjects with a wide variety of solid tumors, demonstrated that the drug was well tolerated and that several subjects experienced disease stabilization. The companies are planning additional phase I safety studies involving the drug in combination with currently approved chemotherapies. Phase II clinical trials examining ISIS-5132 as a single agent therapy in subjects with breast, lung, colon, pancreatic, and prostate cancers are under way.

INDICATION(S) AND RESEARCH PHASE
Breast Cancer – Phase II
Cancer/Tumors (Unspecified) – Phase II
Colon Malignancies – Phase II
Lung Cancer – Phase II
Pancreatic Cancer – Phase II
Prostate Cancer – Phase II

LDI-200
unknown

MANUFACTURER
Milkhaus Laboratory

DESCRIPTION
Clinical trials are testing a subcutanous formulation of LDI-200 for at least three indications: leukemia, myelodysplastic syndrome, and prostate cancer. Results demonstrated that LDI-200 showed both efficacy and safety in a small phase II/III open label crossover trial in subjects with myelodysplastic syndrome. The control consisted of subjects given supportive therapy, consisting of transfusions and antibiotics, who became eligible for treatment if their disease progressed more rapidly than anticipated. A total of 23 subjects were treated using LDI-200, and seven showed significant clinical response.

INDICATION(S) AND RESEARCH PHASE
Leukemia – Phase II completed
Prostate Cancer – Phase II/III
White Blood Cell Disorders – Phase II/III
Myelodysplastic Syndrome – Phase III completed

leuprolide acetate
30-day Leuprogel

MANUFACTURER
Atrix Laboratories

DESCRIPTION
30-day Leuprogel is a new Atrigel formulation that contains leuprolide acetate. The product is injected subcutaneously as a liquid, where it solidifies and releases a predetermined amount of leuprolide. The sustained levels of leuprolide result in decreased testosterone levels, which in turn suppress tumor growth in subjects with hormone-responsive prostate cancer. Leuprogel has an advantage over current treatments due to its delivery by subcutaneous injection and small volume (compared to commonly used large volume intramuscular injection).

INDICATION(S) AND RESEARCH PHASE
Prostate Cancer – NDA submitted

leuprolide acetate
3-month Leuprogel

MANUFACTURER
Atrix Laboratories

DESCRIPTION
Atrix recently announced the early completion of enrollment for a Leuprogel 3-month 22.5 mg phase III trial. This drug is in development for the treatment of prostate cancer.

INDICATION(S) AND RESEARCH PHASE
Prostate Cancer – Phase III

liposomal ether lipid
TLC ELL-12

MANUFACTURER
The Liposome Company

DESCRIPTION
TLC ELL-12 is a liposomal ether lipid that may have efficacy in the treatment of several cancers. This drug has exhibited significant anti-tumor activity, but did not have the hemolytic side effects common to this type of ether lipid when therapeutic doses were used in experimental models. It does not appear to be myelosuppressive.

TLC ELL-12 is currently being developed

in phase I trials for the treatment of lung cancer, multiple myeloma, leukemia, and prostate cancer.

INDICATION(S) AND RESEARCH PHASE
Lung Cancer – Phase I
Multiple Myeloma – Phase I
Leukemia – Phase I
Prostate Cancer – Phase I

MDX-210
unknown

MANUFACTURER
Medarex

DESCRIPTION
MDX-210 is a bispecific (target-trigger) monoclonal antibody (MAb)-based treatment being developed for cancers with specific markers (HER-2/*neu* positive), including renal cell, non-small cell lung, pancreatic, and prostate cancer. Phase II trials have been completed for kidney, prostate, and ovarian cancer. Phase III trials for ovarian cancer have commenced in Europe.

INDICATION(S) AND RESEARCH PHASE
Prostate Cancer – Phase II completed
Renal Cell Carcinoma – Phase II completed
Colon Malignancies – Phase II
Breast Cancer – Phase II
Gastric Cancer – Phase II
Pancreatic Cancer – Phase II
Lung Cancer – Phase II
Ovarian Cancer – Phase III

MDX-220
unknown

MANUFACTURER
Medarex

DESCRIPTION
MDX-220 is a bispecific (target-trigger) monoclonal antibody (MAb) that targets Tag-72 in the treatment of a variety of cancers, including lung, colon, prostate, ovarian, endometrial, pancreatic, and gastric cancer.

INDICATION(S) AND RESEARCH PHASE
Endometrial Cancer – Phase I/II
Gastric Cancer – Phase I/II
Lung Cancer – Phase I/II
Ovarian Cancer – Phase I/II
Pancreatic Cancer – Phase I/II
Prostate Cancer – Phase II
Colorectal Cancer – Phase II

MGI-114, hydroxymethylacylfulvene, HMAF
Irofulven

MANUFACTURER
MGI Pharma

DESCRIPTION
Irofulven (MGI-114) is the first product candidate being developed by MGI Pharma from its family of anti-cancer compounds called acylfulvenes. Early trials demonstrated that Irofulven is absorbed rapidly by tumor cells, and once inside binds to DNA and protein targets. The binding interferes with DNA replication and cell division, leading to tumor-specific cell death. The drug is being tested in a series of trials for a variety of cancers.

In November 2000, results from a phase II trial of Irofulven indicated that the drug produced anti-tumor activity in subjects with advanced pancreatic cancer who were refractory to gemcitabine (Gemzar). Ten of the 53 subjects enrolled achieved six-month survival and two subjects demonstrated objective responses: one subject experienced tumor shrinkage of 100% and another subject experienced an 84% decrease in tumor mass. A phase III trial was initiated in February 2001.

INDICATION(S) AND RESEARCH PHASE
Breast Cancer – Phase II
Colon Malignancies – Phase II
Renal Cell Carcinoma – Phase II
Cervical Dysplasia/Cancer – Phase II
Lung Cancer – Phase II
Ovarian Cancer – Phase I/II
Colorectal Cancer – Phase II
Prostate Cancer – Phase I/II
Cancer/Tumors (Unspecified) – Phase I/II
Pancreatic Cancer – Phase III
Liver Cancer – Phase II

phenoxodiol
unknown

MANUFACTURER
Novogen

DESCRIPTION
Phenoxodiol is a novel, cytotoxic, anit-cancer drug that arrests cancer cell growth and restores apoptosis. It acts through a variety of mechanisms including the inhibition of a number of cellular enzyme systems, including topoiosomerase II and protein tyrosine kinases, which are integral to the development of cancer. Inhibiting these enzyme systems is recognized as a key factor in preventing the growth of cancerous cells. Additionally, the novelty of phenoxodiol lies in its ability to combine a high degree of potency with no known adverse effects on normal cells. Phenoxodiol also possesses a number of other anti-cancer mechanisms that appear to contribute to the overall anti-cancer effect.

Phenoxodiol is currently undergoing a phase Ib trial in an Australian hospital in subjects with solid malignant tumors, including prostate cancer. This study, which commenced in the final quarter of 2000, is investigating the safety and anti-cancer efficacy of phenoxodiol when injected intravenously once weekly for 12 weeks.

Novogen has received approval to commence a second phase Ib trial, which will be conducted at a major Sydney teaching hospital. This new study will measure the safety and anti-cancer effectiveness of phenoxodiol when administered by continuous intravenous infusion over seven days. The study will involve subjects with solid cancers whose cancers have become unresponsive to standard treatment.

INDICATION(S) AND RESEARCH PHASE
Cancer/Tumors (Unspecified) – Phase Ib
Prostate Cancer – Phase Ib

p53 gene therapy
unknown

MANUFACTURER
Aventis

DESCRIPTION
Aventis' p53 gene therapy is an anti-cancer treatment that produces an increased expression of the p53 protein. The p53 protein has the ability to activate other proteins to stop the cell cycle until damage to the cell may be repaired. Additionally, the p53 protein may stop growth in response to additional stimuli, such as reduced nutritional resources or high cell density.

According to scientists, the p53 gene is one of the most frequently altered genes in human cancer, with 50% of all cancers having distorted forms of p53. This p53 gene therapy is delivered by an intraprostatic injection that may result in the suppression of prostate cancer growth. It is currently being tested in a phase I/II trial. Additionally, p53 gene therapy is being tested in phase III trials for head and neck cancer.

INDICATION(S) AND RESEARCH PHASE
Prostate Cancer – Phase I/II
Head and Neck Cancer – Phase III

PSMA – P1/P2
unknown

MANUFACTURER
Northwest Biotherapeutics

DESCRIPTION
Prostate specific membrane antigen (PSMA) is a substance found on a high proportion of prostate cancer cells. PSMA – P1/P2 is in phase I development.

INDICATION(S) AND RESEARCH PHASE
Prostate Cancer – Phase I

samarium Sm 153 lexidronam pentasodium
Quadramet

MANUFACTURER
Cytogen Corporation

DESCRIPTION
Quadramet is a radiopharmaceutical agent containing the radioisotope samarium-153. It is currently in phase II development for the treatment of prostate cancer that has metastasized.

INDICATION(S) AND RESEARCH PHASE
Prostate Cancer – Phase II

SGN-15/Taxotere
unknown

MANUFACTURER
Seattle Genetics

DESCRIPTION
SGN-15 is an antibody drug conjugate composed of the chimeric monoclonal antibody BR96 chemically linked to the drug doxorubicin with an average of eight drug molecules per each mAb molecule. SGN-15 works by binding to a cell surface Ley-related antigen expressed on many tumor types, rapidly internalizing, and then releasing its payload of drug at the low pH present within the cell through acid catalyzed hydrolysis in the endosome. This mechanism of targeted drug delivery allows for relative sparing of tissues normally affected by non-specific chemotherapy, and represents an attractive strategy for the treatment of tumors expressing the BR96 antigen.

SGN-15 is being tested in a combination therapy with Aventis' drug Taxotere in a phase I/II trial in subjects with breast or colon cancer. This trial is being co-funded by Aventis. Additionally, a phase II trial is testing SGN/Taxotere in hormone refractory prostate cancer.

INDICATION(S) AND RESEARCH PHASE
Breast Cancer – Phase I/II
Prostate Cancer – Phase II
Colon Malignancies – Phase I/II

SPD 424
unknown

MANUFACTURER
Shire Pharmaceuticals

DESCRIPTION
SPD 424 (previously RL0903) is a subcutaneous implant that contains a gonadotropin releasing hormone (GnRH) agonist for the treatment of prostate cancer. The hydrogel implant delivers therapeutic agents at a controlled constant release for over one year. Phase III trials are under way.

INDICATION(S) AND RESEARCH PHASE
Prostate Cancer – Phase III

SR-48692
unknown

MANUFACTURER
Sanofi-Synthelabo Pharmaceuticals

DESCRIPTION
SR-48692 is an orally formulated neurotensin antagonist being tested for several indications, including colon cancer, prostate cancer and schizophrenia.

INDICATION(S) AND RESEARCH PHASE
Colon Malignancies – Phase II
Prostate Cancer – Phase II
Schizophrenia and Schizoaffective Disorders – Phase IIa
Psychosis – Phase IIa
Depression – Phase II

strontium-89 chloride injection
Metastron

MANUFACTURER
Nycomed Amersham Imaging

DESCRIPTION
Metastron is an injectable radiopharmaceutical currently indicated for the relief of bone pain in subjects with painful skeletal metastases. Results of a phase II trial demonstrated that subjects with advanced prostate cancer treated with bone-targeted therapy consisting of Metastron in combination with chemotherapy survived longer than those who did not receive the Metastron therapy.

INDICATION(S) AND RESEARCH PHASE
Prostate Cancer – Phase II completed

SU-101
unknown

MANUFACTURER
Sugen

DESCRIPTION
SU-101 is a synthetic, platelet-derived growth factor receptor, which blocks the essential enzyme tyrosine kinase. This drug may be helpful for the treatment of end-stage malignant glioma, a tumor of nerve tissue. The drug is being tested in phase III trials for refractory brain and prostate cancers, and phase II studies for non-small cell lung and ovarian cancers.

INDICATION(S) AND RESEARCH PHASE
Brain Cancer – Phase III
Prostate Cancer – Phase III
Lung Cancer – Phase II
Ovarian Cancer – Phase II

---

tretinoin
Atragen

MANUFACTURER
Aronex Pharmaceuticals

DESCRIPTION
Atragen is a liposomal, intravenous formulation of tretinoin or all-trans retinoic acid. Tretinoin induces cell differentiation in rapidly proliferating cells, such as those observed in malignant diseases. Additionally, Atragen appears to affect the cellular signaling mechanisms that become unbalanced in cancer cells. Results of a phase II trial of Atragen monotherapy for acute promyelocytic leukemia (APL) indicated its potential to induce complete remission. The trial was conducted in Peru, and included 16 subjects with newly-diagnosed or previously-untreated APL who were treated with Atragen every other day as a single agent for a maximum of 28 doses. Fourteen subjects (87.5%) achieved morphologic remission, and 28.6% of these subjects also attained molecular remission. The safety profile observed in the subject population is similar to that reported with the currently approved oral formulation of Atra.

In addition to investigating the safety and efficacy of Atragen as a treatment for APL, the company is conducting trials to evaluate the compound for the treatment of non-Hodgkin's lymphoma, hormone-resistant prostate cancer, acute myelogenous leukemia (AML), and renal cell carcinoma in combination with interferon alpha.

In January 2001, Aronex announced that the FDA has denied approval of the company's NDA for Atragen as a treatment for subjects with APL, for whom therapy with tretinoin (all-trans-retinoic acid or Atra) is necessary but for whom an intravenous administration is required.

INDICATION(S) AND RESEARCH PHASE
Lymphoma, Non-Hodgkin's – Phase II
Prostate Cancer – Phase II
Renal Cell Carcinoma – Phase I/II
Leukemia, APL (Intravenous) – NDA denied
Leukemia, APL (Monotherapy) – Phase II
Leukemia, AML – Phase II

---

troxacitabine, BCH-4556
Troxatyl

MANUFACTURER
BioChem Pharma

DESCRIPTION
Troxatyl is a dioxolane nucleoside analog being investigated as an anticancer agent. The drug is a complete DNA chain terminator and DNA polymerase inhibitor. It acts by incorporating itself into the growing DNA chain of cancer cells, interfering with their ability to replicate further. Troxatyl is being evaluated as a single agent or in combination therapy in a number of ongoing trials in hematologic malignancies, including acute myeloid leukemia and chronic myeloid leukemia (blastic phase), and in lymphoproliferative disorders such as lymphoma, chronic lymphocytic leukemia, and myeloma. It is also being evaluated as a single agent in pancreatic cancer and in combination therapy in a number of solid tumors. Troxatyl is currently in phase II development.

INDICATION(S) AND RESEARCH PHASE
Cancer/Tumors (Unspecified) – Phase II
Colorectal Cancer – Phase II
Head and Neck Cancer – Phase II
Leukemia – Phase II
Lung Cancer – Phase II
Malignant Melanoma – Phase II
Ovarian Cancer – Phase II
Pancreatic Cancer – Phase II
Prostate Cancer – Phase II
Renal Cell Carcinoma – Phase II

---

unknown
Prinomastat

MANUFACTURER
Agouron Pharmaceuticals

DESCRIPTION
Prinomastat is an orally active, synthetic molecule designed to potently and selectively inhibit certain members of a family of enzymes known as a matrix metalloproteases, which are believed to be involved in tumor angiogenesis, invasion, and metastasis. The drug is in trials for various indications, including osteoarthritis, brain cancer, and macular degeneration.

Two phase III trials for advanced non-small cell lung cancer and prostate cancer were halted in August 2000 due to the drug's lack of effectiveness in subjects with late-stage disease.

The most common side effects of Prinomastat have been observed in the joints, and include stiffness, joint swelling, and in a few subjects, some limits on the mobility of certain joints, most often in the shoulders and hands. All these effects were reported to be reversible and were effectively managed by treatment rests and dose reductions.

INDICATION(S) AND RESEARCH PHASE
Lung Cancer – Phase III halted
Prostate Cancer – Phase III halted
Osteoarthritis – Phase II
Brain Cancer – Phase II
Macular Degeneration – Phase II

---

unknown
CyPat

MANUFACTURER
Barr Laboratories

DESCRIPTION

CyPat is a prostate cancer therapy in a phase III clinical trial. The trial is expected to include over 1,000 subjects and more than 40 sites. The drug is expected to be indicated for the treatment of hot flashes experienced by prostate cancer subjects with surgical or chemical castration.

INDICATION(S) AND RESEARCH PHASE
Prostate Cancer – Phase III

---

unknown
Leuvectin

MANUFACTURER
Vical

DESCRIPTION
The active ingredient in the DNA-based drug Leuvectin is a gene encoding interleukin-2 (IL-2), a naturally occurring protein that stimulates the immune system. Administration occurs by direct injection into a tumor, leading to uptake by the tumor cells and subsequent expression of the IL-2 protein. The company anticipates that local expression of IL-2 by cancer cells may stimulate the subject's immune system to attack and destroy the tumor cells. Leuvectin is being evaluated in phase II trials in subjects with kidney and prostate cancer.

INDICATION(S) AND RESEARCH PHASE
Renal Cell Carcinoma – Phase II
Prostate Cancer – Phase II

---

unknown
Abetafen

MANUFACTURER
Bioenvision

DESCRIPTION
Abetafen is a derivative of Modrefen, the company's marketed drug for breast cancer. Modrefen acts on the second estrogen receptor, which may be present in breast cancer and prostate cancer cells. This estrogen receptor is known to play some part in controlling normal prostate growth and may also influence growth of prostate cancer. New trials are under way to test effects of the drug on ERb in prostate cancer. Preclinical tests have shown that Modrefen decreases prostate growth in animals and modulates ligand binding to ERb in prostate cancer cell lines. Abetafen is currently in phase II trials for prostate cancer.

INDICATION(S) AND RESEARCH PHASE
Prostate Cancer – Phase II

---

unknown
Norelin

MANUFACTURER
YM Biosciences

DESCRIPTION
Norelin is an immunopharmaceutical product based on a proprietary recombinant antigen. It utilizes the subject's immune system to stimulate the development of antibodies to gonadotropin-releasing hormone (GnRH). The antibodies block the action of GnRH, which has therapeutic benefits for certain hormone-dependent cancers, such as prostate, breast, ovarian and uterine cancer. The cancer vaccine has been shown to induce an immune response to GnRH in preclinical models, and a significant antitumor effect has been demonstrated.

A formulation with an aluminum-salt based adjuvant was shown to be safe in a phase I/II trial in subjects with hormone-sensitive prostate cancer; however, this formulation did not elicit a satisfactory immune response to GnRH. The company is in the process of commencing immunogenicity studies and testing a variety of formulations, following which it intends to resume clinical testing—phase I/II trials are expected in 2001 for the treatment of prostate cancer.

INDICATION(S) AND RESEARCH PHASE
Prostate Cancer – Phase I/II

---

unknown
Combidex

MANUFACTURER
Advanced Magnetics

DESCRIPTION
Combidex MRI contrast agent was developed to help in the detection, diagnosis, and staging of various cancers. The first indication is for the diagnosis of metastatic cancer to assist in directing biopsy and surgery as well as to aid in the staging of a variety of cancers, including breast and prostate cancer. In clinical studies, Combidex significantly reduced the number of false diagnoses (both false positive and false negative nodes) compared to unenhanced MRI exams. The second indication is for the detection, diagnosis, and characterization of benign versus malignant lesions of the liver and spleen.

In phase III clinical trials, post-Combidex MRI showed clear differentiation between normal and metastatic lymph nodes, while a post-gadolinium image showed no differentiation in normal and metastatic nodes when compared with pre-dose images.

INDICATION(S) AND RESEARCH PHASE
Breast Cancer – Phase III/IV
Liver Cancer – Phase III
Prostate Cancer – Phase III/IV

---

unknown
Tesmilifene

MANUFACTURER
YM Biosciences

DESCRIPTION
Tesmilifene is an intracellular histamine antagonist being developed as a chemopotentiator for the treatment of malignant solid tumors. The compound is cytotoxic to tumor cells and cytoprotective to the gut and normal bone marrow progenitor cells. Studies have indicated its ability to augment the invivo anti-tumor activity of cytotoxic drugs routinely used in the treatment of cancer, such as doxorubicin, cyclophosphamide, 5-fluorouracil (5-FU), cisplatin, and mitoxantrone.

Interim analysis of data from a North American phase II pilot study in hormone refractory metastatic prostate cancer has shown promising results. The company hopes to conclude this phase II trial in 2001 and initiate a randomized pivotal study.

INDICATION(S) AND RESEARCH PHASE
Prostate Cancer – Phase II

---

unknown
GnRH Pharmaccine

MANUFACTURER
Aphton Corporation

DESCRIPTION
Aphton's novel GnRH Pharmaccine is an anti-gonadotropin releasing hormone (GnRH) immunogen, which neutralizes the hormone GnRH. Study results indicate that it induces and maintains castration levels of testosterone and reduced levels of prostate-specific antigen (PSA). Chemical castration of this type is a standard therapy to extend the survival of subjects with advanced prostate cancer. GnRH Pharmaccine is also involved in trials for breast cancer, endometrial cancer, and endometriosis, in addition to prostate cancer.

INDICATION(S) AND RESEARCH PHASE
Prostate Cancer – Phase I/II
Breast Cancer – Phase I/II
Endometrial Cancer – Phase I/II
Endometriosis – Phase I/II

---

unknown
Leuplin 3M DPS

MANUFACTURER
Takeda Chemical Industries

DESCRIPTION
Leuplin 3M DPS is a luteinizing hormone releasing factor being developed for the treatment of prostate cancer. It is currently in phase II trials in Japan.

INDICATION(S) AND RESEARCH PHASE
Prostate Cancer – Phase II

---

unknown
Apomine

MANUFACTURER
ILEX Oncology

DESCRIPTION
Apomine is a potent, orally active bisphosphonate estrogen derivative being developed to treat prostate cancer. Apomine induces apoptosis, which is a normal biological process involving a genetically programmed series of events that leads to cell death. Apomine activates the farnesoid X receptor (FXR) and a cascade of biological signals within the cell that rapidly induces apoptosis without affecting normal cells.

Apomine is being tested in phase II clinical trials in Lyon, France. It is currently being developed by ILEX and Symphar S.A. of Geneva, Switzerland.

INDICATION(S) AND RESEARCH PHASE
Prostate Cancer – Phase II

---

unknown
DCVax

MANUFACTURER
Northwest Biotherapeutics

DESCRIPTION
DCVAx is Northwest Biotherapeutics' proprietary dendritic cell-based immunotherapy. In October 2000, the company announced that no serious side effects had been reported following the first 40 injections of DCVax, and that company immunologists were encouraged by early immunology and PSA data from treated subjects. DCVax is being evaluated as a treatment for late-stage prostate cancer at M.D. Anderson Cancer Center, Houston and the University of California, Los Angeles (UCLA).

INDICATION(S) AND RESEARCH PHASE
Prostate Cancer – Phase I/II

---

vaccine
Onyvax P

MANUFACTURER
Onyvax

DESCRIPTION
Onyvax P is an allogeneic whole-cell vaccine being developed for the treatment of prostate cancer. Phase I/II trials have been completed, and the vaccine is scheduled to enter phase II development in the first quarter of 2001. The phase I/II trial involved 60 subjects with advanced disease. Results showed the vaccine to be safe and capable of generating cancer-specific immune responses.

INDICATION(S) AND RESEARCH PHASE
Prostate Cancer – Phase I/II completed
Vaccines – Phase I/II completed

---

vaccine, adjuvant
AdjuVax-100a

MANUFACTURER
Jenner BioTherapies

DESCRIPTION
AdjuVax-100a is a proprietary emulsion formulation being tested with OncoVax-P prostate cancer vaccine. The combination therapy is in phase II trials.

INDICATION(S) AND RESEARCH PHASE
Prostate Cancer – Phase II
Vaccines – Phase II

---

vaccine, cancer
Gvax

MANUFACTURER
Cell Genesys

DESCRIPTION
Gvax is an allogenric compound that involves the genetic modification of prostate cancer cell lines. These cancer cells have been irradiated and modified to secrete granulocyte-macrophage colony stimulating factor (GM-CSF), a hormone that plays a key role in stimulating the body's immune response to vaccines. The compound is in trials for prostate cancer, pancreatic cancer, lung cancer, leukemia, and malignant melanoma.

The Gvax prostate cancer vaccine demonstrated anti-tumor activity in an initial phase II trial in subjects with advanced metastatic prostate cancer who have not responded to hormone therapy. Prior to initiating a phase III trial, Cell Genesys plans to initiate further trials of Gvax prostate cancer vaccine in 2001 that will employ a higher potency version of the same product. Additionally, future phase III trials in hormone refractory prostate cancer subjects may compare Gvax vaccine in combination with chemotherapy to chemotherapy alone.

INDICATION(S) AND RESEARCH PHASE
Prostate Cancer – Phase II
Lung Cancer – Phase I/II completed
Malignant Melanoma – Phase I/II
Vaccines – Phase I/II
Pancreatic Cancer – Phase II
Leukemia – Phase I/II

vaccine, cancer
GeneVax

MANUFACTURER
Centocor

DESCRIPTION
GeneVax is a DNA-based vaccine technology in phase I development for the treatment of breast and prostate cancer.

INDICATION(S) AND RESEARCH PHASE
Vaccines – Phase I
Breast Cancer – Phase I
Prostate Cancer – Phase I

vaccine, prostate cancer, (rV-psa)
Prostvac

MANUFACTURER
Therion Biologics

DESCRIPTION
Prostvac is a genetically engineered vaccine that is derived from the poxvirus. This immunotherapeutic is being tested in phase II trials for the treatment of prostate cancer.

INDICATION(S) AND RESEARCH PHASE
Prostate Cancer – Phase II
Vaccines – Phase II

YM-598
unknown

MANUFACTURER
Yamanouchi Pharmaceutical

DESCRIPTION
YM-598 is an orally administered endothelin type A receptor (ETA) antagonist being evaluated for the treatment of advanced prostate cancer. It is being developed in Europe and has reached phase II trials.

INDICATION(S) AND RESEARCH PHASE
Prostate Cancer – Phase II

ZD-0473/AMD 473
unknown

MANUFACTURER
AstraZeneca

DESCRIPTION
ZD-0473 is a new platinum-based anticancer agent designed to deliver an extended spectrum of activity and overcome resistance to currently approved platinum drugs, such as cisplatin and carboplatin. It is being evaluated for the treatment of a range of solid-tumor cancers, including colorectal, non-small cell lung, and bladder cancer, which are resistant to carboplatin. ZD-0473 is being tested in both intravenous and oral formulations. The intravenous formulation is in phase II trials and the oral formulation is in preclinical development.

INDICATION(S) AND RESEARCH PHASE
Bladder Cancer – Phase II
Cancer/Tumors (Unspecified) – Phase II
Colorectal Cancer – Phase II
Lung Cancer – Phase II
Ovarian Cancer – Phase II
Prostate Cancer – Phase II
Breast Cancer – Phase II
Cervical Dysplasia/Cancer – Phase II

ZD-1839
Iressa

MANUFACTURER
AstraZeneca

DESCRIPTION
Iressa binds to the epidermal growth factor receptor (EGFR) and inhibits tyrosine kinase, thereby blocking signals for cancer growth and survival. The company reported encouraging results from phase I trials in a variety of tumors, but particularly in non-small cell lung cancer (NSCLC). Iressa is being investigated both as a monotherapy and in combination with other anti-tumor drugs in NSCLC, gastric, colorectal, and hormone-resistant prostate cancers. In 1999, the FDA gave Iressa fast track status. The drug is currently in phase III studies for solid tumors.

INDICATION(S) AND RESEARCH PHASE
Cancer/Tumors (Unspecified) – Phase III
Colorectal Cancer – Phase III
Gastric Cancer – Phase III
Lung Cancer – Phase III
Prostate Cancer – Phase III

Prostate Disorders

lomefloxacin HCl
Maxaquin

MANUFACTURER
Unimed Pharmaceuticals

DESCRIPTION
Maxaquin is currently on the market for the treatment of uncomplicated urinary tract infections and lower respiratory tract infections. The antibiotic drug is in phase III trials for a new indication, chronic bacterial prostatitis. Maxaquin is given as an oral tablet. Additional indications may include metabolic disorders, and benign prostatic hypertrophy.

INDICATION(S) AND RESEARCH PHASE
Bacterial Infection – Phase III
Prostate Disorders – Phase III

pygeum africanum
Tadenan

MANUFACTURER
Fournier Research

DESCRIPTION

Tadenan is an herb that may improve the symptoms of an enlarged prostate. It is currently in phase II trials for benign prostatic hypertrophy. As men age, their prostates enlarge, probably due to the cumulative effects of the male hormone testosterone that acts on prostate tissue. Prostate cells are stimulated to grow and divide by testosterone, leading to gland enlargement, or in some cases, prostate cancer. An enlarged prostate gland may produce symptoms such as difficulty urinating, frequent nocturnal urination, and problems completely voiding the bladder contents.

Pygeum africanum is thought to act by reducing the amount of active testosterone (DHT) in the body. It works by inhibiting an enzyme that converts the testosterone molecule to the active molecule DHT, which is directly responsible for stimulating prostate cells. Recently, there was a preliminary three center trial that tested the efficacy of Tadenan on 85 men with enlarged prostates. After two months of treatment, the men had a 32% decrease in nocturnal urination frequency and a significant improvement in urinary flow. These effects persisted for a month after the drug was discontinued. There was no effect on sexual function and no serious side effects were reported. This medication may be an alternative to existing medications that do cause sexual side effects. It also may be used in conjunction with current medications in order to maximize clinical effect.

INDICATION(S) AND RESEARCH PHASE
Prostate Disorders – Phase II

Renal Cell Carcinoma

AE-941
Neovastat

MANUFACTURER
AEterna Laboratories

DESCRIPTION
Neovastat is an angiogenesis inhibitor being tested for the treatment of non-small cell lung cancer, psoriasis, multiple myeloma, and kidney cancer, among other indications.

A phase II trial for multiple myeloma was initiated in October 2000 and will treat 120 subjects and include approximately 20 sites across North America and Europe. Trial results are expected in the summer of 2002.

In addition, a phase III trial was initiated in May 2000 for kidney cancer, which will include 270 subjects at sites in North America and Europe.

INDICATION(S) AND RESEARCH PHASE
Lung Cancer – Phase III
Psoriasis and Psoriatic Disorders – Phase I/II completed
Cancer/Tumors (Unspecified) – Phase I/II completed
Multiple Myeloma – Phase II
Renal Cell Carcinoma – Phase III
Macular Degeneration – Phase I completed

aldesleukin, interleukin-2 (IL-2)
Proleukin

MANUFACTURER
Chiron Corporation

DESCRIPTION
Proleukin is a genetically engineered (recombinant) form of interleukin-2, which is a naturally occurring immune modulator. Proleukin is being evaluated in trials for acute myelogenous leukemia, non-Hodgkin's lymphoma, and HIV infection. In addition, Proleukin was approved in July 2000 for advanced-stage kidney cancer and melanoma.

INDICATION(S) AND RESEARCH PHASE
HIV Infection – Phase III
Leukemia – Phase III
Lymphoma, Non-Hodgkin's – Phase III
Renal Cell Carcinoma – FDA approved
Melanoma – FDA approved

arsenic trioxide (ATO)
Trisenox

MANUFACTURER
Cell Therapeutics

DESCRIPTION
Trisenox is believed to kill cancer cells through apoptosis, or programmed cell death. The mechanism of action of Trisenox is not fully understood, but the drug appears to induce apoptosis in a different manner than other anti-cancer agents such as retinoids.

Trisenox is FDA approved to treat acute promyelocytic leukemia (APL), and it is also in numerous trials in the United States for indications including other types of leukemia, prostate cancer, multiple myeloma, renal cell cancer, cervical cancer, and bladder cancer.

INDICATION(S) AND RESEARCH PHASE
Leukemia – Phase I
Lymphoma, Non-Hodgkin's – Phase II
Leukemia – Phase II
Multiple Myeloma – Phase II
Prostate Cancer – Phase II
Renal Cell Carcinoma – Phase II
Cervical Dysplasia/Cancer – Phase II
Bladder Cancer – Phase II

CD40 ligand
Avrend

MANUFACTURER
Immunex Corporation

DESCRIPTION
Avrend is a manufactured CD40 ligand product. CD40 ligand is a glycoprotein found primarily on the surface of activated T cells, while its receptor (CD40) is found on immune system cells and cancer cells. Avrend binds directly to CD40 on many tumor cell types, generating a signal for the tumor cell to either stop growing or undergo apoptosis. Avrend also works by stimulating specific immune responses to the tumor.

INDICATION(S) AND RESEARCH PHASE
Renal Cell Carcinoma – Phase II

diarysulfonylurea, ILX-295501
unknown

MANUFACTURER
ILEX Oncology

DESCRIPTION
ILX-295501 belongs to a novel class of antitumor compounds known as diarysulfonylureas. This orally formulated drug is in phase II trials for renal cell carcinoma, malignant melanoma, lung, and ovarian cancers.

INDICATION(S) AND RESEARCH PHASE
Renal Cell Carcinoma – Phase II
Malignant Melanoma – Phase II
Lung Cancer – Phase II
Ovarian Cancer – Phase II

diethylnorspermine
DENSPM

MANUFACTURER
GelTex Pharmaceuticals

DESCRIPTION
DENSPM (diethylnorspermine) is similar to a naturally produced polyamine, except that it may interrupt the rapid growth of tumor cells that need polyamines for growth. The drug is in phase II trials for renal cell carcinoma, pancreatic cancer, malignant melanoma, and non-small cell lung cancer. Additional indications may include ovarian and colon cancers.

INDICATION(S) AND RESEARCH PHASE
Renal Cell Carcinoma – Phase II
Pancreatic Cancer – Phase II
Malignant Melanoma – Phase II
Lung Cancer – Phase II

EMD 82633
unknown

MANUFACTURER
Merck KgaA

DESCRIPTION
EMD 82633 is a humanized and bispecific monoclonal antibody derived from mice. These antibodies are altered in such a way that they no longer appear different from human antibodies. This genetic modification prevents immune reactions against foreign substances of animal origin used in humans. In this bispecific drug, one component binds to tumor cells, while the other activates the body's own CD8 "killer cells" to attack cancer cells.

This new drug is being given as an adjuvant therapy to subjects who have not been adequately helped by conventional forms of treatment, such as chemotherapy. EMD 82633 is being tested in trials for the treatment of renal cancer, head and neck cancer, breast cancer, bladder cancer, and ovarian cancer.

INDICATION(S) AND RESEARCH PHASE
Bladder Cancer – Phase II
Breast Cancer – Phase II
Cancer/Tumors (Unspecified) – Phase II
Head and Neck Cancer – Phase II
Ovarian Cancer – Phase II
Renal Cell Carcinoma – Phase II

GL-331
unknown

MANUFACTURER
Genelabs Technologies

DESCRIPTION
GL-331 is an inhibitor of topoisomerase II. It is a semi-synthetic derivative of podophyllotoxin, which is a chemotherapeutic agent designed to overcome multidrug resistant (MDR) cancers. At this time, development has been discontinued.

INDICATION(S) AND RESEARCH PHASE
Colon Malignancies – Trial discontinued
Leukemia – Trial discontinued
Lung Cancer – Trial discontinued
Renal Cell Carcinoma – Trial discontinued

histamine dihydrochloride
Ceplene

MANUFACTURER
Maxim Pharmaceuticals

DESCRIPTION
Ceplene (formally Maxamine) is a histamine-2 (H_2) receptor stimulator that is being co-administered with immunotherapies, including cytokines and interleukin-2 (IL-2). Clinical testing includes treatment of acute myelogenous leukemia (AML), chronic hepatitis C, malignant melanoma, multiple myeloma, and renal cell carcinoma.

Results from a phase III trial in stage IV malignant melanoma subjects indicated that Ceplene used in combination with a lower dose of interleukin-2 (IL-2) improved survival rates compared to treatment with the same doses of IL-2 alone. Treatment with Ceplene and IL-2 improved overall survival, increased survival rates at 12, 18, and 24 months, and improved time-to-disease progression compared to treatment with IL-2 alone. Twenty-five percent of subjects treated with Ceplene and lower-dose IL-2 survived for a 24-month period. Overall response was achieved in 38% of the subjects treated with Ceplene and lower-dose IL-2. The company received an NDA nonapprovable letter in January 2001 because the FDA stated that the phase III trial forming the basis of the NDA would not be adequate as a single study to support approval.

INDICATION(S) AND RESEARCH PHASE
Hepatitis – Phase II
Leukemia – Phase III completed
Malignant Melanoma – NDA denied
Multiple Myeloma – Phase II
Renal Cell Carcinoma – Phase II

HSPPC-96
Oncophage

MANUFACTURER
Antigenics

DESCRIPTION
Oncophage cancer vaccine is an injectable protein that contains the unique profile ("antigenic fingerprint") of each subject's cancer. The antigens activate the immune system to elicit an anti-tumor response. Oncophage is in clinical trials for several indications, including renal cell carcinoma (phase III), melanoma (phase II), colorectal cancer (phase II), gastric cancer (phase I/II), pancreatic cancer (phase I/II completed), and non-Hodgkin's lymphoma (phase II).

In October 2000, Antigenics announced that it had initiated a phase II trial of Oncophage in subjects who have been diagnosed with sarcoma, also known as soft tissue cancer. The study is expected to initially enroll 20 subjects diagnosed with recurrent metastatic or unresectable soft tissue sarcoma and may be expanded to include an additional 15 subjects depending on preliminary results.

INDICATION(S) AND RESEARCH PHASE
Renal Cell Carcinoma – Phase III
Malignant Melanoma – Phase II
Colorectal Cancer – Phase II
Gastric Cancer – Phase I/II
Pancreatic Cancer – Phase I/II completed
Lymphoma, Non-Hodgkin's – Phase II
Sarcoma – Phase II

IMC-C225, CPT-11
unknown

MANUFACTURER
ImClone Systems

DESCRIPTION
IMC-C225 is a chimerized (part mouse, part human) monoclonal antibody that may help fight cancer cells when used in conjunction with radiation therapy or other chemotherapy agents. This antibody selectively blocks the epidermal growth factor receptor (EGFr), which may be present in greater amounts on actively growing tumor cells. Since many cancers use specific growth factors to stimulate tumor cell growth, blocking this receptor may inhibit the cancer from increasing in size and spreading throughout the body.

The company is conducting phase III clinical trials evaluating IMC-C225 in combination with radiotherapy and with chemotherapy in subjects with advanced squamous cell head and neck carcinoma. IMC-C225 is in trials for several other indications in combination with various anti-cancer agents.

INDICATION(S) AND RESEARCH PHASE
Breast Cancer – Phase I/II
Head and Neck Cancer – Phase III
Lung Cancer – Phase III
Prostate Cancer – Phase I/II
Renal Cell Carcinoma – Phase II
Pancreatic Cancer – Phase II
Colorectal Cancer – Phase II

interleukin-12 (IL-12)
unknown

MANUFACTURER
Genetics Institute

DESCRIPTION
Interleukin-12 (IL-12) is a novel, genetically engineered human immune modulator. It is being tested in phase II trials for the treatment of hepatitis C, chronic liver disease due to hepatitis infection, AIDS, and renal cell carcinoma.

INDICATION(S) AND RESEARCH PHASE
Acquired Immune Deficiency Syndrome (AIDS) and AIDS-Related Infections – Phase II
Hepatitis – Phase II
Renal Cell Carcinoma – Phase II

MDX-210
unknown

MANUFACTURER
Medarex

DESCRIPTION
MDX-210 is a bispecific monoclonal antibody (MAb)-based treatment being developed for cancers with specific markers (HER-2/*neu* positive), including renal cell, non-small cell lung, pancreatic, and prostate cancer. Phase II trials have been completed for kidney, prostate, and ovarian cancer. Phase III trials for ovarian cancer have commenced in Europe.

INDICATION(S) AND RESEARCH PHASE
Prostate Cancer – Phase II completed
Renal Cell Carcinoma – Phase II completed
Colon Malignancies – Phase II
Breast Cancer – Phase II
Gastric Cancer – Phase II
Pancreatic Cancer – Phase II
Lung Cancer – Phase II
Ovarian Cancer – Phase III

MGI-114, hydroxymethylacylfulvene, HMAF
Irofulven

MANUFACTURER
MGI Pharma

DESCRIPTION
Irofulven (MGI-114) is the first product candidate being developed by MGI Pharma from its family of anti-cancer compounds called acylfulvenes. Early trials demonstrated that Irofulven is absorbed rapidly by tumor cells, and once inside binds to DNA and protein targets. The binding interferes with DNA replication and cell division, leading to tumor-specific cell death (apoptosis). The drug is being tested in a series of trials for a variety of cancers.

In November 2000, results from a phase II trial of Irofulven indicated that the drug produced anti-tumor activity in subjects with advanced pancreatic cancer who were refractory to gemcitabine (Gemzar). Ten of the 53 subjects enrolled achieved six-month survival and two subjects demonstrated objective responses: one subject experienced tumor shrinkage of 100% and another subject experienced an 84% decrease in tumor mass. A phase III trial was initiated in February 2001.

INDICATION(S) AND RESEARCH PHASE
Breast Cancer – Phase II
Colon Malignancies – Phase II
Renal Cell Carcinoma – Phase II
Cervical Dysplasia/Cancer – Phase II
Lung Cancer – Phase II
Ovarian Cancer – Phase I/II
Colorectal Cancer – Phase II
Prostate Cancer – Phase I/II
Cancer/Tumors (Unspecified) – Phase I/II
Pancreatic Cancer – Phase III
Liver Cancer – Phase II

peginterferon alfa-2a
Pegasys

MANUFACTURER
Hoffmann-La Roche

DESCRIPTION
Pegasys is a longer-lasting form of interferon, which is a naturally produced immune boosting substance. This drug is in trials for

hepatitis B and C, malignant melanoma, renal cell carcinoma, and chronic myelogenous leukemia.

INDICATION(S) AND RESEARCH PHASE
Hepatitis – Phase III
Malignant Melanoma – Phase II
Renal Cell Carcinoma – Phase II
Leukemia – Phase III

poly I:poly C-12-U
Ampligen

MANUFACTURER
Hemispherx Biopharma

DESCRIPTION
Ampligen is a novel therapeutic treatment composed of polyribonucleotide and synthetic nucleic acid. This intravenous drug is being evaluated in trials for renal carcinoma, malignant melanoma, chronic fatigue syndrome, and HIV.

INDICATION(S) AND RESEARCH PHASE
Renal Cell Carcinoma – Phase II/III
Malignant Melanoma – Phase I/II
Chronic Fatigue Syndrome – Phase III
HIV Infection – Phase III

T cells/Xcellerate technology
unknown

MANUFACTURER
Xcyte Therapies

DESCRIPTION
Xcellerate is a new technology that activates helper T cells exvivo and causes them to proliferate. T cells are isolated from the subjects' blood, activated with the Xcellerate technology, and eventually injected back into the subject. Phase I trials are under way for the treatment of metastatic kidney cancer. Other indications may include various cancers and infectious disease.

INDICATION(S) AND RESEARCH PHASE
Renal Cell Carcinoma – Phase I

tretinoin
Atragen

MANUFACTURER
Aronex Pharmaceuticals

DESCRIPTION
Atragen is a liposomal, intravenous formulation of tretinoin or all-trans retinoic acid. Tretinoin induces cell differentiation in rapidly proliferating cells, such as those observed in malignant diseases. Additionally, Atragen appears to affect the cellular signaling mechanisms that become unbalanced in cancer cells.

Results of a phase II trial of Atragen monotherapy for acute promyelocytic leukemia (APL) indicated its potential to induce complete remission. The trial was conducted in Peru, and included 16 subjects with newly diagnosed or previously untreated APL who were treated with Atragen every other day as a single agent for a maximum of 28 doses. Fourteen subjects (87.5%) achieved morphologic remission, and 28.6% of these subjects also attained molecular remission. The safety profile observed in the subject population is similar to that reported with the currently approved oral formulation of Atra.

In addition to investigating the safety and efficacy of Atragen as a treatment for APL, the company is conducting trials to evaluate the compound for the treatment of non-Hodgkin's lymphoma, hormone-resistant prostate cancer, acute myelogenous leukemia (AML), and renal cell carcinoma in combination with interferon alpha.

In January 2001, Aronex announced that the FDA has denied approval of the company's NDA for Atragen as a treatment for subjects with APL, for whom therapy with tretinoin (all-trans retinoic acid or Atra) is necessary but for whom an intravenous administration is required.

INDICATION(S) AND RESEARCH PHASE
Lymphoma, Non-Hodgkin's – Phase II
Prostate Cancer – Phase II
Renal Cell Carcinoma – Phase I/II
Leukemia, APL (Intravenous) – NDA denied
Leukemia, APL (Monotherapy) – Phase II
Leukemia, AML – Phase II

troxacitabine, BCH-4556
Troxatyl

MANUFACTURER
BioChem Pharma

DESCRIPTION
Troxatyl is a dioxolane nucleoside analog being investigated as an anticancer agent. The drug is a complete DNA chain terminator and DNA polymerase inhibitor. It acts by incorporating itself into the growing DNA chain of cancer cells, interfering with their ability to replicate further. Troxatyl is being evaluated as a single agent or in combination therapy in a number of ongoing trials in hematologic malignancies, including acute myeloid leukemia and chronic myeloid leukemia (blastic phase), and in lymphoproliferative disorders such as lymphoma, chronic lymphocytic leukemia, and myeloma. It is also being evaluated as a single agent in pancreatic cancer and in combination therapy in a number of solid tumors. Troxatyl is currently in phase II development.

INDICATION(S) AND RESEARCH PHASE
Cancer/Tumors (Unspecified) – Phase II
Colorectal Cancer – Phase II
Head and Neck Cancer – Phase II
Leukemia – Phase II
Lung Cancer – Phase II
Malignant Melanoma – Phase II
Ovarian Cancer – Phase II
Pancreatic Cancer – Phase II
Prostate Cancer – Phase II
Renal Cell Carcinoma – Phase II

unknown
Leuvectin

MANUFACTURER
Vical

DESCRIPTION
The active ingredient in the DNA-based drug Leuvectin is a gene encoding interleukin-2 (IL-2), a naturally occurring protein that stimulates the immune system. Administration occurs by direct injection into a tumor, leading to uptake by

the tumor cells and subsequent expression of the IL-2 protein. The company anticipates that local expression of IL-2 by cancer cells may stimulate the subject's immune system to attack and destroy the tumor cells. Leuvectin is being evaluated in phase II trials in subjects with kidney and prostate cancer.

INDICATION(S) AND RESEARCH PHASE
Renal Cell Carcinoma – Phase II
Prostate Cancer – Phase II

unknown
Aroplatin

MANUFACTURER
Aronex Pharmaceuticals

DESCRIPTION
Platinum is a chemotherapeutic agent widely used in the treatment of solid tumors. Aroplatin is a liposomal formulation of a novel platinum product designed to overcome the toxicity and drug resistance associated with platinum use. It is currently in phase II trials for both mesothelioma and renal cell carcinoma.

INDICATION(S) AND RESEARCH PHASE
Mesothelioma – Phase II
Renal Cell Carcinoma – Phase II

vaccine, kidney cancer
unknown

MANUFACTURER
Genzyme Molecular Oncology

DESCRIPTION
This kidney cancer vaccine is currently in a phase I/II trial using proprietary cell fusion technology licensed to Genzyme Molecular Oncology from the Dana-Farber Cancer Institute.

INDICATION(S) AND RESEARCH PHASE
Renal Cell Carcinoma – Phase I/II

Sexual Dysfunction

alprostadil
Topiglan

MANUFACTURER
MacroChem Corporation

DESCRIPTION
Topiglan is a topical gel being evaluated in phase II and phase III studies for the treatment of male erectile dysfunction. Topiglan is a naturally occurring compound that may relax disease-constricted penile blood vessels in impotent men. This drug is a specific type of biochemical called prostaglandin E-1 (PGE-1), that increases blood flow and may help males to produce an erection.

Topiglan is formulated with a special drug delivery technology, known as SEPA (Soft Enhancement of Percutaneous Absorption), which increases absorption across the skin. Previous administrations of Topiglan included injection into the penis with a hypodermic syringe, or insertion into the urethra as a suppository.

MacroChem Corporation reported a preliminary review for a phase IIB double-blind study in which half of the subjects received placebo and the other half received either the active drug plus the SEPA-formulated gel, or only the SEPA gel without the drug. The test article was applied topically to the head of the penis in 60 subjects with known erectile dysfunction. Many of the subjects were reported to have previously failed to respond to available therapies, including Viagra, MUSE, and surgical revascularization.

Results indicated that Topiglan application was associated with a statistically greater penile rigidity and swelling as compared to placebo, as assessed by physicians. Patients' assessment also rated Topiglan results as better. Six times as many subjects stated that the erection produced by using Topiglan was sufficient for vaginal intercourse compared to placebo treated subjects. Treatment was associated with transient, minor to mild symptoms of localized warmth, occasionally mild burning or tingling in some subjects, with no difference observed between the drug and placebo treatments.

A pivotal phase III trial was initiated in July 2000 for impotence and will be conducted with 400 subjects at 20 sites. An additional phase III trial was initiated in January 2001 for the treatment of male erectile dysfunction.

INDICATION(S) AND RESEARCH PHASE
Erectile Dysfunction – Phase III
Impotence – Phase III
Sexual Dysfunction – Phase III

apomorphine HCl
unknown

MANUFACTURER
Nastech Pharmaceutical

DESCRIPTION
Intranasal apomorphine HCl is currently undergoing evaluation for the treatment of sexual dysfunction in women. The formulation works by acting on receptors in the central nervous system that may improve sexual arousal and dyspareunia. In October 2000 positive phase I results were announced. The study involved 48 nasal administrations of apomorphine at dosages of 0.1 mg to 0.75 mg, followed by blood sampling from five to 180 minutes. Clinical safety measurements included clinical nasal examination, blood pressure, heart rate, respiration rate, and side effects. There were no significant changes recorded in blood pressure, heart rate, respiration rate, or nasal mucosa. No serious side effects were observed, including dizziness, sweating, vomiting, hypotension, or syncope, that other companies have seen in the development of non-nasal apomorphine products. A phase II at home study will be the next step in evaluating efficacy. In addition, a phase II trial for male erectile dysfunction was initiated in November 2000.

INDICATION(S) AND RESEARCH PHASE
Erectile Dysfunction – Phase II
Sexual Dysfunction – Phase I completed

estrogens/methyltestosterone
Estratest

MANUFACTURER
Solvay Pharmaceuticals

DESCRIPTION

Estratest consists of esterified estrogens and methyltestosterone and is administered as an oral tablet. It is already approved by the FDA for moderate to severe vasomotor symptoms associated with menopause. Estratest is currently being evaluated in phase III trials for the treatment of sexual dysfunction in women.

INDICATION(S) AND RESEARCH PHASE
Sexual Dysfunction – Phase III
Menopause – FDA approved

IC351
Cialis

MANUFACTURER
Eli Lilly

DESCRIPTION

Cialis (IC351) is an orally administered phosphodiesterase type-5 (PDE-5) inhibitor that has been tested in more than 20 phase I and II trials. Cialis targets PDE-5, an enzyme involved in controlling blood flow to the penis. When PDE-5 is inhibited, natural sexual stimuli produce a more pronounced effect, facilitating the ability of men with erectile dysfunction (ED) to attain and maintain an erection.

In November 2000, results of a phase II trial indicated that up to 88% of men taking Cialis reported improved erections relative to placebo. Subjects with mild-to-severe ED were randomized to receive either placebo or Cialis at doses up to 25 mg over an eight week period. Data obtained from sexual encounter profile diaries showed increased reports from both men and their partners of successful intercourse attempts.

Eli Lilly has initiated a global phase III trial for treatment of ED, as well as phase II trials for female sexual dysfunction (FSD).

INDICATION(S) AND RESEARCH PHASE
Erectile Dysfunction – Phase III
Sexual Dysfunction – Phase II

midodrine HCl
ProAmatine

MANUFACTURER
Shire Pharmaceuticals

DESCRIPTION

ProAmatine is being tested in clinical trials for the relief of urinary incontinence, a serious problem that causes disability and erosion of quality of life for many people. ProAmatine acts to stimulate alpha-1 adrenergic receptors in the sphincter and bladder that increase muscle tone. This action strengthens the tone of the bladder sphincter and delays bladder emptying, giving people more control over urination. Since this medication cannot cross from the bloodstream into the brain or nervous system, it is thought that ProAmatine may cause fewer side effects compared to other drugs used for urinary incontinence.

In addition to urinary incontinence, other indications undergoing phase II clinical testing include ejaculation disorders and hypotension caused by kidney dialysis, infection, or drugs. Roberts Pharmaceutical has licensed ProAmantine from Nycomed Pharma.

INDICATION(S) AND RESEARCH PHASE
Kidney Disease – Phase II
Urinary Incontinence – Phase II
Sexual Dysfunction – Phase II

NMI-870
unknown

MANUFACTURER
NitroMed

DESCRIPTION

NMI-870 is a nitric oxide derivative of the alpha-2 blocker yohimbine, which is being tested in post-menopausal woman experiencing sexual dysfunction.

Results of a randomized, double-blind, placebo-controlled phase II, three-way crossover trial of orally administered NMI-870 showed that the compound demonstrated the ability to increase vaginal blood flow in post-menopausal women diagnosed with female sexual arousal disorder.

INDICATION(S) AND RESEARCH PHASE
Sexual Dysfunction – Phase II completed

TA-1790
unknown

MANUFACTURER
Vivus

DESCRIPTION

TA-1790 is a highly selective phosphodiesterase type 5 (PDE5) inhibitor. The compound is being developed for the treatment of male and female sexual dysfunction. Vivus has a licensing agreement with Tanabe Seiyaku regarding this product.

INDICATION(S) AND RESEARCH PHASE
Sexual Dysfunction – Phase I
Erectile dysfunction – Phase I

testoterone
unknown

MANUFACTURER
Watson Pharmaceuticals

DESCRIPTION

Testosterone is a naturally produced hormone that is responsible for proper development of male secondary sex characteristics. The hormone, which has been formulated in the MTX transdermal patch, is being tested in phase II trials for treatment of sexual dysfunction in surgically menopausal subjects, for use in menopause associated hormone replacement therapy, and treatment of osteoporosis. Additionally, it is in phase III clinical trials for treatment of male hormonal deficiencies and abnormalities.

This hormone regime is also being evaluated in phase II trials for treatment of AIDS wasting in females. Testosterone is an anabolic steroid that may help build up muscle mass in subjects suffering from AIDS.

INDICATION(S) AND RESEARCH PHASE
Acquired Immune Deficiency Syndrome (AIDS) and AIDS-Related Infections – Phase II
Hormone Replacement Therapy-Menopause – Phase II
Male Hormonal Deficiencies/Abnormalities – Phase III

Osteoporosis – Phase II
Sexual Dysfunction – Phase II completed

transdermal testosterone gel
Tostrelle

MANUFACTURER
Cellegy Pharmaceuticals

DESCRIPTION
Tostrelle, in a transdermal testosterone gel formulation, is indicated for the treatment of low levels of testosterone in menopausal women. Testosterone deficiency in women frequently causes diminished libido or low sex drive. Based on phase I trial results, Cellegy plans to begin an expanded phase I/II study to determine the optimal dosing of Tostrelle in surgically induced menopausal women.

INDICATION(S) AND RESEARCH PHASE
Menopause – Phase I/II
Hormone Replacement Therapy:
    Menopause – Phase II
Sexual Dysfunction – Phase I/II

unknown
Alista

MANUFACTURER
Vivus

DESCRIPTION
Alista is a synthetic derivative of a naturally occurring vasodilating agent. It is believed to increase blood flow to the female genitalia, thereby promoting engorgement and other natural processes that occur during sexual stimulation. Alista is a proprietary formulation of alprostadil that is applied locally to female genitalia. Alista is in a phase II multicenter, double-blind, placebo-controlled trial for women with a primary diagnosis of female sexual arousal disorder.

INDICATION(S) AND RESEARCH PHASE
Sexual Dysfunction – Phase II

unknown
Vasofem

MANUFACTURER
Zonagen

DESCRIPTION
Vasofem is a vaginal suppository being developed for the treatment of female sexual dysfunction (FSD). Phase II trials are currently under way.

INDICATION(S) AND RESEARCH PHASE
Sexual Dysfunction – Phase II

unknown
Daproxetine

MANUFACTURER
PPD Genupro

DESCRIPTION
Daproxetine is a selective serotonin reuptake inhibitor for the treatment of premature ejaculation. Daproxetine recently completed a phase II trial in 13 centers throughout the United States. The double-blind, placebo-controlled, three way cross-over study enrolled 155 subjects. It evaluated two different dose levels of the oral drug and placebo. In each period of the study, subjects took the medication one to three hours prior to intercourse, and their partner then recorded ejaculatory latency in a diary. Each period included four attempts over four weeks. Results showed that Daproxetine therapy resulted in a significant prolongation of ejaculatory latency compared to the placebo.

INDICATION(S) AND RESEARCH PHASE
Impotence – Phase II completed
Sexual Dysfunction – Phase II completed

Shingles

vaccine, zoster
unknown

MANUFACTURER
Merck & Co.

DESCRIPTION
The zoster vaccine is in a phase III trial for the treatment of shingles.

INDICATION(S) AND RESEARCH PHASE
Shingles – Phase III

Sjogren's Syndrome

interferon alpha
IFNalpha

MANUFACTURER
Amarillo Biosciences

DESCRIPTION
Interferon (IFN) alpha is a naturally occurring protein with immunomodulatory, antiproliferative, and antiviral properties. IFNalpha is thought to reduce pain and stiffness in subjects with fibromyalgia. Fibromyalgia is characterized by pain and stiffness in the soft tissues, including the muscles, tendons, and ligaments. A phase II study at the University of Texas Health Science Center in San Antonio has completed recruiting subjects with fibromyalgia as of November 2000.

A phase III trial to increase saliva production in subjects with Sjogren's Syndrome has been completed.

INDICATION(S) AND RESEARCH PHASE
Fibromyalgia – Phase II
Sjogren's Syndrome – Phase III completed

Systemic Lupus Erythematosus

5c8 (Anti CD-40 ligand antibody)
Antova

MANUFACTURER
Biogen

DESCRIPTION
Biogen has engineered 5c8 (Anti CD-40 ligand antibody), a humanized monoclonal antibody for the potential treatment of a number of autoimmune disorders. These include idiopathic thrombocytopenia purpura (ITP), systemic lupus erythematosus,

kidney transplantation, and Factor VIII antibody inhibition.

In the aforementioned autoimmune diseases, it is thought that activated white blood cells, called T cell lymphocytes, bind to other tissue cells through a cell surface receptor, the CD-40 ligand. Abnormal antibodies are produced that will then recognize healthy body tissues as foreign, and thereby cause an inflammatory response. The 5c8 antibody may stop this abnormal immune cycle by binding to the CD-40 ligand and inhibiting its ability to bind with its receptor on a variety of other normal cells.

INDICATION(S) AND RESEARCH PHASE
Thrombocytopenia – Phase II discontinued
Systemic Lupus Erythematosus – Phase II discontinued
Kidney Transplant Surgery – Phase II discontinued
Factor VIII antibody inhibition – Phase II discontinued

GL-701, prasterone
Aslera

MANUFACTURER
Genelabs Technologies

DESCRIPTION
The active ingredient in Aslera is prasterone, the synthetic equivalent of the androgenic hormone dehydroepiandrosterone (DHEA). Products containing DHEA are currently marketed as dietary supplements. Aslera is in development for the treatment of systemic lupus erythematosus (SLE). SLE subjects, primarily women, often develop low levels of DHEA. Phase III trials have been completed and an NDA was submitted in October 2000. The FDA is planning to review the NDA in April 2001.

INDICATION(S) AND RESEARCH PHASE
Systemic Lupus Erythematosus – NDA submitted

IDEC-131
unknown

MANUFACTURER
IDEC Pharmaceuticals

DESCRIPTION
IDEC-131 is a humanized monoclonal antibody (Mab) developed for the treatment of systemic lupus erythematosus (SLE). By inhibiting the action of the CD40 ligand molecule, a communication link between the immune helper T cells and B cells, IDEC-131 may reduce excessively abnormal antibody production. This biologic drug may help restore a more normal immune response in subjects with a variety of autoimmune and inflammatory conditions. A phase II trial for SLE has been completed and IDEC-131 is currently in phase II trials for treatment of psoriasis.

INDICATION(S) AND RESEARCH PHASE
Systemic Lupus Erythematosus – Phase II completed
Psoriasis and Psoriatic Disorders – Phase II

LJP-394
unknown

MANUFACTURER
La Jolla Pharmaceutical

DESCRIPTION
LJP-394 is a novel compound derived from La Jolla's proprietary tolerance technology. The mechanism of action of LJP-394 is thought to involve inhibition of B cell antibody production. Antibodies are thought to be important in the pathogenesis of systemic lupus erythematosus (SLE).
In a phase II/III trial, LPJ-394 reduced renal flares in lupus subjects with poor renal function. In subjects with high-affinity antibodies to LJP 394, time to renal flare, the primary endpoint of the trial, was significantly increased in the drug treated population as compared to the placebo treated group. In the high-affinity group, there were one-third as many renal flares in LJP 394 treated subjects compared to placebo treated subjects. A phase III trial for LJP 394 is currently in progress.

INDICATION(S) AND RESEARCH PHASE
Kidney Disease – Phase III
Systemic Lupus Erythematosus – Phase III

Urinary Incontinence

ABT-232, NS-49
unknown

MANUFACTURER
Abbott Laboratories

DESCRIPTION
ABT-232, acting as an alpha agonist, selectively stimulates the adrenergic nerves. It is being evaluated in a phase I trial for the treatment of uncontrollable urination due to stress.

INDICATION(S) AND RESEARCH PHASE
Urinary Incontinence – Phase I

chondrocyte-alginate gel suspension
Chondrogel

MANUFACTURER
Curis

DESCRIPTION
Chondrogel is a tissue augmentation product created from autologous cartilage cells taken from the ear and expanded in a culture. The cells are then injected into the bladder to treat pediatric vesicoureteral reflux disease (VUR). VUR is a congenital condition in children possibly leading to a urinary tract infection and kidney damage. Phase III trials have been completed, and a phase II trial is currently being planned for the treatment of Grade II VUR in pediatric subjects.

A phase II trial for stress urinary incontinence (SUI) is also under way.

INDICATION(S) AND RESEARCH PHASE
Pediatric, Vesicoureteral Reflux Disease – Phase III completed
Urinary Incontinence – Phase II

darifenacin
unknown

MANUFACTURER

Pfizer

DESCRIPTION

Darifenacin is a selective muscarinic antagonist being evaluated for the treatment of overactive bladder. Muscarinic antagonists competitively block the action of acetylcholine. Scientists are trying to develop drugs that will block acetylcholine action on the problematic organ, while minimizing action on other organs and reducing side effects such as blurry vision, dry mouth, and decreased cognitive function. Pfizer believes that because darifenacin is directed at a particular subset of the muscarinic receptor found to be more active in the bladder, it acts more specifically on the neurologic instability of overactive bladders. Darifenacin is currently in phase III development.

INDICATION(S) AND RESEARCH PHASE
Urinary Incontinence – Phase III

duloxetine HCl, LY-248686
unknown

MANUFACTURER
Eli Lilly

DESCRIPTION

Duloxetine hydrochloride is an antidepressant that works by inhibiting the reuptake of norepinephrine and serotonin. This reuptake inhibitor blocks the neurotransmitters from re-entering the nerve cells, and thereby allows a longer period of synaptic stimulation in the brain. Duloxetine is being tested in phase III studies for the treatment of depression as well as for treatment of urinary incontinence. An NDA filing is planned for late 2001 or early 2002.

INDICATION(S) AND RESEARCH PHASE
Depression – Phase III
Urinary Incontinence – Phase III

HCT 1026
unknown

MANUFACTURER
NicOx SA

DESCRIPTION

HCT 1026 is a novel nitric oxide-releasing derivative of the non-steroidal anti-inflammatory drug (NSAID) flurbiprofen. While flurbiprofen has demonstrated effectiveness in the treatment of urinary incontinence, its use has been complicated by gastric toxicity. Because HCT 1026 may provide increased gastric tolerability, it can be administered for extended periods at effective doses. In phase I trials, results indicated that HCT 1026 produced fewer and less severe gastric lesions compared to flurbiprofen.

HCT 1026 produces anti-inflammatory effects through the inhibition of prostaglandin synthesis, while nitric oxide controls inflammatory cell activation. These two factors suggest that HCT 1026 may be an effective treatment for dermatology disorders such as psoriasis. HCT 1026 is in phase II trials for the treatment of urinary incontinence, osteoporosis, and skin disorders.

INDICATION(S) AND RESEARCH PHASE
Urinary Incontinence – Phase II
Osteoporosis – Phase II
Skin Infections/Disorders – Phase II

I-OXY/ UROS Infusor
unknown

MANUFACTURER
Situs Corporation

DESCRIPTION

The UROS Infusor is a novel intravesical drug delivery device designed to provide continuous flow of medicated solution over various lengths of time. This device offers an alternative treatment method for subjects who cannot take oral medication. Situs has initiated a phase I/II trial to test the UROS Infusor with a proprietary intravesical solution, I-OXY, for the treatment of overactive bladder. The trial includes 20 subjects randomized into two groups, one receiving the drug I-OXY and the another receiving a placebo.

INDICATION(S) AND RESEARCH PHASE
Urinary Incontinence – Phase I/II

midodrine HCl
ProAmatine

MANUFACTURER
Shire Pharmaceuticals

DESCRIPTION

ProAmatine is being tested in clinical trials for the relief of urinary incontinence, a serious problem that causes disability and erosion of quality of life for many people. ProAmatine acts to stimulate alpha-1 adrenergic receptors in the sphincter and bladder that increase muscle tone. This action strengthens the tone of the bladder sphincter and delays bladder emptying, giving people more control over urination. Since this medication cannot cross from the bloodstream into the brain or nervous system, it is thought that ProAmatine may cause fewer side effects compared to other drugs used for urinary incontinence.

In addition to urinary incontinence, other indications undergoing phase II clinical testing include ejaculation disorders and hypotension caused by kidney dialysis, infection, or drugs. Roberts Pharmaceutical has licensed ProAmatine from Nycomed Pharma.

INDICATION(S) AND RESEARCH PHASE
Kidney Disease – Phase II
Urinary Incontinence – Phase II
Sexual Dysfunction – Phase II

oxybutynin
unknown

MANUFACTURER
Watson Pharmaceuticals

DESCRIPTION

Oxybutynin reduces urinary bladder and urethra spasms that cause frequent urination and incontinence. The drug exerts its effect by blocking nerve impulses at parasympathetic nerve endings, preventing muscle contractions and gland secretions of the organs involved. Watson is testing oxybutynin in a skin delivery system using the TheraDerm-MTX transdermal patch.

In October 2000, results of a double-blind

phase II trial indicated that transdermally delivered oxybutynin reduces the incidence of incontinent episodes as effectively as the immediate-release orally administered form of the drug. The trial also showed that transdermally delivered oxybutynin significantly reduced the unwanted side effects that can occur with oral treatment.

INDICATION(S) AND RESEARCH PHASE
Urinary Incontinence – Phase II completed

S-oxybutynin
unknown

MANUFACTURER
Sepracor

DESCRIPTION
S-oxybutynin is a single-isomer version of Ditropan. Isomers are molecules that are non-superimposable mirror images of one another. In many cases, only one isomer of a racemic drug, a one to one mixture of two isomers, may be responsible for the drug's effectiveness. The other isomer may be an unnecessary component and may even cause undesirable or severe side effects. S-oxybutynin, in tablet form, is being tested in a phase III trial for treatment of involuntary and stress-related urinary incontinence.

INDICATION(S) AND RESEARCH PHASE
Urinary Incontinence – Phase III

(S)-sibutramine
unknown

MANUFACTURER
Sepracor

DESCRIPTION
According to in vitro studies, (S)-sibutramine is a potent inhibitor of both dopamine and norepinephrine. This dual pharmacology may improve both erectile and ejaculatory dysfunction, and a preclinical model has shown that the (S)-sibutramine metabolite facilitates sexual performance. Sepracor is developing (S)-sibutramine as a treatment for both sexual dysfunction and stress urinary incontinence.

INDICATION(S) AND RESEARCH PHASE
Erectile dysfunction – Phase I
Urinary Incontinence – Phase I

SB 223412
unknown

MANUFACTURER
GlaxoSmithKline

DESCRIPTION
SB 223412 is a tachykinin (NK$_3$) receptor antagonist. It is currently in phase I development for the treatment of urinary incontinence and chronic obstructive pulmonary disease (COPD).

INDICATION(S) AND RESEARCH PHASE
Urinary Incontinence – Phase I
Chronic Obstructive Pulmonary Disease (COPD) – Phase I

TAK-637
unknown

MANUFACTURER
Takeda Chemical Industries

DESCRIPTION
TAK-637 is an NK$_1$ receptor antagonist being developed for the treatment of various indications. It is currently in phase I trials in Japan for urinary incontinence. Additionally, TAK-637 is in phase II trials in Europe and the United States for urinary incontinence, depression, and irritable bowel syndrome.

INDICATION(S) AND RESEARCH PHASE
Urinary Incontinence (Japan) – Phase I
Urinary Incontinence (Europe and United States) – Phase II
Depression – Phase II
Irritable Bowel Syndrome – Phase II

trospium chloride
Trospium

MANUFACTURER
Interneuron Pharmaceuticals

DESCRIPTION
Trospium is being evaluated in phase III trials for the treatment of urinary incontinence. This drug is a muscarinic compound antagonist that relaxes smooth muscle tissue, such as that found in the bladder. Results from the phase III trial are expected at the end of 2001, with NDA filing planned shortly after. Trospium is licensed from Madaus AG, in Germany.

INDICATION(S) AND RESEARCH PHASE
Urinary Incontinence – Phase III

YM-905
unknown

MANUFACTURER
Yamanouchi Pharmaceutical

DESCRIPTION
YM-905 is an orally-administered muscarinic M3 antagonist. It is being evaluated in phase III trials for the treatment of urinary frequency, urgency, and incontinence associated with overactive bladder. The drug is being developed in the United States and Europe.

INDICATION(S) AND RESEARCH PHASE
Urinary Incontinence – Phase III

Urinary Tract Infections

amikacin
Mikasome

MANUFACTURER
Gilead Sciences

DESCRIPTION
Mikasome, an aminoglycoside antibiotic, is in phase II trials for treatment of serious bacterial and mycobacterial infections, including nosocomial *Pseudomonas* pneumonia, complicated urinary tract infections, and *Pseudomonas*-colonized subjects with cystic fibrosis. The drug is delivered in a liposomal formulation.

INDICATION(S) AND RESEARCH PHASE

Bacterial Infection – Phase II
Pneumonia – Phase II
Urinary Tract Infections – Phase II

chondrocyte-alginate gel suspension
Chondrogel

MANUFACTURER
Curis

DESCRIPTION
Chondrogel is a tissue augmentation product created from autologous cartilage cells taken from the ear and expanded in a culture. The cells are then injected into the bladder to treat pediatric vesicoureteral reflux disease (VUR). VUR is a congenital condition in children possibly leading to a urinary tract infection and kidney damage. Phase III trials have been completed, and a phase II trial is currently being planned for the treatment of Grade II VUR in pediatric subjects. A phase II trial for stress urinary incontinence (SUI) is also under way.

INDICATION(S) AND RESEARCH PHASE
Pediatric, Vesicoureteral Reflux Disease – Phase III completed
Urinary Incontinence – Phase II

ciprofloxacin
CIPRO

MANUFACTURER
Bayer Corporation

DESCRIPTION
CIPRO is a fluoroquinolone antibiotic that is currently awaiting FDA approval for the treatment of exposure to aerosolized anthrax bacteria. Without treatment, anthrax infection is usually fatal. Doxycycline and penicillin are approved to treat anthrax, but it is thought that there are strains of anthrax bacteria which have been engineered to be resistant to these antibiotics. CIPRO is already approved for 17 different indications: acute sinusitis, lower respiratory tract infections, nosocomial pneumonia (IV only), urinary tract infections, acute uncomplicated cystitis in females (tablets and oral suspension only), chronic bacterial prostatitis, complicated intra-abdominal infections (in combination with metronidazole), skin and skin structure infections, bone and joint infections, infectious diarrhea, typhoid fever (enteric fever), and uncomplicated cervical and urethral gonorrhea (tablets and oral suspension only).

CIPRO, in intravenous formulation, is also indicated in empirical therapy for febrile neutropenic subjects, in combination with piperacillin sodium. Phase III trials testing CIPRO for the treatment of complicated urinary tract infections in pediatric subjects one to 17 years old are currently under way.

INDICATION(S) AND RESEARCH PHASE
Anthrax Exposure – NDA submitted
Pediatric, Urinary Tract Infections – Phase III
Urinary Tract Infections – Phase III

daptomycin
Cidecin

MANUFACTURER
Cubist Pharmaceuticals

DESCRIPTION
Cidecin is a novel antibiotic lipopeptide, a combination of fatty acids and amino acids, used for the treatment of skin and soft tissue infections, urinary tract infections in hospitalized subjects, and bacteremia, or bacteria in the blood. The drug is made in an intravenous formulation. Cidecin is in trials for skin infections, bacterial infections, and heart disease.

INDICATION(S) AND RESEARCH PHASE
Skin Infections/Disorders – Phase III
Bacterial Infection – Phase II
Urinary Tract Infections – Phase II/III
Heart Disease – Phase II/III

gemifloxacin mesylate
Factive

MANUFACTURER
GlaxoSmithKline

DESCRIPTION
Factive is a broad spectrum fluoroquinolone being developed for the treatment of various bacterial infections. It is in phase III trials in an intravenous formulation for the treatment of respiratory tract infections. Additionally, Factive has been developed in an oral formulation for the treatment of respiratory and urinary tract infections. An NDA and Marketing Authorization Application (MAA) have been submitted for the latter indications.

INDICATION(S) AND RESEARCH PHASE
Bacterial Infection – Phase III
Bacterial Infection – NDA submitted
Bacterial Infection – MAA submitted
Urinary Tract Infections – MAA submitted

MK-826, carbepenem
unknown

MANUFACTURER
Merck & Co.

DESCRIPTION
MK-826 is a broad-spectrum antibiotic being developed in phase III trials for the treatment of bacterial infections including pneumonia, intra-abdominal infections, skin and skin structure infections, urinary tract infections, and obstetric and gynecologic infections.

INDICATION(S) AND RESEARCH PHASE
Pneumonia – Phase III
Skin Infections/Disorders – Phase III
Urinary Tract Infections – Phase III
Gynecological Infections – Phase III
Bacterial Infection – Phase III
Gastrointestinal Diseases and Disorders, miscellaneous – Phase III

vaccine, urinary tract infection
unknown

MANUFACTURER
MedImmune

DESCRIPTION
This is a vaccine for the prevention of urinary tract infection (UTI). More than 80%

of UTIs are caused by *E. coli*.

To test the safety and tolerability of its UTI vaccine, MedImmune immunized 48 healthy subjects in a phase I, randomized, placebo-controlled trial. In this trial, the vaccine was found to be safe, generally well tolerated, and immunogenic. All subjects receiving the vaccine developed serum antibodies and those with the best serum repsonses exhibited antibodies in urine and vaginal secretions. When studied in tissue culture, the antibodies were found to prevent the bacteria from binding to human bladder cells. A phase II trial is now in progress.

INDICATION(S) AND RESEARCH PHASE
Urinary Tract Infections – Phase II

YM-617, tamsulosin
unknown

MANUFACTURER
Yamanouchi Pharmaceutical

DESCRIPTION
YM-617 is an orally administered alpha-1 receptor antagonist being evaluated as a treatment for lower urinary tract disorder. The drug is in phase III trials and is part of Yamanouchi's domestic pipeline.

INDICATION(S) AND RESEARCH PHASE
Urinary Tract Infections – Phase III

11 | Musculoskeletal

Population with illnesses in this category	21 million[1]
Drugs in the development pipeline	281[2]
Number of drugs in preclinical testing	155
Number of drugs in clinical testing	104

Source: 1. World Health Organization, worldwide figures 2. Parexel

Two major therapeutic categories leading the musculoskeletal pipeline are osteoporosis and rheumatoid arthritis. Osteoporosis is the most prevalent of the bone diseases, affecting 10 million people in the United States. More than 18 million people have low bone mass, placing them at risk for fractures. Worldwide, the lifetime risk for a woman to have an osteoporosis related fracture is 30% to 40% and in men it is 13%, according to the International Osteoporosis Foundation. CenterWatch estimates there are approximately 18 drugs in the clinical pipeline and $80 million to $120 million is being spent.

Osteoporosis causes low bone mass and structural deterioration of bone tissue, leading to bone fragility and increased susceptibility to fractures of the hip, spine and wrist. It is known as the "silent disease" because the bone loss occurs without symptoms. The disease will often not be diagnosed until a fracture occurs.

In the past few years, progress has been made in diagnosis, evaluation, treatment and therefore, prognosis of osteoporosis. Effective medications are available for prevention and treatment of the disease and more are being developed.

Two drugs approved in 2000 treat osteoporosis in postmenopausal symptoms; Vivelle (controlled release estradiol), which provides estrogen replacement therapy by releasing estradiol through a controlled release patch, and Activella (estradiol/norethindrone), a once a day combination hormone replacement therapy (HRT) tablet containing both estrogen and progestin. Additionally, a new treatment might soon be available; Fortical Injection, developed by Unigene Laboratories, recently completed phase III trials. Fortical Injection is an injectable version of human parathyroid hormone, a naturally occurring protein, which results in an increase in new bone formation in people with osteoporosis.

Rheumatoid arthritis is another active area in the drug development pipeline. According to PhRMA, approximately 2.1 million people suffer from rheumatoid arthritis including 1.5 million women and 600,000 men. Rheumatoid arthritis usually occurs in middle age, although it often can occur in the 20s and 30s. CenterWatch estimates there are approximately 32 drugs in the pipeline with $140 million to $160 million being spent on drug development.

Rheumatoid arthritis is a chronic disease that causes pain, stiffness, swelling, loss of function in the joints, and inflammation in other body organs. The cause of rheumatoid arthritis is still unknown and so, many of the drugs being tested for the treatment of rheumatoid arthritis are directed at symptomatic treatment.

Several different classes of drugs are used to treat subjects with the various types of rheumatic diseases. Their classes include analgesics to control pain, corticosteroids, uric acid-lowering drugs, immunosuppresive drugs, and nonsteroidal inflammatory drugs (NSAIDs) as well as disease-modifying antirheumatic drugs.

NSAIDs are usually the most commonly used modality for mild-to moderate rheumatoid arthritis because they are well tolerated by the subject and help to control the pain associated with this form of arthritis. Unfortunately, NSAIDs such as aspirin, ibuprofen, idomethacin, naproxen, tolmetin have no effect on the underlying disease and therefore cannot prevent progression of joint destruction or organ damage. Several side effects with these drugs are gastrointestinal tract irritation, including gastric ulcers and gastritis that result in bleeding, skin reactions, decreases in blood coagulation, reversible hepatocellular toxicity and impaired renal function. However, new NSAIDs being developed are designed to have greater cyclooxygenase (COX) specificity, fewer side effects and more desirable dosing regimens. Veldecoxib is a second-generation COX-2 inhibitor expected to be launched in 2001. It is supposed to be more potent than the already approved COX-2 inhibitor, Celeoxib. COX-2 inhibitors are thought to possess less toxicity to the gastric mucosa than non-specific COX inhibitors, but gastrointestinal bleeding is still possible with these new agents.

Disease-modifying antirheumatic drugs (DMARDs) such as antimalarial drugs, gold compounds, penicillamine and sulfasalazine are thought to have some effect on altering the progression of rheumatoid arthritis because they are slower acting and take weeks or months for benefits of the drugs to be noted. In order to be classified as a DMARD, a drug must be shown to improve the symptoms of rheumatoid arthritis for at least one year and must have a different mechanism of action than corticosteriods or NSAIDs. At proper dosage, and with continuous use, a significant reduction in the symptoms of rheumatoid arthritis can occur using DMARDs. However, if a subject discontinues use of the drug, the symptoms will gradually return.

There is now a more complete understanding of the biology of rheumatoid arthritis and some insights into the mechanisms of action of these drugs. As a result, the newer DMARDs are more effective and have fewer side effects than the older agents. Multiple new types of DMARDs are in clinical development, including those that target the manner in which inflammation occurs and others that improve versions of existing DMARDs. Those that target the way inflammation occur focus on the inflammatory proteins such as TNF-alpha inhibitors, interleukin-1 inhibitors, protease inhibitors, chemotaxis inhibitors and complement inhibitors. Other DMARDs target production of basic building block of DNA and RNA.

Acromegaly

pegvisomant
Somavert

MANUFACTURER
Sensus Drug Development

DESCRIPTION
Somavert (pegvisomant), a genetically modified form of human growth hormone, is being tested for the treatment of acromegaly. The drug is designed to block the effects of excessive growth hormone production by a pituitary tumor. Eighty-nine percent of subjects treated in phase III trials experienced normalized serum insulin-like growth factor one (IGF-I) at 12 weeks, compared to 10% receiving placebo. At least 75% of the IGF-I reduction occurred within two weeks of initiating treatment. The Somavert treated group also experienced decreases in soft-tissue swelling, excessive perspiration, and fatigue. The study was conducted by an international team of endocrinologists at centers in both the United States and Europe. Somavert was developed by Sensus Drug Development and Pharmacia is currently collaborating with Sensus to bring Somavert to market.

INDICATION(S) AND RESEARCH PHASE
Acromegaly – Phase III completed

Amyotrophic Lateral Sclerosis (ALS)

AVP-923
unknown

MANUFACTURER
AVANIR Pharmaceuticals

DESCRIPTION
AVP-923 is in a phase II/III trial for the treatment of emotional lability in subjects with Lou Gehrig's disease, the common name for amyotrophic lateral sclerosis (ALS). The trial includes 100 subjects and 11 sites in the United States. The trial is being monitored by INC Research and is expected to continue through July 2001. AVP-923 is also undergoing development in phase II/III trials for pain control and phase II trials for chronic cough. The company plans to initiate another clinical trial this year to be conducted in multiple sclerosis subjects.

INDICATION(S) AND RESEARCH PHASE
Amyotrophic Lateral Sclerosis (ALS) – Phase II/III
Pain, Acute or Chronic – Phase II/III
Emotional Lability – Phase II/III
Chronic Cough – Phase II

brain derived neurotrophic factor, BDNF
unknown

MANUFACTURER
Regeneron Pharmaceuticals

DESCRIPTION
Brain derived neurotrophic factor (BDNF) is a naturally occurring human protein that promotes the survival of spinal neurons. It is being developed for the treatment of amyotrophic lateral sclerosis (ALS), commonly known as Lou Gehrig's disease. ALS is a disease that attacks motor neurons, which are nerve cells that cause muscles to contract. Degeneration of these neurons causes muscle weakness, leading to death due to respiratory insufficiency.

BDNF is currently in phase II/III trials for ALS. Partnerships for development of the protein include Amgen and Sumitomo Pharmaceuticals.

INDICATION(S) AND RESEARCH PHASE
Amyotrophic Lateral Sclerosis (ALS) – Phase II/III

SR-57746
unknown

MANUFACTURER
Sanofi-Synthelabo Pharmaceuticals

DESCRIPTION
SR-57746 is being developed in phase II trials as a treatment for Alzheimer's disease and in phase III trials for amyotrophic lateral sclerosis (ALS), or Lou Gehrig's disease. Both are diseases caused by the death of nerve cells. A substance known as nerve growth factor (NGF) can potentially counteract this destructive process. NGF is responsible for synapse formation between neurons and also protects against neuronal death. In particular, NGF stimulates the growth of cholinergic neurons, the nerve cells that are the first to degenerate in Alzheimer's disease.

Unfortunately, it is very difficult to administer NGF since it cannot cross the blood-brain barrier and gain direct access to brain tissue. Therefore, scientists are developing compounds such as SR-57746 which enhance the effect of existing NGF on cell survival and neuron growth and development. SR-57746 also may lead to increased production of NGF itself. The result may be improvement in several aspects of Alzheimer's disease, including mood disorders, psychosis, aggressiveness, and restlessness. The same NGF-enhancing properties may make SR-57746 an effective therapy for ALS subjects as well, the only difference being the affected cells in ALS are the motor neurons in the spinal cord, not the brain neurons as in Alzheimer's disease.

INDICATION(S) AND RESEARCH PHASE
Amyotrophic Lateral Sclerosis (ALS) – Phase III
Alzheimer's Disease – Phase II

Bone Fractures

synthetic peptide
Chrysalin

MANUFACTURER
OrthoLogic

DESCRIPTION
Chrysalin is a synthetically manufactured peptide being tested to accelerate fracture healing. According to OrthoLogic, Chrysalin represents a portion of the receptor-binding domain of the human thrombin molecule actively involved in the healing process for

both soft tissue and bone. By mimicking specific attributes of the thrombin molecule, Chrysalin stimulates the body's natural healing processes and results in accelerated tissue repair. Chrysalis Bio Technology has licensed U.S. development of this drug to OrthoLogic, who plans to conduct further trials for fresh fracture indications.

Chrysalin is currently being evaluated in a phase I/II trial that includes 90 subjects at three sites. Subjects will receive one injection of Chrysalin or a placebo at the time the fracture is set and will be monitored weekly to evaluate the healing. Preclinical studies showed that a single intrafracture injection of Chrysalin nearly doubled the rate of fracture healing.

INDICATION(S) AND RESEARCH PHASE
Bone Fractures – Phase I/II

TAK-778-SR
unknown

MANUFACTURER
Takeda Chemical Industries

DESCRIPTION
TAK-778-SR is being developed for the treatment of bone fracture. It is being evaluated in an injectable formulation in phase II trials in Europe and Japan.

INDICATION(S) AND RESEARCH PHASE
Bone Fractures – Phase II

Bone Metastases

zoledronate
Zometa

MANUFACTURER
Novartis

DESCRIPTION
Zometa is an intravenous bisphosphonate osteoclast inhibitor. In September 2000, Novartis announced it has received an approvable letter from the FDA for Zometa for the treatment of hypercalcemia of malignancy (HCM), the most common life-threatening metabolic complication associated with cancer. Zometa is also in phase II development for the treatment of postmenopausal osteoporosis and phase III development for bone metastasis treatment and prevention.

INDICATION(S) AND RESEARCH PHASE
Osteoporosis – Phase II
Hypercalcemia – FDA recommend approval letter
Bone Metastases – Phase III

Connective Tissue Diseases

dimethyl sulfoxide, DMSO
unknown

MANUFACTURER
Topical Technologies

DESCRIPTION
Dimethyl sulfoxide (DMSO) is a topical medication being developed in phase III trials for the treatment of palmar-plantar dystensia syndrome, caused by anti-cancer drugs, and in phase II trials for soft-tissue injury following extravasation of cytotoxic drugs. An orphan drug status has been granted for both indications.

Since DMSO penetrates the skin deeply and quickly without apparent damage, it can carry other drugs with it across membranes. It is more successful ferrying some drugs, such as morphine sulfate, penicillin, steroids, and cortisone, than others, such as insulin. What DMSO can carry depends on the molecular weight, shape, and electrochemistry of the molecules. This property may enable DMSO to act as a new drug delivery system that could lower the risk of infection occurring when the skin is penetrated.

DMSO, while approved for topical use over much of the world, has had a long and controversial history with the FDA due to concerns about eye problems and other issues.

INDICATION(S) AND RESEARCH PHASE
Connective Tissue Diseases – Phase II

Effects of Chemotherapy – Phase III
Neurologic Disorders – Phase III

Dupuytren's Disease

collagenase for injection
Cordase

MANUFACTURER
Biospecifics Technologies

DESCRIPTION
Cordase is an injectable formulation of purified collagenase, an enzyme that induces changes in collagen causing it to degrade within the connective tissue. This drug is currently in phase II testing for Dupuytren's disease, a contracture deformity that may cause the fingers to become stuck in a flexed position, as well as for Peyronie's disease and adhesive capsulitis, or frozen shoulder. Cordase is considered an orphan drug due to the limited therapies available for these conditions. Research is under development by Advance Biofactures, a subsidiary of Biospecifics Technologies.

INDICATION(S) AND RESEARCH PHASE
Dupuytren's Disease – Phase II
Peyronie's Disease – Phase II
Adhesive Capsulitis – Phase II

Musculoskeletal Diseases

benzestrom
Esterom

MANUFACTURER
Entropin

DESCRIPTION
Esterom is a topical treatment for impaired range of motion associated with acute lower back sprain and acute painful shoulders. The product name is derived from its chemical identity and medical purpose, it being an ester that improves the range of motion (ROM) of subjects suffering from a painful shoulder sprain/strain. Esterom solution is a mixture of components in a propylene, gly-

col water solution. It contains benzoylecgonine and ecgonine, their hydroxypropyl esters, and other hydrolytic by-products. Its mechanism of action is currently unknown.

In phase II trial testing, Esterom demonstrated effectiveness in the improvement of range of motion associated with impaired shoulder function and acute lower back sprain. Currently, this drug is being tested in a phase III trial that will enroll 600 subjects experiencing only shoulder pain.

INDICATION(S) AND RESEARCH PHASE
Pain, Acute or Chronic – Phase III
Musculoskeletal Diseases – Phase III

botulinum toxin type A, AGN-191622
Botox

MANUFACTURER
Allergan

DESCRIPTION
Botulinum toxin type A, a purified neurotoxin complex, has been used as a therapeutic agent since the 1960s. At a normal neuromuscular junction, a nerve impulse triggers the release of acetylcholine, which causes the muscle to contract. Botox reduces excessive muscle activity by blocking the release of acetylcholine at the neuromuscular junction.

In addition, Botox is being tested in a phase II trial for the prevention of migraine headaches, a phase III trial for lower back pain, and a pediatric phase III trial for juvenile cerebral palsy in subjects two to seven years old.

Botox was FDA approved in December 2000 for the treatment of adults with cervical dystonia. When injected into the affected muscles, Botox decreases the severity of abnormal head position and neck pain associated with this condition by blocking the release of the neurotransmitter acetylcholine from the peripheral nerve terminal to the muscle.

INDICATION(S) AND RESEARCH PHASE
Migraine and Cluster Headaches – Phase II
Musculoskeletal Diseases – FDA approved
Pain, Acute or Chronic – Phase III
Pediatric, Cerebral Palsy – Phase III

recombinant human bone morphogenic protein-2 (rhBMP-2)
unknown

MANUFACTURER
Genetics Institute

DESCRIPTION
According to the Genetics Institute, this recombinant human bone morphogenic protein-2 (rhBMP-2) has shown positive results in accelerating bone and cartilage repair in a variety of situations, including severe orthopedic trauma, oral and maxillofacial surgery, and spinal fusion. This genetically engineered drug works as a growth factor that stimulates new bone development. Genetics Institute, a subsidary of American Home Products, is researching rhBMP-2 in phase III trials through a development partnership with Yamanouchi.

INDICATION(S) AND RESEARCH PHASE
Orthopedics – Phase III
Oral Medicine – Phase III
Musculoskeletal Diseases – Phase III
Spinal Cord Injuries – Phase III

Orthopedic Surgery

hemoglobin glutamer-250 (bovine)
Hemopure

MANUFACTURER
Biopure Corporation

DESCRIPTION
Hemopure is a hemoglobin-based oxygen therapy solution originally derived from cows. Hemoglobin is a naturally produced protein containing iron that red blood cells use to transport oxygen from the lungs to the rest of the body. This blood substitute product is being tested for cases of anemia where more red blood cells and oxygen exchange would be needed. Hemopure is given intravenously and phase III trials are ongoing in the United States and recently have been expanded in Canada. Therapeutic uses may include sickle cell anemia, cardiopulmonary bypass surgery, and trauma. Biopure has completed a phase III trial evaluating Hemopure as an alternative to red blood cell transfusion in orthopedic surgery subjects.

INDICATION(S) AND RESEARCH PHASE
Anemia – Phase III
Orthopedic Surgery – Phase III completed

ORG-31540/SR-90107A
unknown

MANUFACTURER
Organon

DESCRIPTION
ORG-31540/SR-90107A is a synthetic 5-unit multi-sugar (pentasaccharide) that may be used in the prevention and treatment of blood clots, or thrombi, that form in the veins and arteries. According to Organon, the drug is a synthetic antithrombotic with its molecular shape modeled after antithrombin III, a protein molecule involved in blood clotting.

In December 2000, results of an international phase III program demonstrated that ORG-31540/SR90107A provided a superior benefit over enoxaparin in major orthopedic surgery subjects, with an overall relative risk reduction of 50% and a similar safety profile. Four multicenter phase III trials compared the two drugs in the prevention of venous thromboembolism (VTE): EPHESUS (hip replacement surgery), PENTATHLON (hip replacement surgery), PENTHIFRA (hip fracture surgery), and PENTAMAKS (major knee surgery).

Future indications may include prevention and/or treatment of deep vein thrombosis, pulmonary embolism, coronary, and peripheral arterial disease. ORG-31540/SR-90107A is being co-developed by Sanofi-Synthelabo and Organon.

INDICATION(S) AND RESEARCH PHASE
Orthopedic Surgery – Phase III completed
Thrombosis – Phase III completed

Orthopedics

recombinant human bone morphogenic protein-2 (rhBMP-2)
unknown

MANUFACTURER
Genetics Institute

DESCRIPTION
According to the Genetics Institute, this recombinant human bone morphogenic protein-2 (rhBMP-2) has shown positive results in accelerating bone and cartilage repair in a variety of situations, including severe orthopedic trauma, oral and maxillofacial surgery, and spinal fusion. This genetically engineered drug works as a growth factor that stimulates new bone development. Genetics Institute, a subsidiary of American Home Products, is researching rhBMP-2 in phase III trials through a development partnership with Yamanouchi.

INDICATION(S) AND RESEARCH PHASE
Orthopedics – Phase III
Oral Medicine – Phase III
Musculoskeletal Diseases – Phase III
Spinal Cord Injuries – Phase III

Osteoarthritis

asimadoline
unknown

MANUFACTURER
Merck KgaA

DESCRIPTION
Asimadoline is a pain reliever being evaluated in a phase II trial for osteoarthritis. It works by stimulating specific kappa-receptors on nerve cells in the peripheral nervous system. As a peripherally effective opioid or synthetic narcotic, asimadoline may inhibit the pain associated with the inflammatory changes of osteoarthritis.

An additional benefit may be that asimadoline lacks the potential for addiction or substance abuse, since this agent exerts its effect only in the periphery, and has not shown any significant adverse events associated with the central nervous system. According to the company, asimadoline has thus far proved to be well tolerated in clinical investigations.

INDICATION(S) AND RESEARCH PHASE
Osteoarthritis – Phase II
Pain, Acute or Chronic – Phase II

BAY 12-9566
unknown

MANUFACTURER
Bayer Corporation

DESCRIPTION
Scientists believe that cancer cells produce enzymes called matrix metalloproteinases (MMPs) to break down the body's own natural protective barriers, allowing cancer to grow and spread. BAY 12-9566 is an MMP inhibitor designed to interfere with this process.

Bayer Corporation was conducting phase III clinical trials of BAY 12-9566 for the treatment of osteoarthritis, and pancreatic, ovarian, and small and non-small cell lung cancers. However, they announced all clinical trials of BAY 12-9566 have been halted. This action follows a recommendation from an independent Data Safety Monitoring Board that the trial for small cell lung cancer be stopped. It was found that in this trial the drug was performing worse than the placebo.

INDICATION(S) AND RESEARCH PHASE
Cancer/Tumors (Unspecified) – Phase Trial halted
Lung Cancer – Trial halted
Ovarian Cancer – Trial halted
Osteoarthritis – Trial halted

CI-1004
unknown

MANUFACTURER
Parke-Davis Division

DESCRIPTION
CI-1004 is a dual enzyme inhibitor of both cyclooxygenase-2 (COX-2) and 5-lipoxygenase developed to treat inflammatory diseases. CI-1004 may have potential advantages and a cleaner adverse event profile compared to current non-steroidal anti-inflammatory drug (NSAID) therapies, especially for the gastrointestinal tract.

Currently, CI-1004 is in a phase III trial for both arthritis and osteoarthritis.

INDICATION(S) AND RESEARCH PHASE
Arthritis and Arthritic Pain – Phase III
Osteoarthritis – Phase III

COX 189
unknown

MANUFACTURER
Novartis

DESCRIPTION
COX 189 is an oral, non-steroidal anti-inflammatory analgesic belonging to the cyclooxygenase-2 (COX-2) inhibitor class. COX 189 has yielded promising results in dental pain relief, in addition to demonstrating relief of pain due to osteoarthritis and rheumatoid arthritis, comparable to that seen with Voltaren (diclofenac). It is currently in phase III development.

INDICATION(S) AND RESEARCH PHASE
Rheumatoid Arthritis – Phase III
Osteoarthritis – Phase III
Pain, Acute or Chronic – Phase III

etodolac
Lodine

MANUFACTURER
Elan Pharmaceutical Research

DESCRIPTION
Lodine is a non-steroidal anti-inflammatory drug (NSAID) pain reliever that has been on the market in an oral tablet formulation since 1991 for acute and long-term treatment of osteoarthritis and rheumatoid arthritis. Lodine is currently being tested in a once daily intestinal protective drug absorption system (IPDAS) for controlled

release delivery. This new formulation is currently in phase III developemnt. Elan Pharmaceutical Research has a development and marketing agreement with Wyeth-Ayerst for this agent.

INDICATION(S) AND RESEARCH PHASE
Osteoarthritis – Phase III
Rheumatoid Arthritis – Phase III
Pain, Acute or Chronic – Phase III

ibuprofen
Benefen

MANUFACTURER
MacroChem Corporation

DESCRIPTION
Benefen is a topically applied formulation of ibuprofen indicated for the treatment of osteoarthritis pain. Phase II trials are complete but no further studies are currently being conducted. Ibuprofen is a commonly used non-steroidal anti-inflammatory drug (NSAID) for relief of mild to moderate pain, and relief of the symptoms of rheumatoid arthritis and osteoarthritis. It is available over the counter (OTC) at many drug stores in tablet or caplet formulation.

INDICATION(S) AND RESEARCH PHASE
Osteoarthritis – Phase II completed

insulin-like growth factor-I (IGF-I)
unknown

MANUFACTURER
Chiron Corporation

DESCRIPTION
This hormone is a genetically engineered, insulin-like growth factor-I (IGF-I). Citron has decided to halt the trials of the drug due to unfavorable results seen in two 13 week phase II proof of concept trials for the treatment of osteoarthritis of the knee. Subjects reported no statistically differences between receiving IGF-1 and the placebo. The first trial treated subjects undergoing arthroscopy, who were injected with IGF-1 or the placebo directly into the cartilage. The second treated knee-replacement subjects with the protein or the placebo before surgery. It is thought that IGF-I may help slow down the degradation of bones and joints.

INDICATION(S) AND RESEARCH PHASE
Osteoarthritis – Phase halted

ketoprofen
Ketotop

MANUFACTURER
United Therapeutics

DESCRIPTION
Ketotop is a patented transdermal formulation of ketoprofen, a nonsteroidal anti-inflammatory drug (NSAID). Ketoprofen has previously been marketed in an oral formulation for the treatment of headaches and post-operative pain.

In December 2000, phase III trial results of Ketotop for osteoarthritis of the knee prompted United Therapeutics to discontinue development. While individual endpoints in the 500 subject trial achieved statistical significance, the key clinical and regulatory endpoint related to pain reduction did not meet the company's expectations.

INDICATION(S) AND RESEARCH PHASE
Osteoarthritis – Phase III discontinued

matrix metalloprotease inhibitor (MMP)
Prinomastat

MANUFACTURER
Agouron Pharmaceuticals

DESCRIPTION
Prinomastat is an orally active, synthetic molecule designed to potently and selectively inhibit certain members of a family of enzymes known as a matrix metalloproteases (MMPs) that are believed to be involved in tumor angiogenesis, invasion, and metastasis. According to the company, based on their mechanism of action, MMP inhibitors may prove to have potential in reducing the invasiveness of malignant brain tumor cells.

The most common side effects of Prinomastat have been observed in the joints, including stiffness, joint swelling, and in a few subjects, some limits on mobility, most often in the shoulders and hands. All these effects were reported reversible and were effectively managed by treatment rests and dose reductions.

Two phase III trials for advanced non-small cell lung cancer and prostate cancer were halted in August 2000 due to the drug's lack of effectiveness in subjects with late-stage disease.

Prinomastat is in phase II trials for treatment of hormone-refractory prostate cancer combined with mitoxantrone and prednisone, as well as for treatment of osteoarthritis and macular degeneration.

In addition, Prinomastat in combination with chemotherapy for subjects with newly diagnosed glioblastoma multiforme following surgery with radiation therapy, is in a phase II trial.

INDICATION(S) AND RESEARCH PHASE
Lung Cancer – Phase halted
Prostate Cancer – Phase halted
Osteoarthritis – Phase II
Brain Cancer – Phase II
Macular Degeneration – Phase II

MK-663
unknown

MANUFACTURER
Merck & Co.

DESCRIPTION
MK-663 belongs to a relatively new class of non-steroidal anti-inflammatory drugs (NSAIDs) called COX-2 inhibitors. MK-663 is designed to specifically inhibit cyclo-oxygenase-2 (COX-2), which is one of several enzymes that leads to the production of substances that cause acute or chronic discomfort in joints with the associated pain and inflammation of arthritis.

Clinical studies have shown that COX-2 inhibitors work with the body to help it strengthen the system and prevent activation of several enzymes of the arachidonic acid metabolism. Consequently, the inhibitors prevent the formulation of eicosanoides, which are short-lived chemical agents that control a large number of physiological functions. COX-2 inhibitors counteract the formation of prostaglandins, which are responsible for short-term joint discomfort, and leukotrienes, which are responsible for long-term joint discomfort. By inhibiting prostaglandin synthesis and counteracting the destructive changes in healthy joints caused by leukotrienes, the extract COX-2 is the first dual inhibitor available.

Merck reported favorable results from a phase II trial that showed MK-663 relieved pain better than the placebo in 617 subjects with osteoarthritis of the knee. Currently, MK-663 is being tested in phase III trials for the treatment and relief of pain associated with rheumatoid arthritis and osteoarthritis.

INDICATION(S) AND RESEARCH PHASE
Pain, Acute or Chronic – Phase III
Rheumatoid Arthritis – Phase III
Osteoarthritis – Phase III

ML3000
unknown

MANUFACTURER
Forest Laboratories

DESCRIPTION
ML3000 is part of a novel class of dual-acting, anti-inflammatory drugs called COX/LO inhibitors that simultaneously inhibit the enzymes cyclooxygenase (COX) and 5-lipoxygenase (LO). In October 2000, positive results were announced for two double-blind, randomized, placebo-controlled phase II trials. ML3000 provided significantly more pain relief than a placebo in subjects with osteoarthritis and produced fewer side effects in normal volunteers. At doses of 200 and 400 mg, subjects given ML3000 reported fewer symptoms compared to when given a placebo. In both studies, treatment with ML3000 was well tolerated across the entire dose range. Additionally, fewer gastric lesions were observed in ML3000 treated subjects compared to those receiving naproxen treatment. Forest Laboratories has signed a licensing agreement with Merckle GmbH for the development and marketing of ML3000 in the United States. Phase III trials should begin in 2001.

INDICATION(S) AND RESEARCH PHASE
Osteoarthritis – Phase II completed

nabumetone Q
unknown

MANUFACTURER
GlaxoSmithKline

DESCRIPTION
Nabumetone Q is a non-steroidal anti-inflammatory drug (NSAID). It is currently in phase III trials for the treatment of osteoarthritis and pain.

INDICATION(S) AND RESEARCH PHASE
Osteoarthritis – Phase III
Pain, Acute or Chronic – Phase III

propiram
Dirame

MANUFACTURER
Roberts Pharmaceutical

DESCRIPTION
Dirame is an orally administered analgesic that works through the central nervous system to reduce pain. This agent acts as a mixed agonist/antagonist, binding to opioid receptors and blocks painful stimuli. Dirame is being tested in phase III trials for the treatment of moderate to severe pain, especially in osteoarthritis.

INDICATION(S) AND RESEARCH PHASE
Pain, Acute or Chronic – Phase III
Osteoarthritis – Phase III

recombinant salmon calcitonin
Fortical Injection

MANUFACTURER
Unigene Laboratories

DESCRIPTION
Fortical Injection is an ijectable version of human parathyroid hormone, a naturally occurring protein, which results in an increase in new bone formation in people with osteoporosis. The drug has completed phase III trials.

INDICATION(S) AND RESEARCH PHASE
Osteoporosis – Phase III completed

topical testosterone gel
unknown

MANUFACTURER
Auxilium A2

DESCRIPTION
In March 2001, Auxilium A2 initiated phase III trials of a new topical gel formulation of testosterone based upon partnering company Bentley's drug delivery technology and anticipates an NDA filing later in 2001. This is being tested as a treatment for management of severe pain associated with osteoporosis on males.

INDICATION(S) AND RESEARCH PHASE
Pain, Acute or Chronic – Phase III
Osteoporosis – Phase III

unknown
Orthovisc

MANUFACTURER
Anika Therapeutics

DESCRIPTION
Orthovisc is a highly purified, high molecular weight, high viscosity injectable form of hyaluronic acid. It is being developed to relieve pain and improve joint mobility and range of motion in patients with osteoarthritis of the knee. In May 2000, an initial analysis of results from a phase III trial did not show sufficient efficacy to support the filing of a pre-market approval (PMA) application for FDA approval. The company has commenced a new phase III trial for Orthovisc designed to include 360 subjects at up to 20 centers in the United States and Canada, with monitoring for six months after initial treatment.

INDICATION(S) AND RESEARCH PHASE

Osteoarthritis – Phase III

valdecoxib
unknown

MANUFACTURER
Pfizer

DESCRIPTION
Valdecoxib is a second generation cyclooxygenase-2 (COX-2) inhibitor that Pfizer is jointly developing with Pharmacia as a treatment for pain associated with arthritis, osteoarthritis, and rheumatoid arthritis. It offers a rapid onset and prolonged efficacy with once-a-day dosing. The drug is currently in phase III testing and an NDA submission is planned for 2001.

INDICATION(S) AND RESEARCH PHASE
Arthritis and Arthritic Pain – Phase III
Osteoarthritis – Phase III
Rheumatoid Arthritis – Phase III

VX-740, pralnacasan
unknown

MANUFACTURER
Vertex Pharmaceuticals

DESCRIPTION
VX-740 is Vertex's most advanced ICE inhibitor. ICE is an enzyme that regulates the production of IL-1 and IFN gamma, intercellular mediators that initiate and sustain the process of inflammation. Inhibiting ICE may be an effective strategy for curtailing damaging inflammatory processes common to a number of acute and chronic conditions, such as rheumatoid arthritis and osteoarthritis. VX-740 is currently in phase II trials.

INDICATION(S) AND RESEARCH PHASE
Rheumatoid Arthritis – Phase II
Osteoarthritis – Phase II

YM-177, celecoxib
unknown

MANUFACTURER
Yamanouchi Pharmaceutical

DESCRIPTION
YM-177 is an orally administered cyclooxygenase-2 (COX-2) inhibitor being evaluated for the treatment of rheumatoid arthritis and osteoarthritis. It is in phase II trials and is part of Yamanouchi's domestic pipeline. The company is developing the drug with Pharmacia.

INDICATION(S) AND RESEARCH PHASE
Rheumatoid Arthritis – Phase II
Osteoarthritis – Phase II

Osteomyelitis

radiolabeled monoclonal antibody
LeuTech

MANUFACTURER
Palatin Technologies

DESCRIPTION
LeuTech is a monoclonal antibody used for imaging various sites of infection. Researchers participating in a phase III clinical trial of LeuTech concluded that the drug is safe and effective in diagnosing cases of equivocal appendicitis. LeuTech also demonstrated a significant positive impact on the management of these subjects. The trial included 200 subjects at ten sites across the United States. LeuTech demonstrated a 90% sensitivity and 87% specificity, as well as a negative predictive value of 95%. The FDA recommended approval of LeuTech for treatment of appendicitis in July 2000.

In addition, LeuTech is in multiple phase II trials for various infections including such as osteomyelitis and ulcerative colitis.

INDICATION(S) AND RESEARCH PHASE
Gastrointestinal Diseases and Disorders, miscellaneous – FDA approval letter
Ulcerative Colitis – Phase II
Osteomyelitis – Phase II

Osteoporosis

17-beta estradiol/trimegestone
unknown

MANUFACTURER
Wyeth-Ayerst

DESCRIPTION
17-beta estradiol/trimegestone is being evaluated in phase III clinical trials for the treatment of menopausal symptoms and osteoporosis.

INDICATION(S) AND RESEARCH PHASE
Menopause – Phase III
Hormone Replacement Therapy: Menopause – Phase III
Osteoporosis – Phase III

ALX1-11
unknown

MANUFACTURER
NPS Allelix Corp

DESCRIPTION
ALX1-11 is being developed by NPS Allelix for the treatment of osteoporosis. ALX1-11 is a recombinant version of human parathyroid hormone (PTH) and is identical to the naturally occurring protein produced by the parathyroid gland. Unlike agents such as bisphosphonates and hormone replacement therapy, which act by preventing further bone loss, ALX1-11 acts on bone generating cells called osteoblasts to stimulate new bone formation.

Results of phase II trial indicated a significant, dose-related effect of ALX1-11 on bone mineral density after one year of treatment in subjects suffering from postmenopausal osteoporosis. ALX1-11 is currently in phase III trials.

INDICATION(S) AND RESEARCH PHASE
Osteoporosis – Phase III

calcitonin
Macritonin

MANUFACTURER
Provalis

DESCRIPTION
Macritonin is the oral formulation of salmon calcitonin, a calcium regulator for the treatment of postmenopausal osteoporosis. Macritonin uses the Macromol oral drug delivery system. Calcitonin is a well tolerated treatment for osteoporosis currently available in injectable and intranasal formulations. Clinical trials testing the oral formulation are currently in phase II.

INDICATION(S) AND RESEARCH PHASE
Osteoporosis – Phase II
Menopause – Phase II

estradiol/norethisterone acetate
Estalis

MANUFACTURER
Novartis

DESCRIPTION
Estalis, a combination of norethindrone acetate and estradiol-17(B), is a hormone replacement therapy. It is manufactured as a small, transdermal patch designed to be worn continuously and changed twice a week. An application has been filed overseas for the prevention of osteoporosis.

INDICATION(S) AND RESEARCH PHASE
Osteoporosis – Application filed overseas

estradiol/progestin
unknown

MANUFACTURER
Watson Pharmaceuticals

DESCRIPTION
Watson Laboratories has conducted phase III trials for a combination estradiol/progestin hormone replacement therapy (HRT) patch using their transdermal delivery system. The patch administers a continuous dose of both estrogen and progestin through the adhesive into the skin for body absorption. The company received an FDA non-approvable letter in November 2000 due to lack of sufficient evidence to support the safety and efficacy of the patch for the treatment of osteoporosis, and required that an additional endometrial protection trial be submitted. Watson anticipates filing an amendment.

INDICATION(S) AND RESEARCH PHASE
Hormone Replacement Therapy:
  Menopause – FDA denied
Osteoporosis – FDA denied

estrogen
Vivelle-Dot

MANUFACTURER
Noven Pharmaceuticals

DESCRIPTION
Vivelle-Dot is an estrogen transdermal system designed to be exceptionally small and to provide hormone replacement therapy for the treatment of menopausal symptoms. Vivelle-Dot utilizes Dot Matrix adhesive technology to deliver 17B-estradiol through the skin and into the bloodstream. It is FDA approved for the treatment of menopausal symptoms, and an NDA has been filed for the treatment of osteoporosis.

INDICATION(S) AND RESEARCH PHASE
Menopause – FDA approved
Osteoporosis – NDA submitted

estrogen
Vivelle, Menorest

MANUFACTURER
Noven Pharmaceuticals

DESCRIPTION
Vivelle/Menorest is an estradiol transdermal system to be used as hormone replacement therapy (HRT) for the treatment of menopausal symptoms and the prevention of osteoporosis. The product delivers 17-beta estradiol, the primary estrogen produced by the ovaries, through a patch that is applied twice weekly. It has been approved by the FDA for menopausal symptoms, and an application has been filed and results are pending for approval as a treatment for osteoporosis.

Marketing rights have been licensed to Novogyne in the United States, to Novartis in Canada, and to Aventis in all other territories. The product is being sold as Menorest in 19 foreign countries, including France, Germany, and the United Kingdom, while being marketed as Vivelle in the United States and Canada.

INDICATION(S) AND RESEARCH PHASE
Osteoporosis – NDA submitted
Menopause – FDA approved

HCT 1026
unknown

MANUFACTURER
NicOx SA

DESCRIPTION
HCT 1026 is a novel nitric oxide-releasing derivative of the non-steroidal anti-inflammatory drug (NSAID) flurbiprofen. While flurbiprofen has demonstrated effectiveness in the treatment of urinary incontinence, its use has been complicated by gastric toxicity. Because HCT 1026 may provide increased gastric tolerability, it can be administered for extended periods at effective doses. In phase I trials, HCT 1026 produced fewer and less severe gastric lesions compared to flurbiprofen.

HCT 1026 produces anti-inflammatory effects through the inhibition of prostaglandin synthesis, while nitric oxide controls inflammatory cell activation. These two factors suggest that HCT 1026 may be an effective treatment for dermatology disorders, such as psoriasis. HCT 1026 is in phase II trials for the treatment of urinary incontinence, osteoporosis, and skin disorders.

INDICATION(S) AND RESEARCH PHASE
Urinary Incontinence – Phase II
Osteoporosis – Phase II
Skin Infections/Disorders – Phase II

ibandronate
Bonviva

MANUFACTURER
Hoffmann-La Roche

DESCRIPTION
Bonviva (ibandronate) is a third generation of a relatively new class of drugs known as bisphosphonates that are being tested in the treatment of osteoporosis. Bisphosphonates are drugs that inhibit bone turnover by decreasing the resorption of bone. They work both directly by inhibiting the recruitment and function of osteoclasts, the bone-resorbing cells, and indirectly, by stimulating osteoblasts, the bone forming cells, in order to produce an inhibitor of osteoclast formation. Bonviva is currently in phase III trials for treatment of osteoporosis and breast cancer. Other formulations of bisphosphonates have previously been approved for the treatment of Paget's disease and hypercalcemia of cancer.

INDICATION(S) AND RESEARCH PHASE
Osteoporosis – Phase III
Breast Cancer – Phase III

lasofoxifene
unknown

MANUFACTURER
Pfizer

DESCRIPTION
Lasofoxifene is a non-steroidal, potent estrogen mixed agonist/antagonist that binds selectively to the human estrogen receptor-alpha. Lasofoxifene is currently being tested in a phase III trial for the prevention of osteoporosis.

INDICATION(S) AND RESEARCH PHASE
Osteoporosis – Phase III

NE-58095, risedronate sodium
unknown

MANUFACTURER
Takeda Chemical Industries

DESCRIPTION
NE-58095 is a bone resorption inhibitor being developed for the treatment of osteoporosis. The drug is currently under application in Japan.

INDICATION(S) AND RESEARCH PHASE
Osteoporosis – Application submitted in Japan

parathyroid hormone, PTH
unknown

MANUFACTURER
Eli Lilly

DESCRIPTION
Eli Lilly is developing a synthetic form of parathyroid hormone (PTH), that is naturally found in the body. The synthetic hormone is to be given in daily subcutaneous injections for the treatment of osteoporosis. It is currently being tested in phase III clinical trials. Normally, PTH is secreted by the four parathyroid glands, which are located on the back of the thyroid gland in the neck. Studies have shown that PTH acts on bone building cells called osteoblasts to stimulate new bone growth and improve density. Unlike agents already in use that prevent further bone loss, like estrogen and bisphosphonate, synthetic PTH may have the potential to replace depleted bone stores in the body.

Preliminary studies have demonstrated that PTH can increase both bone mass and the amount of new bone produced, especially in the spinal column. All the women who received the drug had higher measures of bone density compared to those subjects given the placebo. Taking bisphosphonate, a medication that decreases the rate of bone resorption, seems to enhance the effect of the PTH.

INDICATION(S) AND RESEARCH PHASE
Osteoporosis – Phase III

SB 273005
unknown

MANUFACTURER
GlaxoSmithKline

DESCRIPTION
SB 273005 is a novel small-molecule, orally active vitronectin antagonist. It is currently in phase I development for osteoporosis and rheumatoid arthritis.

INDICATION(S) AND RESEARCH PHASE
Osteoporosis – Phase I
Rheumatoid Arthritis – Phase I

sodium fluoride
Neosten

MANUFACTURER
Mission Pharmacal

DESCRIPTION
Neosten is a slow releasing oral formulation of sodium flouride that has been developed for the treatment of osteoporosis. Neosten works by stimulating osteoblasts, which are cells responsible for building new bone.

Mission Pharmacal reported that the second phase III trial for osteoporosis was completed, and that an NDA was submitted. Pending FDA approval, the company may initiate a subsequent phase IV trial.

INDICATION(S) AND RESEARCH PHASE
Osteoporosis – NDA submitted

testosterone
unknown

MANUFACTURER
Watson Pharmaceuticals

DESCRIPTION
Testosterone is a naturally produced hormone that is responsible for proper development of male secondary sex characteristics. The hormone, which has been formulated in the MTX transdermal patch, is being tested in phase II trials for treatment of sexual dysfunction in surgically menopausal subjects, for use in menopause associated hormone replacement therapy, and treatment of osteoporosis. Additionally, it is in phase III clinical trials for treatment of male hormonal deficiencies and abnormalities.

This hormone regime is also being evaluated in phase II trials for treatment of AIDS wasting in females. Testosterone is an anabolic steroid that may help build up muscle mass in subjects suffering from AIDS.

INDICATION(S) AND RESEARCH PHASE
Acquired Immune Deficiency Syndrome (AIDS) and AIDS-Related Infections – Phase II
Hormone Replacement Therapy: Menopause – Phase II
Male Hormonal Deficiencies/Abnormalities – Phase III
Osteoporosis – Phase II
Sexual Dysfunction – Phase II completed

TSE-424
unknown

MANUFACTURER
Wyeth-Ayerst

DESCRIPTION
TSE-424 is a selected estrogen receptor modulator (SERM) designed to mimic the beneficial qualities of estrogens, while blocking estrogen in tissues where it can be harmful. A SERM is a partial agonist that binds with high affinity to the estrogen receptor, but has tissue specific effects distinct from estradiol. SERMs are designed to act selectively, by eliminating some of the risks of estrogen, such as undesirable effects on the uterus or breast tissue, while supplementing inadequate estrogen supplies in post-menopausal women.

TSE-424 is being tested in phase II trials for the prevention and treatment of post-menopausal osteoporosis. Wyeth-Ayerst and Ligand Pharmaceuticals have a cooperative agreement for the development of TSE-424.

INDICATION(S) AND RESEARCH PHASE
Osteoporosis – Phase II
Menopause – Phase II

zoledronate
Zometa

MANUFACTURER
Novartis

DESCRIPTION
Zometa is an intravenous bisphosphonate osteoclast inhibitor. In September 2000, Novartis announced it has received an approvable letter from the FDA for Zometa for the treatment of hypercalcemia of malignancy (HCM), the most common life-threatening metabolic complication associated with cancer. Zometa is also in phase II development for the treatment of post-menopausal osteoporosis and phase III development for bone metastasis treatment and prevention.

INDICATION(S) AND RESEARCH PHASE
Osteoporosis – Phase II
Hypercalcemia – FDA recommend approval letter
Bone Metastases – Phase III

Pain, Acute or Chronic

ABT-594, epibatidine
unknown

MANUFACTURER
Abbott Laboratories

DESCRIPTION
In 1976, scientists with the National Institutes of Health isolated a compound from the skin of Epipedobates tricolor, an Ecuadorian frog. Named epibatidine, this alkaloid was found to block pain 200 times more effectively than morphine, without morphine's addictive and harmful side effects. A potent anti-nociceptive agent for acute and persistent pain, this compound works predominately by an action at central neuronal acetylcholine receptors.

Now that the paralyzing effects of the poison can be eliminated, epibatidine is being evaluated in phase II trials for treatment of hepatic encephalopathy in subjects with advanced liver disease. Most analgesics modulate the feeling of pain by binding to opiate receptors. Epibatidine has a very low affinity for the nicotine receptors in the neuromuscular junction that cause the paralysis effect, but a high affinity for the nicotine receptors in the central nervous system that regulate pain perception.

INDICATION(S) AND RESEARCH PHASE
Hepatic Encephalopathy – Phase II
Pain, Acute or Chronic – Phase II

acetaminophen/ dextromethorphan
HydrocoDex

MANUFACTURER
Algos Pharmaceutical

DESCRIPTION
HydrocoDex is a novel *N*-methyl-D-aspartate (*N*MDA) enhanced narcotic combination of acetaminophen and dextromethorphan. This *N*MDA combination with antagonist drugs has been approved for human use in other applications. HydrocoDex is currently being tested in phase II/III trials in an oral formulation for treatment of acute and chronic pain.

INDICATION(S) AND RESEARCH PHASE
Pain, Acute or Chronic – Phase II/III

ADX-153
unknown

MANUFACTURER
Andrx

DESCRIPTION
ADX-153 is being engineered to deliver pain relieving medications to affected areas in a more efficient, targeted manner. Currently, one of the most active areas of drug development is the formulation of new drug delivery systems, including new methods of controlled-release and targeted action. The goal is to ensure that drugs are delivered to their particular target sites without being inactivated or destroyed, leaving their potency intact.

ADX-153 is a chemical union of the active analgesic medication and a protein container. When this container comes into contact with fluids in the digestive tract, it changes shape and begins to allow the slow release of the pain medication. Because of this slower, more controlled release, this drug can be given in a once daily dose, which may result in fewer side effects.

Drugs already in clinical use could potentially become more effective if their transport system to affected sites in the body were improved. More precise delivery of pain medications could result in better pain relief and the ability to use smaller dosages of the drug to achieve equivalent effects, thus minimizing the drug's potential side effects. ADX-153 is currently in phase II development for pain relief.

INDICATION(S) AND RESEARCH PHASE
Pain, Acute or Chronic – Phase II

---

asimadoline
unknown

MANUFACTURER
Merck KgaA

DESCRIPTION
Asimadoline is a pain reliever being evaluated in a phase II trial for osteoarthritis. It works by stimulating specific kappa-receptors on nerve cells in the peripheral nervous system. As a peripherally effective opioid or synthetic narcotic, asimadoline may inhibit the pain associated with the inflammatory changes of osteoarthritis.

An additional benefit may be that asimadoline lacks the potential for addiction or substance abuse, since this agent exerts its effect only in the periphery, and has not shown any significant adverse events associated with the central nervous system. According to the company, asimadoline has thus far proved to be well tolerated in clinical investigations.

INDICATION(S) AND RESEARCH PHASE
Osteoarthritis – Phase II
Pain, Acute or Chronic – Phase II

AVP-923
unknown

MANUFACTURER
AVANIR Pharmaceuticals

DESCRIPTION
AVP-923 is in a phase II/III trial for the treatment of emotional lability in subjects with Lou Gehrig's disease, the common name for amyotrophic lateral sclerosis (ALS). The trial includes 100 subjects and 11 sites in the United States. The trial is being monitored by INC Research and is expected to continue through July 2001. AVP-923 is also undergoing development in phase II/III trials for pain control and phase II trials for chronic cough. The company plans to initiate another clinical trial this year to be conducted in multiple sclerosis subjects.

INDICATION(S) AND RESEARCH PHASE
Amyotrophic Lateral Sclerosis (ALS) – Phase II/III
Pain, Acute or Chronic – Phase II/III
Emotional Lability – Phase II/III
Chronic Cough – Phase II

BCH-3963, LEF576
unknown

MANUFACTURER
BioChem Pharma

DESCRIPTION
BCH-3963 is an injectable delivery form of a new class of pain relievers that work by binding selectively to peripherally located pain, or mu-opioid receptors. This drug does not enter the central nervous system to treat pain. Therefore, BCH-3963 may cause fewer neurological adverse effects, such as the physical dependence associated with morphine, making it potentially suitable for treatment of chronic as well as acute pain. Although BioChem and Astra have a collaborative research agreement, Astra is primarily responsible for the global clinical development of BCH-3963.

INDICATION(S) AND RESEARCH PHASE
Pain, Acute or Chronic – Phase II

---

benzestrom
Esterom

MANUFACTURER
Entropin

DESCRIPTION
Esterom is a topical treatment for impaired range of motion associated with acute lower back sprain and acute painful shoulders. The product name is derived from its chemical identity and medical purpose, it being an ester that improves the range of motion (ROM) of subjects suffering from a painful shoulder sprain/strain. Esterom solution is a mixture of components in a propylene, glycol water solution. It contains benzoylecgonine and ecgonine, their hydroxypropyl esters, and other hydrolytic by-products. Its mechanism of action is currently unknown.

In phase II trial testing, Esterom demonstrated effectiveness in the improvement of range of motion associated with impaired shoulder function and acute lower back sprain. Currently, this drug is being tested in a phase III trial that will enroll 600 subjects experiencing only shoulder pain.

INDICATION(S) AND RESEARCH PHASE
Pain, Acute or Chronic – Phase III
Musculoskeletal Diseases – Phase III

---

botulinum toxin type A, AGN-191622
Botox

MANUFACTURER
Allergan

DESCRIPTION
Botulinum toxin type A, a purified neurotoxin complex, has been used as a therapeutic agent since the 1960s. At a normal neuromuscular junction, a nerve impulse triggers the release of acetylcholine, which causes the muscle to contract. Botox reduces excessive muscle activity by blocking the release of acetylcholine at the neuromuscular junction.

In addition, Botox is being tested in a phase II trial for the prevention of migraine headaches, a phase III trial for lower back pain, and a pediatric phase III trial for juvenile cerebral palsy in subjects two to seven years old.

Botox was FDA approved in December 2000 for the treatment of adults with cervical dystonia. When injected into the affected muscles, Botox decreases the severity of abnormal head position and neck pain associated with this condition by blocking the release of the neurotransmitter acetylcoline from the peripheral nerve terminal to the muscle.

INDICATION(S) AND RESEARCH PHASE
Migraine and Cluster Headaches – Phase II
Musculoskeletal Diseases – FDA approved
Pain, Acute or Chronic – Phase III
Pediatric, Cerebral Palsy – Phase III

bupivacaine
DepoBupivacaine

MANUFACTURER
Skye Pharma

DESCRIPTION
Bupivacaine, an amino-amide compound that causes reversible blockade of nerve impulses to control pain, is classified as a local anesthetic. DepoBupivacaine is administered via injection and provides sustained release using the DepoFoam slow release, lipid-based delivery system. It is thought that the local anesthetic receptors are protein bound receptors located near the sodium channel. Bupivacaine is highly protein bound, which results in a slower dissociation from the receptor and a subsequent prolonged effect. Reported side effects include tremors, cardiovascular abnormalities, and drug hypersensitivity. DepoBupivacaine is being tested in phase II trials for the relief of pain.

INDICATION(S) AND RESEARCH PHASE
Pain, Acute or Chronic – Phase II

clonadine gel
unknown

MANUFACTURER
Curatek

DESCRIPTION
Clonadine gel is in phase III trials testing 600 subjects for the treatment of peripheral neuropathic pain and painful diabetic neuropathy at 20 sites in the United States.

Although clonadine is widely prescribed in both a transdermal patch and an oral formulation, it has also been shown to act as a potent local analgesic. According to Curateck, the gel formulation is being designed to provide concentrated, site-specific therapy over the complete painful area without blocking motor or sensory nerve function. Results from early trials using clonadine gel showed it to be effective with minimal side effects.

INDICATION(S) AND RESEARCH PHASE
Pain, Acute or Chronic – Phase III
Neuropathy – Phase III
Neuropathy, Diabetic – Phase III

COX 189
unknown

MANUFACTURER
Novartis

DESCRIPTION
COX 189 is an oral, non-steroidal anti-inflammatory analgesic belonging to the cyclooxygenase-2 (COX-2) inhibitor class. COX 189 has yielded promising results in dental pain relief, in addition to demonstrating relief of pain due to osteoarthritis and rheumatoid arthritis, comparable to that seen with Voltaren (diclofenac). It is currently in phase III development.

INDICATION(S) AND RESEARCH PHASE
Rheumatoid Arthritis – Phase III
Osteoarthritis – Phase III
Pain, Acute or Chronic – Phase III

CT-3
unknown

MANUFACTURER
Atlantic Pharmaceuticals

DESCRIPTION
CT-3 is an analgesic and anti-inflammatory drug that is a synthetic derivative of tetrahydrocannabinol (THC), the active ingredient in marijuana. CT-3 is in phase I trials in Paris, France.

Results from animal studies demonstrated CT-3 has analgesic and anti-inflammatory properties at microgram doses without the neurological and gastrointestinal side effects, commonly seen with current anti-inflammatory drugs.

INDICATION(S) AND RESEARCH PHASE
Inflammation – Phase I
Pain, Acute or Chronic – Phase I

dexamethasone
IontoDex

MANUFACTURER
Iomed

DESCRIPTION
IontoDex is being developed in phase III trials for the treatment of acute local inflammation, ocular disease, and for systemic pain control. IontoDex is comprised of the drug dexamethasone, an anti-inflammatory steroid, delivered by the proprietary iontophoretic drug delivery device Phoresor. Iontophoresis is a needle-free method of delivering medication directly into and through the skin using a mild, low-level electric current. By programming the system's electric current levels to achieve the desired dose, delivery rate, or pattern of delivery can control the amount of drug delivered.

INDICATION(S) AND RESEARCH PHASE
Eye Disorders/Infections – Phase III
Pain, Acute or Chronic – Phase III
Inflammation – Phase III

diclofenac
unknown

MANUFACTURER
Pharmos Corporation

DESCRIPTION
Diclofenac is a non-steroidal anti-inflammatory drug (NSAID) developed for the treatment of local pain and inflammation. This topically formulated drug is in phase I/II trials.

INDICATION(S) AND RESEARCH PHASE
Pain, Acute or Chronic – Phase I/II
Inflammation – Phase I/II

DPI-3290
unknown

MANUFACTURER
Delta Pharmaceutical Group

DESCRIPTION
DPI-3290 is an analgesic agent that works by stimulating both delta- and mu-receptors. This intravenous drug is being developed for the treatment of severe post-operative pain. Current strong analgesics, such as morphine, act on mu-receptors to suppress pain. These opioids also produce many unwanted side effects, such as nausea, vomiting, constipation, and respiratory depression.

The Delta Pharmaceutical Group has developed DPI-3290 based on a novel class of delta opioid receptors, which have the promise of providing strong analgesia without the serious side effects caused by currently approved drugs, such as respiratory depression, nausea, and vomiting.

In early clinical trials, DPI-3290 showed that it could potentially deliver potent analgesia exceeding that of morphine. Currently, this mixed delta/mu agonist is being tested in a phase II trial for the relief of severe pain, immediately following surgery.

INDICATION(S) AND RESEARCH PHASE
Pain, Acute or Chronic – Phase II

etodolac
Lodine

MANUFACTURER
Elan Pharmaceutical Research

DESCRIPTION
Lodine is a non-steroidal anti-inflammatory (NSAID) pain reliever that has been on the market in an oral tablet formulation since 1991 for acute and long-term treatment of osteoarthritis and rheumatoid arthritis. Lodine is currently being tested in a once daily intestinal protective drug absorption system (IPDAS) for controlled release delivery. This new formulation is currently in phase III development. Elan Pharmaceutical Research has a development and marketing agreement with Wyeth-Ayerst for this agent.

INDICATION(S) AND RESEARCH PHASE
Osteoarthritis – Phase III
Rheumatoid Arthritis – Phase III
Pain, Acute or Chronic – Phase III

fentanyl
unknown

MANUFACTURER
Elan Pharmaceutical Research

DESCRIPTION
Fentanyl is a well-regarded opioid, or synthetic narcotic, that has 75 to 100 times the analgesic potency of morphine, as well as a more rapid onset of action and shorter duration of effect. Unlike morphine, it does not provoke histamine release and is therefore not as commonly associated with vascular dilatation and systemic hypotension. Phase I/II trials are currently testing the administration of fentanyl through the Medipad Continuous System. As a unique pump in a patch system, Medipad provides controlled injectable delivery in a simple, subject friendly format. It is a low-cost, disposable, single-use system that combines microinfusion technology with an integral subcutaneous probe. An adhesive backing fixes the system against the subject's chest or abdomen, where it continuously dispenses a drug for up to 48 hours.

INDICATION(S) AND RESEARCH PHASE
Pain, Acute or Chronic – Phase I/II

fentanyl transdermal system
Duragesic

MANUFACTURER
Alza (Sequus Pharmaceuticals)

DESCRIPTION
Duragesic is a 72 hour transdermal system for management of chronic pain in subjects requiring continuous opioid, or synthetic narcotic, pain relief that cannot be managed by lesser means, such as acetaminophen-opioid combinations or non-steroidal analgesics. Duragesic is marketed by Janssen Pharmaceutica and is currently in phase III trials for the treatment of chronic pain in pediatric subjects ages two to sixteen.

INDICATION(S) AND RESEARCH PHASE
Pain, Acute or Chronic – Phase III
Pediatric, Pain, Acute or Chronic – Phase III

GW 406381
unknown

MANUFACTURER
GlaxoSmithKline

DESCRIPTION
GW 406381 is a second generation cyclooxygenase-2 (COX-2) inhibitor being developed for the treatment of pain, including inflammatory pain. It is currently in phase I trials.

INDICATION(S) AND RESEARCH PHASE
Pain, Acute or Chronic – Phase I
Inflammation – Phase I

HCT 3012
unknown

MANUFACTURER
NicOx SA

DESCRIPTION
HCT 3012 is a nitric-oxide derivative of the non-steroidal anti-inflammatory drug (NSAID) naproxen. In animal models of rheumatoid inflammatory disorders, pain, and arthritis, HCT 3012 exhibited significantly lower gastric toxicity than naproxen. NicOx SA is developing HCT 3012 with AstraZeneca. A phase II trial has been initiated in Europe for treatment of pain and inflammation.

INDICATION(S) AND RESEARCH PHASE
Pain, Acute or Chronic – Phase II
Inflammation – Phase II

hydromorphone
unknown

MANUFACTURER
Alza (Sequus Pharmaceuticals)

DESCRIPTION
A phase III trial is testing hydromorphone, a synthetic narcotic analgesic, with a new 24-hour OROS controlled-release delivery system for treatment of pain caused by severe chronic conditions. The main benefit of combining an analgesic with this delivery system may be continuous, around the clock pain relief.

INDICATION(S) AND RESEARCH PHASE
Pain, Acute or Chronic – Phase III

ketoprofen patch
unknown

MANUFACTURER
Noven Pharmaceuticals

DESCRIPTION
Noven Pharmaceuticals is developing a ketoprofen transdermal patch for the treatment of joint pain. Ketoprofen is a non-steroidal anti-inflammatory drug (NSAID) that works by reducing hormones that cause inflammation and pain in the body. The transdermal patch technology allows ketoprofen to be delivered directly to the site of pain, instead of initially passing through the gastrointestinal tract. According to Noven, this is expected to reduce gastrointestinal toxicity. The ketoprofen patch is currently in phase II trials.

INDICATION(S) AND RESEARCH PHASE
Pain, Acute or Chronic – Phase II

LEF
unknown

MANUFACTURER
AstraZeneca

DESCRIPTION
LEF is a peripheral μ-agonist in an intravenous formulation. It is currently in phase II trials for the treatment of acute or chronic pain.

INDICATION(S) AND RESEARCH PHASE
Pain, Acute or Chronic – Phase II

MH-200, morphine hydrochloride
unknown

MANUFACTURER
Takeda Chemical Industries

DESCRIPTION
MH-200 is a high content/concentration preparation being evaluated as an analgesic for severe pain due to cancer. The drug is currently under application in Japan.

INDICATION(S) AND RESEARCH PHASE
Pain, Acute or Chronic – Under application in Japan

MK-663
unknown

MANUFACTURER
Merck & Co.

DESCRIPTION
MK-663 belongs to a relatively new class of non-steroidal anti-inflammatory drugs (NSAID) called COX-2 inhibitors. MK-663 is designed to specifically inhibit cyclo-oxygenase-2 (COX-2), which is one of several enzymes that leads to the production of substances that cause acute or chronic discomfort in joints with the associated pain and inflammation of arthritis.

Clinical studies have shown that COX-2 inhibitors work with the body to help it strengthen the system and prevent activation of several enzymes of the arachidonic acid metabolism. Consequently, the inhibitors prevent the formulation of eicosanoids, which are short-lived chemical agents that control a large number of physiological functions. COX-2 inhibitors counteract the formation of prostaglandins, that are responsible for short-term joint discomfort, and leukotrienes, that are responsible for long-term joint discomfort. By inhibiting prostaglandin synthesis and counteracting the destructive changes in healthy joints caused by leukotrienes, the extract COX-2 is the first dual inhibitor available.

Merck reported favorable results from a phase II trial that showed MK-663 relieved pain better than the placebo in 617 subjects with osteoarthritis of the knee. Currently, MK-663 is being tested in phase III trials for the treatment and relief of pain associated with rheumatoid arthritis and osteoarthritis.

INDICATION(S) AND RESEARCH PHASE
Pain, Acute or Chronic – Phase III
Rheumatoid Arthritis – Phase III
Osteoarthritis – Phase III

morphine
unknown

MANUFACTURER
Nastech Pharmaceutical

DESCRIPTION
Nastech's intranasal morphine formulation is being evaluated for the treatment of breakthrough pain. The intranasal formulation allows the opioid to be absorbed directly into systemic circulation for a faster therapeutic effect. Results of a phase II trial showed the product to be safe and efficacious in the treatment of eight episodes of breakthrough pain. The treatment group consisted of 13 subjects suffering from moderate to severe chronic pain with daily episodes of breakthrough pain. Sixty-six percent of breakthrough pain episodes were treated successfully within 20 minutes with the nasal formulation. Significantly, five treatments resulted in a total pain score that was below the baseline level of medication used for chronic therapy, meaning that subjects experienced less pain than they feel on a chronic basis. Pain relief typically began within five minutes, and six subjects sustained their total pain score below baseline up to the period of discharge from the study. A broader phase II study is now in progress.

INDICATION(S) AND RESEARCH PHASE
Pain, Acute or Chronic – Phase II

morphine sulfate
Morphelan

MANUFACTURER
Ligand Pharmaceuticals

DESCRIPTION
Morphelan is a once-daily oral morphine presentation that utilizes Elan's SODAS release technology. The controlled release beads produced by the SODAS technology range from one to two mm in diameter. Each bead begins as an inert core onto which the drug is applied, followed by a number of layers of soluble and insoluble polymers combined with other excipients to produce the rate controlling layer. Within the gastrointestinal tract, the soluble polymers dissolve leaving pores within the outer membrane. Fluid then enters the core of the beads and dissolves the drug. The resultant solution then diffuses out in a controlled, pre-determined manner allowing for prolonged invivo dissolution and absorption phases. Morphelan is being tested in phase III trials for pain relief in cancer and AIDS subjects.

Morphelan is also being tested in a transdermal delivery system called MediPad. A pump in a patch system, MediPad provides controlled injectable delivery in a low-cost, disposable, single-use system that combines microinfusion technology with an integral subcutaneous probe. An adhesive backing fixes the system against the user's chest or abdomen, where it continuously dispenses drug for up to 48 hours.

INDICATION(S) AND RESEARCH PHASE
Pain, Acute or Chronic – Phase III

nabumetone Q
unknown

MANUFACTURER
GlaxoSmithKline

DESCRIPTION
Nabumetone Q is a non-steroidal anti-inflammatory drug (NSAID). It is currently in phase III trials for the treatment of osteoarthritis and pain.

INDICATION(S) AND RESEARCH PHASE
Osteoarthritis – Phase III
Pain, Acute or Chronic – Phase III

nasal ketamine
unknown

MANUFACTURER
Innovative Drug Delivery Systems

DESCRIPTION
Nasal ketamine is in phase I/II trials for the treatment of breakthrough episodes in chronic pain.

INDICATION(S) AND RESEARCH PHASE
Pain, Acute or Chronic – Phase I/II

NCX 4016
unknown

MANUFACTURER
NicOx SA

DESCRIPTION
NCX 4016 is a nitric oxide-releasing derivative of acetylsalicylic acid, the active ingredient in aspirin. NCX 4016 may be able to provide the anti-thrombotic effects of aspirin with less gastric damage or toxicity. Also, studies suggest that nitric oxide itself may provide anti-thrombotic activity, and NCX 4016, unlike other treatments, may inhibit almost all phases of the blood clotting process. The compound is in phase I development for pain, inflammation, and prevention of cardiovascular diseases including thrombosis.

INDICATION(S) AND RESEARCH PHASE
Pain, Acute or Chronic – Phase I
Thrombosis – Phase I

NCX 701
unknown

MANUFACTURER
NicOx SA

DESCRIPTION
NCX 701 is a derivative of paracetamol, or acetaminophen, which results in the release of nitric oxide (NO). It is being evaluated for the treatment of pain in a phase I trial in France. This study was initiated in December 2000 and will include 40 subjects.

Preclinical trials demonstrated NCX 701 to have significantly better analgesic activity than paracetamol, and to be a potent anti-inflammatory compound with absence of the liver toxicity characteristic of paracetamol. The anti-inflammatory effect of the NO-compound is a paradoxical finding and one that prompts further investigation.

INDICATION(S) AND RESEARCH PHASE
Pain, Acute or Chronic – Phase I

neurotrophin-3 (NT-3)
unknown

MANUFACTURER
Regeneron Pharmaceuticals

DESCRIPTION
This drug is an injectable formulation of neurotrophin-3 (NT-3), a naturally occurring human protein. It acts on the neurons of the intestinal tract and is being tested for severe constipation and various constipating conditions caused by spinal cord injuries, narcotic analgesics, and Parkinson's disease. NT-3 is currently in phase II development.

INDICATION(S) AND RESEARCH PHASE
Constipation – Phase II
Spinal Cord Injuries – Phase II
Parkinson's Disease – Phase II
Pain, Acute or Chronic – Phase II

NO-naproxen
unknown

MANUFACTURER
AstraZeneca

DESCRIPTION
NO-naproxen is a nitric oxide non-steroidal anti-inflammatory drug (NSAID) derivative. It is currently in phase I trials for the treatment of acute or chronic pain.

INDICATION(S) AND RESEARCH PHASE
Pain, Acute or Chronic – Phase I

oxycodone hydrochloride/

dextromethorphan hydrobromide
OxycoDex

MANUFACTURER
Algos Pharmaceutical

DESCRIPTION
OxycoDex is a novel N-methyl-D-aspartate (NMDA) enhanced narcotic being developed in phase I/II trials for the management of moderate to severe pain. In the nervous system, chemical messengers called neurotransmitters bind to receptors embedded in the cell membranes of neurons. Glutamate, one such neurotransmitter, binds to the NMDA receptor. When activated by glutamate, the NMDA receptor opens a channel in the cell membrane setting off a series of reactions necessary for normal function of the brain.

When impaired, nerve cells are unable control the normal release of neurotransmitters and end up dumping excess glutamate into the extracellular environment. Excess glutamate results in over-excitation of the NMDA receptor, allowing excess calcium to enter the affected neurons. These neurons may then swell and rupture, releasing more glutamate into the surrounding area, which in turn overexcites NMDA receptors on adjacent neurons. This cascade of neuronal injury, referred to as excitotoxicity, follows acute conditions such as stroke and traumatic brain injury. As an NMDA antagonist combined with an analgesic, OxycoDex may significantly improve pain relief over currently available analgesics.

INDICATION(S) AND RESEARCH PHASE
Pain, Acute or Chronic – Phase I/II

pancrelipase
Viokase

MANUFACTURER
Axcan Pharma

DESCRIPTION
Viokase is a pancreatic enzyme preparation containing standardized lipase, protease, and amylase in fixed proportions. It is indicated for the treatment of subjects with exocrine pancreatic enzyme deficiency as is often associated with cystic fibrosis, chronic pancreatitis and post-pancreatectomy. It has been prescribed for years to assist in the digestion and absorption of food. Axcan is currently conducting phase II trials of Viokase at elevated dosages of 8,000 units per day to alleviate pain often associated with pancreatic disorders.

INDICATION(S) AND RESEARCH PHASE
Pain, Acute or Chronic – Phase II
Pancreatic Disorders – Phase II

pregabalin
unknown

MANUFACTURER
Pfizer

DESCRIPTION
Pregabalin is being developed in phase III trials for the treatment of neuropathic pain, epilepsy, a variety of anxiety disorders, and chronic pain syndromes. In February 2001, Pfizer announced it has restricted the use of pregabalin for certain subjects in clinical trials. The restriction follows an analysis by the FDA of previously submitted results from a chronic administration mouse study that showed an increased evidence of a tumor type in the mice. A similar dosing study in rats did not show increases in any tumor type, nor were these results seen in any other toxicological screen or study. The planned submission of the NDA for neuropathic pain and epilepsy is expected to proceed as previously announced.

INDICATION(S) AND RESEARCH PHASE
Pain, Acute or Chronic – Phase III
Epilepsy – Phase III
Anxiety Disorders – Phase III

propiram
Dirame

MANUFACTURER
Roberts Pharmaceutical

DESCRIPTION
Dirame is an orally administered analgesic that works through the central nervous system to reduce pain. This agent acts as a mixed agonist/antagonist, binding to opioid receptors and blocking painful stimuli. Dirame is being tested in phase III trials for the treatment of moderate to severe pain, especially in osteoarthritis.

INDICATION(S) AND RESEARCH PHASE
Pain, Acute or Chronic – Phase III
Osteoarthritis – Phase III

ropivacaine HCl
Naropin

MANUFACTURER
AstraZeneca

DESCRIPTION
Naropin is a sodium channel blocker that is currently in phase III trials for use as a spinal anesthetic in an intra-articular administration. An NDA was submitted in December 2000 for approval for a single-dose administration of Naropin injection for regional anesthesia in pediatric subjects. FDA approval is also sought for Naropin as a treatment for acute pain management in children one to twelve years old. Naropin has been FDA approved as an obstetric anesthesia and regional anesthesia for surgery, as well as for the management of postoperative pain.

INDICATION(S) AND RESEARCH PHASE
Pain, Acute or Chronic – FDA approved
Pediatric, Anesthesia – NDA submitted
Anaesthesia, Regional – FDA approved
Pediatric, Pain, Acute or Chronic – NDA submitted
Anesthesia, Spinal – Phase III

RSD 921
unknown

MANUFACTURER
Nortran Pharmaceuticals

DESCRIPTION
RSD 921 is a novel, sodium channel blocker designed to function as a local anesthetic. An ion channel is a membrane protein that

controls the flow of ions such as sodium, potassium, and calcium in and out of cells. The regulation of these ion concentrations can affect many processes, including nerve signal transmission and muscle contraction. Phase II development was completed in 1998 and upcoming trials have yet to be initiated.

INDICATION(S) AND RESEARCH PHASE
Pain, Acute or Chronic – Phase II completed

topical testosterone gel
unknown

MANUFACTURER
Auxilium A2

DESCRIPTION
In March 2001, Auxilium A2 initiated phase III trials of a new topical gel formulation of testosterone based upon partnering company Bentley's drug delivery technology and anticipates an NDA filing later in 2001. This is being tested as a treatment for management of severe pain associated with osteoporosis on males.

INDICATION(S) AND RESEARCH PHASE
Pain, Acute or Chronic – Phase III
Osteoporosis – Phase III

topiramate tablet
Topamax

MANUFACTURER
R.W. Johnson Pharmaceutical Research Institute

DESCRIPTION
Topamax is being tested in phase III trials for monotherapy in neuropathic pain in a tablet formulation. It is in phase II trials for bipolar mania and was approved by the FDA in May 2000 for epilepsy.

INDICATION(S) AND RESEARCH PHASE
Epilepsy – FDA approved
Pain, Acute or Chronic – Phase III
Bipolar Disorders – Phase II

unknown
Lidocaine

MANUFACTURER
Celltech Chiroscience plc

DESCRIPTION
Lidocaine is in phase II development for the treatment of pain, in a needle free injection formulation. Celltech Chiroscience has established a collaborative venture with PowderJect Pharmaceuticals for the development of local anesthetic products, such as this, delivered via PowderJect's proprietary needle free drug injector technology.

INDICATION(S) AND RESEARCH PHASE
Pain, Acute or Chronic – Phase II

ZD-4953
unknown

MANUFACTURER
AstraZeneca

DESCRIPTION
ZD-4953 is being developed in phase II clinical trials for the treatment of moderate pain. This analgesic drug works through the central nervous system to block painful stimuli.

INDICATION(S) AND RESEARCH PHASE
Pain, Acute or Chronic – Phase II

Rheumatoid Arthritis

5G1.1
unknown

MANUFACTURER
Alexion

DESCRIPTION
5G1.1 is monoclonal antibody that inhibits C5, a major protein in the complement system, important in inflammation. This antibody will result in an anti-inflammatory response. In February 2001, positive interim results were announced for a double-blind, randomized, placebo-controlled phase II trial of 5G1.1 in subjects with rheumatoid arthritis. Additionally, 5G1.1 is in a phase II trial for the treatment of membranous nephritis and in phase Ib pilot studies for the treatment of psoriasis, dermatomyositis, and pemphigoid.

INDICATION(S) AND RESEARCH PHASE
Rheumatoid Arthritis – Phase II
Kidney Disease – Phase II
Skin Infections/Disorders – Phase Ib

ABX-IL8
unknown

MANUFACTURER
Abgenix

DESCRIPTION
ABX-IL8 is a fully humanized antibody developed with Abgenix's XenoMouse technology. ABX-IL8 targets interleukin-8 (IL-8), a cytokine that can cause unwanted inflammation by first enabling immune cells, including neutrophils, to migrate to inflammatory sites and then activating them. There is substantial evidence that IL-8 contributes to a number of inflammatory diseases, including psoriasis, rheumatoid arthritis, and inflammatory bowel disease.

ABX-IL8 is being studied in a phase IIb trial for treatment of psoriasis, a disease that causes a thickening and scaling of the skin accompanied by local inflammation. Studies have shown that IL-8 levels can be elevated 150-fold in psoriatic tissue when compared to normal tissue. In addition to contributing to the inflammation process, IL-8 is also a growth factor for skin cells that are proliferating in psoriatic tissue. IL-8 is a potent angiogenesis factor, so it may be contributing to the ingrowth of blood vessels that nourish psoriatic tissue. Additionally, ABX-IL8 is in a phase II a trial for treatment of rheumatoid arthritis. It is administered by intravenous infusion.

INDICATION(S) AND RESEARCH PHASE
Psoriasis and Psoriatic Disorders – Phase IIb
Rheumatoid Arthritis – Phase IIa

AGIX-4207
unknown

MANUFACTURER
AtheroGenics

DESCRIPTION
AGIX-4207 is a novel, orally administered once-daily drug for the treatment of rheumatoid arthritis (RA). Based on the company's proprietary v-protectant technology, AGIX-4207 blocks the generation of certain proteins, including VCAM-1 and MCP-1, that are important in the initiation and progression of chronic inflammatory events associated with RA. By affecting only a portion of the protein activity, this drug may decrease chronic inflammation in RA and may have fewer side effects than current combination treatments of anti-inflammatory agents and disease modifying antirheumatic drugs.

INDICATION(S) AND RESEARCH PHASE
Rheumatoid Arthritis – Phase I

AGT-1
unknown

MANUFACTURER
Advanced Biotherapy

DESCRIPTION
Researchers have found an overproduction of cytokines in subjects with certain autoimmune diseases, such as rheumatoid arthritis (RA). Within these cytokines, alpha interferon, tumor necrosis factor, and gamma interferon are soluble components of the immune system, largely responsible for regulating the immune response and inflammation.

AGT-1, which is composed of a combination of antibody preparations, removes or neutralizes the cytokines' alpha interferon, gamma interferon, and tumor necrosis factor, thereby alleviating the autoimmune activity of these cells. Phase I/II clinical trials are testing AGT-1 for the treatment of autoimmune diseases, including RA.

INDICATION(S) AND RESEARCH PHASE
Autoimmune Diseases – Phase I/II
Rheumatoid Arthritis – Phase I/II

anti-IFNg
unknown

MANUFACTURER
Advanced Biotherapy

DESCRIPTION
Advanced Biotherapy is developing an anti-interferon-gamma (anti-IFN-γ) drug product to be utilized for the treatment of autoimmune diseases, such as multiple sclerosis (MS) and rheumatoid arthritis (RA). According to the company, IFN-γ may play a central, causative role in many autoimmune disorders. As a result, reducing its levels may have a profound effect in minimizing the autoimmune attack on cells and tissues. Anti-IFN-γ is designed to remove or neutralize IFN-γ.

A phase II double-blind, placebo-controlled trial with 30 subjects obtained positive results for anti-IFN-γ treatment of RA. The anti-IFN-γ-treated subjects showed statistically significant improvements after treatment in comparison to placebo-treated subjects. An intra-muscular administered treatment course of anti-IFN-γ was compared with placebo and anti-tumor necrosis factor-alpha (anti-TNF-α) treatment. The subjects were clinically assessed for seven days on a daily basis and then weekly up to 28 days. Measured outcomes included number of swollen and painful joints, duration of morning stiffness, grip strength, pain, and fatigue. Both anti-cytokine groups showed significant improvement at seven and 28 days, with the anti-IFN-γ group demonstrating the more robust effect at day 28.

INDICATION(S) AND RESEARCH PHASE
Rheumatoid Arthritis – Phase II

BB-2827
unknown

MANUFACTURER
British Biotech plc

DESCRIPTION
BB-2827 is in a phase I trial for the treatment of rheumatoid arthritis and periodontal disease.

INDICATION(S) AND RESEARCH PHASE
Rheumatoid Arthritis – Phase I
Periodontal Disease – Phase I

CCR2b
unknown

MANUFACTURER
AstraZeneca

DESCRIPTION
CCR2b is an immunomodulator that is currently in phase I development for the treatment of rheumatoid arthritis.

INDICATION(S) AND RESEARCH PHASE
Rheumatoid Arthritis – Phase I

CDC 801
SelCID

MANUFACTURER
Celgene Corporation

DESCRIPTION
SelCIDs, selective cytokine inhibitory drugs, are oral immunotherapeutic agents that treat various inflammatory diseases by inhibiting phosphodiesterase type-4 enzyme (PDE-4). The inhibition of PDE-4 decreases production of tumor necrosis factor-alpha (TNF-α), a protein manufactured by cells of the immune system. This inhibition reduces the level of circulating TNF-α and, therefore, its ability to cause inflammation in cells. At normal levels, the protein is essential for effective immune function. However, overproduction of TNF as a result of age, genetic, and other influences contributes to the pathology of numerous diseases.

SelCIDs are in phase II trials for the following indications: inflammatory bowel disease, rheumatoid arthritis, multiple sclerosis, tuberculosis, autoimmune diseases, multiple myeloma, and mycobacterial infections such as leprosy.

INDICATION(S) AND RESEARCH PHASE
Inflammatory Bowel Disease – Phase II
Rheumatoid Arthritis – Phase II
Multiple Sclerosis – Phase II
Asthma – Phase discontinued
Tuberculosis – Phase II
Autoimmune Diseases – Phase II
Bacterial Infection – Phase II
Multiple Myeloma – Phase II

CDP 870
unknown

MANUFACTURER
Celltech Chiroscience plc

DESCRIPTION
CDP 870 is an anti-cytokine antibody fragment indicated for the treatment of rheumatoid arthritis. It works by inhibiting cytokines that are involved in mediating inflammatory responses. The drug is currently in phase IIa trials.

INDICATION(S) AND RESEARCH PHASE
Rheumatoid Arthritis – Phase IIa

CDP-571, BAY 10-356
Humicade

MANUFACTURER
Celltech Chiroscience plc

DESCRIPTION
CDP-571 is a genetically engineered monoclonal antibody (MAb). Specifically, it is a humanized IgG4 antibody that blocks the activity of tumor necrosis factor alpha (TNF-α). TNF-α is an important mediator of inflammation and is naturally produced by the body.

This biological drug is being tested in phase IIb trials for the treatment of various inflammatory conditions, including Crohn's disease, ulcerative colitis, rheumatoid arthritis, and inflammatory bowel disease. The drug is administered by intravenous infusion.

INDICATION(S) AND RESEARCH PHASE
Crohn's Disease – Phase IIb
Inflammatory Bowel Disease – Phase IIb
Rheumatoid Arthritis – Phase IIb
Ulcerative Colitis – Phase IIb

COX 189
unknown

MANUFACTURER
Novartis

DESCRIPTION
COX 189 is an oral, non-steroidal anti-inflammatory analgesic belonging to the cyclooxygenase-2 (COX-2) inhibitor class. COX 189 has yielded promising results in dental pain relief, in addition to demonstrating relief of pain due to osteoarthritis and rheumatoid arthritis, comparable to that seen with Voltaren (diclofenac). It is currently in phase III development.

INDICATION(S) AND RESEARCH PHASE
Rheumatoid Arthritis – Phase III
Osteoarthritis – Phase III
Pain, Acute or Chronic – Phase III

etanercept
Enbrel

MANUFACTURER
Wyeth-Ayerst

DESCRIPTION
Enbrel binds to tumor necrosis factor (TNF), which is one of the dominant cytokines or proteins associated with normal immune function and the series of reactions that cause the inflammatory process of rheumatoid arthritis. Enbrel inhibits the binding of TNF molecules to the TNF receptor (TNFR) sites. The binding of these sites inactivates TNF, resulting in significant reduction in inflammatory cascade. Enbrel has been FDA approved for treatment of rheumatoid arthritis in adults and children.

Results from postmarketing studies demonstrated that Enbrel can have serious adverse effects such as infection, sepsis, and death. According to the company, subjects who are predisposed to infection, such as those with advanced or poorly controlled diabetes, are at greater risk of experiencing side effects. In addition, use of Enbrel should be terminated in subjects with current infections or sepsis. Allergic reactions to Enbrel or its components is also a possibility.

Trial results showed that nearly 75% of children with severe, long-standing juvenile rheumatoid arthritis (JRA) respond to Enbrel. In the first segment of the study, 74% of children (51 of 69) between the ages of four and 17 showed an improvement in disease response when treated with Enbrel for three months. In the second segment, half of these 51 subjects received Enbrel and half received a placebo. Seventy-two percent of those who received Enbrel completed the second segment without worsening of JRA symptoms, compared to 19% who took a placebo.

Enbrel is currently in phase III trials for the treatment of psoriasis and congestive heart failure.

Enbrel is co-marketed by Immunex and Wyeth-Ayerst.

INDICATION(S) AND RESEARCH PHASE
Rheumatoid Arthritis – FDA approved
Pediatric, Juvenile Rheumatoid Arthritis – FDA approved
Psoriasis and Psoriatic Disorders – Phase III
Congestive Heart Failure – Phase III

etodolac
Lodine

MANUFACTURER
Elan Pharmaceutical Research

DESCRIPTION
Lodine is a non-steroidal anti-inflammatory (NSAID) pain reliever that has been on the market in an oral tablet formulation since 1991 for acute and long-term treatment of osteoarthritis and rheumatoid arthritis. Lodine is currently being tested in a once daily intestinal protective drug absorption system (IPDAS) for controlled release delivery. This new formulation is currently in phase III developemnt. Elan Pharmaceutical Research has a development and marketing agreement with Wyeth-Ayerst for this agent.

INDICATION(S) AND RESEARCH PHASE

Osteoarthritis – Phase III
Rheumatoid Arthritis – Phase III
Pain, Acute or Chronic – Phase III

HuMax-CD4
unknown

MANUFACTURER
Genmab A/S

DESCRIPTION
HuMax-CD4 is a human antibody that targets the CD4 receptor on T-cells. These cells are implicated early in the cascade of inflammatory events that cause rheumatoid arthritis (RA). Therefore, blocking the activity of these cells may effectively halt the inflammatory process.

Positive results from a single-dose phase I/II trial of HuMax-CD4 for treatment of RA were announced in November 2000. HuMax-CD4 was well tolerated in the dose-escalating, placebo-controlled trial, and there was no evidence of depletion of subjects' CD4 positive T cells. In the four highest doses, 0.5, 1.0, 2.0, and 4.0 mg/kg, 50% of the treated subjects achieved favorable responses to the antibody.

In addition, a phase II trial was initiated in January 2000 to evaluate HuMax-CD4 in subjects with severe psoriasis. The trial will include four different dose levels along with a placebo.

INDICATION(S) AND RESEARCH PHASE
Rheumatoid Arthritis – Phase I/II completed
Psoriasis and Psoriatic Disorders – Phase II

IDEC-151
unknown

MANUFACTURER
IDEC Pharmaceuticals

DESCRIPTION
IDEC-151 is a humanized anti-CD4 monoclonal antibody that targets CD4 receptors on helper T cells. It is thought to help regulate helper T cell function without affecting other immune functions. It is currently in phase II trials for treatment of rheumatoid arthritis.

INDICATION(S) AND RESEARCH PHASE
Rheumatoid Arthritis – Phase II

IL-1ra/Anakinra
Kineret

MANUFACTURER
Amgen

DESCRIPTION
A phase II/III trial is currently evaluating the injectable formulation of Kineret (Anakinra, IL-1ra) in combination with the FDA approved drug methotrexate, to help treat subjects with rheumatoid arthritis (RA). Interleukin-1 (IL-1) is a mediator of joint inflammation and destruction. The body's natural supply of IL-1ra directly and selectively blocks the deleterious effects of IL-1, a substance released as part of the disease process in people with RA. Initial data indicate that Kineret has the potential to reduce both inflammation and bone and cartilage destruction, thereby slowing disease progression.

Methotrexate is an anti-metabolite drug that has been adopted as a slow acting drug for RA and psoriatic arthritis. It has been widely used for these indications in the United States for the past 20 years, and there is ample evidence to support its efficacy and relative safety in low dosage. It is used to delay the progression of the arthritis, and it is normally taken alongside common analgesic and anti-inflammatory drugs. Its mechanism of action is largely unknown.

INDICATION(S) AND RESEARCH PHASE
Rheumatoid Arthritis – Phase II/III

interleukin-1 (IL-1) trap
unknown

MANUFACTURER
Regeneron Pharmaceuticals

DESCRIPTION
Interleukin-1 (IL-1) is a cytokine antagonist produced by macrophages, a type of white blood cell. IL-1 is a mediator of the joint inflammation that occurs with rheumatoid arthritis (RA), and may be responsible for cartilage and bone damage. According to Regeneron, their IL-1 trap has been shown to block the activity of IL-1 in animal models. A phase I trial of IL-1 for treatment of RA was initiated in December 2000.

INDICATION(S) AND RESEARCH PHASE
Rheumatoid Arthritis – Phase I

IR501
Ravax

MANUFACTURER
Immune Response Corporation

DESCRIPTION
Ravax is a therapeutic vaccine being evaluated for the treatment of rheumatoid arthritis (RA) in individuals with stage II or III disease. This T-cell receptor vaccine consists of three synthetic peptides (VB3, VB14, and VB17) combined with a potent immune system stimulant known as Incomplete Freund's Adjuvant. The vaccine is designed to cause the immune system to inhibit T-cells attacking the joints and causing abnormal cellular damage.

Phase II results showed the drug to be well tolerated in 99 rheumatoid arthritis subjects and demonstrated clinically meaningful improvement after 24 weeks of treatment. However, results also showed that Ravax may be more effective in subjects with early-stage disease, and that continued monthly injections of the vaccine may be required in order to maintain a positive clinical response. Ravax is currently in phase II/III trials.

INDICATION(S) AND RESEARCH PHASE
Rheumatoid Arthritis – Phase II/III
Vaccines – Phase II/III

ISAtx247
Unknown

MANUFACTURER
Isotechnika

DESCRIPTION

ISAtx247 is a novel immunosuppressant for prevention of organ rejection after transplantation and for treatment of autoimmune diseases such as rheumatoid arthritis and psoriasis.

INDICATION(S) AND RESEARCH PHASE
Psoriasis and Psoriatic Disorders – Phase I
Rheumatoid Arthritis – Phase I
Immunosuppressant – Phase I

LF 15-0195
unknown

MANUFACTURER
Fournier Research

DESCRIPTION
Fournier Research is working on a new oral medication for the treatment of rheumatoid arthritis (RA). RA is an autoimmune disease in which the body produces antibodies that attack the collagen tissue that makes up the structure of the joints. This disease can lead to joint destruction, bone erosion, joint dislocation, and narrowing and destruction of the spinal column. Scientists currently believe that the release of two types of immune cells, IgG2A and IL-10, are responsible for most of this joint destruction. IgG2A acts by mistakenly recognizing collagen cells as foreign, and then releasing chemicals that signal the immune system to release more substances to destroy the tissue. IL-10 is a toxic substance marshaled by IgG2A that is capable of exerting direct injury to collagen cells.

LF 15-0195 is an immunosuppressive drug which may inhibit anti-collagen IgG2A production. This inhibition of IgG2A results in less IL-10 being released. By blocking the release of IgG2A and IL-10, LF 15-0195 may improve clinical symptoms of RA and also may halt the progression of the disease. In addition, by targeting specific immune molecules rather than suppressing the entire immune system, as is done with steroid administration, the use of this medication may result in fewer systemic side effects. LF 15-0195 is currently in phase II development.

INDICATION(S) AND RESEARCH PHASE
Rheumatoid Arthritis – Phase II

micellar paclitaxel
unknown

MANUFACTURER
Angiotech Pharmaceuticals

DESCRIPTION
Micellar paclitaxel is being developed for the treatment of secondary progressive multiple sclerosis, rheumatoid arthritis, and severe psoriasis. A double-blind, placebo-controlled, phase I trial produced positive results in the treatment of rheumatoid arthritis (RA). Enrolled patients were between 21 and 75 years of age, presented Class I to III of RA severity, and had failed treatment with at least one disease-modifying anti-rheumatic drug, such as methotrexate. The drug was determined to be safe and well-tolerated in all 15 patients enrolled in the study. Of those patients treated with micellar paclitaxel that completed the study, 25% had a clinical response defined by a series of measures consistent with the American College of Rheumatology (ACR) 20% improvement criteria. A larger phase II study may be initiated in 2001. Trials for multiple sclerosis and psoriasis are currently in phase II.

INDICATION(S) AND RESEARCH PHASE
Multiple Sclerosis – Phase II
Rheumatoid Arthritis – Phase I completed
Psoriasis and Psoriatic Disorders – Phase II

MK-663
unknown

MANUFACTURER
Merck & Co.

DESCRIPTION
MK-663 belongs to a relatively new class of non-steroidal anti-inflammatory drugs (NSAID) called COX-2 inhibitors. MK-663 is designed to specifically inhibit cyclo-oxygenase-2 (COX-2), which is one of several enzymes that leads to the production of substances that cause acute or chronic discomfort in joints with the associated pain and inflammation of arthritis.

Clinical studies have shown that COX-2 inhibitors work with the body to help it strengthen the system and prevent activation of several enzymes of the arachidonic acid metabolism. Consequently, the inhibitors prevent the formulation of eicosanoids, which are short-lived chemical agents that control a large number of physiological functions. COX-2 inhibitors counteract the formation of prostaglandins, that are responsible for short-term joint discomfort, and leukotrienes, that are responsible for long-term joint discomfort. By inhibiting prostaglandin synthesis and counteracting the destructive changes in healthy joints caused by leukotrienes, the extract COX-2 is the first dual inhibitor available.

Merck reported favorable results from a phase II trial that showed MK-663 relieved pain better than the placebo in 617 subjects with osteoarthritis of the knee. Currently, MK-663 is being tested in phase III trials for the treatment and relief of pain associated with rheumatoid arthritis and osteoarthritis.

INDICATION(S) AND RESEARCH PHASE
Pain, Acute or Chronic – Phase III
Rheumatoid Arthritis – Phase III
Osteoarthritis – Phase III

pentostatin
Nipent

MANUFACTURER
SuperGen

DESCRIPTION
Nipent (pentostatin) belongs to a group of drugs called antimetabolites. Nipent inhibits the enzyme adenosine deaminase, leading to cytotoxicity and cell death. This drug is in phase II trials for rheumatoid arthritis and non-Hodgkin's lymphoma. Nipent is also being tested in phase III trials for chronic lymphocytic leukemia.

In December 2000, results of a phase II trial of Nipent indicated the drug has significant 75% overall response rate in the treatment of graft versus host disease (GVHD). Twelve subjects with steroid refractory GVHD received Nipent as salvage therapy after each had previously failed all other treatments. A phase III trial is now under way.

INDICATION(S) AND RESEARCH PHASE
Leukemia – Phase III
Lymphoma, Non-Hodgkin's – Phase II
Rheumatoid Arthritis – Phase II
Immunosuppressive – Phase III

r-hTBP-1, recombinant human tumor necrosis factor-binding protein 1
unknown

MANUFACTURER
Serono Laboratories

DESCRIPTION
This drug is a recombinant human tumor necrosis factor-binding protein (r-hTBP-1). It is currently in phase II development for rheumatoid arthritis, Crohn's disease, and cardiac reperfusion injury.

INDICATION(S) AND RESEARCH PHASE
Rheumatoid Arthritis – Phase II
Crohn's Disease – Phase II
Cardiac Reperfusion Injury – Phase II

recombinant human interferon beta-1a
Rebif

MANUFACTURER
Serono Laboratories

DESCRIPTION
Rebif is an interferon beta-1a product being developed for a variety of indications, including non-small cell lung cancer, neurological disorders, chronic hepatitis C, Crohn's disease, ulcerative colitis, Guillain-Barré syndrome, and rheumatoid arthritis. Rebif has been approved in several countries for the treatment of relapsing-remitting multiple sclerosis (MS). It is currently being evaluated in phase III trials as an early treatment of MS and an NDA has been filed for use as in secondary progressive MS.

INDICATION(S) AND RESEARCH PHASE
Multiple Sclerosis, Early Treatment – Phase III
Multiple Sclerosis, Secondary Progressive – NDA submitted
Lung Cancer – Phase III
Hepatitis – Phase II
Crohn's Disease – Phase II
Ulcerative Colitis – Phase II
Neurologic Disorders – Phase II
Rheumatoid Arthritis – Phase II

SB 273005
unknown

MANUFACTURER
GlaxoSmithKline

DESCRIPTION
SB 273005 is a novel small-molecule, orally active vitronectin antagonist. It is currently in phase I development for osteoporosis and rheumatoid arthritis.

INDICATION(S) AND RESEARCH PHASE
Osteoporosis – Phase I
Rheumatoid Arthritis – Phase I

SB 683698, TR 14035
unknown

MANUFACTURER
GlaxoSmithKline

DESCRIPTION
SB 683698 is a dual alpha4 integrin antagonist (VLA4). It is currently in phase II trials for the treatment of asthma and rheumatoid arthritis.

INDICATION(S) AND RESEARCH PHASE
Asthma – Phase II
Rheumatoid Arthritis – Phase II

SCIO-469
unknown

MANUFACTURER
Scios

DESCRIPTION
SCIO-469 inhibits p38 kinase, a stimulatory modulator of pro-inflammatory cytokines, including tumor necrosis factor-alpha (TNF-α), interleukin-1 (IL-1), and cyclooxygenase-2 (COX-2). These cytokines are known to contribute to both symptoms and disease progression in rheumatoid arthritis (RA). Existing protein-based products that antagonize TNF-α have been shown to markedly relieve the symptoms and retard the progression of RA. As an oral inhibitor of TNF-α, SCIO-469 would offer more convenient dosing over the existing products that must be injected or infused intravenously. This new compound also has the potential for additional benefits associated with its inhibition of IL-1 and COX-2. Scios initiated a phase I b multi-dose trial in healthy subjects in February 2001.

INDICATION(S) AND RESEARCH PHASE
Rheumatoid Arthritis – Phase Ib

sTNF-RI, soluble tumor necrosis factor-a receptor type I
unknown

MANUFACTURER
Amgen

DESCRIPTION
Tumor necrosis factor (TNF) is a protein that is a key messenger in the body's chemical chain reaction that leads to inflammation seen in diseases such as rheumatoid arthritis (RA). By stopping the activation of TNF or absorbing the signals TNF sends to other molecules, it may be possible to stop the process leading to inflammation. People with RA appear to overproduce TNF, which appears to be linked to the swelling, pain, and damage of joints they may experience.

Soluble tumor necrosis factor-α receptor-type 1 (sTNF-R1) is a second-generation TNF binding protein drug that has been developed for RA. Researchers are testing sTNF-R1 in phase II clinical trials to determine whether it will counteract the effects of TNF by binding to the protein and therefore interrupt the inflammatory process in RA.

INDICATION(S) AND RESEARCH PHASE
Rheumatoid Arthritis – Phase II

T-cell receptor vaccine
unknown

MANUFACTURER
Immune Response Corporation

DESCRIPTION
Immune Response has developed a vaccine of T-cell receptor (TCR) peptides which may induce the immune system to suppress the aberrant T cells that are active in rheumatoid arthritis, psoriasis, and multiple sclerosis. While these cells are suppressed, the other normal cells should not be affected. The vaccine is designed to treat the presumed cause of the disease, not just the symptoms. Three trials have recently been completed with the TCR vaccine for treatment of multiple sclerosis (phase I), rheumatoid arthritis (phase IIb), and psoriasis (phase II).

INDICATION(S) AND RESEARCH PHASE
Multiple Sclerosis – Phase I completed
Psoriasis and Psoriatic Disorders – Phase II completed
Rheumatoid Arthritis – Phase IIb completed

tacrolimus hydrate
Prograf

MANUFACTURER
Fujisawa Healthcare

DESCRIPTION
Prograf is a novel immunosuppressant for the treatment of dermatological autoimmune diseases, including atopic dermatitis and rheumatoid arthritis. The drug is administered as a topical ointment and it is being tested in phase III trials.

INDICATION(S) AND RESEARCH PHASE
Atopic Dermatitis – Phase III
Rheumatoid Arthritis – Phase III

thalidomide
Thalomid

MANUFACTURER
Celgene Corporation

DESCRIPTION
Thalomid is an oral formulation of the immunomodulatory agent thalidomide. Thalidomide has a notorious history of having caused birth defects when the medical profession unsuspectingly prescribed it for pregnant women as a treatment for nausea and insomnia. Celgene is investigating new applications for the drug, while being particularly mindful of the potential risks of thalidomide treatment. Thalomid is currently being tested for numerous indications in the areas of oncology and immunology.

INDICATION(S) AND RESEARCH PHASE
Multiple Myeloma – Phase II
Myelodysplastic Syndrome – Phase II
Leukemia – Phase II
Brain Cancer – Phase II
Liver Cancer – Phase II
Kidney Cancer – Phase II
Prostate Cancer – Phase II
Kaposi's Sarcoma – Phase II
Cachexia – Phase II
Recurrent Aphthous Stomatitis – Phase III
Crohn's Disease – Phase II
Inflammatory Bowel Disease – Phase II
Sarcoidosis – Phase II
Scleroderma – Phase II

vaccine, rheumatoid arthritis
AnergiX.RA

MANUFACTURER
Corixa Corporation

DESCRIPTION
AnergiX.RA complexes consist of molecules containing disease specific auto-antigenic peptides. The complexes may reduce autoimmune disease by binding to and deactivating T-cells, which are activated against one's own body during rheumatoid arthritis (RA). In November 2000, results of a randomized, placebo-controlled dose escalation phase I/II trial of AnergiX.RA indicated that it was well tolerated and suggested the compound had biological activity and provided clinical improvements in subjects with RA. Trials are currently in phase IIa.

In January 2001, Corixa Corporation announced it has amended its agreement with Organon to include the continued development of the recombinant form of Corixa's AnergiX.RA complex for the treatment of RA.

INDICATION(S) AND RESEARCH PHASE
Rheumatoid Arthritis – Phase IIa

valdecoxib
unknown

MANUFACTURER
Pfizer

DESCRIPTION
Valdecoxib is a second generation cyclooxygenase-2 (COX-2) inhibitor that Pfizer is jointly developing with Pharmacia as a treatment for pain associated with arthritis, osteoarthritis, and rheumatoid arthritis. It offers a rapid onset and prolonged efficacy with once-a-day dosing. The drug is currently in phase III testing and an NDA submission is planned for 2001.

INDICATION(S) AND RESEARCH PHASE
Arthritis and Arthritic Pain – Phase III
Osteoarthritis – Phase III
Rheumatoid Arthritis – Phase III

VX-740, pralnacasan
unknown

MANUFACTURER
Vertex Pharmaceuticals

DESCRIPTION
VX-740 is Vertex's most advanced ICE inhibitor. ICE is an enzyme that regulates the production of IL-1 and IFN gamma, intercellular mediators that initiate and sustain the process of inflammation. Inhibiting ICE may be an effective strategy for curtailing damaging inflammatory processes common to a number of acute and chronic conditions, such as rheumatoid arthritis and osteoarthritis. VX-740 is currently in phase II trials.

INDICATION(S) AND RESEARCH PHASE
Rheumatoid Arthritis – Phase II
Osteoarthritis – Phase II

VX-745
unknown

MANUFACTURER
Vertex Pharmaceuticals

DESCRIPTION
VX-745 is a p38 MAP kinase inhibitor in development for the treatment of rheumatoid arthritis (RA). p38 MAP kinase is an enzyme that regulates the production of interleukin-1 beta, interleukin-6 (IL-6), and tumor necrosis factor (TNF) alpha, all of which are involved in acute and chronic inflammatory responses. Inhibition of p38 MAP kinase may be an effective strategy for slowing the progression of acute and chronic inflammatory reactions. As of October 2000, VX-745 is in phase II development, in collaboration with Kissei, for the treatment of RA.

INDICATION(S) AND RESEARCH PHASE
Rheumatoid Arthritis – Phase II

YM-177, celecoxib
unknown

MANUFACTURER
Yamanouchi Pharmaceutical

DESCRIPTION
YM-177 is an orally administered cyclooxygenase-2 (COX-2) inhibitor being evaluated for the treatment of rheumatoid arthritis and osteoarthritis. It is in phase II trials and is part of Yamanouchi's domestic pipeline. The company is developing the drug with Pharmacia.

INDICATION(S) AND RESEARCH PHASE
Rheumatoid Arthritis – Phase II
Osteoarthritis – Phase II

ZD2315
unknown

MANUFACTURER
AstraZeneca

DESCRIPTION
ZD2315 is an immuno modulator indicated for the treatment of rheumatoid arthritis. It is currently in phase I development.

INDICATION(S) AND RESEARCH PHASE
Rheumatoid Arthritis – Phase I

Spinal Cord Injuries

fampridine
Neurelan

MANUFACTURER
Acorda Therapeutics

DESCRIPTION
Neurelan is a 4-aminopyridine potassium channel blocker that is being tested in a phase II/III trial for the treatment of multiple sclerosis (MS). In this trial, Neurelan is delivered using the intestinal protective drug absorption system (IPDAS) in a sustained-release formulation. Neurelan has an orphan indication status for the symptomatic relief of MS. The drug is also in phase II trials for treatment of spinal cord injuries.

INDICATION(S) AND RESEARCH PHASE
Multiple Sclerosis – Phase II/III
Spinal Cord Injuries – Phase II

leteprinim potassium, AIT-082
Neotrofin

MANUFACTURER
NeoTherapeutics

DESCRIPTION
Neotrofin is composed of the purine compound hypoxanthine, which is linked with procainamide, an antiarrhythmic drug. Results of a double-blind, dose-escalating phase II trial of Neotrofin indicated that the compound facilitated brain activity in Alzheimer's disease subjects, leading to improvements in memory, attention, and judgement. The improvements were dose-related, with 500 mg and 1,000 mg doses producing more benefit than a 150 mg dose. NeoTherapeutics will initiate further trials in 2001 at doses of 500 mg and 1,000 mg in subjects with moderate Alzheimer's disease.

Neotrofin is in preclinical development for Parkinson's disease, spinal cord injury, and peripheral neuropathy.

INDICATION(S) AND RESEARCH PHASE
Alzheimer's Disease – Phase II completed
Parkinson's Disease – Phase Preclinical
Spinal Cord Injuries – Phase Preclinical
Neuropathy – Phase Preclinical

neurotrophin-3 (NT-3)
unknown

MANUFACTURER
Regeneron Pharmaceuticals

DESCRIPTION
This drug is an injectable formulation of neurotrophin-3 (NT-3), a naturally occurring human protein. It acts on the neurons of the intestinal tract and is being tested for severe constipation and various constipating conditions caused by spinal cord injuries, narcotic analgesics, and Parkinson's disease. NT-3 is currently in phase II development.

INDICATION(S) AND RESEARCH PHASE
Constipation – Phase II
Spinal Cord Injuries – Phase II
Parkinson's Disease – Phase II
Pain, Acute or Chronic – Phase II

recombinant human bone morphogenic protein-2 (rhBMP-2)
unknown

MANUFACTURER
Genetics Institute

DESCRIPTION
According to the Genetics Institute, this recombinant human bone morphogenic protein-2 (rhBMP-2) has shown positive results in accelerating bone and cartilage repair in a variety of situations, including severe orthopedic trauma, oral and maxillofacial surgery, and spinal fusion. This genetically engineered drug works as a growth factor that stimulates new bone development. Genetics Institute, a subsidary of American Home Products, is researching rhBMP-2 in

phase III trials through a development partnership with Yamanouchi.

INDICATION(S) AND RESEARCH PHASE
Orthopedics – Phase III
Oral Medicine – Phase III
Musculoskeletal Diseases – Phase III
Spinal Cord Injuries – Phase III

12 Dermatology

Population with illnesses in this category	900,000[1]
Drugs in the development pipeline	384[2]
Number of drugs in preclinical testing	173
Number of drugs in clinical testing	179

Source: 1. World Health Organization, worldwide figures 2. Parexel

It is estimated that more than seven million Americans have psoriasis, with more than 150,000 cases reported each year. Psoriasis is a chronic and often painful skin disease that can be difficult to treat. Epithelial cells reproduce faster than normal, resulting in round, reddish, thick skin patches with silvery scales that develop on the scalp, knees, elbows, hands and feet. Although psoriasis in not life threatening, it can severely threaten the quality of life.

There is no cure for psoriasis. However the number of treatment options has doubled in the past few years. CenterWatch estimates there are approximately 75 drugs in clinical testing with $400 million to $450 million being spent on clinical development.

Two drugs that have recently been approved by the FDA as promising new treatments for psoriasis are clobetasol propionate and tacrolimus ointment. Clobetasol propionate, currently one of the most effective topical corticosteriods used to treat psorsias, is now available as a foam, specifically for the treatment of psoriatic lesions on the scalp. The foam formulation is more effective than other topical medications since it penetrates the skin easily and is more acceptable to use on skin that is covered with hair.

Tacrolimus ointment is approved for the treatment of atopic dermatitis and shows promise for the treatment of psoriasis on the face and other areas prone to sensitivity and side effects from other topical agents. Tacrolimus is an immunosupressive agent that is currently used to prevent rejection of organ transplants when the drug is given orally or intravenously.

There are also many new promising combination therapies for the treatment of psoriasis. Calcipotriene, a topical synthetic vitamin D derivative, which has been available for years and has shown promising results in the treatment of psoriasis when combined with ultraviolet light therapy (UVB). Additionally, when combined with psoralen and exposure to ultraviolet-A light (PUVA), calcipotriene increases the effectiveness of PUVA and decreases time to remission. Also, results have demonstrated when calcipotriene is combined with halobestasol propionate, a topical steroid, their combined effect is superior to either treatment alone when used twice daily.

Tazarotene, a retinoid vitamin A derivative, also has positive interactions with other treatments for psoriasis. It is compatible when mixed with most topical corticosteroids, resulting in less irritation and greater efficacy.

Clinical trials are just beginning in 2001 for the evaluation of topical calcitriol, another synthetic vitamin D compound. It has been proven safe and effective for the treatment of psoriasis, but is being tested for its efficacy before and after phototherapy, since it blocks transmission of UVB, narrow-band UVB, and PUVA.

Another popular area in the dermatology pipeline is eczema. This term is used to describe all kinds of red, blistering, oozing, scaly, brownish, thickened, and/or itching skin conditions. Examples include atopic dermatitis, allergic contact eczema, seborrheic eczema, and nummular eczema. CenterWatch estimates there are approximately six drugs being tested for the treatment of eczema and atopic dermatitis with $25 million to $43 million being spent on clinical research.

According to the American Academy of Dermatology, since 1970 the incidences of eczema have nearly tripled. Environmental factors, irritants, allergens that trigger the immune system and emotional factors such as stress are contributing to the increased number of people suffering from eczema.

Current treatments used for eczema are topical steroid creams or ointments, antihistamines to control itching, oral antibiotics for bacterial superinfection, oral cyclosporine, topical tar-based gels and ultraviolet therapy for severe cases. However, new treatments are being evaluated in clinical studies.

A new class of drugs called topical immunomodulators (TIMs) show promise in treating eczema. TIMs work differently than steroids to relieve itching, redness and pain associated with many skin infections, especially atopic dermatitis. Two TIMs currently in development are tacrolimus hydrate and ascomycin, which are both steroid-free. Based on clinical trial results, it is believed that TIMs will improve and even completely clear the majority of people suffering from atopic dermatitis.

Acne

5-aminolevulinic acid
Levulan Photodynamic Therapy

MANUFACTURER
DUSA Pharmaceuticals

DESCRIPTION
Levulan photodynamic therapy (PDT) is being evaluated for the treatment of certain conditions such as early cancers, pre-cancers, and acne vulgaris. Levulan is preferentially absorbed by abnormal cells and is converted into protoporphyrin IX (PpIX), a potent photosensitizer. PpIX can then be activated by an appropriate light source, producing singlet oxygen, which causes cell membrane damage to the abnormal cells.

Positive trial results of Levulan PDT for the treatment of dysplastic Barrett's esophagus (BE) were reported. The double-blind, placebo-controlled trial involved 36 subjects and was conducted by independent investigators in the United Kingdom. Sixteen of 18 (89%) subjects in the Levulan group experienced a response, with a median decrease in area of BE averaging 30%. In the placebo group, a median area decrease of 0% was observed. The company reported the initiation of a new phase I/II trial of Levulan PDT for the treatment of acne vulgaris in November 2000.

INDICATION(S) AND RESEARCH PHASE
Acne – Phase I/II

clindamycin
ResiDerm, Zindaclin

MANUFACTURER
Access Pharmaceuticals

DESCRIPTION
ResiDerm is an anti-acne compound that uses a topical zinc delivery system to deliver the antibiotic clindamycin. The company claims that the zinc ion technology produces a reservoir of drug in the skin that increases efficacy. Phase III trials of the drug for the treatment of acne have been completed. Additional indications may include other dermatological diseases. ResiDerm will be developed and marketed under the trade name of Zindaclin in the United Kingdom.

In November 2000, positive results of a phase III European trial of ResiDerm for the treatment of acne were announced. The trial was conducted at ten European centers and the primary clinical endpoint, change in total facial inflammatory lesion counts from the initial visit to the end of 16 weeks of treatment, was achieved. Based on the trial results, Strakan, who has co-developed ResiDerm, is expected to file a product license application in the United Kingdom.

INDICATION(S) AND RESEARCH PHASE
Acne – Phase III completed (Europe)

dadsone topical gel
Atrisone

MANUFACTURER
Atrix Laboratories

DESCRIPTION
Atrisone, dadsone topical gel, is in phase II trials for moderate to severe acne. A phase III trial is planned for early 2001.

INDICATION(S) AND RESEARCH PHASE
Acne – Phase II

levonorgestrel/ethinyl estradio
Alesse

MANUFACTURER
Wyeth-Ayerst

DESCRIPTION
Alesse is a combination formulation of 0.1 mg levonorgesterel and 20 mcg ethinyl estradiol. It is used in the treatment of moderate acne vulgaris in women of reproductive age who have no known contraindications to oral contraceptive use and who are unresponsive to topical anti-acne medications. An NDA was submitted January 2001 for this indication.

INDICATION(S) AND RESEARCH PHASE
Acne – NDA submitted

MBI 594AN
unknown

MANUFACTURER
Micrologix

DESCRIPTION
MBI 594AN is a novel topical compound in phase II trials for the treatment of acne. The phase II trial is a randomized, double-blind, placebo-controlled, dose-ranging efficacy study in 75 acne subjects over the age of 13.

Results of a phase I trial demonstrated MBI 594AN was safe, well tolerated and has antimicrobial activity against the acne-causing bacterium, *Propionibacterium acnes*. The two part trial consisted of a five-day, open-label study in 17 acne subjects, and a randomized double-blind study over six weeks in 36 healthy volunteers colonized with the bacterium but free of active acne.

INDICATION(S) AND RESEARCH PHASE
Acne – Phase II

tazarotene
Tazorac

MANUFACTURER
Allergan

DESCRIPTION
Tazorac is a receptor-selective retinoid for the treatment of psoriasis and photodamage to the skin. A retinoid is a compound with vitamin A-like properties that may be prescribed for severe cases of psoriasis that do not respond to other therapies. Because systemic treatment with retinoids may cause birth defects, this drug was approved for psoriasis and psoriatic disorders in a topical cream formulation .05% and .1% in October 2000. Additionally, an NDA has been submitted for the treatment of acne.

INDICATION(S) AND RESEARCH PHASE
Psoriasis and Psoriatic Disorders – FDA approved
Acne – NDA submitted

Alopecia

GI 198745
unknown

MANUFACTURER
GlaxoSmithKline

DESCRIPTION
GI 198745 is a dual inhibitor of 5-alpha-reductase type 1 and 2 isozymes. GlaxoSmithKline has developed the drug for the treatment of benign prostatic hyperplasia (BPH). An NDA was submitted for this indication in December 2000. Additionally, GI 198745 is in phase II trials for the treatment of alopecia.

INDICATION(S) AND RESEARCH PHASE
Alopecia – Phase II
Benign Prostatic Hyperplasia – NDA submitted

Anal Fissures

nitroglycerin ointment
Anogesic

MANUFACTURER
Cellegy Pharmaceuticals

DESCRIPTION
Anogesic is a nitroglycerin-based ointment applied topically for the treatment of anal fissures and hemorrhoids. Although used for more than a century for the treatment of certain cardiovascular diseases, nitroglycerin has only recently been tested in this proprietary formulation for anal fissures, which are tears in the anal canal caused by involuntary contraction of the anal sphincter, and hemorrhoids, which are enlarged veins in the anal area.

Phase III results show that Anogesic (nitroglycerin ointment) demonstrated a statistically significant reduction in pain associated with chronic anal fissures. Three hundred and four subjects with chronic anal fissures were randomly assigned to one of eight treatment regimens utilizing several concentrations of nitroglycerin or placebo for up to eight weeks. Statistical significance was not achieved with the primary endpoint, but treatment with 0.4% nitroglycerin ointment resulted in a highly significant decrease in pain intensity compared with placebo. In a second study, 34 hemorrhoidectomy subjects were randomly assigned to 0.2% nitroglycerin ointment or placebo applied three times daily following surgery. It was found that use of oral narcotic drug was higher in the placebo group than the nitroglycerin group, indicating that the ointment promoted pain relief.

INDICATION(S) AND RESEARCH PHASE
Anal Fissures – Phase III completed
Hemorrhoids – Phase II

Atopic Dermatitis

ADL 2-1294
unknown

MANUFACTURER
Adolor

DESCRIPTION
ADL2-1294 is a peripheral opiate (synthetic narcotic) being tested for the treatment of pain and itching associated with burns, abrasions, eczema, and dermatitis. The drug, in a topical formulation, is in phase II trials for atopic dermatitis, burns and burn infections, herpes zoster infections, psoriasis and psoriatic disorders, and for eye disorders and infections.

INDICATION(S) AND RESEARCH PHASE
Atopic Dermatitis – Phase II
Burns and Burn Infections – Phase II
Herpes Zoster Infections – Phase II
Psoriasis and Psoriatic Disorders – Phase II
Eye Disorders/Infections – Phase II
Skin Infections/Disorders – Phase II

bexarotene
Targretin-capsule

MANUFACTURER
Ligand Pharmaceuticals

DESCRIPTION
Targretin, which selectively stimulates a (retinoid subtype) receptor, is being developed in an oral capsule formulation for the treatment of lung and breast cancer, head and neck cancer, cutaneous T-cell lymphoma (CTCL), psoriasis and psoriatic disorders, and atopic dermatitis. The drug is in phase II trials for head and neck cancer, phase II/III trials for breast cancer, CTCL, and psoriasis and psoriatic disorders, and phase III trials for non-small cell lung cancer.

INDICATION(S) AND RESEARCH PHASE
Atopic Dermatitis – Phase II
Psoriasis and Psoriatic Disorders – Phase II/III
Lung Cancer – Phase III
Breast Cancer – Phase II/III
Head and Neck Cancer – Phase II

HCT 1026
unknown

MANUFACTURER
NicOx SA

DESCRIPTION
HCT 1026 is a novel nitric oxide-releasing derivative of the non-steroidal anti-inflammatory drug (NSAID) flurbiprofen. While flurbiprofen has demonstrated effectiveness in the treatment of urinary incontinence, its use has been complicated by gastric toxicity. Because HCT 1026 may provide increased gastric tolerability, it can be administered for extended periods at effective doses. In Phase I trials, results indicated that HCT 1026 produced fewer and less severe gastric lesions compared to flurbiprofen.

HCT 1026 produces anti-inflammatory effects through the inhibition of prostaglandin synthesis, while nitric oxide controls inflammatory cell activation. These two factors suggest that HCT 1026 may be an effective treatment for dermatology disorders such as psoriasis. HCT 1026 is in phase II trials for the treatment of urinary incontinence, osteoporosis, and skin disorders such as atopic dermatitis and psoriasis.

INDICATION(S) AND RESEARCH PHASE

Atopic Dermatitis – Phase II
Urinary Incontinence – Phase II
Osteoporosis – Phase II
Psoriasis and Psoriatic Disorders – Phase II
Skin Infections/Disorders – Phase II

pimecrolimus, ASM 981
Elidel

MANUFACTURER
Novartis

DESCRIPTION
Elidel is an ascomycin derivative being studied for the treatment of inflammatory skin disease. It produces a therapeutic effect through the inhibition of T-cells and mast cells. Elidel is being developed in both an oral and topical (cream) formulation. The oral formulation is in phase II trials, while an NDA has been filed for the cream formulation. Phase III trials involving more than 2,000 subjects ages three months to adult have recently been completed. The majority of the subjects in the phase III studies were pediatric.

Data presented from two previous vehicle-controlled trials demonstrated that ASM 981 cream was safe and effective for the treatment of atopic dermatitis. The two trials involved a total of 403 (267 ASM 981 and 136 vehicle) pediatric subjects ages two to 17 years old with mild to moderate atopic dermatitis. Both studies consisted of a 6-week randomized, multicenter, double-blind, parallel-group phase followed by a 20-week open-label phase to assess safety and efficacy. Thirty-seven percent of ASM subjects were clear or almost clear of the signs of atopic dermatitis, significantly more than in the vehicle control group. Over 65% of subjects achieved some degree of improvement. Of those who showed improvement, over 85% were cleared of the disease.

INDICATION(S) AND RESEARCH PHASE
Atopic Dermatitis – Phase II
Pediatric, Atopic Dermatitis – Phase III completed
Atopic Dermatitis – NDA submitted

tacrolimus hydrate
Prograf

MANUFACTURER
Fujisawa Healthcare

DESCRIPTION
Prograf is a novel immunosuppressant for the treatment of dermatological (skin) autoimmune diseases, including atopic dermatitis. The drug is administered as a topical ointment and it is being tested in phase III trials.

INDICATION(S) AND RESEARCH PHASE
Atopic Dermatitis – Phase III
Rheumatoid Arthritis – Phase III

Burns and Burn Infections

ADL 2-1294
unknown

MANUFACTURER
Adolor

DESCRIPTION
ADL2-1294 is a peripheral opiate (synthetic narcotic) being tested for the treatment of pain and itching associated with burns, abrasions, eczema, and dermatitis. The drug, in a topical formulation, is in phase II trials for atopic dermatitis, burns and burn infections, herpes zoster infections, psoriasis and psoriatic disorders, and for eye disorders and infections.

INDICATION(S) AND RESEARCH PHASE
Atopic Dermatitis – Phase II
Burns and Burn Infections – Phase II
Herpes Zoster Infections – Phase II
Psoriasis and Psoriatic Disorders – Phase II
Eye Disorders/Infections – Phase II
Skin Infections/Disorders – Phase II

unknown
Fibrostat

MANUFACTURER
Procyon Biopharma

DESCRIPTION
Fibrostat is a topical therapeutic cream of transglutaminase inhibitor being developed in a phase III trial for burns and scar healing following surgery. The phase III trial is being conducted in Canada.

INDICATION(S) AND RESEARCH PHASE
Burns and Burn Infections – Phase III
Scar Tissue – Phase III

VM-301, OAS 1000
unknown

MANUFACTURER
Nexell Therapeutics

DESCRIPTION
VM-301 is a topical wound healing agent that is being tested in phase II trials. Indications include treatment of skin graft donor sites of both partial and full thickness wounds, including burns, surgical wounds, diabetic skin ulcers, and decubitus ulcers.

INDICATION(S) AND RESEARCH PHASE
Burns and Burn Infections – Phase II
Decubitus Ulcers (Bed Sores) – Phase II
Diabetic Foot Ulcers – Phase II
Wounds – Phase II

Decubitus Ulcers (Bed Sores)

VM-301, OAS 1000
unknown

MANUFACTURER
Nexell Therapeutics

DESCRIPTION
VM-301 is a topical wound healing agent that is being tested in phase II trials. Indications include treatment of skin graft donor sites of both partial and full thickness wounds, including burns, surgical wounds, diabetic skin ulcers, and decubitus ulcers.

INDICATION(S) AND RESEARCH PHASE

Diabetic Foot Ulcers

becaplermin
Regranex

MANUFACTURER
Chiron Corporation

DESCRIPTION
Regranex is a wound healing therapeutic for pressure ulcers. These skin ulcers may develop in weight-bearing areas due to many different disease conditions, especially diabetes. The drug is currently being tested in phase III trials. Chiron Corporation has a licensing agreement with R.W. Johnson Pharmaceutical Research Institute for developing Regranex.

INDICATION(S) AND RESEARCH PHASE
Diabetic Foot Ulcers – Phase III
Skin Wounds – Phase III

therapeutic, wound healing
unknown

MANUFACTURER
Mylan

DESCRIPTION
This drug is an unspecified therapeutic being tested in phase III trials for both wound healing and diabetic foot ulcers.

INDICATION(S) AND RESEARCH PHASE
Diabetic Foot Ulcers – Phase III
Wounds – Phase III

transforming growth factor beta-2 (TGF-b2)
unknown

MANUFACTURER
Genzyme Tissue Repair

DESCRIPTION
This synthetic drug is known as transforming growth factor-beta2 (TGF-β2). It is normally made in the body to help stimulate the formation of granulation tissue for treating chronic skin ulcers. The company, Genzyme Tissue Repair, reported the results of a completed phase II trial for diabetic foot ulcers. The data for this double blinded, randomized trial were collected over a three year period with testing at 15 study centers with diabetic foot ulcer subjects. Both safety and dose ranging efficacy were evaluated. The two important criteria used to study TGF-β2 were the frequency of complete wound closure and time to wound closure.

Genzyme stated that the study subjects were randomly assigned to one of five groups. The first group of 24 subjects received standard care only which consisted of surgical debridement, compression dressing, and off-loading of weight from the wound site. The remainder of the subjects were enrolled in the blinded part of the trial. One group of 22 subjects received placebo sponges and standardized care. The remaining 131 subjects were evenly divided among three doses in addition to standardized care. All the subjects were treated twice a week for 20 weeks or until their ulcer healed.

Study results from the phase II trial suggested that TGF-β2 was safe and effective at all dose levels tested. The subject group which received the highest dosage of TGF-β2 (5 µg/cm^2) demonstrated statistically significant improvement compared to placebo in both the efficacy endpoints, frequency of complete closure and time to closure. Subjects in the groups which received the middle or low doses of TGF-β2 also showed improvements in both endpoints but did not consistently achieve statistical significance.

The company, Genzyme Tissue Repair is actively seeking a partner to work with them in the final stages of development and commercialization for the TGF-β2 drug.

INDICATION(S) AND RESEARCH PHASE
Diabetic Foot Ulcers – Phase II completed
Skin Infections/Disorders – Phase II completed

VM-301, OAS 1000
unknown

MANUFACTURER
Nexell Therapeutics

DESCRIPTION
VM-301 is a topical wound healing agent that is being tested in phase II trials. Indications include treatment of skin graft donor sites of both partial and full thickness wounds, including burns, surgical wounds, diabetic skin ulcers and decubitus ulcers.

INDICATION(S) AND RESEARCH PHASE
Burns and Burn Infections – Phase II
Decubitus Ulcers (Bed Sores) – Phase II
Diabetic Foot Ulcers – Phase II
Wounds – Phase II

Fungal Infections

amphotericin B
AmBisome

MANUFACTURER
Fujisawa Healthcare

DESCRIPTION
AmBisome is a novel antifungal agent for the treatment of histoplasmosis, a fungus infection caused by *Histoplasma capsulatum*. The drug is in phase III trials for this orphan indication.

INDICATION(S) AND RESEARCH PHASE
Fungal Infections – Phase III

BMS-207147
unknown

MANUFACTURER
Bristol-Myers Squibb

DESCRIPTION
BMS-207147 is an antifungal agent being tested for the treatment of aspergillosis, mucosal candidiasis, endemic mycosis, and onychomycosis. The drug is in phase II trials. Future indications may include certain

infectious diseases and viral diseases.

INDICATION(S) AND RESEARCH PHASE
Fungal Infections – Phase II

C319-14/6
Oramed

MANUFACTURER
Biosyn

DESCRIPTION
Oramed is an antifungal oral rinse for treatment of azole-resistant strains of oral candidiasis in HIV positive subjects. The drug completed phase II. Testing for other indications may include acquired immune deficiency syndrome (AIDS) related diseases, infectious diseases and viral diseases, antifungal applications, and candidiasis.

INDICATION(S) AND RESEARCH PHASE
Acquired Immune Deficiency Syndrome (AIDS) and AIDS-Related Infections – Phase II completed
Fungal Infections – Phase II completed

ciclopirox olamine
Loprox

MANUFACTURER
Aventis

DESCRIPTION
Loprox is a broad spectrum antifungal in phase III trials for the treatment of seborrheic dermatitis, an inflammatory, scaling disease of the scalp and face.

INDICATION(S) AND RESEARCH PHASE
Seborrhea – Phase III
Fungal Infections – Phase III

FK463, echinocandin
unknown

MANUFACTURER
Fujisawa Healthcare

DESCRIPTION
Echinocandin is a novel antifungal agent for the treatment of systemic fungal infections. The drug is used as prophylaxis, empirical therapy, and second line treatment for candidiasis and aspergillosis. Echinocandin is in phase II/III trials for these indications as well as other fungal infections.

INDICATION(S) AND RESEARCH PHASE
Aspergillosis – Phase II/III
Candidiasis – Phase II/III
Fungal Infections – Phase II/III

liposomal amphotericin B
AmBisome

MANUFACTURER
Gilead Sciences

DESCRIPTION
AmBisome is currently in phase II trials for pediatric subjects 13 years and older. AmBisome is a liposomal formulation of amphotericin B, the active ingredient of AmBisome and acts by binding to the ergostrol in the fungal cell membrane, which leads to alterations in cell permeability and cell death. Amphotericin B has a higher affinity for the ergosterol component of the fungal cell membrane but can also bind to the cholesterol component of the mammalian cell leading to cytotoxicity. AmBisome, the liposomal formulation of amphotericin B, has been shown to penetrate the cell wall of both extracellular and intracellular forms of susceptible fungi. It has been approved in the United States and Europe for the prophylaxis and treatment of certain fungal infections in adults.

INDICATION(S) AND RESEARCH PHASE
Pediatric, Fungal Infections – Phase II

posaconazole
unknown

MANUFACTURER
Schering-Plough Corporation

DESCRIPTION
Posaconazole is an orally administered triazole antifungal. It was developed to treat opportunistic fungal infections that may thrive when a subject's immune system becomes rundown or compromised by another disease. The drug is currently in phase III trials.

INDICATION(S) AND RESEARCH PHASE
Fungal Infections – Phase III

unknown
Vfend

MANUFACTURER
Pfizer

DESCRIPTION
Vfend is a broad spectrum antifungal compound that blocks the synthesis of erosterol in major sterol in the fungal cell membrane. It is active against the fungi most commonly causing invasive fungal infections, including *Candida* and *Aspergillus* species. Vfend will be available in both oral and intravenous forms. An NDA has been filed for this drug.

INDICATION(S) AND RESEARCH PHASE
Fungal Infections – NDA submitted

V-Echinocandin
unknown

MANUFACTURER
Versicor

DESCRIPTION
V-Echinocandin is a novel intravenous drug being developed for the treatment of fungal infections. The drug selectively inhibits an enzyme in fungi involved in cell wall synthesis. V-Echinocandin has shown invtro activity against various fungi including *Candida* and *Aspergillus*.

V-Echinocandin has been well tolerated in five trials involving over 100 individuals. In one phase II trial of subjects with esophagitis, over 80% of evaluable subjects were cured or improved (as defined by endoscopy) by the end of the treatment. Twenty-nine evaluable subjects were treated with daily intravenous infusions of V-Echinocandin for up to 21 days. Phase III trials in subjects with *Candida esophagitis* are scheduled to begin in the first quarter of 2001. In these trials, an increased dose of V-Echinocandin will be compared to fluconazole.

INDICATION(S) AND RESEARCH PHASE
Fungal Infections – Phase II completed
Esophageal Disorders – Phase II completed

Genital Herpes

APL400-024Px
Genevax - HSV-Px

MANUFACTURER
Wyeth-Lederle Vaccines

DESCRIPTION
HSV-Px is a novel facilitated DNA vaccine for prevention of herpes simplex virus-2 (HSV-2) infection that causes genital herpes. This vaccine uses injected GENEVAX delivery technology and it is in phase II trials.

INDICATION(S) AND RESEARCH PHASE
Genital Herpes – Phase II

GW 419458, DISC-HSV
unknown

MANUFACTURER
GlaxoSmithKline

DESCRIPTION
DISC (disabled infectious single cycle)-HSV is an immunotherapeutic vaccine using a disabled live virus for treatment and prevention of genital herpes. Since the drug therapy induces a natural immune response and may promote immunologic memory, the chance of disease recurrence is drastically reduced. It also eliminates the need for constant dosing, thereby increasing subject compliance and improving lifestyle. The drug is in phase II trials for genital herpes. GlaxoSmithKline has worldwide development and marketing rights.

INDICATION(S) AND RESEARCH PHASE
Genital Herpes – Phase II

resiquimod
unknown

MANUFACTURER
3M Pharmaceuticals

DESCRIPTION
Resiquimod is in phase III trials for recurrent genital herpes in both the United States and Europe. In November 2000, positive phase II results of a double-blind, placebo-controlled trial were reported. In the six month follow-up, the time to the first recurrence was significantly increased and the total number of recurrences was significantly decreased for subjects on active study medication compared to a placebo gel.

INDICATION(S) AND RESEARCH PHASE
Genital Herpes – Phase III

TA-HSV
unknown

MANUFACTURER
Cantab Pharmaceuticals plc

DESCRIPTION
TA-HSV (Therapeutic Antigen-Herpes Simplex Virus) is a genetically disabled vaccine containing HSV that allows only a single cycle of replication within a host cell. It is in phase II trials for the treatment of genital herpes.

INDICATION(S) AND RESEARCH PHASE
Genital Herpes – Phase II

unknown
Docosanol

MANUFACTURER
AVANIR Pharmaceuticals

DESCRIPTION
Docosanol is approved as a treatment for cold sores and fever blisters. It is in phase III trials for the treatment of genital herpes. Docosanol works by inhibiting fusion between the plasma membrane and the herpes simplex virus (HSV) envelope, thereby preventing viral entry into cells and subsequent viral replication. Since the compound doesn't act directly on the virus, it is unlikely it will produce drug resistant mutants of HSV. All known competitive Rx products work by inhibition of viral DNA replication and, as such, carry risk of mutating the virus.

INDICATION(S) AND RESEARCH PHASE
Genital Herpes – Phase III

vaccine, genital herpes
unknown

MANUFACTURER
Corixa Montana

DESCRIPTION
This immunostimulant vaccine uses monophosphoryl lipid A (MPL) adjuvant for prevention and treatment of herpes simplex virus types 1 and 2 that causes genital herpes. The vaccine is in phase III trials.

INDICATION(S) AND RESEARCH PHASE
Genital Herpes – Phase III
Herpes Simplex Infections – Phase III

vaccine, genital herpes
Simplirix

MANUFACTURER
GlaxoSmithKline

DESCRIPTION
Simplirix is a recombinant vaccine being developed for genital herpes prophylaxis. Simplirix consists of a recombinant glycoprotein from herpes simplex virus 2 (HSV-2), in combination with an adjuvant "derivative endotoxin." Results of two large, placebo-controlled, randomized international trials were presented at the 40th annual Interscience Conference on Antimicrobials and Chemotherapy in 2000. Both were "discordant partner studies," in which one of the partners had genital herpes and the other did not. The first trial included 847 subjects who tested negative for HSV-1 and HSV-2 at baseline, and the second trial involved 1867 subjects who were negative

for HSV-2. The vaccine had absolutely no effect in the men in either group; however, a notable effect was observed in the women. In the first study, the vaccine efficacy in women was 73%. Similarly, among the seronegative women in the second study, the vaccine efficacy was 74%. The vaccine was not protective in the women who were HSV-1-positive and HSV-2-negative.

INDICATION(S) AND RESEARCH PHASE
Genital Herpes – Phase II
Vaccines – Phase II

Genital Warts

HspE7
unknown

MANUFACTURER
StressGen

DESCRIPTION
HspE7 is a recombinant fusion product composed of the heat shock protein 65 (Hsp65) from *Mycobacterium bovis* BCG and the protein E7. The E7 protein is derived from the human papillomavirus (HPV) and is involved in the malignant transformation of anal and cervical epithelial cells. E7 is a tumor-specific antigen and represents a precise target for immune system attack on abnormal cells.

StressGen has initiated subjects, treatment in a phase III trial to investigate HspE7 as a novel immunotherapeutic for anal dysplasia (AIN) caused by HPV. The company also has phase II HspE7 trials in women with HPV-related cervical dysplasia and cervical cancer. In January 2001, a phase II trial was initiated to test HspE7 on 52 subjects suffering from genital warts caused by HPV.

INDICATION(S) AND RESEARCH PHASE
Cervical Dysplasia/Cancer – Phase II
Anal Dysplasia – Phase III
Genital Warts – Phase II

interferon (IFN), alfa-n3
Alferon N Gel

MANUFACTURER
Interferon Sciences

DESCRIPTION
Alferon N Gel is a human leukocyte-derived natural interferon (IFN) treatment being tested for vaginal infections in phase II trials. Interferons are naturally produced chemicals that modulate and boost the immune system. These trials are testing the drug in a topical gel formulation.

Already on the market, interferon alfa-n3 (human leukocyte derived) is an injectable formulation of Natural Alpha Interferon, approved by the FDA in 1989 for the intralesional treatment of refractory or recurring external condylomata acuminata in subjects 18 years of age or older.

INDICATION(S) AND RESEARCH PHASE
Genital Warts – Phase II
Vaginal Infection – Phase II
Viral Infection – Phase II

PEN203
unknown

MANUFACTURER
Pentose Pharmaceuticals

DESCRIPTION
PEN203 represents a novel class of small molecule pharmaceuticals with broad spectrum antiviral activity. These compounds are designed to act through a natural antiviral pathway induced by interferon. Like interferon, they are believed to work by enhancing the body's natural mechanism for protection against viruses. Unlike injectable interferon or ablative topical therapies, PEN203 can be topically applied and is designed to be well tolerated by subjects, providing a key advantage over currently available treatments for HPV infections.

Forty eight subjects are being treated in a phase I/II trial for genital warts.

INDICATION(S) AND RESEARCH PHASE
Genital Warts – Phase I/II

TA-GW pharmaccine
unknown

MANUFACTURER
Cantab Pharmaceuticals plc

DESCRIPTION
TA-GW pharmaccine is a novel therapeutic vaccine for genital warts. The compound, in an intravenous formulation, combines an HPV (human papillomavirus) protein with an adjuvant to produce an immune reaction directed against the virus. SmithKline Beecham (now GlaxoSmithKline), who have been responsible for funding development, have decided to discontinue investment in TA-GW. This decision was based on results of a phase II trial, which showed that at six months there was no significant difference in the wart recurrence rate between subjects who received TA-GW and those in the control group.

INDICATION(S) AND RESEARCH PHASE
Genital Warts – Phase II discontinued

unknown
Polyphenon E

MANUFACTURER
MediGene AG

DESCRIPTION
Polyphenon E consists of polphenols, which inhibit viruses causing genital warts. In addition, polphenols have anti-tumor and anti-inflammatory properties. Polyphenon E is in a phase III trial to treat genital warts caused by human papillomaviruses and will enroll 260 subjects, 50% male and 50% female, at 30 sites throughout Germany and Russia. The trial will be randomized, double blinded, and placebo controlled.

INDICATION(S) AND RESEARCH PHASE
Genital Warts – Phase III

Herpes Labialis Infections

ME-609
unknown

MANUFACTURER

Herpes Labialis Infections

Medivir

DESCRIPTION
ME-609 is a cream currently in development for the treatment of oral herpes simplex infections. In December 2000, preliminary results of a phase II trial demonstrated that the cream reduced the healing time of cold sores by 15% compared to placebo. The double-blind, placebo-controlled, randomized trial was carried out by university clinics in North America. Subjects with a history of sun-induced herpes simplex virus infections around the mouth were irradiated with UV light. Treatment began after 48 hours; half of the subjects were treated with ME-609 and half with an inactive placebo cream. Medivir has conducted phase I and II trials in collaboration with AstraZeneca; however, this partnership will not be continued for the remainder of development.

INDICATION(S) AND RESEARCH PHASE
Herpes Labialis Infections – Phase II completed

Herpes Simplex Infections

AG-701
unknown

MANUFACTURER
Antigenics

DESCRIPTION
AG-701 is a recombinant human HSP complexed to a synthetic peptide derived from HSV-2 being tested in a phase I trial in subjects diagnosed with herpes simplex virus type 2 (HSV-2).

INDICATION(S) AND RESEARCH PHASE
Herpes Simplex Infections – Phase I

vaccine, genital herpes
unknown

MANUFACTURER
Corixa Montana

DESCRIPTION
This immunostimulant vaccine uses monophosphoryl lipid A (MPL) adjuvant for prevention and treatment of herpes simplex virus types 1 and 2 that causes genital herpes. The vaccine is in phase III trials.

INDICATION(S) AND RESEARCH PHASE
Genital Herpes – Phase III
Herpes Simplex Infections – Phase III

valaciclovir
Valtrex, Zelitrex

MANUFACTURER
GlaxoSmithKline

DESCRIPTION
Valtrex (valaciclovir) is a nucleoside analogue in phase III development. It is being tested for three new indications: the prevention of herpes simplex virus (HSV) transmission, HSV suppression in immunocompromised subjects, and cold sores. Valtrex is also marketed under the trade name Zelitrex.

INDICATION(S) AND RESEARCH PHASE
Herpes Simplex Infections – Phase III
Cold Sores – Phase III
HSV Suppression – Phase III

Herpes Zoster Infections

ADL 2-1294
unknown

MANUFACTURER
Adolor

DESCRIPTION
ADL 2-1294 is a peripheral opiate (synthetic narcotic) being tested for the treatment of pain and itching associated with burns, abrasions, eczema, and dermatitis. The drug, in a topical formulation, is in phase II trials for atopic dermatitis, burns and burn infections, herpes zoster infections, psoriasis and psoriatic disorders, and for eye disorders and infections.

INDICATION(S) AND RESEARCH PHASE
Atopic Dermatitis – Phase II
Burns and Burn Infections – Phase II
Herpes Zoster Infections – Phase II
Psoriasis and Psoriatic Disorders – Phase II
Eye Disorders/Infections – Phase II
Skin Infections/Disorders – Phase II

Ichthyosis

glyceryl monolaurin, T-100
Glylorin

MANUFACTURER
Cellegy Pharmaceuticals

DESCRIPTION
Glylorin is a lipid-based treatment (containing a monocarboxylic acid ester) being tested for certain skin diseases, such as atopic dermatitis and impetigo. The drug, in a transdermal delivery formulation, completed phase II trials for ichthyosis vulgaris, which did not show statistical significance.

INDICATION(S) AND RESEARCH PHASE
Ichthyosis – Phase II completed

Keratoses

bexarotene
Targretin-gel

MANUFACTURER
Ligand Pharmaceuticals

DESCRIPTION
Targretin, topical gel formulation, which selectively stimulates a (retinoid subtype) receptor, is being developed for the treatment of actinic keratosis. The drug has just completed phase I/II trials.

INDICATION(S) AND RESEARCH PHASE
Keratoses – Phase I/II

Mycosis Fungoides

HOE-351
unknown

MANUFACTURER
Aventis

DESCRIPTION
HOE-351 is a novel compound being developed in a topical formulation for the treatment of superficial fungal infections of the skin (dermatomycoses). The company discontinued testing the drug against mycosis fungoides in phase II trials. It may be indicated for other dermatological conditions.

INDICATION(S) AND RESEARCH PHASE
Mycosis Fungoides – Phase II discontinued

terbinafine
Lamisil

MANUFACTURER
Novartis

DESCRIPTION
Lamasil inhibits squalene epoxidase, a key enzyme in sterol biosynthesis in fungi, causing a decrease in ergosterol and a corresponding accumulation of sterol within the fungal cells. The drug is being evaluated in phase III trials in an oral formulation for the treatment of both systemic mycoses and tinea capitis.

INDICATION(S) AND RESEARCH PHASE
Pediatric, Tinea Capitis – Phase II
Tinea Capitis – Phase III
Mycosis Fungoides – Phase III

Pressure Ulcers

oxandrolone, CO221
unknown

MANUFACTURER
Bio-Technology General

DESCRIPTION
Oxandrolone is an anabolic (converts simple compounds into complex such as protoplasm) steroid for treatment of chronic obstructive pulmonary disease (COPD) and pressure ulcers. The drug, in oral tablet formulation, is in phase II trials for both indications.

INDICATION(S) AND RESEARCH PHASE
Chronic Obstructive Pulmonary Disease (COPD) – Phase II
Pressure Ulcers – Phase II

Psoriasis and Psoriatic Disorders

ABX-IL8
unknown

MANUFACTURER
Abgenix

DESCRIPTION
ABX-IL8 is a fully humanized antibody developed with the company's XenoMouse technology. It targets interleukin-8 (IL-8), which is a cytokine that can cause unwanted inflammation by first enabling immune cells, including neutrophils, to migrate to inflammatory sites and subsequently activating them. There is substantial evidence that IL-8 contributes to a number of inflammatory diseases, including psoriasis, rheumatoid arthritis, and inflammatory bowel disease.

ABX-IL8 is being studied in a phase II trial for psoriasis, which is a disease that causes a thickening and scaling of the skin accompanied by local inflammation, because of the drug's potential to intervene at multiple steps in the disease pathology by blocking IL-8. Scientific studies have shown that IL-8 levels can be elevated 150-fold in psoriatic tissue when compared to normal tissue. In addition to contributing to the inflammation process, IL-8 is also a growth factor for skin cells that are proliferating in psoriatic tissue.

Additionally, IL-8 is a potent angiogenesis factor, so it may be contributing to the ingrowth of blood vessels that nourish psoriatic tissue. ABX-IL8 is administered by intravenous infusion.

INDICATION(S) AND RESEARCH PHASE
Psoriasis and Psoriatic Disorders – Phase IIb
Rheumatoid Arthritis – Phase IIa

ADL 2-1294
unknown

MANUFACTURER
Adolor

DESCRIPTION
ADL2-1294 is a peripheral opiate (synthetic narcotic) being tested for the treatment of pain and itching associated with burns, abrasions, eczema, and dermatitis. The drug, in a topical formulation, is in phase II trials for atopic dermatitis, burns and burn infections, herpes zoster infections, psoriasis and psoriatic disorders, and for eye disorders and infections.

INDICATION(S) AND RESEARCH PHASE
Atopic Dermatitis – Phase II
Burns and Burn Infections – Phase II
Herpes Zoster Infections – Phase II
Psoriasis and Psoriatic Disorders – Phase II
Eye Disorders/Infections – Phase II
Skin Infections/Disorders – Phase II

AE-941
Neovastat

MANUFACTURER
AEterna Laboratories

DESCRIPTION
Neovastat is an angiogenesis inhibitor being tested in two phase II trials to treat subjects with non-small cell lung cancer, subjects with moderate to severe psoriasis, multiple myeloma, kidney cancer, and macular degeneration.

A phase II trial for multiple myeloma was initiated in October 2000 and will treat 120 subjects and include approximately 20 sites across North America and Europe. Trial results are expected summer 2002.

Additionally, a phase III trial was initiated in May 2000 for kidney cancer and will include 270 subjects at sites in North America and Europe.

INDICATION(S) AND RESEARCH PHASE
Lung Cancer – Phase III
Psoriasis and Psoriatic Disorders – Phase I/II completed
Cancer/Tumors (Unspecified) – Phase I/II completed
Multiple Myeloma – Phase II
Renal Cell Carcinoma – Phase III
Macular Degeneration – Phase I completed

alitretinoin, ALRT-1057
Panretin

MANUFACTURER
Ligand Pharmaceuticals

DESCRIPTION
This product is 9-cis-retinoic acid and is chemically related to vitamin A. It activates all known retinoid receptors. Activation of retinoid receptors regulates the expression of genes controlling processes related to cell differentiation and proliferation. A topical gel formulation of Panretin has been on the market since February 1999 for the treatment of lesions associated with Kaposi's sarcoma.

These new trials are evaluating the effects of the oral capsule formulation for the following new indications: treatment of breast and pediatric cancers (phase II), myelodysplastic syndrome, bronchial metaplasia, and psoriasis and psoriatic disorders (phase II/III).

INDICATION(S) AND RESEARCH PHASE
Breast Cancer – Phase II
Lung Cancer – Phase II/III
Pediatric, Cancer/Tumors (Unspecified) – Phase II
Psoriasis and Psoriatic Disorders – Phase II/III
White Blood Cell Disorders – Phase II/III

anti-CD11a, hu1124
unknown

MANUFACTURER
XOMA Corporation

DESCRIPTION
This drug is a monoclonal antibody (the fusion of 2 types of cells, an antibody producing cell and a myeloma cell) for the treatment of moderate to severe plaque psoriasis. It works by inhibiting a specific type of white blood cell, known as a T-cell, and targets a specific cell marker, CD11a, on the T-cell surface to inhibit it. Anti-CD11a then potentially turns off the abnormal autoimmune response in psoriasis subjects. The drug is given intravenously.

These T-cell lymphocytes play a large role in the immune system to help the body fight off infection and recognize foreign materials. Sometimes the immune system becomes short-circuited and the body starts attacking itself. This widely diverse group of problems is called autoimmune diseases. Psoriasis is one type of the autoimmune disease in which the immune system sends lymphocytes to attack parts of the skin around the hands, elbows, and other areas. The skin becomes chronically inflamed and then red, scaly plaques form. Drugs that suppress this abnormal immune response may provide new therapies for autoimmune diseases like psoriasis.

The phase II placebo-controlled clinical trial conducted in Canada tested the Anti-CD11a antibody in 145 moderate-to-severe psoriasis subjects who received an 8-week course of therapy with either the antibody or placebo. XOMA claims that a preliminary analysis of the data, demonstrated a clinical response of 75% or better improvement over baseline as measured by physician's global assessment (what the doctors thought even though they were study blinded), in 25% of the subjects treated with the drug versus 2% of the subjects in the placebo group. Side effects included a temporary hearing loss in one subject that may or may not be related to the drug. The more common adverse effects were mild headaches and low body temperature increases, usually after the first dose.

INDICATION(S) AND RESEARCH PHASE
Psoriasis and Psoriatic Disorders – Phase III
Kidney Transplant Surgery – Phase I/II

bexarotene
Targretin-capsule

MANUFACTURER
Ligand Pharmaceuticals

DESCRIPTION
Targretin, which selectively stimulates a (retinoid subtype) receptor, is being developed in an oral capsule formulation for the treatment of lung and breast cancer, head and neck cancer, cutaneous T-cell lymphoma (CTCL), psoriasis and psoriatic disorders, and atopic dermatitis. The drug is in phase II trials for head and neck cancer, phase II/III trials for breast cancer, CTCL, and psoriasis and psoriatic disorders, and phase III trials for non-small cell lung cancer.

INDICATION(S) AND RESEARCH PHASE
Atopic Dermatitis – Phase II
Psoriasis and Psoriatic Disorders – Phase II/III
Lung Cancer – Phase III
Breast Cancer – Phase II/III
Head and Neck Cancer – Phase II

BMS-188667, CTLA4Ig
unknown

MANUFACTURER

DESCRIPTION
CTLA4Ig is a modified antibody molecule/antibody fusion protein with selective immunosuppressive activity. The drug is being evaluated in phase II trials for the treatment of psoriasis.

INDICATION(S) AND RESEARCH PHASE
Psoriasis and Psoriatic Disorders – Phase II

BTI-322, MEDI-507
unknown

MANUFACTURER
BioTransplant

DESCRIPTION
MEDI-507 is a novel, humanized monoclonal antibody which binds specifically to the CD2 surface antigen receptor found on T-cells and natural killer (NK) cells. MEDI-507 was engineered from BTI-322, a murine

antibody, in order to reduce potential immunogenicity and allow for long-term administration. Laboratory studies have suggested that MEDI-507 and BTI-322 primarily inhibit the response of specific activated T-cells while subsequently allowing other immune cells to respond normally. Therefore, these drugs may be able to prevent the host rejection of a transplanted organ without compromising the entire immune system. MEDI-501 may prove to induce long-term functional transplantation tolerance in humans, increase the therapeutic benefit of bone marrow transplants, and reduce or eliminate the need for lifelong immunosuppressive therapy.

The drug is currently in multiple phase II clinical trials for treatment of graft versus host disease, a frequent and often fatal outcome of bone marrow transplantation, caused when donor white blood cells in a bone marrow transplant attack the tissue of the recipient. Clinical manifestations include skin rash, severe diarrhea, liver abnormalities, and jaundice.

Phase II trials for kidney transplant rejection are also in progress. MEDI-507 is also being evaluated for treatment of psoriasis as a proof of concept for its use in autoimmune diseases.

INDICATION(S) AND RESEARCH PHASE
Graft Versus Host Disease – Phase II
Kidney Transplant Surgery – Phase II
Psoriasis and Psoriatic Disorders – Phase II
Liver Transplant Rejection – Phase I/II completed

efalizumab monoclonal antibody
Xanelim

MANUFACTURER
Genentech

DESCRIPTION
Xanelim is an anti-CD11a recombinant humanized monoclonal antibody (Mab)/T cell activatiom inhibitor being tested in weekly subcutaneous injection formulation. It is currently in phase III trials for treatment of moderate to severe psoriasis.

INDICATION(S) AND RESEARCH PHASE
Psoriasis and Psoriatic Disorders – Phase III

etanercept
Enbrel

MANUFACTURER
Wyeth-Ayerst

DESCRIPTION
Enbrel binds to tumor necrosis factor (TNF), which is one of the dominant cytokines or proteins associated with normal immune function and the series of reactions that cause the inflammatory process of rheumatoid arthritis. Enbrel inhibits the binding of TNF molecules to the TNF receptor (TNFR) sites. The binding of these sites inactivates TNF, resulting in significant reduction in inflammatory cascade.

Results from postmarketing studies demonstrated that Enbrel can have serious adverse effects such as infection, sepsis, and death. According to the company, subjects who are predisposed to infection, such as those with advanced or poorly controlled diabetes, are at greater risk of experiencing side effects. In addition, use of Enbrel should be terminated in subjects with current infections or sepsis. Allergic reactions to Enbrel or its components is also a possibility.

Additionally, in pediatric trial results show that nearly 75% of children with severe, long-standing juvenile rheumatoid arthritis (JRA) respond to Enbrel. In the first segment of the study, 74% of children (51 of 69) between the ages of four and 17 showed an improvement in disease response when treated with Enbrel for three months. In the second segment, half of these 51 subjects received Enbrel and half received a placebo. Seventy-two percent of those who received Enbrel completed the second segment without worsening of JRA symptoms, compared to 19% who took a placebo.

Trials are also under way for the treatment of psoriasis and congestive heart failure.

INDICATION(S) AND RESEARCH PHASE
Rheumatoid Arthritis – FDA approved
Pediatric, Rheumatoid Arthritis – FDA approved
Psoriasis and Psoriatic Disorders – Phase III
Congestive Heart Failure – Phase III

HCT 1026
unknown

MANUFACTURER
NicOx SA

DESCRIPTION
HCT 1026 is a novel nitric oxide-releasing derivative of the non-steroidal anti-inflammatory drug (NSAID) flurbiprofen. While flurbiprofen has demonstrated effectiveness in the treatment of urinary incontinence, its use has been complicated by gastric toxicity. Because HCT 1026 may provide increased gastric tolerability, it can be administered for extended periods at effective doses. In Phase I trials, results indicated that HCT 1026 produced fewer and less severe gastric lesions compared to flurbiprofen.

HCT 1026 produces anti-inflammatory effects through the inhibition of prostaglandin synthesis, while nitric oxide controls inflammatory cell activation. These two factors suggest that HCT 1026 may be an effective treatment for dermatology disorders such as psoriasis. HCT 1026 is in phase II trials for the treatment of urinary incontinence, osteoporosis, and skin disorders such as atopic dermatitis and psoriasis.

INDICATION(S) AND RESEARCH PHASE
Atopic Dermatitis – Phase II
Urinary Incontinence – Phase II
Osteoporosis – Phase II
Psoriasis and Psoriatic Disorders – Phase II
Skin Infections/Disorders – Phase II

HuMax-CD4
unknown

MANUFACTURER
Genmab A/S

DESCRIPTION
HuMax-CD4 is a human antibody that targets the CD4 receptor on T-cells. These cells are implicated early in the cascade of inflammatory events that cause rheumatoid arthritis (RA). Therefore, blocking the activ-

ity of these cells may effectively halt the inflammatory process.

Positive results from a single-dose phase I/II trial of HuMax-CD4 for rheumatoid arthritis were announced in November 2000. HuMax-CD4 was well tolerated in the dose-escalating, placebo-controlled trial, and there was no evidence of depletion of subjects' CD4 positive T cells. Furthermore, in the four highest doses, 0.5, 1.0, 2.0, and 4.0 mg/kg, 50% of the treated subjects achieved favorable responses to the antibody.

In addition, a phase II trial was initiated in January 2001 test HuMax-CD4 in subjects with severe psoriasis. The trial will include four different dose levels plus a placebo arm.

INDICATION(S) AND RESEARCH PHASE
Rheumatoid Arthritis – Phase I/II
Psoriasis and Psoriatic Disorders – Phase II

hypericin
VIMRxyn

MANUFACTURER
Nexell Therapeutics

DESCRIPTION
VIMRxyn (hypericin) is a light-activated and topically applied formulation of aromatic polycyclic dione, (APD-1) which is a synthetic agent directed against retroviruses. This drug is being tested for treatment of specific skin diseases including psoriasis, cutaneous T-cell lymphoma, and warts.

VIMRx Pharmaceuticals has also manufactured an oral, once-daily formulation of aromatic polycyclic dione (APD-1). This drug form is being evaluated for the treatment of malignant gliomas.

INDICATION(S) AND RESEARCH PHASE
Brain Cancer – Phase I/II
Lymphomas – Phase I/II
Psoriasis and Psoriatic Disorders – Phase I/II
Skin Infections/Disorders – Phase I/II

IDEC-114
Primatized

MANUFACTURER
IDEC Pharmaceuticals

DESCRIPTION
IDEC-114 (anti-B7-1 (CD80) monoclonal antibody) selectively targets an important co-stimulatory molecule on antigen-presenting cells. The antibody inhibits the binding of the B7-1 ligand on these cells to the CD28 receptor on T-cells, thus blocking the second signal for inflammatory T-cell activation. Inappropriately activated T-cells are implicated in many autoimmune disorders, making IDEC-114 potentially useful in a wide variety of diseases.

The company has initiated a phase I/II clinical trial of IDEC-114 for the treatment of psoriasis. The study will evaluate the safety, tolerability, pharmacokinetics, and potential activity of multiple doses of this investigational agent.

INDICATION(S) AND RESEARCH PHASE
Psoriasis and Psoriatic Disorders – Phase I/II

IDEC-131
unknown

MANUFACTURER
IDEC Pharmaceuticals

DESCRIPTION
IDEC-131 is a humanized monoclonal antibody (Mab) developed for the treatment of systemic lupus erythematosus (SLE). By inhibiting the action of the CD40 ligand molecule, a communication link between the immune helper T-cells and B-cells, IDEC-131 may reduce excessively abnormal antibody production. This biologic drug may help restore a more normal immune response in subjects with a variety of autoimmune and inflammatory conditions. The drug is in trials for SLE and and psoriasis.

INDICATION(S) AND RESEARCH PHASE
Systemic Lupus Erythematosus – Phase II completed
Psoriasis and Psoriatic Disorders – Phase II

interleukin-10
Tenovil

MANUFACTURER
Schering-Plough

DESCRIPTION
Tenovil is an immunomodulator being developed in an injectable formulation. It is currently being evaluated for the treatment of ischemia reperfusion injury, hepatic fibrosis, hepatitis C, and psoriasis.

INDICATION(S) AND RESEARCH PHASE
Liver Disease – Phase II
Hepatitis – Phase I
Ischemia Reperfusion Injury – Phase I
Psoriasis and Psoriatic Disorders – Phase II

IR502
Zorcell

MANUFACTURER
Immune Response Corporation

DESCRIPTION
IR502 is a therapeutic vaccine consisting of synthetic peptides combined with a potent immune system stimulant called incomplete Freund's adjuvant (IFA). This T-cell receptor (TCR) vaccine is designed to cause the immune system to shut down activated T-cells attacking the joints and causing tissue damage. It is being tested for the treatment of moderate-to-severe psoriasis.

INDICATION(S) AND RESEARCH PHASE
Psoriasis and Psoriatic Disorders – Phase II
Vaccines – Phase II

ISAtx247
Unknown

MANUFACTURER
Isotechnika

DESCRIPTION
ISAtx247 is a novel immunosuppressant for prevention of organ rejection after transplantation and for treatment of autoimmune diseases such as rheumatoid arthritis

and psoriasis.

INDICATION(S) AND RESEARCH PHASE
Psoriasis and Psoriatic Disorders – Phase I
Rheumatoid Arthritis – Phase I
Immunosuppressant – Phase I

ISIS-2302
unknown

MANUFACTURER
Isis Pharmaceuticals

DESCRIPTION
ISIS-2302 is an inhibitor of antisense intracellular adhesion molecule-1 (ICAM-1), which is a chemical that plays a central role in inflammation. Antisense drugs work at the genetic level to interrupt the process by which disease-causing proteins are produced. Proteins play a central role in virtually every aspect of human metabolism. Many human diseases are the result of inappropriate protein production (or disordered protein performance). This is true of both host diseases (such as cancer) and infectious diseases (such as AIDS).

Traditional drugs are designed to interact with protein molecules throughout the body that support or cause diseases. Antisense drugs are designed to inhibit the production of disease-causing proteins. They can be designed to treat a wide range of diseases including infectious, inflammatory, and cardiovascular diseases, and cancer.

ISIS-2302 is being tested in a phase II trial using an enema formulation to treat subjects with ulcerative colitis. This method of administration allows potentially therapeutic amounts of the drug to be absorbed by the lining of the intestine, which is inflamed in subjects with ulcerative colitis.

In addition, ISIS-2302 is in trials for kidney transplant, psoriasis, and Crohn's disease.

INDICATION(S) AND RESEARCH PHASE
Crohn's Disease – Phase III
Psoriasis and Psoriatic Disorders – Phase II
Inflammatory Bowel Disease – Phase II
Kidney Transplant Surgery – Phase II

maxacalcitol
unknown

MANUFACTURER
Schering-Plough

DESCRIPTION
Maxacalcitol is a vitamin D3 analog being developed in phase II trials for the treatment of psoriasis. The drug is in topical formulation.

INDICATION(S) AND RESEARCH PHASE
Psoriasis and Psoriatic Disorders – Phase II

MEDI-507
unknown

MANUFACTURER
MedImmune

DESCRIPTION
MEDI-507 is a humanized form of the murine monoclonal antibody, BTI-322. It binds specifically to the CD2 receptor found on T cells and natural killer (NK) cells and has the ability to inhibit the response of T cells directed at transplant antigens, while still allowing immune cells to respond normally to other antigens.

The compound is in development for the treatment of steroid-resistant, severe graft-versus-host disease (GvHD) in adult and pediatric subjects. Additionally, MEDI-507 is in phase I/II development for psoriasis. Development for the prevention of acute renal transplant rejection has been discontinued.

INDICATION(S) AND RESEARCH PHASE
Psoriasis and Psoriatic Disorders – Phase II
Pediatric, Graft Versus Host Disease – Phase I/II
Graft Versus Host Disease – Phase I/II

micellar paclitaxel
unknown

MANUFACTURER
Angiotech Pharmaceuticals

DESCRIPTION
Micellar paclitaxel is being developed for the treatment of secondary progressive multiple sclerosis, rheumatoid arthritis, and severe psoriasis. A double-blind, placebo-controlled, phase I trial produced positive results in the treatment of rheumatoid arthritis (RA). Enrolled patients were between 21 and 75 years of age, presented Class I to III of RA severity, and had failed treatment with at least one disease-modifying anti-rheumatic drug, such as methotrexate. The drug was determined to be safe and well-tolerated in all 15 patients enrolled in the study. Of those patients treated with micellar paclitaxel that completed the study, 25% had a clinical response defined by a series of measures consistent with the American College of Rheumatology (ACR) 20% improvement criteria. A larger phase II study may be initiated in 2001. Trials for multiple sclerosis and psoriasis are currently in phase II.

INDICATION(S) AND RESEARCH PHASE
Multiple Sclerosis – Phase II
Rheumatoid Arthritis – Phase I completed
Psoriasis and Psoriatic Disorders – Phase II

NCX 1022
unknown

MANUFACTURER
NicOx SA

DESCRIPTION
NCX 1022 is a nitric oxide-releasing derivative of hydrocortisone in a topical formulation. It is being evaluated in a phase I trial for the treatment of psoriasis. The trial is being conducted in France and will enroll 36 subjects. Three doses of NCX 1022 will be studied along with a placebo. The objectives of this study are to assess the local tolerability of NCX 1022 and compare the pharmacological blanching effect due to vasoconstriction with reference steroids.

INDICATION(S) AND RESEARCH PHASE
Psoriasis and Psoriatic Disorders – Phase I

paclitaxel

unknown

MANUFACTURER
Angiotech Pharmaceuticals

DESCRIPTION
Paclitaxel is an anti-microtubule agent that inhibits cell division and blocks the AP-1 cellular pathway. It inhibits several blood processes including cell migration, angiogenesis, and the production of enzymes responsible for tissue destruction. The substance also aids in reducing inflammation. Paclitaxel is being tested in a topical gel formulation for the treatment of mild to moderate psoriasis. The drug has completed phase I testing.

INDICATION(S) AND RESEARCH PHASE
Psoriasis and Psoriatic Disorders – Phase I completed

PEN203
unknown

MANUFACTURER
CoPharma

DESCRIPTION
PEN203 represents a novel class of small molecule pharmaceuticals with broad spectrum antiviral activity. These anti-proliferative compounds are designed to act through a natural antiviral pathway induced by interferon. Like interferon, they are believed to work by enhancing the body's natural mechanism for protection against viruses. Unlike injectable interferon or ablative topical therapies, however, PEN203 can be topically applied and is designed to be well tolerated by patients.
  PEN203 is currently in phase IIb trials for treatment of basal cell carcinoma, psoriasis, and genital warts.

INDICATION(S) AND RESEARCH PHASE
Genital Warts – Phase IIb
Psoriasis and Psoriatic Disorders – Phase IIb
Basal Cell Carcinoma – Phase IIb

PVAC
unknown

MANUFACTURER
Corixa Corporation

DESCRIPTION
PVAC is an immunomodulator currently in phase II trials for the treatment of moderate to severe psoriasis. PVAC is based on a proprietary process and formulation derived from heat-killed *Mycobacterium vaccae*.

INDICATION(S) AND RESEARCH PHASE
Psoriasis and Psoriatic Disorders – Phase II

recombinant human lactoferrin (rhLF)
unknown

MANUFACTURER
Agennix

DESCRIPTION
Recombinant human lactoferrin is being tested in a topical formulation in phase I/II trials for the treatment of psoriasis and contact allergic dermatitis. Lactoferrin is a multi-functional protein naturally found in human milk. It plays an essential role in stimulating the body's immune system and also works as a natural antioxidant, helping to control cell and tissue damage caused by oxidation. Agennix's breakthrough technology has made it possible to manufacture human lactoferrin in commercial quantities for the first time.

INDICATION(S) AND RESEARCH PHASE
Psoriasis and Psoriatic Disorders – Phase I/II
Skin Infections/Disorders – Phase I/II

recombinant LFA-3/IgG1 Human Fusion Protein
Amevive

MANUFACTURER
Biogen

DESCRIPTION
Amevive (LFA-3/IgG1) is an injectable formulation of a recombinant fusion protein designed to modulate the immune response by blocking the cellular pathway that activates T-cells, the specialized white blood cells that play a critical role in inflammation. Amevive has a unique selectivity for memory-effector T-cells. The aim of treatment with Amevive is to reduce the number of these memory-effector T cells, which play an important role in the progression of psoriasis, without reducing naive T-cells that affect important immune functions. This drug is being tested in phase III trials for the treatment of moderate to severe psoriasis.

INDICATION(S) AND RESEARCH PHASE
Psoriasis and Psoriatic Disorders – Phase III

SMART anti-CD3
Nuvion

MANUFACTURER
Protein Design Labs

DESCRIPTION
Nuvion is an IgG2 monoclonal antibody that targets the CD3 antigen present on all T-cells. Nuvion is an immunosuppressive drug in phase I/II trials for the treatment of psoriasis and phase I trials for graft vs. host disease and t-cell malignancies.

INDICATION(S) AND RESEARCH PHASE
Psoriasis and Psoriatic Disorders – Phase I/II
Immunosuppressant – Phase I

ST630
unknown

MANUFACTURER
Bertek

DESCRIPTION
ST630 is a hexafluoronated steroid. This vitamin D analogue is being developed, using the TopiCare liquid polymer topical delivery system, for the treatment of psoriasis. Phase II trials have been completed and pending analysis of the results, Bertek will decide if development of ST630 will be continued.

INDICATION(S) AND RESEARCH PHASE
Psoriasis and Psoriatic Disorders – Phase II

completed

T-cell receptor vaccine
unknown

MANUFACTURER
Immune Response Corporation

DESCRIPTION
Immune Response has developed a vaccine of T-cell receptor (TCR) peptides which may induce the immune system to suppress the aberrant T cells that are active in rheumatoid arthritis, psoriasis, and multiple sclerosis. While these cells are suppressed, the other normal cells should not be affected. The vaccine is designed to treat the presumed cause of the disease, not just the symptoms. Three trials have recently been completed with the TCR vaccine for treatment of multiple sclerosis (phase I), rheumatoid arthritis (phase IIb), and psoriasis (phase II).

INDICATION(S) AND RESEARCH PHASE
Multiple Sclerosis – Phase I completed
Psoriasis and Psoriatic Disorders – Phase II completed
Rheumatoid Arthritis – Phase IIb completed

tazarotene
Tazorac

MANUFACTURER
Allergan

DESCRIPTION
Tazorac is a receptor-selective retinoid for the treatment of psoriasis and photodamage to the skin. A retinoid is a compound with vitamin A-like properties that may be prescribed for severe cases of psoriasis that do not respond to other therapies. Because systemic treatment with retinoids may cause birth defects, this drug was approved for psoriasis and psoriatic disorders in a topical cream formulation .05% and .1% in October 2000.

Additionally, an NDA has been submitted for the treatment of acne.

INDICATION(S) AND RESEARCH PHASE
Psoriasis and Psoriatic Disorders – FDA approved
Acne – NDA submitted

unknown
Birex

MANUFACTURER
Verex Laboratories

DESCRIPTION
Birex has been evaluated in phase II trials for the treatment of psoriasis. The drug is given in an oral formulation. Birex works well in treating plaque-type psoriasis, but not the punctated (gutta) type. The company has decided not to pursue further development of Birex at this time.

INDICATION(S) AND RESEARCH PHASE
Psoriasis and Psoriatic Disorders – Phase II discontinued

VAS 972
unknown

MANUFACTURER
Vasogen

DESCRIPTION
VAS 972 therapy is designed to target disease-causing processes in psoriasis by altering immune responses that lead to destructive inflammation. In October 2000, results of a phase I/II trial of VAS972 therapy for moderate to severe psoriasis suggested the drug is safe and effective. The randomized, double-blind, placebo-controlled, feasibility trial was conducted in Toronto, and consisted of 20 subjects with moderate to severe psoriasis. Of the subjects receiving VAS972 therapy, 70% reported symptomatic improvement by the end of their first course of therapy. Additionally, using the PASI (psoriasis area severity index) score, 50% of subjects receiving VAS972 experienced a clinically significant benefit, and of these, 80% had a greater than 50% improvement—double that seen in the placebo group.

INDICATION(S) AND RESEARCH PHASE
Psoriasis and Psoriatic Disorders – Phase II

verteporfin
unknown

MANUFACTURER
QLT Inc.

DESCRIPTION
Verteporfin is a second generation porhyrin derivative that is administered through intravenous injection and is then activated by a laser. This combination causes the disruption of biological processes in target cells. These cells are destroyed while surrounding cells are left intact. Phase I/II trials for the treatment of moderate to severe psoriasis have been completed.

INDICATION(S) AND RESEARCH PHASE
Psoriasis and Psoriatic Disorders – Phase I/II

VX-148
unknown

MANUFACTURER
Vertex Pharmaceuticals

DESCRIPTION
VX-148 is an inhibitor of inosine monophosphate dehydrogenase (IMPDH), a cellular enzyme essential for production of guanine nucleotides, one of the building blocks of RNA and DNA. Inhibiting IMPDH may be an effective strategy for blocking the growth of lymphocytes and the replication of viruses, since both depend on nucleotide synthesis for replication. Vertex's IMPDH inhibitors have the potential to treat viral infections, autoimmune diseases, and psoriasis. These three indications are currently being tested in phase I trials.

INDICATION(S) AND RESEARCH PHASE
Viral Infection – Phase I
Autoimmune Diseases – Phase I
Psoriasis and Psoriatic Disorders – Phase I

Scar Tissue

unknown
Fibrostat

MANUFACTURER
Procyon Biopharma

DESCRIPTION
Fibrostat is a topical therapeutic cream of transglutaminase inhibitor being developed in a phase III trial for burns and scar healing following surgery. The phase III trial is being conducted in Canada.

INDICATION(S) AND RESEARCH PHASE
Burns and Burn Infections – Phase III
Scar Tissue – Phase III

Seborrhea

ciclopirox olamine
Loprox

MANUFACTURER
Aventis

DESCRIPTION
Loprox is a broad spectrum antifungal in phase III trials for the treatment of seborrheic dermatitis, an inflammatory, scaling disease of the scalp and face.

INDICATION(S) AND RESEARCH PHASE
Seborrhea – Phase III
Fungal Infections – Phase III

Skin Infections/Disorders

5G1.1
unknown

MANUFACTURER
Alexion

DESCRIPTION
5G1.1 is monoclonal antibody, which inhibits C5, a major protein in the complement system, which is important in inflammation. This antibody will result in an anti-inflammatory response. In February 2001, positive interim results were announced for a double-blind, randomized, placebo-controlled phase II trial of 5G1.1 in subjects with rheumatoid arthritis. In addition to rheumatoid arthritis, 5G1.1 is in a phase II trial for the treatment of membranous nephritis and in phase Ib pilot studies for the treatment of psoriasis, dermatomyositis, and pemphigoid.

INDICATION(S) AND RESEARCH PHASE
Rheumatoid Arthritis – Phase II
Kidney Disease – Phase II
Skin Infections/Disorders – Phase Ib

ADL 2-1294
unknown

MANUFACTURER
Adolor

DESCRIPTION
ADL2-1294 is a peripheral opiate (synthetic narcotic) being tested for the treatment of pain and itching associated with burns, abrasions, eczema, and dermatitis. The drug, in a topical formulation, is in phase II trials for atopic dermatitis, burns and burn infections, herpes zoster infections, psoriasis and psoriatic disorders, and for eye disorders and infections.

INDICATION(S) AND RESEARCH PHASE
Atopic Dermatitis – Phase II
Burns and Burn Infections – Phase II
Herpes Zoster Infections – Phase II
Psoriasis and Psoriatic Disorders – Phase II
Eye Disorders/Infections – Phase II
Skin Infections/Disorders – Phase II

ALT-711
unknown

MANUFACTURER
Alteon

DESCRIPTION
ALT-711 is an advanced glycosylation end-product (AGE) crosslink breaker being developed for the treatment of cardiovascular disorders including isolated systolic hypertension. AGEs are permanent bonds between glucose and the native surface protein of cells. These structures interact with adjacent proteins to form pathological links called AGE crosslinks. The formation of AGE crosslinks is a natural part of the aging process that can lead to stiffening of proteins and loss of function in tissues, organs, and vessels including large arteries. Diabetic individuals form excessive amounts of AGEs earlier in life than non-diabetic individuals.

In January 2001, results of a phase IIa trial indicated that ALT-711 produced a statistically significant decrease in arterial pressure and an increase in large artery compliance (flexibility). The double-blind, placebo-controlled trial included 93 subjects over the age of 50 with measurably stiffened cardiovasculature including systolic blood pressure of at least 140 mm Hg and pulse pressure of at lease 60 mm Hg. Alteon plans to initiate phase IIb trials to further assess ALT-711 as a treatment for isolated systolic hypertension, in addition to evaluating the compound for other therapeutic applications.

INDICATION(S) AND RESEARCH PHASE
Cardiovascular disorders – Phase II
Eye Disorders/Infections – Phase I/II
Skin Infections/Disorders – Phase I/II

daptomycin
Cidecin

MANUFACTURER
Cubist Pharmaceuticals

DESCRIPTION
Daptomycin is a novel antibiotic lipopeptide for the treatment of skin and soft tissue infections, urinary tract infections in hospitalized subjects, and bacteremia. The drug is made in an intravenous formulation. Daptomycin is in trials for skin infections, urinary tract infections, heart disease and for bacterial infections.

INDICATION(S) AND RESEARCH PHASE
Skin Infections/Disorders – Phase III
Bacterial Infection – Phase II
Urinary Tract Infections – Phase III

Heart Disease – Phase II/III

HCT 1026
unknown

MANUFACTURER
NicOx SA

DESCRIPTION
HCT 1026 is a novel nitric oxide-releasing derivative of the non-steroidal anti-inflammatory drug (NSAID) flurbiprofen. While flurbiprofen has demonstrated effectiveness in the treatment of urinary incontinence, its use has been complicated by gastric toxicity. Because HCT 1026 may provide increased gastric tolerability, it can be administered for extended periods at effective doses. In Phase I trials, results indicated that HCT 1026 produced fewer and less severe gastric lesions compared to flurbiprofen.

HCT 1026 produces anti-inflammatory effects through the inhibition of prostaglandin synthesis, while nitric oxide controls inflammatory cell activation. These two factors suggest that HCT 1026 may be an effective treatment for dermatology disorders such as psoriasis. HCT 1026 is in phase II trials for the treatment of urinary incontinence, osteoporosis, and skin disorders such as atopic dermatitis and psoriasis.

INDICATION(S) AND RESEARCH PHASE
Atopic Dermatitis – Phase II
Urinary Incontinence – Phase II
Osteoporosis – Phase II
Psoriasis and Psoriatic Disorders – Phase II
Skin Infections/Disorders – Phase II

hypericin
VIMRxyn

MANUFACTURER
Nexell Therapeutics

DESCRIPTION
VIMRxyn (hypericin) is a light-activated and topically applied formulation of aromatic polycyclic dione (APD-1), which is a synthetic agent directed against retroviruses. This drug is being tested for treatment of specific skin diseases including psoriasis, cutaneous T-cell lymphoma and warts.

VIMRx Pharmaceuticals has also manufactured an oral, once-daily formulation of aromatic polycyclic dione (APD-1). This drug form is being evaluated for the treatment of malignant gliomas. Subject enrollment has now completed for this trial.

INDICATION(S) AND RESEARCH PHASE
Brain Cancer – Phase I/II
Lymphomas – Phase I/II
Psoriasis and Psoriatic Disorders – Phase I/II
Skin Infections/Disorders – Phase I/II

MK-826, carbepenem
unknown

MANUFACTURER
Merck & Co.

DESCRIPTION
Carbapenem is a broad-spectrum antibiotic being developed for the treatment of bacterial infections including pneumonia, intra-abdominal infections, skin and skin structure infections, urinary tract infections, and obstetric and gynecological infections.

INDICATION(S) AND RESEARCH PHASE
Pneumonia – Phase III
Skin Infections/Disorders – Phase III
Urinary Tract Infections – Phase III
Gynecological Infections – Phase III
Bacterial Infection – Phase III
Gastrointestinal Diseases and Disorders, miscellaneous – Phase III

quinupristin/dalfopristin
Synercid

MANUFACTURER
Aventis

DESCRIPTION
Synercid is a combination therapy of two semi-synthetic antibacterial agents, quinupristin and dalfopristen. The antibiotic blocks bacterial protein synthesis.

Synercid has been FDA approved for the treatment of bloodstream infections due to vancomycin-resistant *Enterococcus faecium* (VREF) and skin and skin structure infections (SSTI) caused by methicillin-susceptible *Staphylococcus aureus* or *Streptococcus pyogenes*. It is in intravenous formulation. It is currently in pediatric trials for pneumonia.

INDICATION(S) AND RESEARCH PHASE
Bacterial Infection – FDA approved
Skin Infections/Disorders – FDA approved
Pediatric, Pneumonia – Phase III

transforming growth factor beta-2 (TGF-b2)
unknown

MANUFACTURER
Genzyme Tissue Repair

DESCRIPTION
This synthetic drug is known as transforming growth factor-beta2 (TGF-β2). It is normally made in the body to help stimulate the formation of granulation tissue for treating chronic skin ulcers. The company, Genzyme Tissue Repair, reported the results of a completed phase II trial for diabetic foot ulcers. The data for this double blinded, randomized trial were collected over a three-year period with testing at 15 study centers with diabetic foot ulcer subjects. Both safety and dose ranging efficacy were evaluated. The two important criteria used to study TGF-β2 were the frequency of complete wound closure and time to wound closure.

Genzyme stated that the study subjects were randomly assigned to one of five groups. The first group of 24 subjects received standard care only which consisted of surgical debridement, compression dressing, and off-loading of weight from the wound site. The remainder of the subjects were enrolled in the blinded part of the trial. One group of 22 subjects received placebo sponges and standardized care. The remaining 131 subjects were evenly divided among three doses in addition to standardized care. All the subjects were treated twice a week for 20 weeks or until their ulcer healed.

Study results from the phase II trial suggested that TGF-β2 was safe and effective at all dose levels tested. The subject group which received the highest dosage of TGF-β2 (5 μg/cm²) demonstrated statistically significant improvement compared to placebo in both the efficacy endpoints, frequency of complete closure, and time to closure. Subjects in the groups which received the middle or low doses of TGF-β2 also showed improvements in both endpoints but did not consistently achieve statistical significance.

The company, Genzyme Tissue Repair is actively seeking a partner to work with them in the final stages of development and commercialization for the TGF-β2 drug.

INDICATION(S) AND RESEARCH PHASE
Diabetic Foot Ulcers – Phase II completed
Skin Infections/Disorders – Phase II completed

Unknown
AIC

MANUFACTURER
Dynavax

DESCRIPTION
AIC is Dynavax's proprietary conjugate of purified ragweed allergen. ISS (immunostimulatory DNA) administered with allergens is thought to enhance immune response. ISS is attached to specific allergens so that they are presented to the immune system simultaneously. ISS, when linked to an allergen, "hides" the allergen from the immune system, thereby preventing the symptoms of an allergy attack. AIC ragweed immunotherapy is currently in phase II development.

INDICATION(S) AND RESEARCH PHASE
Skin Infections/Disorders – Phase II
Allergy – Phase II

Unknown
Merrem

MANUFACTURER
AstraZeneca

DESCRIPTION
Merrem is a carbapenem antibiotic currently in numerous phase III line extension studies. The indications being tested include hospital- and community-acquired pneumonia, cystic fibrosis, skin and soft tissue infections, abdominal infections, and for use in neutropenics.

INDICATION(S) AND RESEARCH PHASE
Skin Infections/Disorders – Phase III
Cystic Fibrosis – Phase III
Pneumonia – Phase III
Neutropenics – Phase III
Abdominal infections – Phase III

Skin Wounds

becaplermin
Regranex

MANUFACTURER
Chiron Corporation

DESCRIPTION
Regranex is a wound healing therapeutic for pressure ulcers. These skin ulcers may develop in weight-bearing areas due to many different disease conditions, especially diabetes. The drug is currently being tested in phase III trials. Chiron Corporation has a licensing agreement with R.W. Johnson Pharmaceutical Research Institute for developing Regranex.

INDICATION(S) AND RESEARCH PHASE
Diabetic Foot Ulcers – Phase III
Skin Wounds – Phase III

dexamethasone
IontoDex

MANUFACTURER
Iomed

DESCRIPTION
IontoDex is being developed for the treatment of acute local inflammation, for the treatment of ocular disease and for systemic pain control. IontoDex is comprised of the drug dexamethasone, an anti-inflammatory steroid, delivered by the proprietary iontophoretic drug delivery device Phoresor. Iontophoresis is a needle-free method of delivering certain types of medication directly into and through the skin using a mild, low-level electric current. Programming the system's electric current levels to achieve the desired dose, delivery rate or pattern of delivery can control the amount of drug delivered. This drug is in phase III trials and the company plans to file for the NDA.

INDICATION(S) AND RESEARCH PHASE
Eye Disorders/Infections – Phase III
Pain, Acute or Chronic – Phase III
Skin Wounds – Phase III

keratinocyte growth factor-2 (KGF-2)
Repifermin

MANUFACTURER
Human Genome Sciences

DESCRIPTION
Repifermin is a genomics-derived therapeutic protein drug, also known as keratinocyte growth factor-2 (KGF-2). It is in a phase II study for the treatment of mucositis associated with bone marrow transplantation for the treatment of cancer. This phase II trial is a randomized, double-blind, placebo-controlled, dose-escalation study that is being conducted at several sites in the United States. In addition, Repifermin is in trials for topical wound healing treatment of venous ulcers and for inflammatory bowel disease (IBD).

Results for phase I clinical trials showed that systemically-administered Repifermin is safe and well tolerated in healthy human subjects at doses proposed for subsequent clinical studies. None of the subjects withdrew from the study or required dose modification because of adverse effects.

KGF-2 stimulates the growth of keratinocyte cells, which make up 95% of the epidermal (skin) cells. Together, keratinocyte and melanocyte cells form the epidermis of the body. The company claims that KGF-2 has demonstrated beneficial effects on both the dermal and epidermal tissues of the skin, healing full-thickness wounds in a short period of time. In mucositis, Repifermin may stimulate the creation of new mucosal tissue.

INDICATION(S) AND RESEARCH PHASE
Bone Marrow Transplant – Phase II
Effects of Chemotherapy – Phase II
Oral Medicine – Phase II
Skin Wounds – Phase IIb
Inflammatory Bowel Disease – Phase II

Systemic Fungal Infections

nystatin, AR-121
Nyotran

MANUFACTURER
Aronex Pharmaceuticals

DESCRIPTION
Nyotran is an intravenous liposomal formulation of nystatin being developed for the treatment of serious systemic, opportunistic fungal infections. Phase III trials have been completed for systemic fungal infections and confirmed cryptococcal meningitis. Additionally, phase II trials have been completed for candidiasis and aspergillosis.

Nyotran is under agreement with Abbott Laboratories for worldwide commercialization. Abbott will fund clinical development and will submit marketing registration outside the United States.

INDICATION(S) AND RESEARCH PHASE
Aspergillosis – Phase II completed
Candidiasis – Phase II completed
Systemic Fungal Infections – Phase III completed
Meningitis – Phase III completed

Systemic Lupus Erythematosus

5c8 (anti CD-40 ligand antibody)
Antova

MANUFACTURER
Biogen

DESCRIPTION
Biogen has engineered 5c8 (Anti CD-40 ligand antibody), a humanized monoclonal antibody for the potential treatment of a number of autoimmune disorders. These include idiopathic thrombocytopenia purpura (ITP), systemic lupus erythematosus, kidney transplantation, and factor VIII antibody inhibition.

In the aforementioned autoimmune diseases, it is thought that activated white blood cells, called T-cell lymphocytes, bind to other tissue cells through a cell surface receptor, the CD-40 ligand. Abnormal antibodies are produced that will then recognize healthy body tissues as foreign, and thereby cause an inflammatory response. The 5c8 antibody may stop this abnormal immune cycle by binding to the CD-40 ligand and inhibiting its ability to bind with its receptor on a variety of other normal cells.

INDICATION(S) AND RESEARCH PHASE
Thrombocytopenia – Phase II discontinued
Systemic Lupus Erythematosus – Phase II discontinued
Kidney Transplant Surgery – Phase II discontinued
Factor VIII antibody inhibition – Phase II discontinued

GL-701, prasterone
Aslera

MANUFACTURER
Genelabs Technologies

DESCRIPTION
The active ingredient in Aslera is prasterone, the synthetic equivalent of the androgenic hormone dehydroepiandrosterone (DHEA). Products containing DHEA are currently marketed as dietary supplements. Aslera is currently in development for the treatment of systemic lupus erythematosus (SLE). SLE sufferers often develop low levels of DHEA and are primarily women. Phase III trials have been completed and an NDA was submitted in October 2000. The FDA is planning to review the NDA on April 19, 2001.

INDICATION(S) AND RESEARCH PHASE
Systemic Lupus Erythematosus – NDA submitted

IDEC-131
unknown

MANUFACTURER
IDEC Pharmaceuticals

DESCRIPTION
IDEC-131 is a humanized monoclonal antibody (Mab) developed for the treatment of systemic lupus erythematosus (SLE). By inhibiting the action of the CD40 ligand molecule, a communication link between the immune helper T-cells and B-cells, IDEC-131 may reduce excessively abnormal antibody production. This biologic drug may help restore a more normal immune response in subjects with a variety of autoimmune and inflammatory conditions. The drug is in trials for SLE and and psoriasis.

INDICATION(S) AND RESEARCH PHASE
Systemic Lupus Erythematosus – Phase II completed
Psoriasis and Psoriatic Disorders – Phase II

LJP-394
unknown

MANUFACTURER
La Jolla Pharmaceutical

DESCRIPTION
LJP-394 is a novel compound derived from the company's proprietary tolerance technology. The mechanism of action of LJP-394 is thought to involve inhibition of B-cell antibody production. Antibodies are thought to be important in the pathogenesis of systemic lupus erythematosus (SLE). In a phase II/III trial, LPJ-394 reduced renal flares in lupus subjects with poor renal function. In subjects with high-affinity antibodies to LJP 394 (89% of subjects), time to renal flare—the primary endpoint of the trial—was significantly increased in the drug-treated population when compared to the placebo-treated group. In the high-affin-

ity group, there were one-third as many renal flares in LJP 394-treated subjects compared to placebo-treated subjects. A phase III trial for LJP 394 is currently in progress.

INDICATION(S) AND RESEARCH PHASE
Kidney Disease – Phase III
Systemic Lupus Erythematosus – Phase III

Tinea Capitis

terbinafine
Lamisil

MANUFACTURER
Novartis

DESCRIPTION
Lamasil inhibits squalene epoxidase, a key enzyme in sterol biosynthesis in fungi, causing a decrease in ergosterol and a corresponding accumulation of sterol within the fungal cells. The drug is being evaluated in phase III trials in an oral formulation for the treatment of both systemic mycoses and tinea capitis.

INDICATION(S) AND RESEARCH PHASE
Pediatric, Tinea Capitis – Phase II
Tinea Capitis – Phase III
Mycosis Fungoides – Phase III

Venous Leg Ulcers

ifetroban sodium, BMS-180291
unknown

MANUFACTURER
Bristol-Myers Squibb

DESCRIPTION
BMS-180291 is ifetroban sodium, an oral drug that may prevent the formation of blood clots. It works much like aspirin by inhibiting the clumping of platelets, which are elements in the blood that promote coagulation. Ifetroban was designed to be given once a day to prevent blood clotting and interruption of the blood flow.

Results from in animal studies showed to ifetroban reduces the tissue injury caused by inadequate blood flow related to coronary artery obstruction. If it is successful it could replace current treatments for acute and chronic ischemic heart disease, such as calcium channel blockers and beta-blockers.

BMS-180291-02 is currently in a phase II trial for venous ulcers, with studies run jointly by PRI and ConvaTec. Phase II trials are also ongoing in the United States and Europe for cardiovascular indications. In addition, an exploratory Phase II trial is taking place to evaluate ifetroban as a treatment for subjects with intermittent from peripheral arterial disease.

INDICATION(S) AND RESEARCH PHASE
Peripheral Vascular Disease – Phase II
Venous Leg Ulcers – Phase II
Cardiovascular – Phase II

Wounds

imaging agent, entire body
unknown

MANUFACTURER
Mallinckrodt

DESCRIPTION
The original drug, a nonionic magnetic resonance imaging (MRI) contrast agent for the central nervous system, has passed phase III trials and is awaiting FDA approval. The company has begun phase II trials of the agent for the entire body. MRI can be particularly useful in emergency room situations where an immediate assessment of a subject's condition or wounds is critical. Related areas of application may include diagnostics, radiopharmaceuticals, and contrast agents.

INDICATION(S) AND RESEARCH PHASE
Wounds – Phase II

P53
unknown

MANUFACTURER
Phytopharm plc

DESCRIPTION
P53 is in phase IIa clinical trials for the treatment of the itching that accompanies skin disorders such as eczema and psoriasis.

INDICATION(S) AND RESEARCH PHASE
Wounds – Phase IIa

therapeutic, wound healing
unknown

MANUFACTURER
Mylan

DESCRIPTION
This drug is an unspecified therapeutic being tested in phase III trials for both wound healing and diabetic foot ulcers.

INDICATION(S) AND RESEARCH PHASE
Diabetic Foot Ulcers – Phase III
Wounds – Phase III

Unknown
Apligraf

MANUFACTURER
Novartis

DESCRIPTION
Apligraf is a topical living skin equivalent. The lower dermal layer combines bovine type 1 collagen and human fibroblasts, while the upper epidermal layer is formed by promoting human keratinocytes to multiply and differentiate to replicate the structure of the human epidermis. Apligraf differs from human skin in that it does not contain melanocytes, Langerhans cells, macrophages, lymphocytes, and other structures.

Apligraf is currently in phase III trials for wound healing. It is being developed under and agreement between Organogenesis and Novartis.

INDICATION(S) AND RESEARCH PHASE
Wounds – NDA submitted

VM-301, OAS 1000
unknown

MANUFACTURER
Nexell Therapeutics

DESCRIPTION
VM-301 is a topical wound healing agent that is being tested in phase II trials. Indications include treatment of skin graft donor sites of both partial and full thickness wounds, including burns, surgical wounds, diabetic skin ulcers, and decubitus ulcers.

INDICATION(S) AND RESEARCH PHASE
Burns and Burn Infections – Phase II
Decubitus Ulcers (Bed Sores) – Phase II
Diabetic Foot Ulcers – Phase II
Wounds – Phase II

13 | Ophthalmology

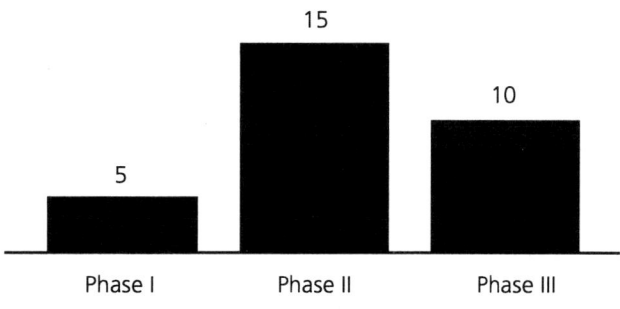

Drugs in the development pipeline

Phase I: 5
Phase II: 15
Phase III: 10

Source: CenterWatch, 2001

Glaucoma is the second leading cause of blindness in America. According to the World Health Organization, an estimated 67 million people worldwide have glaucoma, including three million Americans. Glaucoma is one of a number of diseases that are associated with an increased pressure within the eye that eventually damages the optic nerve. The exact cause is unknown; the end result however, is that the aqueous humor, which occupies the anterior chamber of the eye, does not drain properly. Only a comprehensive eye examination, including determination of intraocular pressure, can detect the presence of elevated pressures within the eye with certainty. Once vision has deteriorated, the vision loss can not be reversed.

CenterWatch estimates approximately six drugs are in clinical development with approximately $40 million to $45 million being spent annually. The search for a cure has brought promising new treatment options that help slow or stop the disease from progressing.

Current new treatments differ according to the type of glaucoma present, and include eye drops, tablets, surgery, or lasers, but most have the goal of either reducing the amount of fluid entering the eye or draining it once it is there, to spare the optic nerve any further damage from the elevated pressures. There are some drawbacks with available treatments including straining of the iris, uncomfortable administration, fluid drainage problems and side effects of adrenaline and beta-blockers.

Two prostaglandin-related drugs were approved in March 2001 for the treatment of glaucoma. There are Travatan, marketed by Alcon, and Lumingan, marketed by Allergan. Both drugs work by increasing the drainage of intraocular fluid, thereby decreasing intraocular pressure. According to study results, Travatan may work best for treating African-Americans with glaucoma, thus making Travatan the first treatment approved by the FDA to be marketed to a specific population at high risk for glaucoma. Additionally, both drugs might be considered for subjects who have not had success with, or cannot tolerate other drugs, which decrease intraocular pressure.

Two new breakthroughs in the treatment of glaucoma have also been reported. Copaxone, a vaccine used to treat multiple sclerosis, has been shown in preclinical data to possibly protect the optic nerve even in the presence of elevated intraocular pressures. The second drug, amionguanidine, has demonstrated inhibition of nitric oxide synthetase (NOS-2), an enzyme that synthesizes nitric oxide, a compound that decreases and possibly prevents the loss of retinal ganglion cells (RGCs)—the crucial nerve cells so important to sight. Researchers hope that both drugs will advance to clinical testing in the next few years.

Another area of intense drug development in the ophthalmology pipeline is age-related macular degeneration. Age-related macular degeneration is either "wet," denoting "leaking" of the blood vessels around the macula, or "dry," denoting a decrease in the macula's function wherein parts of it become less sensitive to light.

The leading cause of blindness is the neovascular "wet" form of age-related macular degeneration, which is responsible for 90% of severe loss of vision in Americans. It is an incurable eye disease that affects 10 million Americans aged 55 or older. There are approximately 200,000 new cases of wet macular degeneration in the United States each year and the number is only on the rise as life expectancy increases. CenterWatch estimates there are approximately 18 drugs in the clinical pipeline with as much as $90 million to $100 million being spent annually on clinical development.

Visudyne (verteporfin for injection) was approved in April 2000 as a photodynamic therapy for the treatment of "wet" form of age-related macular degeneration in subjects with predominantly classic subfoveal choroidal neovascularization (CNV). Visudyne is injected into the blood vessels and it is activated by a light beam, thus focusing the active moiety in the retina, and preventing damage to the surrounding normal tissue. Another popular photodynamic therapy in the pipeline is Miravant (purlytin), which works by a similar mechanism.

Cataracts

MDX-RA
unknown

MANUFACTURER
Medarex

DESCRIPTION
MDX-RA is a monoclonal antibody based immunotoxin for the prevention of secondary cataracts. The drug is in phase III clinical trials. Additional indications may include other eye diseases or disorders.

INDICATION(S) AND RESEARCH PHASE
Cataracts – Phase III

Cytomegalovirus (CMV) Retinitis

ganciclovir
Cytovene

MANUFACTURER
Hoffmann-La Roche

DESCRIPTION
Cytovene is currently on the market for treatment and prevention of cytomegalovirus (CMV) retinitis in AIDS subjects. This drug is in phase III trials for a new indication; treatment and prevention of cytomegalovirus in transplant subjects. Additional indications may include infectious diseases and viral diseases.

INDICATION(S) AND RESEARCH PHASE
Cytomegalovirus (CMV) Retinitis – Phase III

ISIS-13312
unknown

MANUFACTURER
Isis Pharmaceuticals

DESCRIPTION
ISIS-13312 is a genetically engineered complex (second-generation antisense compound). This drug is being tested in phase I/II trials for the treatment of cytomegalovirus (CMV) retinitis.

INDICATION(S) AND RESEARCH PHASE
Cytomegalovirus (CMV) Retinitis – Phase I/II

vaccine, cytomegalovirus
unknown

MANUFACTURER
Aviron

DESCRIPTION
A cytomegalovirus(CMV) vaccine is in a phase I trial and will test four live attenuate injectable vaccine candidates developed by Aviron. The trial is being conducted by the National Insititute of Allergy and Infectious Disease and is taking place at Saint Louis University and will include 25 subjects. Currently, there is no vaccine available for CMV.

INDICATION(S) AND RESEARCH PHASE
Cytomegalovirus (CMV) Retinitis – Phase I

valganciclovir
Cymeval

MANUFACTURER
Hoffmann-La Roche

DESCRIPTION
Cymeval is an antiviral agent being evaluated for the prevention of cytomegalovirus (CMV) retinitis in subjects with AIDS. Valganciclovir is a pro-drug of Roche's existing anti-CMV treatment, ganciclovir (Cytovene) and is manufactured by adding a valine amino acid to ganciclovir. This allows the drug to be given orally, rather than intravenously. In addition, absorption is much better than that of the present compound, ganciclovir. The company submitted an NDA in October 2000.

In addition, a phase III trial is comparing valganciclovir to oral Cytovene for prevention of cytomegalovirus disease in solid organ transplant recipients.

INDICATION(S) AND RESEARCH PHASE
Cytomegalovirus (CMV) Retinitis – NDA submitted

Eye Disorders/Infections

ADL 2-1294
unknown

MANUFACTURER
Adolor

DESCRIPTION
ADL2-1294 is a peripheral opiate (synthetic narcotic) being tested for the treatment of pain and itching associated with burns, abrasions, eczema, and dermatitis. The drug, in a topical formulation, is in phase II trials for atopic dermatitis, burns and burn infections, herpes zoster infections, psoriasis and psoriatic disorders, as well as for eye disorders and infections.

INDICATION(S) AND RESEARCH PHASE
Atopic Dermatitis – Phase II
Burns and Burn Infections – Phase II
Herpes Zoster Infections – Phase II
Psoriasis and Psoriatic Disorders – Phase II
Eye Disorders/Infections – Phase II
Skin Infections/Disorders – Phase II

ALT-711
unknown

MANUFACTURER
Alteon

DESCRIPTION
ALT-711 is an advanced glycosylation end-product (AGE) crosslink breaker being developed for the treatment of cardiovascular disorders including isolated systolic hypertension. AGEs are permanent bonds between glucose and the native surface protein of cells. These structures interact with adjacent proteins to form pathological links called AGE crosslinks. The formation of AGE crosslinks is a natural part of the aging process that can lead to stiffening of proteins and loss of function in tissues, organs, and vessels including large arteries. Diabetic

individuals form excessive amounts of AGEs earlier in life than non-diabetic individuals.

In January 2001, results of a phase IIa trial indicated that ALT-711 produced a statistically significant decrease in arterial pressure and an increase in large artery compliance (flexibility). The double-blind, placebo-controlled trial included 93 subjects over the age of 50 with measurably stiffened cardiovasculature including systolic blood pressure of at least 140 mm Hg and pulse pressure of at lease 60 mm Hg. Alteon plans to initiate phase IIb trials to further assess ALT-711 as a treatment for isolated systolic hypertension, in addition to evaluating the compound for other therapeutic applications.

INDICATION(S) AND RESEARCH PHASE
Cardiovascular Disorders – Phase II
Eye Disorders/Infections – Phase I/II
Skin Infections/Disorders – Phase I/II

batimastat, ISV-120
unknown

MANUFACTURER
InSite Vision

DESCRIPTION
ISV-120 is an ophthalmic formulation of batimastat for the prevention of post-surgical recurrence of pterygium, a vascular overgrowth that occurs on the eye and may impair vision. ISV-120 is a non-toxic matrix metalloproteinase (MMP) inhibitor using DuraSite delivery.

InSite finished a phase II trial for the recurrence of pterygium. However, plans for conducting a phase III trial have been on hold since 1998.

INDICATION(S) AND RESEARCH PHASE
Eye Disorders/Infections – Phase II/III completed

cidofovir
unknown

MANUFACTURER
Gilead Sciences

DESCRIPTION
Cidofovir is a broad-spectrum antiviral for the treatment of a variety of ophthalmic viruses, including adenovirus and viral keratoconjunctivitis. The drug, which is made in a topical ophthalmic formulation, is in phase II trials.

INDICATION(S) AND RESEARCH PHASE
Eye Disorders/Infections – Phase II
Viral Infection – Phase II

cysteamine hydrochloride
Cystavision

MANUFACTURER
Sigma-Tau Pharmaceuticals

DESCRIPTION
Cysteamine hydrochloride eye drops are being tested for the treatment of corneal cystine accumulation, a rare disorder affecting approximately 1,000 subjects. Corneal cystine accumulation is the formation of crystals in the cornea of the eye as a result of the build up of cystine, a naturally occurring amino acid. This condition is a related consequence of cystinosis, a rare and serious genetic disease that primarily affects kidney function. Phase III trials for pediatric subjects to 18 years of age have been completed.

INDICATION(S) AND RESEARCH PHASE
Pediatric, Eye Disorders/Infections – Phase III completed

dexamethasone
IontoDex

MANUFACTURER
Iomed

DESCRIPTION
IontoDex is being developed for the treatment of acute local inflammation, for the treatment of ocular disease and for systemic (whole body) pain control. IontoDex is comprised of the drug dexamethasone, an anti-inflammatory steroid, delivered by the proprietary iontophoretic drug delivery device Phoresor. Iontophoresis is a needle-free method of delivering certain types of medication directly into and through the skin using a mild, low-level electric current. Programming the system's electric current levels to achieve the desired dose, delivery rate, or pattern of delivery can control the amount of drug delivered. This drug is in phase III trials. The company plans to file for the NDA in 2001.

INDICATION(S) AND RESEARCH PHASE
Eye Disorders/Infections – Phase III
Pain, Acute or Chronic – Phase III
Skin Wounds – Phase III

dexamethasone
Surodex

MANUFACTURER
Oculex Pharmaceuticals

DESCRIPTION
Surodex is a biodegradable polymer implant that can deliver drugs continuously inside the eye (sustained release, intraocular drug delivery system). The device can be implanted in the front or rear chamber of the eye. Any drug bound to this polymer is gradually released at a programmed rate as the polymer dissolves. Depending on the formulation, this release can occur over a period of one week, or over as long a period as one year.

For the treatment of inflammation following cataract surgery, dexamethasone, an anti-inflammatory steroid, is bound to a polymer and put into the front (anterior) chamber of the eye to reduce subsequent pain and swelling. Surodex has completed phase III trials for the treatment of inflammation following cataract surgery.

INDICATION(S) AND RESEARCH PHASE
Eye Disorders/Infections – Phase III completed

diclofenac, ISV-205
unknown

MANUFACTURER
InSite Vision

DESCRIPTION
This drug is a special formulation of

diclofenac, a non-steroidal anti-inflammatory drug (NSAID) delivered to the eye using an extended-release eye-drop based delivery system. This technology may allow the effective treatment of glaucoma by protecting the trabecular meshwork and preventing disease progression through higher concentrations and longer residence time of diclofenac inside the eye.

A previous phase II study showed that diclofenac was safe and effective in reducing by 75% the number of subjects with clinically significant intraocular pressure elevations. The drug was given to subjects over a six-week dosing period. This study included 136 first-degree relatives of glaucoma subjects who were challenged with corticosteroids. A second phase II study including a larger subject population is planned.

INDICATION(S) AND RESEARCH PHASE
Glaucoma – Phase II
Eye Disorders/Infections – Phase II

INS365 ophthalmic
unknown

MANUFACTURER
Inspire Pharmaceuticals

DESCRIPTION
INS365 ophthalmic is in development for the treatment of dry eye disease. It is a small-molecule drug that stimulates the P2Y(2) receptor, a key mediator of mucosal hydration and lubrication. INS365 ophthalmic eye drops are expected to enhance the eye's natural cleansing and protective systems by stimulating the release of salt, water, mucus, and other natural tear components, providing lubrication of the eye's surface.

In November 2000, Inspire Pharmaceuticals announced positive results from a phase II, multicenter, placebo-controlled, dose-ranging trial of INS365 ophthalmic for the treatment of dry eye disease. The trial was conducted at 12 ophthalmology centers in the United States, and compared several concentrations of INS365 ophthalmic and placebo in 158 moderate-to-severe subjects. The trial indicated improvements in objective and subjective measurements, and supported the usefulness of the P2Y(2) receptor agonist approach. Inspire is planning to initiate a phase III program.

INDICATION(S) AND RESEARCH PHASE
Eye Disorders/Infections – Phase II completed

INS37217 respiratory
unknown

MANUFACTURER
Inspire Pharmaceuticals

DESCRIPTION
INS37217 respiratory is a second-generation P2Y (2) agonist being tested in a phase I clinical trial for cystic fibrosis as an inhalation. INS37217 is designed to enhance the lung's innate mucosal hydration and mucociliary clearance mechanisms, which are seriously impaired in cystic fibrosis subjects due to genetic defect. Preclinical results demonstrated INS37217 respiratory has extended duration of action. Inspire Pharmaceuticals is co-developing INS37217 with Genentech.

In addition, a phase II/III trial will be initiated in early 2001 for testing INS37217 for the treatment of retinal detachment and retinal edema.

INDICATION(S) AND RESEARCH PHASE
Cystic Fibrosis – Phase I
Eye Disorders/Infections – Phase II/III

intravitreal hyaluronidase
Vitrase

MANUFACTURER
Advanced Corneal Systems

DESCRIPTION
Vitrase (intravitreal hyaluronidase) is being tested in a phase III trial for the treatment of vitreous hemorrhage or bleeding into the back portion of the eye and a phase II trial for diabetic retinopathy. It has received FDA fast track designation.

INDICATION(S) AND RESEARCH PHASE
Hemorrhage – Phase III
Eye Disorders/Infections – Phase II

ketotifen fumarate
Zaditen

MANUFACTURER
Novartis

DESCRIPTION
Zaditen is a topical selective H1-receptor antagonist, mast cell stabilizer, eosinophil infiltration inhibitor. An application has been filed overseas and the drug is in registration as an anti-allergic eyedrop.

INDICATION(S) AND RESEARCH PHASE
Allergy – MAA submitted
Eye Disorders/Infections – MAA submitted

LY-333531
unknown

MANUFACTURER
Eli Lilly

DESCRIPTION
LY-333531 is an enzyme inhibitor (of PKC). It is being tested in diabetes subjects in a phase II trial for the treatment of neuropathy and macular edema, which are pathological diabetic complications.

INDICATION(S) AND RESEARCH PHASE
Neuropathy, Diabetic – Phase II
Eye Disorders/Infections – Phase II

octreotide acetate
Sandostatin LAR

MANUFACTURER
Novartis

DESCRIPTION
Sandostatin LAR (octreotide acetate) is a combination of growth hormone and IGF-1 inhibitor. It is being tested in an intramuscular formulation for the treatment of diabetic retinopathy and other indications. It is currently in phase III development.

INDICATION(S) AND RESEARCH PHASE

Eye Disorders/Infections – Phase III

piroxicam
unknown

MANUFACTURER
Akorn

DESCRIPTION
Piroxicam is a non-steroidal anti-inflammatory drug (NSAID) currently on the market for the treatment of osteoarthritis and rheumatoid arthritis. The drug is in phase III trials for a new indication, eye inflammation, in an ophthalmic formulation. Pfizer and Akorn Ophthalmics are developing this drug indication.

INDICATION(S) AND RESEARCH PHASE
Eye Disorders/Infections – Phase III completed

PKC 412
unknown

MANUFACTURER
Novartis

DESCRIPTION
PKC 412, an oral anti-sense drug, inhibits the action of protein kinase C (PKC). Anti-sense technology is a method for disrupting the expression of a specific protein or proteins within cells. This technology involves the introduction of an anti-sense DNA that is complementary to the messenger RNA (mRNA) that encodes the target protein. This anti-sense DNA binds specifically to the mRNA and inhibits its translation into protein. Thus, this technology may disrupt the specific production of a single protein within cells. PKC plays a role in signal processes that regulate cell growth and differentiation. It is one of a family of enzymes thought to have an important function in the development of some solid tumors. An oral formulation of PKC 412 is being tested in phase II trials for a variety of solid tumors and macular edema.

INDICATION(S) AND RESEARCH PHASE
Solid Tumors – Phase II

Eye Disorders/Infections – Phase II

proparacaine
ToPreSite

MANUFACTURER
InSite Vision

DESCRIPTION
ToPreSite is a topical anesthetic for supplemental (adjunctive) use in ophthalmic surgery using the DuraSite sustained-release delivery system. The partnering company, Ciba Vision, put development of the ToPreSite product on hold at phase II.

INDICATION(S) AND RESEARCH PHASE
Eye Disorders/Infections – Phase II on hold

unknown
Keraform

MANUFACTURER
Advanced Corneal Systems

DESCRIPTION
Keraform is in a phase II trial for refractive correction.

INDICATION(S) AND RESEARCH PHASE
Eye Disorders/Infections – Phase II

unknown
Dehydrex

MANUFACTURER
Holles Laboratories

DESCRIPTION
Dehydrex is an eye treatment being developed for recurrent corneal erosion. The drug is in ongoing phase III trials and it has an orphan drug status.

INDICATION(S) AND RESEARCH PHASE
Eye Disorders/Infections – Phase III

unknown
Posurdex

MANUFACTURER
Oculex Pharmaceuticals

DESCRIPTION
Posurdex is in a phase II trial for the treatment of acute inflammation following posterior segment surgery (eyes). Phase I data demonstrated safety in severe back of the eye diseases, specifically uveitis and proliferative vitreoretinopathy (PVR).

INDICATION(S) AND RESEARCH PHASE
Eye Disorders/Infections – Phase II

Glaucoma

AGN 192024
Lumigan

MANUFACTURER
Allergan

DESCRIPTION
AGN 192024 is a member of a new class of pharmacologically unique intraocular pressure (IOP) lowering agents called prostamides. Prostamides are naturally occurring substances found in the eye, representing newly discovered intrinsic factors that regulate IOP. As a synthetic analogue, AGN 192024 mimics the strong IOP-lowering activity of prostamides.

Results of a phase III trial demonstrated that AGN 192024 0.03%, dosed once daily (QD), significantly lowered IOP in comparison to timolol 0.5%, dosed twice daily (BID), in subjects with ocular hypertension or glaucoma. In the randomized, double-masked trial, 596 subjects were assigned to one of three groups: AGN 192024 once daily (QD), AGN 192024 twice daily (BID), or timolol twice daily (BID). Subjects receiving either AGN 192024 regimen achieved greater IOP lowering at all timepoints throughout the day than those receiving timolol, with the once-a-day dosing of AGN 192024 proving the most effective. In September 2000, Allergan submitted an NDA for AGN 192024.

INDICATION(S) AND RESEARCH PHASE
Ocular Hypertension – NDA submitted

Glaucoma – NDA submitted

brimonidine tartrate
Alphagan

MANUFACTURER
Allergan

DESCRIPTION
Alphagan is a 0.2% ophthalmic solution of brimonidine tartrate. Brimonidine tartrate is an alpha2-adrenergic agonist indicated for lowering intra-ocular pressure in subjects with primary open angle glaucoma or ocular hypertension. The drug is currently in phase III trials for pediatric glaucoma in subjects two to seven years of age.

INDICATION(S) AND RESEARCH PHASE
Pediatric, Glaucoma – Phase III

CAT-152
unknown

MANUFACTURER
Cambridge Antibody Technology Group plc

DESCRIPTION
CAT-152 is a human monclonal antibody that neutralizes transforming growth factor-beta2 (TGF-β2). TGF-β2 is a protein produced in response to an injury to the eye, such as is endured following surgery for glaucoma. During surgery, increased pressure in the eye is lowered by improving fluid drainage. The ocular fluid in glaucoma patients has increased levels of TGF-β2. TGF-β2 is believed to be responsible for the formulation of excessive scar tissue, which is the main reason glaucoma surgery may fail. Trial results show less pressure in the eye and a trend for reduced post-operative intervention in patients who received CAT-152, which may lead to reduce failure of surgery. CAT-152 is currently being tested in phase II trials.

INDICATION(S) AND RESEARCH PHASE
Glaucoma – Phase II

diclofenac, ISV-205
unknown

MANUFACTURER
InSite Vision

DESCRIPTION
This drug is a special formulation of diclofenac, a non-steroidal anti-inflammatory drug (NSAID) delivered to the eye using an extended-release eye-drop based delivery system. This technology may allow the effective treatment of glaucoma by protecting the trabecular meshwork and preventing disease progression through higher concentrations and longer residence time of diclofenac inside the eye.

A previous phase II study showed that diclofenac was safe and effective in reducing by 75% the number of subjects with clinically significant intraocular pressure elevations. The drug was given to subjects over a six-week dosing period. This study included 136 first-degree relatives of glaucoma subjects who were challenged with corticosteroids. A second phase II study including a larger subject population is planned.

INDICATION(S) AND RESEARCH PHASE
Glaucoma – Phase II
Eye Disorders/Infections – Phase II

latanoprost
Xalatan

MANUFACTURER
Pharmacia Corporation

DESCRIPTION
Xalatan contains latanoprost, a prostanoid selective FP receptor agonist believed to reduce intraocular pressure by increasing the outflow of aqueous humor. Studies suggest that the main mechanism of action is increased uveoscleral outflow. Xalatan Fixed Flow Device is currently in phase II trials to evaluate its effectiveness for glaucoma.

INDICATION(S) AND RESEARCH PHASE
Glaucoma - Phase II

memantine
unknown

MANUFACTURER
Allergan

DESCRIPTION
Memantime is an *N*-methyl-D-aspartate receptor antagonist that has been successfully used to treat dementia. The drug is currently in phase III trials in oral formulation for treatment of glaucoma. Its neuroprotective ability may limit damage caused by open-angle glaucoma and ocular hypertension.

Memantine is licensed to Allergan from Merz.

INDICATION(S) AND RESEARCH PHASE
Glaucoma – Phase III

Macular Degeneration

AE-941
Neovastat

MANUFACTURER
AEterna Laboratories

DESCRIPTION
Neovastat is an angiogenesis inhibitor being tested in two phase II trials to treat subjects with non-small cell lung cancer, subjects with moderate to severe psoriasis, multiple myeloma, kidney cancer, and macular degeneration.

A phase II trial for multiple myeloma was initiated in October 2000 and will treat 120 subjects and include approximately 20 sites across North America and Europe. Trial results are expected in summer 2002.

In addition, a phase III trial was initiated in May 2000 for kidney cancer and will include 270 subjects at sites in North America and Europe.

INDICATION(S) AND RESEARCH PHASE
Lung Cancer – Phase III
Psoriasis and Psoriatic Disorders – Phase I/II completed
Cancer/Tumors (Unspecified) – Phase I/II completed
Multiple Myeloma – Phase II
Renal Cell Carcinoma – Phase III
Macular Degeneration – Phase I completed

AMD Fab
unknown

MANUFACTURER
Genentech

DESCRIPTION
AMD Fab is a customized fragment of an anti-VEGF antibody. In age-related macular degeneration, excessive blood vessel growth occurs in the retina of the eye. VEGF appears to play a role in inducing this growth of new blood vessels; by blocking it, AMD Fab may prove an effective therapeutic.

A phase Ia trial has been completed in subjects with age-related macular degeneration. Plans for a phase Ib trial are underway.

INDICATION(S) AND RESEARCH PHASE
Macular Degeneration – Phase I

anecortave acetate
unknown

MANUFACTURER
Alcon

DESCRIPTION
Anecortave acetate is a steroid with anti-angiogenic properties. In wet age-related macular degeneration, abnormal blood vessel growth occurs in the back of the eye. In various preclinical models, anecortave acetate has been shown to prevent such blood vessel growth. The compound is currently in phase II development.

INDICATION(S) AND RESEARCH PHASE
Macular Degeneration – Phase II

EYE-001, NX-1838
unknown

MANUFACTURER
EyeTech Pharmaceuticals

DESCRIPTION
EYE-001 is an inhibitor of vascular endothelial growth factor (VEGF), which has been implicated in the development of age-related macular degeneration (AMD) and diabetic retinopathy. EYE-001 has been shown to target and block VEGF, and as a result may prevent the abnormal growth of ocular blood vessels and vessel leakage in the eye.

EyeTech has signed an agreement with Gilead Sciences for the worldwide rights to all therapeutic uses of the investigational compound. EYE-001 is currently in early clinical trials.

INDICATION(S) AND RESEARCH PHASE
Macular Degeneration – Phase I

matrix metalloprotease inhibitor (MMP)
Prinomastat

MANUFACTURER
Agouron Pharmaceuticals

DESCRIPTION
Prinomastat is an orally active, synthetic molecule designed to potently and selectively inhibit certain members of a family of enzymes known as a matrix metalloproteases that are believed to be involved in tumor angiogenesis, invasion, and metastasis. Based on their mechanism of action, MMP inhibitors may prove to have potential in reducing the invasiveness of malignant brain tumor cells.

The most common side effects of Prinomastat have been observed in the joints, and include stiffness, joint swelling, and in a few subjects, some limits on the mobility of certain joints, most often in the shoulders and hands. All these effects were reported reversible and were effectively managed by treatment rests and dose reductions.

Two phase III trials for advanced non-small cell lung cancer and prostate cancer were halted in August 2000 due to the drug's lack of effectiveness in subjects with late-stage disease.

Additionally, matrix metalloprotease inhibitors are also in a phase II trial for treatment of hormone-refractory prostate cancer combined with mitoxantrone prednisone, osteoarthritis, and Prinomastat in combination with chemotherapy for subjects with newly diagnosed glioblastoma multiforme following surgery with radiation therapy.

Subjects who are interested in finding more information on the drug Prinomastat can call the toll free number 888-849-6482.

INDICATION(S) AND RESEARCH PHASE
Lung Cancer – Phase II Halted
Prostate Cancer – Phase II Halted
Osteoarthritis – Phase II
Brain Cancer – Phase II
Macular Degeneration – Phase II

motexafin lutetium
Optrin

MANUFACTURER
Alcon

DESCRIPTION
Optrin belongs to a group of synthetic molecules called texaphyrins. The drug works by accumulating in specific diseased tissue, where it can then be activated by 732nm light to produce cytotoxic effects. In 1997, Pharmacyclics and Alcon entered into an evaluation and license agreement for the commercialization of Optrin for ophthalmology indications.

INDICATION(S) AND RESEARCH PHASE
Macular Degeneration – Phase II

SnET2
PhotoPoint - SnET2

MANUFACTURER
Miravant

DESCRIPTION
PhotoPoint SnET2 (photodynamic therapy) is in a phase III study for age-related macular degeneration (AMD). The phase III trial has closed subject enrollment with a total of 934 recruited subjects that were treated at 59 ophthalmology centers in the United States.

AMD is the leading cause of blindness in Americans over age 50. Due to limited therapeutic options for this debilitating disease, the FDA has granted this clinical trial a fast tracking status.

INDICATION(S) AND RESEARCH PHASE
Macular Degeneration – Phase III

Ocular Hypertension

AGN 192024
Lumigan

MANUFACTURER
Allergan

DESCRIPTION
AGN 192024 is a member of a new class of pharmacologically unique intraocular pressure (IOP) lowering agents called prostamides. Prostamides are naturally occurring substances found in the eye, representing newly discovered intrinsic factors that regulate IOP. As a synthetic analogue, AGN 192024 mimics the strong IOP-lowering activity of prostamides.

Results of a phase III trial demonstrated that AGN 192024 0.03%, dosed once daily (QD), significantly lowered IOP in comparison to timolol 0.5%, dosed twice daily (BID), in subjects with ocular hypertension or glaucoma. In the randomized, double-masked trial, 596 subjects were assigned to one of three groups: AGN 192024 once daily (QD), AGN 192024 twice daily (BID), or timolol twice daily (BID). Subjects receiving either AGN 192024 regimen achieved greater IOP lowering at all timepoints throughout the day than those receiving timolol, with the once-a-day dosing of AGN 192024 proving the most effective. In September 2000, Allergan submitted an NDA for AGN 192024.

INDICATION(S) AND RESEARCH PHASE
Ocular Hypertension – NDA submitted
Glaucoma – NDA submitted

14 Otolaryngology

Drugs in the development pipeline

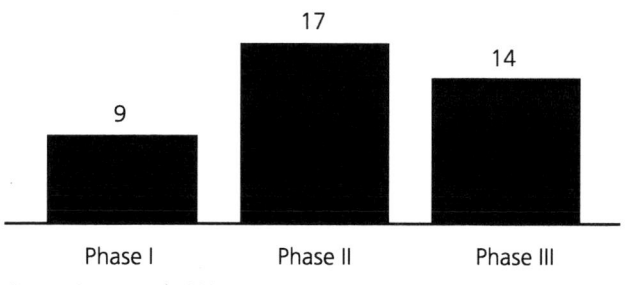

Source: CenterWatch, 2001

Popular drug development areas in the field of otolaryngology include rhinitis, allergies such as hayfever, and otitis media.

Rhinitis is an inflammation of the mucous membranes of the nose and is characterized by nasal congestion, rhinorrhea, sneezing, itching of the nose and/or postnasal drainage. Rhinitis is often accompanied by symptoms involving the eyes, ears and throat. Often times, causes of rhinitis go unrecognized by both physicians and subjects, which can lead to suboptimal control of the disease. CenterWatch estimates eight drugs are in the clinical pipeline with $35 million to $55 million being spent annually.

Allergic rhinitis is the most common form and affects between 20 million and 40 million people annually in the United States. Allergic rhinitis occurs when the immune system reacts to pollens and other allergens. The FDA recently approved Tri-Nasal Spray, administered intranasally, for the treatment of nasal symptoms of seasonal and perennial allergic rhinitis in adults and children 12 years or older. These symptoms include sneezing, stuffiness, discharge, and itching.

More effective and easily administered treatments are being developed to treat allergies. CenterWatch estimates there are 11 drugs in the pipeline for the treatment of allergies with $60 million to $80 million spent annually on treatments in clinical development. There are a number of drugs in the late stage development pipeline. For example, a phase III trial has been completed for Sepracor's levocetirizine, a single isomer version of the Pfizer's already approved drug Zyrtec, for the relief of symptoms associated with seasonal allergic rhinitis. Zyrtec is also in phase III trials for pediatric subjects six months to two years of age suffering from allergic rhinitis. Additionally, an NDA has been submitted for Sepracor's Desloratadine, an active metabolite of Claritin, a non-sedating antihistamine, and phase III trials are under way for norastemizole, a noncardiotoxic metabolite of astemizole (Hismanal) in a once-daily formulation.

Rhinitis is a common predisposing cause of otitis media. Otitis media is an inflammatory condition of the middle ear that is initiated by functional or mechanical obstruction of the eustachian tube, which leads to changing pressures of the gases in the middle ear. It is a common childhood disease and primarily affects infants and preschoolers. Almost all children experience one or more episodes of otitis media before age six. CenterWatch estimates there are three drugs in the pipeline with between $5 million and $10 million spent annually in clinical development.

Otitis media needs to be treated immediately to prevent it from becoming chronic and causing complications. Amoxicillin is the antibiotic most commonly used but other choices are Zithromax (azithromycin), cefaclor, Omnicef (cefdinir), ceftibuten, Rocephin (ceftriaxone), erythromycin, (Biaxin) clarithromycin or the combination drug Bactrim (trimethoprim/sulfamethoxazole). The infection usually begins to clear within 48 to 72 hours after starting a course of antibiotics. A relatively new option is the use of ofloxacin otic solution (Floxin) applied as ear drops through drainage tubes that are inserted through the eardrum.

Two popular drugs in the pipeline for the treatment of pediatric otitis media are Neose Technologies' NE-1530, which is a complex carbohydrate that is produced naturally in the human breast milk and functions as an antibacterial agent, and R.W. Johnson's Levaquin, a quinolone antibiotic, which is available in the United States for oral and intravenous administration.

Allergy

brompheniramine/pseudoephedrine HCl
Conquer-A

MANUFACTURER
Verex Laboratories

DESCRIPTION
Conquer-A is a once daily tablet formulation of brompheniramine/pseudoephedrine, which is a combination of an antihistamine plus a vasoconstrictor. This drug was being developed for the treatment of allergies and other minor respiratory problems. However, Conquer-A has stalled in a phase II trial due to low interest from the industry, but the company hopes it will soon be restarted. The company believes that Conquer-A is unique compared to other antihistamines because only the low dosage of 12-16 mg of brompheniramine appears to be needed to provide relief of allergies.

INDICATION(S) AND RESEARCH PHASE
Allergy – Phase II

cetirizine HCl
Zyrtec

MANUFACTURER
Pfizer

DESCRIPTION
Zyrtec (cetirizine HCl) is an orally active and selective H1-receptor antagonist. It has been approved by the FDA for the relief of symptoms associated with seasonal allergic rhinitis in adults and children two years of age and older. Zyrtec is currently in phase III trials for pediatric subjects ages six months to two years.

INDICATION(S) AND RESEARCH PHASE
Pediatric, Allergy – Phase III
Allergy – FDA approved

CpG compound
unknown

MANUFACTURER
Coley Pharmaceutical

DESCRIPTION
CpG compound is a novel immune modulator designed to redirect hypersensitivity reactions (allergic and asthmatic) into more normal responses, thereby eliminating or reducing the appearance of symptoms. CpG molecules simultaneously suppress Th2-type (allergic) immune responses that can result in airway inflammation and bronchial spasm, and induce Th1-type (normal) immune responses that promote antibody and cellular responses. In October 2000, Coley Pharmaceutical initiated a phase II trial for the treatment of allergic asthma. The study will be conducted in the United Kingdom, and is designed to evaluate the safety and efficacy of CpG.

INDICATION(S) AND RESEARCH PHASE
Asthma – Phase II
Allergy – Phase I

desloratadine, descarboethoxyloratadine
unknown

MANUFACTURER
Sepracor

DESCRIPTION
Desloratadine is an active metabolite of Claritin, a non-sedating antihistamine, for the treatment of seasonal allergic rhinitis. The drug selectively blocks histamine-1 receptors in the bloodstream, and thereby prevents the release of histamine by inflammatory cells. Desloratadine is being developed under an agreement between Sepracor and Schering-Plough Corporation.

INDICATION(S) AND RESEARCH PHASE
Allergy – NDA submitted
Rhinitis – NDA submitted

Hu-901
unknown

MANUFACTURER
Tanox

DESCRIPTION
Hu-901 is an anti-IgE monoclonal antibody currently being tested for the prevention of anaphylactic reactions to peanuts (PIA). Anti-IgE is a genetically-engineered humanized monoclonal antibody that has been developed to target the source of allergy symptoms for all allergens. Anti-IgE inhibits the allergic response by binding to IgE, thereby blocking the consequent release of inflammatory mediators such as histamine, prostaglandins, and leukotrienes. In general, these inflammatory mediators play a role in the pathology of a variety of allergic diseases including allergic asthma, allergic rhinitis, atopic dermatitis, and anaphylactic shock.

INDICATION(S) AND RESEARCH PHASE
Allergy – Phase I/II

IDEC-152
unknown

MANUFACTURER
IDEC Pharmaceuticals

DESCRIPTION
IDEC-152 is an anti-CD23 monoclonal antibody, which targets the CD23 receptor on immune cells. The anti-CD23 antibody is part of IDEC's "Primatized Antibody" technology that may be useful in treating allergic conditions such as allergic asthma, allergic rhinitis, and atopic conditions. This antibody enables the treatment of specific allergy conditions because it combines with the CD23 factor to regulate the production of the allergy-triggering immuno-globulin (IgE), and generates no further immuno-globulin production. In February 2000, IDEC initiated a phase I trial in allergic asthma to evaluate safety, tolerability, and pharmacokinetics. IDEC-152 is being developed by IDEC Pharmaceuticals and Seikagaku Corporation of Japan.

INDICATION(S) AND RESEARCH PHASE
Asthma – Phase I
Allergy – Phase I

ketotifen fumarate
Zaditen

MANUFACTURER
Novartis

DESCRIPTION
Zaditen is a topical selective H1-receptor antagonist, mast cell stabilizer, eosinophil infiltration inhibitor. An application has been filed overseas and the drug is in registration as an anti-allergic eyedrop.

INDICATION(S) AND RESEARCH PHASE
Allergy – In registration overseas
Eye Disorders/Infections – In registration overseas

levocetirizine
unknown

MANUFACTURER
Sepracor

DESCRIPTION
Levocetirizine is the single-isomer version of Zyrtec, which contains both isomers of cetirizine. All development and marketing rights have been licensed to UCB Pharma for Europe. UCB intends to file a MAA, the European equivalent of an NDA for levocetirizine. This isomer offers the possibility of an improved treatment for subjects with allergies.

INDICATION(S) AND RESEARCH PHASE
Allergy – Phase III completed

norastemizole
unknown

MANUFACTURER
Sepracor

DESCRIPTION
Norastemizole, a noncardiotoxic metabolite of astemizole (Hismanal), is in phase III trials for the treatment of seasonal and perennial allergic rhinitis in a once-daily formulation. The company claims that the drug is nonsedating and has no harmful effects on the heart, which are improvements over previous generations of antihistamines.

INDICATION(S) AND RESEARCH PHASE
Allergy – Phase III
Rhinitis – Phase III

unknown
MPL vaccine adjuvant

MANUFACTURER
Corixa Corporation

DESCRIPTION
MPL, a vaccine adjuvant, is currently undergoing phase III trials in Europe for use in allergy vaccines marketed by Allergy Therapeutics.

Allergies caused by grasses, trees, and house dust mites afflict an estimated 20% of the population in developed countries. While most allergy medications offer some relief to sufferers, the company believes that adding MPL adjuvant may allow the development of more effective and easily administered allergy treatments.

INDICATION(S) AND RESEARCH PHASE
Allergy – Phase III
Vaccines – Phase III

unknown
AIC

MANUFACTURER
Dynavax

DESCRIPTION
AIC is Dynavax's proprietary conjugate of purified ragweed allergen. ISS (immunostimulatory DNA) administered with allergens is thought to enhance immune response. ISS is attached to specific allergens so that they are presented to the immune system simultaneously. ISS, when linked to an allergen, "hides" the allergen from the immune system, thereby preventing the symptoms of an allergy attack. AIC ragweed immunotherapy is currently in phase II development.

INDICATION(S) AND RESEARCH PHASE
Skin Infections/Disorders – Phase II
Allergy – Phase II

vaccines, allergy
unknown

MANUFACTURER
Corixa Montana

DESCRIPTION
MPL-containing allergy vaccines are being developed to be more potent and effective treatments for common allergic reactions. One-fifth of the population of developed countries suffers from allergies to grasses, pollen, dust mites, animal dander, and other causes. Current methods of treating this pervasive problem include desensitization methods that involve a series of allergy injections over a period of weeks to years; the frequency of these injections initially is weekly, and then tapers down to monthly shots. This therapy can last up to three years.

MPL is a supplemental molecule (adjuvant) that could make allergy injections stronger and more effective. Phase II studies have shown that it may potentially reduce the total amount of injections necessary for desensitization to foreign material (allergens). MPL is formulated from a protein found in a certain species of bacteria. This bacteria and the proteins that compose it provoke a strong immune reaction in humans. By adding this protein to an allergy vaccine, MDL stimulates the body to react more strongly than it would have to the vaccine components alone.

If clinical studies demonstrate the effectiveness of the MDL adjuvant molecule, a chemical that signals the immune system to further boost its response to foreign material, this technology may be useful not only with allergy vaccines, but with cancer and infectious disease therapies as well. Testing of this vaccine is currently in phase III.

INDICATION(S) AND RESEARCH PHASE
Allergy – Phase III
Vaccines – Phase III

Aspergillosis

FK463, echinocandin
unknown

MANUFACTURER
Fujisawa Healthcare

DESCRIPTION
Echinocandin is a novel antifungal agent for the treatment of systemic fungal infections. The drug is used as prophylaxis, empirical therapy, and second line treatment for candidiasis and aspergillosis. Echinocandin is in phase II/III trials for these indications as well as other fungal infections.

INDICATION(S) AND RESEARCH PHASE
Aspergillosis – Phase II/III
Candidiasis – Phase II/III
Fungal Infections – Phase II/III

nystatin, AR-121
Nyotran

MANUFACTURER
Aronex Pharmaceuticals

DESCRIPTION
Nyotran is an intravenous liposomal formulation of nystatin being developed for the treatment of serious systemic, opportunistic fungal infections. Phase III trials have been completed for systemic fungal infections and confirmed cryptococcal meningitis. Additionally, phase II trials have been completed for candidiasis and aspergillosis.

Nyotran is under agreement with Abbott Laboratories for worldwide commercialization. Abbott will fund clinical development and will submit marketing registration outside the United States.

INDICATION(S) AND RESEARCH PHASE
Aspergillosis – Phase II completed
Candidiasis – Phase II completed
Systemic Fungal Infections – Phase III completed
Meningitis – Phase III completed

Ear Infections

NE-1530
unknown

MANUFACTURER
Neose Technologies

DESCRIPTION
NE-1530, a complex carbohydrate that is produced naturally in human breast milk, is an antibacterial agent being evaluated for the prevention and treatment of pediatric middle ear infections, or otitis media. The drug is in phase II trials for ear infections and otitis media. Additional indications may include infectious diseases and viral diseases associated with the nose, throat, and lungs, including pneumonia.

INDICATION(S) AND RESEARCH PHASE
Pediatric, Ear Infections – Phase II
Pediatric, Otitis Media – Phase II

vaccine, Streptococcus pneumoniae
unknown

MANUFACTURER
GlaxoSmithKline

DESCRIPTION
This conjugated pediatric vaccine is currently in phase III trials for Streptococcus pneumoniae disease prophylaxis. The vaccine contains antigens for prevention of pneumonia, middle ear infections, and meningitis in pediatric patients.

INDICATION(S) AND RESEARCH PHASE
Pediatric, Bacterial Infection—Phase III
Pediatric, Ear Infections —Phase III
Pediatric, Meningitis —Phase III
Pediatric, Pneumonia— Phase III

Laryngeal Tumors/Disorders

cidofovir
Vistide

MANUFACTURER
Gilead Sciences

DESCRIPTION
Vistide is being tested as an injectable formulation for treatment of central nervous system infections and hepatitis B virus respiratory tumors, and tumors or disorders of the larynx. The drug is in phase I/II trials for HBV respiratory tumors, laryngeal papillomatosis, and progressive multifocal leukoencephalopathy.

INDICATION(S) AND RESEARCH PHASE
Hepatitis – Phase I/II
Laryngeal Tumors/Disorders – Phase I/II
Viral Infection – Phase I/II
Brain Cancer – Phase I/II

cidofovir
Vistide

MANUFACTURER
Gilead Sciences

DESCRIPTION
Vistide is being tested as an injectable formulation for treatment of central nervous system infections and hepatitis B virus respiratory tumors, and tumors or disorders of the larynx. The drug is in phase I/II trials for HBV respiratory tumors, laryngeal papillomatosis, and progressive multifocal leukoencephalopathy.

INDICATION(S) AND RESEARCH PHASE
Hepatitis – Phase I/II
Laryngeal Tumors/Disorders – Phase I/II
Viral Infection – Phase I/II
Brain Cancer – Phase I/II

Otitis Media

gatifloxacin
Tequin

MANUFACTURER
Bristol-Myers Squibb

DESCRIPTION
Tequin is a broad-spectrum 8-methoxy fluoroquinolone antibiotic in a phase II trial for the treatment of recurrent otitis media in subjects 6 months to 17 years old. Tequin is primarily excreted through the kidneys and less than 1% is metabolized by the liver. Tequin has been approved by the FDA for the treatment of certain infections in adults.

INDICATION(S) AND RESEARCH PHASE
Pediatric, Otitis Media – Phase II

levofloxacin
Levaquin

MANUFACTURER
R.W. Johnson Pharmaceutical Research Institute

DESCRIPTION
Levaquin (levofloxacin tablets/injection) is an anti-infective currently in phase I development for pediatric subjects with otitis media. Levaquin was FDA approved in 1991 for the treatment of adults with community-acquired pneumonia, acute maxillary sinusitis or acute bacterial exacerbation of chronic bronchitis. Levaquin is licensed from the Daiichi Seiyaku Co.

INDICATION(S) AND RESEARCH PHASE
Pediatric, Otitis Media – Phase I

NE-1530
unknown

MANUFACTURER
Neose Technologies

DESCRIPTION
NE-1530, a complex carbohydrate that is produced naturally in human breast milk, is an antibacterial agent being evaluated for the prevention and treatment of pediatric middle ear infections, or otitis media. The drug is in phase II trials for ear infections and otitis media. Additional indications may include infectious diseases and viral diseases associated with the nose, throat, and lungs, including pneumonia.

INDICATION(S) AND RESEARCH PHASE
Pediatric, Ear Infections – Phase II
Pediatric, Otitis Media – Phase II

Pneumonia

amikacin
Mikasome

MANUFACTURER
Gilead Sciences

DESCRIPTION
Mikasome, an aminoglycoside antibiotic, is in phase II trials for treatment of serious bacterial and mycobacterial infections including nosocomial *Pseudomonas* pneumonia, complicated urinary tract infections and *Pseudomonas*-colonized subjects with cystic fibrosis. The drug is delivered in a liposomal formulation.

INDICATION(S) AND RESEARCH PHASE
Bacterial Infection – Phase II
Pneumonia – Phase II
Urinary Tract Infections – Phase II

cefditoren pivoxil
unknown

MANUFACTURER
Abbott Laboratories

DESCRIPTION
Cefditoren is an advanced generation oral cephalosporin that has a broad spectrum of activity against gram-positive and gram-negative pathogens. It is being tested in phase III trials as a first-line agent for respiratory tract infections, including pneumonia.

INDICATION(S) AND RESEARCH PHASE
Pediatric, Pneumonia – Phase III

DB-289
unknown

MANUFACTURER
Immtech International/NextEra Therapeutics

DESCRIPTION
DB-289 is currently in development for the treatment of *Pneumocystis carinii* pneumonia (PCP) and trypanosomiasis. DB-289 is effective due to neutralized positive charges that enable it to cross the digestive membranes. Once DB-289 enters the circulatory system, naturally occurring enzymes remove the patented masking or neutralizing charges to expose the active drug. The drug is in a phase I/II trial in Germany. The company has hired Parexel International to manage the study in Berlin.

INDICATION(S) AND RESEARCH PHASE
Pneumonia – Phase I/II

HMR-3647, RU-64,004
unknown

MANUFACTURER
Aventis

DESCRIPTION
HMR-3647 is an anti-infective drug which was being tested against a broad range of bacteria, including drug-resistant, susceptible strains of *Streptococcus pneumoniae* and other common pathogens. The company reported that development on this antibiotic was discontinued.

INDICATION(S) AND RESEARCH PHASE
Bacterial Infection – Trial discontinued
Pneumonia – Trial discontinued

MK-826, carbepenem
unknown

MANUFACTURER
Merck & Co.

DESCRIPTION

Carbapenem is a broad-spectrum antibiotic being developed for the treatment of pneumonia, skin infections and disorders, urinary tract infections, gynecological infections, bacterial infection, gastrointestinal diseases and disorders, bacterial infections including pneumonia, intra-abdominal infections, skin and skin structure infections, urinary tract infections, and obstetric and gynecological infections. Phase III trials are in progress for all indications.

INDICATION(S) AND RESEARCH PHASE
Pneumonia – Phase III
Skin Infections/Disorders – Phase III
Urinary Tract Infections – Phase III
Gynecological Infections – Phase III
Bacterial Infection – Phase III
Gastrointestinal Diseases and Disorders, miscellaneous – Phase III

opebecan, rBPI-21, recombinant human bactericidal/permeability-increasing protein
Neuprex

MANUFACTURER
XOMA Corporation

DESCRIPTION

Neuprex is a systemic formulation of recombinant bactericidal/permeability-increasing protein; rBPI-21, for the treatment of severe meningococcemia, a rare systemic gram-negative bacterial infection that primarily affects children. The active molecule in Neuprex, rBPI-21, binds to endotoxin molecules (LOS and LPS, lipopolysaccharide) in living bacteria, disrupting their cell walls, killing the bacteria or making them more susceptible to antibiotics. Phase III data were released in Sept. 2000 for both pediatric and adult trials.

XOMA is pursuing various indications for Neuprex: One indication is severe meningococcemia in children who become infected with these harmful bacteria that attack their brain and spinal cord's protective sheathing after entering the bloodstream. The gram-negative bacteria, called *Neisseria meningitidis*, cause meningococcemia and produce spiking high fever and a classic rigid stiff neck. Shock and death may occur in just a few hours after infection. Other indications are the preventions of serious lung complications (pneumonia and acute respiratory distress syndrome (ARDS)), acute intra-abdominal infection (Neuprex in combination with other antibiotics) and subjects who have had part of their liver removed during surgery. Neuprex may prevent infection and complications after this major surgery.

INDICATION(S) AND RESEARCH PHASE
Bacterial Infection – Phase III
Pediatric, Meningococcemia – Phase III completed
Meningitis – Phase III
Acute Respiratory Distress Syndrome (ARDS) – Phase III
Pneumonia – Phase III
Liver Disease – Phase II
Intra-abdominal infection – Phase I/II

Protegrin IB-367, rinse, gel
unknown

MANUFACTURER
IntraBiotics Pharmaceuticals

DESCRIPTION

Protegrin IB-367 is a synthetic antimicrobial peptide molecule that belongs to a new class of agents called protegrins. Studies suggest that Protegrin IB-367 kills bacteria by integrating with and disrupting the integrity of bacterial cell membranes. The antibiotic has a broad spectrum of microbicidal activity against gram-positive and gram-negative bacteria that are frequent pathogens in ventilator-associated pneumonia.

Results of a single-dose phase I trial indicated that Protegrin IB-367 safely reduces bacterial levels in the mouths of subjects at risk of experiencing ventilator-associated pneumonia. A rinse and gel formulation of Protegrin IB-367 was topically applied to the mouth to reduce the number of oral and oropharyngeal bacteria of intubated subjects. A single administration of 9 milligrams of the rinse formulation safely and rapidly reduced the total bacteria in orally intubated subjects compared to placebo. The magnitude and duration of effect after a single 9-milligram dose of Protegrin IB-367 rinse were similar to the response measured after a single 30-milligram dose. In November 2000, IntraBiotics began subject enrollment in a phase IIa trial.

The rinse formulation of Protegrin IB-367 is also undergoing evaluation in two phase III trials for the prevention of oral mucositis. As of February 2001, one trial had completed enrollment of subjects receiving high-dose chemotherapy, while the other continues to enroll subjects receiving radiotherapy.

INDICATION(S) AND RESEARCH PHASE
Effects of Chemotherapy – Phase III
Bacterial Infection – Phase IIa completed
Pneumonia – Phase IIa completed
Oral Medicine – Phase III

quinupristin/dalfopristin
Synercid

MANUFACTURER
Aventis

DESCRIPTION

Synercid is a combination therapy of two semi-synthetic antibacterial agents, quinupristin and dalfopristen. The antibiotic blocks bacterial protein synthesis.

Synercid has been FDA approved for the treatment of bloodstream infections due to vancomycin-resistant *Enterococcus faecium* (VREF) and skin and skin structure infections (SSTI) caused by methicillin-susceptible *Staphylococcus aureus* or *Streptococcus pyogenes*. It is in intravenous formulation. It is currently in pediatric trials for pneumonia.

INDICATION(S) AND RESEARCH PHASE
Bacterial Infection – FDA approved
Skin Infections/Disorders – FDA approved
Pediatric, Pneumonia – Phase III
Pneumonia – Phase III

unknown
Merrem

MANUFACTURER
AstraZeneca

DESCRIPTION
Merrem is a carbapenem antibiotic currently in numerous phase III line extension studies. The indications being tested include hospital and community acquired pneumonia, cystic fibrosis, skin and soft tissue infections, abdominal infections and for use in neutropenics.

INDICATION(S) AND RESEARCH PHASE
Skin Infections/Disorders – Phase III
Cystic Fibrosis – Phase III
Pneumonia – Phase III
Neutropenics – Phase III
Abdominal infections – Phase III

vaccine, pneumococcal infections
Quilimmune-P

MANUFACTURER
Aquila Biopharmaceuticals

DESCRIPTION
Quilimmune-P is designed to enhance the immune response to *Streptococcus pneumoniae*, a prominent bacterial pathogen, and to provide improved protection in the elderly against diseases such as pneumonia, bacteremia, and meningitis. *S. pneumoniae* is a leading cause of morbidity and mortality in the United States and in the world, especially among the very young and the elderly.

A phase IIb study initiated in 1999 involves 30 elderly subjects who have received a single immunization of Quilimmune-P in the original Phase IIa trial. The subjects will receive a second immunization of Quilimmune-P approximately 12 months after the first one. The primary end-point of the study is safety. The secondary objectives are to evaluate the immune response to two immunizations given one year apart, and the persistence of the immune response at 12 months following the first immunization.

INDICATION(S) AND RESEARCH PHASE
Pneumonia – Phase II
Vaccines – Phase II

vaccine, respiratory syncytial virus
unknown

MANUFACTURER
Aventis Pasteur

DESCRIPTION
Respiratory syncytial virus (RSV), a common cause of winter outbreaks of acute respiratory disease, may cause an estimated 90,000 hospitalizations and 4,500 deaths each year from lower respiratory tract disease in both infants and young children. RSV is a common, but preventable cause of hospital-acquired (nosocomial) infection. The source of this virus transmission may include other infected subjects, staff, and visitors.

Most severe manifestations of infection with RSV (e.g., pneumonia and bronchiolitis) occur in infants aged 2-6 months; however, children of any age with underlying cardiac or pulmonary disease or who are immunocompromised are at risk for serious complications from this infection. Because natural infection with RSV provides limited protective immunity, RSV causes repeated symptomatic infections throughout life. In adults, RSV usually causes upper respiratory tract manifestations but may cause lower respiratory tract disease, especially in the elderly and in immunocompromised persons.

The company has an RSV-mediated lower respiratory disease vaccination for at-risk children and the elderly being tested in phase I/II trials in various indications.

INDICATION(S) AND RESEARCH PHASE
Bronchitis – Phase I/II
Lung Disease – Phase I/II
Pediatric, Respiratory Syncytial Virus – Phase I/II
Pneumonia – Phase I/II
Vaccines – Phase I/II
Viral Infection – Phase I/II

vaccine, Streptococcus pneumoniae
unknown

MANUFACTURER
GlaxoSmithKline

DESCRIPTION
This conjugated pediatric vaccine is currently in phase III trials for Streptococcus pneumoniae disease prophylaxis. The vaccine contains antigens for prevention of pneumonia, middle ear infections, and meningitis in pediatric patients.

INDICATION(S) AND RESEARCH PHASE
Pediatric, Bacterial Infection—Phase III
Pediatric, Ear Infections —Phase III
Pediatric, Meningitis —Phase III
Pediatric, Pneumonia— Phase III

Rhinitis

AG7088, anti-rhinoviral agent
unknown

MANUFACTURER
Agouron Pharmaceuticals

DESCRIPTION
AG7088 is a small synthetic molecule designed to inhibit the rhinovirus 3C protease and presents a broad spectrum of potent antirhinoviral activity in preclinical testing.

The company reported that in a phase II study volunteers were administered multiple daily intranasal doses of AG7088 starting 24 hours after exposure to human rhinovirus. Results showed that AG7088 was well tolerated and it significantly reduced total cold symptoms and respiratory symptoms. Based on these results the company initiated a larger phase II/III trial in more than 50 sites throughout the United States.

INDICATION(S) AND RESEARCH PHASE
Rhinitis – Phase II/III
Sinus Infections – Phase II/III

desloratadine, descarboethoxyloratadine
unknown

MANUFACTURER
Sepracor

DESCRIPTION

Desloratadine is an active metabolite of Claritin, a non-sedating antihistamine, for the treatment of seasonal allergic rhinitis (inflammation of the mucous membranes causing a runny nose). The drug selectively blocks histamine-1 receptors in the bloodstream, and thereby prevents the release of histamine by inflammatory cells. Desloratadine is being developed under an agreement between Sepracor and Schering-Plough Corporation.

INDICATION(S) AND RESEARCH PHASE
Allergy – NDA submitted
Rhinitis – NDA submitted

DNK 333
unknown

MANUFACTURER
Novartis

DESCRIPTION
DNK 333 is a dual NK1/NK2 antagonist being developed in an oral formulation. It is in phase II development for rhinitis, asthma, and chronic obstructive pulmonary disease.

INDICATION(S) AND RESEARCH PHASE
Asthma – Phase II
Rhinitis – Phase II
Chronic Obstructive Pulmonary Disease (COPD) – Phase II

fluticasone/salmeterol
unknown

MANUFACTURER
GlaxoSmithKline

DESCRIPTION
This combination product includes a beta2-adrenergic agonist (salmeterol) and an inhaled corticosteroid (fluticasone) to be administered by intranasal inhilation. It is currently in phase I development for the treatment of rhinitis.

INDICATION(S) AND RESEARCH PHASE
Rhinitis – Phase I

loratadine/montelukast sodium
Claritin/Singulair

MANUFACTURER
Schering-Plough Corporation

DESCRIPTION
Schering-Plough and Merck are collaborating for the development of a once-daily fixed-combination tablet containing Claritin (loratadine) and Singulair (montelukast sodium). Claritin is a once-daily nonsedating antihistamine indicated for the treatment of seasonal allergic rhinitis, while Singulair is a once-daily leukotriene receptor antagonist for the treatment of asthma. The combination drug is currently being developed for the treatment of seasonal allergic rhinitis.

INDICATION(S) AND RESEARCH PHASE
Allergy – Phase III
Rhinitis – Phase III

norastemizole
unknown

MANUFACTURER
Sepracor

DESCRIPTION
Norastemizole, a noncardiotoxic metabolite of astemizole (Hismanal), is in phase III trials for the treatment of seasonal and perennial allergic rhinitis in a once-daily formulation. The company claims that the drug is nonsedating and has no harmful effects on the heart, which are improvements over previous generations of antihistamines.

INDICATION(S) AND RESEARCH PHASE
Allergy – Phase III
Rhinitis – Phase III

omalizumab
Xolair

MANUFACTURER
Genentech

DESCRIPTION
Xolair is a recombinant humanized monoclonal antibody to immunoglobulin (Ig) E. It is being developed for the treatment of asthma and the prevention of seasonal allergic rhinitis. A BLA has been submitted for the two above indications and for pediatric subjects ages 6-12. This drug is being developed in partnership with Novartis and Tanox. It is currently awaiting FDA approval.

INDICATION(S) AND RESEARCH PHASE
Asthma – NDA submitted
Rhinitis – NDA submitted
Pediatric, Asthma, Rhinitis – NDA submitted

rofleponide palmitate
unknown

MANUFACTURER
AstraZeneca

DESCRIPTION
Rofleponide palmitate is an intranasal steroid indicated for the treatment of rhinitis. It is currently in phase II trials.

INDICATION(S) AND RESEARCH PHASE
Rhinitis – Phase II

Sinus Infections

AG7088, anti-rhinoviral agent
unknown

MANUFACTURER
Agouron Pharmaceuticals

DESCRIPTION
AG7088 is a small synthetic molecule designed to inhibit the rhinovirus 3C protease and presents a broad spectrum of potent antirhinoviral activity in preclinical testing.

The company reported that in a phase II trials, study volunteers were administered multiple daily intranasal doses of AG7088 starting 24 hours after exposure to human rhinovirus. Results showed that AG7088 was well tolerated and it significantly reduced total cold symptoms and respiratory symptoms. Based on these results the company plans to initiate a larger phase II/III trial in more than 50 sites throughout the United States.

INDICATION(S) AND RESEARCH PHASE
Rhinitis – Phase II/III
Sinus Infections – Phase II/III

mupirocin
Bactroban

MANUFACTURER
GlaxoSmithKline

DESCRIPTION
Bactroban is an antibiotic that is currently marketed in a topical cream formulation for the treatment of secondarily infected traumatic skin lesions due to susceptible strains of *Staphylococcus aureus* and *Streptococcus pyogenes*. Bactroban is also being developed for the prevention of recurrent sinusitis; phase II trials are under way.

INDICATION(S) AND RESEARCH PHASE
Sinus Infections – Phase II

SB 275833
unknown

MANUFACTURER
GlaxoSmithKline

DESCRIPTION
SB 275833 is a bacterial protein synthesis inhibitor being developed for the prevention of recurrent sinusitis. It is currently in phase I development.

INDICATION(S) AND RESEARCH PHASE
Sinus Infections – Phase I

Vestibular Hypofunction

scopolamine
unknown

MANUFACTURER
Elan Transdermal Technologies

DESCRIPTION
Scopolamine acts as a central nervous system depressant. It is an alkaloid derived from plants of the Solanaceae family (Deadly Nightshade), particularly Datura metel and Scopolia carniolica. The drug is in phase II trials for the prevention of motion sickness and for treatment of gastrointestinal disorders, central and peripheral nervous system disorders, and vertigo. It is administered in a transdermal patch formulation.

INDICATION(S) AND RESEARCH PHASE
Gastrointestinal Diseases and Disorders, miscellaneous – Phase II
Vestibular Hypofunction – Phase II

15 | Women's Disorders

Population with illnesses in this category	27 million*
Drugs in the development pipeline	52

Source: World Health Organization, worldwide figures

Research on diseases specific to women focuses mainly on female sexual disorders, hormonal replacement therapy, contraception, cervical dysplasia and endometriosis. While not specifically a disease confined to a given gender, osteoporosis is more common among post-menopausal women. More information on this condition can be found in the Musculoskeletal Diseases and Connective Tissue Diseases chapter.

It is estimated that approximately 47 million American women suffer from female sexual arousal disorder: 25% who are pre-menopausal and 75% who are post-menopausal. Symptoms include the lack of lubrication, inability to experience sexual arousal, or to achieve orgasm. CenterWatch estimates that there are nine drugs in the clinical pipeline and $40 million to $50 million spent on these clinical development projects each year.

Currently, there are no drugs approved for treating female sexual arousal disorder. However, there are several drugs in the pipeline that may eventually be approved by the FDA, some indicated for the treatment of women's lack of desire and others to assist in helping women's sexual arousal.

Phase III trials of NexMed's Femprox cream were completed in May 2000. Femprox incorporates alprostadil (progstalandin E1), a vasodilator useful in the treatment of erectile dysfunction. It works by enhancing blood flow to the genital area and restoring the natural ability of genital tissues to engorge with blood and produce lubricating secretions during sexual stimulation, thus improving sexual arousal and pleasure. Another drug in the clinical pipeline containing alprostadil is Vivus' Alistra.

After menopause, testosterone levels decrease significantly in many women and this may cause a lack of interest in sexual activity. It is estimated that 11 million to 16 million women suffer from testosterone deficiency in the U.S. but only 5% to 10% of these women are receiving treatment for this deficiency. Numerous drugs in the pipeline focus on testosterone replacement and use a variety of forms such as tablets, injections, patches and implants. Many of the new patches in the pipeline aim to mimic serum testosterone concentrations similar to those present in young healthy women.

In November 2000, Watson Pharmaceuticals received a non-approvable letter from FDA for its estradiol/progestin hormone replacement therapy patch because of lack of sufficient evidence to support its safety and efficacy. The company anticipates filing an amendment to the FDA in the near future.

Female contraception is also another active area in the drug development pipeline. CenterWatch estimates 17 drugs are under investigation with $70 million to $90 million being spent annually on these drugs in clinical trials. The drugs in the pipeline are being tested in a variety of formulations and are designed to prevent the transmission of sexually transmitted diseases (STDs) including HIV, chlamydia and gonorrhea, in addition to providing contraception.

Ortho-McNeil Pharmaceuticals submitted an NDA in December 2000 for Ortho EVRA, a transdermal patch typically worn for three weeks on the lower abdomen or buttocks. These patches need to be changed every seven days. This represents a new method of combination hormonal contraception designed to deliver norelgestomin and ethinyl estradiol. If approved, it will be the world's first transdermal contraception.

In 2000, Pharmacia and UpJohn's Lunelle, an injectable formulation of estradiol cypionate and medroxyprogesterone acetate for the prevention of pregnancy, was approved. Lunelle's monthly contraception injection inhibits the secretion of gonadotropins, which, in turn, prevents follicular maturation and ovulation. Although the primary mechanism of action is inhibition of ovulation, other possible mechanisms of action include the thickening and a reduction in volume of cervical mucus (which decreases sperm penetration) and thinning of the endometrium (which may reduce the likelihood of embryo implantation).

Disorders affecting female reproduction organs represent major health concerns in the U.S. Nearly one quarter of American women of reproductive age may be affected by cervical dysplasia or endometriosis. Both are significant causes of infertility in women, which effects about 5.3 million Americans. CenterWatch estimates that $50 million to $60 million is being spent each year on cervical dysplasia with 12 drugs in the pipeline. Another $15 million to $25 million is being spent annually on endometriosis with four drugs being developed.

Cervical dysplasia is a premalignant condition. There are three stages of cervical dysplasia: mild, moderate and severe. Mild dysplasia is by far the most common and probably is not a true malignant disease. Moderate and severe dysplasia is treated when discovered because of the higher rates of malignant transformation. The majority of the drugs in the pipeline are still in phase I and II clinical trials with only Maxia Pharmaceuticals' MX6 being in phase III. MX6 is a naphtholic acid derivative, in a topical formulation, which inhibits cancer cell proliferation and promotes cell apoptosis.

Roughly 5.5 million women throughout North America have endometriosis, a disease caused by ectopic growth of uterine cells. Infertility is a complication that occurs in approximately 30% to 40% of patients with endometriosis. Most of the drugs currently in preclinical and clinical development block the effects of gonadatropin releasing hormone which is also currently used to treat infertility.

Cervical Dysplasia/Cancer

difluoromethylornithine (DFMO)
unknown

MANUFACTURER
Aventis

DESCRIPTION
Difluoromethylornithine (DFMO) is a potent, irreversible inhibitor of ornithine decarboxylase (OCD), an enzyme that is elevated in most tumors and pre-malignant lesions. Eflornithine is currently in a phase III clinical trial to determine the effectiveness of the drug in treating subjects who have newly-diagnosed or recurrent bladder cancer. The drug is administered orally in tablet form.

DFMO is also in trials for the prevention and treatment of HIV infections, skin, breast, prostate and cervical dysplasia/cancer.

INDICATION(S) AND RESEARCH PHASE
Bladder Cancer – Phase III
Breast Cancer – Phase II/III
Cervical Dysplasia/Cancer – Phase II
HIV Infection – Phase II
Prostate Cancer – Phase II
Skin Cancer – Phase III

arsenic trioxide (ATO)
Trisenox

MANUFACTURER
Cell Therapeutics

DESCRIPTION
Trisenox is believed to act by killing cancer cells through apoptosis, or programmed cell death. The mechanism of action for Trisenox is not fully understood, but it is believed that the drug induces apoptosis in ways different from other anti-cancer agents such as retinoids.

Trisenox is currently FDA approved to treat acute promyelocytic leukemia (APL) but is currently in fourteen different trials in the United States for other types of leukemia such as refractory lymphoma, relapsed and refractory non-Hodgkins lymphoma, relapsed or refractory chronic myelogenous leukemia, and relapsed and refractory Hodgkin's disease. Additionally, trials are being conducted for prostate cancer, multiple myeloma, renal cell cancer, cervical cancer, and bladder cancer.

INDICATION(S) AND RESEARCH PHASE
Leukemia – Phase I
Lymphoma, Non-Hodgkin's – Phase II
Leukemia – Phase II
Leukemia – Phase III
Multiple Myeloma – Phase I/II
Prostate Cancer – Phase II
Renal Cell Carcinoma – Phase II
Cervical Dysplasia/Cancer – Phase II
Bladder Cancer – Phase II
Leukemia – FDA approved

CI-1042, ONYX-015
unknown

MANUFACTURER
Onyx Pharmaceuticals

DESCRIPTION
CI-1042 (ONYX-015) is a tumor-selective, modified adenovirus that has been genetically engineered to replicate in and kill cancer cells that possess a mutated oncogene called p53, while sparing normal cells with functioning p53. p53 Is a tumor suppressor gene that is mutated in approximately 50% of all human cancers. CI-1042 is in development for several indications, including pancreatic cancer, liver metastases of colorectal cancer, and lung cancer.

Results of a phase II trial demonstrated that CI-1042 administered as a single-agent replicates and causes tumor regression in refractory head and neck cancer. CI-1042 was shown to selectively target cancer cells containing a mutant p53 gene, while sparing normal cells with a functioning p53 gene. Of the 19 subjects who received the standard dosing regimen, four (21%) had an objective response, including two complete responses and two partial responses. CI-1042 is being co-developed with Pfizer.

INDICATION(S) AND RESEARCH PHASE
Colorectal Cancer – Phase II
Pancreatic Cancer – Phase II
Head and Neck Cancer – Phase III
Cervical Dysplasia/Cancer – Phase I completed
Lung Cancer – Phase II
Bladder Cancer – Phase I completed
Brain Cancer – Phase I completed

HspE7
unknown

MANUFACTURER
StressGen

DESCRIPTION
HspE7 is a recombinant fusion product composed of the heat shock protein 65 (Hsp65) from *M. bovis* BCG and the protein E7. The E7 protein is derived from the human papillomavirus (HPV) and is involved in the malignant transformation of anal and cervical epithelial cells. E7 is a tumor-specific antigen and represents a precise target for immune system attack on abnormal cells.

StressGen has initiated a phase III trial to investigate HspE7 as a novel immunotherapeutic for anal dysplasia (AIN) caused by HPV. The company also has phase II HspE7 trials in women with HPV-related cervical dysplasia and cervical cancer. In January 2001, a phase II trial was initiated to test HspE7 on 52 subjects suffering from genital warts caused by HPV.

INDICATION(S) AND RESEARCH PHASE
Cervical Dysplasia/Cancer – Phase II
Anal Dysplasia – Phase III
Genital Warts – Phase II

LGD-1550
unknown

MANUFACTURER
Ligand Pharmaceuticals

DESCRIPTION
LGD-1550 is being formulated to limit the proliferation and spread of head, neck, and cervical cancers; it is to be given orally and is currently in phase II trials. Retinoids are a group of substances, one of which is vita-

min A, that are thought to be responsible for growth, bone development, vision, and skin integrity. It is thought that retinoids act against cancer by regulating the process by which cells reproduce themselves (gene transcription regulation). Studies have shown that subjects with metastatic cancer have lower levels of retinoid activity in their bodies. LGD-1550 works by binding to retinoid receptors in cells, thereby stimulating retinoid activity.

Preliminary studies have shown that retinoids may inhibit cell proliferation and promote cell differentiation. Cancer arises when there is uncontrolled growth of immature cells. Retinoids act to slow cell division and stimulates cell maturation, making it less likely that these mature cells will be transformed into cancerous cells. Retinoids have also been shown in early studies to boost the effects of other anti-cancer medications.

Phase II trials of LGD-1550 for head and neck cancer and cervical cancer are currently under way. Also, studies investigating solid and hematological tumors will begin phase II testing.

INDICATION(S) AND RESEARCH PHASE
Blood Cancer – Phase II
Cancer/Tumors (Unspecified) – Phase II
Cervical Dysplasia/Cancer – Phase II
Head and Neck Cancer – Phase II

MEDI-517
unknown

MANUFACTURER
MedImmune

DESCRIPTION
MEDI-517 is a virus-like particle vaccine designed to elicit an immune response against the Human papilloma virus (HPV). HPVs have been implicated in the development of genital warts and cervical cancer, with specific types of HPV associated with each condition. HPV-6 and HPV-11 cause the majority of genital warts, while HPV-16 and HPV-18 cause the majority of cervical cancers. MEDI-517 is currently in phase II trials for the prevention of cervical cancer.

INDICATION(S) AND RESEARCH PHASE
Viral Infection – Phase II
Cervical Dysplasia/Cancer – Phase II

MGI-114, hydroxymethylacylfulvene, HMAF
Irofulven

MANUFACTURER
MGI Pharma

DESCRIPTION
Irofulven (MGI-114) is the first product candidate being developed by MGI Pharma from its family of anti-cancer compounds called acylfulvenes. Early trials demonstrated that Irofulven is absorbed rapidly by tumor cells, and once inside binds to DNA and protein targets. The binding interferes with DNA replication and cell division, leading to tumor-specific cell death. The drug is being tested in a series of phase I and II trials for a variety of cancers.

Results from a phase II trial of Irofulven indicated that the drug produced anti-tumor activity in subjects with advanced pancreatic cancer who were refractory (resistant) to gemcitabine (Gemzar). Ten of the 53 subjects enrolled achieved six-month survival and two subjects demonstrated objective responses: one subject experienced tumor shrinkage of 100% and another subject experienced an 84% decrease in tumor mass. A phase III trial was initiated in February 2001.

INDICATION(S) AND RESEARCH PHASE
Breast Cancer – Phase II
Colon Malignancies – Phase II
Renal Cell Carcinoma – Phase II
Cervical Dysplasia/Cancer – Phase II
Lung Cancer – Phase II
Ovarian Cancer – Phase I/II
Colorectal Cancer – Phase II
Prostate Cancer – Phase I/II
Cancer/Tumors (Unspecified) – Phase I/II
Pancreatic Cancer – Phase III
Liver Cancer – Phase II

MX6
unknown

MANUFACTURER
Maxia Pharmaceuticals

DESCRIPTION
MX 6 is a naphthoic acid derivative, which inhibits cancer cell proliferation and promotes cell apoptosis. The drug is in phase III trials for treatment of cervical dysplasia using a topical gel formulation.

INDICATION(S) AND RESEARCH PHASE
Cervical Dysplasia/Cancer – Phase III

TA-CIN
unknown

MANUFACTURER
Cantab Pharmaceuticals plc

DESCRIPTION
TA-CIN is a novel vaccine in phase I trials for the treatment of cervical dysplasia. TA-CIN is based on a genetically engineered fusion protein derived from HPV, and it is designed to stimulate the immune system to destroy cervical cells infected with HPV-16, the most common HPV type found in advanced stages of cervical dyplasia. A phase I trial is being conducted in 40 subjects at a center in the Netherlands.

INDICATION(S) AND RESEARCH PHASE
Cervical Dysplasia/Cancer – Phase I

TA-HPV
unknown

MANUFACTURER
Cantab Pharmaceuticals plc

DESCRIPTION
TA-HPV is a vaccine for the treatment of cervical cancer. It is designed to initiate a natural immune response to cancer cells, eliminating tumor growth or metastatic spread. A phase II study held by the company in collaboration with the European Organization for the Research and Treatment of Cancer (EORTC) showed efficacy in treating subjects with cervical cancer. Two additional phase II studies are under way in Europe.

INDICATION(S) AND RESEARCH PHASE
Cervical Dysplasia/Cancer – Phase II

---

vaccine, cervical cancer
unknown

MANUFACTURER
MediGene AG

DESCRIPTION
MediGene's HPV16-L1E7-CVLP vaccine is being developed for the treatment of precancerous lesions of the cervix (CIN) caused by human papillomaviruses (HPV). The company's CVLP-technology is based on chimeric virus-like particles (CVLPs), which induce an immune response against HPV, both preventing infection and killing already infected cells. Phase I/II testing is under way.

INDICATION(S) AND RESEARCH PHASE
Cervical Dysplasia/Cancer – Phase I/II

ZD-0473/AMD 473
unknown

MANUFACTURER
AstraZeneca

DESCRIPTION
ZD-0473 is a new platinum-based anticancer agent designed to deliver an extended spectrum of activity and overcome resistance to currently approved platinum drugs, such as cisplatin and carboplatin. It is being evaluated for the treatment of a range of solid-tumor cancers, including colorectal, non-small cell lung, and bladder cancer, which are resistant to carboplatin. ZD-0473 is formulated in both intravenous and oral forms. The intravenous formulation is in phase II trials and the oral form is in preclinical development.

INDICATION(S) AND RESEARCH PHASE
Bladder Cancer – Phase II
Cancer/Tumors (Unspecified) – Phase II
Colorectal Cancer – Phase II
Lung Cancer – Phase II
Ovarian Cancer – Phase II
Prostate Cancer – Phase II

Breast Cancer – Phase II
Cervical Dysplasia/Cancer – Phase II

Contraception

Contraceptive Patch
Amylin

MANUFACTURER
Levotech

DESCRIPTION
The 7-day transdermal contraceptive patch consisting of levonorgestrel (LNG) and ethinyl estradiol (EE) may be considered a safer alternative to oral contraceptives since results from a phase IIb trial showed the patch to have fewer side effects.

The phase IIb trial tested three skin patches of different sizes on 86 women in a five month study sponsored by the National Research Institute for Family Planning. According to the company, dose proportionality was obtained. Serum levels of LNG and EE were in ranges required for effective contraception. Nine ultrasounds per menstrual cycle, plus hormone and drug levels, were done on each subject. Follicular size and endometrial thickening indicated that all patches were potentially similar in efficacy to oral contraceptive pills. The company plans to initiate a phase III.

INDICATION(S) AND RESEARCH PHASE
Contraception – Phase III

---

ethinyl estradiol/trimegestrone
unknown

MANUFACTURER
Wyeth-Ayerst

DESCRIPTION
Ethinyl estradiol/trimegestrone is a combination female oral contraceptive being evaluated in phase II trials. It has beeb shown to have improved side effects compared to other oral contraceptives.

INDICATION(S) AND RESEARCH PHASE
Contraception – Phase II

---

glyminox vaginal gel
Savvy

MANUFACTURER
Biosyn

DESCRIPTION
Savvy (glyminox vaginal gel) is a broad spectrum microbicide designed to prevent the transmission of sexually transmitted diseases (STDs) including HIV, chlamydia, and gonorrhea, and to provide contraception. Topical microbicides work by killing the STD pathogen upon entering the body, or by creating a barrier to the pathogen, blocking its ability to enter or bind with cells. The active ingredient in Savvy is C31G, which has a high affinity for bacteria, fungi, yeast, and viruses while offering low cell toxicity. Savvy is undergoing an expanded phase I program to fully evaluate its formulation prior to entering combined phase II/III trials in 2001.

INDICATION(S) AND RESEARCH PHASE
Contraception – Phase I completed
Prevention of STD's – Phase I completed

---

immunocontraception
unknown

MANUFACTURER
Aphton Corporation

DESCRIPTION
Immunocontraception is a prophylactic vaccine that neutralizes the hormone, human chorionic gonadotropin (HCG). Using vaccine-like technology, immunocontraception is being developed for use as a female contraceptive to prevent pregnancy. Currently, this agent is being tested in a phase I/II trial.

INDICATION(S) AND RESEARCH PHASE
Contraception – Phase I/II

Implanon
etonogestrel

MANUFACTURER

Organon

DESCRIPTION

Implanon is an implantable one-rod female contraceptive that is administered by dedicated injector. The four cm long, 2 mm thick rod is implanted in the inside upper arm. The rod is a soft plastic containing the hormone etonogestrel, that is released daily. Implanon prevemts pregnancy for three years with high reliability levels. It has been approved in Europe since 1999 and is currently in phase III testing in the United States with NDA filing planned for 2001.

INDICATION(S) AND RESEARCH PHASE
Contraception – Phase III

levonorgestrel/ethinyl estradiol
unknown

MANUFACTURER
Agile

DESCRIPTION

The seven-day transdermal contraceptive patch is a combination progestin and estrogen treatment being evaluated in an eight month phase II trial in the United States and Australia. Positive phase I/II trial results were obtained from studies conducted in China.

INDICATION(S) AND RESEARCH PHASE
Contraception - Phase II

norgestimate/ethinyl estradiol transdermal patch
Evra

MANUFACTURER
R.W. Johnson Pharmaceutical Research Institute

DESCRIPTION

Evra is a norgestimate/ethinyol estradiol transdermal patch in phase III trials for contraception.

INDICATION(S) AND RESEARCH PHASE
Contraception – Phase III
Pregnancy, Labor and Delivery – Phase III

norgestimate/ethinyl estradiol tablet
Ortho-Eldose

MANUFACTURER
R.W. Johnson Pharmaceutical Research Institute

DESCRIPTION

Ortho-Eldose is being tested in phase III trials for a low dose of contraception in tablet formulation.

INDICATION(S) AND RESEARCH PHASE
Contraception – Phase III

Ortho EVRA
unknown

MANUFACTURER
Ortho-McNeil Pharmaceutical

DESCRIPTION

Ortho EVRA is a new method of combination hormonal contraception designed to deliver norelgestromin and ethinyl estradiol (progestin and estrogen) for a seven day period. This transdermal patch is typically worn on the lower abdomen or buttocks. It is worn for one week at a time and is changed on the same day of the week for three weeks. No patch is worn the fourth week. An NDA was filed in December 2000 and if approved, Ortho EVRA will be the world's first transdermal contraceptive.

INDICATION(S) AND RESEARCH PHASE
Contraceptive – NDA submitted

polyacrylic acid
BufferGel

MANUFACTURER
ReProtect, LLC

DESCRIPTION

BufferGel is a spermicidal microbicide for vaginal protection against pregnancy. It is designed to block the alkaline action of semen. This pH neutralizing action of semen abolishes the protective acidity of the vagina for several hours after intercourse, and thereby helps bring about fertilization since the acidity of the vagina would otherwise quickly immobilize and kill sperm. By blocking this alkaline action of semen, BufferGel maintains the protective acidity of the vagina and this acidity (pH4) kills sperm and may prevent both unwanted pregnancy and sexually transmitted diseases. BufferGel is a non-irritating lubricant gel with no taste or odor, it also does not contain detergents, such as nonoxynol-9.

The company plans to initiate a phase II/III trial for contraception and phase III trial for HIV prevention in Zimbabwe and Malawi (by the National Institutes of Health).

INDICATION(S) AND RESEARCH PHASE
Contraception – Phase II/III
HIV Prevention – Phase III

PREVEN2
levonorgestrel

MANUFACTURER
Gynetics

DESCRIPTION

PREVEN2 is an emrgency contraception kit currently in phase III trials. Like the original PREVEN kit, the pills must be administered within 72 hours of intercourse. PREVEN2 contains only the hormone levonorgestrel, unlike PREVEN, which contains ethinyl estradiol as well. Being a progestin-only treatment, PREVEN2 is thought to cause reduced nausea and vomiting that is associated with emergency contraception.

INDICATION(S) AND RESEARCH PHASE
Contraception - Phase III

PRO 2000 Gel
unknown

MANUFACTURER
Procept

DESCRIPTION

PRO 2000 gel is a synthetic naphthalene sulfonate polymer of approximately 5,000 molecular weight. Its high solubility and lack of color and odor make it well suited for topical use. Thus, PRO 2000 gel, a topical microbicide can be used for the prevention of human immunodeficiency virus (HIV) infection and sexually transmitted diseases (STDs).

Results from pre-clinical studies showed PRO 2000 gel reduced the infection rate in female rhesus macaques exposed to a high dose of an HIV-like virus, protected mice completely from vaginal HSV-2 infection as well as being a contraceptive in rabbits.

Phase I/II trials in the United States and South Africa; testing the safety and acceptability of PRO 2000 gel in healthy, sexually active women and in sexually abstinent, asymptomatic, HIV-seropositive women; were completed and phase II/III trials will begin in Africa and India in late 2001.

INDICATION(S) AND RESEARCH PHASE
HIV Infection – Phase I/II completed
Contraception – Phase I/II completed

progestin
unknown

MANUFACTURER
Watson Pharmaceuticals

DESCRIPTION
Using a patented transdermal TheraDerm-MTX delivery technology, Watson Laboratories is testing the effects of administering progestin alone for birth control. Progestin has traditionally been administered with estrogen. Although the company discontinued phase II trials for the treatment of osteoporosis and hormone replacement therapy (HRT), this drug is being evaluated in phase II trials for the prevention of pregnancy.

INDICATION(S) AND RESEARCH PHASE
Contraception – Phase II

progestin, ethynylestradiol
Nestorone

MANUFACTURER
Population Council Center for Biomedical Research

DESCRIPTION
Nestorone is a synthetic female hormone (progestin) similar to progesterone that is naturally produced by the body. This drug is not active when given orally, but many other delivery forms are being developed, such as patches, rings, gels, and implants, either combined with estrogen or used alone.

Nestorone is being tested in phase II clinical trials as an intravaginal ring for contraception. This flexible vaginal ring is a doughnut-shaped drug-delivery system. It may slowly release hormones to be absorbed into the bloodstream at a lower dosage than oral contraceptives, which may advantageously decrease drug side events.

Clinical trials are being designed using single and combination therapy of female hormones using the ring delivery device. Combination therapy may include Nestorone plus the synthetic estrogen, ethynylestradiol. Other tests include a one-year progestin-only ring for lactating women, which may be used up to 12 months. Also in development is a progesterone ring for breastfeeding mothers, which may extend the contraceptive effectiveness of nursing. The Council conducted previous clinical studies using the ring in 900 women in eight countries. Effective contraceptive results were reported.

INDICATION(S) AND RESEARCH PHASE
Contraception – Phase II

trimegestone/ethinyl estradiol
unknown

MANUFACTURER
Wyeth-Ayerst

DESCRIPTION
Trimegestone/Ethinyl estradiol is being evaluated as a new oral contraceptive. It is designed to have improved side effects when compared to other oral contraceptives and is currently in phase II trials.

INDICATION(S) AND RESEARCH PHASE
Contraception – Phase II

unknown
Protectaid

MANUFACTURER
Axcan Pharma

DESCRIPTION
Gephar Pharmaceuticals is developing a new contraceptive sponge, which is being developed both to provide effective contraception and to prevent the contraction of sexually transmitted diseases (STDs), including HIV. The Protectaid sponge is made of a foam material that is saturated with a formulation called F-5 Gel, which is a combination of three sperm-killing (spermicidal) chemicals. This sponge acts in three ways: it creates a physical barrier against sperm entering the uterus, it absorbs the semen, preventing its progression, and it destroys sperm because of its spermicidal chemicals. The company reported that initial studies demonstrated high contraceptive efficacy with few side effects.

The sponge may cause less vaginal irritation because instead of using large amounts of one potentially irritating spermicidal ingredient, it contains smaller amounts of three synergistically acting spermicidal compounds. Its sperm-killing ingredients and the gel that composes the sponge's structure all contribute to limiting the amount of vaginal irritation. Therefore, this product has the potential to limit the transmission of sexually transmitted diseases that are more easily spread when there is vaginal lining irritation.

Early studies also show that the spermicidal components in Protectaid could destroy STDs such as viruses, fungi, and HIV. The F-5 Gel has been shown to destroy organisms such as HIV, *Chlamydia*, and *Neisseria gonorrhea*. From a contraceptive standpoint, Protectaid has been demonstrated to be 90% effective when used correctly at preventing pregnancy. The sponge can be inserted any time prior to sexual intercourse and should not be removed for at least six hours after intercourse. Protectaid is currently being evaluated in phase II trials.

INDICATION(S) AND RESEARCH PHASE
Acquired Immune Deficiency Syndrome

(AIDS) and AIDS-Related Infections – Phase II
HIV Infection – Phase II
Contraception – Phase II

unknown
Seasonale

MANUFACTURER
Barr Laboratories

DESCRIPTION
Seasonale is an oral contraceptive that is being developed for the prevention of pregnancy. Currently it is being evaluated in a phase III study. If approved, the company plans to launch the product in late 2002 or early 2003.

INDICATION(S) AND RESEARCH PHASE
Contraception – Phase III

Endometriosis

abarelix, PPI-149
unknown

MANUFACTURER
Praecis Pharmaceuticals

DESCRIPTION
Abarelix is a synthetic peptide for the treatment of hormonally responsive prostate cancer. Prostate cancer develops when glandular cells of the prostate multiply abnormally. The drug acts through a complex series of actions to inhibit the production of testosterone, which, in turn, inhibits the growth of prostate cells. An NDA was submitted in January 2001 for Abarelix to block the effect of gonadatropin releasing hormone (GnRH), which is also called leutinizing hormone-releasing hormone (LHRH), on the pituitary gland.

The company is also conducting phase III trials testing abarelix on the treatment of endometriosis, which may be responsive to inhibition of LHRH. The company is in sales and marketing partnership with Amgen.

INDICATION(S) AND RESEARCH PHASE
Prostate Cancer – NDA submitted
Endometriosis – Phase III

unknown
Abarelix-Depot F

MANUFACTURER
Amgen

DESCRIPTION
Abarelix-Depot F is a peptide antagonist that inhibits the action of lutenizing hormone releasing hormone (LHRH). The action of this drug on the pituitary gland results in the reduction of estrogen production in women. Estrogen significantly increases the symptoms of endometriosis. The drug is currently in phase II trials for endometriosis.

INDICATION(S) AND RESEARCH PHASE
Endometriosis – Phase II

unknown
GnRH Pharmaccine

MANUFACTURER
Aphton Corporation

DESCRIPTION
Aphton's novel GnRH Pharmaccine is an anti-gonadotropin releasing hormone (GnRH) immunogen, which neutralizes the hormone GnRH. Study results indicate that it induces and maintains castration levels of testosterone and reduced levels of prostate-specific antigen (PSA). Chemical castration of this type is a standard therapy to extend the survival of subjects with advanced prostate cancer. GnRH Pharmaccine will also be involved in trials for breast cancer, endometrial cancer, endometriosis, and prostate cancer.

INDICATION(S) AND RESEARCH PHASE
Prostate Cancer – Phase I/II
Breast Cancer – Phase I/II
Endometrial Cancer – Phase I/II
Endometriosis – Phase I/II

YM-511
unknown

MANUFACTURER
Yamanouchi Pharmaceutical

DESCRIPTION
YM-511 is an aromatase inhibitor, which is administered in an oral formulation. The drug is being developed in Europe and is currently in phase II trials for the treatment of breast cancer, endometriosis, and uterine fibroids.

INDICATION(S) AND RESEARCH PHASE
Breast Cancer – Phase II
Endometriosis – Phase II
Uterine Fibroids – Phase II

Genital Herpes

APL400-024Px
Genevax - HSV-Px

MANUFACTURER
Wyeth-Lederle Vaccines

DESCRIPTION
HSV-Px is a novel facilitated DNA vaccine for prevention of herpes simplex virus-2 (HSV-2) infection that causes genital herpes. This vaccine uses injected Genevax delivery technology and it is in phase II trials.

INDICATION(S) AND RESEARCH PHASE
Genital Herpes – Phase II

GW 419458, DISC-HSV
unknown

MANUFACTURER
GlaxoSmithKline

DESCRIPTION
DISC (disabled infectious single cycle)-HSV is an immunotherapeutic vaccine using a disabled live virus for treatment and prevention of genital herpes. Since the drug therapy induces a natural immune response and

may promote immunologic memory, the chance of disease recurrence is drastically reduced. It also eliminates the need for constant dosing, thereby increasing subject compliance and improving lifestyle. The drug is in phase II trials for genital herpes. GlaxoSmithKline has worldwide development and marketing rights.

INDICATION(S) AND RESEARCH PHASE
Genital Herpes – Phase II

---

resiquimod
unknown

MANUFACTURER
3M Pharmaceuticals

DESCRIPTION
Resiquimod is in phase III trials for recurrent genital herpes in both the United States and Europe. Positive phase II results of a double-blind, placebo-controlled trial were reported. In the six-month follow-up, the time to the first recurrence was significantly increased and the total number of recurrences was significantly decreased for subjects on active study medication compared to a placebo gel.

INDICATION(S) AND RESEARCH PHASE
Genital Herpes – Phase III

TA-HSV
unknown

MANUFACTURER
Cantab Pharmaceuticals plc

DESCRIPTION
TA-HSV (therapeutic antigen-herpes simplex virus) is a genetically disabled vaccine containing HSV that allows only a single cycle of replication within a host cell. It is in phase II trials for the treatment of genital herpes.

INDICATION(S) AND RESEARCH PHASE
Genital Herpes – Phase II

---

unknown

Docosanol

MANUFACTURER
AVANIR Pharmaceuticals

DESCRIPTION
Docosanol is approved as a treatment for cold sores and fever blisters. It is in phase III trials for the treatment of genital herpes. Docosanol works by inhibiting fusion between the plasma membrane and the herpes simplex virus (HSV) envelope, thereby preventing viral entry into cells and subsequent viral replication. Since the compound doesn't act directly on the virus, it is unlikely it will produce drug resistant mutants of HSV. All known competitive Rx products work by inhibition of viral DNA replication and, as such, carry risk of mutating the virus.

INDICATION(S) AND RESEARCH PHASE
Genital Herpes – Phase III

---

vaccine, genital herpes
unknown

MANUFACTURER
Corixa Montana

DESCRIPTION
This immunostimulant vaccine uses monophosphoryl lipid A (MPL) adjuvant for prevention and treatment of herpes simplex virus types 1 and 2 that causes genital herpes. The vaccine is in phase III trials.

INDICATION(S) AND RESEARCH PHASE
Genital Herpes – Phase III
Herpes Simplex Infections – Phase III

---

vaccine, genital herpes
Simplirix

MANUFACTURER
GlaxoSmithKline

DESCRIPTION
Simplirix is a recombinant vaccine being developed for genital herpes prophylaxis. Simplirix consists of a recombinant glycoprotein from herpes simplex virus 2 (HSV-2), in combination with an adjuvant "derivative endotoxin." Results of two large, placebo-controlled, randomized international trials were reported. The two trials were "discordant partner studies," in which one of the partners had genital herpes and the other did not. The first trial included 847 subjects who tested negative for HSV-1 and HSV-2 at baseline, and the second trial involved 1867 subjects who were negative for HSV-2. The vaccine had absolutely no effect in the men in either group; however, a notable effect was observed in the women. In the first study, the vaccine efficacy in women was 73%. Similarly, among the seronegative women in the second study, the vaccine efficacy was 74%. The vaccine was not protective in the women who were HSV-1-positive and HSV-2-negative.

INDICATION(S) AND RESEARCH PHASE
Genital Herpes – Phase II
Vaccines – Phase II

Gynecological Infections

MK-826, carbepenem
unknown

MANUFACTURER
Merck & Co.

DESCRIPTION
Carbapenem is a broad-spectrum antibiotic being developed for the treatment of bacterial infections including pneumonia, intra-abdominal infections, skin and skin structure infections, urinary tract infection and obstetric and gynecologic infections. Phase III trials are in progress for pneumonia, skin infections and disorders, urinary tract infections, gynecological infections, bacterial infection, gastrointestinal diseases and disorders.

INDICATION(S) AND RESEARCH PHASE
Pneumonia – Phase III
Skin Infections/Disorders – Phase III
Urinary Tract Infections – Phase III
Gynecological Infections – Phase III
Bacterial Infection – Phase III
Gastrointestinal Diseases and Disorders, miscellaneous – Phase III

Hormone Replacement Therapy

17-beta estradiol/trimegestone
unknown

MANUFACTURER
Wyeth-Ayerst

DESCRIPTION
17-beta estradiol/trimegestone is being evaluated in late clinical trials for the treatment of menopausal symptoms and osteoporosis.

INDICATION(S) AND RESEARCH PHASE
Menopause – Phase III
Hormone Replacement Therapy:
  Menopause – Phase III
Osteoporosis – Phase III

conjugated estrogen tablets
Premarin/trimegestone

MANUFACTURER
Wyeth-Ayerst

DESCRIPTION
Premarin/trimegestone is being evaluated in phase III trials for relieving menopausal symptoms as well as decreasing the incidence of endometrial hyperplasia seen with estrogen-alone therapy. Premarin for oral administration contains a mixture of estrogens obtained exclusively from natural sources. Trimegestone is a progestational molecule originated by Aventis for hormone replacement therapy.

INDICATION(S) AND RESEARCH PHASE
Menopause – Phase III
Hormone Replacement Therapy:
  Menopause – Phase III

estradiol
Estrasorb

MANUFACTURER
Novavax

DESCRIPTION
Estrasorb is an estrogen replacement therapy developed for symptomatic menopausal women. It is applied as a typical cosmetic lotion, and is designed to deliver 17-beta etradiol through the skin. Estrasorb completed phase III trials in November 2000 on 200 subjects.

Previous results showed that Estrasorb successfully delivered therapeutic doses of estradiol transdermally. No skin irritation was found and no significant fluctuations in blood hormone levels were observed.

INDICATION(S) AND RESEARCH PHASE
Hormone Replacement Therapy:
  Menopause – Phase III completed

estradiol, 17-beta
Estrogel

MANUFACTURER
Solvay Pharmaceuticals

DESCRIPTION
Estrogel is a topical gel steroid (17-beta estradiol) developed for use as an estrogen hormone replacement therapy. The estradiol accumulates in the skin and forms a reservoir, providing a steady release of the drug. Estrogel is under FDA review as a transdermal treatment for vasomotor symptoms of menopause, including hot flashes and night sweats. An NDA was submitted by Unimed Pharmaceuticals, which is a subsidiary of Solvay Pharmaceuticals.

INDICATION(S) AND RESEARCH PHASE
Hormone Replacement Therapy:
  Menopause – NDA submitted

estradiol/progestin
unknown

MANUFACTURER
Watson Pharmaceuticals

DESCRIPTION
Watson Laboratories has conducted phase III trials for a combination estradiol/progestin hormone replacement therapy (HRT) patch using their transdermal (patch) delivery system. The patch administers a continuous dose of both estrogen and progestin through the patch's adhesive into the skin for body absorption. The company received a non-approvable letter in November 2000 because of lack of sufficient evidence to support the safety and efficacy of the estradiol/progestin for the prevention of hyperplasia and required that an additional endometrial protection trial be submitted. The company anticipates filing an amendment.

INDICATION(S) AND RESEARCH PHASE
Hormone Replacement Therapy:
  Menopause – FDA denied
Osteoporosis – Phase III

estrogens/methyltestosterone
Estratest

MANUFACTURER
Solvay Pharmaceuticals

DESCRIPTION
Estratest consists of esterified estrogens and methyltestosterone administered as an oral tablet. It is already approved by the FDA for moderate to severe vasomotor symptoms associated with menopause. Estratest is currently being evaluated in phase III trials for the treatment of sexual dysfunction in women.

INDICATION(S) AND RESEARCH PHASE
Sexual Dysfunction – Phase III
Female Hormonal
  Deficiencies/Abnormalities – Phase III

testosterone
unknown

MANUFACTURER
Watson Pharmaceuticals

DESCRIPTION
Testosterone is a naturally produced hormone, which is responsible for proper development of male secondary sex characteristics. This hormone which has been formulated in the MTX transdermal patch is being tested in phase II trials for several indications, which include the treatment of

sexual dysfunction in surgically menopausal subjects, menopause associated hormone replacement therapy, and osteoporosis. Additionally, this drug is in phase III clinical trials for male hormonal deficiencies and abnormalities.

This hormone regime is also being evaluated in phase II trials for treatment of female AIDS wasting. Testosterone is an anabolic steroid that may help build up muscle mass in subjects suffering from AIDS.

INDICATION(S) AND RESEARCH PHASE
Acquired Immune Deficiency Syndrome (AIDS) and AIDS-Related Infections – Phase II
Hormone Replacement Therapy: Menopause – Phase II
Male Hormonal Deficiencies/Abnormalities – Phase III
Osteoporosis – Phase II
Sexual Dysfunction – Phase II completed

transdermal testosterone gel
Tostrelle

MANUFACTURER
Cellegy Pharmaceuticals

DESCRIPTION
Tostrelle (transdermal testosterone gel) is indicated for the treatment of low levels of testosterone in menopausal women. Testosterone deficiency in women is a frequent cause of diminished libido or low sex drive. Based on previous phase I trial results, the company is planning to begin an expanded phase I/II study to determine the optimal dosing of Tostrelle in surgically induced menopausal women only.

INDICATION(S) AND RESEARCH PHASE
Menopause – Phase I/II
Hormone Replacement Therapy: Menopause – Phase II
Sexual Dysfunction – Phase I/II

Infertility

follitropin alpha
Gonal-F

MANUFACTURER
Serono Laboratories

DESCRIPTION
Gonal-F is a genetically engineered follicle stimulating hormone (FSH) being developed for the treatment of infertility and ovulation disorders. The subcutaneously administered drug is currently marketed in several countries for the treatment of both male and female infertility. An application has been filed for a multi-dose formulation of the drug, and phase III testing is also under way for an improved treatment schedule and delivery systems.

INDICATION(S) AND RESEARCH PHASE
Infertility – FDA approved
Treatment Schedule and Delivery Systems – Phase III

goserelin acetate
Zoladex IVF

MANUFACTURER
AstraZeneca

DESCRIPTION
Zoladex IVF is a luteinizing hormone-releasing hormone (LHRH) analogue for the treatment of invitro fertilization. Currently, Zoladex IVF is being evaluated in a phase III clinical trial for the treatment of infertility and for premenopausal adjuvant breast cancer.

INDICATION(S) AND RESEARCH PHASE
Infertility – Phase III
Breast Cancer – Phase III

LHRH, luteinizing hormone-releasing hormone antagonist
unknown

MANUFACTURER
Serono Laboratories

DESCRIPTION
This is a luteinizing hormone-releasing hormone (LHRH) antagonist for the treatment of female infertility and for use in assisted reproductive technologies. It is currently in phase II development.

INDICATION(S) AND RESEARCH PHASE
Infertility – Phase II

r-hCG
Ovidrel

MANUFACTURER
Serono Laboratories

DESCRIPTION
Ovidrel is a sterile powder that contains recombinant human chorionic gonadotropin (r-hCG). The drug has been approved by the FDA for the induction of final follicular maturation and early luteinization in infertile women who have undergone pituitary desensitization and who have been appropriately pre-treated with follicle stimulating hormones as part of an assisted reproductive technology (ART) program. Ovidrel is also indicated for the induction of ovulation and pregnancy in anovulatory infertile subjects in whom the cause of infertility is functional and not due to primary ovarian failure. Additionally, r-hCG is in phase II trials for the treatment of breast cancer.

INDICATION(S) AND RESEARCH PHASE
Infertility – FDA approved
Breast Cancer – Phase II

r-hLH
unknown

MANUFACTURER
Serono Laboratories

DESCRIPTION
This recombinant human luteinizing hormone (r-hLH) is being developed for the treatment of infertility and related indications. An application has been filed for the

treatment of female infertility/luteinizing hormone deficiency syndrome. The drug is also in trials as an ovulation trigger in female infertility (phase II: ovulation induction, phase III: assisted reproductive technology).

INDICATION(S) AND RESEARCH PHASE
Infertility – Phase II/III

Menopause

17-beta estradiol/trimegestone
unknown

MANUFACTURER
Wyeth-Ayerst

DESCRIPTION
17-beta estradiol/trimegestone is being evaluated in late clinical trials for the treatment of menopausal symptoms and osteoporosis.

INDICATION(S) AND RESEARCH PHASE
Menopause – Phase III
Hormone Replacement Therapy:
    Menopause – Phase III
Osteoporosis – Phase III

calcitonin
Macritonin

MANUFACTURER
Provalis

DESCRIPTION
Macritonin is the oral formulation of salmon calcitonin, a calcium regulator for the treatment of postmenopausal osteoporosis, using Macromol oral drug delivery system. Calcitonin is a well-tolerated treatment for osteoporosis currently available in injectable and intranasal formulations. Clinical trials are currently in phase II testing.

INDICATION(S) AND RESEARCH PHASE
Osteoporosis – Phase II
Menopause – Phase II

conjugated estrogen tablets
Premarin/trimegestone

MANUFACTURER
Wyeth-Ayerst

DESCRIPTION
Premarin/Trimegestone is being evaluated in phase III trials for relieving menopausal symptoms as well as decreasing the incidence of endometrial hyperplasia seen with estrogen-alone therapy. Premarin for oral administration contains a mixture of estrogens obtained exclusively from natural sources. Trimegestone is a progestational molecule originated by Aventis for hormone replacement therapy.

INDICATION(S) AND RESEARCH PHASE
Menopause – Phase III
Hormone Replacement Therapy:
    Menopause – Phase III

estrogen
Vivelle, Menorest

MANUFACTURER
Noven Pharmaceuticals

DESCRIPTION
Vivelle/Menorest is an estradiol transdermal system to be used as hormone replacement therapy (HRT) for the treatment of menopausal symptoms and the prevention of osteoporosis. The product delivers 17-beta estradiol, the primary estrogen produced by the ovaries, through a patch that is applied twice weekly. It has been approved by the FDA for menopausal symptoms, and an application has been filed and results are pending for the osteoporosis indication.

Marketing rights have been licensed to Novogyne in the United States, to Novartis in Canada, and to Aventis in all other territories. The product is being sold as Menorest in 19 foreign countries, including France, Germany, and the United Kingdom, while being marketed as Vivelle in the United States and Canada.

INDICATION(S) AND RESEARCH PHASE
Osteoporosis – NDA submitted
Menopause – FDA approved

estrogen
Vivelle-Dot

MANUFACTURER
Noven Pharmaceuticals

DESCRIPTION
Vivelle-Dot is an estrogen transdermal system designed to be exceptionally small and provide hormone replacement therapy for the treatment of menopausal symptoms. Vivelle-Dot utilizes Dot Matrix adhesive technology to deliver 17-beta estradiol through the skin and into the bloodstream. It is FDA approved for the treatment of menopausal symptoms, and is also in clinical development for the treatment of osteoporosis.

INDICATION(S) AND RESEARCH PHASE
Menopause – FDA approved
Osteoporosis – NDA submitted

testosterone
Androsorb

MANUFACTURER
Novavax

DESCRIPTION
Androsorb is a cream for testosterone replacement therapy in phase II clinical trials for testosterone deficient men and phase I trials for post-menopausal women. A phase I trial will test 21 postmenopausal women at two sites. Androsorb is being developed using Novavax's proprietary micellar nanoparticle technology, a microemulsion drug delivery platform.

INDICATION(S) AND RESEARCH PHASE
Male Hormonal Deficiencies/Abnormalities
    – Phase II
Menopause – Phase I

transdermal testosterone gel
Tostrelle

MANUFACTURER
Cellegy Pharmaceuticals

DESCRIPTION

Tostrelle (transdermal testosterone gel) is indicated for the treatment of low levels of testosterone in menopausal women. Testosterone deficiency in women is a frequent cause of diminished libido or low sex drive. Based on previous phase I trial results, the company is planning to begin an expanded phase I/II study to determine the optimal dosing of Tostrelle in surgically induced menopausal women only. Additionally, trials are under way for sexual dysfunction

INDICATION(S) AND RESEARCH PHASE

Menopause – Phase I/II
Hormone Replacement Therapy:
    Menopause – Phase II
Sexual Dysfunction – Phase I/II

TSE-424
unknown

MANUFACTURER

Wyeth-Ayerst

DESCRIPTION

TSE-424 is a selected estrogen receptor modulator (SERM) designed to mimic the beneficial qualities of estrogens while blocking estrogen in tissues where it can be harmful. A SERM is a partial agonist that binds with high affinity to the estrogen receptor (ER) but has tissue specific effects distinct from estradiol. SERMs are designed to act selectively, eliminating some of the risks of estrogen such as undesirable effects on the uterus or breast tissue while supplementing inadequate estrogen supplies in post-menopausal women.

TSE-424 is being tested in phase II trials for the prevention and treatment of post-menopausal osteoporosis. Wyeth-Ayerst and Ligand Pharmaceuticals have a cooperative agreement for the development of TSE-424.

INDICATION(S) AND RESEARCH PHASE

Osteoporosis – Phase II
Menopause – Phase II

Labor, and Delivery

SR 49059
Unknown

MANUFACTURER

Sanofi-Synthelabo Pharmaceuticals

DESCRIPTION

SR 49059 is a non-peptide arginine-vasopressin V1A receptor antagonist. A phase IIa trial evaluating the compound for the prevention of preterm labor has been completed.

INDICATION(S) AND RESEARCH PHASE

Labor, and Delivery – Phase IIa completed

Premenstrual Syndrome

vomeropherin, PH-80
unknown

MANUFACTURER

Pherin Pharmaceuticals

DESCRIPTION

Vomeropherin, in a nasal spray formulation, is in a phase I trial for the treatment of premenstrual syndrome and for the treatment of anxiety disorders.

INDICATION(S) AND RESEARCH PHASE

Premenstrual Syndrome – Phase I
Anxiety Disorders – Phase I

Sexual Dysfunction

alprostadil
emprox

MANUFACTURER

NexMed

DESCRIPTION

Femprox cream, incorporating the active drug ingredient alprostadil, is in development for the treatment of female sexual dysfunction. Results demonstrated Femprox had a positive effect on increasing blood flow to the clitoris and labia in 18 female subjects. Femprox utilizes NexACT as a drug delivery method. According to the company, NexACT contains skin penetration-enhancing molecules that allow a drug to be quickly absorbed to a localized site.

INDICATION(S) AND RESEARCH PHASE

Sexual Dysfunction – Phase III completed

apomorphine HCl
unknown

MANUFACTURER

Nastech Pharmaceutical

DESCRIPTION

Intranasal apomorphine HCl is currently undergoing evaluation for the treatment of sexual dysfunction in women. The formulation may work by acting on receptors in the central nervous system that may improve sexual arousal and dyspareunia. Positive phase I results were reported by the company. The study involved 48 nasal administrations of apomorphine at dosages from 0.1 mg to 0.75 mg per dose, followed by blood sampling from five to 180 minutes. Clinical safety measurements included clinical nasal examination, blood pressure, heart rate, respiration rate, and side effects. There were no significant changes recorded in blood pressure, heart rate, respiration rate, or nasal mucosa. No serious side effects were observed, including dizziness, sweating, vomiting, hypotension or syncope. Other companies have seen these side effects in the development of non-nasal apomorphine products. A phase II "at home" study will be the next step in evaluating efficacy. In addition, a phase II trial for male erectile dysfunction was initiated in November 2000.

INDICATION(S) AND RESEARCH PHASE

Erectile dysfunction – Phase II
Sexual Dysfunction – Phase I completed

estrogens/methyltestosterone
Estratest

MANUFACTURER
Solvay Pharmaceuticals

DESCRIPTION
Estratest consists of esterified estrogens and methyltestosterone administered as an oral tablet. It is already approved by the FDA for moderate to severe vasomotor symptoms associated with menopause. Estratest is currently being evaluated in phase III trials for the treatment of sexual dysfunction in women.

INDICATION(S) AND RESEARCH PHASE
Sexual Dysfunction – Phase III
Female Hormonal
    Deficiencies/Abnormalities – Phase III

IC351
Cialis

MANUFACTURER
Eli Lilly

DESCRIPTION
Cialis (IC351) is an orally administered phosphodiesterase type 5 (PDE5) inhibitor that has been tested in a global phase III trial for ED, and a phase II trials for female sexual dysfunction (FSD).

INDICATION(S) AND RESEARCH PHASE
Erectile dysfunction – Phase III
Sexual Dysfunction – Phase II

NMI-870
unknown

MANUFACTURER
NitroMed

DESCRIPTION
NMI-870 is a nitric oxide derivative of the alpha2 blocker yohimbine, which is being tested in post-menopausal woman.
  Results of a randomized, double-blind, placebo-controlled phase II, three-way crossover trial of orally-administered NMI-870 showed that the compound demonstrated the ability to increase vaginal blood flow in post-menopausal women diagnosed with female sexual arousal disorder.

INDICATION(S) AND RESEARCH PHASE
Sexual Dysfunction – Phase II

testoterone
unknown

MANUFACTURER
Watson Pharmaceuticals

DESCRIPTION
Testosterone is a naturally produced hormone, which is responsible for proper development of male secondary sex characteristics. This hormone which has been formulated in the MTX transdermal patch is being tested in trials for several indications, which include the treatment of sexual dysfunction in surgically menopausal subjects, menopause associated hormone replacement therapy, osteoporosis and male hormonal deficiencies and abnormalities.
  This hormone regime is also being evaluated in phase II trials for treatment of female AIDS wasting. Testosterone is an anabolic steroid that may help build up muscle mass in subjects suffering from AIDS.

INDICATION(S) AND RESEARCH PHASE
Acquired Immune Deficiency Syndrome
    (AIDS) and AIDS-Related Infections –
    Phase II
Hormone Replacement Therapy:
    Menopause – Phase II
Male Hormonal Deficiencies/Abnormalities
    – Phase III
Osteoporosis – Phase II
Sexual Dysfunction – Phase II completed

transdermal testosterone gel
Tostrelle

MANUFACTURER
Cellegy Pharmaceuticals

DESCRIPTION
Tostrelle (transdermal testosterone gel) is indicated for the treatment of low levels of testosterone in menopausal women. Testosterone deficiency in women is a frequent cause of diminished libido or low sex drive. Based on previous phase I trial results, the company is planning to begin an expanded phase I/II study to determine the optimal dosing of Tostrelle in surgically-induced menopausal women only.

INDICATION(S) AND RESEARCH PHASE
Menopause – Phase I/II
Hormone Replacement Therapy:
    Menopause – Phase II
Sexual Dysfunction – Phase I/II

unknown
Vasofem

MANUFACTURER
Zonagen

DESCRIPTION
Vasofem is a vaginal suppository being developed for the treatment of female sexual dysfunction (FSD). Phase II trials are currently under way.

INDICATION(S) AND RESEARCH PHASE
Sexual Dysfunction – Phase II

unknown
Alista

MANUFACTURER
Vivus

DESCRIPTION
Aprostadil is a synthetic derivative of a naturally occurring vasodilating agent. Alista is believed to increase blood flow to the female genitalia, thereby promoting engorgement and other natural processes that occur during sexual stimulation. Alista is a proprietary formulation of alprostadil, which is applied locally to female genitalia. Alista is in a phase II multi-center, double-blind, placebo-controlled trial for women with a primary diagnosis of female sexual arousal disorder.

INDICATION(S) AND RESEARCH PHASE
Sexual Dysfunction – Phase II

Urinary Tract Infections

amikacin
Mikasome

MANUFACTURER
Gilead Sciences

DESCRIPTION
Mikasome, an aminoglycoside antibiotic, is in phase II trials for treatment of serious bacterial and mycobacterial infections including nosocomial *Pseudomonas* pneumonia, complicated urinary tract infections and *Pseudomonas*-colonized subjects with cystic fibrosis. The drug is delivered in a liposomal formulation.

INDICATION(S) AND RESEARCH PHASE
Bacterial Infection – Phase II
Pneumonia – Phase II
Urinary Tract Infections – Phase II

chondrocyte-alginate gel suspension
Chondrogel

MANUFACTURER
Curis

DESCRIPTION
Chondrogel is a tissue augmentation product created from autologous cartilage cells taken from a subject's ear and expanded in culture. These cells are then injected into the bladder to treat pediatric vesicoureteral reflux disease (VUR). VUR is a congenital condition in children possibly leading to a urinary tract infection and kidney damage. Phase III trials have been completed, and a phase II trial is currently being planned for the treatment of Grade II VUR in pediatric subjects.
  A phase II trial for stress urinary incontinence (SUI) is also under way.

INDICATION(S) AND RESEARCH PHASE
Urinary Tract Infections – Phase III completed
Pediatric, Vesicoureteral Reflux Disease – Phase III completed
Urinary Incontinence – Phase II

ciprofloxacin
CIPRO

MANUFACTURER
Bayer Corporation

DESCRIPTION
CIPRO is a fluoroquinolone antibiotic and is currently awaiting FDA approval for the treatment of exposure to aerosolized anthrax bacteria. Without treatment, anthrax infection is usually fatal. Doxycycline and penicillin are approved to treat anthrax, but it is thought that there are strains of anthrax bacteria, which have been engineered to be resistant to these antibiotics. CIPRO is already approved for 17 different indications: acute sinusitis, lower respiratory tract infections, nosocomial pneumonia (intravenous only), urinary tract infections, acute uncomplicated cystitis in females (tablets and oral suspension only), chronic bacterial prostatitis, complicated intra-abdominal infections (in combination with metronidazole), skin and skin structure infections, bone and joint infections, infectious diarrhea, typhoid fever (enteric fever), and uncomplicated cervical and urethral gonorrhea (tablets and oral suspension only).
  CIPRO intravenous is also indicated in empirical therapy for febrile neutropenic subjects (in combination with piperacillin sodium). Phase III trials testing Cipro for the treatment of complicated urinary tract infections in pediatric subjects 1-17 years old are currently under way.

INDICATION(S) AND RESEARCH PHASE
Anthrax exposure – NDA submitted
Pediatric, Urinary Tract Infections – Phase III

daptomycin
Cidecin

MANUFACTURER
Cubist Pharmaceuticals

DESCRIPTION
Daptomycin is a novel antibiotic lipopeptide for the treatment of skin and soft tissue infections, urinary tract infections in hospitalized subjects, and bacteremia. The drug is made in an intravenous formulation. Daptomycin is in trials for skin infections, urinary tract infections and for bacterial infections.

INDICATION(S) AND RESEARCH PHASE
Skin Infections/Disorders – Phase III
Bacterial Infection – Phase II
Urinary Tract Infections – Phase II/III
Heart Disease – Phase II/III

gemifloxacin mesylate
Factive

MANUFACTURER
GlaxoSmithKline

DESCRIPTION
Factive is a broad spectrum fluoroquinolone being developed for the treatment of various bacterial infections. It is in phase III trials in an intravenous formulation for the treatment of respiratory tract infections. Additionally, Factive has been developed in an oral formulation for the treatment of respiratory and urinary tract infections. An NDA and Marketing Authorization Application (MAA) have been submitted for the latter indications.

INDICATION(S) AND RESEARCH PHASE
Bacterial Infection – Phase III
Bacterial Infection – NDA submitted
Bacterial Infection – MAA submitted
Urinary Tract Infections – MAA submitted

MK-826, carbepenem
unknown

MANUFACTURER
Merck & Co.

DESCRIPTION
Carbapenem is a broad-spectrum antibiotic being developed for the treatment for pneumonia, skin infections and disorders, urinary tract infections, gynecological infections, bacterial infection, and gastrointestinal diseases and disorders. Phase III trials are under way for all indications.

572/Urinary Tract Infections

INDICATION(S) AND RESEARCH PHASE
Pneumonia – Phase III
Skin Infections/Disorders – Phase III
Urinary Tract Infections – Phase III
Gynecological Infections – Phase III
Bacterial Infection – Phase III
Gastrointestinal Diseases and Disorders, miscellaneous – Phase III

vaccine, urinary tract infection
unknown

MANUFACTURER
MedImmune

DESCRIPTION
This is a vaccine for the prevention of urinary tract infection (UTI). More than 80% of UTIs are caused by *E. coli*.

To test the safety and tolerability of its UTI vaccine, MedImmune immunized 48 healthy, female volunteers in a phase I, randomized, placebo-controlled trial. In this trial, the vaccine was found to be safe, generally well tolerated and immunogenic. There was also evidence of a clear dose response: all volunteers receiving the vaccine developed serum antibodies and those with the best serum repsonses exhibited antibodies in urine and vaginal secretions. When studied in tissue culture, the antibodies were found to prevent the bacteria from binding to human bladder cells.

INDICATION(S) AND RESEARCH PHASE
Urinary Tract Infections – Phase II

YM-617, tamsulosin
unknown

MANUFACTURER
Yamanouchi Pharmaceutical

DESCRIPTION
YM-617 is an orally administered alpha-1 receptor antagonist being evaluated as a treatment for lower urinary tract disorder. The drug is in phase III trials and is part of Yamanouchi's domestic pipeline.

INDICATION(S) AND RESEARCH PHASE
Urinary Tract Infections – Phase III

Uterine Fibroids

goserelin acetate
Zoladex FIB

MANUFACTURER
AstraZeneca

DESCRIPTION
Uterine leiomyomas are the most common pelvic tumors in women and they cause significant problems including excessive menstrual bleeding and an enlarged uterine size. Because fibroids are dependent on estrogen for their development and growth, induction of a low estrogen state causes reduction of tumor and uterine mass, resolving pressure symptoms. The most effective medications for the treatment of fibroids are gonadotropin releasing hormone agonists (GnRHa), because they induce a low-estrogen (menopause-like) state. GnRHs are a form of luteinizing hormone-releasing hormone.

Zoladex FIB is an implant delivery system for a luteinizing hormone-releasing hormone (LHRH) analogue being tested in phase III trials for the treatment of uterine fibroids.

INDICATION(S) AND RESEARCH PHASE
Uterine Fibroids – Phase III

YM-511
unknown

MANUFACTURER
Yamanouchi Pharmaceutical

DESCRIPTION
YM-511 is an aromatase inhibitor, which is administered in an oral formulation. The drug is being developed in Europe and is currently in phase II trials for the treatment of breast cancer, endometriosis, and uterine fibroids.

INDICATION(S) AND RESEARCH PHASE
Breast Cancer – Phase II
Endometriosis – Phase II
Uterine Fibroids – Phase II

Vaginal Infection

interferon (IFN), alfa-n3
Alferon N Gel

MANUFACTURER
Interferon Sciences

DESCRIPTION
Alferon N Gel is a human leukocyte-derived natural interferon (IFN) treatment being tested for vaginal infections in phase II trials. Interferons are naturally produced chemicals that modulate and boost the immune system. These trials are testing the drug in a topical gel formulation.

Already on the market, interferon alfa-n3 (human leukocyte derived) is an injectable formulation of Natural Alpha Interferon, approved by the U.S. Food and Drug Administration (FDA) in 1989 for the intralesional treatment of refractory or recurring external condylomata acuminata in subjects 18 years of age or older.

INDICATION(S) AND RESEARCH PHASE
Genital Warts – Phase II
Vaginal Infection – Phase II
Viral Infection – Phase II

16 | Men's Disorders

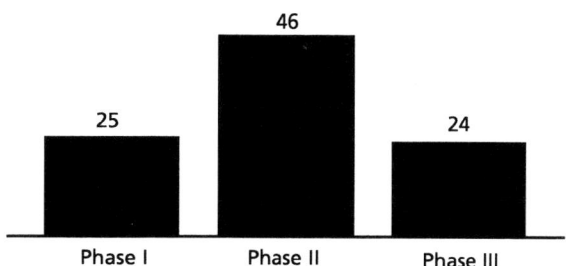

Drugs in the development pipeline

Phase I: 25
Phase II: 46
Phase III: 24

Source: CenterWatch, 2001

Two major indications make up most of the drug development research in the area of men's disorders: sexual dysfunction and prostate cancer.

Male sexual dysfunction can be divided into two types: erectile dysfunction (historically called impotence) and ejaculatory dysfunction, which includes premature, retarded, and retrograde ejaculation.

Erectile dysfunction affects an estimated 52 million men worldwide. It is characterized by the inability to achieve or maintain an erect penis sufficient for sexual intercourse. The inability to maintain an erect penis can be caused by medical conditions such as diabetes, heart disease, hypertension, or situational conditions such as smoking, excessive alcohol consumption or depression. The incidence of impotence rises with age; about 5% of men suffer from it by the age of 40 and between 15% to 20% by the age of 65. CenterWatch estimates that there are 20 drugs in the pipeline for erectile dysfunction and between $90 and $110 million being spent on clinical development projects each year.

Since the approval of Viagra in 1999, research on drugs for treating erectile dysfunction has expanded. Drugs being developed for treating erectile dysfunction can be taken orally, injected directly into the penis or inserted into the urethra. It is hoped that these new treatments will have fewer side effects than drugs currently on the market.

Most drugs in the development pipeline can be categorgized into three mechanisms of action for the treatment of erectile dysfunction: dopamine agonists, ejaculatory agents and pro-erectile agents.

In June 2000, TAP Pharmaceuticals withdrew the NDA they submitted for Uprima (apomorphine) because of concerns from the FDA. Uprima works directly by improving blood flow to the penis and is a fast-acting drug (leading to an erection within 30 minutes after administration), thus allowing for more natural sex as well as faster return to normal postcoital status. The FDA felt the major area of concern using Uprima was the occurrence of serious adverse events including syncope, hypotension and bradycardia. The FDA also questioned if Uprima should be indicated for all subjects suffering from erectile dysfunction. Clinical trials only included subjects who had erectile dysfunction and a normal (nocturnal penile tumescence) test, representing only a select group of subjects suffering from erectile dysfunction. The company plans to resubmit the NDA at a later date. If approved, Uprine will be a major competitor to Viagra. Additionally, several other companies are testing apomorphine in a variety of formulations such as a pill, a liquid, nasal spray or as an injection for erectile dysfunction.

Two other drugs that have completed phase III trials as treatments for erectile dysfunction are Zonagen's VasoMax (phentolamine mesylate), in an oral formulation, and Lilly Icos' Cialis. Zonagen blocks alpha-receptors, which are located on the vascular endothelium and may produce an effect in as little as 15 to 20 minutes. Cialis is a new PDE5 inhibitor for diabetes-related erectile dysfunction.

Prostate cancer is another major focus of drug development for men's disorders. It is the most common cancer diagnosed in men in the United States and is the second leading cause of mortality due to cancer in men after lung cancer. In 2000, an estimated 180,000 new cases were diagnosed and almost 32,000 deaths occurred. Between 1989 and 1992, incidence rates dramatically rose, but they are now declining. This large increase was most likely due to earlier diagnosis in men without any symptoms through the increased use of prostate-specific antigen (PSA) blood test screenings. In patients with localized prostate cancers with metastases only to regional structures, the five-year survival rate is 100%. For all stages combined, the survival rate has now reached 92%.

These impressive survival rates are largely due to the numerous treatment options for men suffering from prostate cancer. This progress is evident from the close to 70 drugs currently in development. CenterWatch estimates that as much as $300 million will be spent on this research each year. Current prostate cancer research focuses on hormone therapy, gene therapy, immunologic agents, vaccines, anti-angiogenesis, and drug delivery.

Most cancers treated with hormone therapy become resistant to the hormone within months or years. Therefore, researchers are now focusing on intermittent hormone administration or second line agents to decrease such resistance. Gene therapy is among the most active arenas in prostate cancer research, with several gene-directed biologics in the pipeline. Scientists have located the genes responsible for some forms of hereditary prostate cancer and now are determining in what way each one is responsible for cancer development and how to manipulate these genes to achieve prevention or cure. The potential of antiangiogenesis drugs to arrest the growth of cancerous tissue is currently under intense investigation. By blocking blood vessel growth, these drugs may prevent the tissue from receiving nutrients and oxygen. With many new agents in the pipeline, prostate cancer treatment is progressing rapidly and the chance of survival is greatly improved.

Benign Prostatic Hyperplasia

alfuzosin
Xatral

MANUFACTURER
Sanofi-Synthelabo Pharmaceuticals

DESCRIPTION
Alfuzosin is a new medication being developed to treat benign prostatic hypertrophy (BPH), a condition that impacts the quality of life for many older men.

Treatments for BPH include surgical removal of part of the enlarged prostate gland, drugs that lower the active hormone (DHT) that is causing excessive prostate growth, and alpha receptor blockers which prevent abnormal prostate muscular contraction. By relaxing prostate tissue, alpha receptor blockers open up urine passageways. Alpha receptors are located throughout the body, and have many actions, including cardiac and respiratory effects. Because of their widespread activity, current alpha blocker medications can produce serious cardiac and respiratory side effects. Alfuzosin works on blocking a specific type of alpha receptor that is primarily located in the urinary tract and prostate gland. This allows the drug to act only where it is needed—in the urinary tract. This specificity of action may lead to fewer side effects than seen with drugs that block alpha receptors throughout the body.

INDICATION(S) AND RESEARCH PHASE
Benign Prostatic Hyperplasia – Phase III

GI 198745
unknown

MANUFACTURER
GlaxoSmithKline

DESCRIPTION
GI 198745 is a dual inhibitor of 5-alpha-reductase type 1 and 2 isozymes. An NDA was submitted for this indication in December 2000. Additionally, GI 198745 is in phase II trials for the treatment of alopecia.

INDICATION(S) AND RESEARCH PHASE
Alopecia – Phase II
Benign Prostatic Hyperplasia – NDA submitted

S-doxazosin
unknown

MANUFACTURER
Sepracor

DESCRIPTION
S-doxazosin is the single-isomer version of Cardura, developed and marketed by Pfizer. S-doxazosin has the potential to significantly reduce orthostatic hypotension with a greater potency than Cardura. This drug could reduce the cost of treatment by reducing the number of doctor's visits required for dosage titration. S-doxazosin is currently in phase I study for benign prostatic hyperplasia, BPH.

INDICATION(S) AND RESEARCH PHASE
Benign Prostatic Hyperplasia – Phase I

Erectile Dysfunction

alprostadil
Topiglan

MANUFACTURER
MacroChem Corporation

DESCRIPTION
Topiglan is a topical gel that is being evaluated in phase II and phase III studies for the treatment of male erectile dysfunction. Topiglan is a naturally occurring compound that may relax disease-constricted penile blood vessels in impotent men. This drug is a specific type of biochemical called prostaglandin E-1 (PGE-1), which increases blood flow and may help males to produce an erection.

Topiglan is formulated with a special drug delivery technology, known as SEPA (soft enhancement of percutaneous absorption), that increases absorption across the skin. Previous administrations of Topiglan included injection into the penis with a hypodermic syringe, or insertion into the urethra as a suppository.

Macrochem Corporation reported a preliminary review for a phase IIB double-blind study in which half of the subjects received placebo, and the other half received either the active drug plus the SEPA-formulated gel, or only the SEPA-gel without the drug. The test article was applied topically to the head of the penis in sixty subjects with known erectile dysfunction. Many of the subjects were reported to have previously failed to respond to available therapies, including Viagra, MUSE, and surgical revascularization.

According to the company, the results indicated that Topiglan application was associated with a statistically greater penile rigidity and swelling (tumescence) as compared to placebo, as assessed by physicians. Subject's assessment also rated Topiglan results as better. Six times more subjects stated that the erection produced by using Topiglan was sufficient for vaginal intercourse compared to placebo treated subjects. Treatment was associated with transient, minor to mild symptoms of localized warmth, occasionally mild burning or tingling in some subjects, with no difference observed between the drug and placebo treatments.

A pivotal phase III trial was initiated in July 2000 for impotence and will be conducted at 20 sites and will include 400 subjects. In addition, a phase III trial was initiated in January 2001 for the treatment of male erectile dysfunction.

INDICATION(S) AND RESEARCH PHASE
Impotence – Phase III
Sexual Dysfunction – Phase III
Erectile Dysfuction – Phase III

alprostadil
Alprox-TD, Befar

MANUFACTURER
NexMed

DESCRIPTION

Erectile Dysfunction

Alprox-TD is a topical treatment that contains alprostadil, which has been used for the treatment of erectile dysfunction (ED). Alprostadil is a vasodilator that relaxes blood vessels and increases blood flow. NexMed's Alprox-TD combines alprostadil with the NexACT transdermal penetration enhancing technology. According to NexMed, NexACT contains skin penetration-enhancing molecules that allow a drug to be quickly absorbed to a localized disease site.

Results of a phase II trial of Alprox-TD indicated that three different dose levels of the drug were more effective than placebo in the treatment of mild to moderate ED. The randomized, double-blind, placebo-controlled trial was conducted at 12 clinical sites in the United States. The response to the Global Assessment Questionnaire, which measures improvement in erectile function, indicated an effectiveness rate of 73% in the highest dose group compared to 23% in the placebo group.

Additionally, phase III trials have been completed in China, where Alprox-TD will be marketed as Befar. The company has a New Drug Application for marketing approval pending with the State Drug Administration of China.

INDICATION(S) AND RESEARCH PHASE
Erectile Dysfunction – Phase II completed
Erectile Dysfunction – Application submitted (China)

alprostadil/prazosin hydrochloride
Alibra

MANUFACTURER
Vivus

DESCRIPTION
Alibra is a urethral microsuppository of alprostadil and prazosin hydrochloride and is indicated for the treatment of male erectile dysfunction. An NDA was withdrawn in October 2000 because additional information is needed by the FDA.

INDICATION(S) AND RESEARCH PHASE
Erectile Dysfunction – NDA withdrawn

apomorphine HCl
Uprima

MANUFACTURER
Abbott Laboratories

DESCRIPTION
Uprima is a dopamine receptor agonist being developed in a novel sublingual formulation. This formulation allows for the specific stimulation of parts of the brain involved in the erectile process, thereby replicating the way the body naturally produces an erection.

Uprima has had a somewhat troubled history in terms of safety concerns; however, in January 2001 Abbott Laboratories reported that the European Union's Committee for Proprietary Medicinal Products (CPMP) has adopted a positive opinion on Uprima for the treatment of erectile dysfunction. The CPMP opinion will be considered by the European Commission, which will make a final decision regarding the issue of marketing authorization.

Abbott Laboratories holds non-exclusive rights to Uprima in markets outside the United States and Canada. Abbott licensed the drug from TAP Pharmaceuticals.

INDICATION(S) AND RESEARCH PHASE
Erectile Dysfunction – Phase III

BMS-193884
unknown

MANUFACTURER
Bristol-Myers Squibb

DESCRIPTION
BMS-193884 is an endothelin-A receptor stimulator for both congestive heart failure and male erectile dysfunction. It is made in an oral formulation. Clinical testing is in phase II.

INDICATION(S) AND RESEARCH PHASE
Congestive Heart Failure – Phase II
Erectile Dysfunction – Phase II

BMS-223131
unknown

MANUFACTURER
Bristol-Myers Squibb

DESCRIPTION
BMS-223131 is being developed for the treatment of erectile dysfunction. It is currently in phase I/II development.

INDICATION(S) AND RESEARCH PHASE
Erectile Dysfunction – Phase I/II

IC351
Cialis

MANUFACTURER
Eli Lilly

DESCRIPTION
Cialis (IC351) is an orally administered phosphodiesterase type 5 (PDE5) inhibitor that has been tested in more than 20 phase I and II trials. Cialis targets PDE5, which is an enzyme involved in controlling blood flow to the penis. When PDE5 is inhibited, natural sexual stimuli produce a more pronounced effect, facilitating the ability of men with erectile dysfunction (ED) to attain and maintain an erection.

In November 2000, results of a phase II trial indicated that up to 88% of men taking Cialis reported improved erections relative to placebo. Subjects with mild-to-severe ED were randomized to receive either placebo or Cialis at doses up to 25 mg over an eight-week period. Data obtained from sexual encounter profile diaries showed increased reports from both men and their partners of successful intercourse attempts.

Lilly ICOS has initiated a global phase III trial for ED, and Cialis is also in phase II trials for female sexual dysfunction (FSD).

INDICATION(S) AND RESEARCH PHASE
Erectile Dysfunction – Phase III
Sexual Dysfunction – Phase II

phentolamine mesylate
Vasomax

MANUFACTURER

Zonagen

DESCRIPTION
Vasomax is an oral drug being developed for the treatment of male erectile dysfunction. This drug works by blocking alpha-receptors, which are located on the interior of blood vessels. An NDA has been submitted for Vasomax, which has been approved in Mexico under the name Z-Max. The drug has been developed under and agreement between Schering-Plough and Zonagen.

INDICATION(S) AND RESEARCH PHASE
Erectile Dysfunction – NDA submitted

PT-141
unknown

MANUFACTURER
Palatin Technologies

DESCRIPTION
PT-141 is a synthetic modification of PT-14, which is an analogue of a naturally occurring peptide hormone called alpha MSH. A phase I trial was initiated in January 2001 testing PT-141 as a nasal spray for erectile dysfunction. Results from a small pilot study found PT-141 was approximately 80% effective in treating men with erectile dysfunction.

INDICATION(S) AND RESEARCH PHASE
Erectile Dysfunction – Phase I

(S)-sibutramine
unknown

MANUFACTURER
Sepracor

DESCRIPTION
According to in vitro studies, (S)-sibutramine is a potent inhibitor of both dopamine and norepinephrine. This dual pharmacology may improve both erectile and ejaculatory dysfunction, and a preclinical model has shown that the (S)-sibutramine metabolite facilitates sexual performance. Sepracor is developing (S)-sibutramine as a treatment for both sexual dysfunction and stress urinary incontinence.

INDICATION(S) AND RESEARCH PHASE
Erectile Dysfunction – Phase I
Urinary Incontinence – Phase I

TA-1790
unknown

MANUFACTURER
Vivus

DESCRIPTION
TA-1790 is a highly selective phosphodiesterase type 5 (PDE5) inhibitor. The compound is being developed for the treatment of male and female sexual dysfunction. Vivus has a licensing agreement with Tanabe Seiyaku regarding this product.

INDICATION(S) AND RESEARCH PHASE
Sexual Dysfunction – Phase I
Erectile Dysfunction – Phase I

TAK-251, apomorphine
unknown

MANUFACTURER
Takeda Chemical Industries

DESCRIPTION
TAK-251 is a dopamine receptor agonist in testing for the treatment of erectile dysfunction. The drug is in phase I trials in Japan, phase III trials in the United States and an application has been filed in Europe.

INDICATION(S) AND RESEARCH PHASE
Erectile Dysfunction (Japan) – Phase I
Erectile Dysfunction – Phase III
Erectile Dysfunction – MAA submitted

testosterone
unknown

MANUFACTURER
MacroChem Corporation

DESCRIPTION
This drug product is a SEPA enhanced formulation of testosterone that is being developed for the treatment of male erectile dysfunction. The phase II trial is completed, and the phase III study is pending protocol design modifications.

INDICATION(S) AND RESEARCH PHASE
Erectile Dysfunction – Phase II completed

Transdermal testosterone gel
Tostrex

MANUFACTURER
Cellegy Pharmaceuticals

DESCRIPTION
This transdermal testosterone gel is currently in phase III trials for the treatment of male hormone hypogonadism, a disorder frequently characterized by diminished libido and reduced muscle mass. This hormonal gel is a more convenient treatment than injections and a less irritating alternative to the current patch products.

INDICATION(S) AND RESEARCH PHASE
Male Hormonal Deficiencies/Abnormalities – Phase III
Erectile Dysfunction – Phase II/III

unknown
Daproxetine

MANUFACTURER
PPD Genupro

DESCRIPTION
Daproxetine is a selective serotonin reuptake inhibitor for the treatment of premature ejaculation. Daproxetine has recently completed a phase II trial in thirteen centers throughout the United States. The double-blind, placebo-controlled, three way cross-over study enrolled 155 subjects. It evaluated two different dose levels of the oral drug and placebo. In each period of the study, each subject took the medication 1-3 hours prior to intercourse, and the subject's partner recorded ejaculatory latency in a diary. Each period included four attempts over four weeks. Results showed that daproxetine therapy resulted in a significant prolongation of ejaculatory latency compared to

placebo.

INDICATION(S) AND RESEARCH PHASE
Erectile Dysfunction – Phase II
Sexual Dysfunction – Phase II

unknown
Invicorp

MANUFACTURER
Senetek PLC

DESCRIPTION
Invicorp is a combination of vasoactive intestinal peptide (VIP) and 1 to 2 mg of phentolamine mesylate (PMS). The drug is administered using a novel drug delivery system that makes the self-injection process pain free.

In phase III trials in the United Kingdom, Denmark, Ireland and Australia, an efficacy of 83% was achieved without serious side effects. The most frequent side effect was transient facial flushing which resolved minutes after using Invicorp.

Invicorp has received approval for the treatment of erectile dysfunction in the United Kingdom, Denmark and New Zealand. In the United States, the FDA has upgraded the status of the Invicorp IND to a partial clinical hold.

INDICATION(S) AND RESEARCH PHASE
Erectile Dysfunction – Phase III

vardenafil
unknown

MANUFACTURER
Bayer Corporation

DESCRIPTION
Vardenafil is a phosphodiesterase type 5 (PDE5) inhibitor being developed for the treatment of erectile dysfunction (ED). Phase II results indicated that men with ED reported a significant increase in their ability to achieve erection and complete intercourse with ejaculation after vardenafil treatment. The drug is currently in phase III trials.

INDICATION(S) AND RESEARCH PHASE
Erectile Dysfunction – Phase III

Genital Herpes

APL400-024Px
Genevax - HSV-Px

MANUFACTURER
Wyeth-Lederle Vaccines

DESCRIPTION
HSV-Px is a novel facilitated DNA vaccine for prevention of herpes simplex virus-2 (HSV-2) infection that causes genital herpes. This vaccine uses injected Genevax delivery technology and it is in phase II trials.

INDICATION(S) AND RESEARCH PHASE
Genital Herpes – Phase II

GW 419458, DISC-HSV
unknown

MANUFACTURER
GlaxoSmithKline

DESCRIPTION
DISC (disabled infectious single cycle)-HSV is an immunotherapeutic vaccine using a disabled live virus for treatment and prevention of genital herpes. Since the drug therapy induces a natural immune response and may promote "immunologic memory," the chance of disease recurrence is drastically reduced. It also eliminates the need for constant dosing, thereby increasing subject compliance and improving lifestyle. The drug is in phase II trials for genital herpes. GlaxoSmithKline has worldwide development and marketing rights.

INDICATION(S) AND RESEARCH PHASE
Genital Herpes – Phase II

resiquimod
unknown

MANUFACTURER
3M Pharmaceuticals

DESCRIPTION
Resiquimod is in phase III trials for recurrent genital herpes in both the United States and Europe. In November 2000, positive phase II results of a double-blind, placebo-controlled trial were reported. In the six month follow-up, the time to the first recurrence was significantly increased and the total number of recurrences was significantly decreased for subjects on active study medication compared to a placebo gel.

INDICATION(S) AND RESEARCH PHASE
Genital Herpes – Phase III

TA-HSV
unknown

MANUFACTURER
Cantab Pharmaceuticals plc

DESCRIPTION
TA-HSV (therapeutic antigen-herpes simplex virus) is a genetically disabled vaccine containing HSV that allows only a single cycle of replication within a host cell. It is in phase II trials for the treatment of genital herpes.

INDICATION(S) AND RESEARCH PHASE
Genital Herpes – Phase II

unknown
Docosanol

MANUFACTURER
AVANIR Pharmaceuticals

DESCRIPTION
Docosanol is approved as a treatment for cold sores and fever blisters. It is in phase III trials for the treatment of genital herpes. Docosanol works by inhibiting fusion between the plasma membrane and the herpes simplex virus (HSV) envelope, thereby preventing viral entry into cells and subsequent viral replication. Since the compound doesn't act directly on the virus, it is unlikely it will produce drug resistant mutants of HSV. All known competitive Rx products

work by inhibition of viral DNA replication and, as such, carry risk of mutating the virus.

INDICATION(S) AND RESEARCH PHASE
Genital Herpes – Phase III

vaccine, genital herpes
Simplirix

MANUFACTURER
GlaxoSmithKline

DESCRIPTION
Simplirix is a recombinant vaccine being developed for genital herpes prophylaxis. Simplirix consists of a recombinant glycoprotein from herpes simplex virus 2 (HSV-2), in combination with an adjuvant "derivative endotoxin." Results of two large, placebo-controlled, randomized international trials were reported; both were "discordant partner studies," in which one of the partners had genital herpes and the other did not. The first trial included 847 subjects who tested negative for HSV-1 and HSV-2 at baseline, and the second trial involved 1867 subjects who were negative for HSV-2. The vaccine had "absolutely no effect" in the men in either group; however, a notable effect was observed in the women. In the first study, the vaccine efficacy in women was 73%. Similarly, among the seronegative women in the second study, the vaccine efficacy was 74%. The vaccine was not protective in the women who were HSV-1-positive and HSV-2-negative.

INDICATION(S) AND RESEARCH PHASE
Genital Herpes – Phase II
Vaccines – Phase II

vaccine, genital herpes
unknown

MANUFACTURER
Corixa Montana

DESCRIPTION
This immunostimulant vaccine uses monophosphoryl lipid A (MPL) adjuvant for prevention and treatment of herpes simplex virus types I and II that causes genital herpes. The vaccine is in phase III trials.

INDICATION(S) AND RESEARCH PHASE
Genital Herpes – Phase III
Herpes Simplex Infections – Phase III

Male Hormonal Deficiencies/ Abnormalities

dihydrotestosterone
Andractim

MANUFACTURER
Unimed Pharmaceuticals

DESCRIPTION
Andractim is a hormone replacement therapy for the treatment of male testosterone deficiency. It is being tested in phase III trials for geriatric hypogonadism, a condition characterized by abnormally decreased sexual function of the testes in elderly males. Additionally, this anabolic steroid is also being tested in phase II trials for the treatment of weight loss associated with HIV wasting in AIDS subjects. Andractim is a clear, odorless, non-irritating, topical gel that delivers dihydrotestosterone transdermally to the bloodstream. Dihydrotestosterone is a natural male hormone that can assist in building muscle mass. Unimed Pharmaceuticals has a collaborative agreement with BioChem Pharma to develop Andractim, which is licensed from Laboratoires Besins Iscovesco S.A., France.

INDICATION(S) AND RESEARCH PHASE
Acquired Immune Deficiency Syndrome (AIDS) and AIDS-Related Infections – Phase II
Male Hormonal Deficiencies/Abnormalities – Phase III

testosterone
Androsorb

MANUFACTURER
Novavax

DESCRIPTION
Androsorb is a cream for testosterone replacement therapy in phase II clinical trials for testosterone deficient men and phase I trials for post-menopausal women. Phase phase I trial will test 21 postmenopausal women at two sites. Androsorb is being developed using Novavax's proprietary micellar nanoparticle technology, a microemulsion drug delivery platform.

INDICATION(S) AND RESEARCH PHASE
Male Hormonal Deficiencies/Abnormalities – Phase II
Menopause – Phase I

testosterone
unknown

MANUFACTURER
Watson Pharmaceuticals

DESCRIPTION
Testosterone is a naturally produced hormone, which is responsible for proper development of male secondary sex characteristics. This hormone which has been formulated in the MTX transdermal patch is being tested in phase II trials for several indications, which include the treatment of sexual dysfunction in surgically menopausal subjects, menopause associated hormone replacement therapy, and osteoporosis. Additionally, this drug is in phase III clinical trials for male hormonal deficiencies and abnormalities and treatment of female AIDS wasting.

INDICATION(S) AND RESEARCH PHASE
Acquired Immune Deficiency Syndrome (AIDS) and AIDS-Related Infections – Phase II
Hormone Replacement Therapy: Menopause – Phase II
Male Hormonal Deficiencies/Abnormalities – Phase III
Osteoporosis – Phase II
Sexual Dysfunction – Phase II completed

transdermal testosterone gel
Tostrex

MANUFACTURER
Cellegy Pharmaceuticals

DESCRIPTION
This transdermal testosterone gel is currently in phase III trials for the treatment of male hormone hypogonadism, a disorder frequently characterized by diminished libido and reduced muscle mass. This hormonal gel is a more convenient treatment than injections and a less irritating alternative to the current patch products.

INDICATION(S) AND RESEARCH PHASE
Male Hormonal Deficiencies/Abnormalities – Phase III
Impotence – Phase II/III

Peyronie's Disease

collagenase for injection
Cordase

MANUFACTURER
Biospecifics Technologies

DESCRIPTION
Cordase is an injectable formulation of purified collagenase, an enzyme that induces changes in collagen causing it to degrade within the connective tissue. This drug is currently in phase II testing for Dupuytren's disease, a contracture deformity that may cause the fingers to become stuck in a flexed position. Cordase is considered an orphan drug since there are limited therapies for this uncommon condition. Research is under development by Advance Biofactures, a subsidiary of Biospecifics Technologies.

INDICATION(S) AND RESEARCH PHASE
Dupuytren's Disease – Phase II
Peyronie's Disease – Phase II
Adhesive Capsulitis – Phase II

Premature Ejaculation

paroxetine HCl
unknown

MANUFACTURER
Pentech Pharmaceuticals

DESCRIPTION
Paroxetine HCl is a selective serotonin reuptake inhibitor (SSRI) being tested by Pentech for the treatment of premature ejaculation. The drug is currently in phase III trials.

INDICATION(S) AND RESEARCH PHASE
Premature Ejaculation – Phase III

Prostate Cancer

abarelix depot, PPI-149
unknown

MANUFACTURER
Praecis Pharmaceuticals

DESCRIPTION
Approximately 85% of newly diagnosed prostate cancers are hormone-dependent tumors that require the male hormone testosterone for their continued growth. Lowering the body's normal production of testosterone, therefore, is the primary goal of hormonal treatment. However, available hormonal therapies may cause an initial surge or increase in the level of testosterone before the desired effect of lowering testosterone occurs. Abarelix depot is designed to rapidly block the production of testosterone and avoid the initial testosterone level surge. An NDA was submitted in December 2000.
  Additionally, a multisite, blinded phase II/III trial of abarelix depot for the treatment of endometriosis is under way. Subject enrollment in this study is complete, with 365 subjects enrolled. Praecis is developing abarelix depot under an agreement with Amgen and Sanofi-Synthelabo.

INDICATION(S) AND RESEARCH PHASE
Prostate Cancer – NDA submitted
Endometriosis – Phase II/III

abiraterone acetate
unknown

MANUFACTURER
BTG International

DESCRIPTION
Abiraterone acetate, an approved drug in the United Kingdom, inhibits both testicular and adrenal androgen production by selective inhibition of 17 alpha-hydroxylase/C17-20 lyase, the key enzyme in the androgen biosynthetic pathway. Due to abiraterone acetate's high inhibitory potency, a phase I trial for the treatment of prostate cancer was conducted. The trial examined the effects of single or multiple doses of abiraterone acetate in chemically castrated or untreated subjects. Results indicated that the drug is a potent inhibitor of testosterone production and can itself reduce testosterone to sub-castrate levels.

INDICATION(S) AND RESEARCH PHASE
Prostate Cancer – Phase I completed

ABT-627
unknown

MANUFACTURER
Abbott Laboratories

DESCRIPTION
ABT-627 is a drug that is being developed to halt the progression of late-stage, metastatic prostate cancer. Cancer requires the growth of blood vessels that will nourish the cancer cells as they grow and divide. If there is a limited blood supply, the cancer cells will die and the growth of the tumor will be slowed. ABT-627 acts to restrict the blood supply to newly forming cancer cells.
  ABT-627 blocks the action of a potent substance in the body (endothelin-A). This substance is a strong constrictor of blood vessels that also stimulates cell proliferation. By preventing the action of endothelin-A, it is thought that blood vessel and cancer cell growth will be slowed or halted altogether.

In initial trials, ABT-627 decreased the amount of a prostate protein (PSA) that is used to monitor the progression of prostate cancer therapy. Additionally, the drug decreased pain resulting from cancerous spread to the bone, and it enabled subjects to decrease their narcotic use.

This new medication has shown that it can stabilize the progression of prostate cancer for up to fifteen months and improve the quality of life of prostate cancer subjects. Phase II studies are currently under way.

INDICATION(S) AND RESEARCH PHASE
Prostate Cancer – Phase II

APC8015
Provenge

MANUFACTURER
Dendreon Corporation

DESCRIPTION
Provenge is a dendritic exvivo cell therapy being tested for the treatment of advanced prostate cancer. The aim of the therapy is to heighten the immunologic response to cancer cells by removing dendritic cells from a subject, pulsing them with a prostate cancer antigen, and reinjecting them into the subject. The dendritic cells help the immune system by attaching pieces of the tumor proteins to their own surface and presenting them to lymphocytes, which then learn to recognize the antigens as foreign matter and attack them.

Phase II trial results published in December 2000 indicated that Provenge was safe, well tolerated, and stimulated an immune response in subjects with prostate cancer. Phase III trials are under way throughout the United States.

INDICATION(S) AND RESEARCH PHASE
Prostate Cancer – Phase III

arsenic trioxide (ATO)
Trisenox

MANUFACTURER
Cell Therapeutics

DESCRIPTION
Trisenox is believed to kill cancer cells through apoptosis. The mechanism of action of Trisenox is not fully understood, but the drug appears to induce apoptosis in a different manner than other anti-cancer agents such as retinoids.

Trisenox is FDA approved to treat acute promyelocytic leukemia (APL), and it is also in numerous trials in the United States for indications including other types of leukemia, prostate cancer, multiple myeloma, renal cell cancer, cervical cancer, and bladder cancer.

INDICATION(S) AND RESEARCH PHASE
Leukemia – Phase I
Lymphoma, Non-Hodgkin's – Phase II
Leukemia – Phase II
Multiple Myeloma – Phase II
Prostate Cancer – Phase II
Renal Cell Carcinoma – Phase II
Cervical Dysplasia/Cancer – Phase II
Bladder Cancer – Phase II

bicalutimide
Casodex

MANUFACTURER
AstraZeneca

DESCRIPTION
Casodex is a non-steroidal anti-androgen for the treatment of advanced prostate cancer. Prostate cancer is known to be sensitive to androgen—it responds to treatment that counteracts the effects of androgen and/or removes the source of androgen. Data suggest that this oral hormonal medication shows no statistical difference in overall survival or time-to-progression when compared to castration in subjects with non-metastatic, locally advanced prostate cancer. The company has submitted a supplemental NDA for this indication. Casodex is given in an oral tablet form.

INDICATION(S) AND RESEARCH PHASE
Prostate Cancer – Phase sNDA submitted

CEP-2563
unknown

MANUFACTURER
Cephalon

DESCRIPTION
CEP-2563 is an orally active inhibitor of tyrosine kinase. It is currently in phase I development for the treatment of prostate cancer. Cephalon has CEP-2563 development agreements with TAP Pharmaceuticals and Abbott Laboratories.

INDICATION(S) AND RESEARCH PHASE
Prostate Cancer – Phase I

CEP-701
unknown

MANUFACTURER
Cephalon

DESCRIPTION
CEP-701 is an orally active inhibitor of the enzyme tyrosine kinase. It is being evaluated in phase II studies for prostate cancer and pancreatic ductal adenocarcinoma.

INDICATION(S) AND RESEARCH PHASE
Pancreatic Cancer – Phase II
Prostate Cancer – Phase II

CT-2584
Apra

MANUFACTURER
Cell Therapeutics

DESCRIPTION
Apra is a novel synthetic inhibitor of phosphatidic acid metabolism in tumor cells. This antineoplastic agent kills cancer cells without having to depend on cell division to exert its effect. Additionally, Apra may also help inhibit multi-drug resistance of certain cancers. The drug is in trials for the treatment of prostate cancer and sarcomas. Additional indications may include cancers of the colon, breast, and female reproductive system including the ovaries.

INDICATION(S) AND RESEARCH PHASE
Prostate Cancer – Phase II
Sarcoma – Phase II

CTP-37
Avicine

MANUFACTURER
AVI BioPharma

DESCRIPTION
Avicine is a hormone vaccine derived from human chorionic gonadotropin peptide that is being tested for prevention of colorectal, pancreatic, and prostate cancer. The drug is in phase II trials for prostate cancer, and phase III trials for colorectal and pancreatic cancer. AVI BioPharma has partnered with SuperGen and under the terms of the agreement, SuperGen will be responsible for U.S. marketing and sales of Avicine, and AVI will be responsible for product manufacturing.

INDICATION(S) AND RESEARCH PHASE
Colorectal Cancer – Phase III
Pancreatic Cancer – Phase III
Prostate Cancer – Phase II

CV706
unknown

MANUFACTURER
Calydon

DESCRIPTION
CV706 is an oncolytic virus that is able to replicate in and kill targeted cancer cells, leaving non-cancer cells unharmed. It is currently in development for the treatment of prostate cancer. In October 2000, phase I/II trial results indicated that CV706 displayed anti-tumor activity and that the drug was well tolerated. Subjects showing the greatest anti-tumor response were treated at one of the top two doses evaluated; four of these 11 subjects exhibited a prostate specific antigen (PSA) partial response, defined as a 50% or greater reduction in serum PSA for at least four weeks. In three of the subjects, their partial response lasted at least nine months. PSA levels decreased from baseline in nine of the 11 subjects (80%) treated in the top two dose groups. A study of post-treatment biopsy samples demonstrated that adenoviral replication—the mechanism upon which CV706 has been designed to both target and kill prostate cancer cells—had occurred in subjects.

INDICATION(S) AND RESEARCH PHASE
Prostate Cancer – Phase I/II completed

CV787
unknown

MANUFACTURER
Calydon

DESCRIPTION
CV787 is a genetically engineered adenovirus type 5 that is cytolytic to cells expressing prostate specific antigen (PSA). It is being evaluated in a phase I/II trial in subjects with locally recurrent prostate cancer following definitive radiotherapy and/or brachytherapy. The phase I/II trial is an open-label, dose finding study designed to determine the safety and tolerance of an injection of CV787 directly into the prostate. The trial is being conducted at six hospitals in the United States.

INDICATION(S) AND RESEARCH PHASE
Prostate Cancer – Phase I/II

cVax-Pr
unknown

MANUFACTURER
Jenner BioTherapies

DESCRIPTION
cVax-Pr is a vaccine designed from DNA pieces from a protein (prostate-specific antigen, PSA) found in both healthy and cancerous prostate cancer cells. Scientists add molecules to this DNA that stimulate the body's immune system. In this manner, the body is manipulated into recognizing PSA-DNA as foreign material. Consequently, this immune response attacks both normal and cancerous prostate cells.

In preliminary studies, administration of cVax-Pr stimulated antibody and white blood cell production. cVax-Pr is being tested in phase II trials.

INDICATION(S) AND RESEARCH PHASE
Prostate Cancer – Phase II

doxorubicin HCl
Doxil, Caelyx

MANUFACTURER
Alza (Sequus Pharmaceuticals)

DESCRIPTION
Doxil is a liposomal formulation of doxorubicin hydrochloride, an intravenous chemotherapy agent. This anthracycline anti-tumor agent is currently on the market for the treatment of Kaposi's sarcoma. The drug uses a novel, targeted delivery system to help evade recognition and uptake by the immune system so that the liposomes can circulate in the body longer. A long circulation time increases the likelihood that the liposomes and their pharmaceutical contents will reach their targeted tumor site. Doxil may act through its ability to bind DNA and inhibit nucleic acid synthesis.

Doxil is being tested in trials for the treatment of breast, liver, lung, and prostate cancers, as well as for unspecified cancers and tumors.

Alza markets this product in the United States under the tradename Doxil; however, it is marketed under the name Caelyx in other areas. Schering-Plough has exclusive international marketing rights to Caelyx, excluding Japan and Israel, through a distribution agreement with Alza.

INDICATION(S) AND RESEARCH PHASE
Breast Cancer – Phase II/III
Liver Cancer – Phase II/III
Lung Cancer – Phase II/III
Prostate Cancer – Phase II/III
Cancer/Tumors (Unspecified) – Phase II

DPPE
unknown

MANUFACTURER
Bristol-Myers Squibb

DESCRIPTION
DPPE is being developed to potentiate the effects of chemotherapy in subjects with late-stage prostate cancer. There are many

substances in the body that play a role in the regulation of cell growth. When there is an imbalance or problem with one of these regulatory substances, uncontrolled cell growth or cancer may result.

An example of one such substance is histamine, which acts as a growth factor in both normal and cancer cells. It spurs cell growth by stimulating growth receptors located within the cell.

DPPE is a drug designed to block these receptors for histamine. By blocking the effects of histamine, it is proposed that unregulated cell growth will decrease. When given with standard chemotherapy agents, DPPE may help these agents better destroy cancer cells.

INDICATION(S) AND RESEARCH PHASE
Prostate Cancer – Phase II

eflornithine, DFMO (difluoromethylornydil)
unknown

MANUFACTURER
Aventis

DESCRIPTION
Eflornithine is a potent, irreversible inhibitor of ornithine decarboxylase (OCD), an enzyme that is elevated in most tumors and pre-malignant lesions. Eflornithine is currently in a phase III clinical trial to determine the effectiveness of the drug in treating subjects who have newly diagnosed or recurrent bladder cancer. The drug is administered orally in tablet form.

Eflornithine is also in trials for the prevention and treatment of HIV infections, skin cancer, breast cancer, prostate cancer and cervical dysplasia/cancer.

INDICATION(S) AND RESEARCH PHASE
Bladder Cancer – Phase III
Breast Cancer – Phase II/III
Cervical Dysplasia/Cancer – Phase II
HIV Infection – Phase II
Prostate Cancer – Phase II
Skin Cancer – Phase III

exisulind
Aptosyn/LHRH agonist

MANUFACTURER
Cell Pathways

DESCRIPTION
Aptosyn (exisulind) belongs to a novel class of compounds called selective apoptotic anti-neoplastic drugs (SAANDs). SAANDs inhibit a form of cyclic GMP phosphodiesterase and selectively induce apoptosis in abnormally growing precancerous and cancerous cells. Aptosyn is being tested with LHRH agonist hormone therapy for the treatment of prostate cancer. The objective of this study is to determine the preliminary efficacy of Aptosyn in subjects who are receiving LHRH agonist hormone therapy and have rising prostate specific antigen (PSA) levels. This open-label, 12-month phase II trial will include 15 subjects.

INDICATION(S) AND RESEARCH PHASE
Prostate Cancer – Phase II

exisulind
Aptosyn

MANUFACTURER
Cell Pathways

DESCRIPTION
Aptosyn (exisulind) belongs to a novel class of compounds called selective apoptotic anti-neoplastic drugs (SAANDs). SAANDs inhibit a form of cyclic GMP phosphodiesterase and selectively induce apoptosis in abnormally growing precancerous and cancerous cells. Aptosyn is being tested for several indications and is in five different trials for adenomatous polyposis coli (APC) and familial adenomatous polyposis coli; two of these trials are specifically for pediatric subjects.

The company received a non-approvable letter from the FDA in September 2000 for one of the trials for familial adenomatous polyposis. The company intends to amend the NDA and request a meeting to address the deficiencies and the possible requirement for additional clinical data.

Additionally, Aptosyn is being tested in trials for the treatment of prostate cancer, lung cancer, breast cancer, sporadic colonic polyps, and Barrett's esophagus disease.

INDICATION(S) AND RESEARCH PHASE
Adenomatous Polyposis Coli – Phase non-approvable letter
Pediatric, Familial Adenomatous Polyposis Coli – Phase II
Adenomatous Polyposis Coli – Phase I/II
Barrett's Esophagus Disease – Phase II
Prostate Cancer – Phase II/III
Breast Cancer – Phase II/III
Lung Cancer – Phase Ib
Colon Polyps – Phase II/III

exisulind/docetaxel
Aposyn/Taxotere

MANUFACTURER
Cell Pathways

DESCRIPTION
Aptosyn (exisulind) belongs to a novel class of compounds called selective apoptotic anti-neoplastic drugs (SAANDs). SAANDs inhibit a form of cyclic GMP phosphodiesterase and selectively induce apoptosis in abnormally growing precancerous and cancerous cells. Because SAANDs do not induce apoptosis in normal cells, they do not produce the serious side effects normally associated with traditional chemotherapeutic agents. They also do not inhibit cyclooxygenase (COX I or COX II) and have not exhibited the gastric and renal toxicities associated with non-steroidal anti-inflammatory drugs (NSAIDs), including the COX II inhibitors.

Aptosyn is being tested with Rhone-Poulenc Rorer's Taxotere for the treatment of prostate, lung, and breast cancer as well as for solid tumors. Both companies will jointly share the cost of the trials and will retain all marketing rights to its respective products.

INDICATION(S) AND RESEARCH PHASE
Prostate Cancer – Phase I/II
Breast Cancer – Phase I/II
Lung Cancer – Phase I/II
Lung Cancer – Phase III
Cancer/Tumors (Unspecified) – Phase I

FK-317
unknown

MANUFACTURER
Fujisawa Healthcare

DESCRIPTION
Fujisawa has developed a new anti-cancer medication, FK-317, that originally was developed as an antibiotic. The molecule, known as a dihydrobenzoxazine, underwent preliminary testing in thirty-one subjects with solid tumors that were refractory to other chemotherapeutic treatments. The company reported that tumor reduction was observed in four subjects, two of whom achieved complete remission. Side effects and other toxicities such as leukopenia (decreased white blood cells) and neutropenia were modest in comparison to other established treatments.

It is unclear how exactly this compound works to limit the growth of cancer, but it seems to influence the process by which cells reproduce themselves. Currently, FK-317 is given at a dose of 24mg/day intravenously and it is being evaluated in phase II trials. Scientists are testing it in a variety of solid tumors such as prostate, breast, and skin cancer.

INDICATION(S) AND RESEARCH PHASE
Breast Cancer – Phase II
Cancer/Tumors (Unspecified) – Phase II
Prostate Cancer – Phase II
Skin Cancer – Phase II

G3139/mitoxantrone
Genasense/mitoxantrone

MANUFACTURER
Genta

DESCRIPTION
Genasense (G3139) is designed to reduce levels of bcl-2, a protein that contributes to the resistance of cancer cells to current forms of cancer treatment. Treatment with Genasense may markedly improve the effectiveness of standard anticancer therapies; it is being tested in combination with mitoxantrone for treatment of prostate and colorectal cancers.

INDICATION(S) AND RESEARCH PHASE
Colorectal Cancer – Phase II
Prostate Cancer – Phase I/II

G3139/docetaxel
Genasense/Taxotere

MANUFACTURER
Genta

DESCRIPTION
Genasense (G3139) attacks Bcl-2, a protein that is over-expressed in many forms of cancer. Bcl-2 appears to contribute to the resistance of these diseases to standard treatment. Genta is using its proprietary antisense approach to first decrease the expression of Bcl-2, and then to administer state-of-the-art anticancer therapy in an effort to improve subject outcome. Genasense in combination with docetaxel is in trials for treatment of breast and prostate cancer.

INDICATION(S) AND RESEARCH PHASE
Breast Cancer – Phase I/II
Prostate Cancer – Phase II

G3139/androgen blockade
Genasense/androgen blockade

MANUFACTURER
Genta

DESCRIPTION
Genasense (G3139) is designed to reduce levels of bcl-2, a protein that contributes to the resistance of cancer cells to current forms of cancer treatment. Genasense in combination with androgen blockade is in phase I/II trials for the treatment of androgen-insensitive metastatic prostate cancer.

INDICATION(S) AND RESEARCH PHASE
Prostate Cancer – Phase I/II

GBC-590
unknown

MANUFACTURER
Safe Sciences

DESCRIPTION
GBC-590 belongs to a new class of drugs called lectin inhibitors that specifically interfere with cellular interactions. GBC-590 competitively binds to unique lectins (special protein cell-surface receptors) on cancer cells and disrupts the metastatic process. GBC-590's affinity for cancer lectins is the core reason for its significant biological activity and specificity.

GBC-590 is being tested in phase II studies for pancreatic and colorectal cancer, and the company plans to test it in phase II trials for prostate cancer.

INDICATION(S) AND RESEARCH PHASE
Colorectal Cancer – Phase II
Pancreatic Cancer – Phase II
Prostate Cancer – Phase I/II

gallium maltolate
unknown

MANUFACTURER
Titan Pharmaceuticals

DESCRIPTION
Gallium is a semi-metallic element that has shown some therapeutic activity in metabolic bone disease, hypercalcemia of malignancy and cancer. Gallium maltolate can displace divalent iron from the iron transporting protein, transferrin; thus gallium maltolate causes interference with iron metabolism with inhibition of enzymes requiring divalent iron. The most important of these in the cancer setting appears to be ribonucleotide reductase (RNR). Additionally, gallium appears to form salts with calcium and phosphate and become incorporated into bone. The bone that is created with incorporated gallium appears to be at least as strong as normal bone, and it appears to be more resistant to degradation by osteoclasts and tumor cells.

INDICATION(S) AND RESEARCH PHASE
Prostate Cancer – Phase I/II
Lymphomas – Phase I/II
Myeloma – Phase I/II
Bladder Cancer – Phase I/II

HIV Infection – Phase I/II

IM862
unknown

MANUFACTURER
Cytran

DESCRIPTION
IM862 is a small peptide comprised of two amino acids that may inhibit new blood vessel formation (angiogenesis). When there is excessive growth of new blood vessels, a number of pathological conditions result, including malignant tumors, age-related macular degeneration, and vascular diseases. Limiting the growth of new blood vessels in tumors deprives them of nourishment and can ultimately kill these cancers. This drug is being developed in phase III trials for Kaposi's sarcoma and phase I/II trials for ovarian cancer.

INDICATION(S) AND RESEARCH PHASE
Kaposi's Sarcoma – Phase III
Ovarian Cancer – Phase I/II
Malignant Melanoma – Preclinical
Prostate Cancer – Preclinical

IMC-C225, CPT-11
unknown

MANUFACTURER
ImClone Systems

DESCRIPTION
IMC-C225 is a chimerized (part mouse, part human) monoclonal antibody that may help fight cancer cells when used in conjunction with radiation therapy or other chemotherapy agents. This antibody selectively blocks the epidermal growth factor receptor (EGFr), which may be present in greater amounts on actively growing tumor cells. Since many cancers use specific growth factors to stimulate tumor cell growth, blocking this receptor may inhibit the cancer from increasing in size and spreading throughout the body.

The company is conducting phase III clinical trials evaluating IMC-C225 in combination with radiotherapy and with chemotherapy in subjects with advanced squamous cell head and neck carcinoma. IMC-C225 is in trials for several other indications in combination with various anticancer agents.

INDICATION(S) AND RESEARCH PHASE
Breast Cancer – Phase I/II
Head and Neck Cancer – Phase III
Lung Cancer – Phase III
Prostate Cancer – Phase I/II
Renal Cell Carcinoma – Phase II
Pancreatic Cancer – Phase II
Colorectal Cancer – Phase II

INGN-201, adenoviral p53
unknown

MANUFACTURER
Introgen Therapeutics

DESCRIPTION
INGN-201 is a p53 gene therapy product. It has been tested as a treatment for a variety of solid tumor cancers with administration via intratumoral injection. The drug was well tolerated according to the company, and additional trials are under way using an intravenous infusion in order to reach more types of cancers. The tumor-suppressing p53 gene encodes a protein that responds to damage involving cellular DNA by terminating cell division. Normal p53 genes are delivered into cancer cells of the subject through an adenoviral vector.

The developers of INGN-201 have signed a Cooperative Research and Development Agreement (CRADA) with the National Cancer Institute to evaluate the potential effectiveness and superiority of the drug over other treatments against breast, ovarian, bladder, prostate, and brain cancers in phase I and phase II trials. A phase III trial in head and neck cancer was initiated in March 2000.

INDICATION(S) AND RESEARCH PHASE
Head and Neck Cancer – Phase III
Bladder Cancer – Phase I
Brain Cancer – Phase I
Breast Cancer – Phase I
Bronchoalveolar Cancer – Phase I
Ovarian Cancer – Phase I
Prostate Cancer – Phase I
Lung Cancer – Phase II
Cancer/Tumors (Unspecified) – Phase I

interleukin (IL)
MultiKine

MANUFACTURER
CEL-SCI Corporation

DESCRIPTION
MultiKine is a multiple combination therapy made from a natural, cytokine cocktail (which includes Interleukin-2 (IL-2), IL-β, TNF-α, Gm-CSF and an IFN-γ/immunomodulator). It is being tested for the treatment of advanced head and neck cancer in subjects who have previously failed standard therapy, and for head and neck cancer treatment prior to surgery.

MultiKine has just completed two phase II trials for head and neck cancer. The first trial consisted of 16 subjects and tested four different doses of MultiKine in four subjects each. To qualify for the trial, the subjects must have had a recurrence of the cancer and failed conventional therapy.

The company reported that in an earlier and still ongoing study conducted in newly diagnosed head and neck cancer subjects, 10 subjects had tumor reductions prior to surgery within a short time period. Three of ten subjects had tumor reductions exceeding 50%, and one additional subject with a tumor that was nearly three inches in diameter had a complete clinical response. Lastly, two subjects refused surgery because they were satisfied with their condition after treatment with MultiKine.

INDICATION(S) AND RESEARCH PHASE
Head and Neck Cancer – Phase II
HIV Infection – Phase II
Breast Cancer – Phase I
Prostate Cancer – Phase I/II

ISIS-5132, CGP-69846A
unknown

MANUFACTURER
Isis Pharmaceuticals

DESCRIPTION

ISIS-5132 is a potent antisense inhibitor of the enzyme c-Raf-1 kinase. Antisense drugs inhibit the production of disease-causing proteins by altering the genetic information that messenger RNA uses to produce new protein. c-Raf kinase plays a role in signal processes that regulate cell growth and proliferation. It is one of a family of Raf genes thought to play an important role in the development of some solid tumors. The company reports that activated-Raf has also been detected in a substantial variety of human cancers including small cell lung carcinoma and breast cancer. For example, it has been reported that 60% of all lung carcinoma cells express unusually high levels of normal c-Raf mRNA and protein.

The sponsor companies reported that results from phase I studies, which examined subjects with a wide variety of solid tumors, demonstrated that the drug was well tolerated and that several subjects experienced disease stabilization. The companies are planning additional phase I safety studies involving the drug in combination with currently approved chemotherapies. Phase II clinical trials examining ISIS-5132 as a single agent therapy in subjects with breast, lung, colon, pancreatic, and prostate cancers are under way.

INDICATION(S) AND RESEARCH PHASE

Breast Cancer – Phase II
Cancer/Tumors (Unspecified) – Phase II
Colon Malignancies – Phase II
Lung Cancer – Phase II
Pancreatic Cancer – Phase II
Prostate Cancer – Phase II

LDI-200
unknown

MANUFACTURER
Milkhaus Laboratory

DESCRIPTION
Clinical trials are testing a subcutanous formulation of LDI-200 for at least three indications: leukemia, myelodysplastic syndrome, and prostate cancer. Results demonstrated that LDI-200 showed both efficacy and safety in a small phase II/III open label crossover trial in subjects with myelodysplastic syndrome. The control consisted of subjects given supportive therapy, consisting of transfusions and antibiotics, who became eligible for treatment if their disease progressed more rapidly than anticipated. A total of 23 subjects were treated using LDI-200, and 7 showed significant clinical response.

INDICATION(S) AND RESEARCH PHASE
Leukemia – Phase II completed
Prostate Cancer – Phase II/III
White Blood Cell Disorders – Phase II/III
Myelodysplastic Syndrome – Phase III completed

leuprolide acetate
30-day Leuprogel

MANUFACTURER
Atrix Laboratories

DESCRIPTION
30-day Leuprogel is a new Atrigel formulation that contains leuprolide acetate. The product is injected subcutaneously as a liquid, where it solidifies and releases a predetermined amount of leuprolide. The sustained levels of leuprolide result in decreased testosterone levels, which in turn suppress tumor growth in subjects with hormone-responsive prostate cancer. Leuprogel has an advantage over current treatments due to its delivery by subcutaneous injection and small volume (compared to commonly used large volume intramuscular injection).

INDICATION(S) AND RESEARCH PHASE
Prostate Cancer – Phase III

leuprolide acetate
3-month Leuprogel

MANUFACTURER
Atrix Laboratories

DESCRIPTION
Atrix recently announced the early completion of enrollment for a Leuprogel 3-month 22.5 mg phase III trial. This drug is in development for the treatment of prostate cancer.

INDICATION(S) AND RESEARCH PHASE
Prostate Cancer – Phase III

liposomal ether lipid
TLC ELL-12

MANUFACTURER
The Liposome Company

DESCRIPTION
TLC ELL-12 is a liposomal ether lipid that may have efficacy in the treatment of several cancers. This drug has exhibited significant anti-tumor activity, but did not have the hemolytic side effects common to this type of ether lipid when therapeutic doses were used in experimental models. It does not appear to be myelosuppressive.

TLC ELL-12 is currently being developed in phase I trials for the treatment of lung cancer, multiple myeloma, leukemia, and prostate cancer.

INDICATION(S) AND RESEARCH PHASE
Lung Cancer – Phase I
Multiple Myeloma – Phase I
Leukemia – Phase I
Prostate Cancer – Phase I

unknown
Prinomastat

MANUFACTURER
Agouron Pharmaceuticals

DESCRIPTION
Prinomastat is an orally active, synthetic molecule designed to potently and selectively inhibit certain members of a family of enzymes known as a matrix metalloproteases, which are believed to be involved in tumor angiogenesis, invasion, and metastasis. The drug is in trials for various indications, including osteoarthritis, brain cancer, and macular degeneration.

Two phase III trials for advanced non-small cell lung cancer and prostate cancer were halted in August 2000 due to the drug's lack of effectiveness in subjects with late-stage disease.

The most common side effects of Prinomastat have been observed in the joints, and include stiffness, joint swelling, and in a few subjects, some limits on the mobility of certain joints, most often in the shoulders and hands. All these effects were reported to be reversible and were effectively managed by treatment rests and dose reductions.

INDICATION(S) AND RESEARCH PHASE
Lung Cancer – Phase III halted
Prostate Cancer – Phase III halted
Osteoarthritis – Phase II
Brain Cancer – Phase II
Macular Degeneration – Phase II

MDX-210
unknown

MANUFACTURER
Medarex

DESCRIPTION
MDX-210 is a bispecific (target-trigger) monoclonal antibody (MAb)-based treatment being developed for cancers with specific markers (HER-2/*neu* positive), including renal cell, non-small cell lung, pancreatic and prostate cancer. Phase II trials have been completed for kidney, prostate, and ovarian cancer. Phase III trials for ovarian cancer have have commenced in Europe.

INDICATION(S) AND RESEARCH PHASE
Prostate Cancer – Phase II completed
Renal Cell Carcinoma – Phase II completed
Colon Malignancies – Phase II
Breast Cancer – Phase II
Gastric Cancer – Phase II
Pancreatic Cancer – Phase II
Lung Cancer – Phase II
Ovarian Cancer – Phase III

MDX-220
unknown

MANUFACTURER
Medarex

DESCRIPTION
MDX-220 is a bispecific (target-trigger) monoclonal antibody (MAb) that targets Tag-72 in the treatment of a variety of cancers, including lung, colon, prostate, ovarian, endometrial, pancreatic, and gastric cancer.

INDICATION(S) AND RESEARCH PHASE
Endometrial Cancer – Phase I/II
Gastric Cancer – Phase I/II
Lung Cancer – Phase I/II
Ovarian Cancer – Phase I/II
Pancreatic Cancer – Phase I/II
Prostate Cancer – Phase II
Colorectal Cancer – Phase II

MGI-114, hydroxymethylacylfulvene, HMAF
Irofulven

MANUFACTURER
MGI Pharma

DESCRIPTION
Irofulven (MGI-114) is the first product candidate being developed by MGI Pharma from its family of anti-cancer compounds called acylfulvenes. Early trials demonstrated that Irofulven is absorbed rapidly by tumor cells, and once inside binds to DNA and protein targets. The binding interferes with DNA replication and cell division, leading to tumor-specific cell death. The drug is being tested in a series of trials for a variety of cancers.

In November 2000, results from a phase II trial of Irofulven indicated that the drug produced anti-tumor activity in subjects with advanced pancreatic cancer who were refractory to gemcitabine (Gemzar). Ten of the 53 subjects enrolled achieved six-month survival and two subjects demonstrated objective responses: one subject experienced tumor shrinkage of 100% and another subject experienced an 84% decrease in tumor mass. A phase III trial was initiated in February 2001.

INDICATION(S) AND RESEARCH PHASE
Breast Cancer – Phase II
Colon Malignancies – Phase II
Renal Cell Carcinoma – Phase II
Cervical Dysplasia/Cancer – Phase II
Lung Cancer – Phase II
Ovarian Cancer – Phase I/II
Colorectal Cancer – Phase II
Prostate Cancer – Phase I/II
Cancer/Tumors (Unspecified) – Phase I/II
Pancreatic Cancer – Phase III
Liver Cancer – Phase II

phenoxodiol
unknown

MANUFACTURER
Novogen

DESCRIPTION
Phenoxodiol is a novel, cytotoxic, anit-cancer drug that arrests cancer cell growth and restores apoptosis. It acts through a variety of mechanisms including the inhibition of a number of cellular enzyme systems, including topoiosomerase 2 and protein tyrosine kinases, which are integral to the development of cancer. Inhibiting these enzyme systems is recognized as a key factor in preventing the growth of cancerous cells. Additionally, the novelty of phenoxodiol lies in its ability to combine a high degree of potency with no known adverse effects on normal cells. Phenoxodiol also possesses a number of other anti-cancer mechanisms that appear to contribute to the overall anti-cancer effect.

Phenoxodiol is currently undergoing a phase Ib trial in an Australian hospital in subjects with solid malignant tumors, including prostate cancer. This study, which commenced in the final quarter of 2000, is investigating the safety and anti-cancer efficacy of phenoxodiol when injected intravenously once weekly for 12 weeks.

Novogen has received approval to commence a second phase Ib trial, which will be conducted at a major Sydney teaching hospital. This new study will measure the safety and anti-cancer effectiveness of phenoxodiol when administered by continuous intravenous infusion over seven days. The study will involve subjects with solid cancers whose cancers have become unresponsive to standard treatment.

INDICATION(S) AND RESEARCH PHASE
Cancer/Tumors (Unspecified) – Phase Ib
Prostate Cancer – Phase Ib

p53 gene therapy
unknown

MANUFACTURER
Aventis

DESCRIPTION
Aventis' p53 gene therapy is an anti-cancer treatment that produces an increased expression of the p53 protein. The p53 protein has the ability to activate other proteins to stop the cell cycle until damage to the cell may be repaired. Additionally, the p53 protein may stop growth in response to additional stimuli, such as reduced nutritional resources or high cell density.

According to scientists, the p53 gene is one of the most frequently altered genes in human cancer, with 50% of all cancers having distorted forms of p53. This p53 gene therapy is delivered by an intraprostatic injection that may result in the suppression of prostate cancer growth. It is currently being tested in a phase I/II trial. Additionally, p53 gene therapy is being tested in phase III trials for head and neck cancer.

INDICATION(S) AND RESEARCH PHASE
Prostate Cancer – Phase I/II
Head and Neck Cancer – Phase III

PSMA - P1/P2
unknown

MANUFACTURER
Northwest Biotherapeutics

DESCRIPTION
Prostate specific membrane antigen (PSMA) is a substance found on a high proportion of prostate cancer cells. PSMA - P1/P2 is in phase I development.

INDICATION(S) AND RESEARCH PHASE
Prostate Cancer – Phase I

samarium Sm 153 lexidronam pentasodium
Quadramet

MANUFACTURER
Cytogen Corporation

DESCRIPTION
Quadramet is a radiopharmaceutical agent containing the radioisotope samarium-153. It is currently in phase II development for the treatment of prostate cancer that has metastasized.

INDICATION(S) AND RESEARCH PHASE
Prostate Cancer – Phase II

SGN-15/Taxotere
unknown

MANUFACTURER
Seattle Genetics

DESCRIPTION
SGN-15 is an antibody drug conjugate composed of the chimeric monoclonal antibody BR96 chemically linked to the drug doxorubicin with an average of eight drug molecules per each mAb molecule. SGN-15 works by binding to a cell surface Ley-related antigen expressed on many tumor types, rapidly internalizing, and then releasing its payload of drug at the low pH present within the cell through acid catalyzed hydrolysis in the endosome. This mechanism of targeted drug delivery allows for relative sparing of tissues normally affected by non-specific chemotherapy, and represents an attractive strategy for the treatment of tumors expressing the BR96 antigen.

SGN-15 is being tested in a combination therapy with Aventis' drug Taxotere in a phase I/II trial in subjects with breast or colon cancer. This trial is being co-funded by Aventis. Additionally, a phase II trial is testing SGN/Taxotere in hormone refractory prostate cancer.

INDICATION(S) AND RESEARCH PHASE
Breast Cancer – Phase I/II
Prostate Cancer – Phase II
Colon Malignancies – Phase I/II

SPD 424
unknown

MANUFACTURER
Shire Pharmaceuticals

DESCRIPTION
SPD 424 (previously RL0903) is a subcutaneous implant that contains a gonadotropin releasing hormone (GnRH) agonist for the treatment of prostate cancer. The hydrogel implant delivers therapeutic agents at a controlled constant release for over one year. Phase III trials are under way.

INDICATION(S) AND RESEARCH PHASE
Prostate Cancer – Phase III

SR-48692
unknown

MANUFACTURER
Sanofi-Synthelabo Pharmaceuticals

DESCRIPTION
SR-48692 is an orally formulated neurotensin antagonist being tested for several indications, including colon cancer, prostate cancer, and schizophrenia.

INDICATION(S) AND RESEARCH PHASE
Colon Malignancies – Phase II
Prostate Cancer – Phase II
Schizophrenia and Schizoaffective Disorders – Phase IIa
Psychosis – Phase IIa
Depression – Phase II

strontium-89 chloride injection
Metastron

MANUFACTURER
Nycomed Amersham Imaging

DESCRIPTION
Metastron is an injectable radiopharmaceutical currently indicated for the relief of bone pain in subjects with painful skeletal metastases. Results of a phase II trial demonstrated that subjects with advanced prostate cancer treated with bone-targeted therapy consisting of Metastron in combination with chemotherapy survived longer than those who did not receive the Metastron therapy.

INDICATION(S) AND RESEARCH PHASE
Prostate Cancer – Phase II completed

SU-101
unknown

MANUFACTURER
Sugen

DESCRIPTION
SU-101 is a synthetic, platelet-derived growth factor receptor, which blocks the essential enzyme tyrosine kinase. This drug may be helpful for the treatment of end-stage malignant glioma, a tumor of nerve tissue. The drug is being tested in phase III trials for refractory brain and prostate cancers, and phase II studies for non-small cell lung and ovarian cancers.

INDICATION(S) AND RESEARCH PHASE
Brain Cancer – Phase III
Prostate Cancer – Phase III
Lung Cancer – Phase II
Ovarian Cancer – Phase II

tretinoin
Atragen

MANUFACTURER
Aronex Pharmaceuticals

DESCRIPTION
Atragen is a liposomal, intravenous formulation of tretinoin or all-trans retinoic acid. Tretinoin induces cell differentiation in rapidly proliferating cells, such as those observed in malignant diseases. Additionally, Atragen appears to affect the cellular signaling mechanisms that become unbalanced in cancer cells. Results of a phase II trial of Atragen monotherapy for acute promyelocytic leukemia (APL) indicated its potential to induce complete remission. The trial was conducted in Peru, and included 16 subjects with newly diagnosed or previously untreated APL who were treated with Atragen every other day as a single agent for a maximum of 28 doses. Fourteen subjects (87.5%) achieved morphologic remission, and 28.6% of these subjects also attained molecular remission. The safety profile observed in the subject population is similar to that reported with the currently approved oral formulation of Atra.

In addition to investigating the safety and efficacy of Atragen as a treatment for APL, the company is conducting trials to evaluate the compound for the treatment of non-Hodgkin's lymphoma, hormone-resistant prostate cancer, acute myelogenous leukemia (AML), and renal cell carcinoma in combination with interferon alpha.

In January 2001, Aronex announced that the FDA has denied approval of the company's NDA for Atragen as a treatment for subjects with APL, for whom therapy with tretinoin (all-trans retinoic acid or Atra) is necessary but for whom an intravenous administration is required.

INDICATION(S) AND RESEARCH PHASE
Lymphoma, Non-Hodgkin's – Phase II
Prostate Cancer – Phase II
Renal Cell Carcinoma – Phase I/II
Leukemia, APL (intravenous) – NDA denied
Leukemia, APL (monotherapy) – Phase II
Leukemia, AML – Phase II

troxacitabine, BCH-4556
Troxatyl

MANUFACTURER
BioChem Pharma

DESCRIPTION
Troxatyl is a dioxolane nucleoside analog being investigated as an anticancer agent. The drug is a complete DNA chain terminator and DNA polymerase inhibitor. It acts by incorporating itself into the growing DNA chain of cancer cells, interfering with their ability to replicate further. Troxatyl is being evaluated as a single agent or in combination therapy in a number of ongoing trials in hematologic malignancies, including acute myeloid leukemia and chronic myeloid leukemia (blastic phase), and in lymphoproliferative disorders such as lymphoma, chronic lymphocytic leukemia and myeloma. It is also being evaluated as a single agent in pancreatic cancer and in combination therapy in a number of solid tumors. Troxatyl is currently in phase II development.

INDICATION(S) AND RESEARCH PHASE
Cancer/Tumors (Unspecified) – Phase II
Colorectal Cancer – Phase II
Head and Neck Cancer – Phase II
Leukemia – Phase II
Lung Cancer – Phase II
Malignant Melanoma – Phase II
Ovarian Cancer – Phase II
Pancreatic Cancer – Phase II
Prostate Cancer – Phase II
Renal Cell Carcinoma – Phase II

unknown
CyPat

MANUFACTURER
Barr Laboratories

DESCRIPTION
CyPat is a prostate cancer therapy in a phase III clinical trial. The trial is expected to include over 1,000 subjects and more than 40 sites. The drug is expected to be indicated for the treatment of hot flashes experienced by prostate cancer subjects with surgical or chemical castration.

INDICATION(S) AND RESEARCH PHASE
Prostate Cancer – Phase III

unknown
Leuvectin

MANUFACTURER
Vical

DESCRIPTION
The active ingredient in the DNA-based drug Leuvectin is a gene encoding interleukin-2 (IL-2), a naturally occurring protein that stimulates the immune system. Administration occurs by direct injection into a tumor, leading to uptake by the tumor cells and subsequent expression of the IL-2 protein. The company anticipates that local expression of IL-2 by cancer cells may stimulate the subject's immune system to attack and destroy the tumor cells. Leuvectin is being evaluated in phase II

trials in subjects with kidney and prostate cancer.

INDICATION(S) AND RESEARCH PHASE
Renal Cell Carcinoma – Phase II
Prostate Cancer – Phase II

unknown
Abetafen

MANUFACTURER
Bioenvision

DESCRIPTION
Abetafen is a derivative of Modrefen, the company's marketed drug for breast cancer. Modrefen acts on the second estrogen receptor, which may be present in breast cancer and prostate cancer cells. This estrogen receptor is known to play some part in controlling normal prostate growth and may also influence growth of prostate cancer. New trials are under way to test effects of the drug on ERb in prostate cancer. Preclinical tests have shown that Modrefen decreases prostate growth in animals and modulates ligand binding to ERb in prostate cancer cell lines. Abetafen is currently in phase II trials for prostate cancer.

INDICATION(S) AND RESEARCH PHASE
Prostate Cancer – Phase II

unknown
Norelin

MANUFACTURER
YM Biosciences

DESCRIPTION
Norelin is an immunopharmaceutical product based on a proprietary recombinant antigen. It utilizes the subject's immune system to stimulate the development of antibodies to gonadotropin-releasing hormone (GnRH). The antibodies block the action of GnRH, which has therapeutic benefits for certain hormone-dependent cancers, such as prostate, breast, ovarian, and uterine cancer. The cancer vaccine has been shown to induce an immune response to GnRH in preclinical models, and a significant anti-tumor effect has been demonstrated.

A formulation with an aluminum-salt based adjuvant was shown to be safe in a phase I/II trial in subjects with hormone-sensitive prostate cancer; however, this formulation did not elicit a satisfactory immune response to GnRH. The company is in the process of commencing immunogenicity studies and testing a variety of formulations, following which it intends to resume clinical testing—phase I/II trials are expected in 2001 for the treatment of prostate cancer.

INDICATION(S) AND RESEARCH PHASE
Prostate Cancer – Phase I/II

unknown
Combidex

MANUFACTURER
Advanced Magnetics

DESCRIPTION
Combidex MRI contrast agent was developed to help in the detection, diagnosis, and staging of various cancers. The first indication is for the diagnosis of metastatic cancer to assist in directing biopsy and surgery as well as to aid in the staging of a variety of cancers, including breast and prostate cancer. In clinical studies, Combidex significantly reduced the number of false diagnoses (both false positive and false negative nodes) compared to unenhanced MRI exams. The second indication is for the detection, diagnosis, and characterization of benign versus malignant lesions of the liver and spleen.

In phase III clinical trials, post-Combidex MRI showed clear differentiation between normal and metastatic lymph nodes, while a post-gadolinium image showed no differentiation in normal and metastatic nodes when compared with pre-dose images.

INDICATION(S) AND RESEARCH PHASE
Breast Cancer – Phase III/IV
Liver Cancer – Phase III
Prostate Cancer – Phase III/IV

unknown
Tesmilifene

MANUFACTURER
YM Biosciences

DESCRIPTION
Tesmilifene is an intracellular histamine antagonist being developed as a chemopotentiator for the treatment of malignant solid tumors. The compound is cytotoxic to tumor cells and cytoprotective to the gut and normal bone marrow progenitor cells. Studies have indicated its ability to augment the invivo anti-tumor activity of cytotoxic drugs routinely used in the treatment of cancer, such as doxorubicin, cyclophosphamide, 5-fluorouracil (5-FU), cisplatin, and mitoxantrone.

Interim analysis of data from a North American phase II pilot study in hormone refractory metastatic prostate cancer has shown promising results. The company hopes to conclude this phase II trial in 2001 and initiate a randomized pivotal study.

INDICATION(S) AND RESEARCH PHASE
Prostate Cancer – Phase II

unknown
GnRH Pharmaccine

MANUFACTURER
Aphton Corporation

DESCRIPTION
Aphton's novel GnRH Pharmaccine is an anti-gonadotropin releasing hormone (GnRH) immunogen, which neutralizes the hormone GnRH. Study results indicate that it induces and maintains castration levels of testosterone and reduced levels of prostate-specific antigen (PSA). Chemical castration of this type is a standard therapy to extend the survival of subjects with advanced prostate cancer. GnRH Pharmaccine is also involved in trials for breast cancer, endometrial cancer, and endometriosis, in addition to prostate cancer.

INDICATION(S) AND RESEARCH PHASE
Prostate Cancer – Phase I/II
Breast Cancer – Phase I/II
Endometrial Cancer – Phase I/II
Endometriosis – Phase I/II

unknown
Leuplin 3M DPS

MANUFACTURER
Takeda Chemical Industries

DESCRIPTION
Leuplin 3M DPS is a luteinizing hormone releasing factor being developed for the treatment of prostate cancer. It is currently in phase II trials in Japan.

INDICATION(S) AND RESEARCH PHASE
Prostate Cancer – Phase II

unknown
Apomine

MANUFACTURER
ILEX Oncology

DESCRIPTION
Apomine is a potent, orally active bishphosphonate estrogen derivative being developed to treat prostate cancer. Apomine induces apoptosis, which is a normal biological process involving a genetically programmed series of events that leads to cell death. Apomine activates the farnesoid X receptor (FXR) and a cascade of biological signals within the cell that rapidly induces apoptosis without affecting normal cells.

Apomine is being tested in phase II clinical trials in Lyon, France. It is currently being developed by ILEX and Symphar S.A. of Geneva, Switzerland.

INDICATION(S) AND RESEARCH PHASE
Prostate Cancer – Phase II

unknown
DCVax

MANUFACTURER
Northwest Biotherapeutics

DESCRIPTION
DCVAx is Northwest Biotherapeutics' proprietary dendritic cell-based immunotherapy. In October 2000, the company announced that no serious side effects had been reported following the first 40 injections of DCVax, and that company immunologists were encouraged by early immunology and PSA data from treated subjects. DCVax is being evaluated as a treatment for late-stage prostate cancer at M.D. Anderson Cancer Center, Houston, and the University of California, Los Angeles (UCLA).

INDICATION(S) AND RESEARCH PHASE
Prostate Cancer – Phase I/II

vaccine
Onyvax P

MANUFACTURER
Onyvax

DESCRIPTION
Onyvax P is an allogeneic whole-cell vaccine being developed for the treatment of prostate cancer. Phase I/II trials have been completed, and the vaccine is scheduled to enter phase II development in the first quarter of 2001. The phase I/II trial involved 60 subjects with advanced disease. Results showed the vaccine to be safe and capable of generating cancer-specific immune responses.

INDICATION(S) AND RESEARCH PHASE
Prostate Cancer – Phase I/II completed
Vaccines – Phase I/II completed

vaccine, adjuvant
AdjuVax-100a

MANUFACTURER
Jenner BioTherapies

DESCRIPTION
AdjuVax-100a is a proprietary emulsion formulation being tested with OncoVax-P prostate cancer vaccine. The combination therapy is in phase II trials.

INDICATION(S) AND RESEARCH PHASE
Prostate Cancer – Phase II
Vaccines – Phase II

vaccine, cancer
Gvax

MANUFACTURER
Cell Genesys

DESCRIPTION
Gvax is an allogeneic compound that involves the genetic modification of prostate cancer cell lines. These cancer cells have been irradiated and modified to secrete granulocyte macrophage-colony stimulating factor (GM-CSF), a hormone which plays a key role in stimulating the body's immune response to vaccines. The compound is in trials for prostate cancer, pancreatic cancer, lung cancer, leukemia, and malignant melanoma.

The Gvax prostate cancer vaccine demonstrated anti-tumor activity in an initial phase II trial in subjects with advanced metastatic prostate cancer who have not responded to hormone therapy. Prior to initiating a phase III trial, Cell Genesys plans to initiate further trials of Gvax prostate cancer vaccine in 2001 that will employ a higher potency version of the same product. Additionally, future phase III trials in hormone refractory prostate cancer subjects may compare Gvax vaccine in combination with chemotherapy to chemotherapy alone.

INDICATION(S) AND RESEARCH PHASE
Prostate Cancer – Phase II
Lung Cancer – Phase I/II completed
Malignant Melanoma – Phase I/II
Vaccines – Phase I/II
Pancreatic Cancer – Phase II
Leukemia – Phase I/II

vaccine, cancer
GeneVax

MANUFACTURER
Centocor

DESCRIPTION
GeneVax is a DNA-based vaccine technology in phase I development for the treatment of breast and prostate cancer.

INDICATION(S) AND RESEARCH PHASE

Vaccines – Phase I
Breast Cancer – Phase I
Prostate Cancer – Phase I

vaccine, prostate cancer, (rV-psa)
Prostvac

MANUFACTURER
Therion Biologics

DESCRIPTION
Prostvac is a genetically engineered vaccine that is derived from the poxvirus. This immunotherapeutic is being tested in phase II trials for the treatment of prostate cancer.

INDICATION(S) AND RESEARCH PHASE
Prostate Cancer – Phase II
Vaccines – Phase II

YM-598
unknown

MANUFACTURER
Yamanouchi Pharmaceutical

DESCRIPTION
YM-598 is an orally administered endothelin type A receptor (ETA) antagonist being evaluated for the treatment of advanced prostate cancer. It is being developed in Europe and has reached phase II trials.

INDICATION(S) AND RESEARCH PHASE
Prostate Cancer – Phase II

ZD-0473/AMD 473
unknown

MANUFACTURER
AstraZeneca

DESCRIPTION
ZD-0473 is a new platinum-based anticancer agent designed to deliver an extended spectrum of activity and overcome resistance to currently approved platinum drugs, such as cisplatin and carboplatin. It is being evaluated for the treatment of a range of solid-tumor cancers, including colorectal, non-small cell lung, and bladder cancer, which are resistant to carboplatin. ZD-0473 is being tested in both intravenous and oral formulations. The intravenous formulation is in phase II trials and the oral formulation is in preclinical development.

INDICATION(S) AND RESEARCH PHASE
Bladder Cancer – Phase II
Cancer/Tumors (Unspecified) – Phase II
Colorectal Cancer – Phase II
Lung Cancer – Phase II
Ovarian Cancer – Phase II
Prostate Cancer – Phase II
Breast Cancer – Phase II
Cervical Dysplasia/Cancer – Phase II

ZD-1839
Iressa

MANUFACTURER
AstraZeneca

DESCRIPTION
Iressa binds to the epidermal growth factor receptor (EGFR) and inhibits tyrosine kinase, thereby blocking signals for cancer growth and survival. The company reported encouraging results from phase I trials in a variety of tumors, but particularly in non-small cell lung cancer (NSCLC). Iressa is being investigated both as a monotherapy and in combination with other anti-tumor drugs in NSCLC, gastric, colorectal and hormone-resistant prostate cancers. In 1999, the FDA gave Iressa fast track status. The drug is currently in phase III studies for solid tumors.

INDICATION(S) AND RESEARCH PHASE
Cancer/Tumors (Unspecified) – Phase III
Colorectal Cancer – Phase III
Gastric Cancer – Phase III
Lung Cancer – Phase III
Prostate Cancer – Phase III

Prostate Disorders

lomefloxacin HCl
Maxaquin

MANUFACTURER
Unimed Pharmaceuticals

DESCRIPTION
Maxaquin is currently on the market for the treatment of subjects with uncomplicated urinary tract infections and lower respiratory tract infections. The antibiotic drug is in phase III trials for a new indication, chronic bacterial prostatitis. Maxaquin is given as an oral tablet. Additional indications may include metabolic disorders, benign prostatic hypertrophy.

INDICATION(S) AND RESEARCH PHASE
Bacterial Infection – Phase III
Prostate Disorders – Phase III

pygeum africanum
Tadenan

MANUFACTURER
Fournier Research

DESCRIPTION
Pygeum africanum is an herb than may improve the symptoms of an enlarged prostate. It is currently in Phase II trials for benign prostatic hypertrophy. As men age, their prostates enlarge, probably due to the cumulative effects of the male hormone testosterone that acts on prostate tissue. Prostate cells are stimulated to grow and divide by testosterone, leading to gland enlargement, or in some cases, prostate cancer. An enlarged prostate gland may produce symptoms such as difficulty urinating, which may include frequent nocturnal urination and problems completely voiding the bladder contents.

Pygeum africanum is thought to act by reducing the amount of active testosterone (DHT) in the body. It works by inhibiting an enzyme that converts the testosterone molecule to the active molecule DHT. It is DHT which is directly responsible for stimulating prostate cells. Recently, there was a preliminary three center trial that tested the efficacy of tadenan on eighty-five men with enlarged prostates. After two months of treatment, the men had a 32% decrease in nocturnal urination frequency and a significant improvement in urinary flow. These effects persisted for a month after the drug was discontinued. There also was no effect on the men's sexual function and no serious side effects produced. This medication may be an alternative to existing medications which may cause sexual side effects. It also may be used in conjunction with current medications in order to maximize clinical effect. Further studies are under way.

INDICATION(S) AND RESEARCH PHASE
Prostate Disorders – Phase II

17 Pediatric Illnesses

Drugs in the development pipeline	217
Drugs approved in 2000	25

In the past century, the medical community has made tremendous progress in improving the health of children through pediatric clinical trials. Recently developed vaccines and approved drugs have significantly reduced the number of pediatric deaths. In 1997, Congress granted drug companies an additional six months of patent exclusivity if a company has successfully met the criteria established by the FDA for pediatric clinical trials. This decision enables drug companies to generate millions of incremental, patent-protected drug sales. In turn, this has driven the current boom in the testing of pediatric drugs.

Previously, prescribing drugs for children was more art than science as 80% of the drugs given to children had only been tested among adults. The FDA allowed all approved drugs to be given to children; however, doctors largely had to guess the dosage levels. For the past 20 years, there has been ongoing debate among doctors and healthcare professionals with regard to the safety to children in prescribing drugs approved for adults. One side believed that children's immature organs and different metabolic and immune systems could lead to unforeseen adverse reactions. The other side argued that fatally ill children were being deprived of life-saving treatments, especially with some AIDS drugs and other breakthrough therapies.

Then, in 1998, the FDA announced new pediatric regulations. The regulations required that all new drugs be therapeutically evaluated in children (from newborns to adolescents) and have specific dosing information for children based on scientific research. In addition, the creation of special formulations, such as liquid or chewable tablets, was encouraged to facilitate children being able to take the drugs. The FDA also required pediatric trials for already marketed drugs commonly prescribed for use in children.

Activity in the pipeline continued to snowball when the FDA announced that, by December 2000, all newly approved drugs and new formulations of existing drugs would require testing in children. A recent survey conducted by Pharmaceutical Research and Manufacturers of America (PhRMA) reported 217 medicines and vaccines currently in development for children. In addition, the survey found that the FDA approved 25 drugs for children in the past year, with an additional 52 potential drugs expected to soon begin clinical trials. CenterWatch estimates that as much as $850 million is currently being spent on drugs that may involve pediatric clinical trials.

The majority of pediatric clinical trials focus on treatments for cancer, asthma, bacterial infections, AIDS, cystic fibrosis, genetic disorders and psychiatric disorders.

In the year 2000, 12,400 children will be diagnosed with cancer. Cancer is considered the leading killer of children under the age of 15 and claims 2,300 lives each year. CenterWatch has identified 30 drugs being tested by the National Cancer Institute and 16 other drugs being tested by pharmaceutical companies. A total of 22 of these drugs currently undergoing trials have already been approved by the FDA for use in adults and are now being tested in children. Researchers are testing drugs in the areas of refractory or relapsed CNS leukemia and lymphoma, refractory or relapsed pediatric malignancies and allogenic bone marrow transplants.

Asthma, the most common cause of chronic illness in children, affects five million American children. An estimated $3.2 billion is spent on treating asthma in children under 18. CenterWatch identified 14 drugs in the pipeline. Two drugs approved this year specifically for pediatric use are AstraZeneca's pulmicort respules in children as young as 12 months old and Singulair, manufactured by Merck, for prophylaxis of asthma in children ages two to five. In addition, Glaxo Wellcome submitted an NDA in August 2000 for Advanir Diskus a long-term, twice daily maintenance treatment in patients 12 years or older.

AIDS and related disorders is another large area involving pediatric patients. There are 14 drugs in the development pipeline. A once-a-day pill used in combination therapy for children with AIDS was approved this past year. Cystic fibrosis, which occurs in approximately one in every 3,900 live births and is the most fatal genetic disease in the United States, has 11 drugs in the pipeline. There are 13 drugs in the pipeline targeting bacterial infections.

There are 10 drugs in the pipeline for genetic disorders and 10 for psychiatric disorders. Furthermore, new drugs are being developed for diabetes, epilepsy, gastrointestinal disorders, growth disorders, viral and fungal infections, neurological disorders, respiratory disorders, rheumatoid arthritis, skin disorders, drugs to increase the effectiveness of transplants and vaccines to prevent a variety of diseases.

A few other popular drugs that have been approved recently for pediatric patients are: Wallace Laboratories' Astelin Nasal Spray for symptoms of seasonal allergic sneezing for children five years and older, Pharmacia's Azulfidine EN-tabs Tablets for the treatment of juvenile rheumatoid arthritis, and Roxanne Laboratories' Cafict Oral Solution for the short-term treatment of apnea of prematurity in infants between 20 and 33 weeks. The list also includes Concerta, manufactured by Alza, for Attention Deficit disorder, Novartis' Trileptal for epilepsy in children ages four to 16, and Glaxo Wellcome's Curtivate for the relief of the inflammatory and pruritic manifestations of corticosteroid-responsive dermatoses in children ages three months or older.

Despite the practical, legal and ethical difficulties of testing drugs in children, research and development can only expand in the years to come. The FDA estimates that an additional 375 pediatric studies will be conducted annually.

Acute Pharyngitis

cefditoren pivoxil
Spectracef

MANUFACTURER
TAP Pharmaceuticals

DESCRIPTION
Sprectracef (cefditoren pivoxil) is a broad-spectrum cephalosporin antibiotic. Studies have indicated the drug is effective in treating maxillary sinusitis, streptococcal pharyngitis and exacerbations from acute chronic bronchitis. It is in phase III trials for the treatment of acute pharyngitis, bronchitis and tonsillitis in children ages one month to 18 years.

INDICATION(S) AND RESEARCH PHASE
Pediatric, Acute Pharyngitis – Phase III
Pediatric, Tonsillitis – Phase III
Pediatric, Bronchitis – Phase III

Allergy

cetirizine HCl
Zyrtec

MANUFACTURER
Pfizer

DESCRIPTION
Zyrtec (cetirizine HCl) is an orally active and selective H1-receptor antagonist. It has been approved by the FDA for the relief of symptoms associated with seasonal allergic rhinitis in adults and children two years of age and older. Zyrtec is currently in phase III trials for pediatric subjects ages six months to two years old.

INDICATION(S) AND RESEARCH PHASE
Pediatric, Allergy – Phase III
Allergy – FDA approved

Anesthesia

ropivacaine HCl
Naropin

MANUFACTURER
AstraZeneca

DESCRIPTION
Naropin is a sodium channel blocker that is currently in phase III trials for use as a spinal anesthetic in an intra-articular administration. An NDA was submitted in December 2000 for approval of a single-dose administration of Naropin injection for regional anesthesia in pediatric subjects. FDA approval is also sought for Naropin as a treatment for acute pain management in children one to twelve years old. Naropin has been FDA approved as an obstetric anesthesia and regional anesthesia for surgery, as well as for the management of post-operative pain.

INDICATION(S) AND RESEARCH PHASE
Anesthesia, Regional – FDA approved
Anesthesia, Spinal – Phase III
Pain, Acute or Chronic – FDA approved
Pediatric, Anesthesia – NDA submitted
Pediatric, Pain, Acute or Chronic – NDA submitted

Asthma

albuterol
Pediavent

MANUFACTURER
Ascent Pediatrics

DESCRIPTION
Pediavent is a prescription product indicated for the treatment of asthma. This drug is for twice a day dosage. It is formulated specifically to decrease the bitter taste of albuterol, which should increase the chances that children will use it as directed. Pediavent is a suspension in the form of granules which contain albuterol within a special coating. This coating allows the drug to be released at a controlled rate and masks the unpleasant taste. This controlled release technology allows the compound to be administered to a child only twice a day, alleviating the need to wake a child at night to administer medicine. A phase III trial has been completed, but currently development of this drug has been suspended due to lack of financial resources.

INDICATION(S) AND RESEARCH PHASE
Pediatric, Asthma – Phase III completed

beclomethasone dipropionate
Qvar Oral Inhalation

MANUFACTURER
3M Pharmaceuticals

DESCRIPTION
Qvar Oral Inhalation is an aerosol metered dose inhaler (MDI) used for the preventative management of asthma. The inhaler contains beclomethasone dipropionate (BDP) in a solution and does not contain a chlorofluorocarbon (CFC) propellant. It is designed to deliver small-particle-sized medication to the large, intermediate, and small airways.

Qvar Oral Inhalation is FDA approved for use in subjects ages 12 and over, and is currently in a phase III trial for pediatric subjects ages six and over.

INDICATION(S) AND RESEARCH PHASE
Asthma – FDA Approved
Pediatric, Asthma – Phase III

cromolyn sodium
Intal HFA-227

MANUFACTURER
Aventis

DESCRIPTION
Intal, in its original formulation, is currently on the market for the treatment of asthma. The active ingredient, cromolyn sodium, inhibits both the immediate and non-immediate bronchoconstrictive reactions to inhaled antigen. Cromolyn sodium also decreases bronchospasm caused by exercise,

toluene diisocyanate, aspirin, cold air, sulfur dioxide, and environmental pollutants. Although the exact mechanism of action of cromolyn sodium is unknown, its effects are mediated through the secondary messenger, cyclic-AMP. The drug has no intrinsic bronchodilator or antihistamine activity. This new non-CFC formulation, Intal HFA-227, is in phase III trials for the treatment of asthma in both adults and children.

INDICATION(S) AND RESEARCH PHASE
Asthma – Phase III
Pediatric, Asthma – Phase III

flunisolide
Aerobid

MANUFACTURER
Forest Laboratories

DESCRIPTION
Aerobid, a steroid inhaler containing flunisolide, may be more effective than currently prescribed steroid inhalers and may also produce fewer side effects. In preliminary trials, Aerobid has been shown to have strong anti-inflammatory and anti-allergic action on airways. In addition, after Aerobid is absorbed into the body, it is quickly converted into a conjugate that has little or no effect on other organs in the body. Aerobid is in phase III trials for the treatment of asthma in both children and adults.

INDICATION(S) AND RESEARCH PHASE
Asthma – Phase III
Pediatric, Asthma – Phase III

formoterol
Budoxis, Oxis

MANUFACTURER
AstraZeneca

DESCRIPTION
Oxis combines a long-acting beta-2 agonist, formoterol, with budesonide, an inhaled glucocorticoid. Formoterol has been approved by the FDA for use in the Oxis Turbuhaler, which administers the drug through a multi-dose dry powder inhalation device. Clinical documentation of the Oxis Turbuhaler demonstrated the combination of a rapid onset of symptom relief and long-lasting bronchodilation.

The Oxis Turbuhaler is currently in three phase III trials for the treatment of asthma, both in children and adults, and for chronic obstructive pulmonary disease (COPD).

INDICATION(S) AND RESEARCH PHASE
Asthma – Phase III
Chronic Obstructive Pulmonary Disease (COPD) – Phase III
Pediatric, Asthma – Phase III

formoterol
Foradil

MANUFACTURER
Novartis

DESCRIPTION
Foradil (formoterol), a long-acting beta-2 agonist, is a bronchodilator for the treatment of asthma and chronic obstructive pulmonary disease. It is currently being tested in phase II trials in a multi-dose dry powder inhaler. It has been approved for twice-daily use via the aerolizer inhaler (a single-dose powder inhalation device) in adults and children ages five and older.

In February 2001, Foradil Aerolizer was approved by the FDA for long-term, twice daily administration in the maintenance treatment of asthma and in the prevention of bronchospasm in adults and children five years of age and older with reversible obstructive airways disease.

INDICATION(S) AND RESEARCH PHASE
Asthma – Phase II
Asthma – FDA approved
Reversible Obstructive Airways Disease – FDA approved
Pediatric, Asthma – FDA approved

levalbuterol HCl
Xopenex

MANUFACTURER

DESCRIPTION
Xopenex (levalbuterol HCl) is indicated for the treatment or prevention of bronchospasm (narrowing of the airways) in adults and adolescents 12 years of age and older with reversible obstructive airway disease (asthma). Levalbuterol is a beta-adrenergic receptor agonist that relaxes the smooth muscles of all airways, from the trachea to the terminal bonchioles. A four-week, multicenter, placebo-controlled trial was conducted in 362 adult and adolescent patients 12 years of age and older with mild-to-moderate asthma. Efficacy was demonstrated for all active treatment regimens compared with placebo on Day 1 and Day 29. In some patients, the duration of effect was as long as eight hours. Xopenex is currently in phase III trials treating newborns and children ages 11 years old for asthma.

INDICATION(S) AND RESEARCH PHASE
Pediatric, Asthma – Phase II

omalizumab
Xolair

MANUFACTURER
Genentech

DESCRIPTION
Xolair is a recombinant humanized monoclonal antibody to immunoglobulin E. It is being developed for the treatment of asthma and the prevention of seasonal allergic rhinitis. A BLA has been submitted for the two above indications and for pediatric subjects ages six to 12 years old. This drug is being developed in partnership with Novartis and Tanox. It is currently awaiting FDA approval.

INDICATION(S) AND RESEARCH PHASE
Asthma – NDA submitted
Pediatric, Asthma – NDA submitted
Rhinitis – NDA submitted

theophylline
Theolan

MANUFACTURER
Elan Pharmaceutical Research

DESCRIPTION

Theolan is one of many formulations of theophylline used in the treatment of asthma. It causes the relaxation of bronchial smooth muscle and the modulation of mediator release by inhibiting cyclic-AMP degradation. The drug is in phase III trials in a pediatric liquid suspension formulation, using twice-daily proprietary PharmaZome oral delivery technology.

INDICATION(S) AND RESEARCH PHASE
Asthma – Phase III
Pediatric, Asthma – Phase III

unknown
MSI-Albuterol

MANUFACTURER
Zambon S.p.A.

DESCRIPTION

The metered solution inhaler (MSI) system is a small, portable hand-held nebulizer designed to combine the therapeutic benefits of nebulization with the convenience of pressurized metered dose inhalers (MDIs).

In June 2000, Zambon Group and Sheffield Pharmaceuticals announced the successful completion and preliminary results of the second phase II trial evaluating the MSI-Albuterol system. The randomized, cross over, cumulative dose trial demonstrated that it was comparable to the market-leading albuterol product delivered through an MDI. Both the MSI-Albuterol and MDI-Albuterol were given as cumulative doses to 24 adult subjects with moderate, persistent asthma. A phase I trial in pediatric subjects is currently in progress.

INDICATION(S) AND RESEARCH PHASE
Asthma – Phase II completed
Pediatric, Asthma – Phase I

unknown
Pulmicort Respules

MANUFACTURER
AstraZeneca

DESCRIPTION

Pulmicort Respules, budesonide nebulizing suspension, is an inhaled steroid. An NDA has been filed for the treatment of asthma in subjects one year and older.

INDICATION(S) AND RESEARCH PHASE
Pediatric, Asthma – NDA Submitted

zafirlukast
Accolate

MANUFACTURER
AstraZeneca

DESCRIPTION

Accolate (zafirlukast) is a synthetic, selective leukotriene receptor antagonist (LTRA) that inhibits bronchoconstriction. It is available in tablet form, and is indicated for the chronic treatment of asthma in adults and children seven years of age and older.

Three U.S. double-blind, randomized, placebo-controlled, 13-week trials were conducted in 1,380 adults and children 12 years of age and older with mild-to-moderate asthma. The trials demonstrated that Accolate improved daytime asthma symptoms, nighttime awakenings, mornings with asthma symptoms, and rescue beta-agonist use among other outcomes. Improvement in asthma symptoms occurred within one week of initiating treatment with Accolate. Adverse reactions reported by subjects included headache, infection, and nausea.

Additionally, phase III trials for children ages five for 11 years have also been completed. An NDA was submitted in December 2000.

INDICATION(S) AND RESEARCH PHASE
Asthma – FDA Approved
Pediatric, Asthma – NDA Submitted

Atopic Dermatitis

LDP-392
unknown

MANUFACTURER
LeukoSite

DESCRIPTION

LDP-392 is formulated as a topical product designed to block two biochemical pathways involving inflammation. It is a dual function, 5-lipoxygenase (5-LO) inhibitor and platelet activating factor (PAF) antagonist. It treats inflammation by targeting the two critical pathways that form leukotrienes and mediate PAF activity, respectively. These pro-inflammatory pathways have been implicated in dermatological conditions such as psoriasis and atopic dermatitis.

Early trials indicate that LDP-392 may help subjects to avoid the toxicities associated with steroid treatment. This drug is being tested in phase II trials for the treatment of atopic dermatitis in children and psoriasis and psoriatic disorders in adults.

INDICATION(S) AND RESEARCH PHASE
Pediatric, Atopic Dermatitis – Phase II
Psoriasis and Psoriatic Disorders – Phase II

pimecrolimus, ASM 981
Elidel

MANUFACTURER
Novartis

DESCRIPTION

Elidel is an ascomycin derivative being studied for the treatment of inflammatory skin disease. It produces a therapeutic effect through the inhibition of T-cells and mast cells. Elidel is being developed in both an oral and topical (cream) formulation. The oral formulation is in phase II trials, while an NDA has been filed for the cream formulation. Phase III trials involving more than 2,000 subjects ages three months to adult have recently been completed. The majority of the subjects in the phase III studies were pediatric.

Data presented from two previous vehicle-controlled trials demonstrated that ASM 981 cream was safe and effective for the treatment of atopic dermatitis. The two trials involved a total of 403 (267 ASM 981 and 136 vehicle) pediatric subjects ages two to 17 years old with mild to moderate atopic dermatitis. Both studies consisted of a six-week randomized, multicenter, double-blind, parallel-group phase followed by a

20-week open-label phase to assess safety and efficacy. Thirty-seven percent of ASM subjects were clear or almost clear of the signs of atopic dermatitis, significantly more than in the vehicle-control group. Over 65% of subjects achieved some degree of improvement. Of those who showed improvement, over 85% were cleared of the disease.

INDICATION(S) AND RESEARCH PHASE
Atopic Dermatitis – Phase II
Pediatric, Atopic Dermatitis – Phase III completed
Atopic Dermatitis – NDA submitted

Attention Deficit/Hyperactivity Disorder (ADHD)

CNS stimulant
unknown

MANUFACTURER
Elan Pharmaceutical Research

DESCRIPTION
This central nervous system (CNS) stimulant is being developed for the treatment of attention deficit/hyperactivity disorder (ADHD) in pediatric subjects. This drug is being tested in a phase II trial using the CODAS delivery technology.

INDICATION(S) AND RESEARCH PHASE
Pediatric, Attention Deficit/Hyperactivity Disorder (ADHD) – Phase II

d-methylphenidate HCl
unknown

MANUFACTURER
Celgene Corporation

DESCRIPTION
D-methylphenidate hydrochloride (d-MPH) is a chirally pure, single isomer version of Ritalin in an oral formulation. It is being tested in a phase III study for the treatment of attention deficit/hyperactivity disorder (ADHD) in children.

INDICATION(S) AND RESEARCH PHASE
Pediatric, Attention Deficit/Hyperactivity Disorder (ADHD) – Phase III

donepezil hydrochloride, E2020
Aricept

MANUFACTURER
Eisai

DESCRIPTION
Aricept is an acetylcholinesterase inhibitor. The enzyme acetylcholinesterase breaks down acetylcholine—by inhibiting this process, Aricept increases the concentration of acetylcholine. Acetylcholine is a neurotransmitter associated with memory, which means that greater concentrations of it could significantly improve the conditions of Alzheimer's disease. In addition, Aricept is in phase II trials in children seven to 16 years old who are suffering from attention deficit/hyperactivity disorder.

Aricept is currently in development in Japan, Europe and the United States. Aricept is being co-promoted by Pfizer.

INDICATION(S) AND RESEARCH PHASE
Alzheimer's Disease – NDA submitted in Japan
Dementia – Phase III
Pediatric, Attention Deficit/Hyperactivity Disorder – Phase II

mecamylamine HCl
Inversine

MANUFACTURER
Layton Bioscience

DESCRIPTION
Inversine is being evaluated in phase III trials for the treatment of Tourette's syndrome in young adult subjects. Additionally it is being tested in trials for the treatment of attention deficit/hyperactivity disorder (ADHD) in pediatric subjects.

INDICATION(S) AND RESEARCH PHASE
Pediatric, Tourette's Syndrome – Phase III
Pediatric, Attention Deficit/Hyperactivity Disorder – Phase III

methylphenidate
MethyPatch

MANUFACTURER
Noven Pharmaceuticals

DESCRIPTION
MethyPatch, a transdermal methylphenidate patch, is in phase III development. Methylphenidate is the active ingredient found in Ritalin, Novartis Pharmaceuticals' approved drug for attention deficit/hyperactivity disorder (ADHD). The patch is being developed to address the social concerns of children needing to take an oral pill each day. The company hopes that a discreet patch will eliminate the stigma children suffer from taking an oral medication during the school day, as well as eliminate drug diversion and abuse issues that affect the pill formulation. The company expects to file an NDA in the first half of 2001.

INDICATION(S) AND RESEARCH PHASE
Pediatric, Attention Deficit/Hyperactivity Disorder (ADHD) – Phase III

methylphenidate
Ritalin LA

MANUFACTURER
Novartis

DESCRIPTION
Ritalin LA, a time-release product, is an NK-1 substance P antagonist. Ritalin is an established treatment for attention deficit/hyperactivity disorder (ADHD) that works by increasing attention and decreasing restlessness in children and adults who are overactive, cannot concentrate for very long or are easily distracted, and are impulsive. An application has been submitted overseas for Ritalin LA for the treatment of attention deficit disorders.

INDICATION(S) AND RESEARCH PHASE
Attention Deficit/Hyperactivity Disorder (ADHD) – MAA submitted
Pediatric, Attention Deficit/Hyperactivity Disorder (ADHD) – MAA submitted

methylphenidate
Ritalin QD

MANUFACTURER
Novartis

DESCRIPTION
Ritalin QD (methylphenidate) is a central nervous system stimulant. Ritalin is an established treatment for Attention Deficit Hyperactivity Disorder (ADHD) that works by increasing attention and decreasing restlessness in children and adults who are overactive, cannot concentrate for very long or are easily distracted, and are impulsive. This formulation allows for once daily administration. Ritalin QD is in phase III trials for the treatment of ADHD in children six to 16 years old.

INDICATION(S) AND RESEARCH PHASE
Pediatric, Attention Deficit Hyperactivity Disorder – Phase III

methylphenidate HCl
unknown

MANUFACTURER
Medeva plc

DESCRIPTION
Methylphenidate is a stimulant used for the treatment of attention deficit/hyperactivity disorder (ADHD). Methylphenidate HCl modified release capsules utilize Eurand's novel Diffucaps technology, a multi-particulate bead delivery system with each bead acting as a drug reservoir. Each bead is coated with a chosen polymer to provide a unique release profile. Customized release profiles can then be achieved by incorporating different types of beads into each capsule.

Phase III trial results of the formulation demonstrated that the capsules control the symptoms of ADHD throughout the school day without the need for a second midday dose. Three hundred and fourteen children with ADHD between the ages of six and 15 were evaluated in the randomized, double-blind, placebo-controlled trial. The primary efficacy measure was the difference from baseline on the teacher's version of the Conners' Global Index (CGI). The estimated mean improvement from baseline was 7.9 for methylphenidate modified release capsules compared to 1.2 for placebo.

INDICATION(S) AND RESEARCH PHASE
Pediatric, Attention Deficit/Hyperactivity Disorder (ADHD) – Phase III

modafinil
Provigil

MANUFACTURER
Cephalon

DESCRIPTION
Provigil (modafinil) is a dopamine-releasing agent that increases excitatory glutamatergic transmission. It is being developed in phase III trials for the prevention of daytime sleepiness associated with obstructive sleep apnea, hypersomnia, and shift work. Phase II trials are being conducted for the prevention of excessive daytime sleepiness associated with Alzheimer's disease and Parkinson's disease.

A phase II trial has been completed using Provigil as a treatment for sleep apnea and fatigue associated with multiple sclerosis. This drug is also in a phase III trial for the treatment of sleepiness regardless of cause, with an NDA filing planned for late 2001.

Additionally, Provigil is currently in phase I/II trials for ADHD in pediatric subjects.

INDICATION(S) AND RESEARCH PHASE
Multiple Sclerosis – Phase II completed
Sleep Disorders – Phase III
Pediatric, Attention Deficit/Hyperactivity Disorder – Phase I/II
Parkinson's Disease – Phase II
Alzheimer's Disease – Phase II

SPD 420
unknown

MANUFACTURER
Shire Pharmaceuticals

DESCRIPTION
Ampakine CX516 (designated as SPD 420) is being evaluated for the treatment of attention deficit/hyperactivity disorder (ADHD). The drug is being developed for worldwide use in both adult and pediatric subjects.

INDICATION(S) AND RESEARCH PHASE
Attention Deficit/Hyperactivity Disorder (ADHD) – Phase I completed
Pediatric, Attention Deficit/Hyperactivity Disorder (ADHD) – Phase I completed

SPD 503
unknown

MANUFACTURER
Shire Pharmaceuticals

DESCRIPTION
SPD 503 is being evaluated for the treatment of both adult and pediatric Attention Deficit Hyperactivity Disorder (ADHD). SPD 503 is in phase I trials, and a proof of concept study is expected to begin in the first half of 2001.

INDICATION(S) AND RESEARCH PHASE
Attention Deficit Hyperactivity Disorder (ADHD) – Phase I
Pediatric, Attention Deficit Hyperactivity Disorder (ADHD) – Phase I

tomoxetine
unknown

MANUFACTURER
Eli Lilly

DESCRIPTION
Tomoxetine, a noradrenergic compound, is in development for the treatment of attention deficit/hyperactivity disorder (ADHD). It is being tested in phase III trials in children ages six and older.

INDICATION(S) AND RESEARCH PHASE
Pediatric, Attention Deficit/Hyperactivity Disorder (ADHD) – Phase III

Autism

secretin
unknown

MANUFACTURER
Repligen Corporation

DESCRIPTION
Secretin is a hormone that stimulates the pancreas as part of normal digestion. It is currently approved by the FDA for the diagnosis of gastrinoma and the assessment of pancreatic function. Anecdotal off-label use of secretin in pediatric autism has led to interest in its potential as a treatment.

In March 2000, Repligen initiated a phase II trial that will evaluate three doses of secretin over nine weeks in more than 100 children. In November 2000, the company announced it has completed subject recruitment for the phase II trial of secretin for pediatric autism. Data should be available during the first quarter of 2001.

INDICATION(S) AND RESEARCH PHASE
Pediatric, Autism – Phase II
Gastrointestinal Diseases and Disorders, Miscellaneous – FDA approved

Bacterial Infection

ABT-773
unknown

MANUFACTURER
Abbott Laboratories

DESCRIPTION
ABT-773 is a novel ketolide antibiotic, which has the potential to fight drug resistant respiratory infections. ABT-773 is in a phase II trial treating subjects two years and older.

INDICATION(S) AND RESEARCH PHASE
Pediatric, Bacterial Infection – Phase II

amoxicillin/clavulanate
Augmentin ES

MANUFACTURER
GlaxoSmithKline

DESCRIPTION
Augmentin ES is a new formulation of Augmentin, a penicillin derivative already approved for use around the world. Results presented in September 2000 demonstrated that it is highly effective in eradicating the three most common bacteria (Streptococcus pneumoniae, Haemophilus influenzae, and Moraxella catarrhalis) that cause middle ear infections in children, including drug-resistant strains, while maintaining the typical safety profile of the currently marketed Augmentin. An NDA has been submitted for Augmentin ES for the treatment of acute otitis media, including penicillin-resistant S. pneumoniae.

INDICATION(S) AND RESEARCH PHASE
Pediatric, Bacterial Infection – NDA Submitted
Pediatric, Otitis Media – NDA Submitted

galasomite
Synsorb Pk

MANUFACTURER
Synsorb Biotech

DESCRIPTION
Synsorb Pk is an orally delivered gastroenteric product designed for the prevention of hemolytic uremic syndrome (HUS) in children caused by *E. coli* toxins. Development of Synsorb Pk has been discontinued as of the first quarter of 2001. The company intends to concentrate resources on aggressive development of its lead product, Synsorb Cd, which management believes offers a more significant market opportunity.

INDICATION(S) AND RESEARCH PHASE
Pediatric, Bacterial Infection – Phase II trial discontinued

gatifloxacin
Tequin

MANUFACTURER
Bristol-Myers Squibb

DESCRIPTION
Tequin is a broad-spectrum 8-methoxy fluoroquinolone antibiotic in a phase II trial for the treatment of recurrent otitis media in subjects six months to 17 years old. Tequin is primarily excreted through the kidneys and less than 1% is metabolized by the liver. Tequin has been approved by the FDA for the treatment of certain infections in adults.

INDICATION(S) AND RESEARCH PHASE
Pediatric, Bacterial Infection – Phase II

Linezolid
Zyvox

MANUFACTURER
Pharmacia

DESCRIPTION
Zyvox is an antibiotic in the oxazolidinone family. The drug blocks bacterial protein synthesis so that bacteria cannot multiply. Zyvox was FDA approved for adults on April 18th, 2000 for the treatment of nosocomial pneumonia, community-acquired pneumonia, complicated and uncomplicated skin and skin structure infections caused by vancomycin-resistant Enterococcus (VRE). Zyvox is available in either IV or oral formulations. Zyvox has been tested in over 4,000 subjects with efficacy in treating gram-positive infections. It is currently in phase III trials for pediatric subjects.

INDICATION(S) AND RESEARCH PHASE
Pediatric, Bacterial Infection – Phase III

streptogamin
unknown

MANUFACTURER
Aventis

DESCRIPTION
Streptogamin is an antibiotic treatment for community-acquired (non-hospital) infections, including those due to multi-resistant

gram-positive bacteria. The drug was being evaluated in phase II/III trials against bacterial infections in an oral formulation for adult and pediatric subjects. Development has been discontinued.

INDICATION(S) AND RESEARCH PHASE
Bacterial Infection – Phase II/III discontinued
Pediatric, Bacterial Infection – Phase II/III discontinued

telithromycin
Ketek

MANUFACTURER
Aventis

DESCRIPTION
Ketek is a novel antibiotic that fights resistant bacteria by inhibiting the protein synthesis necessary for bacterial reproduction. Invitro data suggest that it has a low propensity to induce bacterial resistance.

Phase III data from ten multinational studies found that Ketek tablets may provide a convenient, once-daily, short-course treatment option for select respiratory tract infections (RTIs), including those infections caused by bacteria resistant to available therapies. The ten phase III studies were comprised of data from almost 2,500 subjects treated with Ketek and almost 1,800 subjects treated with comparator antibiotics. Ketek showed a high level of activity against *Streptococcus pneumoniae*, *Streptococcus pyogenes*, *Staphylococcus aureus*, *Haemophilus influenzae*, and *Moraxella catarrhalis*, as well as against atypical bacteria such as *Chlamydia pneumoniae*, *Mycoplasma pneumoniae*, and *Legionella pneumoniae*. An NDA was submitted in March 2000 for adults. A phase III trial for pediatric subjects is ongoing in the United States.

INDICATION(S) AND RESEARCH PHASE
Bacterial Infection – NDA submitted
Pediatric, Bacterial Infection – Phase III

vaccine, DPT/Haemophilus influenzae type B
unknown

MANUFACTURER
Chiron Corporation

DESCRIPTION
Chiron Corporation has formulated a combination vaccine that might effectively immunize children against four serious diseases: *Haemophilus influenzae* type B, diphtheria, pertussis, and tetanus—with a single injection. This vaccine has the potential to simplify pediatric vaccination schedules, thereby lowering costs, increasing convenience, and improving compliance. The vaccine is composed of inactive molecules of diphtheria toxin, pertussis toxin, and tetanus toxin. The vaccine also contains inactivated *H. influenza* proteins.

INDICATION(S) AND RESEARCH PHASE
Pediatric, Bacterial Infection – Phase III
Pediatric, Influenza – Phase III
Pediatric, Vaccines – Phase III
Pediatric, Viral Infection – Phase III

vaccine, Group B streptococcus
unknown

MANUFACTURER
Amvax/Baxter Highland Immuno

DESCRIPTION
Group B streptococci (GBS) are the leading infectious cause of illness and death among newborn infants fewer than 28 days old.

Because some foreign bodies or antigens (e.g., in capsule form) are not easily recognized by the immature immune system, conjugate vaccines link them to a recognizable carrier so that they act together to develop immunity. The company's proprietary technology links polysaccharides to carrier proteins for an enhanced immune response. A unique application of this technology couples antigens from the same organism. This vaccine is in phase II clinical trials.

INDICATION(S) AND RESEARCH PHASE
Pediatric, Bacterial Infection – Phase II
Vaccines – Phase II

vaccine, Group C Meningococcus
unknown

MANUFACTURER
Amvax/Bacter Highland Immuno

DESCRIPTION
Amvax Pharmaceuticals is working on a new vaccine for meningococcal bacterial infections. The bacteria known as Neisseria meningitidis produce these types of infections. This organism can cause everything from benign upper respiratory infections to serious blood infections, which can lead to rashes, muscle and joint aches, and meningitis. Meningococcal meningitis begins when the organism crosses the meninges, which are the membranes surrounding the brain and spinal cord. This bacterial invasion into the central nervous system can result in fever, neck stiffness, headache and coma. In a third of affected subjects, overwhelming infection causes the body to go into shock with associated blood clotting problems, lung and heart infections, and death. If patients survive, they could experience residual problems such as deafness, paralysis, and mental retardation.

Approximately half of all cases of meningococcal meningitis occur in children under the age of 15 years, with most cases of meningitis occurring among infants three to eight months of age. Amvax Pharmaceuticals has developed a vaccine to immunize against one important subtype of this bacteria (N. meningitidis serotype C). This new vaccine is composed of inactivated meningococcal proteins combined with tetanus proteins. The tetanus proteins stimulate a stronger immunization response than if the patient were vaccinated with the meningococcal proteins alone. This is especially important in young children whose immune systems are not fully mature and might not respond adequately to an unenhanced vaccine. Even though further study is needed, this vaccine may be an improvement on vaccines already in use, since it may be used in very young children and might result in a longer, more complete immunization from the disease.

The company reported that an NDA has been filed with the FDA and is awaiting approval. This vaccine was formulated as an intramuscular injection. Clinical testing indications for this vaccine may include meningococcal infection for children older than twelve months of age, adults with immune deficiencies, complement deficiencies, asplenia, and HIV infection/AIDS subjects.

INDICATION(S) AND RESEARCH PHASE
Pediatric, Bacterial Infections – NDA Submitted
Acquired Immune Deficiency Syndrome (AIDS) and AIDS-Related Infections – Phase III
White Blood Cell Disorders – Phase III
Meningitis – Phase III

vaccine, meningococcal conjugate
unknown

MANUFACTURER
Aventis Pasteur

DESCRIPTION
Meningococcus is a bacterium that can invade the bloodstream causing septicaemia and the lining of the brain causing meningitis. This vaccine is in development for the treatment of meningococcal infections. It is currently in phase II/III trials for children ages two, four, and six months.

INDICATION(S) AND RESEARCH PHASE
Pediatric, Bacterial Infections – Phase II/III

vaccine, S. pneumoniae
unknown

MANUFACTURER
GlaxoSmithKline

DESCRIPTION
This pediatric conjugated vaccine is currently in phase III trials for *S. pneumoniae* disease prophylaxis.

INDICATION(S) AND RESEARCH PHASE
Pediatric, Bacterial Infection – Phase III

vaccine, DPT/ Haemophilus influenzae type B
unknown

MANUFACTURER
Chiron Corporation

DESCRIPTION
Chiron Corporation has formulated a combination vaccine to immunize children against *Haemophilus influenzae* type B, diphtheria, pertussis, and tetanus in a single injection formulation. This vaccine has the potential to simplify pediatric vaccination schedules, thereby lowering costs, increasing convenience and improving compliance. The vaccine is composed of inactive molecules of diphtheria toxin, pertussis toxin, and tetanus toxin. The vaccine also contains inactivated *H. influenzae* proteins.

This combination vaccine, given as an intramuscular injection, is currently in phase III trials.

INDICATION(S) AND RESEARCH PHASE
Pediatric, Bacterial Infection – Phase III
Pediatric, Influenza – Phase III
Pediatric, Vaccines – Phase III
Pediatric, Viral Infection – Phase III

Bone Marrow Transplant

palivizumab
Synagis

MANUFACTURER
MedImmune

DESCRIPTION
Synagis (palivizumab) is a humanized monoclonal antibody (IgG1k) produced by recombinant DNA technology, directed to an epitope in the A antigenic site of the F protein of respiratory syncytial virus (RSV). It has been approved for the prevention of serious lower respiratory tract disease caused by RSV in pediatric subjects at high risk of RSV disease.

It is currently being tested in a phase IV trial for pediatric subjects with cystic fibrosis. It is also in phase III trials for pediatric subjects for prevention of RSV disease in subjects with congenital heart disease. Finally, it is in phase III testing for treatment of RSV disease in bone marrow transplant subjects. This trial is being conducted by the collaborative antiviral study group (CASG) of the NIH.

INDICATION(S) AND RESEARCH PHASE
Pediatric, Congenital Heart Disease – Phase III
Pediatric, Bone Marrow Transplant – Phase III
Pediatric, Cystic Fibrosis – Phase IV

Bronchitis

cefditoren pivoxil
Spectracef

MANUFACTURER
TAP Pharmaceuticals

DESCRIPTION
Sprectracef (cefditoren pivoxil) is a broad-spectrum cephalosporin antibiotic. Studies have indicated the drug is effective in treating maxillary sinusitis, streptococcal pharyngitis and exacerbations from acute chronic bronchitis. It is in phase III trials for the treatment of acute pharyngitis, bronchitis and tonsillitis in children ages one month to 18 years.

INDICATION(S) AND RESEARCH PHASE
Pediatric, Acute Pharyngitis – Phase III
Pediatric, Tonsillitis – Phase III
Pediatric, Bronchitis – Phase III

Campylobacter Infection

vaccine, campylobacter
Campyvax

MANUFACTURER
Antex Biologics

DESCRIPTION
This orally administered vaccine, developed under a Cooperative Research

and Development Agreement (CRADA) with the U.S. Navy and Army, is designed to prevent gastroenteritis and traveler's diarrhea caused by *Campylobacter jejuni*. A novel proprietary technology combines the vaccine, consisting of inactivated whole cells, with an adjuvant. While vaccines typically provide protection after bacteria enter the body, this new genetic engineering technology provides the platform for vaccines that prevent bacterial infection.

According to the companies involved, phase II trials showed encouraging results for continued development of the vaccine.

INDICATION(S) AND RESEARCH PHASE
Bacterial Infection – Phase II completed
Diarrhea – Phase II completed
Gastroenteritis – Phase II completed
Pediatric, Campylobacter Infection – Phase II completed

Cancer/Tumors

alitretinoin, ALRT-1057
Panretin

MANUFACTURER
Ligand Pharmaceuticals

DESCRIPTION
Panretin, 9-cis retinoic acid, is chemically related to vitamin A. It activates all known retinoid receptors, which regulates the expression of genes controlling processes related to cell differentiation and proliferation. A topical gel formulation of Panretin has been on the market since February 1999 for the treatment of lesions associated with Kaposi's sarcoma.

Currently, Panretin in oral capsule formulation is being evaluated for the treatment of breast cancer, pediatric cancers, myelodysplastic syndrome, bronchial metaplasia, and psoriasis.

INDICATION(S) AND RESEARCH PHASE
Breast Cancer – Phase II
Lung Cancer – Phase II/III
Pediatric, Cancer – Phase III
Psoriasis and Psoriatic Disorders – Phase II/III
White Blood Cell Disorders, Myelodysplastic Syndrome – Phase II/III
Kaposi's Sarcoma – FDA approved

BNP 1350
Karenitecin

MANUFACTURER
BioNumerik Pharmaceuticals

DESCRIPTION
BNP 1350 belongs to a novel class of orally active highly lipophilic topoisomerase I inhibitors called karenitecins. The compound has demonstrated potent antitumor activity in several preclinical models including human cancer cell lines and animal bearing human tumor models.

BioNumerik is planning to proceed with phase II trials in solid tumors and leukemias. Additionally, a pediatric phase I trial has been initiated in individuals ages one to 20 years of age with solid tumors.

INDICATION(S) AND RESEARCH PHASE
Cancer/Tumors (Unspecified) – Phase I completed
Pediatric, Solid Tumors – Phase I

farnesyl transferase inhibitor
unknown

MANUFACTURER
Janssen Pharmaceutica

DESCRIPTION
Farnesyl transferase inhibitors (FTIs) are chemotherapeutic agents being evaluated in phase II trials for the treatment of refractory solid tumors in children ages two to 18. FTIs are a novel class of antitumor drugs that block the oncogenic activity of Ras proteins. Certain Ras proteins are responsible for turning cell growth on and off. Mutant forms of Ras protein signal the "on" switch to remain permanently activated, such that abnormal cell growth and proliferation continue uninterrupted. Effective Ras signaling requires the attachment of Ras proteins to the plasma membrane, and it is initiated by the enzyme farnesyl protein transferase.

FTIs inhibit oncogenic Ras signaling by interfering with the action of the P21 proteins. According to the company research shows that FTIs are potent activators of apoptosis in Ras-transformed cells, if the cells are prevented from attaching to a substratum surface. Further results indicate that FTIs revert cells to a state in which cell-substratum attachment is necessary for viability, and this data suggests that apoptosis forms the basis for drug-induced tumor regression.

INDICATION(S) AND RESEARCH PHASE
Cancer/Tumors (Unspecified) – Phase II
Pediatric, Cancer/Tumors (Unspecified) – Phase II

multiple-drug resistance inhibitor
unkown

MANUFACTURER
Eli Lilly

DESCRIPTION
Multiple-drug resistance inhibitor is being tested in a phase II pediatric trial for children of all ages suffering from cancer.

INDICATION(S) AND RESEARCH PHASE
Pediatric, Cancer – Phase II

R115777
unknown

MANUFACTURER
Janssen Pharmaceutica

DESCRIPTION
R115777 is an anticancer drug that inhibits the transformation of normal cells to cancer cells. It is belongs to a group of drugs called farnesyl transferase inhibitors (FTIs), which are signal transduction inhibitors that may suppress Ras function. Ras proteins play key roles in cell growth and survival, and in activating mutations of the proteins, which are common in human cancer. R115777 is currently in phase III trials for the treatment of solid tumors in adults and is in phase I pediatric studies for refractory solid tumors in children two to 18 years of age.

INDICATION(S) AND RESEARCH PHASE
Cancer/Tumors (Unspecified) – Phase III
Pediatric, Cancer/Tumors (Unspecified) – Phase I

squalamine
unknown

MANUFACTURER
Genaera Corporation

DESCRIPTION
Squalamine is an aminosterol compound isolated from the tissues of the dogfish shark. This drug inhibits salt-and-acid-regulating pumps on endothelial cells that normally line blood vessels, which prevents growth factors from stimulating the cells to form capillaries. It is thought that this activity results in anti-angiogenisis, anti-inflammatory and anti-tumor effects.

The company is conducting several trials testing squalamine against certain cancers, such as non-small cell lung cancer and ovarian cancer. Additional trials for squalamine are being planned in pediatric solid tumors, other solid adult tumors and small cell lung cancer.

INDICATION(S) AND RESEARCH PHASE
Breast Cancer – Phase II
Lung Cancer – Phase II a
Cancer/Tumors (Unspecified) – Phase II
Ovarian Cancer – Phase II
Pediatric, Solid Tumors – Phase II

TNP-470
unknown

MANUFACTURER
Takeda Chemical Industries

DESCRIPTION
TNP-470 is a synthetically modified form of the antibiotic fumagillin. This drug inhibits new blood vessel growth and is being tested in phase II trials for treatment of adults with malignant solid tumors. It is also being evaluated in a phase I trial in children with solid tumors, lymphomas, and acute leukemias.

INDICATION(S) AND RESEARCH PHASE
Cancer/Tumors (Unspecified) – Phase II
Pediatric, Solid Tumors – Phase I
Pediatric, Leukemia – Phase I
Pediatric, Lymphomas – Phase I

unknown
Cereport

MANUFACTURER
Alkermes

DESCRIPTION
Cereport is a bradykinin agonist, which temporarily increases the permeability of the blood-brain barrier by activating B2 receptors on endothelial cells. The ability to transiently open the junctions between the tightly joined endothelial cells allows for the selective transport of drug molecules across the blood-brain barrier into the brain.

Cereport's safety, tolerability in combination with other drugs, and preliminary efficacy have been tested in a series of clinical trials in more than 600 subjects. Alkermes has completed four phase II trials of Cereport in combination with carboplatin in subjects with recurrent, malignant brain tumors. Additionally, Cereport is in a pediatric phase II trial for the treatment of brain tumors in children six to 18 years old. Alkermes is in a partnership with ALZA Corporation for the development and commercialization of Cereport.

INDICATION(S) AND RESEARCH PHASE
Brain Cancer – Phase II completed
Pediatric, Brain Tumors – Phase II

vincristine
Onco TCS

MANUFACTURER
Inex Pharmaceuticals

DESCRIPTION
Onco TCS consists of the cancer drug vincristine encapsulated in Inex's patented drug delivery technology, Transmembrane Carrier System (TCS). The TCS technology provides prolonged blood circulation, tumor accumulation and extended drug release at the cancer site. These characteristics are designed to increase the effectiveness and reduce the toxicities of the encapsulated drug.

Inex has begun enrolling subjects in a phase II trial to evaluate Onco TCS as part of a first-line treatment for aggressive non-Hodgkin's lymphoma (NHL). Additionally, a pivotal phase II/III trial is underway at 74 medical centers in Canada and the United States evaluating the drug as a treatment for second or later relapsed aggressive NHL. This trial is designed to provide sufficient data to apply in late 2002 or early 2003 for marketing approval. Lastly, Onco TCS is being evaluated in two phase II trials as a treatment for small cell lung cancer and for pediatric malignancies.

INDICATION(S) AND RESEARCH PHASE
Lymphoma, Non-Hodgkin's – Phase II/III
Lung Cancer – Phase II
Pediatric, Cancer – Phase II

Cardiac Surgery

TP10
unknown

MANUFACTURER
AVANT Immunotherapeutics

DESCRIPTION
TP10 is a genetically engineered (recombinant) soluble complement receptor-1 (sCR1). Complement-1 is a naturally occurring substance that binds to antibodies as part of the immune response to infection or foreign bodies. Clinical trials are testing TP10 in an intravenous formulation for a variety of disorders including the treatment of acute respiratory distress syndrome (ARDS), reperfusion injury, heart attack, cardiac surgery, organ reperfusion, xenotransplantation, allotransplantation, and post-surgical complications in infants.

A phase IIb trial was initiated in January 2001 in approximately 30 infants undergoing high risk cardiac surgery utilizing cardiopulmonary bypass. The trial will be conducted at seven sites in the United States.

INDICATION(S) AND RESEARCH PHASE
Acute Respiratory Distress Syndrome (ARDS) – Phase II/III
Cardiac Ischemia – Phase I/II
Cardiac Surgery – Phase IIb
Myocardial Infarction – Phase I/II
Pediatric, Post-surgical Complications – Phase I/II
Pediatric, Cardiac Surgery – Phase IIb

unknown
CV Seprafilm Adhesive Barrier

MANUFACTURER
Genzyme Surgical

DESCRIPTION
CV Seprafilm Adhesive Barrier is a seprafilm bioresorbable membrane, which works as an adhesion prevention for pediatric cardiac surgery.

INDICATION(S) AND RESEARCH PHASE
Pediatric, Cardiac Surgery – Phase III

Cataplexy

sodium oxybate (GHB)
Xyrem

MANUFACTURER
Orphan Medical

DESCRIPTION
Sodium oxybate (GHB) is a naturally occurring neurotransmitter in the brain that is involved in sleep regulation. Xyrem is administered as an oral solution for the treatment of narcolepsy and cataplexy. Cataplexy is a form of narcolepsy, characterized by loss of muscle control in response to strong emotion. Other treatments for narcolepsy do not address this syndrome and their effectiveness can be diminished over time due to drug tolerance. They may also have unpleasant side effects such as weight gain, palpitations, dry mouth, and loss of sense of self. Xyrem offers an alternative to these treatments. A phase IIIb trial is under way to assess the drug's efficacy in controlling excessive daytime sleepiness (EDS). The company submitted an NDA in October 2000. In addition, phase III trials for children 12 years and older have been completed.

INDICATION(S) AND RESEARCH PHASE
Sleep Disorders – NDA submitted
Pediatric, Cataplexy – Phase III completed

Cerebral Palsy

botulinum toxin type A, AGN-191622
Botox

MANUFACTURER
Allergan

DESCRIPTION
Botulinum toxin type A, a purified neurotoxin complex, has been used as a therapeutic agent since the 1960s. At a normal neuromuscular junction, a nerve impulse triggers the release of acetylcholine, which causes the muscle to contract. Botox reduces excessive muscle activity by blocking the release of acetylcholine at the neuromuscular junction.

Botox is being tested in a phase II trial for the prevention of migraine headaches, a phase III trial for lower back pain, and a pediatric phase III trial for juvenile cerebral palsy in subjects two to seven years old.

Botox was FDA approved in December 2000 for the treatment of adults with cervical dystonia. When injected into the affected muscles, Botox decreases the severity of abnormal head position and neck pain associated with this condition by blocking the release of the neurotransmitter acetylcoline from the peripheral nerve terminal to the muscle.

INDICATION(S) AND RESEARCH PHASE
Migraine and Cluster Headaches – Phase II
Musculoskeletal Diseases – FDA approved
Pain, Acute or Chronic – Phase III
Pediatric, Cerebral Palsy – Phase III

Cholesterol (High Levels)

cerivastatin sodium
Baycol

MANUFACTURER
Bayer Corporation

DESCRIPTION
Baycol (cerivastatin sodium tablets) is indicated as an adjunct to diet for patients with primary hypercholesterolemia and mixed dyslipidemia. Baycol reduces elevated levels of total cholesterol, low-density-lipoprotein cholesterol (LDL-C), apolipoprotein B (apo B), and triglycerides (TG). Cerivastatin is a competitive inhibitor of HMG-CoA reductase, an enzyme important for cholesterol synthesis. The inhibition of cholesterol synthesis reduces the level of cholesterol in hepatic cells, which stimulates the synthesis of LDL receptors, thereby increasing the uptake of cellular LDL particles. The end result of these biochemical processes is a reduction of the plasma cholesterol concentration.

Baycol has been studied in controlled trials in North America, Europe, Israel, and South Africa, and has been shown to be effective in reducing plasma cholesterol. Baycol tablets (0.4 mg) were approved by the FDA in 1999. The drug is currently in phase II/III trials for hypercholesterolemia for children ages 10 to 17 years.

INDICATION(S) AND RESEARCH PHASE
Pediatric, Cholesterol (High Levels) – Phase II/III

lovastatin
Mevacor

MANUFACTURER
Merck & Co.

DESCRIPTION
Mevacor is a statin cholesterol-lowering drug that is in a phase IV trial testing children between the ages of 10-17 years old suffering from heterozygous familial hypercholesterolemia.

Chronic Obstructive Pulmonary Disease

oxandrolone, CO221
unknown

MANUFACTURER
Bio-Technology General

DESCRIPTION
Oxandrolone is an anabolic steroid for treatment of chronic obstructive pulmonary disease (COPD) and pressure ulcers. The drug, in oral tablet formulation, is in phase II trials for both indications.

INDICATION(S) AND RESEARCH PHASE
Chronic Obstructive Pulmonary Disease (COPD) – Phase II
Pressure Ulcers – Phase II
Pediatric, Chronic Obstructive Pulmonary Disease (COPD) – Phase III
Pediatric, Pressure Ulcers – Phase III

Clostridium difficile

Saccharomyces boulardii
unknown

MANUFACTURER
Biocodex

DESCRIPTION
Saccharomyces boulardii is a yeast that appears to have an inhibitory effect against a type of bacteria (*Clostridium difficile*) that causes severe diarrhea in a variety of subjects. Sixty-one percent of neonates are colonized with this bacteria, and in a study at the Children's Hospital in Philadelphia, one-third of the children tested were found to have the destructive chemicals (toxins) made by *C. difficile* bacteria in their stools.

Scientists are not certain how exactly this yeast exerts its destructive effect against bacterial infection, but it might produce an enzyme that destroys one of the toxins produced by the bacteria. It also may prevent invading bacteria from binding to the intestinal walls, or it might stimulate the production of immune cells by the body that helps attack the invading bacteria. One French study showed that subjects who were producing four to eight liters of diarrhea a day had normal stools after an eight-day course of *Saccharomyces boulardii*.

People taking antibiotics for infections are susceptible to *C. difficile* infection, since antibiotics strip the intestinal walls of normal bacteria that are protective against infection. In a study of people taking antibiotics for various reasons, the group receiving *Saccharomyces boulardii* experienced a lower incidence of *C. difficile* diarrhea than those receiving other anti-diarrheal therapies. Further study is under way to determine exactly how effective this yeast may be in treating infection and what subjects might receive the most benefit from it.

INDICATION(S) AND RESEARCH PHASE
Bacterial Infection – Phase II
Diarrhea – Phase II
Pediatric, Clostridium difficile – Phase II

Conduct Disorder

risperidone
Risperdal

MANUFACTURER
Janssen Pharmaceutica

DESCRIPTION
Risperdal is an antipsychotic medication that belongs to a new chemical class, the benzisoxazole derivatives. As with other antipsychotic drugs, the exact mechanism of action is unknown, but researchers believe that Risperdal works as a receptor antagonist for a combination of neurotransmitters, including dopamine type 2 (D_2) and serotonin type 2 ($5-HT_2$).

Risperdal has already been FDA approved in tablet and oral solutions to treat schizophrenia and schizoaffective disorder, though the company is conducting further studies for first-break treatment and relapse prevention for these indications.

Risperdal is currently in phase III trials for the treatment of conduct disorder in pediatric subjects ages five to 16 years old in both an oral and tablet formulation. It is also in trials for the treatment of schizophrenia in an intramuscular depot formulation.

Janssen Pharmaceutica terminated their collaborative agreement for development and marketing with SmithKline Beecham in 1999.

INDICATION(S) AND RESEARCH PHASE
Bipolar Disorders – Phase III
Pediatric, Conduct Disorder – Phase III
Schizophrenia and Schizoaffective Disorders – Phase III

Congenital Heart Disease

palivizumab
Synagis

MANUFACTURER
MedImmune

DESCRIPTION
Synagis (palivizumab) is a humanized monoclonal antibody (IgG1k) produced by recombinant DNA technology, directed to an epitope in the A antigenic site of the F protein of respiratory syncytial virus (RSV). It has been approved for the prevention of serious lower respiratory tract disease caused by RSV in pediatric subjects at high risk of RSV disease.

It is currently being tested in a phase IV trial for pediatric subjects with cystic fibrosis. It is also in phase III trials for pediatric subjects for prevention of RSV disease in subjects with congenital heart disease. Finally, it is in phase III testing for treatment of RSV disease in bone marrow transplant subjects. This trial is being conducted by the collaborative antiviral study group (CASG) of the NIH.

INDICATION(S) AND RESEARCH PHASE
Pediatric, Congenital Heart Disease – Phase III

Pediatric, Bone Marrow Transplant – Phase III
Pediatric, Cystic Fibrosis – Phase IV

Congestive Heart Failure

carvedilol
Coreg

MANUFACTURER
GlaxoSmithKline

DESCRIPTION
Coreg is a nonselective beta-adrenergic blocking agent with alpha1-blocking activity. It is administered in tablet formulation and is rapidly and extensively absorbed by the body. An international study of Coreg in subjects with advanced chronic heart failure, called COPERNICUS (Carvedilol Prospective Randomized Cumulative Survival Trial), was stopped early by its steering committee due to a significant survival benefit seen with the drug. The study, which was conducted in over 300 medical centers in 21 countries, enrolled more than 2,200 subjects with advanced heart failure who had symptoms at rest or on minimal exertion but who did not require hospitalization in the intensive care unit or intravenous pharmacologic support. The mortality rate in the Coreg group was significantly lower than in the placebo group, and there were fewer serious adverse effects with Coreg treatment.

The drug was approved in May 1997 for the treatment of mild or moderate heart failure. It is currently in phase III trials for severe heart failure, and pediatric phase III trials are under way for congestive heart failure in children ages one to 18 years old.

INDICATION(S) AND RESEARCH PHASE
Heart Failure – Phase III
Pediatric, Congestive Heart Failure – Phase III

Crohn's Disease

infliximab
Remicade

MANUFACTURER
Centocor

DESCRIPTION
Remicade (infliximab) is a monoclonal antibody that binds to a key inflammatory mediator called tumor necrosis factor alpha (TNF-alpha). Overproduction of TNF-alpha leads to inflammation in conditions such as Crohn's disease, rheumatoid arthritis and other autoimmune diseases. Research suggests that TNF-alpha may also cause the inflammation associated with psoriasis. Remicade reduces inflammation by binding to and neutralizing TNF-alpha on the cell membrane and in the blood.

Trial results of Remicade have demonstrated that children with active, severe Crohn's disease showed significant improvement and were able to decrease steroid usage within four weeks of infusion. Data also showed that children with early disease had a markedly prolonged response to the drug compared with those who were diagnosed with Crohn's disease for longer than two years.

Remicade is in phase III trials for the treatment of Crohn's disease in pediatric subjects. Remicade has been approved by the FDA for the treatment of Crohn's disease and rheumatoid arthritis.

Centocor markets Remicade in the United States. Schering-Plough Corporation has rights to market Remicade in all other countries throughout the world, except in Japan and parts of the Far East, where Remicade will be marketed by Tanabe Seiyaku.

INDICATION(S) AND RESEARCH PHASE
Crohn's Disease – FDA Approved
Pediatric, Crohn's Disease – Phase III
Rheumatoid Arthritis – FDA Approved
Psoriasis and Psoriatic Disorders – Phase II completed

Cystic Fibrosis

HP-3
unknown

MANUFACTURER
Milkhaus Laboratory

DESCRIPTION
HP-3 is a nucleic acid medication in an oral formulation. It is a novel therapeutic agent being tested in phase II and III trials for the treatment of chronic bronchitis (CB), chronic obstructive pulmonary disease (COPD), and cystic fibrosis (CF). HP-3 is also being tested in pediatric subjects, ages six to 21 years old.

Results from a phase II trial for CF showed significant improvement in pulmonary function and an increase in sputum clearance.

Results for all three indications showed that HP-3 increased sputum expectoration and significantly improved pulmonary function. The company believes that the drug evokes such responses through a mechanism common to all three diseases. Consequently, HP-3 may have a broad potential utility in relieving the debilitating symptoms of respiratory distress, which afflict more than 15 million individuals.

INDICATION(S) AND RESEARCH PHASE
Bronchitis – Phase III
Chronic Obstructive Pulmonary Disease (COPD) – Phase II completed
Cystic Fibrosis – Phase II completed
Pediatric, Cystic Fibrosis – Phase II completed

palivizumab
Synagis

MANUFACTURER
MedImmune

DESCRIPTION
Synagis (palivizumab) is a humanized monoclonal antibody (IgG1k) produced by recombinant DNA technology, directed to an epitope in the A antigenic site of the F

protein of respiratory syncytial virus (RSV). It has been approved for the prevention of serious lower respiratory tract disease caused by RSV in pediatric subjects at high risk of RSV disease.

It is currently being tested in a phase IV trial for pediatric subjects with cystic fibrosis. It is also in phase III trials for pediatric subjects for prevention of RSV disease in subjects with congenital heart disease. Finally, it is in phase III testing for treatment of RSV disease in bone marrow transplant subjects. This trial is being conducted by the collaborative antiviral study group (CASG) of the NIH.

INDICATION(S) AND RESEARCH PHASE
Pediatric, Congenital Heart Disease – Phase III
Pediatric, Bone Marrow Transplant – Phase III
Pediatric, Cystic Fibrosis – Phase IV

tgAAV-CF
unknown

MANUFACTURER
Targeted Genetics

DESCRIPTION
tgAAV-CF is a gene therapy compound administered in an aerosol formulation. It is thought to decrease the amount of IL-8, an inflammatory cytokine, present in the lungs of cystic fibrosis (CF) subjects. A phase I trial was completed at the Stanford University Medical Center in collaboration with the Cystic Fibrosis Foundation's Therapeutics Development Network. The drug was well tolerated, with a greater distribution area than other formulations. A phase IIa trial was initiated November 2000 for adults. In addition, a phase II trial is testing tgAAV-CF in CF subjects 15 years and older. tgAAV-CF is being co-developed with Celltech Chiroscience.

INDICATION(S) AND RESEARCH PHASE
Cystic Fibrosis – Phase II a
Pediatric, Cystic Fibrosis – Phase II

tyloxapol
SuperVent

MANUFACTURER
Discovery Laboratories

DESCRIPTION
SuperVent Aerosol Solution is a potent antioxidant that has anti-inflammatory activity through the inhibition of NF-(Kappa)B. A phase IIa clinical trial will evaluate this mechanism of action in cystic fibrosis subjects and examine the benefits of SuperVent Aerosol Solution on pulmonary function. In addition, a phase II trial is being run in pediatric subjects.

According to the company, SuperVent Aerosol Solution was shown to be safe and well tolerated at concentrations up to 1.25% in a phase I study with 20 subjects. The phase II trials are being conducted at the Intermountain Cystic Fibrosis Center at the University of Utah in Salt Lake City.

INDICATION(S) AND RESEARCH PHASE
Cystic Fibrosis – Phase IIa
Pediatric, Cystic Fibrosis – Phase II

Depression

Mirtazapine
Remeron Tablets

MANUFACTURER
Organon

DESCRIPTION
Remeron is the first NaSSA—Noradrenergic and Specific Serotonergic Antidepressant. It enhances the release of the neurotransmitter noradrenaline in certain areas in the brain. It also increases the release of another neurotransmitter, serotonin. Such dual action is increasingly being recognized as beneficial for effectiveness in treating depression. It is FDA approved for the treatment of depression in adults and is currently in phase III trials in pediatric subjects suffering from depression.

INDICATION(S) AND RESEARCH PHASE
Pediatric, Depression – Phase III

sertraline HCl
Zoloft

MANUFACTURER
Pfizer

DESCRIPTION
Zoloft (sertraline HCl) is a selective serotonin reuptake inhibitor in an oral formulation. It is currently being marketed by Pfizer for multiple indications including post-traumatic stress disorder, depression, obsessive compulsive disorder and panic disorder. Additionally, Zoloft is in phase III trials for the treatment of depression and post-traumatic stress disorder in children ages six to 17 years.

INDICATION(S) AND RESEARCH PHASE
Pediatric, Depression – Phase III
Pediatric, Post-Traumatic Stress Disorder – Phase III

unknown
TritAb

MANUFACTURER
Protherics

DESCRIPTION
TritAb is an antibody product made to offset the toxic effects of overdoses of tricyclic antidepressants (TCAs). This antidote is made from specialized monoclonal antibodies that target TCAs. TritAb is being tested in both pediatric and adult subjects. Phase III development is scheduled to be initiated. The TritAb program for reversal of antidepressant toxicity has an orphan drug status.

INDICATION(S) AND RESEARCH PHASE
Depression – Phase II/III
Overdose/Drug Toxicity – Phase II/III
Pediatric, Depression – Phase II

venlafaxine HCl
Effexor XR

MANUFACTURER
Wyeth-Ayerst

DESCRIPTION

Effexor XR is a serotonin/norepinephrine reuptake inhibitor developed for once-a-day administration. It has been approved by the FDA for the treatment of depression and generalized anxiety disorder. Additional efforts are under way to extend the base of indications for the product. A phase III pediatric trial is underway in children ages eight to 16 years old.

INDICATION(S) AND RESEARCH PHASE
Pediatric, Depression – Phase III

Diabetes Mellitus Types 1 and 2

glyburide/metformin
Glucovance

MANUFACTURER
Bristol-Myers Squibb

DESCRIPTION

Glucovance is a novel oral antidiabetic that combines the two leading oral antidiabetic agents, metformin and glyburide, in a single pill. It has been approved as a first line therapy for type 2 diabetes patients who cannot manage their condition with diet and exercise alone. It has also been approved as a second line therapy for people taking sulfonylurea and who blood sugar levels are still inadequately controlled. Glucovance is currently in phase I trials in pediatric patients for the treatment of type 2 diabetes.

This drug will be available in three dosing strengths; 1.25mg/250mg (glyburide/metformin), 2.5mg/500mg, and 5mg/500mg tablets.

INDICATION(S) AND RESEARCH PHASE
Diabetes Mellitus Types I and II – FDA Approved
Pediatric, Diabetes Mellitus Types I and II – Phase I

inhaled insulin
unknown

MANUFACTURER
Pfizer

DESCRIPTION

Pfizer is currently developing inhaled insulin, a new route of administration for the treatment of diabetes, in collaboration with Aventis and Inhale Therapeutic Systems. The inhaled insulin system has been as effective as subcutaneous injections of short-acting insulin in the treatment of insulin-dependent or type 1 diabetes in preliminary studies. Inhaled insulin is currently being tested in phase III trials; the NDA and MAA will be filed in late 2001.

INDICATION(S) AND RESEARCH PHASE
Pediatric, Diabetes Mellitus Types 1 and 2 – Phase III
Diabetes Mellitus Types 1 and 2 – Phase III

NBI-6024
unknown

MANUFACTURER
Neurocrine Biosciences

DESCRIPTION

NBI-6024 is an altered peptide ligand that is designed to induce an immune response that could result in preservation of beta-cell function and endogenous insulin production in diabetic subjects. Phase I/II trials are currently underway and a phase IIb will be initiated in the third quarter of 2001 in 600 adult and pediatric subjects, for type I diabetes.

INDICATION(S) AND RESEARCH PHASE
Diabetes Mellitus Types I and II – Phase I/II
Pediatric, Diabetes Mellitus Types I and II – Phase II b

Ear Infections

NE-1530
unknown

MANUFACTURER
Neose Technologies

DESCRIPTION

NE-1530, a complex carbohydrate that is produced naturally in human breast milk, is an antibacterial agent being evaluated for the prevention and treatment of pediatric middle ear infections, or otitis media. The drug is in phase II trials for ear infections and otitis media. Additional indications may include infectious diseases and viral diseases associated with the nose, throat, and lungs, including pneumonia.

INDICATION(S) AND RESEARCH PHASE
Pediatric, Ear Infections – Phase II
Pediatric, Otitis Media – Phase II

Epilepsy

fosphenytoin sodium injection
unknown

MANUFACTURER
Pfizer

DESCRIPTION

Fosphenytoin is a phosphate ester of phenytoin that has been classified "1S" (new molecular entity) by the FDA. It is freely soluble in aqueous solutions, including standard intravenous solutions. After administration, fosphenytoin is rapidly converted (within eight to 15 minutes) to phenytoin by phosphatases found in a number of tissues. Unlike phenytoin, fosphenytoin can be given rapidly intravenously and promptly achieves therapeutic levels. It is rapidly absorbed when given intramuscularly, and is well tolerated. The drug is 100% bioavailable, and it is bioequivalent to phenytoin (10 mL fosphenytoin is equivalent to 5 mg intravenous phenytoin). Side effects are minor and transient. Unlike benzodiazepines and barbiturates, fosphenytoin does not cause respiratory or CNS depression; thus subjects can breathe well enough to compensate for metabolic acidosis, and think well enough after recovery to cooperate with diagnostic evaluation.

Fosphenytoin sodium injection has been approved for the treatment of seizures in adults and currently an NDA has been submitted to treat pediatric subjects.

INDICATION(S) AND RESEARCH PHASE
Epilepsy – FDA approved
Pediatric, Epilepsy – NDA submitted

gabapentin
Neurontin

MANUFACTURER
Pfizer

DESCRIPTION
Neurontin is an anticonvulsant used with other medications to treat certain types of seizures, including elementary partial and complex partial seizures, with and without secondary generalization. This drug has been approved by the FDA for the treatment of epilepsy in adults. An NDA has been submitted for Neurontin as a treatment for epilepsy in pediatric subjects. In addition, Neurontin may be used in the future for the treatment of generalized and social anxiety disorders, panic disorder, and bipolar disorder.

INDICATION(S) AND RESEARCH PHASE
Epilepsy – FDA approved
Pediatric, Epilepsy – NDA submitted

ganaxolone, CCD-1042
unknown

MANUFACTURER
CoCensys

DESCRIPTION
Ganaxolone is a synthetic epalon-based compound that works as an allosteric receptor modulator of the neurotransmitter, gamma-amino butyric acid (GABA). Epalons are naturally occurring neuroactive compounds.

Ganaxolone is being tested as both an oral suspension and tablet formulation. The company reported that phase II trials are completed for migraine prophylaxis.

In addition, ganaxolone is being evaluated in a phase II trial for the treatment of catamenial (related to menstruation) epilepsy. Seizure research includes the orphan indication of infantile spasms and the treatment of adult subjects experiencing complex partial seizures. Furthermore, a phase II trial is being conducted in pediatric subjects from two months to 15 years of age suffering from epilepsy.

INDICATION(S) AND RESEARCH PHASE
Epilepsy – Phase II
Migraine and Cluster Headaches – Phase II completed
Pediatric, Epilepsy – Phase II

rufinamide, RUF 331
unknown

MANUFACTURER
Novartis

DESCRIPTION
Rufinamide is an anticonvulsant being evaluated in phase III trials for the treatment of epilepsy. It acts as a sodium-dependent action potential inhibitor and is made in an oral formulation. It is being tested in children two to 18 years of age with epilepsy.

INDICATION(S) AND RESEARCH PHASE
Pediatric, Epilepsy – Phase III

vigabatin
Sabril

MANUFACTURER
Aventis

DESCRIPTION
Sabril was in a phase III trial for epilepsy in children three to 16 years old. Development has been discontinued.

INDICATION(S) AND RESEARCH PHASE
Pediatric, Epilepsy – Phase III Discontinued

Esophageal Infections

Lansoprazole
Prevacid

MANUFACTURER
TAP Pharmaceuticals

DESCRIPTION
Prevacid (lansoprazole) is a proton pump inhibitor (PPI) indicated for the relief of heartburn symptoms in patients with erosive esophagitis. PPIs relieve heartburn through interaction with the gastric acid pump, H+, K+-adenosine triphosphatase (ATPase). The drugs accumulate in the acid space of the parietal cell and block the final step of acid secretion by inhibiting H+, K+-ATPase. Prevacid is currently in phase I trials for pediatric subjects one to 17 years old. The drug is approved for use in adults for the same indication.

INDICATION(S) AND RESEARCH PHASE
Pediatric, Esophageal Disorders – Phase I

Eye Disorders/Infections

cysteamine hydrochloride
Cystavision

MANUFACTURER
Sigma-Tau Pharmaceuticals

DESCRIPTION
Cysteamine hydrochloride eye drops are being tested for the treatment of corneal cystine accumulation, a rare disorder affecting approximately 1,000 individuals. Corneal cystine accumulation is the formation of crystals in the cornea of the eye as a result of the build up of cystine, a naturally occurring amino acid. This condition is a consequence of cystinosis, a rare and serious genetic disease that primarily affects kidney function. Phase III trials for pediatric subjects up to 18 years of age have been completed.

INDICATION(S) AND RESEARCH PHASE
Pediatric, Eye Disorders/Infections – Phase III completed

povidone-iodine
unknown

MANUFACTURER
Escalon Medical

DESCRIPTION
Povidone-iodine is a 2.5% solution for the prevention of neonatal conjunctivitis. The Company is currently searching for a development partner before continuing with clinical trials. Providone-iodine is available for topical use as a disinfectant.

INDICATION(S) AND RESEARCH PHASE
Pediatric, Eye Disorders/Infections – Phase III

---

unknown
Azelastine

MANUFACTURER
ASTA Medica AG

DESCRIPTION
Azelastine eye drops are indicated for the treatment of allergic conjunctivitis and rhinoconjunctivitis. This product alleviates tearing and redness without the side effects of other treatments. An NDA was submitted to the FDA in August of 1999. In Europe, an extension of the approval was granted allowing the company to sell the product for children four to 12 years. An extension to include the new indication, treatment and prophylaxis of perennial allergic conjunctivitis, is now being prepared for approval in Europe. If approval is granted, new trials will be initiated to test for this indication.

INDICATION(S) AND RESEARCH PHASE
Pediatric, Eye Disorders/Infections – NDA Submitted

Fabry Disease

agalsidase beta
Fabrazyme

MANUFACTURER
Genzyme

DESCRIPTION
Fabrazyme is an enzyme replacement therapy for subjects with Fabry disease, which is an inherited disorder caused by a deficiency of the enzyme alpha-galactosidase. This deficiency results in the body's inability to break down certain glycolipids, primarily globotriaosylceramide (GL-3), which then accumulate in the lining of the blood vessels within the kidney, heart, skin and other organs. This accumulation can result in kidney failure, stroke, and cardiac disease.

Results of a pivotal phase III trial of Fabrazyme demonstrated that it has a significant effect in clearing GL-3 from major organs affected by Fabry disease. The trial's primary endpoint — a nearly complete clearance of GL-3 from the blood vessels of the kidney — was met with high statistical significance. The double-blinded, randomized, and placebo-controlled study enrolled 58 subjects at eight medical centers in the United States and Europe. In addition to meeting its primary endpoint, the trial met two of its secondary efficacy endpoints, and positive trends were observed within the trial's nine tertiary endpoints.

Fabrazyme is being tested in a phase III trial for pediatric subjects.

INDICATION(S) AND RESEARCH PHASE
Fabry Disease – Phase III
Pediatric, Fabry Disease – Phase III

Familial Adenomatous Polyposis Coli

exisulind
Aptosyn

MANUFACTURER
Cell Pathways

DESCRIPTION
Aptosyn (exisulind) belongs to a novel class of compounds called selective apoptotic anti-neoplastic drugs (SAANDs). SAANDs inhibit a form of cyclic GMP phosphodiesterase and selectively induce apoptosis in abnormally growing precancerous and cancerous cells. Aptosyn is being tested for several indications and is in five different trials for adenomatous polyposis coli (APC) and familial adenomatous polyposis coli; two of these trials are specifically for pediatric subjects.

The company received a non-approvable letter from the FDA in September 2000 for one of the trials for familial adenomatous polyposis. The company intends to amend the NDA and request a meeting to address the deficiencies and the possible requirement for additional clinical data.

Additionally, Aptosyn is being tested in trials for the treatment of prostate cancer, lung cancer, breast cancer, sporadic colonic polyps, and Barrett's esophagus disease.

INDICATION(S) AND RESEARCH PHASE
Adenomatous Polyposis Coli – Non-approvable letter
Pediatric, Familial Adenomatous Polyposis Coli – Phase II
Adenomatous Polyposis Coli – Phase I/II
Barrett's Esophagus Disease – Phase II
Prostate Cancer – Phase II/III
Breast Cancer – Phase II/III
Lung Cancer – Phase Ib
Colon Polyps – Phase II/III

Gastroesophageal Reflux Disease (GERD)

rabeprazole sodium, E3810
Aciphex

MANUFACTURER
Eisai

DESCRIPTION
Rabeprazole has been characterized as a gastric proton-pump inhibitor that blocks the final step of gastric acid secretion. Aciphex has been approved for the following indications: healing of erosive or ulcerative gastroesophageal reflux disease (GERD); maintenance of healing of erosive or ulcerative GERD; healing of duodenal ulcer; and treatment of pathological hypersecretory conditions, including Zollinger-Ellison Syndrome.

Results of an eight-week, open-label, multicenter trial of Aciphex indicated that it provides symptom relief for both daytime and nighttime heartburn after the first day of treatment. The trial involved more than 2,500 subjects with endoscopically confirmed GERD. By day seven, 91.2% of subjects reported satisfactory symptom relief for daytime heartburn, and 91.7% reported satisfactory symptom relief for nighttime heartburn. Research was sponsored by Janssen Pharmaceutica and Eisai.

It is currently in phase I trials for GERD in pediatric patients seven to 16 years of age.

INDICATION(S) AND RESEARCH PHASE
Gastroesophageal Reflux Disease (GERD) – FDA Approved
Pediatric, Gastroesophageal Reflux Disease (GERD) – Phase I
Helicobacter Pylori – Phase III
Ulcers – FDA Approved

Glaucoma

brimonidine tartrate
Alphagan

MANUFACTURER
Allergan

DESCRIPTION
Alphagan is a 0.2% ophthalmic solution of brimonidine tartrate. Brimonidine tartrate is an alpha2-adrenergic agonist indicated for lowering intraocular pressure in subjects with primary open angle glaucoma or ocular hypertension. The drug is currently in phase III trials for pediatric glaucoma in subjects two to seven years of age.

INDICATION(S) AND RESEARCH PHASE
Pediatric, Glaucoma – Phase III

Graft Versus Host Disease

MEDI-507
unknown

MANUFACTURER
MedImmune

DESCRIPTION
MEDI-507 is a humanized form of the murine monoclonal antibody, BTI-322. It binds specifically to the CD2 receptor found on T cells and natural killer (NK) cells and has the ability to inhibit the response of T cells directed at transplant antigens, while still allowing immune cells to respond normally to other antigens.

The compound is in development for the treatment of steroid-resistant, severe graft-versus-host disease (GvHD) in adult and pediatric subjects. Additionally, MEDI-507 is in phase II development for psoriasis. Development for the prevention of acute renal transplant rejection has been discontinued.

INDICATION(S) AND RESEARCH PHASE
Psoriasis and Psoriatic Disorders – Phase II
Pediatric, Graft Versus Host Disease – Phase I/II
Graft Versus Host Disease – Phase I/II

Growth Hormone Deficiencies/ Abnormalities

pralmorelin
unknown

MANUFACTURER
Fujisawa Healthcare

DESCRIPTION
Pralmorelin is a growth hormone releasing factor that is being developed for treatment of growth retardation. The releasing factor may activate the anterior lobe of the pituitary gland to secrete growth hormone into the bloodstream. Pralmorelin is being tested in phase II/III clinical trials. Fujisawa Healthcare has a licensing agreement with ICN Pharmaceuticals for this drug product.

INDICATION(S) AND RESEARCH PHASE
Pediatric, Growth Hormone Deficiencies/Abnormalities – Phase II/III

Somatropin
Genotropin

MANUFACTURER
Pharmacia

DESCRIPTION
Genotropin is currently in phase III trials for pediatric subjects 2 years and older for the treatment of growth retardation in SGA (small for gestational age) children. In addition, an NDA has been submitted for pediatric subjects 2 years and older for growth retardation in Prader-Willi syndrome.

INDICATION(S) AND RESEARCH PHASE
Pediatric, Growth Hormone Deficiencies/Abnormalities – Phase III

Helicobacter Pylori Infection

vaccine, Helicobacter pylori
Helivax

MANUFACTURER
Antex Biologics

DESCRIPTION
This vaccine/adjuvant combination is designed for the prevention and treatment of peptic ulcers and gastrointestinal disorders caused by the bacterium, *Helicobacter pylori*. The vaccine is given in an oral liquid formulation.

INDICATION(S) AND RESEARCH PHASE
Helicobacter Pylori – Phase II
Pediatric, Helicobacter Pylori Infection – Phase I/II

Hepatitis

hepatitis B immune globulin
HBVIg

MANUFACTURER
Nabi

DESCRIPTION
HBVIg is a human hepatitis B immune globulin in development for the treatment of acute exposure to blood containing hepatitis B virus surface antigen. It is also being developed in an intravenous formulation to prevent hepatitis B virus re-infection of transplanted livers in subjects with hepatitis B. A Biologics License Application has been

submitted for the first indication, and the drug is in phase III trials regarding liver transplants.

INDICATION(S) AND RESEARCH PHASE
Liver Transplant – Phase III
Pediatric, Hepatitis – NDA submitted

hepatitis vaccine
Twinrix-2 doses

MANUFACTURER
GlaxoSmithKline

DESCRIPTION
Twinrix (2 doses) is a recombinant vaccine that immunizes recipients against both hepatitis A and hepatitis B. Benefits of this vaccine may include greater convenience and protection for subjects, since immunization against two diseases can be achieved with one injection. Twinrix (two doses) is in phase III trials for combined hepatitis A and B prophylaxis in children and adolescents.

INDICATION(S) AND RESEARCH PHASE
Pediatric, Hepatitis – Phase III
Vaccines – Phase III

HeXa-HepB-IPV/Hib
Infanrix

MANUFACTURER
GlaxoSmithKline

DESCRIPTION
This conjugated, recombinant pediatric vaccine is being developed for a variety of indications. It has been approved by the European Union (EU) as a vaccine for the prevention of diphtheria, tetanus, pertussis, hepatitis B, polio prophylaxis and Haemophilus influenzae type B. An estimated NDA filing date has yet to be determined by the company.

INDICATION(S) AND RESEARCH PHASE
Vaccines – EU Approved
Pediatric, Viral Infection- EU Approved
Pediatric, Hepatitis – EU Approved

lamivudine
Zeffix

MANUFACTURER
GlaxoSmithKline

DESCRIPTION
Zeffix (lamivudine) is a reverse transcriptase inhibitor designed for the treatment of hepatitis B. Lamivudine is phosphorylated into its active 5'-triphosphate metabolite, which inhibits HIV reverse transcription via viral DNA chain termination. It also inhibits the RNA- and DNA-dependent DNA polymerase activities of reverse transcriptase. Zeffix has been approved by the FDA for use in the United States. It is also in phase III trials for the treatment of hepatitis B in pediatric subjects.

INDICATION(S) AND RESEARCH PHASE
Hepatitis – FDA Approved
Pediatric, Hepatitis – Phase III

vaccine, Hepatitis A
unknown

MANUFACTURER
Aventis Pasteur

DESCRIPTION
This vaccine is currently in phase III pediatric trials for the treatment of hepatitis A.

INDICATION(S) AND RESEARCH PHASE
Pediatric, Hepatitis – Phase III

vaccine, HIB/Hep B/IPV/DtaP
unknown

MANUFACTURER
Aventis Pasteur

DESCRIPTION
This vaccine is in development for the treatment of Haemophilus influenzae b, hepatitis B, polio, diphtheria, tetanus, and pertussis. It is in phase II/III trials in children ages two, four, and six months.

INDICATION(S) AND RESEARCH PHASE
Pediatric, Diptheria, Tetanus, Pertussis, Polio – Phase II/III
Pediatric, Hepatitis – Phase II/III

HIV/AIDS

abacavir
Ziagen

MANUFACTURER
GlaxoSmithKline

DESCRIPTION
Ziagen is a nucleoside reverse transcriptase inhibitor (NRTI) approved by the FDA for the treatment of HIV-1 infection in adults and children (ages three months and above). It is also in phase II trials in combination with the reverse transcriptase inhibitor Epivir for the treatment of HIV infection.

INDICATION(S) AND RESEARCH PHASE
HIV Infection – Phase II
Pediatric, HIV Infection – FDA approved

emivirine
Coactinon

MANUFACTURER
Triangle Pharmaceuticals

DESCRIPTION
Coactinon is a nucleoside analogue derivative that functions as a non-nucleoside reverse transcriptase inhibitor (NNRTI). In August 2000, the company announced its intention to continue developing Coactinon for the treatment of HIV infection, following notification in 1999 that additional phase III trials may be necessary to prove that regimens containing Coactinon are equivalent or superior to current first-line therapies. MKC-401 is currently ongoing and has been amended to enroll an additional 280 subjects.

INDICATION(S) AND RESEARCH PHASE
Acquired Immune Deficiency Syndrome (AIDS) and AIDS-Related Infections – Phase III

HIV Infection – Phase III
Pediatric, AIDS/HIV – Phase III

emtricitabine
Coviracil

MANUFACTURER
Triangle Pharmaceuticals

DESCRIPTION
Coviracil, a nucleoside reverse transcript inhibitor (NRTI), has been shown to be a potent inhibitor of hepatitis B virus (HBV) replication. In October 2000, results of a phase I/II trial of Coviracil involving subjects chronically infected with HBV indicated that a daily dose of 200 mg was most effective. As a result, the 200 mg/day dosage was selected for a phase III trial, which was initiated in October 2000. Coviracil is also in phase III trials for the treatment of HIV infection in adult and pediatric subjects.

INDICATION(S) AND RESEARCH PHASE
HIV Infection – Phase III
Hepatitis – Phase III
Pediatric, AIDS/HIV – Phase III

delavirdine mesylate
Rescriptor

MANUFACTURER
Agouron Pharmaceuticals

DESCRIPTION
Rescriptor belongs to the class of anti-HIV drugs called non-nucleoside reverse transcriptase inhibitors (NNRTIs). Rescriptor is approved for the treatment of HIV infection in adults. The drug is currently in a phase II pediatric trial for the treatment of HIV/AIDS.

INDICATION(S) AND RESEARCH PHASE
Pediatric, HIV Infection – Phase II

HIV-1 immunogen
Remune

MANUFACTURER
Immune Response Corporation

DESCRIPTION
Remune (HIV-1 immunogen) is designed to stimulate an individual's immune system to attack HIV-infected cells and slow the progression of the disease. Trial results have indicated the drug produces a favorable impact on important indicators of HIV disease progression including CD4 cell levels, viral burden, weight gain, and the stimulation of cell-mediated immune responses to HIV.

Immune Response is conducting a phase I trial, in collaboration with the National Institutes of Health, in up to 32 HIV-infected children. The trial is designed to demonstrate the safety and immunogenicity of the product in a pediatric population.

Remune is co-developed by the Immune Response Corporation and Agouron Pharmaceuticals.

INDICATION(S) AND RESEARCH PHASE
HIV Infection – Phase III
Pediatric, HIV Infection – Phase I

pentafuside, T-20
unknown

MANUFACTURER
Trimeris

DESCRIPTION
Pentafuside (T-20) belongs to a new class of investigational anti-HIV treatments called fusion inhibitors. Unlike existing anti-retroviral drugs that work in the cell to target enzymes involved in viral replication, T-20 inhibits fusion of HIV with host cells before the virus can begin replicating and infecting other cells.

Results of an open-label, randomized phase II trial of T-20 in combination with oral antiretrovirals suggested that the addition of T-20 to a standard antiretroviral regimen was well tolerated and provided additional decreases in viral load compared to the antiretroviral control regimen alone in HIV subjects.

Preliminary results of a phase I/II trial suggested that short-term (up to 12 weeks) subcutaneous dosing with T-20 was well tolerated by children with HIV. Additionally, in the highest dose group (60 mg/m^2), T-20 caused rapid suppression of HIV RNA of approximately 10-fold average reduction from baseline levels in seven days. The trial evaluated 12 treatment-experienced or treatment-naïve children ages three to 12. It was conducted in collaboration with the Pediatric AIDS Clinical Trials Group (PACTG) of the National Institute of Allergy and Infectious Diseases.

T-20 is co-developed by Trimeris and Hoffmann-La Roche.

INDICATION(S) AND RESEARCH PHASE
HIV Infection – Phase II
Pediatric, HIV Infection – Phase II

PRO 542
unknown

MANUFACTURER
Progenics Pharmaceuticals

DESCRIPTION
PRO 542, a novel fusion protein, incorporates the HIV-binding region of the human cell surface receptor (CD4) into a human antibody molecule. This complex binds to the HIV surface glycoprotein and blocks the virus from attaching itself to human host cells. This mechanism of action is unique among antiretrovirals that are either approved or in late stage clinical development.

Additionally, PRO 542 is being evaluated in a multi-dose phase II pediatric trial sponsored by the AIDS Clinical Trials Group of the National Institutes of Health. Engineered to provide a different strategy for treating and preventing HIV infection, subjects have been able to tolerate PRO 542 in early clinical testing.

Results from a phase I trial demonstrated PRO 542 had strong antiviral effects and was considered safe and effective in subjects who were infected with HIV. The subjects received a single injection of PRO 542 at one of four dose levels. Subjects receiving high doses of PRO 542 showed a statistically significant acute reduction in plasma HIV RNA or viral load, which is considered an accepted clinical endpoint for antiretroviral therapies. Phase II testing is under way.

INDICATION(S) AND RESEARCH PHASE
Acquired Immune Deficiency Syndrome (AIDS) and AIDS-Related Infections – Phase II
HIV Infection – Phase II
Pediatric, HIV Infection – Phase II

---

rifapentine, MDL-473
Priftin

MANUFACTURER
Aventis

DESCRIPTION
Priftin is an antibiotic prophylactic treatment of Mycobacterium avium complex in patients with AIDS and a CD4+ count less than or equal to 75/mm3. The drug was formerly in phase III trials for this indication and is also indicated for other bacterial infections. Priftin is an orphan indication because there are relatively few cases of this particular condition. Currently development of this drug has been discontinued.

INDICATION(S) AND RESEARCH PHASE
Acquired Immune Deficiency Syndrome (AIDS) and AIDS-Related Infections – Phase III Discontinued
Pediatric, Acquired Immune Deficiency Syndrome (AIDS) and AIDS-Related Infections – Phase III Discontinued

---

saquinavir
Fortovase

MANUFACTURER
Hoffman-La Roche

DESCRIPTION
Fortovase brand of saquinavir is an inhibitor of the human immunodeficiency virus (HIV) protease. The drug is indicated for use in combination with other antiretroviral agents for the treatment of HIV infection. Fortovase in combination with nucleoside analogues and/or protease inhibitors is being tested in a phase III pediatric trial in children six months to 13 years old.

INDICATION(S) AND RESEARCH PHASE
Pediatric, HIV Infection – Phase III

Hormone Deficiencies

somatropin
Nutropin Depot

MANUFACTURER
Genentech

DESCRIPTION
Nutropin Depot is a long-acting dosage formulation of Genetech's human growth hormone, which employs Alkermes' ProLease injectable extended-release drug delivery system. The drug is currently indicated for the long-term treatment of growth failure in pediatric subjects due to a lack of adequate endogenous growth hormone secretion. Nutropin Depot entered a phase II/III trial in January 2001 for treatment of adults with growth hormone deficiencies. Genentech is co-developing Nutropin Depot with Alkermes.

INDICATION(S) AND RESEARCH PHASE
Hormone Deficiencies – Phase II/III
Pediatric, Hormone Deficiencies – FDA approved

Hyperlipidemia

atorvastatin calcium
Lipitor

MANUFACTURER

DESCRIPTION
Lipitor (atorvastatin calcium) is a selective, competitive inhibitor of 3-hydroxy-3-methylglutaryl-coenzyme A (HMG-CoA) reductase, the enzyme that converts HMG-CoA to mevalonate, a precursor of sterols including cholesterol. By blocking or inhibiting the action of HMG-CoA reductase, a link is broken in the chain of reactions that produces cholesterol. When less cholesterol is produced, the liver takes up more cholesterol from the bloodstream, which results in lower levels of cholesterol circulating in the blood. Lipitor has been approved by the FDA for the reduction of LDL cholesterol and triglyceride levels in adults. It is currently in phase III trials for children 10-17 years old for the treatment of hyperlipidemia.

INDICATION(S) AND RESEARCH PHASE
Pediatric, Hyperlipidemia – Phase III

Hypertension

amlodipine besylate
Norvasc

MANUFACTURER
Pfizer

DESCRIPTION
Norvasc is the besylate salt of amlodipine, a long acting calcium channel blocker. The drug blocks the flow of calcium ions across the cell membrane into vascular smooth muscle and cardiac muscle. Additionally, Norvasc is a peripheral arterial vasodilator that acts directly on vascular smooth muscle to reduce peripheral vascular resistance and blood pressure.

Norvasc has been approved by the FDA for the treatment of hypertension, chronic stable angina, and vasospastic angina in adults.

It is currently in phase III trials for hypertension in children between the ages of six and 17 years.

INDICATION(S) AND RESEARCH PHASE
Pediatric, Hypertension – Phase III
Hypertension – FDA approved
Angina – FDA approved

---

benazepril hydrochloride
Lotensin

MANUFACTURER
Novartis

DESCRIPTION
Lotensin (benazepril) is an angiotensin converting enzyme inhibitor (ACEI). ACE inhibitors block the conversion of angiotensin I to the vasoconstrictor angiotensin II. Without this vasoconstric-

tion, the heart does not have to work against as much resistance when pumping blood throughout the body. Angiotensin II also stimulates the release of aldosterone, which causes the kidney to reabsorb sodium and increases fluid retention. The increased fluid results in more work for the heart, as it has to pump a larger overall volume. The overall effects of ACE on the vasculature and kidneys can result in hypertension. ACEI have been successfully used as anti-hypertensives in adults.

Lotensin has been approved by the FDA for the treatment of hypertension in adults. It is currently in a phase III trial for pediatric subjects ages one month to 16 years for hypertension.

INDICATION(S) AND RESEARCH PHASE
Hypertension – FDA Approved
Pediatric, Hypertension – Phase III

candesartan cilexetil
Atacand

MANUFACTURER
AstraZeneca

DESCRIPTION
Atacand (candesartan cilexetil) is an angiotensin II receptor blocker (ARB) being tested for the treatment of hypertension. Results of two multicenter, double-blind, randomized studies in more than 1,200 hypertensive subjects demonstrated Atacand to be significantly more effective in lowering both diastolic and systolic blood pressure than the most prescribed ARB, Cozaar (losartan). During the double-blind treatment period, subjects were randomized to receive either 16 mg of Atacand or 50 mg of losartan. At week two, all subjects were titrated to double their current dose to 32 mg of Atacand or 100 mg of losartan. Duration of treatment was eight weeks unless a subject was discontinued due to an adverse event, had an insufficient therapeutic response, or withdrew consent. The incidence of discontinuation was only 2.7% for Atacand and 1.8% for losartan. The most commonly reported adverse events for both medications were headache, dizziness, sinusitis, and respiratory infection.

The drug is currently being tested in phase III trials for hypertension outcomes (SCOPE study), congestive heart failure outcomes (CHARM study), and diabetic retinopathy. Pediatric phase III trials for hypertension are ongoing. Atacand Plus (a diuretic formula) is FDA approved for hypertension in adults.

INDICATION(S) AND RESEARCH PHASE
Hypertension – Phase III
Pediatric, Hypertension – Phase III
Congestive Heart Failure – Phase III
Diabetic Retinopathy – Phase III

felodipine
Plendil

MANUFACTURER
AstraZeneca

DESCRIPTION
Plendil is in a phase III trial for pediatric subjects for hypertension.

INDICATION(S) AND RESEARCH PHASE
Pediatric, Hypertension – Phase III

lisinopril
Zestril

MANUFACTURER
AstraZeneca

DESCRIPTION
Zestril (lisinopril) is an oral long-acting angiotensin converting enzyme(ACE) inhibitor that is currently in a phase III trial in pediatric subjects for hypertension.

INDICATION(S) AND RESEARCH PHASE
Pediatric, Hypertension – Phase III

metoprolol succinate
Toprol-XL

MANUFACTURER
AstraZeneca

DESCRIPTION
Toprol- XL (metoprolol succinate) has been FDA approved for angina, hypertension and congestive heart failure. The MERIT-HF study has been completed and trial results showed that study volunteers taking Toprol-XL beta-blockers along with standard treatment for congestive heart failure had an increased survival rate. It is given orally once daily.

In addition, Toprol-XL is being tested in phase III trials for pediatric subjects suffering from hypertension.

INDICATION(S) AND RESEARCH PHASE
Pediatric, Hypertension – Phase III
Angina – FDA Approved
Hypertension – FDA Approved
Congestive Heart Failure – FDA Approved

quinapril hydrochloride
Accupril

MANUFACTURER
Accupril

DESCRIPTION
Accupril is an inhibitor of ACE, a peptidyl dipeptidase that catalyzes the conversion of angiotensin I to the vasoconstrictor angiotensin II. The drug has been approved by the FDA for the treatment of hypertension and as adjunctive therapy for the management of heart failure. Accupril (tablet) is also in phase III trials for hypertension in infants up to 24 months old.

INDICATION(S) AND RESEARCH PHASE
Pediatric, Hypertension – Phase III

Hyperuricemia

SR 29142, rasburicase
Unknown

MANUFACTURER
Sanofi-Synthelabo Pharmaceuticals

DESCRIPTION
SR 29142 (rasburicase) is a recombinant urate oxidase developed for the prevention and treatment of hyperuricemia in subjects receiving chemotherapy. Rapid destruction of cancer cells can result in the release of

uric acid into the blood. Rasburicase acts by converting uric acid to alantoin, which can be excreted by the kidney. An NDA has been submitted for SR 29142 for pediatric subjects.

INDICATION(S) AND RESEARCH PHASE
Pediatric, Hyperuricemia – NDA submitted

Ileus

prucalopride
Resolor

MANUFACTURER
Janssen Pharmaceutica

DESCRIPTION
Resolor is a colonic motility agent for the treatment of chronic constipation. The drug is administered in an oral capsule formulation, and it is currently in phase III trials. Resolor is also being tested in an injectable subcutaneous formulation in phase I/II trials for post-operative ileus. Pediatric trials for this drug have been discontinued.

INDICATION(S) AND RESEARCH PHASE
Constipation – Phase III
Ileus – Phase I/II
Pediatric, Ileus – Trial discontinued

Influenza

unknown
FluMist

MANUFACTURER
Wyeth-Ayerst

DESCRIPTION
FluMist is an investigational cold-adapted intranasal influenza vaccine. It is designed to be effective in children by inducing immunity via the nasal mucosa. In October 2000, Aviron and American Home Products Corporation announced that a Biologics License Application for FluMist has been submitted to the FDA. Wyeth-Ayerst is the pharmaceutical division of American Home Products.

INDICATION(S) AND RESEARCH PHASE
Influenza – Phase III
Pediatric, Influenza – Phase III
Vaccines – Phase III

vaccine, DPT/ Haemophilus influenzae type B
unknown

MANUFACTURER
Chiron Corporation

DESCRIPTION
Chiron Corporation has formulated a combination vaccine that might effectively immunize children against four serious diseases: *Haemophilus influenzae* type B, diphtheria, pertussis, and tetanus—with a single injection. This vaccine has the potential to simplify pediatric vaccination schedules, thereby lowering costs, increasing convenience, and improving compliance. The vaccine is composed of inactive molecules of diphtheria toxin, pertussis toxin, and tetanus toxin. The vaccine also contains inactivated *H. influenza* proteins.

INDICATION(S) AND RESEARCH PHASE
Pediatric, Bacterial Infection – Phase III
Pediatric, Influenza – Phase III
Pediatric, Vaccines – Phase III
Pediatric, Viral Infection – Phase III

vaccine, influenza
unknown

MANUFACTURER
BioChem Pharma

DESCRIPTION
In order to improve vaccination rates, BioChem Pharma is developing an influenza vaccine to be taken as a nasal spray. This method of vaccination may create a helpful systemic immune response in the blood and throughout the body, and may stimulate a local immune response in the mucosal lining of the nose, mouth, and throat, which would create an additional barrier to influenza infection and increase efficacy. Phase I results have shown comparable immunization responses to that of the injectable vaccine. Clinical testing is in phase II for the influenza virus in both children and adults.

INDICATION(S) AND RESEARCH PHASE
Influenza – Phase II
Vaccines – Phase II
Pediatric, Influenza – Phase II

vaccine, parainfluenza
unknown

MANUFACTURER
Wyeth-Lederle Vaccines

DESCRIPTION
This product is a novel vaccine for prevention of parainfluenza virus (PIV), a mediated serious respiratory illness in children. The vaccine is made from live attenuated influenza A virus and is administered as a nasal spray. These live attenuated vaccines stimulate local antibody production more efficiently than conventional inactivated vaccines. The drug is in phase II testing in adults and phase I/II testing in infants and toddlers.

INDICATION(S) AND RESEARCH PHASE
Influenza – Phase II
Pediatric, Influenza – Phase I/II

Kidney Transplant Surgery

mycophenylate mofetil
CellCept

MANUFACTURER
Hoffman-La Roche

DESCRIPTION
CellCept is an orally formulated drug that inhibits inflammation caused by abnormal immunological responses. Clinical trials are testing CellCept in phase III for the treatment for kidney transplant surgery in pediatric subjects.

INDICATION(S) AND RESEARCH PHASE
Pediatric, Kidney Transplant Surgery – Phase III

Leukemia

Busulfan
Busulfex

MANUFACTURER

DESCRIPTION
Busulfex is an alkylating agent that interferes with the function of bone marrow. In February 1999, the FDA approved Busulfex Injection for use in combination with cyclophosphamide as a conditioning regimen prior to allogenic hematopoietic progenitor cell transplantation for chronic myelogenous leukemia. Currently, Busulfex is being evaluated for ages newborn to 16 years; trials have been completed, however an NDA has not yet been submitted.

INDICATION(S) AND RESEARCH PHASE
Pediatric, Leukemia – Phase III completed

clofarabine
unknown

MANUFACTURER
Bioenvision

DESCRIPTION
Clofarabine, a 2-fluoro-2-chloro substituted purine nucleoside analog, is currently undergoing phase II trials at the M.D. Anderson Cancer Center in Houston. The drug is being given to fludarabine-resistant subjects with acute lymphocytic leukemia and subjects with acute myelogenous leukemia. Trials are being conducted in both adult and pediatric subjects.

Clofarabine's unique mechanism of action stems from its nulcleoside structural features, where both the purine and ribose rings are halogenated. This purine analog inhibits DNA synthesis at two critical junctures, DNA polymerse I and RNA reductase.

INDICATION(S) AND RESEARCH PHASE
Leukemia – Phase II
Pediatric, Leukemia – Phase II

gemtuzumab ozogamicin
Mylotarg

MANUFACTURER
Celltech Chiroscience plc

DESCRIPTION
Mylotarg (gemtuzumab ozogamicin) is a chemotherapeutic agent targeted directly to cancerous cells using monoclonal antibody technology. It consists of a recombinant antibody linked with an anti-tumor antibiotic called calicheamicin. The antibody portion of Mylotarg binds specifically to the CD33 antigen, a protein commonly found on leukemic cells. Mylotarg is indicated for the treatment of acute myeloid leukemia (AML) in first relapse subjects who are 60 years of age or older and who are not considered candidates for cytoxic chemotherapy. The product was approved by the FDA under accelerated approval provisions due to a lack of current products for subjects with relapse of AML. It is also in pediatric phase I trials for subjects 18 years of age and younger. Mylotarg has been jointly developed by Wyeth-Ayerst and Celltech Group.

INDICATION(S) AND RESEARCH PHASE
Leukemia – FDA Approved
Pediatric, Leukemia – Phase I

imatinib, STI 571
Glivec

MANUFACTURER
Novartis

DESCRIPTION
Glivec is a Bcr-Abl tyrokinase inhibitor. The drug works by blocking signals within cancer cells that express the Bcr-Abl protein, thus preventing a series of chemical reactions that elicit cell proliferation. Glivec is currently in phase III trials for acute lymphocytic leukemia and an NDA has been submitted for chronic myeloid leukemia. It is also in a phase I trial for Philadelphia-positive leukemia for newborns to children 16 years old.

INDICATION(S) AND RESEARCH PHASE
Leukemia – NDA submitted
Leukemia – Phase III
Pediatric, Leukemia – Phase I

TNP-470
unknown

MANUFACTURER
Takeda Chemical Industries

DESCRIPTION
TNP-470 is a synthetically modified form of the antibiotic fumagillin. This drug inhibits new blood vessel growth and is being tested in phase II trials for the treatment of adults with malignant solid tumors. It is also being evaluated in a phase I trial in children with solid tumors, lymphomas, and acute leukemias.

INDICATION(S) AND RESEARCH PHASE
Cancer/Tumors (Unspecified) – Phase II
Pediatric, Solid Tumors – Phase I
Pediatric, Leukemia – Phase I
Pediatric, Lymphomas – Phase I

Lung Disease

recombinant human superoxide dismutase (rhSOD)
Oxsodrol

MANUFACTURER
Bio-Technology General

DESCRIPTION
Oxsodrol is indicated for the treatment of bronchopulmonary dysplasia. It is currently in phase II trials in premature infants.

INDICATION(S) AND RESEARCH PHASE
Pediatric, Lung Disease – Phase II

Lymphomas

TNP-470
unknown

MANUFACTURER
Takeda Chemical Industries

DESCRIPTION
TNP-470 is a synthetically modified form of the antibiotic fumagillin. This drug inhibits new blood vessel growth and is being tested in phase II trials for the treatment of adults with malignant solid tumors. It is also being evaluated in a phase I trial in children with solid tumors, lymphomas, and acute leukemias.

INDICATION(S) AND RESEARCH PHASE
Cancer/Tumors (Unspecified) – Phase II
Pediatric, Solid Tumors – Phase I
Pediatric, Leukemia – Phase I
Pediatric, Lymphomas – Phase I

Meconium Aspiration Syndrome

lucinactant
Surfaxin

MANUFACTURER
Discovery Laboratories

DESCRIPTION
Surfaxin has been granted a fast track designation by the FDA for development as a treatment for meconium aspiration syndrome (MAS), acute respiratory distress syndrome (ARDS), and acute lung injury (ALI). The drug is currently in late stage phase III trials in premature babies.

Surfactant is a surface-active agent secreted by alveolar type II cells that decreases the surface tension of pulmonary fluids and increases elasticity of lung tissue. Surfaxin is a novel surfactant, containing a peptide mimic of the human protein B. It cleanses the lung and restores surfactant inactivated by MAS.

INDICATION(S) AND RESEARCH PHASE
Pediatric, Meconium Aspiration Syndrome and Acute Lung Injury – Phase III

Meningitis

cytarabine liposome injection
DepoCyt

MANUFACTURER
Skye Pharma

DESCRIPTION
DepoCyt is an injectable sustained-release formulation that gradually releases cytarabine into the cerebral spinal fluid (CSF). Cytarabine is a cell cycle phase-specific drug that stops or slows the maturation and spread of tumor cells, affecting cells only during the S-phase of cell division. DepoCyt was approved by the FDA in 1999 for the treatment of lymphomatous meningitis. It is currently in phase I pediatric trials for newborns to children 18 years old.

DepoCyt is being co-developed by DepoTech Corporation (a wholly owned subsidiary of SkyPharma) and Chiron for the U.S. market; Pharmacia & Upjohn will market the product internationally.

INDICATION(S) AND RESEARCH PHASE
Meningitis – FDA approved
Pediatric, Meningitis – Phase I

vaccine, meningitis B
unknown

MANUFACTURER
GlaxoSmithKline

DESCRIPTION
This subunit vaccine has been designed for prevention of *Neisseria meningitides* type B in children. It is in phase II development.

INDICATION(S) AND RESEARCH PHASE
Pediatric, Meningitis – Phase II
Pediatric, Vaccines – Phase II

vaccine, meningococcal C conjugate
Meningitec

MANUFACTURER
Wyeth-Ayerst

DESCRIPTION
Meningitec is a conjugate vaccine for the prevention of meningococcal Group C disease. In October 1999, the vaccine was approved for use in the United Kingdom. Meningitec is being evaluated in clinics in combination with the pneumococcal conjugate vaccine.

INDICATION(S) AND RESEARCH PHASE
Meningitis – Phase III
Pediatric, Meningococcal Group C Meningitis – Phase III
Vaccines – Phase III

vaccine, meningococcus C
unknown

MANUFACTURER
Chiron Corporation

DESCRIPTION
Chiron Corporation is working on a new vaccine for meningococcal bacterial infections. The bacteria known as *Neisseria meningitidis* produce these infections. This organism can cause a variety of diseases ranging from benign upper respiratory infections to serious blood infections, which can lead to rashes, muscle and joint aches, and meningitis.

INDICATION(S) AND RESEARCH PHASE
Pediatric, Meningitis – Phase III
Pediatric, Vaccines – Phase III

vaccine, N. meningitidis A/C
unknown

MANUFACTURER
GlaxoSmithKline

DESCRIPTION
N. meningitidis A/C is a conjugated vaccine in phase II trials for meningitis prophylaxis in children.

INDICATION(S) AND RESEARCH PHASE
Pediatric, Meningitis – Phase II
Vaccines – Phase II

Meningococcemia

opebecan, rBPI-21, recombinant human bactericidal/permeability-increasing protein
Neuprex

MANUFACTURER
XOMA Corporation

DESCRIPTION
Neuprex is a systemic formulation of recombinant bactericidal/permeability-increasing protein being developed for the treatment of severe meningococcemia, meningitis, pneumonia, liver disease, intra-abdominal infection and acute respiratory distress syndrome. The active molecule in Neuprex, rBPI-21, binds to the endotoxin molecules LOS and LPS, lipopolysaccharides in living bacteria, disrupting their cell walls, killing the bacteria, or making them more susceptible to antibiotics.

A 1,650 subject phase III trauma trial evaluating whether Neuprex can prevent pneumonia and acute respiratory distress syndrome (ARDS) is under way. Subjects are enrolled after experiencing a severe accident, in which they have lost at least two units of blood. More than 800 subjects are currently enrolled.

INDICATION(S) AND RESEARCH PHASE
Bacterial Infection – Phase III
Pediatric, Meningococcemia – Phase III completed
Meningitis – Phase III
Acute Respiratory Distress Syndrome (ARDS) – Phase III
Pneumonia – Phase III
Liver Disease – Phase II
Intra-abdominal Infection – Phase I/II

Metabolic Disease

alpha-1-iduronidase
Aldurazyme

MANUFACTURER
Genzyme

DESCRIPTION
Aldurazyme is an enzyme replacement therapy being evaluated for the treatment of mucopolysaccaridosis-I (MPS-I). In January 2001, results of an open-label trial indicated that Aldurazyme has the potential to alleviate the primary symptoms of MPS-I. The trial included ten MPS-I subjects ages five to 22 years, collectively exhibiting a wide range of clinical severity. Significantly decreased liver or spleen size was recorded in all subjects, with eight of 10 subjects showing a normal liver size by 26 weeks. Subjects experienced reduced excretion of complex carbohydrates in the urine within three to four weeks, reaching near normal excretions in nine of 10 subjects. Improved range of motion in the shoulder was observed, and subjects showed clinically significant improvements in sleep apnea. Finally, near double increases in height growth velocity and more than double weight growth velocity were reported in the six prepubertal subjects.

A phase III trial was initiated in December 2000, which BioMarin expects to conclude in the third quarter of 2001. Aldurazyme is being developed by BioMarin Pharmaceutical and Genzyme.

INDICATION(S) AND RESEARCH PHASE
Metabolic Disease – Phase III
Pediatric, Metabolic Disease – Phase III

Migraine and Cluster Headaches

sumatriptan
Imigran, Imitrex

MANUFACTURER
GlaxoSmithKline

DESCRIPTION
Imigran (sumatriptan) is a 5-hydroxytryptamine ($5HT_1$) agonist for the treatment of migraine headaches. $5HT_1$ receptors are found on the cells of cranial artery endothelia. When the receptors are activated by sumatriptan, the resulting vasoconstriction provides relief of migraine symptoms. A needle-free injection formulation of the drug is in phase II trials. Additionally, an MAA and an NDA have been submitted for a nasal formulation for the treatment of adolescent migraine. Imigran is also marketed under the trade name Imitrex.

INDICATION(S) AND RESEARCH PHASE
Pediatric, Adolescent Migraine – NDA submitted, MAA submitted
Migraine and Cluster Headaches – Phase II

zolmitriptan
Zomig

MANUFACTURER
AstraZeneca

DESCRIPTION
Zomig is an agent belonging to a new class of drugs known as "triptans," which target specific subtype receptors of the neurotransmitter, serotonin. Tripans are considered "abortive" drugs, since they stop the pain before it has started by constricting blood vessels in the brain associated with serotonergic nerve projections. It is thought that migraine headaches may occur due to dilation of these blood vessels. These triptans may also reduce inflammation in the nerves that signal the pain of a migraine headache.

Zomig capsules are currently FDA approved for treating adult migraines, an NDA has been submitted to include pediatric subjects who experience migraine headaches.

INDICATION(S) AND RESEARCH PHASE
Migraine and Cluster Headaches – FDA approved
Pediatric, Migraine – NDA submitted

zolmitriptan

Zomig Aura

MANUFACTURER
AstraZeneca

DESCRIPTION
Zomig Aura is an oral formulation of a second generation, selective serotonin ($5HT_1$ agonist) receptor stimulator in a phase III trial for the treatment of aura headaches due to migraines.

INDICATION(S) AND RESEARCH PHASE
Migraine and Cluster Headaches – Phase III
Pediatric, Migraine and Cluster Headaches – Phase III

Muscular Dystrophy

oxandrolone
Oxandrin

MANUFACTURER
Bio-Technology General

DESCRIPTION
Oxandrin is indicated for the treatment of Duchenne's muscular dystophy. Phase II studies have been completed in pediatric subjects five to 10 years of age.

INDICATION(S) AND RESEARCH PHASE
Pediatric, Muscular Dystrophy – Phase II completed

Neuroblastoma

vaccine, allogenic and autologous neuroblastoma cells
unknown

MANUFACTURER
St. Jude Children's Research Hospital

DESCRIPTION
Currently, phase II/III clinical trials are evaluating gene-modified cancer vaccines using autologous and allogenic tumor cells from interleukin-2 (IL-2) secreting neuroblastomas after autologous bone marrow transplant in first remission. Researchers are conducting parallel clinical trials in children with recurrent neuroblastoma who are receiving either allogenic or autologous tumor cells that are gene modified to secrete small amounts of IL-2.

In the autologous trial, one subject had a complete tumor response, one had a partial response, and three had stable disease following the tumor immunogen alone. Four of the five subjects with tumor responses had coexisting neuroblastoma-specific cytotoxic T-lymphocyte activity, as opposed to only one of the subjects with non-responsive disease. These results show a promising correlation between immune response and clinical outcome with autologous vaccines.

In the allogenic group, one child had a partial response, five had stable disease, and four had progressive disease. Although immunization with autologous vaccine produced superior immune responses, these results offer encouragement for the continued pursuit of allogenic vaccine strategies in human cancer.

INDICATION(S) AND RESEARCH PHASE
Pediatric, Neuroblastoma – Phase II/III
Pediatric, Vaccines – Phase II/III

Obesity

orlistat
Xenical

MANUFACTURER
Hoffmann-La Roche

DESCRIPTION
Xenical (orlistat) is a lipase inhibitor that inhibits the absorption of dietary fats. It is currently being marketed by Hoffmann-La Roche in the United States for the treatment of obesity. It is in phase III trials for children 12 to 16 years of age for obesity and phase III trials for diabetes in adult subjects.

INDICATION(S) AND RESEARCH PHASE
Obesity – FDA approved
Pediatric, Obesity – Phase III
Diabetes Mellitus Type 2 – Phase III

Otitis Media

amoxicillin/clavulanate
Augmentin ES

MANUFACTURER
GlaxoSmithKline

DESCRIPTION
Augmentin ES is a new formulation of Augmentin, a penicillin derivative already approved for use around the world. Results presented in September 2000 demonstrated that it is highly effective in eradicating the three most common bacteria (Streptococcus pneumoniae, Haemophilus influenzae, and Moraxella catarrhalis) that cause middle ear infections in children, including drug-resistant strains, while maintaining the typical safety profile of the currently marketed Augmentin. An NDA has been submitted for Augmentin ES for the treatment of acute otitis media, including penicillin-resistant S. pneumoniae.

INDICATION(S) AND RESEARCH PHASE
Pediatric, Bacterial Infection – NDA Submitted
Pediatric, Otitis Media – NDA Submitted

gatifloxacin
Tequin

MANUFACTURER
Bristol-Myers Squibb

DESCRIPTION
Tequin is a broad-spectrum 8-methoxy fluoroquinolone antibiotic in a phase II trial for the treatment of recurrent otitis media in subjects 6 months to 17 years old. Tequin is primarily excreted through the kidneys and less than 1% is metabolized by the liver. Tequin has been approved by the FDA for the treatment of certain infections in adults.

INDICATION(S) AND RESEARCH PHASE
Pediatric, Otitis Media – Phase II

levofloxacin

Levaquin

MANUFACTURER
R.W. Johnson Pharmaceutical Research Institute

DESCRIPTION
Levaquin (levofloxacin tablets/injection) is an anti-infective currently in phase I development for pediatric subjects with otitis media. Levaquin was FDA approved in 1991 for the treatment of adults with community-acquired pneumonia, acute maxillary sinusitis or acute bacterial exacerbation of chronic bronchitis. Levaquin was licensed from the Daiichi Seiyaku Company.

INDICATION(S) AND RESEARCH PHASE
Pediatric, Otitis Media – Phase I

NE-1530
unknown

MANUFACTURER
Neose Technologies

DESCRIPTION
NE-1530, a complex carbohydrate that is produced naturally in human breast milk, is an antibacterial agent being evaluated for the prevention and treatment of pediatric middle ear infections, or otitis media. Additional indications may include infectious diseases and viral diseases associated with the nose, throat, and lungs, including pneumonia.

INDICATION(S) AND RESEARCH PHASE
Pediatric, Otitis Media – Phase II

vaccine, Haemophilus influenzae
unknown

MANUFACTURER
Antex Biologics

DESCRIPTION
Haemophilus influenzae vaccine is currently in phase I/II trials in infants for the treatment of otitis media.

INDICATION(S) AND RESEARCH PHASE
Pediatric, Otitis Media – Phase I/II

Pain, Acute or Chronic

fentanyl transdermal system
Duragesic

MANUFACTURER
Alza (Sequus Pharmaceuticals)

DESCRIPTION
Duragesic is a 72-hour transdermal system for management of chronic pain in subjects requiring continuous opioid or synthetic narcotic pain relief that cannot be managed by lesser means, such as acetaminophen-opioid combinations or non-steroidal analgesics.

Duragesic is marketed by Janssen Pharmaceutica, and it is currently in phase III trials for the treatment of chronic pain in pediatric subjects ages two to sixteen years old.

INDICATION(S) AND RESEARCH PHASE
Pediatric, Pain, Acute or Chronic – Phase III

ropivacaine HCl
Naropin

MANUFACTURER
AstraZeneca

DESCRIPTION
Naropin is a sodium channel blocker that is currently in phase III trials for use as a spinal anesthetic in an intra-articular administration. An NDA was submitted in December 2000 for a single-dose administration of Naropin injection for regional anesthesia in pediatric subjects. FDA approval is also sought for Naropin as a treatment for acute pain management in children one to twelve years old. Naropin has been FDA approved as an obstetric anesthesia and regional anesthesia for surgery, as well as for the management of postoperative pain.

INDICATION(S) AND RESEARCH PHASE
Pain, Acute or Chronic – FDA approved
Pediatric, Anesthesia – NDA submitted
Anesthesia, Regional – FDA approved
Pediatric, Pain, Acute or Chronic – NDA submitted
Anesthesia, Spinal – Phase III

tramadol hydrochloride
Ultram

MANUFACTURER
R.W. Johnson Pharmaceutical Research Institute

DESCRIPTION
Ultram, tramadol hydrochloride, is a centrally acting synthetic analgesic. While the mode of action of ultram is not completely understood, laboratory studies suggest that at least two complementary mechanisms appear applicable: binding of parent and M1 metabolite to opioid receptors and weak inhibition of the reuptake of norephinephrine and serotonin

The drug was FDA approved in March, 1995 for the management of moderate to moderately severe pain in adults. An NDA has been submitted for the approval of the drug for pediatric subjects.

INDICATION(S) AND RESEARCH PHASE
Pediatric, Pain, Acute or Chronic – NDA submitted

Pertussis

immune globulin (IG-IV)
unknown

MANUFACTURER
Massachusettts Biologic Laboratories

DESCRIPTION
Immune globulin (a class of proteins involved in producing an immune response) or IG-IV is in phase II for the treatment of pertussis (whooping cough) using an intravenous formulation.

INDICATION(S) AND RESEARCH PHASE
Pertussis – Phase II
Pediatric, Pertussis – Phase II

vaccine, acellular pertussis
unknown

MANUFACTURER
Amvax/Baxter Highland Immuno
Amvax Pharmaceuticals is formulating a new pertussis vaccine that may improve efficacy and have fewer side effects compared to the current pertussis vaccine. The bacteria known as Bordetella pertussis is responsible for the serious upper respiratory disease known as whooping cough

The damage that the pertussis bacterium causes in the body occurs due to the release of a destructive toxin by the organism. Current vaccines are composed of inactived versions of this toxin that stimulate an immunization response by the body. The new vaccine by Amvax uses only a small part of the inactive toxin molecule, and by not using the entire inactivated toxin molecule, scientists theorize that side effects may be reduced and stronger immunization may be achieved. The new vaccine might also have a longer duration of action and be appropriate for use in older children and adults. These improvements are important since in recent years, there has been a resurgence of pertussis infection in older children and adults. This acellular pertussis vaccine is being tested in phase II trials in an intramuscular injection.

INDICATION(S) AND RESEARCH PHASE
Pertussis – Phase II
Pediatric, Pertussis – Phase II
Vaccines – Phase II

Pneumonia

cefditoren pivoxil
unknown

MANUFACTURER
Abbott Laboratories

DESCRIPTION
Cefditoren pivoxil is an advanced generation oral cephalosporin that has a broad spectrum of activity against gram-positive and gram-negative pathogens. It is being tested in phase III trials as a first-line agent for pneumonia in adults and children.

INDICATION(S) AND RESEARCH PHASE
Pneumonia – Phase III
Pediatric, Pneumonia – Phase III

quinupristin/dalfopristin
Synercid

MANUFACTURER
Aventis

DESCRIPTION
Synercid is an intravenous combination therapy of two semi-synthetic antibacterial agents, quinupristin and dalfopristen. Synercid has been FDA approved for the treatment of bloodstream infections due to vancomycin-resistant *Enterococcus faecium* (VREF) and skin and skin structure infections (SSTI) caused by methicillin-susceptible *Staphylococcus aureus* or *Streptococcus pyogenes*. Additionally, it is in pediatric phase III trials for pneumonia.

INDICATION(S) AND RESEARCH PHASE
Bacterial Infection – FDA approved
Skin Infections/Disorders – FDA approved
Pediatric, Pneumonia – Phase III
Pneumonia – Phase III

Pompe's Disease

recombinant human alpha-glucosidase
unknown

MANUFACTURER
Genzyme

DESCRIPTION
Genzyme and Pharming are currently developing an enzyme replacement therapy for the treatment of Pompe's disease—a rare genetic disorder caused by the lack of the enzyme alpha-glucosidase. An ongoing phase I/II trial is being conducted in infants with the disease. Results from the first 12 months of the trial showed that infants treated with an enzyme replacement therapy experienced heart-failure-free survival at one year.

The open-label trial includes three infants who have been receiving intravenous infusions of recombinant human alpha-Glucosidase purified from CHO cells for over 18 months. All three infants passed the age of one year, currently remain on therapy, and have reached the ages of 20 months, 22 months and 26 months. Trial results also indicated that the therapy might reduce heart size and improve cardiac function. Improvements in skeletal muscle function have also been observed, although the significance and extent of these improvements have been more variable than with those in cardiac function.

INDICATION(S) AND RESEARCH PHASE
Pediatric, Pompe's Disease – Phase I/II

Post-Surgical Complications

TP10
unknown

MANUFACTURER
AVANT Immunotherapeutics

DESCRIPTION
TP10 is a genetically engineered (recombinant) soluble complement receptor-1 (sCR1). Complement-1 is a naturally occurring substance that binds to antibodies as part of the immune response to infection or foreign bodies. Clinical trials are testing TP10 in an intravenous formulation for a variety of disorders including the treatment of acute respiratory distress syndrome (ARDS), reperfusion injury, heart attack, cardiac surgery, organ reperfusion, xeno-transplantation, allotransplantation, and post-surgical complications in infants.

A phase IIb trial was initiated in January 2001 in approximately 30 infants undergoing high risk cardiac surgery utilizing cardiopulmonary bypass. The trial will be conducted at seven sites in the United States.

INDICATION(S) AND RESEARCH PHASE
Acute Respiratory Distress Syndrome

(ARDS) – Phase II/III
Cardiac Ischemia – Phase I/II
Cardiac Surgery – Phase IIb
Myocardial Infarction – Phase I/II
Pediatric, Post-surgical Complications – Phase I/II
Pediatric, Cardiac Surgery – Phase IIb

Post-Traumatic Stress Disorder

sertraline HCl
Zoloft

MANUFACTURER
Pfizer

DESCRIPTION
Zoloft (sertraline HCl) is a selective serotonin reuptake inhibitor in an oral formulation. It is currently being marketed by Pfizer for multiple indications including post-traumatic stress disorder, depression, obsessive compulsive disorder and panic disorder. Additionally, Zoloft is in phase III trials for the treatment of depression and post-traumatic stress disorder in children ages six to 17 years.

INDICATION(S) AND RESEARCH PHASE
Pediatric, Depression – Phase III
Pediatric, Post-Traumatic Stress Disorder – Phase III

Pressure Ulcers

oxandrolone, CO221
unknown

MANUFACTURER
Bio-Technology General

DESCRIPTION
Oxandrolone is an anabolic steroid for treatment of chronic obstructive pulmonary disease (COPD) and pressure ulcers. The drug, in oral tablet formulation, is in phase II trials for both indications.

INDICATION(S) AND RESEARCH PHASE
Chronic Obstructive Pulmonary Disease (COPD) – Phase II
Pressure Ulcers – Phase II
Pediatric, Chronic Obstructive Pulmonary Disease (COPD) – Phase III
Pediatric, Pressure Ulcers – Phase III

Psychiatric Disorders

paroxetine
Paxil, Seroxat

MANUFACTURER
GlaxoSmithKline

DESCRIPTION
Paxil (paroxetine) is an orally-administered selective serotonin reuptake inhibitor (SSRI) currently approved to treat a variety of mood and anxiety disorders. FDA approval has been received for the treatment of depression, obsessive complusive disorder (OCD), panic disorder, and social anxiety disorder or social phobia. This drug is sold under the brand name Paxil in United States and Seroxat in Europe.

Paxil is currently in phase III trials for the treatment of depression in a dispersible tablet formulation. NDAs have also been submitted for the treatment of generalized anxiety disorders and post-traumatic stress disorder. For pediatric patients, the drug is in phase III trials for the treatment of psychiatric disorders.

INDICATION(S) AND RESEARCH PHASE
Post-Traumatic Stress Disorders – NDA submitted
Anxiety Disorders – NDA submitted
Depression – Phase III
Pediatric, Psychiatric Disorders – Phase III

Pubertal Gynecomastia

anastrozole, ZD-1033
Arimidex

MANUFACTURER
AstraZeneca

DESCRIPTION
Studies suggest that the female hormone estrogen stimulates the growth of some breast cancer tumors. Arimidex, a non-steroidal compound, is a selective oral inhibitor of the enzyme aromatase. Inhibition of aromatase reduces the production of estrogen. Thus, Arimidex reduces serum concentration of estrogen, an effect that has been shown to be of benefit in postmenopausal women with breast cancer.

Arimidex works differently from Tamoxifen, the most popularly prescribed first-line treatment for breast cancer. Tamoxifen works primarily by blocking estrogen receptors in tumor cells. Arimidex works by suppressing the synthesis of estrogen, such that less hormone is available to bind with estrogen receptors.

Arimidex is being tested in phase III trials for first-line treatment of advanced breast cancer in women who have never received hormonal therapy. It is also being tested for the treatment of pubertal gynecomastia.

INDICATION(S) AND RESEARCH PHASE
Breast Cancer – Phase III
Pediatric, Pubertal Gynecomastia – Phase IV

Respiratory Failure

vaccine, respiratory syncytial virus

MANUFACTURER
Unknown

MANUFACTURER
Wyeth-Lederle Vaccines

DESCRIPTION
This novel RSV live attenuated vaccine for prevention of RSV virus-mediated lower respiratory disease in infants uses a subunit or section of the virus that is sufficient to invoke an immune response but not produce the disease itself. The vaccine is targeted for prevention of RSV-mediated lower respiratory disease with at-risk children and the elderly, and it is in being tested in phase II trials.

INDICATION(S) AND RESEARCH PHASE
Pediatric, Respiratory Failure – Phase II

Respiratory Syncytial Virus

vaccine, respiratory syncytial virus
unknown

MANUFACTURER
Aventis Pasteur

DESCRIPTION
Respiratory syncytial virus (RSV), a common cause of winter outbreaks of acute respiratory disease, may cause an estimated 90,000 hospitalizations and 4,500 deaths each year from lower respiratory tract disease in both infants and young children. RSV is a common, but preventable cause of hospital-acquired (nosocomial) infection. The source of this virus transmission may include other infected subjects, staff, and visitors.

Most severe manifestations of infection with RSV (e.g., pneumonia and bronchiolitis) occur in infants aged two to six months; however, children of any age with underlying cardiac or pulmonary disease or who are immunocompromised are at risk for serious complications from this infection. Because natural infection with RSV provides limited protective immunity, RSV causes repeated symptomatic infections throughout life. In adults, RSV usually causes upper respiratory tract manifestations but may cause lower respiratory tract disease, especially in the elderly and in immunocompromised persons.

Aventis has an RSV-mediated lower respiratory disease vaccination for at-risk children and the elderly being tested in phase I/II trials.

INDICATION(S) AND RESEARCH PHASE
Bronchitis – Phase I/II
Lung Disease – Phase I/II
Pediatric, Respiratory Syncytial Virus – Phase I/II
Pneumonia – Phase I/II
Vaccines – Phase I/II
Viral Infection – Phase I/II

Reversible Obstructive Airways Disease

formoterol
Foradil

MANUFACTURER
Novartis

DESCRIPTION
Foradil (formoterol), a long-acting beta2-agonist, is a bronchodilator for the treatment of asthma and chronic obstructive pulmonary disease. It is currently being tested in phase II trials in a multi-dose dry powder inhaler. It has been approved for twice-daily use via the Aerolizer inhaler (a single-dose powder inhalation device) in adults and children ages five and older.

The multi-dose dry powder formulation is being tested in phase II trials for the treatment of asthma. In February 2001, Foradil Aerolizer was approved by the FDA for long-term, twice daily administration in the maintenance treatment of asthma and in the prevention of bronchospasm in adults and children five years of age and older with reversible obstructive airways disease.

INDICATION(S) AND RESEARCH PHASE
Asthma – Phase II
Asthma – FDA approved
Reversible Obstructive Airways Disease – FDA approved
Pediatric, Asthma – FDA approved
Pediatric, Reversible Obstructive Airways Disease – FDA approved

Rheumatoid Arthritis

DMP-777
Unknown

MANUFACTURER
DuPont

DESCRIPTION
DMP 777 is a neutrophil elastase inhibitor currently in phase II trials for juvenile rheumatoid arthritis. The drug is being tested for children 12 years of age and older.

INDICATION(S) AND RESEARCH PHASE
Pediatric, Juvenile Rheumatoid Arthritis – Phase II

etanercept
Enbrel

MANUFACTURER
Wyeth-Ayerst

DESCRIPTION
Enbrel binds to tumor necrosis factor (TNF), which is one of the dominant cytokines associated with normal immune function and the series of reactions that cause the inflammatory process of rheumatoid arthritis. Enbrel inhibits the binding of TNF molecules to the TNF receptor (TNFR) sites. The binding of these sites inactivates TNF, resulting in a significant reduction of the inflammatory cascade. Enbrel has been FDA approved for treatment of rheumatoid arthritis in adults and children.

Results from postmarketing studies demonstrated that Enbrel can have serious adverse effects such as infection, sepsis, and death. According to the company, subjects who are predisposed to infection, such as those with advanced or poorly controlled diabetes, are at greater risk of experiencing side effects. In addition, use of Enbrel should be terminated in subjects with current infections or sepsis. Allergic reactions to Enbrel or its components are also a possibility.

Pediatric trial results showed that nearly 75% of children with severe, long-standing juvenile rheumatoid arthritis (JRA) respond to Enbrel. In the first segment of the study, 74% of children (51 of 69) between the ages of four and 17 showed an improvement in disease response when treated with Enbrel for three months. In the second segment, half of these 51 subjects received Enbrel and half received a placebo. Seventy-two percent of those who received Enbrel completed the second segment without worsening of JRA symptoms, compared to 19% who took a placebo.

Enbrel is currently in phase III trials for the treatment of psoriasis and congestive heart failure in Adults.

Enbrel is co-marketed by Immunex and Wyeth-Ayerst.

INDICATION(S) AND RESEARCH PHASE
Rheumatoid Arthritis – FDA approved
Pediatric, Juvenile Rheumatoid Arthritis – FDA approved
Psoriasis and Psoriatic Disorders – Phase III
Congestive Heart Failure – Phase III

leflunomide
Arava

MANUFACTURER
Aventis

DESCRIPTION
Arava (leflunomide) is a disease-modifying antirheumatic drug (DMARD) approved for the treatment of rheumatoid arthritis. It is also in phase II trials for children ages four to 16 years.

INDICATION(S) AND RESEARCH PHASE
Pediatric, Juvenile Rheumatoid Arthritis – Phase II

Rhinitis

budesonide
Rhinocort Aqua

MANUFACTURER
AstraZeneca

DESCRIPTION
Rhinocort Aqua is indicated for the treatment of allergic rhinitis. It is currently in phase III trials in pediatric subjects.

INDICATION(S) AND RESEARCH PHASE
Pediatric, Rhinitis – Phase III

ebastine
Kestine

MANUFACTURER
Aventis

DESCRIPTION
Kestine (ebastine) is a non-sedating antihistamine in development for the treatment of seasonal and perennial rhinitis. An NDA has been submitted for children 12 to 17 years of age.

INDICATION(S) AND RESEARCH PHASE
Pediatric, Rhinits – NDA Submitted

omalizumab
Xolair

MANUFACTURER
Genentech

DESCRIPTION
Xolair is a recombinant humanized monoclonal antibody to immunoglobulin E. It is being developed for the treatment of asthma and the prevention of seasonal allergic rhinitis. A BLA has been submitted for the two above indications and pediatric subjects ages six to 12. This drug is being developed in partnership with Novartis and Tanox. It is currently awaiting FDA approval.

INDICATION(S) AND RESEARCH PHASE
Pediatric, Asthma – NDA submitted
Pediatric, Rhinitis – NDA submitted

Rotavirus Prophylaxis

rotavirus vaccine
Rotarix

MANUFACTURER
GlaxoSmithKline

DESCRIPTION
Rotarix is an oral pediatric live attenuated vaccine derived from a naturally occurring isolate of rotavirus found in children. Roatrix is currently in phase II development for rotavirus prophylaxis.

INDICATION(S) AND RESEARCH PHASE
Pediatric, Rotavirus Prophylaxis – Phase II
Vaccines – Phase II

Sarcoma

disaccharide tripeptide glycerol dipalmitoyl
ImmTher

MANUFACTURER
Endorex Corporation

DESCRIPTION
ImmTher, a bone cancer drug candidate, stimulates human macrophages to exhibit broad tumoricidal activity against a variety of human cancer cells. ImmTher is a novel muramyl dipeptide immunomodulator formulated in liposomes. The drug acts by activating macrophages to attack micrometastatic cancer cells that have evaded chemotherapy or surgery. These activated macrophages kill cancer cells by engulfing them or by secreting lethal factors.

Trials are under way for the treatment of subjects with osteosarcoma and Ewing's sarcoma. Additionally, a phase II trial is under way for children six to 18 years of age for the treatment of Ewing's sarcoma. The FDA has designated ImmTher as an Orphan Drug for the treatment of the primary types of bone cancers, Ewing's sarcoma and osteosarcoma.

INDICATION(S) AND RESEARCH PHASE
Pediatric, Sarcoma – Phase II
Sarcoma – Phase II

Sepsis

recombinant human activated protein C (rhAPC)
unknown

MANUFACTURER
Eli Lilly

DESCRIPTION
Recombinant human activated protein C (rhAPC) is a genetically engineered biological drug. Clinical trials are in phase III test-

ing for the treatment of severe sepsis.

INDICATION(S) AND RESEARCH PHASE
Sepsis and Septicemia – Phase III
Pediatric, Sepsis – Phase III

Sickle Cell Disease

CPC-111
Cordox

MANUFACTURER
Questcor

DESCRIPTION
Cordox is a fructose-1,6-diphosphate, a naturally occurring small molecule that has a protective effect on cells, especially red blood cells. This drug is being evaluated in a phase III trial for its ability to improve the biochemical and physical characteristics of stored human red blood cells. According to Questcor, Cordox is expected to increase the shelf-life of blood from the current maximum level of 42 days to eight to ten weeks.

In 2000, a trial evaluating Cordox as an analgesic agent for the treatment of sickle cell disease painful crises was terminated. As of January 2001, the data from enrolled subjects is under review. A pediatric phase II trial for treatment of sickle cell disease has been completed.

INDICATION(S) AND RESEARCH PHASE
Anemia, Sickle cell – Phase Discontinued
Blood Preservative – Phase III
Pediatric, Sickle Cell Disease – Phase II completed

poloxamer 188 N.F., CRL-5861
Flocor

MANUFACTURER
CytRx Corporation

DESCRIPTION
Flocor is an injectable drug that may improve blood flow. It is a purified form of poloxamer 188, which is a surface-active agent that helps reduce surface tension on blood cells to keep fluids flowing.

Flocor is in a phase I/II study in subjects with acute lung injury. This clinical trial is being conducted at Vanderbilt University Medical Center in Nashville, Tennessee. In acute lung injury, arterial and venous microvascular obstructions contribute to the severity of pulmonary dysfunction. Flocor is being evaluated for the prevention of secondary platelet aggregation and stasis-related capillary obstruction, and the development and propagation of dynamic blood clots, or thrombi.

Flocor is also being evaluated in a pivotal phase III study for the treatment of the acute painful crisis in sickle cell subjects ages ten and over, and a phase I study in sickle cell subjects with acute chest syndrome.

INDICATION(S) AND RESEARCH PHASE
Anemia, Sickle Cell – Phase III
Anemia, Sickle Cell – Phase I
Lung Injury – Phase I/II
Thrombosis – Phase I/II
Pediatric, Sickle Cell Disease – Phase III

Staph Bacterial Infections

hyperimmune globulin
Nabi-Altastaph

MANUFACTURER
Nabi

DESCRIPTION
Nabi-Altastaph is an antibody-based product that contains high levels of antibodies against *Staphylococcus aureus*. It is currently in development for the prevention of *Staphylococcus aureus* infections in subjects who are unable to respond to a vaccine, or who are at immediate risk of infection (i.e., trauma subjects, low birth weight newborns). Nabi-Altastaph is currently in phase II trials in neonates, and Nabi also plans to evaluate the product as a therapeutic drug for the treatment of diagnosed *Staphylococcus aureus* infections.

INDICATION(S) AND RESEARCH PHASE
Staph Bacterial Infections – Phase II
Pediatric, Staph Bacterial Infections – Phase II

Surgery

rapacuronium bromide
Raplon

MANUFACTURER
Organon

DESCRIPTION
Raplon is a neuromuscular blocking agent as adjunct to anesthesia to facilitate tracheal intubation and to provide skeletal muscle relaxation during surgery. An NDA has been submitted for the pediatric indication.

INDICATION(S) AND RESEARCH PHASE
Pediatric, Muscle Relaxation During Surgery – NDA submitted

Thrombocytopenia

thrombopoietin
Unknown

MANUFACTURER
Pharmacia

DESCRIPTION
Thrombopoietin (TPO) is a protein being developed for the potential treatment of thrombocytopenia in cancer subjects receiving chemotherapy. The protein binds to receptors on primitive blood cells and megakaryocytes, which are cells in the bone marrow that produce platelets. Cell growth is stimulated, and primitive blood cells can differentiate into platelet-producing megakaryocytes.

Thrombopoietin is being tested in phase III trials. Pharmacia and Genentech will jointly develop thrombopoietin, and Pharmacia will have exclusive rights to market it worldwide.

INDICATION(S) AND RESEARCH PHASE
Pediatric, Thrombocytopenia – Phase III

Thrombosis

enoxaprarin sodium
Lovenox Injection

MANUFACTURER
Aventis

DESCRIPTION
Lovenox injection, a low-molecular-weight heparin, is an anticoagulant that is used to help prevent the formation of blood clots in subjects at risk. It is a sterile solution containing enoxaparin sodium, a low molecular weight heparin. Lovenox injection is in a phase III trial for children up to 11 years old for deep vein thrombosis. It was approved for use in adults for the prevention of deep vein thrombosis in 1997.

INDICATION(S) AND RESEARCH PHASE
Pediatric, Thrombosis – Phase III

Tinea Capitis

terbinafine
Lamisil

MANUFACTURER
Novartis

DESCRIPTION
Lamasil inhibits squalene epoxidase, a key enzyme in sterol biosynthesis in fungi, causing a decrease in ergosterol and a corresponding accumulation of sterol within the fungal cells. The drug is being evaluated in phase III trials in an oral formulation for the treatment of both systemic mycoses and tinea capitis.

INDICATION(S) AND RESEARCH PHASE
Pediatric, Tinea Capitis – Phase II
Tinea Capitis – Phase III
Mycosis Fungoides – Phase III

Tonsillitis

cefditoren pivoxil
Spectracef

MANUFACTURER
TAP Pharmaceuticals

DESCRIPTION
Sprectracef (cefditoren pivoxil) is a broad-spectrum cephalosporin antibiotic. Studies have indicated the drug is effective in treating maxillary sinusitis, streptococcal pharyngitis and exacerbations from acute chronic bronchitis. It is in phase III trials for the treatment of acute pharyngitis, bronchitis and tonsillitis in children ages one month to 18 years.

INDICATION(S) AND RESEARCH PHASE
Pediatric, Acute Pharyngitis – Phase III
Pediatric, Tonsillitis – Phase III
Pediatric, Bronchitis – Phase III

Tourette's Syndrome

mecamylamine HCl
Inversine

MANUFACTURER
Layton Bioscience

DESCRIPTION
Inversine is being evaluated in phase III trials for the treatment of Tourette's syndrome and attention deficit/hyperactivity disorder (ADHD) in pediatric subjects.

INDICATION(S) AND RESEARCH PHASE
Pediatric, Tourette's Syndrome – Phase III
Pediatric, Attention Deficit/Hyperactivity Disorder (ADHD) – Phase III

Transplantation

SDZ RAD
unknown

MANUFACTURER
Novartis

DESCRIPTION
SDZ RAD is a potent immunosuppressive that inhibits growth factor-driven cell proliferation. It is currently in development for kidney, liver, and lung transplantation, including a pediatric phase II/III trial in children ages two through 16 years.

INDICATION(S) AND RESEARCH PHASE
Immunosuppressive – Phase II/III
Pediatric, Transplantation – Phase II/III

Turner's Syndrome

human growth hormone
unknown

MANUFACTURER
Cangene Corporation

DESCRIPTION
Natural human growth hormone is a protein produced by the pituitary gland that acts on the long bones of the body until the onset of puberty and promotes growth to normal stature. A deficiency of this hormone during childhood results in abnormally small stature. This drug is being tested in a phase III European trial for the treatment of Turner's syndrome in girls, as well as to combat short stature in children with growth hormone deficiency.

INDICATION(S) AND RESEARCH PHASE
Pediatric, Turner's Syndrome – Phase III

Urinary Incontinence

Tolterodine
Detrol

MANUFACTURER
Pharmacia

DESCRIPTION
Detrol Once-Daily is a new formulation of a drug currently on the market for overactive bladder. This drug form is taken once-a-day, whereas the current formulation is taken twice-a-day. The drug is in phase III trials for children five to 10 years of age.

INDICATION(S) AND RESEARCH PHASE
Pediatric, Urinary Incontinence – Phase III

Urinary Tract Infections

ciprofloxacin
CIPRO

MANUFACTURER
Bayer Corporation

DESCRIPTION
CIPRO is a fluoroquinolone antibiotic that is currently awaiting FDA approval for the treatment of exposure to aerosolized anthrax bacteria. Without treatment, anthrax infection is usually fatal. Doxycycline and penicillin are approved to treat anthrax, but it is thought that there are strains of anthrax bacteria resistant to these antibiotics. CIPRO is already approved for 17 different indications: acute sinusitis, lower respiratory tract infections, nosocomial pneumonia (IV only), urinary tract infections, acute uncomplicated cystitis in females (tablets and oral suspension only), chronic bacterial prostatitis, complicated intra-abdominal infections (in combination with metronidazole), skin and skin structure infections, bone and joint infections, infectious diarrhea, typhoid fever (enteric fever), and uncomplicated cervical and urethral gonorrhea (tablets and oral suspension only).

CIPRO, in intravenous formulation, is also indicated in empirical therapy for febrile neutropenic subjects, in combination with piperacillin sodium. Phase III trials testing CIPRO for the treatment of complicated urinary tract infections in pediatric subjects one to 17 years old are currently under way.

INDICATION(S) AND RESEARCH PHASE
Anthrax Exposure – NDA submitted
Pediatric, Urinary Tract Infections – Phase III
Urinary Tract Infections – Phase III

Vaccines

PeNta-HepB-IPV, vaccine
Infanrix

MANUFACTURER
GlaxoSmithKline

DESCRIPTION
This recombinant vaccine has been developed to address several indications. It has been approved by the European Union for diphtheria, tetanus, pertussis, hepatitis B, and polio. An NDA has also been submitted for these indications.

INDICATION(S) AND RESEARCH PHASE
Pediatric, Diptheria, Tetanus, Pertussis, Polio, and Hepatitis – NDA submitted

vaccine, allogenic and autologous neuroblastoma cells
unknown

MANUFACTURER
St. Jude Children's Research Hospital

DESCRIPTION
Currently, phase II/III clinical trials are evaluating gene-modified cancer vaccines using autologous and allogenic tumor cells from interleukin-2 (IL-2) secreting neuroblastomas after autologous bone marrow transplant in first remission. Researchers are conducting parallel clinical trials in children with recurrent neuroblastoma who are receiving either allogenic or autologous tumor cells that are gene modified to secrete small amounts of IL-2.

In the autologous trial, one subject had a complete tumor response, one had a partial response, and three had stable disease following the tumor immunogen alone. Four of the five subjects with tumor responses had coexisting neuroblastoma-specific cytotoxic T-lymphocyte activity, as opposed to only one of the subjects with non-responsive disease. These results show a promising correlation between immune response and clinical outcome with autologous vaccines.

In the allogenic group, one child had a partial response, five had stable disease, and four had progressive disease. Although immunization with autologous vaccine produced superior immune responses, these results offer encouragement for the continued pursuit of allogenic vaccine strategies in human cancer.

INDICATION(S) AND RESEARCH PHASE
Pediatric, Neuroblastoma – Phase II/III
Pediatric, Vaccines – Phase II/III

vaccine, Campylobacter
Campyvax

MANUFACTURER
Antex Biologics

DESCRIPTION
This vaccine, developed under a Cooperative Research and Development Agreement (CRADA) with the U.S. Navy and Army, is designed to prevent gastroenteritis and traveler's diarrhea caused by the enteropathogenic *Campylobacter jejuni*. A novel proprietary technology combines the vaccine, consisting of inactivated whole cells, with an adjuvant. While vaccines typically provide protection after bacteria enter the body, this new genetic engineering technology is the platform for vaccines that prevent infection before bacteria can penetrate tissue. The vaccine is given orally in liquid form.

INDICATION(S) AND RESEARCH PHASE
Bacterial Infection – Phase II completed
Diarrhea – Phase II completed

Gastroenteritis – Phase II completed
Pediatric, Campylobacter Infection – Phase II completed

vaccine, DPT/Haemophilus influenzae tyype B
unknown

MANUFACTURER
Chiron Corporation

DESCRIPTION
Chiron Corporation has formulated a combination vaccine that might effectively immunize children against four serious diseases—*Haemophilus influenzae* type B, diphtheria, pertussis, and tetanus—with a single injection. This vaccine has the potential to simplify pediatric vaccination schedules, thereby lowering costs, increasing convenience and improving compliance. The vaccine is composed of inactive molecules of diptheria toxin, pertussis toxin, and tetanus toxin. The vaccine also contains inactivated *H. influenzae* proteins.

The combination vaccine given as an intramuscular injection is currently in phase III trials.

INDICATION(S) AND RESEARCH PHASE
Pediatric, Bacterial Infection – Phase III
Pediatric, Influenza – Phase III
Pediatric, Vaccines – Phase III
Pediatric, Viral Infection – Phase III

vaccine, influenza
unknown

MANUFACTURER
BioChem Pharma

DESCRIPTION
In order to improve vaccination rates, BioChem Pharma is developing an influenza vaccine that can be taken as a nasal spray. This method of vaccination might not only create a helpful systemic immune response, but also stimulate a local immune response in the mucosal lining of the nose, mouth, and throat, which would create an additional barrier to influenza infection and increase efficacy. Phase I results demonstrated comparable immunization responses to that of the injectable vaccine. Clinical testing is in phase III for this nasal inhalation vaccination against the influenza virus in adult and pediatric subjects.

INDICATION(S) AND RESEARCH PHASE
Influenza – Phase III
Vaccines – Phase III
Pediatric, Influenza – Phase III
Pediatric, Vaccines – Phase III

vaccine, meningitis B
unknown

MANUFACTURER
GlaxoSmithKline

DESCRIPTION
This subunit vaccine has been designed for prevention of *Neisseria meningitides* type B meningitis in children. It is in phase II development.

INDICATION(S) AND RESEARCH PHASE
Pediatric, Meningitis – Phase II
Pediatric, Vaccines – Phase II

vaccine, meningococcus C
unknown

MANUFACTURER
Chiron Corporation

DESCRIPTION
Chiron Corporation is developing a new vaccine for meningococcal bacterial infections. The bacteria known as *Neisseria meningitidis* produce these infections. This organism can cause a variety of diseases ranging from benign upper respiratory infections to serious blood infections, which can lead to rashes, muscle and joint aches, and meningitis.

INDICATION(S) AND RESEARCH PHASE
Meningitis – Phase III
Vaccines – Phase III
Pediatric, Meningitis – Phase III
Pediatric, Vaccines – Phase II

vaccine, MMR-varicella
unknown

MANUFACTURER
GlaxoSmithKline

DESCRIPTION
This is a live attenuated vaccine for the prevention of measles, mumps, rubella, and varicella. It is currently in phase III trials for pediatric subjects.

INDICATION(S) AND RESEARCH PHASE
Vaccines – Phase III
Pediatric, Measles, Mumps, Rubella, and Varicella Prophylaxis – Phase III

Vesicoureteral Reflux Disease

chondrocyte-alginate gel suspension
Chondrogel

MANUFACTURER
Curis

DESCRIPTION
Chondrogel is a tissue augmentation product created from autologous cartilage cells taken from the ear and expanded in a culture. The cells are then injected into the bladder to treat pediatric vesicoureteral reflux disease (VUR). VUR is a congenital condition in children that may lead to a urinary tract infection and kidney damage. Phase III trials have been completed, and a phase II trial is currently being planned for the treatment of Grade II VUR in pediatric subjects. A phase II trial for stress urinary incontinence (SUI) is also under way.

INDICATION(S) AND RESEARCH PHASE
Pediatric, Vesicoureteral Reflux Disease – Phase III completed
Urinary Incontinence – Phase II

Viral Infection

PeNta-HepB-IPV, vaccine
Infanrix

MANUFACTURER
GlaxoSmithKline

DESCRIPTION
This recombinant vaccine has been developed to address several indications. It has been approved by the European Union for diphtheria, tetanus, pertussis, hepatitis B, and polio. An NDA has also been submitted for these indications in pediatric subjects.

INDICATION(S) AND RESEARCH PHASE
Pediatric, Diphtheria, Tetanus, Pertussis, Polio, and Hepatitis – NDA submitted

vaccine, HIB/Hep B/IPV/DtaP
unknown

MANUFACTURER
Aventis Pasteur

DESCRIPTION
This vaccine is in development for the treatment of Haemophilus influenzae b, hepatitis B, polio, diphtheria, tetanus, and pertussis. It is in phase II/III trials in children ages two, four, and six months.

INDICATION(S) AND RESEARCH PHASE
Pediatric, Diptheria, Tetanus, Pertussis, Polio – Phase II/III
Pediatric, Hepatitis – Phase II/III

HeXa-HepB-IPV/Hib
Infanrix

MANUFACTURER
GlaxoSmithKline

DESCRIPTION
This conjugated, recombinant pediatric vaccine is being developed for a variety of indications. It has been approved by the European Union (EU) as a vaccine for the prevention of diphtheria, tetanus, pertussis, hepatitis B, polio prophylaxis and Haemophilus influenzae type B. An estimated NDA filing date has yet to be determined by the company.

INDICATION(S) AND RESEARCH PHASE
Vaccines – EU Approved
Pediatric, Viral Infection – EU Approved
Pediatric, Hepatitis – EU Approved

vaccine, DPT and Polio
Certiva-IPV

MANUFACTURER
Amvax/Baxter Highland Immuno

DESCRIPTION
Amvax has formulated a combination vaccine that might effectively immunize children with a single injection against four serious diseases: polio, diphtheria, pertussis, and tetanus. This vaccine has the potential to simplify pediatric vaccination schedules, thereby lowering costs, increasing convenience and improving compliance. The vaccine is composed of inactivated molecules of diphtheria toxin, pertussis toxin, tetanus toxin, and polio toxin. Toxins are the destructive molecules that cause most of the pathology seen in these diseases. Phase II trials are being conducted for all these indications.

INDICATION(S) AND RESEARCH PHASE
Pediatric, Viral Infection – Phase II
Vaccines – Phase II

vaccine, DPT/Haemophilus influenzae type B
unknown

MANUFACTURER
Chiron Corporation

DESCRIPTION
Chiron Corporation has formulated a combination vaccine to immunize children against *Haemophilus influenzae* type B, diphtheria, pertussis, and tetanus in a single injection formulation. This vaccine has the potential to simplify pediatric vaccination schedules, thereby lowering costs, increasing convenience and improving compliance. The vaccine is composed of inactive molecules of diphtheria toxin, pertussis toxin, and tetanus toxin. Toxins are the destructive molecules that cause most of the pathology seen in these diseases. The vaccine also contains inactivated *H. influenzae* proteins.

This combination vaccine, given as an intramuscular injection, is currently in phase III trials.

INDICATION(S) AND RESEARCH PHASE
Pediatric, Bacterial Infection – Phase III
Pediatric, Influenza – Phase III
Pediatric, Bacterial Infection, Influenza, Viral Infection – Phase III
Pediatric, Viral Infection – Phase III
Vaccines – Phase III

vaccine, MMR-varicella
unknown

MANUFACTURER
GlaxoSmithKline

DESCRIPTION
This is a live attenuated vaccine for the prevention of measles, mumps, rubella, and varicella. It is currently in phase III trials for pediatric subjects.

INDICATION(S) AND RESEARCH PHASE
Vaccines – Phase III
Pediatric, Measles, Mumps, Rubella, and Varicella Prophylaxis – Phase III

von Willebrand's Disease

antihemophilic factor
Alphanate

MANUFACTURER
Alpha Therapeutic

DESCRIPTION
Alphanate is a heat-treated human blood factor approved by the FDA to treat hemophilia A. It is a highly purified Factor VIII, which is normally responsible for clotting blood to prevent hemorrhage. A phase IV trial is being conducted to further expand

the safety and pharmacology characteristics.

A phase III study was completed in children seven years and older for the treatment of von Willebrand's disease, a bleeding disorder.

INDICATION(S) AND RESEARCH PHASE
Hemophilia – Phase IV/FDA approved
Pediatric, von Willebrand's disease – Phase III completed

Indexes

Manufacturers Index 637

Therapeutic Indications Index 673

Generic and Trade Name Index 697

Pediatric Manufacturer's Index 710

Pediatric Therapeutic Indications Index 718

Pediatric Generic and Trade Name Index 723

Manufacturers Index

Contained in this index are sponsor companies and contact information followed by a listing of the drugs they are manufacturing. Scientific names are set in standard type and potential trade names are set in italics.

3M Pharmaceuticals
3M Center
Building 275-3W-01
St. Paul, MN 55144-1000
651-733-1100
651-736-2133 fax
www.mmm.com

resiquimod 307, 520, 565, 578

Abbott Laboratories
100 Abbott Park Rd.
Abbot Park, IL 60064-3537
847-937-6100
847-937-1511 fax
www.abbott.com

Abbokinase *39, 119*
ABT-232, NS-49 480
ABT-594, epibatidine 104, 426, 496
ABT-627 ....263, 461, 580
ABT-773 298
apomorphine HCl 451, 576
cefditoren pivoxil 372, 552
HMFG1 ....*257*
Norvir/ABT-378 ....*431*
NPS 1776, alifatic amide 89, 132
prourokinase 39 119
ritonavir 431
Uprima *451, 576*

Abgenix
7601 Dumbarton Circle
Fremont, CA 94555
510-608-6500
510-608-6565 fax
www.abgenix.com

ABX-EGF 175
ABX-IL8 ....503, 523
monoclonal antibody, ABX-CBL 326

Academic Pharmaceuticals
21 North Skokie Valley Highway
Suite G3
Lake Bluff, IL 60044
847-735-1170
847-735-1173 fax

Amio-Aqueous IV *15*
amiodarone HCl 15

Acambis
38 Sidney Street
Cambridge, Massachusetts 02139
617-494-1339
617-494-1741 fax
www.acambis.com

Arilvax *347, 351*
C. difficile vaccine, CdVax ..298, 337, 422
ChimeriVax JE *340, 349*
ETEC vaccine 299, 337, 415
H. pylori vaccine 300, 338, 423
typhoid vaccine 303, 340
yellow fever vaccine 347, 351

Access Pharmaceuticals
2600 Stemmons Freeway
Suite 176
Dallas, TX 75207
214-905-5100
214-905-5101 fax
axcs@accesspharma.com
www.accesspharma.com

amlexanox liquid 202
clindamycin 515
OraRinse 202
polymer platinate, AP5280 193
ResiDerm, Zindaclin 515

Achillion Pharmaceuticals
300 George Street
New Haven, CT 06511
203-624-7000
203-624-7003 fax
www.biospace.com

ACH-126,443 ....308, 316, 426

Acorda Therapeutics
15 Skyline Drive
Hawthorne, NY 10532
914-347-4300
914-347-4560 fax
info@acorda.com
www.acorda.com

fampridine 98, 116, 510
Neurelan *98, 116, 510*

Actelion Pharmaceuticals
16 Gewerbestrasse
CH-4123 Allschwil
Switzerland
41-61-487-4545
41-61-487-4500 fax
www.actelion.com

bosentan 32, 453
Tracleer *32, 453*

Acusphere
University Park at MIT
38 Sidney St.
Cambridge, MA 02139-4169
617-577-8800
617-577-0233 fax

AI-700 26

Adolor
371 Phoenixville Pike
Malverne, PA 19355
610-889-5779
610-889-2203 fax
www.adolor.com

ADL 2-1294 ....296, 316, 516,
  517, 522, 523, 530, 539
ADL 8-2698 422

Advanced Biotherapy
802 Rollins Avenue
Rockville, MD 20852
760-431-4282
760-431-7408 fax
www.advancedbiotherapy.com

AGT-1 ....297, 504
anti-IFNg 504

Advanced Corneal Systems
15279 Alton Parkway
Suite 100
Irvine, CA 92618
949-788-6000
949-789-7744 fax
www.sanderling.com/port.html

intravitreal hyaluronidase 541
Keraform *542*
Vitrase *541*

Advanced Magnetics
61 Mooney St.
Cambridge, MA 02138-1038
617-497-2070
617-547-2445 fax
www.advancedmagnetics.com

Combidex *173, 222, 273, 470, 590*

Advanced Plant Pharmaceuticals
17 John St.
3rd Floor
New York, NY 10038
212-402-7878
212-402-7879 fax
IR@advancedplantpharm.com
www.advancedplantpharm.com

perthon/abavca 291
Perthon *291*

AEterna Laboratories
1405 Parc-Technologique
Quebec City, PQ G1P 4P5
Canada
418-652-8525
418-523-0881 fax
www.aeterna.com

AE-941 ....64, 175, 223, 247,
  275, 473, 523, 543
Neovastat *64, 175, 223, 247,*
  275, 473, 523, 543

Agennix
8 Greenway Plaza
Suite 710
Houston, TX 77046
713-552-1091
713-552-0795 fax
www.agennix.com

recombinant human
  lactoferrin (rhLF) 528
levonorgestrel/ethinyl estradiol 562

Agouron Pharmaceuticals
10350 No. Torrey Pines Rd.
La Jolla, CA 92037
800-585-6050
858-622-3298 fax
www.agouron.com

AG7088, anti-rhinoviral
  agent 332, 376, 554, 555
matrix metalloprotease
  inhibitor (MMP) 85, 491, 544
nelfinavir, AG1661 290
Prinomastat *85, 159, 231, 269,*
  469, 491, 544, 586
Remune *290*

Akorn
2500 Millbrook Drive
Buffalo Grove, IL 60089
847-279-6100
847-279-6123 fax
www.akorn.com

piroxicam 542

Alcon
6201 S. Freeway
Ft. Worth, TX 76134
817-293-0450
817-568-7128 fax
www.alconlabs.com

anecortave acetate 544
motexafin lutetium 544
Optrin *544*

Alexion
25 Science Park
Suite 360
New Haven, CT 06511
203-776-1790
203-772-3655 fax
www.alxn.com

5G1.1 ....456, 503, 530
pexelizumab 19, 37

Alfacell
225 Belleville Ave.
Bloomfield, NJ 07003
973-748-8082
973-748-9788 fax
www.alfacell.com

Onconase 247
ranpirnase 247

Algos Pharmaceutical
1333 Campus Parkway
Neptune, NJ 07753
732-938-5959
732-938-2825 fax
www.algos.com

acetaminophen/
 dextromethorphan 104, 496
HydrocoDex...................104, 496
methadone/dextromethorphan 148
nicotine addiction product 147, 377
OxycoDex 109, 502
oxycodone hydrochloride/
 dextromethorphan
 hydrobromide 109, 502

Alkermes
64 Sidney St.
Cambridge, MA 02139
617-494-0171
617-621-7856 fax
www.alkermes.com

Albuterol 362
Cereport 161
Medisorb Naltrexone.............148
naltrexone 148
pulmonary insulin 386

Allergan
2525 DuPont Dr.
P.O. Box 19534
Irvine, CA 92623-9534
714-246-4500
714-246-5499 fax
www.allergan.com

AGN 192024 ....542, 545
Alphagan 543
Botox 94, 489. 497
botulinum toxin type A,
 AGN-191622 ....94, 489, 497
brimonidine tartrate 543
Lumigan 542, 545
memantine 543
tazarotene 515, 529
Tazorac 515, 529

Alliance Pharmaceutical
3040 Science Park Rd.
San Diego, CA 92121
858-410-5200
858-410-5201 fax
www.allp.com

Imagent 19, 184
LiquiVent..................355, 375
perflubron 355, 375
perfluorohexane emulsion 19, 184

Allos Therapeutics
7000 N. Broadway
Suite 400
Denver, CO 80221
303-426-6262
303-412-9160 fax
www.allos.com

RSR13 ....15, 17, 86, 160, 233

Alpha Therapeutic
5555 Valley Blvd.
Los Angeles, CA 90032
800-421-0008
323-227-7027 fax
www.alphather.com

alpha-1 proteinase inhibitor 369
Alphanate 31, 52
antihemophilic factor 31, 52
AS-013 ....36, 390
Circulase 36, 390

immune globulin intravenous ...51, 156,
 311, 429
Venoglobulin-S 51, 156, 311, 429

AltaRex
Campus Tower 300
8625 112th St.
Edmonton, Alberta T6G 1K8
Canada
781-672-0138
781-672-0142 fax
www.altarex.com

BrevaRex MAb 66, 249
monoclonal antibody 66, 249
OvaRex 257

Alteon
170 Williams Dr.
Ramsey, NJ 07446
201-934-5000
201-934-8880 fax
www.alteonpharma.com

ALT-711 ....530, 539
pimagedine HCl 385, 458

Alza Corporation
(Sequs Pharmaceuticals)
950 Page Mill Road
Palo Alto, CA 94303
650-494-5000
650-494-5151 fax
info@alza.com
www.alza.com

Doxil, Caelyx 164, 177, 221,
 226, 265, 462, 582
Doxil/Taxotere 164
doxorubicin HCl 164, 177, 221,
 226, 265, 462, 582
doxorubicin/docetaxel 164
Duragesic...................106, 499
fentanyl transdermal system 106, 499
hydromorphone 107, 500
oxycodone 88

Amarillo Biosciences
800 W. 9th Ave.
Amarillo, TX 79101
806-376-1741
806-376-9301 fax
www.amarbio.com

IFNalpha 479
interferon alpha 479

Amgen

One Amgen Center Drive
Thousand Oaks, CA 91320-1789
805-447-1000
805-447-1010 fax
www.amgen.com

Abarelix-Depot F 564
Aranesp .177, 456
calcimimetics .399
darbepoetin alfa 177, 456
IL-1ra/Anakinra 506
keratinocyte growth factor
   (KGF) .202, 423
Kineret 506
leptin 383, 393
novel erythropoiesis stimulating
   protein (NESP) 50, 458
SD/01 .70, 171, 204
sTNF-RI, soluble tumor necrosis
   factor-a receptor type I 508

Amylin Pharmaceuticals
9373 Towne Centre Dr.
Suite 250
San Diego, CA 92121
858-552-2200
858-552-2212 fax
www.amylin.com

AC2993 LAR .381
AC2993 381
AC3056 40
Exendin-4 383
exendin 383
pramlintide 385
Symlin 385

Andrx
4001 SW 47th Ave.
Suite 201
Fort Lauderdale, FL 33314
954-581-7500
954-587-1054 fax
www.andrx.com

ADX-153 . . . . .104, 496
Lovastatin XL .21
metformin hydrochloride, ADX-155 . .384
Metformin XT 384

Angiotech Pharmaceuticals
6660 NW Marine Dr.
Vancouver, BC V6T-1Z4
Canada
604-221-7676
604-221-2330 fax
www.angiotech.com

micellar paclitaxel 99, 507, 527
paclitaxel 528

Anika Therapeutics
236 West Cummings Park
Woburn, MA 01801
781-932-6616
781-932-9735 fax
www.anikatherapeutics.com

Orthovisc 492

Annovis
34 Mount Pleasant Drive
Aston, PA 19014
610-361-9224
610-361-8255 fax
www.annovis.com

amino-cyclopropane carboxylic
   acid 125, 126, 134

AnorMED
20353 64th Ave.
Suite 100
Langley, BC V2Y-1N5
Canada
604-530-1057
604-530-0976 fax
www.anormed.com

AMD-3100 . . . . .287, 317

Antex Biologics
300 Professional Dr.
Gaithersburg, MD 20879
301-590-0129
301-590-1251 fax
www.antexbiologics.com

Campyvax 304, 416, 420
Helivax 425
vaccine, campylobacter 304, 416, 420
vaccine, Helicobacter pylori 425

Anthra Pharmaceuticals
103 Carnegie Center
Suite 102
Princeton, NJ 08540
609-514-1060
609-924-3875 fax
www.anthra.com

valrubicin 155, 257, 449
Valstar 155, 257, 449

Antigenics
630 Fifth Avenue
New York, NY 10111
212-332-4774
212-332-4778 fax
www.antigenics.com

AG-701 .316, 522
HSPPC-96 . . . . .197, 206, 238, 243,
   259, 277, 280, 395, 407, 418, 440, 474
Oncophage 197, 206, 238, 243,
   259, 277, 280, 395, 407, 418, 440, 474

Antisoma plc
West Africa House
Hanger Lane
Ealing, London W5 3QR
United Kingdom
44-0-181-799-8200
44-0-181-799-8201 fax
enquiries@antisoma.co.uk
www.antisoma.co.uk

murine monoclonal antibody 207,
   255, 419
TheraFab 173
Theragyn 207, 255, 419

Apex Bioscience
2810 Meridian Parkway
Suite 120
Durham, NC 27713
919-405-4000
919-405-4010 fax
info@apexbioscience.com
www.apexbioscience.com

pyridoxalated hemoglobin
   polyoxyethylene (PHP) 50, 335

Aphton Corporation
P.O. Box 1049
Woodland, CA 95776
530-668-5100
530-666-1314 fax
www.aphton.com

Gastrimmune 200, 206, 207,

Manufacturers Index/**641**

222, 262, 398, 411, 417, 419, 443
GnRH Pharmaccine *174, 205, 273, 471, 564, 590*
immunocontraception .... .561
vaccine, anti-gastrin II .... .422
vaccine, anti-gastrin 200, 206, 207, 222, 262, 398, 411, 417, 419, 443

Aquila Biopharmaceuticals

175 Crossing Blvd.
Framingham, MA 01702
508-766-2700
508-766-2705 fax
www.aquilabio.com

QS-21 .... .339
Quilimmune-M *332, 345*
Quilimmune-P *346, 374, 554*
vaccine, malaria 332, 345
vaccine, pneumococcal
 infections 346, 374, 554

Aradigm Corporation

3929 Point Eden Way
Hayward, CA 94545
510-265-9000
510-265-0277 fax
investor@aradigm.com
www.aradigm.com

AERx diabetes management system ..381
alfa inhalation solution .... .367

Aronex Pharmaceuticals

8707 Technology Forest Place
The Woodlands, TX 77381-1191
281-367-1666
281-367-1676 fax
www.aronex-pharm.com

Annamycin *54, 162, 215*
AR-522 .... 54, 162, 215
Aroplatin *247, 279, 477*
Atragen *60, 219, 272, 240, 278, 469, 476, 589*
Nyotran *93, 296, 305, 331, 356, 533, 551*
nystatin, AR-121 ..... 93, 296, 305, 331, 356, 533, 551
tretinoin *60, 219, 240, 272, 278, 469, 476, 589*

ASTA Medica AG

Weismellerstrasse 45
Frankfurt-am-Main
Germany
60314
011-0351-25555-0
011-0351-2555-404 fax
www.astamedica.de

retigabine .... .91

AstraZeneca

1800 Concord Pike
P.O. Box 15437
Wilmington, DE 19850-5438
800-456-3669
302-886-2972 fax
www.astrazeneca.com

Ambicin .... .444
anastrozole, ZD-1033 .... .161
AR-C68397AA .... .364
AR-C89855 .... .364
AR-H047108 .... 421, 422
AR-H049020 .... .382
AR69931 .... 13, 42
Arimidex .... .161
Atacand *22, 33, 453*
AZ 242 (AR-H039242) .... .382
AZD 6140 (AR-C126532) .... .42
AZD2563 .... .298
AZD3409 .... .176
AZD6474 .... .176
bicalutimide 264, 461, 581
budesonide 412, 434
Budoxis, Oxis *358, 364*
candesartan cilexetil 22, 33, 453
Casodex *264, 461, 581*
CCR2b .... .504
clomethiazole .... .117
Crestor .... .22
Entocort CR .... .434
Entocort .... .412
Faslodex *167, 205*
formoterol 358, 364
goserelin acetate 166, 567, 572
H376/95 .... 37, 117
ICI-182,780 .... 167, 205
Iressa *190, 201, 208, 236, 275, 411, 420, 472, 592*
LEF 107, 500
melagatran .... .43
Merrem *369, 374, 532, 553*
NAD299 .... 127, 137
Naropin *109, 502*
neurokinin antagonist .... .137

nisin .... .444
NO-naproxen 109, 501
NXY-059 .... 78, 119
quetiapine fumarate 78, 133, 141, 145
raltitrexed, ZD-1694 ... 185, 198, 339, 408
reflux inhibitor .... .421
remacemide 91, 92, 113
rofleponide palmitate 333, 555
rofleponide .... .437
ropivacaine HCl 109, 502
Seroquel *78, 133, 141, 145*
Symbicort pMDI *362, 366*
Symbicort Turbuhaler *361, 366*
T3 .... .361
Tomudex *185, 198, 339, 408*
Viozan *364*
ZD-0101, CM-101 .... .190
ZD-0473/AMD 473 .... 155, 175, 190, 192, 201, 236, 258, 275, 411, 450, 472, 561, 592
ZD-1839 .... 190, 201, 208, 236, 275, 411, 420, 472, 592
ZD-4522, S-4522 .... .22
ZD-4953 .... 110, 503
ZD-8321 .... 356, 366
ZD-9331 .... .190
ZD0473 .... 213, 450
ZD2315 .... .510
ZD4407 .... .367
ZD4927 .... .45
Zendra *117*
Zoladex FIB *572*
Zoladex IVF *166, 567*
zolmitriptan 97, 98
Zomig Aura *98*
Zomig Cluster *97*
Zomig FM *97*
Zomig IN *97*
Zomig *97*

AtheroGenics

8995 Westside Parkway
Altharetta, GA 30004
678-336-2500
678-336-2500 fax
www.atherogenics.com

AGI-1067 .... *20, 35, 40*
AGIX-4207 .... .504

Atlantic Pharmaceuticals

1017 Main Cmpus Dr.
Suite 3900
Raleigh, NC 27606

919-513-7020
www.atlan.com

CT-3 . . . . .105, 498

Atrix Laboratories
2579 Midpoint Dr.
Ft. Collins, CO 80525
970-482-5868
970-482-9735 fax
www.atrixlabs.com

3-month Leuprogel 269, 466, 586
30-day Leuprogel 269, 466, 586
Atrisone 515
dadsone topical gel 515
leuprolide acetate 269, 466, 586

AutoImmune
128 Spring St.
Lexington, MA 02421
781-860-0710
781-860-7075 fax
www.autoimmune.com

AI-401 381
AI-502 325

AVANIR Pharmaceuticals
9393 Towne Centre Drive
Suite 200
San Diego, CA 92121
858-558-0364
858-453-5845 fax
www.avanir.com

AVP-923 . . . . .79, 102, 487, 497
Docosanol 307, 520, 565, 578

AVANT Immunotherapeutics
119 4th Ave.
Needham, MA 02494-2725
781-433-0771
781-433-0626 fax
www.avantimmune.com

CETP vaccine, CETi-1 21
Peru-15 339
TM27, ATM027, TCAR 101
TP10 . . . . .17, 20, 38, 355

AVAX Technologies
4520 Main St.
Suite 930
Kansas City, MO 64111
816-960-1333
816-960-1334 fax
kdoak@avax-tech.com
www.avax-tech.com

B-vax 174
L-Vax 61, 220
M-Vax 245
O-Vax 257
vaccine, cancer 174
vaccine, melanoma 245
vaccine, tumor cell suspension 257

Aventis Pasteur
Discovery Drive
Swiftwater, PA 18370-0187
800-VACCINE
570-839-4287 fax
www.aventispasteur.com

ALVAC-HIV 1 . . . . .287, 317
vaccine, malaria 330, 344
vaccine, respiratory syncytial
    virus 346, 350, 363, 372, 374, 554

Aventis
P. O. Box 9627
Kansas City, MO 64134
800-362-7466
816-231-5804 fax
www.hoechst.com
www.aventis.com

AIDS gene therapy 287, 316
alpha-1-proteinase inhibitor 369
AMP-579 36
antithrombin III 334
cariporide mesylate, HOE-642 . . . .27, 36
ciclopirox olamine 519, 530
cromolyn sodium 357
desirudin/recombinant hirudin 43
difluoromethylornithine
    (DFMO) 191, 318, 559
docetaxel hydrate . .84, 157, 163, 206, 209,
    226, 252, 418
eflornithine, DFMO
    (difluoromethylornydil) 154, 164,
    266, 280, 448, 463, 583
endothelin A receptor antagonist 23
enoxaparin sodium/tirofiban 27
enoxaparin sodium 17, 43
fibrinogen-receptor antagonist 14, 37
flavopiridol, HMR-1275 . . . . .56, 206,
    216, 228, 417
Gliadel 86, 159
HMR-1883/1098 24
HMR-3647, RU-64,004 . . . .300, 373, 552
HMR-4004 . . . . .289, 320
HOE-351 . . . . .250, 523
Intal HFA-227 357
Ketek 303
Loprox 519, 530
Lovenox/Aggrastat 27
Lovenox/Clexane 17, 43
M100907 144
p53 gene therapy 212, 270, 467, 588
Priftin 292, 302
prolifeprosan 20/carmustine 86, 159
propentofylline, HWA-285 . . . . . . .78, 89
quinupristin/dalfopristin 302, 374,
    531, 553
Revasc 43
rifapentine, MDL-473 . . . . .292, 302
Rilutek 113
riluzole 113
roxithromycine, RU-28,965 . . . . .302, 332
salbutamol 360
streptogamin 303
Synercid 302, 374, 531, 553
Taxotere 84, 163, 206, 209,
    226, 252, 418, 157
telithromycin 303
Ultrahaler 360

AVI BioPharma
4575 Southwest Research Way
Suite 200
Corvallis, OR 97333
541-753-3635
541-754-3545 fax
www.AVIBIO.com

Avicine 196, 259, 264, 395,
    406, 439, 462, 582
CTP-37 . . . . .196, 259, 264, 395,
    406, 439, 462, 582
Resten-NG 31

Avigen
1201 Harbor Bay Pkwy.
Ste. 1000
Alameda, CA 94502
510-748-7153
510-748-7155 fax
www.avigen.com

Coagulin-B 32, 53

Manufacturers Index/643

Aviron
297 North Bernardo Ave.
Mt. View, CA 94043
650-919-6500
fax 650-919-6610
www.aviron.com

vaccine, cytomegalovirus 306, 539
vaccine, Epstein-Barr virus 342, 350

Axcan Pharma
597 Laurier Blvd.
Mont-Saint-Hilaire, Quebec J3H-6C4
Canada
450-467-5138
fax 450-464-9979
www.axcan.com

bismuth subcitrate/metronidazole/
    tetracycline 425
Helicide 425
pancrelipase 109, 399, 444, 502
Protectaid 293, 563
Urso 21, 195, 200, 314,
    405, 410, 418, 432
ursodiol 21, 195, 200, 314,
    405, 410, 418, 432
Viokase 109, 399, 444, 502

Axonyx
110 Second St.
Stevenson, WA 98648
509-427-5132
509-427-5694 fax
www.axonyx.com

phenserine 78

Axys Pharmaceuticals
180 Kimball Way
South San Francisco, CA 94080
650-829-1000
650-829-1001 fax
www.axyspharm.com

APC 2059 434

Barr Laboratories
2 Quaker Road
P.O, 2900
Pamona, NY 10970
800-BarrLab
845-353-3843 fax
www.Barlabs.com

CyPat 272, 469, 589
Seasonale 564

Bayer Corporation
400 Morgan Lane
West Haven, CT 06516-4175
203-812-2000
203-812-5554 fax
www.bayer.com

Avelox 301, 363, 371, 373, 376
BAY 12-9566 . . . . .223, 251, 258, 490
BAY 13-9952 .20
CIPRO 483, 571
ciprofloxacin 483, 571
moxifloxacin 301, 363, 371, 373, 376
vardenafil 453, 578

Berlex Laboratories
300 Fairfield Road
Wayne, NJ 07470
888-237-5394
973-276-2005 fax
corpcom@allp.com
www.berlex.com

Ad5FGF4 26
Fludara 238
fludarabine phosphate 238
Generx 26
iloprost 40
Levovist 31
Oncolym 240

Bertek
320 Lakeside Dr.
Suite A
Foster City, CA 94404
650-358-0100
investor_relations@mylan.com
www.penederm.com

ST630 528

Bio-Technology General
70 Wood Ave. South
Second Floor
Iselin, NJ 08830
732-632-8800
732-632-8844 fax
www.btgc.com

oxandrolone, CO221 . . . . .365, 523

BioChem Pharma
275 Armend Frappier
Laval, Quebec H7V 4A7
Canada
450-681-1744
450-978-7755 fax
www.biochempharma.com

BCH-3963, LEF576 . . . . .104, 497
dOTC 287
nitazoxanide (NTZ) 290, 332, 415
troxacitabine, BCH-4556 . . . . . .61, 187,
    199, 212, 219, 234, 244, 256, 262, 272,
    278, 398, 409, 443, 469, 476, 589
Troxatyl 187
Troxatyl 61, 199, 212, 219,
    234, 244, 256, 262, 272, 278, 398, 409,
    443, 469, 476, 589
vaccine, influenza 328, 344, 370

Biocodex
1910 Fairview Ave. E.
Suite 208
Seattle, WA 98102
206-322-5663
206-323-2968 fax
www.biocodex-usa.com

Saccharomyces boulardii 303, 415

BioCryst Pharmaceuticals
2190 Parkway Lake Dr.
Birmingham, AL 35244
205-444-4600
205-444-4640 fax
www.biocryst.com

BCX-1470 18
BCX-34 . . . . .55, 62, 215, 241, 317

Bionenvision Ltd.
Trafalger House
11 Waterloo Place
St. James
London SW1Y 4AU
U.K.
www.bioenvision.co.uk

Abetafen 272, 470, 590
Clofarabine 61, 64, 220
cytostatics 153, 448
gene therapy, leukemia 57, 217

Biogen

644/Manufacturers Index

14 Cambridge Ctr.
Cambridge, MA 02142
617-679-2000
617-679-2617 fax
www.biogen.com

5c8 (Anti CD-40 ligand antibody) 68, 281, 458, 479, 533
Adentri 23, 456
Amevive 528
Antova 68, 281, 458, 479, 533
Avonex 84, 99, 158, 375
CVT-124 .23, 456
interferon beta-1a 84, 99, 158, 375
recombinant LFA-3/
  IgG1 Human Fusion Protein 528
very late antigen-4 inhibitor
  (VLA-4) 362

Biomira
2011 94th St.
Edmonton, Alberta T6N-1H1
Canada
877-234-0444
780-463-0871 fax
www.biomira.com

BLP-25 .224, 337
Theratope 174
vaccine, breast cancer 174

Bioniche Life Sciences
383 Sovereign Rd.
London, ON
Canada, N6M 1A3
519-453-0641
519-453-2418 fax
www.bioniche.com

MCC 155, 449

BioNumerik Pharmaceuticals
8122 Datapoint Dr.
Suite 1250
San Antonio, TX 78229
210-614-1701
210-614-0643
210-614-1701
210-615-8030 fax

BNP 1350 176
Karenitecin .176
MDAM (y-methylene-10-
  deazaaminopterin) 183

Biopure Corporation
11 Hurley Street
Cambridge, MA 02141
617-234-6500
617-234-6830 fax
www.biopure.com

hemoglobin glutamer-250
  (bovine) 49, 489
Hemopure 49, 489

Biospecifics Technologies
35 Wilbur St.
Lynbrook, NY 11563
516-593-7000
516-593-7039 fax
www.biospecifics.com

collagenase for injection 460, 488, 580
Cordase 460, 488, 580

BioStratum
2605 Meridian Parkway
Suite 120
Durham, NC 27713
919-572-6515
919-544-5425 fax
www.biostratum.com

Angiocol 189

Biosyn
3401 Market St
Suite 300
Philadelphia, PA 19104
215-387-5338
215-387-5332 fax
www.biosyn-inc.com

C319-14/6 . . . . .287, 519
glyminox vaginal gel 561
Oramed 287, 519
Savvy 561

BioTransplant
Third Ave.
Building 75, Charlestown Navy Yard
Charlestown, MA 02129
617-241-5200
617-241-8780 fax
www.biotransplant.com

AlloMune 63, 327, 241, 460
BTI-322, MEDI-507 . . . . . . .326, 459, 524

organ transplantation system 63, 241, 327, 460

Biovail Corporation International
2488 Dunwin Dr.
Mississauga, Ontario L5L-1J9
Canada
416-285-6000
416-285-6499 fax
www.biovail.com

buspirone 126

Bone Care International
1 Science Court
Madison, WI 53711
608-236-2500
608-236-0314 fax
www.bonecare.com

doxercalciferol 456
Hectorol Capsules 456

Boston Life Sciences
31 Newbury Street
Suite 300
Boston, MA 02116
617-425-0200
617-425-0996 fax
mariaz1@msn.com
www.bostonlifesciences.com

altropane 80, 110, 129

Bristol-Myers Squibb
345 Park Avenue
New York, NY 10154
212-546-4000
212-546-4020 fax
www.bms.com

A4, prodrug .175
aripiprazole, OPC-14597, OPC-31 . . . .75, 143
Avapro 22, 103, 392
BMS-182751, JM-216 . . . . .225, 252
BMS-186295, SR-47436
  (irbesartan) 22, 103, 392
BMS-186716, omapatrilat 22, 32, 453
BMS-193884 . . . . .22, 451, 576
BMS-200475 . . . . .309, 427, 347
BMS-201038 .32

Manufacturers Index/645

BMS-207147 518
BMS-214778 114
BMS-223131 . . . . .451, 576
BMS-232632 . . . . .287, 317
BuSpar *126*
buspirone HCl 126
Combretastatin *175*
D1927 177
DPPE 265, 463, 582
Entecavir *309, 347, 427*
estrogen/pravastatin 21
expected to be Abilitat *75, 143*
fluoropyrimidine, S-1 . . . . . .179, 206, 418
gatifloxacin 299, 552
ifetroban sodium, BMS-180291 39, 40, 534
paclitaxel/carboplatin/trastuzumab . . .170
Premarin/Pravachol *21*
Taxol/Paraplatin/Herceptin *170*
Tequin 299, 552
UFT/leucovorin calcium 410
Vanlev *22, 32, 453*

Britannia Pharmaceuticals Limited
41-75 Brighton Road
Forum House
Redhill, Surrey, RH1 6YS
United Kingdom
011-44-73-777-3741
011-44-73-776-2672 fax
www.britannia-pharm.co.uk

apomorphine 110
lofexidine .148
pumactant 360

British Biotech plc
Watlington Road
Oxford OX4 5LY
UK
44-0-1865-748747
44-0-1865-781047 fax
webadmin@britishbiotech.com
www.britbio.com

BB-10153 . . . . .29, 116
BB-2827 504
BB-3644 176
E21R 178
marimastat, BB-2516 . . .85, 158, 169, 230, 254, 261, 397, 441

BSD Medical
2188 West 2200 South
Salt Lake City Utah 84119-1326
801-972-5555
801-972-5930 fax
www.bsdmc.com

hyperteria/doxorubicin 253

BTG International
2200 Renaissance Blvd.
Gulph Mills, PA 19406
610-278-1660
610-278-1605 fax
www.btgplc.com

abiraterone acetate 263, 460, 580
Campath *58, 218*
LDP-03 . . . . .58, 218

Calydon
1324 Chesapeake Terrace
Sunnyvale, CA 94089
408-734-0733
408-734-2808 fax
www.calydon.com

CV706 . . . . .265, 462, 582
CV787 . . . . .265, 462, 582

Calyx Therapeutics
3513 Breakwater Avenue
Hayward, CA 94545
510-780-1020
510.780.1025 fax
info@calyxti.com
http://www.calyxtherapeutics.com/

CLX-0901 .382

Cambridge Antibody Technology Group plc
The Science Park Melbourn
Cambridgeshire SG8 6JJ
United Kingdom
44-1763-263-233
44-1763-263-413 fax

CAT-152 543

Cambridge NeuroScience
One Kendall Square
Building 700
Cambridge, MA 02139
617-225-0600
617-225-2741 fax
www.cambneuro.com

Aptiganel *117, 120*
CNS-5161 .94
ion-channel blocker 117, 120

Cangene Corporation
104 Chancellor Matheson Road
Winnipeg, MB R3T 5Y3
Canada
877-226-4363
204-487-4086 fax
www.cangene.com

anti-hepatitis B 309, 426
anti-hepatitis C 309, 427
human growth hormone 400
Leucotropin *52, 156, 203*
recombinant human GM-CSF 52, 156, 203

Cantab Pharmaceuticals plc
310 Cambridge Science Park
Cambridge CB4 0WG
UK
44-0-1223-423413
44-0-1223-423458 fax
www.cantab.co.uk

DISC GM-CSF 246
TA-CD *148*
TA-CIN 192, 560
TA-GW pharmaccine 308, 521
TA-HPV 192, 307, 520, 560, 565, 578
vaccine, cocaine 148

Carrington Laboratories
P.O. Box 168128
2001 Walnut Hill Lane
Irving, TX 75038
800-527-5216
972-518-1020 fax
aloe@carringtonlabs.com
www.carringtonlabs.com

Aliminase *434*
Carn 1000 434
Carn 750 .176
CarraVex *176*

CEL-SCI Corporation
8229 Boone Blvd.
Ste. 802

646/Manufacturers Index

Vienna, VA 22182
703-506-9460
703-506-9471 fax
www.cel-sci.com

HGP-30W 320, 338
interleukin (IL) 168, 210, 268, 321, 465, 585
MultiKine 168, 210, 268, 321, 465, 585

Celgene Corporation
7 Powder Horn Dr.
Warren, NJ 07059
800-890-4619, extension 3905
732-271-4184 fax
www.celgene.com

CDC 801 ....65, 98, 248, 297, 298, 336, 357, 377, 412, 504
d-methylphenidate HCl 81, 130
SelCID 98, 297, 298, 336, 377, 412, 504
SelCIDs 65, 248, 357
thalidomide 66, 87, 101, 160, 187, 214, 293, 327, 414, 509
Thalomid 66, 87, 101, 160, 187, 214, 293, 327, 414, 509

Cell Genesys
342 Lakeside Dr.
Foster City, CA 94404
650-425-4400
650-425-4457 fax
www.cellgenesys.com

Gvax 61, 220, 235, 245, 262, 274, 341, 399, 443, 471, 591
vaccine, cancer 61, 220, 235, 245, 262, 274, 341, 399, 443, 471, 591

Cell Pathways
1300 South Potomac Street
Ste. 110
Aurora, CO 80012
877-231-4567
303-755-2252 fax
trials@cellpathways.com (for patients)
www.cellpathways.com

Aposyn/Taxotere ..165, 179, 227, 266, 463, 583
Apotsyn/Xeloda 165
Aptosyn/Gemzar 227
Aptosyn/LHRH agonist 266, 463, 583
Aptosyn/Navelbine 227

Aptosyn/Taxotere/carboplatin 234
Aptosyn 153, 165, 195, 227, 266, 405, 417, 463. 583
CP-461 177
exisulind/capecitabine 165
exisulind/docetaxel 165, 179, 227, 266, 463, 583
exisulind/gemcitabine HCl 227
exisulind/vinorelbine tartrate injection 227
exisulind 153, 165, 195, 227, 266, 405, 417, 463, 583

Cell Therapeutics
201 Elliott Ave. W.
Ste. 400
Seattle, WA 98119
206-282-7100
206-284-6206 fax
www.cticseattle.com

Apra 264, 279, 462, 581
arsenic trioxide (ATO) 55, 62, 65, 153, 190, 215, 237, 248, 264, 275, 447, 461, 473, 559, 581
CT-2584 ....264, 279, 462, 581
lisofylline, CT-1501R 51, 59
ProTec 51, 59
Trisenox/dexamethasone 60, 66
Trisenox 55, 62, 65, 153, 190, 215, 237, 248, 264, 275, 447, 461, 473, 559, 581

Cellegy Pharmaceuticals
1065 E Hillsdale Blvd.
Ste. 418
Foster City, CA 94404
650-616-2200
650-616-2222 fax
www.cellegy.com

Anogesic 403, 426, 516
glyceryl monolaurin, T-100 522
Glylorin 522
nitroglycerin ointment 403, 426, 516
Tostrelle 390, 392, 479, 567, 568, 570
Tostrex 391, 452, 577, 580
transdermal testosterone gel 390, 391, 392, 452, 479, 568, 570, 567, 577, 580

Celltech Chiroscience plc
216 Bath Road
Slough, Berkshire 5L1 4EN
UK
011-44-753-534655

011-44-753-536632 fax
www.celltech.co.uk

CDP 870 505
CDP-571, BAY 10-356 .....413, 435, 505
D2163, BMS 275291 177
Hepagene 314, 433
Humicade 413, 435, 505
Lidocaine 110, 503
methylphenidate 82, 131
MR Racemate 82, 131
PDE4i, SCH351591 360
SCH55700 361
tetanus/diphtheria booster 340
vaccine, hepatitis B 314, 433

Centaur Pharmaceuticals
484 Oakmead Parkway
Sunnyvale, CA 94086
408-822-1600
408-822-1601 fax
www.centpharm.com

CPI-1189 ....111, 288
nitrone radical trap (NRT) ..112, 118, 290

Centocor
200 Great Valley Pkwy.
Malvern, PA 19355-1307
888-874-3083
610-889-4701 fax
www.centocor.com

abciximab, c7E3 ....13, 29, 36
GeneVax 174, 274, 342, 472, 591
ReoPro 13, 29, 36
vaccine, cancer ...174, 274, 342, 472, 591

Cephalon
145 Brandywine Pkwy.
West Chester, PA 19380
610-344-0200
610-344-0065 fax
www.cephalon.com

CEP-1347 ....75, 111
CEP-2563 ....264, 461, 581
CEP-701 .....258, 264, 394, 439, 461, 581
modafinil 77, 82, 99, 112, 115, 131
Provigil 77, 82, 99, 112, 115, 131

Cerus Corporation
2525 Stanwell Dr.
Suite 300

Manufacturers Index/647

Concord, CA 94520
888-254-9115
925-603-9099 fax
ir@ceruscorp.com
www.ceruscorp.com

psoralen, S-59 . . .67, 69, 70, 282, 302, 349

Chiron Corporation
4560 Horton Street
Emeryville, CA 94608
510-655-8730
510-655-9910 fax
corpcomm@cc.chiron.com
www.chiron.com

adjuvanted influenza 328, 370
aldesleukin, interleukin-2 (IL-2) 54,
    214, 236, 246, 275, 317, 473
becaplermin 387, 518, 532
Betaseron 98
factor VIII gene therapy 32, 53
Fiblast 28, 41
Fluad 328, 370
hepatitis A 310, 428
hepatitis B immunotherapy,
    HBV/MF59 . . . . .310, 428
insulin-like growth factor-I
    (IGF-I) 491
interferon beta-1b 98
MIV-150 321
Nothav .310, 428
Proleukin Interleukin-2 and
    standard anti-HIV therapy 291, 323
Proleukin 54, 214, 236, 246,
    275, 317, 473
Regranex 387, 518, 532
Td-IPV 340
tifacogin 335
trafermin 28, 41
vaccine, DPT/Haemophilus
    influenzae type B 304, 328, 342,
    350, 370
vaccine, HCV/MF59, hepatitis C 314,
    432
vaccine, HIV-1 gp-120 prime-boost . .294,
    325, 343
vaccine, meningococcus C . . .94, 331, 345

CoCensys
201 Technology Dr.
Irvine, CA 92618
949-753-6100
949-790-8710 fax
dslade@cocensys.com

www.cocensys.com

epalon, CCD-3693 . . . . .92, 114
ganaxolone, CCD-1042 . . . . .90, 95
licostinel, ACEA-1021 118

Cogent Pharmaceuticals
One Tower Bridge Suite 1350
100 Front St.
West Conshohocken, PA 19428
610-940-0300
610-940-0301 fax

Arecoline 79

Coley Pharmaceutical
55 William St.
Suite 120
Wellesley, MA 02481
781-431-6400
781-431-6403 fax
www.coleypharma.com

CpG 7909 . . . . .237, 246, 280
CpG compound 295, 357, 549

CollaGenex Pharmaceuticals
301 South State Street
Newtown, PA 18940
215-579-7388
215-579-8577 fax
www.collagenex.com

Col-3 . . . . .214, 329
Metastat 214, 329

Collateral Therapeutics
11622 El Camino Real
San Diego, CA 92130
858-794-3400
858-794-3440 fax
www.collateralTHX.com

Genvascor 39

Columbia Laboratories
2875 Northeast 191 Street
Suite 400
Aventura, FL 33180
800-749-1919
305-493-6142 fax
www.columbialabs.com

Advantage-S .292

SPC3 292

Conjuchem
225, President-Kennedy Avenue
Third floor, Suite 3950
Montreal (Quebec)
H2X 3Y8
Canada
514-844-5558
514-844-1119 fax
www.conjuchem.com

CCI-1004 43

CoPharma
97 South Street
Hopkinton, MA 01748
508-497-0700
508-497-0777 fax

PEN203 .308, 521
PEN203 528

COR Therapeutics
256 E. Grand Ave.
South San Francisco, CA 94080
650-244-6800
650-244-9208 fax
www.corr.com

Cromafiban 14, 27, 117
eptifibatide 27, 37
GP IIb/IIa 14, 27, 117
Integrilin .27, 37

Core Group plc
44-0-1294-848484
44-0-1294-848486 fax

CE-1050 125

Corixa Corporation
1124 Columbia St.
Suite 200
Seattle, WA 98104
206-754-5711
206-754-5715 fax
www.corixa.com

AnergiX.MS .101
AnergiX.RA .509
Detox 173, 340
HER-2/neu dendritic cell vaccine 166,
    253, 338

648/Manufacturers Index

MPL vaccine adjuvant ...... .296, 340, 550
PVAC .... .528
vaccine, allergy .... .341, 550
vaccine, genital herpes .... .307, 316, 520, 522, 565, 579
vaccine, rheumatoid arthritis .... .509

Cortex Pharmaceuticals
15241 Barranca Pkwy.
Irvine, CA 92618
949-727-3157
949-727-3657 fax
www.cortexpharm.com

Ampalex .... .75, 144
CX-516, BDP-12 .... .75, 144
CX-619, ORG-24448 .... .135

Corvas International
3030 Science Park Rd.
San Diego, CA 92121
858-455-9800
858-455-7895 fax
www.corvas.com

rNAPc2 .... .20, 44

Coulter Pharmaceuticals
600 Gateway Boulevard
South San Francisco, CA 94080
650-553-2000
650-553-2028 fax
www.coulterpharm.com

Bexxar .... .239
tositumomab .... .239

Cubist Pharmaceuticals
24 Emily St.
Cambridge, MA 02139
617-576-1999
617-576-0232 fax
ir@cubist.com
www.cubist.com

Cidecin .... .29, 299, 483, 530, 571
daptomycin .... .29, 299, 483, 530, 571

Curatek
1965 Pratt Blvd.
Elk Grove Village, IL 60007
847-806-7680
847-806-7612 fax

clonadine gel .... .105, 498

Curis
45 Moulton St.
Cambridge, MA 02138
617-876-0086
617-876-0866 fax
www.curis.com

chondrocyte-alginate gel
 suspension .... .480, 483, 571
Chondrogel .... .480, 483, 571
Vascugel .... .20

CV Therapeutics
3172 Porter Dr.
Palo Alto, CA 94304
650-812-0585
650-858-0390 fax
www.cvt.com

CVT-510 .... .16
ranolazine, CVT-303 .... .14, 24

Cytogen Corporation
600 College Rd. E.
Princeton, NJ 08540
800-833-3533
609-750-8123 fax
www.cytogen.com

Quadramet .... .271, 468, 588
samarium Sm 153 lexidronam pentasodium .... .271, 468, 588

Cytran
10230 NE Points Dr. #530
Kirkland, WA 98033
425-889-8822
425-822-5343 fax
www.cytran.com

IM862 ..214, 243, 253, 267, 330, 465, 585

CytRx Corporation
154 Technology Pkwy.
Norcross, GA 30092
770-368-9500
770-368-0622 fax
www.cytrx.com

Flocor .... .44, 50, 371
poloxamer 188 N.F., CRL-5861 44, 50, 371

Daiichi Pharmaceutical
11 Philips Parkway
Montvale, NJ 07645
888-727-2500
201-573-7650 fax
www.daiichius.com

DX-8951 .... .178

Dainippon Pharmaceutical
Dainippon Pharmaceutical
Enoki 33-94, Suita
Osaka, Japan 564-0053
81-6-6337-5875
81-6-6338-7656 fax
www.dainippon-pharm.co.jp

AJ-9677, TAK-677 .... .382
blonanserin, AD-5423 .... .144
moclobemide .... .137

Delta Pharmaceutical Group
MCB/HLB Complex, RTI
3040 Cornwallis Road
Research Triangle Park, NC 27709
919-806-1806
919-806-1161 fax

DPI-3290 .... .106, 499

Dendreon Corporation
3005 First Ave.
Seattle, WA 98121
206-256-4545
206-256-0571 fax
webmaster@dendreon.com
www.dendreon.com

APC8015 .... .264, 461, 581
APC8020 .... .64, 248
APC8024 .... .162, 193, 251, 403
Mylovenge .... .64, 248
Provenge .... .264, 461, 581

Diacrin
13th Street
Building 96, Charlestown Navy Yard
Charlestown, MA 02129
617-242-9100
617-242-0070 fax
www.diacrin.com

human liver cells .... .438, 439
 human muscle cells, cardiac disease 30, 37

Manufacturers Index/649

NeuroCell-HD *92, 112*
porcine fetal cells 92, 112
porcine neural cells, focal epilepsy 90
porcine neural cells, stroke 119

Diamyd Medical
Djurgårdsbrunnsv.54
S-115 25 Stockholm
Sweden
(46)-8-661 00 26
(46)-8-661 63 68 fax
www.diamyd.com

Diamyd *387*

Discovery Laboratories
350 South Main Street
Suite 307
Doylestown, PA 18901
215-340-4699
215-340-3940 fax
www.discoverylabs.com

lucinactant 355, 375
SuperVent *368*
Surfaxin *355, 375*
tyloxapol 368

DOV Pharmaceutical
One Parker Plaza
Suite 1500
Fort Lee, NJ 07024
201-968-0980
201-968-0986 fax

DOV 216303 .125
GABA agonist, anxiolytic 90, 114

Draximage
888-633-5343
514-694-9295 fax
info@draximage.com
www.draximage.com/english.htm

Amiscan *38*
Fibrimage *45*
technetium-99m-labeled FBD 45

Du Pont
1007 Market St.
Wilmington, DE 19898
800-441-7515
302-892-8530 fax
www.dupont.com

DMP-450 . . . . .288, 318
DPC-444 .43, 382
DPC-543, DMP-543 76

DUSA Pharmaceuticals
6870 Goreway Dr.
Mississauga, Ontario L4V 1P1
Canada
416-363-5059
416-363-6602 fax

5-aminolevulinic acid 515
Levulan Photodynamic Therapy *515*

Dyax Corporation
1 Kendall Square
Building 600, 5th Floor
Cambridge, MA 02139
617-225-2500
617-225-2501 fax
www.dyax.com

AIC *296, 532, 550*

Eisai
6-10 Koishikawa
4 Chome Bunkyo-ku
Tokyo, 112-88
JAPAN
011-81-03-3817-5015
011-81-03-3811-3077 fax
webmaster@eisai.co.jp
www.eisai.co.jp

Aricept *75, 81, 88, 130*
donepezil hydrochloride, E2020 75, 81, 88, 130
E5531 334
E7010 178

Elan Pharmaceutical Research
1300 Gould Drive
Gainesville, GA 30504
888-638-7605
770-534-8247 fax

AN-1792 75
Antegren *100, 413, 436*
Captelan *23, 33, 453*
captopril 23, 33, 453
Cardizide SR *13*
CNS stimulant 80, 130
Corlopam *24, 457*

diltiazem HCl/hydrochlorothiazide 13
Elangesic *420, 435, 444*
etodolac 106, 490, 499, 505
fenoldopam mesylate, SK&F-8252624, 457
fentanyl .106, 499
frovatriptan 95
ibuprofen 420, 435, 444
isradipine 33, 454
Lodine *106, 490, 499, 505*
natalizumab 100, 413, 436
selegiline 113
Theolan *361*
theophylline .361
Zelapar *113*
ziconotide, SNX-111 88

Elan Transdermal Technologies
3250 Commerce Parkway
Miramar, FL 33025
954-430-3340
954-430-3390 fax
www.elancorp.com

scopolamine 120, 424, 556
therapeutic, substance abuse 148

Eli Lilly
Lilly Corporate Center
Indianapolis, IN 46285
800-545-5979
317-277-6579 fax
www.lilly.com

Cialis *451, 478, 570, 576*
drotrecogin alfa 334
duloxetine HCl, LY-248686 . . . . .135, 481
Evista *28, 171*
fluoxetine HCl 136, 141, 142
fluoxetine/olanzapine 136
gemcitabine HCl .166, 228, 253, 259, 395, 440, 448
Gemzar . .*166, 228, 253, 259, 395, 440, 448*
IC351 . . . . .451, 478, 570, 576
LY-333531 . . . . .103, 392, 541
LY-354740 . . . . .127, 147, 377
LY231514, antifolate 183
LY333328 300
olanzapine 89, 133, 145
Oritavancin *300*
parathyroid hormone, PTH 495
Prozac *136, 141, 142*
raloxifene, LY-139481 . . . . .28, 171
recombinant human activated protein C (rhAPC) 335

650/Manufacturers Index

SERM III 171
tomoxetine 83, 132
Zovant *334*
Zyp/Zac *136*
Zyprexa *89, 133, 145*

Endorex Corporation
28101 Ballard Road
Suite F
Lake Forest, IL 60045
847-573-8990
847-573-9285 fax
TheProTeam@aol.com
www.endorex.com

disaccharide tripeptide glycerol dipalmitoyl 279
ImmTher *279*

Endovasc
15001 Walden Road
Suite 108
Montgomery, TX 77356
409-448-2222
409-582-2250 fax
endovasc@lcc.net
www.usrc.net/endovascltd

liposomal prostaglandin E1, PGE-1 30, 35
Liprostin *30, 35*

EntreMed
9610 Medical Center Dr.
Suite 200
Rockville, MD 20850
301-217-9858
301-217-9594 fax
webmaster@entremed.com
www.entremed.com

Angiostatin with radiation therapy *187*
human endostatin protein 180
rhEndostatin *180*

Entropin
21550 Oxnard St.
Suite 810
Woodland Hills, CA 91367
818-340-2323
818-347-6563 fax
www.entropin.com

benzestrom 105, 488, 497
Esterom *105, 488, 497*

Enzo Biochem
60 Executive Blvd
Farmingdale, NY 11735
516-755-5500
516-755-5561 fax
www.enzo.com

EHT899 .309, 427
hepatitis C protein 310, 428
HGTV-43 320

Enzon
20 Kingsbridge Rd.
Piscataway, NJ 08854-3998
732-980-4500
732-980-5911 fax
www.enzon.com

interferon alfa-2b/ribavirin 311, 430
PEG-camptothecin 184
PEG-Intron/Rebetol *311, 430*
Prothecan *184*

EpiGenesis Pharmaceuticals
3100 Tower Blvd.
Suite 513
Durham, NC 27707
919-419-0389
www.epigene.com

EPI-2010 357

Ergo Science
43 High Street
North Andover, MA 01845
978-974-9474
978-974-0633 fax
www.ergo.com

bromocriptine, ER-230 393
Ergoset *393*

Esperion Therapeutics
695 KMS Place
3621 South State St.
Ann Arbor, MI 48108
734-332-0506
734-443-0516 fax
www.esperion.com

ApoA-I Milano 45

Exocell
3508 Market Street
Suite 420
Philadelphia, PA 19104
215-222-5515
215-222-5325 fax
www.exocell.com

EXO-226 388

EyeTech Pharmaceuticals
10 Hoyt Street
Norwalk, CT 06851
203-838-4401

EYE-001, NX-1838 544

Fabre-Kramer Pharmaceuticals
5847 San Felipe
Suite 3147
Houston, TX 77057
713-975-6900
713-977-1574 fax

gepirone 136
Geppar (proposed to PTO) *136*

Farmacon
1720 Post Road East
Westport, CT 06880
203-255-8898
203-255-3888 fax

flumecinol 67
Zixoryn *67*

FeRx
4330 La Jolla Village Dr.
Suite 250
San Diego, CA 92122
619-677-7788
619-677-9898 fax
www.ferx.com

MTC-DOX 221

First Circle Medical
530 North Third Street
Suite 400
Minneapolis, MN 55401
612-333-4200
512-334-9511 fax
www.fcmedical.com

EWBH treatment 289, 319

Manufacturers Index/651

Forest Laboratories
909 Third Ave.
New York, NY 10022
800-947-5227
212-750-9152 fax
www.frx.com

Aerobid 357
citalopram HBr 134
Dexloxiglumide 438
Escitalopram 134
flunisolide 357
lercanidipine 33, 454
LU 26-054, SSRI 137
Memantine 79
ML3000 492
Siramesine 129

Fournier Research
Nine Law Drive
Fairfield, NJ 07004
973-575-1010
973-575-7374 fax
www.groupe-fournier.com

LF 15-0195 507
pygeum africanum 472, 592
Tadenan 472, 592
tresperimus 52, 157

Fujisawa Healthcare
Three Parkway North
Parkway North Center
Deerfield, IL 60015
800-888-7704
847-317-7296 fax
www.fujisawa.com

AmBisome 518
amphotericin B 518
DTI-0009 16
FK-317 ......165, 179, 266, 281, 464, 584
FK463, echinocandin ..296, 305, 356, 519, 551
FK960 76
pralmorelin 388
Prograf 297, 509, 517
tacrolimus hydrate ...297, 509, 517

GelTex Pharmaceuticals
Nine 4th Ave.
Waltham, MA 02154
800-847-0069
781-290-5890 fax
www.geltex.com

Cholestagel/Zocor 21
colsevelam/simvastatin 21
DENSPM 226, 243, 259, 276, 395, 439, 474
diethylnorspermine 226, 243, 259, 276, 395, 439, 474

Gem Pharmaceuticals
180 Chandalar Place Dr.
Pelham, AL 35124
205-621-9911
205-621-8395 fax
www.gempharm.com

Adriamycin 57, 217
GPX-100 ....57, 166, 180, 217

Genelabs Technologies
505 Penobscot Dr.
Redwood City, CA 94063
650-369-9500
650-368-0709 fax
www.genelabs.com

Aslera 480, 533
GL-331 ...57, 193, 217, 228, 276, 403, 474
GL-701, prasterone 480, 533

Genentech
One DNA Way
South San Francisco, CA 94080
800-225-1000
650-225-6000 fax
webmaster@gene.com
www.gene.com

AMD Fab 544
efalizumab monoclonal antibody 525
Herceptin 173
monoclonal antibody (Mab), anti-VEGF . 28, 184
Nutropin Depot 389
omalizumab 333, 555, 359
Rituxan 239
rituximab/chemotherapy 239
somatropin 389
trastuzumab 173
Xanelim 525
Xolair 333, 555, 359

Generex Biotechnology
33 Harbour Square
Suite 202
Toronto, ON M5J 2G2
Canada
800-391-6755
416-364-9363 fax
info@generex.com
www.generex.com

insulin 383
Oralgen 383

Genetics Institute
87 Cambridge Park Drive
Cambridge, MA 02140
888-446-3344
617-876-0388 fax
info@genetics.com
www.genetics.com

interleukin-12 (IL-12) .277, 289, 312, 430, 475
lanoteplase, BMS-200980 37
recombinant human bone morphogenic protein-2 (rhBMP-2) .116, 489, 490, 510

Genitope Corporation
525 Penobscot Drive
Redwood City, Ca 94063
650-482-2000
650-482-2002 fax
ClinicalInfo@genitope.com
www.genitope.com

subject-specific immunotherapy 238

Genmab A/S
Bredgade 23A
3rd Floor
DK-1260
Copenhagen K
DENMARK
45-7020-2728
45-7020-2729 fax
www.genmab.com

HuMax-CD4 ....506, 525

Genta
99 Hayden Avenue
Suite 200
Lexington, MA 02421
781-860-5150
781-860-5137 fax
info@genta.com
www.genta.com

652/Manufacturers Index

G3139/androgen blockade . .267, 464, 584
G3139/cyclophosphamide 238
G3139/dacarbazine 246
G3139/docetaxel 166, 267, 464, 584
G3139/irinotecan 196, 406
G3139/mitoxantrone . .196, 267, 406, 464, 584
G3139 . . . . .56, 57, 216
Genasense/androgen blockade 267, 464, 584
Genasense/cyclophosphamide *238*
Genasense/dacarbazine *246*
Genasense/Irinotecan *196, 406*
Genasense/Mitoxantrone 196, 267, 406, 464, 584
Genasense/Mylotarg *56, 216*
Genasense/Taxotere *166, 267, 464, 584*
Genasense *57, 216*

GenVec
12111 Parklawn Dr.
Rockville, MD 20852
240-632-0740
240-632-0735 fax
www.genvec.com

BioByPass *28, 42*
vascular endothelial growth factor-121 (VEGF) 28, 42

Genzyme Genetics Division
5 Mountain Road
Framingham, MA 01701
800-357-5744
508-872-5663 fax
www.genzyme.com

antithrombin III, rhATIII 18, 42
vaccine, cancer 64, 67, 242, 250

Genzyme Molecular Oncology
One Mountain Road
Framingham, MA 01701
508-271-2627
508-872-9080 fax
www.genzyme.com

vaccine, kidney cancer 279, 477
vaccine, melanoma 247

Genzyme Tissue Repair
64 Sidney St.
Cambridge, MA 02139-4136
617-494-8484

617-494-6561 fax
www.genzyme.com

transforming growth factor beta-2 (TGF-b2) 387, 518, 531

Gilead Sciences
2860 Wilderness Place
Boulder, CO 80301
800-572-1932
303-546-7812 fax
www.gilead.com

adefovir dipivoxil, GS-840 . . . . . .308, 426
AmBisome *519*
amikacin 298, 372, 482, 552, 571
cidofovir . .83, 214, 309, 348, 427, 540, 551
daunorubicin citrate 55, 62, 216, 237
DaunoXome *55, 62, 216, 237*
liposomal amphotericin B 519
Mikasome *298, 372, 482, 552, 571*
NX 211 . . . . .232, 255
Tenofovir DF *293, 324*
tenofovir disoproxil fumarate . . .293, 324
Vistide *83, 214, 309, 348, 427, 551*

GlaxoSmithKline
New Horizons Ct.
Great West Road
Brentford, Middlesex
United Kingdom
TW89 EP
919-248-2100, 888-825-5249
011-44-181-975-2764 fax
www.gsk.com

abacavir 316
albuterol 356, 363
amoxicillin/clavulante potassium 298
Ariflo *360, 365*
Augmentin SR *298*
Avandia *386*
Bactroban *376, 556*
carvedilol 23
Coreg *23*
Epivir *321*
Epstein-Barr virus vaccine 337, 348
Factive *299, 483, 571*
Flixotide, Flovent *358, 364*
fluticasone propionate 358, 364
fluticasone/salmeterol 333, 555
gemifloxacin mesylate 299, 483, 571
GI 181771 . . . . .393, 417
GI 198745 . . . . .381, 447, 516, 575

GI 262570 .383
GW 150013 127
GW 270773 335
GW 273293 . . . . .90, 133
GW 320659, 1555U88 . . . . .81, 130
GW 328267 . . . . .358, 364
GW 406381 . . . . .106, 499
GW 419458, DISC-HSV 306, 520, 564, 578
GW 427353 . . . . .383, 393
GW 433908 319
GW 468816 . . . . .96, 147, 376
GW 473178 . . . . .16, 43
GW 572016 180
GW 597599 136
GW 650250 136
GW 660511 . . . . .33, 454
GW-650250A, NS-2389 136
hepatitis vaccine 338
Hycamtin *199, 234, 256, 409*
Imigran, Imitrex *97*
Infanrix *313, 339, 431*
lamivudine .321
Lotrafiban *38*
mepolizumab, SB 240563 359
mupirocin 376, 556
N. meningitidis A/C 339
nabumetone Q 108, 492, 501
Naramig, Amerge *96*
naratriptan 96
paroxetine 128, 138, 142
Paxil, Seroxat *128, 138, 142*
PeNta-HepB-IPV, vaccine . .313, 339, 431
Relenza *329, 371*
ReQuip *113*
ropinirole 113
rosiglitazone 386
Rotarix *339*
rotavirus vaccine 339
salmeterol xinafoate 360, 365
salmeterol/fluticasone propionate 360, 365
SB 204269 91
SB 207266 16
SB 207499 . . . . .360, 365
SB 214857 38
SB 217242 25
SB 223412 . . . . .366, 482
SB 243213 .139
SB 249417 . . . . .119, 335
SB 249553 . . . . .233, 246
SB 251353 .204
SB 273005 . . . . .495, 508
SB 275833 . . . . .376, 556
SB 408075 . . . . .199, 409
SB 418790 . . . . .386, 394

Manufacturers Index/653

SB 424323 17
SB 435495 41
SB 596168 186
SB 659746A, EMD 68843 139
SB 683698, TR 14035 . . . . .361, 508
SB M00026 . . . . .313, 431
SB-237376 16
Seretide, Advair 360, 365
Serevent .360, 365
Simplirix 307, 342, 520, 565, 579
sumatriptan 97
tafenoquine, SB 252263 330
telmisartan 34, 455
topotecan HCl 199, 234, 256, 409
Tranilast 31
Twinrix-2 doses 338
Twinrix-three doses 314, 343, 432
vaccine, genital herpes .307, 342, 520, 565, 579
vaccine, hepatitis B 314, 433
vaccine, hepatitis E 314, 432
vaccine, hepatitis 314, 343, 432
vaccine, HIV 324, 343
vaccine, HPV 343, 350
vaccine, influenza 329, 344, 370
vaccine, malaria 330, 344
vaccine, meningitis B 345
vaccine, MMR-varicella 346
vaccine, S. pneumoniae 305
vaccine, Streptococcus pneumoniae . .305, 331, 347, 551, 554
valaciclovir 316, 522
Valtrex, Zelitrex 316, 522
Ventolin 356, 363
YH-1885, SB 641257 422
zanamavir 329, 371
Ziagen 316

Gliatech

23420 Commerce Park Rd.
Cleveland, OH 44122
216-831-3200
216-831-4220 fax
www.gliatech.com

GT-2331 . . . . .76, 81, 114, 130
Perceptin 76, 81, 114, 130

Guilford Pharmaceuticals

6611 Tributary St.
Baltimore, MD 21224
410-631-6300
410-631-6338 fax
ir@guilfordpharm.com
www.guilfordpharm.com

FKBP-neuroimmunophilin ligands . . .111

Gynetics

105 Raider Blvd.
Suite 203
Bell Mead, NJ 08502-1510
908-359-2429
908-359-6660 fax
info@gynetics.com
www.gynetics.com

levonorgestrel 562
PREVEN2 562

H. Lundbeck A/S

H. Lundbeck A/S
Ottiliavej 9
Dk-25000 Valby
Copenhagen, Denmark
45-3630-1311
45-3630-1940 fax
www.lunbeck.com

Gaboxadol 115
Lu 35-139 143

Helsinn Healthcare SA

P.O. Box 357
6915 Pambio-Noranco
Switzerland
41-91-9852121
41-91-9932122 fax
info-hhc@helsinn.com
www.helsinn.com/

Palonosetron 188

Hemispherx Biopharma

1617 JFK Blvd.
One Penn Center, Suite 660
Philadelphia, PA 19103
800-442-3437
215-988-1739 fax
www.hemispherx.com

Ampligen 88, 244, 278, 306, 322, 476
poly I:poly C-12-U .88, 244, 278, 306, 322, 476

Hemosol

115 Skyway Ave.
Etobicoke, Ontario M9W 4Z4
Canada
781-829-9993
781-821-9161 fax
www.hemosol.com

blood substitute 18, 224
Hemolink 18, 224

Hoffmann-La Roche

340 Kingsland St.
Nutley, NJ 07110
800-526-6367
973-562-2206 fax
www.rocheusa.com

Bonviva 167, 495
capecitabine/docetaxel 163
capecitabine 195, 405
Cymeval 306, 539
Cytovene 306, 539
ganciclovir 306, 539
ibandronate 167, 495
NK-1 . . . . .137, 145
orlistat .385, 393
Pegasys . . .59, 218, 244, 278, 313, 431, 475
peginterferon alfa-2a 59, 218, 244, 278, 313, 431, 475
valganciclovir 306, 539
Xeloda/Taxotere 163
Xeloda 195, 385, 393, 405

Holles Laboratories

30 Forest Notch
Cohasset, MA 02025
781-383-0741
781-383-0005 fax

Dehydrex 542

Hollis-Eden Pharmaceuticals

9333 Genesee Ave.
Suite 100
San Diego, CA 92121
858-587-9333
858-558-6470 fax
www.holliseden.com

HE2000 428

Human Genome Sciences

9410 Key West Avenue
Rockville, MD 20850-3838
301-309-8504
301-309-8512 fax

www.hgsi.com

Albuferon *314, 432*
keratinocyte growth factor-2 (KGF-2) .51, 156, 203, 435, 532
myeloid progenitor inhibitory factor (MPIF) .... .203
Repifermin *51, 156, 203, 435, 532*
vascular endothelial growth factor-2 gene therapy (gtVEGF-2) .... .18, 28

Hybridon
155 Fortune Boulevard
Milford, MA 01757
617-679-5582 fax
www.hybridon.com

GEM-231 .... .180
GEM-92 .... .289, 319

IBEX Technologies
5485 Pare Street
Montreal, Quebec H4P 1P7
Canada
514-344-4004
514-344-8827 fax
www.ibex.ca

heparinase I .... .19
Neutralase .... *.19*

ICN Pharmaceuticals
3300 Hyland Ave.
Costa Mesa, CA 92626
800-548-5100
714-556-0131 fax
www.icnpharm.com

growth hormone releasing factor (GRF) . 388
ribavirin .... .349, 372
tiazofurin .... .60, 219
Tiazole .... *.60, 219*
Virazole .... *.349, 372*

ICOS Corporation
22021 20th Ave. SE
Bothell, WA 98021
425-485-1900
425-489-0356 fax
www.icos.com

IC14 .... .335
Pafase .... *.335*

Sitaxsentan .... .34, 454

ID Biomedical
8855 Northbrook Court
Burnaby, British Columbia V5J-5J1
Canada
604-431-9314
604-431-9378 fax
www.idbiomedical.com

A streptococcus vaccine .... .337
StreptAvax .... *.337*

IDEC Pharmaceuticals
11011 Torreyana Rd.
San Diego, CA 92121
858-431-8500
858-431-8750 fax
www.idecpharm.com

IDEC-114 .... .526
IDEC-131 .... .480, 526, 506, 533
IDEC-152 .... .295, 358, 549
IDEC-Y2B8, In2B8 .... .238
Primatized .... *.526*
Zevalin .... *.238*

IDUN Pharmaceuticals
11085 N. Torrey Pines Road
Suite 300
La Jolla, CA 92037
858-623-1330
858-623-2765 fax
www.idun.com

IDN-6556 .... .310, 428

ILEX Oncology
11550 IH-10 West
Suite 300
San Antonio, TX 78230
210-949-8200
210-949-8210 fax
www.ilexoncology.com

aminopterin .... .54, 205, 215
Apomine .... *.274, 471, 591*
diarysulfonylurea, ILX-295501 ..226, 242, 252, 276, 473
ILX-651 .... .181
NM-3 .... .153
piritrexim .... .213

ImClone Systems
180 Varick St.
7th Floor
New York, NY 10014
212-645-1405
212-645-2054 fax
ir@imclone.com
www.imclone.com

BEC2 .... .224
FLT3 ligand ...63, 166, 179, 237, 241, 253
IMC-1C11 .... .197, 407
IMC-C225, CPT-11167, 197, 210, 228, 260, 268, 277, 396, 407, 440, 465, 475, 585
Mobist .... *.63, 166, 179, 237, 241, 253*

Immtech International/ NextEra Therapeutics
1890 Maple Avenue
Suite 110
Evanston, IL 60201
888-463-7850
847-573-0045 fax
www.immtech.org

DB-075 .... .415
DB-289 .... .373, 552

ImmuCell Corporation
56 Evergreen Dr.
Portland, ME 04103
207-878-2770
207-878-2117 fax
www.immucell.com

DiffGAM .... *.300, 415*
immune globulin (IgG) .... .300, 415

Immune Response Corporation
5935 Darwin Court
Carlsbad, CA 92008
800-491-0153
760-431-8636 fax
www.imnr.com

HIV-1 immunogen .... .320
IR208 .... .99, 338
IR501 .... .338, 506
IR502 .... .338, 526
NeuroVax .... *.99, 338*
Ravax .... *.338, 506*
Remune .... *.320*
T-cell peptide vaccines .... .339
T-cell receptor vaccine 100, 509, 529
Zorcell .... *.338, 526*

Manufacturers Index/655

Immunex Corporation
51 University St.
Seattle, WA 98101
206-470-4193
206-587-0606 fax
www.immunex.com

Avrend 276, 473
CD40 ligand 276, 473
interleukin-4 (IL-4) 359
Nuvance 359

ImmunoGen
333 Providence Highway
Norwood, MA 02062
781-769-4242
781-255-9679 fax
www.immunogen.com

HuC242-DM1/SB-408075 ..197, 228, 259, 395, 407, 440
HuN901-DM1 228

Immunomedics
300 American Rd.
Morris Plains, NJ 07950
973-605-8200
973-605-8282 fax
www.immunomedics.com

AFP-Scan 221
arcitumomab 162, 223, 283, 399
bectumomab 237
CEA-Cide 167, 181, 198, 229, 253, 260, 396, 408, 441
CEA-Scan 162, 223, 283, 399
epratuzumab 237
imaging agent 221
IMMU-MN14, anti-CEA ..167, 181, 198, 229, 253, 260, 396, 408, 441
LymphoCide 237
LymphoScan 237

Inex Pharmaceuticals
8900 Glanlyon Pkwy.
Suite 100
Burnaby, British Columbia V5J-5J8
Canada
604-419-3200
604-419-3201 fax
www.inexpharm.com

Onco TCS 189, 235, 240
vincristine 189, 235, 240

Inflazyme Pharmaceuticals
5600 Parkwood Way
Suite 425
Richmond, British Columbia V6V 2M2
Canada
800-315-3660
604-279-8711 fax
info@inflazyme.com
www.inflazyme.com

IPL 576,092 359

Inhibitex
8995 Westside Parkway
Alpharetta, GA 30004
678-336-2600
678-335-2626 fax
www.inhibitex.com

SA-IGIV 336

Inkine Pharmaceutical Company
1720 Walton Road
Suite 200
Blue Bell, PA 19422
800-759-9350
610-260-9355 fax
www.inkine.com

CBP-1011 ....412, 435
CBP-1011 ....68, 282
Colirest 68, 282, 412, 435

Innapharma
10 Mountview Road
Suite 301
Upper Saddle River, NJ 07458-1935
914-357-4100
914-369-7899 fax

INN-00835 136

Innovative Drug Delivery Systems, Inc.
787 Seventh Avenue, 48th floor
New York, NY 10019
212-554-4550
212-554-4554 fax
mcarroll@idds.com
www.idds.com

nasal ketamine 501

InSite Vision
965 Atlantic Ave.
Alameda, CA 94501
510-865-8800
510-865-5700 fax
insitemail@insite.com
www.insitevision.com

batimastat, ISV-120 540
diclofenac, ISV-205 ....540, 543
proparacaine 542
ToPreSite 542

Inspire Pharmaceuticals
4222 Emperor Blvd.
Suite 470
Durham, NC 27703
919-941-9777
919-941-9797 fax
www.inspirepharm.com

INS316 229
INS365 ophthalmic 541
INS365 ....363, 368
INS37217 respiratory 368, 541

Integra LifeSciences
P.O. Box 688
Plainsboro, NJ 08536
609-275-0500
609-799-3297 fax
www.integra-ls.com

TP-9201 ....15, 30, 119

Intellivax International
5757 Cavendish Blvd.
Suite 165
Cote Saint-Luc, Quebec H4W 2W8
Canada
514-338-3883
514-334-0606 fax
info@intellivax.com
www.intellivax.com

vaccine, nasal proteosome influenza .329, 371
vaccine, Shigella flexneri and sonneii .305, 347, 416

Interferon Sciences
783 Jersey Ave.
New Brunswick, NJ 08901-3660
888-728-4372
732-249-6895 fax

www.interferonsciences.com

Alferon LDO 321
Alferon N Gel 308, 348, 521, 572
Alferon N Injection 311, 321, 429
interferon (IFN) alfa-n3 308, 311, 321, 348, 429, 521, 572

InterMune
1710 Gilbreth Road
Suite 301
Burlingame, CA 94010-1317
650-843-2855

gamma interferon 367

Interneuron Pharmaceuticals
One Ledgemont Center
99 Hayden Avenue
Lexington, MA 02421
781-861-8444
781-861-3830 fax
www.interneuron.com

CerAxon 116
citicoline sodium 116
IP501 ....125, 312, 430, 438
trospium chloride 482
Trospium 482

IntraBiotics Pharmaceuticals
1245 Terra Bella Ave.
Mountain View, CA 94043
650-526-6800
650-969-0663 fax
info@intrabiotics.com
www.intrabiotics.com

protegrin IB-367, aerosol 368
protegrin IB-367, rinse, gel .203, 301, 374, 553
Ramoplanin Oral 336, 347

INTRACEL Corporation
1330 Picard Drive
Rockville, MD 20850-4396
301-258-5200
301-840-2161 fax
info@intracel.com
www.intracel.com

BCI-Immune Activator 155, 449
HumaRAD-HN 213
HumaSPECT/BR 174

HumaSPECT/Infectious Diseases 351
votumumab 174, 351

Introgen Therapeutics
301 Congress Avenue
Suite 1850
Austin, TX 78701
512-708-9310
512-708-9311 fax
www.introgen.com

Adenoviral p53 ....84, 158
INGN 241 (mda-7) 167, 181, 229
INGN-201, adenoviral p53 .154, 168, 181, 210, 229, 254, 268, 448, 465, 585
INGN-201 ....84, 158

Iomed
3385 West 1820 South
Salt Lake City, UT 84104
800-621-3347
801-972-9072 fax
www.iomed.com

dexamethasone 105, 498, 532, 540
IontoDex 105, 498, 532, 540

Isis Pharmaceuticals
2292 Faraday Avenue
Carlsbad, CA 92008
760-931-9200
760-931-9639 fax
info@isisph.com
www.isip.com

ISIS 2503 168, 193, 229, 260, 396, 403, 441
ISIS 3521 ....168, 230
ISIS 5132, CGP 69846A 169, 182, 193, 230, 260, 286, 396, 403, 441, 466, 585
ISIS-13312 ....306, 539
ISIS-14803 ....312, 430
ISIS-2302 ....413, 435, 459, 527

Isotechnika
17208 -108 Avenue
Edmonton, Alberta
Canada
T5S 1E8
780-487-1600
780 484-4105 fax
www.isotechnika.com

ISAtx247 ....326, 506, 526

Janssen Pharmaceutica
1125 Trenton-Harbourtown Rd.
P.O. Box 200
Titusville, NJ 08560-0200
800-526-7736
609-730-2616 fax
www.jnj.com

(+)-norcisapride 420
prucalopride 412, 434
R 107474 138
R 149524 421
R 115777 185
Resolor 412, 434
Risperdal 133, 134, 145
risperidone 1133, 134, 145
YKP-10A 140

Janssen Research Foundation
1125 Trenton-Harbortown Road
P.O. Box 200
Titusville, NJ 08560-0200
609-730-2000
609-730-2323 fax
www.jrf.com

galantamine hydrobromide 76, 88, 89, 305
Reminyl 76, 88, 89, 305

Jenner BioTherapies
2010 Crow Canyon Place
Suite 100
San Ramon, CA 94583
262-275-0064
262-275-8381 fax
wtrade@hughestech.net
www.jennerbio.com

AdjuVax-100a 274, 341, 471, 591
cVax-Pr 265, 462, 582
vaccine, adjuvant 274, 341, 471, 591

John Wayne Cancer Institute
1328 22nd St.
Three West
Santa Monica, CA 90404
310-449-5250
310-449-5259 fax
www.jwci.org

CancerVax, C-VAX 242

King Pharmaceuticals
501 5th Street

Manufacturers Index/657

Bristol, TN 37620
423-989-8000
423-274-8677 fax
www.kingpharm.com

AMISTAD-II 36
MRE0470 28
Pallacor 36

Knoll Pharmaceutical
3000 Continental Drive North
Mt. Olive, NJ 07828-1234
800-240-3820
973-426-5145 fax
knollcom@knoll-pharma.com
www.knoll-pharma.com

ancrod 18, 42, 116
atelimomab 334
PEG-hirudin 14, 19
Segard 334
Viprinex 18, 42, 116

La Jolla Pharmaceutical
6455 Nancy Ridge Dr.
San Diego, CA 92121
858-452-6600
858-623-0649 fax
investor.relations@ljpc.com
www.ljpc.com

LJP-394 ....457, 480, 533

Layton Bioscience
105 Reservoir Road
Atherton, CA 94027
650-854-6614
650-854-4776 fax
www.laytonbio.com

Inversine 81, 120, 130
LBS-neurons 117
mecamylamine HCl 81, 120, 130

LeukoSite
215 First Street
Cambridge, MA 02142
617-621-9350
617-621-9349 fax
information@leukosite.com
www.leukosite.com

LDP-01 ....30, 118
LDP-392 296

LDP-977 359

Levotech
100 Front St.
Suite 1350
West Conshohocken, PA 19428
610-940-0300
610-940-0301 fax

Amylin 561
Contraceptive Patch 561

LifeTime Pharmaceuticals
387 Technology Drive
College Park, MD 20742
301-314-1480
301-439-7917 fax
www.ltpharma.com

Beta LT 64, 67, 242, 249

Ligand Pharmaceuticals
10275 Science Center Dr.
San Diego, CA 92121
858-550-7500
858-550-7506 fax
www.ligand.com

alitretinoin, ALRT-1057 .69, 161, 223, 524
bexarotene162, 208, 224, 241, 516, 522, 524
denileukin diftitox 56, 62, 216, 241
LGD-1550 ....17, 156, 182, 191, 211, 559
Morphelan 108, 501
morphine sulfate 108, 501
Ontak 56, 62, 216, 241
Panretin 69, 161, 223, 524
Targretin-capsule ..162, 208, 224, 241, 516, 524
Targretin-gel 522

Lipha Pharmaceuticals
1114 Avenue of Americas
41st Floor
New York, NY 10036-7703
800-547-4299
212-398-5026 fax
www.lipha.com

acamprosate 125

Lorus Therapeutics Inc.
1285 Morningside Avenue
Scarborough, Ontario M1B 3W2
Canada

905-305-1100
905-305-1584 fax
www.lorusthera.com

virulizin 263, 443

MacroChem Corporation
110 Hartwell Avenue
Lexington, MA 02421-3134
781-862-4003
781-862-4338 fax
www.macrochem.com

alprostadil 450, 477, 575
Benefen 491
ibuprofen 491
testosterone 452, 577
Topiglan 450, 477, 575

Magainin Pharmaceuticals
5110 Campus Dr.
Plymouth Meeting, PA 19462
800-522-8973
610-941-5399 fax
www.magainin.com

squalamine 172, 186, 233, 256

Mallinckrodt
675 McDonnell Blvd.
P.O. Box 5840
St. Louis, MO 63134
888-744-1414
888-222-9799 fax
www.mallinckrodt.com

AngioMARK 39, 41, 45
imaging agent, entire body 534
MS-325 ....39, 41, 45

Maret Pharmaceuticals
4041 MacArthur Blvd.
Suie 375
Newport Beach, CA 92660
949-225-0005
949-225-0006 fax
maret@maretpharma.com
www.maretpharma.com

MARstem 51, 173

Marnac
8609 NW Plaza Dr.
Suite 435

658/Manufacturers Index

Dallas, TX 75225
214-987-1388
214-692-8510 fax

Deskar *100, 375*
pirfenidone 100, 375

Massachusetts Biologic Laboratories
305 South St.
Jamaica Plain, MA 02130
617-983-6300
617-983-6301 fax

immune globulin (IG-IV) 300

Matrix Pharmaceutical
34700 Campus Drive
Freemont, CA 94555
888-800-2521
510-742-8510 fax
www.matx.com

cisplatin/epinephrine . .163, 176, 195, 205, 208, 220, 242, 406, 416
FMdC 196, 228, 253, 406
IntraDose 163, 176, 195, 205, 208, 220, 242, 406, 416
MPI-5020 170

Maxia Pharmaceuticals
10835 Altman Row
Suite 250
San Diego, CA 92121
858-824-1988
858-824-1967 fax

MX6 . . . . .192, 560

Maxim Pharmaceuticals
8899 University Center Lane
Suite 400
San Diego, CA 92122
888-562-9465
858-552-2263 fax
www.maxim.com

Ceplene *57, 65, 217, 243, 248, 276, 311, 429, 474*
histamine dihydrochloride 65, 217, 243, 248, 276, 474
immunotherapeutic, AML . . .57, 311, 429

Medarex
1545 Route 22 East
Annandale, NJ 08801-0953
908-713-6001
609-430-2850 fax
www.medarex.com

MDX-210169, 194, 207, 231, 254, 261, 270, 277, 397, 404, 419, 442, 467, 475, 587
MDX-220198, 205, 207, 231, 254, 261, 270, 397, 408, 419, 442, 467, 587
MDX-22 . . . . .52, 59, 218
MDX-33 . . . . .49, 68, 282
MDX-447, H-447 . .85, 155, 159, 170, 211, 231, 449
MDX-RA 539

Medeva plc
10 St. James Street
London SW1A 1EF
United Kingdom
44-0-1372-364000
44-0-1372-364167 fax
www.medeva.co.uk

methylphenidate HCl 82, 131

MediGene AG
Lochhamer Str. 11
D-82152
Martinsried/Munich
Germany
011-49-89-89-56-32-0
www.medigene.de

Etomoxir *26*
Polyphenon E *308, 521*
vaccine, cervical cancer 192, 561

MedImmune
35 W. Watkins Mill Road
Gaithersburg, MD 20878
301-417-0770
301-527-4207 fax
www.medimmune.com

amifostine 202
cisplatin/vinblastine/amifostine 225
Ethyol *202*
MEDI-507 527
MEDI-517 . . . . .191, 348, 560
NeuTrexin *199, 409*
paclitaxel/carboplatin/amifostine 232
trimetrexate glucuronate/leucovorin .199, 409

vaccine, urinary tract infection . .483, 572
Vitaxin *188*

Medinox
11575 Sorrento Valley Road
Suite 201
San Diego, CA 92121
858-793-4820
858-793-4823 fax
info@medinox.com
www.medinox.com

NOX-100 . . . .*458*

Medivir
44-1223-275-300
44-1233-416-300 fax
www.medivir.se

ME-609 . . . . .315, 522
MIV-210 . . . . .312, 431

Merck & Co.
1 Merck Dr.
P.O. Box 100
Whitehouse Station, NJ 08889-0100
800-422-9675
908-735-1253 fax
www.merck.com

MK-826, carbapenem 301
vaccine, human papilloma virus .344, 350
vaccine, rotavirus 351
KRP-297 383
MK-663 . . . . .107, 193, 491, 500, 507
MK-826, carbepenem .373, 423, 483, 531, 552, 565, 571
MK-869 . . . . .127, 133, 137, 203
substance P antagonist candidates129, 140
vaccine, zoster 479

Merck KgaA
64721 Darmstadt
Germany
011-49-6151-72-0
011-49-6151727776 fax
www.merck.de

antidepressant 134
asimadoline 104, 490, 497
EGF-receptor specific monoclonal antibody 178
EMD 82633 .154, 164, 178, 209, 252, 276, 448, 474

Manufacturers Index/659

EMD-57445 144
metformin/sulfonylureas 384
neuroleptic .144

Metabolex
3876 Bay Center Place
Hayward, CA 94545
510-293-8800
510-293-9090 fax
info@metabolex.com
www.metabolex.com

MBX-102 384

MGI Pharma
9900 Bren Rd. East
Suite 300E
Minnetonka, MN 55343-9667
800-562-5580
612-346-4800 fax
www.mgipharma.com

Irofulven .170, 183, 192, 194, 198, 221, 232,
255, 261, 270, 277, 397, 442, 404, 408,
467, 475, 560, 587
MG98 211
MGI-114, hydroxymethylacylfulvene,
HMAF 170, 183, 192, 194, 198, 221, 232,
255, 261, 270, 277, 397, 442, 404, 408,
467, 475, 560, 587

Micrologix
3650 Wesbrook Mall
Vancouver BC
Canada
V6S 2L2
800-665-1968
604-221-9688 fax
www.mbiotech.com

MBI 226 301
MBI 594AN 515
MBI 853NL .336

Milkhaus Laboratory
48 Main Street
Boxford, MA 01921
978-887-2086
www.milkhaus.com

2CVV 87, 305
HP-3 . . . . .362, 365, 367
HP-4 180
LDI-200 . . . . . . .58, 69, 218, 269, 466, 586

Millenium Pharmaceuticals
640 Memorial Dr.
Cambridge, MA 02139
617-374-9480
617-374-7788 fax
pr@mlnm.com
www.mlnm.com

LDP-02 .413, 436
LDP-341, PS-341 . . . . .65, 182, 249

Miravant
7408 Hollister Ave
Santa Barbara, CA 93117
888-471-4403
805-685-2959 fax
www.miravant.com

PhotoPoint - SnET2 544
SnET2 544

Mission Pharmacal
1325 E. Durango Blvd.
San Antonio, TX 78210
800-531-3333
210-533-4487 fax
www.missionpharmacal.com

Neosten 495
sodium fluoride 495

ML Laboratories plc
Innovation House, Kelburn Court
Daten Park
Birchwood, Warrington WA3 6UT
United Kingdom
44-1925-844700
44-1925-844702 fax
www.mllabs.co.uk

icodextrin, Extraneal 457
Icodial 457

Molecular Biosystems
10030 Barnes Canyon Road
San Diego, CA 92121
619-452-0681

human albumin microspheres . .14, 27, 30
MB-U820 423
Optison 14, 27, 30
Oralex 423

Mucos Pharma GmbH
Malvenweg 2
D-82538 Geretsried
Germany
49-0-8171-518-0
49-0-8171-52008 fax
www.mucos.de

Wobe-Mugos-E 67, 204, 250

Mylan
1030 Century Bldg.
130-7th St.
Pittsburgh, PA 15222
412-232-0100
412-232-0123 fax
www.mylan.com

dotarizine 95
therapeutic, wound healing .387, 518, 534

Nabi
5800 Park of Commerce Blvd. NW
Boca Raton, FL 33487
800-635-1766
561-989-5890 fax
www.nabi.com

HBVIg 310, 428
hepatitis B immune globulin 310, 428
hyperimmune globulin 335
immune globulin 310, 429
Nabi Civacir 310, 429
Nabi StaphVAX 336, 347
Nabi-Altastaph 335
vaccine, Staphylococcus aureus . .336, 347

Nastech Pharmaceutical
45 Davids Drive
Hauppauge, NY 11788
800-422-6237 (cancer svcs)
516-273-0252 fax
www.nastech.com

apomorphine HCl 477, 569
doxylamine .114
morphine 107, 500
selective serotonergic agent 96

NeoPharma
100 Corporate North
Suite 215
Bannockburn, IL 60015
46-0-18-69-23-83
46-0-18-69-35-95 fax

Duodopa *112*
levodopa/carbidopa 112

NeoRx Corporation
410 W. Harrison St.
Seattle, WA 98119
206-281-7001
206-298-9442 fax
www.neorx.com

Pretarget *240*
skeletal targeted radiotherapy (STR) ..66, 249

Neose Technologies
102 Witmer Road
Horsham, PA 19044
215-441-5890
215-441-5896 fax
info@neose.com
www.neose.com

NE-0080 .... .425
NE-1530 .... .551, 552

NeoTherapeutics
157 Technology Dr.
Irvine, CA 92618
949-788-6700
949-450-6706 fax
info@neotherapeutics.com
www.neotherapeutics.com

leteprinim potassium, AIT-082 ...76, 101, 102, 111, 118, 510
Neotrofin *76, 101, 102, 111, 118, 510*

Neurobiological Technologies
1387 Marina Way South
Richmond, CA 94804
510-215-8000
510-215- 8100 fax
invest@ntii.com
www.ntii.com

memantine .... .77, 103, 290, 392

Neurocrine Biosciences
10555 Science Center Drive
San Diego, CA 92121
619-658-7600
619-658-7601 fax
www.neurocrine.com

CRF receptor antagonist (partnered), NBI-37582 .... 126, 135
CRF receptor antagonist (proprietary)126, 135
interleukin-4 (IL-4) fusion toxin, NBI-3001 .... .85, 158
NBI-34060 .... .92, 115
NBI-5788, MSP-771 .... .100
NBI-6024 .... .384

Neurogen Corporation
35 Northeast Industrial Road
Branford, CT 06405
203-488-8201
203-483-8651 fax
info@nrgn.com
www.neurogen.com

NGD 91-1 .... .127
NGD 91-3 .... .128
NGD 96-1 .... .92
NGD 97-1 .... .77, 89

NeuroSearch A/S
26 B Smedeland
DK-2600
Glostrup
Denmark
011-45-4460-8000
011-45-4460-8080 fax
www.neurosearch.dk/uk

brasofensine, NS-2214, BMS-204756 .111
NS-1209, SPD-502 .... .118
NS-2330 .... .78
NS-2359 .... .125
NS-2389 .... .138
NS-2710 .... .128

Nexell Therapeutics
Nine Parker
Irvine, CA 92618-1605
949-470-9011
949-586-2420 fax
www.nexellinc.com

hypericin .... .63, 84, 526, 531
VIMRxyn *63, 84, 526, 531*
VM-301, OAS 1000 .... .388, 517, 518, 535

NexMed
350 Corporate Blvd.
Robbinsville, NJ 08691
609-208-9688
609-208-1868 fax
NexMedLA@aol.com
www.nexmed.com

alprostadil .... .450, 569, 575
Alprox-TD, Befar *450, 575*
emprox *569*

NicOx SA
1900 Route des Cretes/BP 313
06906 Sophia-Antipolis cedex
France
33-0-4-92387020
33-0-4-92387030 fax
www.nicox.com/uk/company.htm

HCT 1026 .... .481, 494, 516, 525, 531
HCT 3012 .... .107, 499
NCX 1015 .... .436
NCX 1022 .... .527
NCX 4016 .... .44, 108, 501
NCX 701 .... .108, 501

NitroMed
12 Oak Park Dr.
Bedford, MA 01730
781-275-9700
781-275-2282 fax
www.nitromed.com

NMI-870 .... .478, 570

Northfield Laboratories
1560 Sherman Ave.
Suite 1000
Evanston, IL 60201-4422
847-864-3500
847-864-3577 fax
investor@frb.bsmg.com
www.northfieldlabs.com

hemoglobin .... .54
PolyHeme *54*

Northwest Biotherapeutics
120 Northgate Plaza
Suite 200
Seattle, WA 98125
877-606-9246
425-608-3026 fax
www.nwbio.com

DCVax *274, 471, 591*

PSMA - P1/P2 . . . . .271, 468, 588

Nortran Pharmaceuticals
3650 Wesbrook Mall
Vancouver, BC V6S 2L2
Canada
800-330-9928
604-222-6617 fax
www.nortran.com

RSD 921 .110, 502

Novartis
556 Morris Avenue
Summit, NJ 07901
973-781-8300
973-781-8265 fax
www.novartis.com

Amdray 255
Apligraf 534
Certican 326
Comtan 111
COX 189 . . . . .105, 490, 498, 505
Diovan 26, 35, 38, 455
DNK 333 . . . . .333, 357, 364, 555
DPP 728/LAF 237 382
DTA 201 142
Elidel 297, 517
entacapone 111
Estalis 494
estradiol/norethisterone acetate 494
everolimus 326
Femara 169
Foradil .358, 376
formoterol 358, 376
FTY 720 326
Glivec 57, 217
ICL 670 52
imatinib, STI 571 . . . . .57, 217
ketotifen fumarate 295, 541, 550
Lamisil 250, 523, 534
letrozole 169
LTB 019 365
methylphenidate 82, 131
NKP 608 128
octreotide acetate 541
pimecrolimus, ASM 981 . . . . . . .297, 517
PKC 412 . . . . .185, 542
PSC 833, valspodar 255
Ritalin LA 82, 131
Sandostatin LAR 541
SDZ RAD 327
tegaserod 412, 421, 425, 438

terbinafine 250, 523, 534
valsartan 26, 35, 38, 455
Zaditen 295, 541, 550
Zelmac 412, 421, 425, 438
zoledronate 54, 157, 213, 488, 496
Zometa 54, 157, 213, 488, 496

Novavax
8320 Guilford Road
Suite C
Columbia, MD 21046
301-854-3900
301-854-3901 fax
info@novavax.com
www.novavax.com

Androsorb 391, 568, 579
estradiol 389, 566
Estrasorb 389, 566
testosterone 391, 568, 579
vaccine, HPV-16 VLP 344, 350

Novelos Therapeutics
617-244-1616
617-964-6331 fax
www.novelos.com

BAM-002 223

Noven Pharmaceuticals
11960 SW 144th St.
Miami, FL 33186
800-340-7302
305-251-1887 fax
www.noven.com

estrogen 391, 392, 494, 568
ketoprofen patch 107, 500
methylphenidate 81, 130
MethyPatch 81, 130
Vivelle, *Menorest* 392, 494, 568
Vivelle-Dot 391, 494, 568

Novo Nordisk
Krogshojvej 30
2880 Bagsvaerd
Denmark
011-45-4444-8888
212-867-0298 fax
plha@novo.dk
www.novonordisk.com

NN 1215 384
NN 1998, Insulin (r-human) 384

NN 2344, DRF-2593 384
NN 304, insulin detemir 384
NN 414 384
NN 4201, NNC-42-1001 385
NN 622, DRF-2725 385
NN 703, NNC 26-0703, r-Somatropin 388
NNC-90-1170, NN 2211 385
NovoNorm 386
NovoSeven 32, 53, 438
r-FVIIa 32, 53, 438
repaglinide 386

Novogen
140 Wicks Road
North Ryde
New South Wales 2113
Australia
800-668-6436
61 2 9878 0055 fax
www.novogen.com

phenoxodiol 185, 270, 467, 587

NPS Allelix Corp
6850 Goreway Dr.
Mississauga, Ontario L4V-1V7
Canada
905-677-0831
905-677-9595 fax
www.allelix.com

ALX-0600 422
ALX-0646 94
ALX1-11 493
AMG 073 399
NPS 1506 . . . . .118, 138

Nycomed Amersham Imaging
2636 S. Clearbrook Dr.
Arlington Heights, IL 60005
800-633-4123
609-514-6572 fax
www.nycomed-amersham.com

Metastron 271, 468, 588
strontium-89 chloride injection .271, 468, 588

Oculex Pharmaceuticals
639 N. Pastoria Ave.
Sunnyvale, CA 94086-2917
408-481-0424
408-481-0662 fax
oculexinc@aol.com

662/Manufacturers Index

www.oculex.com

dexamethasone .... .540
Posurdex .... *.542*
Surodex .... *.540*

Oncolytics Biotech
301-1211 Kensington Road N.W.
Calgary, AB T2N 3P6
Canada
403-670-7380
403-283-0858 fax
www.oncolyticsbiotech.com

Reolysin .... *.187*

Ontogen Corporation
6451 El Camino Real
Carlsbad, CA 92009
760-930-0100
760-930-0200 fax
www.ontogen.com

OC144-093 .... .184

Onyvax
St. George's Hospital Med. School
P.O. Box 17717/Cranmer Terrace
London
United Kingdom
SW17 0WG
44-0-20-8682-9494
44-0-20-8682-9495 fax
mail@onyvax.com
www.onyvax.com

Onyvax 105 .... *.201, 341, 411*
Onyvax CR .... *.200, 340, 410*
Onyvax P .... *.274, 340, 471, 591*
vaccine, 105AD7 .... .201, 341, 411
vaccine ..200, 274, 410, 340, 410, 471, 591

Onyx Pharmaceuticals
3031 Research Dr., Bldg. A
Richmond, CA 94806
510-222-9700
510-222-9758 fax
www.onyx-pharm.com

CI-1042, ONYX-01583, 153, 157, 190, 195,
   208, 225, 258, 394, 405, 439, 447, 559
Ras pathway inhibitor .... .186

Ophidian Pharmaceuticals
5445 E. Cheryl Pkwy.
Madison, WI 53711
608-271-0878
608-277-2395 fax
www.ophidian.com

OPHE001 .... .415

Organon
375 Mt. Pleasant Ave.
West Orange, NJ 07052
800-241-8812
973-325-4589 fax
r&d@organon.com
www.organon.com

5-HT1A partial agonist .... .134
Ampakine .... *.144*
Ariza .... *.134*
CX-516, BDP-12 .... .144
etonogestrel .... *.562*
Implanon .... .562
ORG-12962 .... .138
ORG-23430 .... .145
ORG-31540/SR-90107A .... .44, 489
ORG-34167 .... .138
ORG-34517 .... .138
ORG-5222 .... .145

Orphan Medical
13911 Ridgedale Dr.
Suite 475
Minnetonka, MN 55305
888-867-7426
612-514-9209 fax
pservices@orphan.com
www.orphan.com

sodium oxybate (GHB) .... .115
Xyrem .... *.115*

Ortho-McNeil Pharmaceutical
1000 U.S. Highway 202 South
Raritan, NJ 08869
800-682-6532
www.orthomcneil.com

Ortho EVRA .... .562

OrthoLogic
1275 W. Washington
Tempe, Arizona 85281
800-937-5520
usinquiries@olgc.com
www.orthologic.com

Chrysalin .... *.487*
synthetic peptide .... .487

OSI Pharmaceuticals
106 Charles Lindberg Blvd.
Uniondale, NY 11553
516-222-0023
516-222-0114 fax
www.osip.com

CP-358,774 .... 163, 209, 225, 252
OSI-774 .... .211, 232

Otsuka America Pharmaceutical
2440 Research Blvd.
Rockville, MD 20850
800-562-3974
301-990-0035 fax
www.otsuka.com

OPC-14523 .... .138
OPC-18790 .... .30
toborinone .... .25

OXiGENE
One Copley Place
Ste. 602
Boston, MA 02116
617-536-9500
617-536-4700 fax
dsherris@oxigene.com
www.oxigene.com

declopramide .... .196, 406

OXO Chemie
601 Gateway Blvd.
Suite 450
South San Francisco, CA 94080
650-635-0110
650-246-2222 fax
www.oxochemie.com

WF10 .... .294, 325

Palatin Technologies
214 Carnegie Center
Suite 100
Princeton, NJ 08540
609-520-1911
609-452-0880 fax
info@palatin.com

www.palatin.com

LeuTech *424, 436, 493*
PT-141 . . . . *452, 577*
radiolabeled monoclonal antibody . . . *424, 436, 493*

Parke-Davis Division
201 Tabor Rd.
Morris Plains, NJ 07950
800-223-0432
973-540-3320 fax
www.warner-lambert.com

CI-1004 490

Pentech Pharmaceuticals
417 Harvester Court
Wheeling, IL 60090
847-459-9122
847-459-5602 fax
pentech@msn.com
www.pentech/inc.com

apomorphine 110
paroxetine HCl 580

Pfizer
235 E. 42nd St.
New York, NY 10017-5755
212-573-2323
860-441-1895 fax
www.pfizer.com

amlodipine besylate 13
avasimibe 40
capravirine 288, 318
cetirizine HCl 549
CI-1033 . . . . .163, 208, 225
corleukin NIF 53, 117
CP-122,721 .135
CP-526,555 . . . . .147, 376
CP-529,414 40
darifenacin .481
eletriptan 95
fosphenytoin sodium injection 90
gabapentin 90
inhaled insulin 383
JO-1784, CI-1019 137
lasofoxifene .495
Neurontin *90*
NGD 91-2 127
NGD 98-1 . . . . .128, 137
Norvasc *13*

pagoclone 128
pagoclone 142
pregabalin 91, 109, 502
Relpax *95*
sunepitron, CP-93,393 129
valdecoxib 493, 509
Vfend *519*
zenarestat 103, 393
Zyrtec *549*

Pharmacia
100 Rte. 206 North
Peapack, NJ 07977
908-901-8000
908-901-8379 fax
www.pharmacia.com

latanoprost .543
Xalatan *543*
Liposomal Encapsulated Paclitaxel . . .419

Pharmacyclics
995 E. Arques Ave.
Sunnyvale, CA 94086-4521
408-774-0330
408-774-0340 fax
info@pcyc.com
www.pcyc.com

Antrin/Photoangioplasty *35, 39*
motexafing adolinium 86, 159
Xcytrin *86, 159*

PharmaMar
C/de la Calero
3 Tres Cantos
Madrid, Spain 28760
918-03-20-00
918-03-11-43 fax
www.pharmamar.com

ecteinascidin, ET-743 178

Pharmos Corporation
33 Wood Avenue South
Suite 466
Iseline, NJ 08830
732-452-9556
732-452-9557 fax
pharmos@compuserve.com
www.pharmoscorp.com

dexanabinol, HU-211 120
diclofenac 106, 498

Pherin Pharmaceuticals
535 Middlefield Road
Suite 240
Menlo Park, CA 94025
650-903-7100
650-903-7101 fax
www.pherin.com

PH94B 128
vomeropherin, PH-80 . . . . .129, 142, 569

PhotoCure ASA
Hoffsveien 48
0377 Oslo
Norway
47 22 06 22 10
47 22 06 22 18 fax
www.photocure.com

Metvix PDT *281*

Phytopharm plc
Corpus Christie House
9 West St.
Godmanchester Huntingdon
Cambridgeshire PE18 8HG
United Kingdom
44-14-80-437697
44-14-80-417090 fax
www.phytopharm.co.uk

P53 534

Population Council Center for Biomedical Research
1230 York Ave.
New York, NY 10021
212-327-8731
www.popcouncil.org

Nestorone *563*
progestin, ethynylestradiol 563

PowderJect Pharmaceuticals
4 Robert Robinson Ave.
Oxford Science Park
Oxford OX44GA
United Kingdom
44-0-1865-332600
44-0-1865-332601 fax
www.powderject.com/

vaccine, hepatitis B DNA 314, 433

664/Manufacturers Index

Pozen
6330 Quadrangle Dr.
Suite 240
Chapel Hill, NC 27514
919-490-0012

MT 100 96
MT 400 96
MT 500 96

PPD Genupro
3151 South 17th Street
Wilmington, NC 28412 USA
910-251-0081
910-762-5820 fax
www.ppdi.com

Daproxetine 452, 479, 577

PPL Therapeutics plc
Roslin, Edinburgh
EH25 9PP Scotland
United Kingdom
44-131-440-4777
44-131-440-4888 fax
www.ppl-therapeutics.com

alpha-1 antitrypsin (AAT) 367

Praecis Pharmaceuticals
One Hampshire St.
Cambridge, MA 02139
877-580-7146
info@praecis.com
www.praecis.com

abarelix depot, PPI-149 ....263, 460, 580
abarelix, PPI-149 564

Procept
840 Memorial Dr.
Cambridge, MA 02139
617-491-1100
www.procept.com

O6-Benzylguanine (BG) 184
PRO 2000 Gel 322, 562

Procter & Gamble Pharmaceuticals
1 Procter & Gamble Plaza
Cincinnati, OH 45202-3314
800-836-0658
www.pg.com/

azimilide 16
Stedicor 16

Procyon Biopharma
746 Baseline Road
Suite 100
London, }Ontario N6C 5Z2
Canada
519-432-8486
519-432-9888 fax
www.procyonbiopharma.com

Fibrostat 517, 530

Progen Industries
Progen Industries Limited
ACN 010 975 612
2806 Ipswich Road
Darra Qld 4076
Australia
61 7 3273 9100
61 7 3275 1168 fax
www.progen.com.au

PI-88 ....68, 185, 282

Progenics Pharmaceuticals
777 Old Saw Mill River Road
Tarrytown, NY 10591
888-425-2122
914-789-2817 fax
clinicaltrials@progneics.com
www.progenics.com

MGV 183
PRO 140 322
PRO 367 ....291, 322
PRO 542 ....291, 322
vaccine, GMK 245, 343

Protarga
1100 E. Hector St.
Suite 450
Conshohocken, PA 19428
800-4-CANCER
610-260-6868 fax
www.protarga.com

DHA-paclitaxel 184
Taxoprexin 184

Protein Design Labs
34801 Campus Dr.
Fremont, CA 94555
510-574-1400
510-574-1500 fax
www.pdl.com

Nuvion 327, 528
OST 577 ....313, 348, 431
Ostavir 313, 348, 431
SMART 1D10 antibody 239
SMART anti-CD3 ....327, 460, 528
SMART Anti-Gamma Interferon Antibody
  414
SMART M195 ....60, 70, 219

Protherics
1207 17th Ave. South
Suite 103
Nashville, TN 37212
888-327-1027
615-320-1212 fax
www.protherics.com

anti-tumor necrosis factor-alpha 333
CytoTAb 333
TritAb 140

Provalis
Newtech Square
Deeside Industrial Park
Deeside CH5 2NT
United Kingdom
44 1244 288888
44 1244 280221 fax
www.provalis.com

calcitonin 494, 568
Macritonin 494, 568
Pseudostat 304, 329, 346, 363, 369, 371
vaccine, Pseudomonas infection .304, 329,
  346, 363, 369, 371

QLT Phototherapeutics Inc.
520 West 6th Avenue
Vancouver, British Columbia V5Z 4H5
Canada
800-663-5486
604-873-0816 fax
www.qlt-pdt.com

verteporfin 529

Questcor
2714 Loker Ave. W.
Carlsbad, CA 92008

Manufacturers Index/665

510-732-5551
510-732-7741 fax
www.questcor.com

Cordox *49*
CPC-111 ....*49*
Emitasol, Pramidin *423, 425*
intranasal metoclopramide 423, 425
Migrastat *96*
propranolol 96

R.W. Johnson Pharmaceutical Research Institute
920 Route 202 South
P.O. Box 300
Raritan, NJ 06689
908-704-4000

RWJ 241947 ....328, 370
RWJ 270201 ....328, 370
erythropoietin 49
Evra *562*
Levaquin *552*
levofloxacin 552
norgestimate/ethinyl estradiol tablet ..562
norgestimate/ethinyl estradiol transdermal
  patch 562
Ortho-Eldose *562*
Procrit *49*
Topamax *91, 110, 134, 503*
topiramate tablet 91, 110, 134, 503

Regeneron Pharmaceuticals
777 Old Saw Mill River Road
Tarrytown, NY 10591
800-637-8322
914-347-2847 fax
Info@regpha.com
www.regeneron.com

Axokine *394*
brain derived neurotrophic factor, BDNF .
  80,487
interleukin-1 (IL-1) trap 506
neurotrophin-3, NT-3 .108, 112, 116, 412,
  501, 510

Repligen Corporation
117 4th Ave.
Needham, MA 02494
800-622-2259
781-453-0048 fax
info@repligen.com
www.repligen.com

CTLA4-Ig 55, 215
secretin 132
triacetyl uridine 458

ReProtect, LLC
703 Stags Head Road
Baltimore, MD 21286
410-337-8377
info@reprotect.com
www.reprotect.com

BufferGel *562*
polyacrylic acid 562

Ribozyme Pharmaceuticals
2950 Wilderness Pl.
Boulder, CO 80301
303-449-6500
303-449-6995 fax
www.rpi.com

Angiozyme *162*
anti-angiogenic ribozyme 162
Heptazyme *312, 430*
LY466700 ....312, 430
ribozyme gene therapy 239, 292, 323

Roberts Pharmaceutical
4 Industrial Way West
Eatontown, NJ 07724
732 389-1182
732 389-1014 fax
www.robertspharm.com

Dirame *109, 492, 502*
propiram 109, 4952, 502
tazofelone 414, 437

Safe Sciences
31 St. James Ave.
Suite 520
Boston, MA 02116
800-260-6843
617-422-0675 fax
www.safesci.com

GBC-590 197, 259, 267, 395, 407, 440, 464,
  584

Salix Pharmaceuticals
3600 W. Bayshore Road
Suite 205
Palo Alto, CA 94303

800-SALIX001
650-856-1555 fax

rifaximin *302, 424*

Samaritan Pharmaceuticals
Steroidogenesis Inhibitors International
Bank of America Center
Convention Center Drive
Suite 310
Las Vegas, NV 89109
702-735-7001
702-737-7016 fax
www.anticort.com

Anticort *291*
procaine HCl 291

SangStat Medical
6300 Dumbarton Circle
Fremont, CA 94555
888-764-7828
510-789-4400 fax
www.sangstat.com

Anti-LFA-1, odulimomab 325, 459

Sankyo
7-12, Ginza 2-chome
Chuo-ku, Tokyo 104
Japan
011-81-3-3562-0411
www.sankyo.co.jp

CS-866 ....33, 454

Sanofi-Synthelabo Pharmaceuticals
90 Park Avenue
New York, NY 10016
212-551-4000
www.sanofi-synthelaboUS.com

alfuzosin *447, 575*
amindarone-best, SR-33589 15
amisulpride, SL 91.1076 143
argatroban 68
befloxatone 134
CP-99142 202
NK-2 antagonist 437
Osanetant *134*
Saredutant *437*
Solian *143*
SR 49059 569

SR-140333 361
SR-141716 ....146, 147, 377, 394
SR-142801, osanetant ..128, 139, 143, 146
SR-27897B 125, 262, 398, 442
SR-31742 146
SR-31747 327
SR-34006 45
SR-46349 ....115, 139, 147
SR-48692 140, 143, 147, 194, 271, 404, 468, 588
SR-57746 ....79, 80, 487
SR-58611 140
tirapazamine/cisplatin 234
Tirazone 234
Xatral 447, 575

Schering-Plough Corporation
110 Allen Road
Liberty Corner, NJ 07938
800-526-4099
www.sch-plough.com

anti-interleukin-5 MAb (Anti-IL-5) ..356
Asmanex 359
Claritin/Singulair 333, 555
ecopipam 393
evernimicin 299
ezetimibe 21
farnesyl protein transferase inhibitor .179
interferon alfa-2b ..58, 181, 218, 244, 311, 429
interleukin-10 (IL-10) 438
loratadine/montelukast sodium ..333, 555
Melacine 245, 345
mometasone furoate 359
NGD 94-4 145
p53 tumor suppressor gene 255
PEG-Intron 58, 181, 218, 244, 311, 429
posaconazole 519
pure anti-estrogen 171
Temodar 87, 160, 187
temozolomide 87, 160, 187
Tenovil 438
vaccine, melanoma 245, 345
Ziracin 299
interleukin-10 ....312, 430, 526
maxacalcitol 527
Tenovil 312, 430, 526

Schwarz Pharma
6140 West Executive Road
Mequon, WI 53092
800-558-5114
414-242-1641 fax

info@schwarzusa.com
www.schwarzusa.com

N-0923 112

SciClone Pharmaceuticals
901 Mariner's Island Blvd.
Suite 205
San Mateo, CA 94404
650-358-3451
650-358-3469 fax
investorrelations@sciclone.com
www.sciclone.com

8-cyclopentyl 1,3-dipropylxanthine, CPX . 367
thymalfasin 222, 244, 313, 349, 431
Zadaxin 222, 244, 313, 349, 431

Scios
2450 Bayshore Parkway
Mountain View, CA 94043
800-522-9586.
408-616-8206 fax
investor_relations@sciosinc.com
www.sciosinc.com

Natrecor 24
nesiritide 24
SCIO-469 508
VEGF121 ....29, 42

Scotia Pharmaceuticals
558 Cathcart Road
Glasgow G42
Scotland
011-44-41-423-1856
011-44-1628-486796 fax

SC-111 146

Seattle Genetics
22215 26th Avenue S.E., Suite 3000
Bothell, Washington 98021
425-489-4990
425-489-4798 fax
www.seattlegenetics.com

SGN-10 188
SGN-15/Taxotere .172, 194, 271, 404, 468, 588

Selectus Pharmaceuticals
100 Front St.

Suite 1350
West Conshohocken, PA 19428
610-940-0300
610-940-0301 fax

esprolol 14, 95, 141

Senetek plc
23 Palace Street
London, SW1E-5HW
United Kingdom
011-44-171-828-4800
011-33-171-828-8081 fax
www.senetekplc.com

Invicorp 452, 578

Sensus Drug Development
98 San Jacinto Blvd.
Suite 430
Austin, TX 78701
512-487-2000
512-487-2045 fax
info@sensuscorp.com

pegvisomant 381, 487
Somavert 381, 487

Sepracor
111 Locke Dr.
Marlborough, MA 01752
800-SEPRACOR
508-357-7490 fax
info@sepracor.com
www.sepracor.com

(R,R)-formoterol 356, 369
(S)-sibutramine 452, 482, 577
+DDMS 81, 102
desloratadine, descarboethoxyloratadine . 295, 332, 549, 554
levocetirizine 295, 550
nefazodone metabolite 137
norastemizole 333, 550, 555
R-fluoxetine 139
racemic zoplicone 93
S-doxazosin 447, 575
s-fluoxetine 96
S-oxybutynin 482
Serzone-ER 137
xyzal, xusal 295, 550
Zopiclone 93

Serono Laboratories

Manufacturers Index/667

100 Longwater Circle
Norwell, MA 02061
781-982-9000
781-871-6754 fax
www.serono.com

follitropin alpha 567
Gonal-F *567*
LHRH, luteinizing hormone-releasing
   hormone antagonist 567
Ovidrel *171*
Ovidrel *567*
r-hCG 171, 567
r-hLH 567
r-hTBP-1 .414, 508
Rebif *102, 233, 313, 414, 431, 437, 508*
recombinant human interferon beta-1a . .
  102, 233, 313, 414, 431, 437, 508
Serostim *25, 292, 389, 424*
somatropin, r-hGH 25, 292, 389, 424

Shaman Pharmaceuticals
213 E. Grand Ave.
South San Francisco, CA 94080
800-546-8622
650-873-8367 fax
www.shamanbotanicals.com

Provir *292, 416*
SP-303 . . . . .292, 416

Shire Pharmaceuticals
East Anton
Andover, Hants SP105RG
UK
240-453-6400
240-453-6404 fax
www.shiregroup.com

Adderall *83, 132*
Balsalazide *437*
Carbatrol *134*
Lambda *457*
lanthanum carbonate 457
mesalamine 436
midodrine HCl 457, 478, 481
Pentasa *436*
ProAmatine *457, 478, 481*
SLI 381 .83, 132
SPD 417, carbamazepine 134
SPD 418 91
SPD 420 . . . . .83, 132
SPD 421 91
SPD 424 . . . . .271, 468, 588

SPD 503 .83, 132

Sibia Neurosciences
505 Coast Blvd. S.
Suite #300
La Jolla, CA 92037
619-452-5892
619-452-9279 fax
www.sibia.com

SIB-1508Y 36, 82, 93, 113, 131
SIB-1553A 78

Sigma-Tau Pharmaceuticals
800 South Frederick Ave.
Suite 300
Gaithersburg, MD 20877
800-447-0169
301-948-3679 fax
aa@sigmatau.com
www.sigmatau.com

acetyl-L-carnitine 75, 387
Alcar *75, 387*
Cystavision *540*
cysteamine hydrochloride 540
Dromos *41*
propionyl-L-carnitine 41

Situs Corporation
201 Lomas Santa Fe Dr.
Suite 400
Solana Beach, CA
858-509-1090
858-509-1091 fax
jshin@situscorp.com
www.uros.com

I-OXY/ UROS Infusor 481

SK Corporation
Bio-Pharmaceutical R&D Center
140 A New Dutch Lane
Fairfield, NJ 07004
973-227-3939
973-227-7942 fax
www.skcorp.com/eng

YKP-10A 141

Skye Pharma
10450 Science Center Drive
Suite 100
San Diego, CA 92121

858-625-2424
858-625-2439 fax
www.depotech.com
amikacin 298
bupivacaine 105, 498
cytarabine liposome injection 330
DepoAmikacin *298*
DepoBupivacaine *105, 498*
DepoCyt *330*
diclofenac 209, 288
Oralease *209, 288*

Solvay Pharmaceuticals
901 Sawyer Road
Marietta, GA 30062
800-354-0026
www.solvay.com

cilansetron .437
DU125530 . . . . .126, 135
DU127090 .142
estradiol, 17-beta 389, 566
Estratest *388, 477, 566, 570*
Estrogel *389, 566*
estrogens/methyltestosterone 388, 477, 566, 570
flesinoxan 127, 136
fluvoxamine maleate 127, 141
Fluvoxamine-CR *127, 141*
KC-11458 421
SLV 305 . . . . .421, 424
SLV 306 . . . . .25, 34, 454
SLV 308 . . . . .113, 139
SLV 311 . . . . .421, 424
tarazepide .425
Tedangin *15, 17*
tedisamil 15, 17

Somerset Pharmaceuticals
5215 W. Laurel Street
Tampa, FL 33607
800-892-8889
www.somersetpharm.com

Eldepryl *113, 139*
selgiline 113, 139

Sonus Pharmaceuticals
111 SW 5th Ave
Suite 2390
Portland, OR 97204
888-333-9152
425-489-0626 fax
www.sonuspharma.com

S-8184 186

Speedel Pharma
Petersgraben 35
CH-4051 Basel
Switzerland
41 61 264 31 00
41 61 264 31 01 fax
www.speedelpharma.com

SPP 100 ....34, 455

St. Jude Children's Research Hospital
332 N. Lauderdale St.
P.O. Box 318
Memphis, TN 38101-0318
901-495-3300
901-495-3122 fax
lin.ballew@stjude.org
www.stjude.org

vaccine, allogenic and autologous neuroblastoma cells 101, 251, 341

Steroidogenesis Inhibitors International
101 Convention Center Dr.
Suite 310
Las Vegas, NV 89109
702-735-7001
702-737-7016 fax
www.anticort.com/index1.htm

Anticort *323*
procaine HCl *323*

StressGen
4243 Glanford Ave.
Suite 350
Victoria, BC V8Z 4B9
Canada
800-661-4978
250-744-2877 fax
www.stressgen.com

HspE7 ....191, 307, 521, 559

Sugen
230 East Grand Ave.
South San Francisco, CA 94080
650-553-8300
650-553-8301 fax
www.sugen.com

SU-101 ...86, 160, 233, 256, 271, 469, 589
SU-101/BCNU 87, 160

SuperGen
2 Annabel Lane
Suite 220
San Ramon, CA 94583
925-327-0200
925-327-7347 fax
investor_relations@supergen.com
www.supergen.com

decitabine 49, 56, 216, 226
Lucanthone *161*
Nipent *59, 218, 239, 327, 507*
pentostatin 59, 218, 239, 327, 507
pyrazinoylguanidine (PZG) 386
RF-1010 50
RF-1012 ....50, 70, 204
RF-1051 ....386, 393
RFS-2000 59, 171, 198, 207, 219, 244, 255, 262, 398, 408, 419, 442
Rubitecan .*59, 171, 198, 207, 219, 244, 255, 262, 398, 408, 419, 442*

Synsorb Biotech
1204 Kensington Road, NW
Calgary, Alberta T2N 3P5
Canada
403-283-5900
403-283-5907 fax
www.synsorb.com

galasomite 299
Synsorb Cd *303*
Synsorb PK *299*

Takeda Chemical Industries
Millbrook Business Center
475 Half Day Road
Suite 500
Lincolnshire, IL 60069
847-383-3000
847-383-3050 fax
www.takeda.com/index-e.html

Actos *385*
AG-1749, lansoprazole 420, 422
Basen *387*
Blopress *23, 382*
candesartan cilexetil 23, 382
cerivastatin sodium 20
Certa *20*
lansoprazole 421, 423
Leuplin 3M DPS *273, 471, 591*
MH-200, morphine hydrochloride107, 500
NE-58095, risedronate sodium 495
pioglitazone HCl 385
TAK-147 ....79, 89
TAK-251, apomorphine 452, 577
TAK-637 ....140, 438, 482
TAK-778-SR 488
Takepron *421, 423*
TCV-116, candesartan cilexetil 25
TCV-116C 34, 455
TNP-470 ....60, 63, 187
voglibose 387

Tanox Biosystems
10301 Stella Link
Houston, TX 77025
713-664-2288
713-664-8914 fax
dduncan@tanox.com
www.tanox.com

5D12 412
Hu-901 ....295, 549

Targeted Genetics
1100 Olive Way
Suite 100
Seattle, WA 98101
206-623-7612
206-223-0288 fax
targen@targen.com
www.targen.com

tgAAV-CF 368
tgDCC-E1A, RGG 0853 ....173, 212, 256

Telik
750 Gateway Blvd.
South San Francisco, CA 94080
650-244-9303
650-244-9388 fax
INQUIRY@TELIK.COM
www.telik.com

TLK286 405

Telluride Pharmaceutical
146 Flanders Drive
Hillsborough, NJ 08876-4656
908-359-1375

Manufacturers Index/669

908-359-8236 fax
tpcorp@tellpharm.com
www.halcyon.com/tpcorp

Cachexon 182, 290, 416
L-glutathione 182, 290, 416
Memex 77
nicotinamide adenine dinucleotide (NAD) 77

Teva Pharmaceutical Industries
5 Basel St.
P.O. Box 3190
Petah Tiqva 49131
Israel
011-972-03-926-7267
011-972-03-923-4050 fax
www.tevapharmusa.com

Copaxone 98
etilevodopa, TV-1203 111
glatiramer acetate 98
TVP-1012, rasagiline mesylate 79, 114
TVP-1901 92

Texas Biotechnology
7000 Fannin Street
Suite 1920
Houston, TX 77030
713-796-8822
713-796-8232 fax
www.tbc.com

Argatroban 45, 119
TBC-11251 . . . . .25, 366, 372
TBC-1269 361
TBC-3711 . . . . .25, 34, 455

The Liposome Company
One Research Way
Princeton, NJ 08540-6619
609-452-7060
609-452-1890 fax
www.lipo.com

liposomal ether lipid 58, 66, 218, 230, 249, 269, 466, 586
TLC ELL-12 58, 66, 218, 230, 249, 269, 466, 586

The Medicines Company
One Cambridge Center
Cambridge, MA 02142
617-225-9099

617-225-2397 fax
www.themedicinescompany.com

Angiomax .13, 43
bivalirudin 13, 43

Theratechnologies
630 Rene-Levesque West
5th Floor
Montreal, Quebec H3B-1S6
Canada
514-877-0077
514-877-3177 fax
www.theratech.com

thGRF 1-44 . . . . .115, 366

Therion Biologics
76 Rogers St.
Cambridge, MA 02142
617-876-7779
617-876-9391 fax
www.therionbio.com

Cea-Tricom 200, 410
Prostvac 274, 346, 472, 592
TBA-CEA 199, 409
vaccine, prostate cancer (rV-psa) 274, 346, 472, 592

Titan Pharmaceuticals
400 Oyster Point Blvd.
Suite 505
South San Fransisco, CA 94080-1921
650-244-4990
650-244-4956 fax
www.titanpharm.com

CeaVac/TriAb 200, 235, 410
CeaVac 200, 410
gallium maltolate . .63, 154, 250, 267, 319, 448, 465, 584
iloperidone 144
pivaloyloxymethylbutyrate 222, 232
Pivanex .222, 232
spheramine .114
TriAb/TriGem 235
TriAb 174
TriGem 245
vaccine, anti-cancer 174, 200, 235, 245, 410
Zomaril 144

Topical Technologies
7301 E. 22nd St.

Tucson, AZ 85710
520-571-6029

dimethyl sulfoxide, DMSO . .102, 202, 488

Transkaryotic Therapies
195 Albany St.
Cambridge, MA 02139
617-349-0200
617-349-0599 fax
www.tktx.com

Dynepo 49
factor VIII gene therapy 31, 53
gene-activated erythropoietin 49

Triangle Pharmaceuticals
4 University Place
4611 University Drive
Durham, NC 27707
919-493-5980
919-493-5925 fax
www.tripharm.com

clevudine 309, 427
Coactinon 288, 318
Coviracil 309, 318, 427
DAPD 318
emivirine 288, 318
emtricitabine 309, 318, 427
immunostimulatory sequences (ISS) candidate 311, 429
mozenavir dimesylate 321

Trimeris
4727 University Drive
Suite 100
Durham, NC 27707
919-419-6050
919-419-1816 fax
info@trimeris.com
www.trimeris.com

pentafuside, T-20 321
T-1249 .292, 323

Tularik
2 Corporate Drive
South San Francisco, CA 94080
650-825-7000
650-825-7303 fax
www.tularik.com

T607 186

Manufacturers Index

T611 349
T64 .87, 160, 172, 186, 199, 212, 233, 234, 247, 280, 409

Unigene Laboratories
110 Little Falls Rd.
Fairfield, NJ 07004
973-882-0860
973-227-6088 fax
www.unigene.com

Fortical Injection 492
recombinant salmon calcitonin 492

Unimed Pharmaceuticals
2150 E. Lake Cook Rd.
Ste. 210
Buffalo Grove, IL 60089-1862
847-541-2525
847-541-2569 fax
www.unimed.com

Anadrol-50 291
Andractim 288, 390, 579
dihydrotestosterone 288, 390, 579
dronabinol 76, 88
lomefloxacin HCl 300, 472, 592
Marinol 76, 88
Maxaquin 300, 472, 592
oxymetholone 291

United Therapeutics
68 T.W. Alexander Drive
Research Triangle Park, NC 27709
919-485-8350
919-485-8352 fax
tbongartz@unither.com
www.unither.com

Beraprost 34, 41, 455
ketoprofen 491
Ketotop 491
UT-15 .... 35, 42, 455

V.I. Technologies
155 Duryea Road
Melville, NY 11747
516-752-7314
516-752-8768 fax
www.vitechnologies.com

fibrin sealant 54

Valentis
863 A Mitten Road
Burlingame, CA 94010
650-697-1900
650-652-1990 fax
www.valentis.com

CFTR, GR-213487B 367
gene therapy, IL-2 and superantigen gene (SEB) 243, 337
gene therapy, interleukin-2 ..... 209, 243
interleukin-12 gene therapy 210, 281

Vasogen
2155 Dunwin Dr.
Suite 10
Mississauga, Ontario L5L 4M1
Canada
905-569-2265
905-569-9231 fax
www.vasogen.com

VAS 972 529
VAS 991 26
VAS 981 328
VasoCare 41
Vasogen IMT 61, 220

VaxGen
1000 Marina Boulevard
Suite 200
Brisbane, CA 94005
650-624-1000
650-624-1001 fax
www.vaxgen.com

Aidsvax 294, 324, 343
vaccine, HIV 294, 324, 343

Verex Laboratories
14 Inverness Drive East
Suite D-100
Englewood, CO 80112
303-799-4499
303-799-1734 fax
verex@verex.com
www.verex.com

Birex 529
brompheniramine/pseudoephedrine HCl 294, 549
Conquer-A 294, 549
diltiazem HCl 33, 454
Verzem 33, 454

Vernalis
P.O. Box 106
Surrey Research Park
Guildford, Surrey GU2 5ZH
United Kingdom
44-0-118-977-3133
www.vanguardmedica.com

VML 600, R-848 .... 315, 433
VML-670 204

Versicor
34790 Ardentech Court
Freemont, CA 94555
510-739-3000
510-739-3003 fax
info@versicor.com
www.versicor.com

V-Echinocandin 417, 519
V-Glycopeptide, BI-397 304

Vertex Pharmaceuticals
130 Waverly St.
Cambridge, MA 02139-4242
617-577-6000
617-577-6680 fax
webmaster@vpharm
www.vpharm.com

biricodar dicitrate, VX-710 ..... 224, 251
Incel 224, 236, 251, 257, 280
timcodar dimesylate 103, 392
Timcodar 103, 392
VX-148 .... 298, 351, 529
VX-175 325
VX-497 .... 315, 433
VX-710 .... 236, 257, 280
VX-740, pralnacasan 493, 509
VX-745 510
VX-853 189

Vical
9373 Towne Centre Dr.
Suite 100
San Diego, CA 92121
858-646-1100
858-646-1151 fax
www.vical.com

Allovectin-7 .... 213, 247, 251
Leuvectin 272, 279, 470, 476, 589
vaccine, lymphoma 64, 242
Vaxid 64, 242

Manufacturers Index/671

Vion Pharmaceuticals
4 Science Park
New Haven, CT 06511
203-498-4210
203-498-4211 fax
www.vionpharm.com

porfiromycin 212
Promycin *212*
Tapet *189*
Triapine *188*
VNP 20009 .189
VNP 40101M 201, 411

Viragen
865 SW 78th Ave.
Suite 100
Plantation, FL 33324
954-233-8746
954-233-1414 fax
www.viragen.com

Omniferon *313, 432*

Virax Holdings Limited
ACN 006 569 106
Suite 220, Kew Junction Tower
89 High Street, Kew
Vic 3101 Australia
61 3 9854 6230
61 3 9853 5134 fax
www.virax.com.au

VIR201 . . . .*324*

ViroPharma
405 Eagleview Boulevard
Exton, PA 19341
610-458-7300
610-458-7380 fax
www.viropharma.com

pleconaril 349
VP 14637 351
VP 50406 . . . . .315, 433

Viventia Biotech
30 Novopharm Court
Toronto, Ontario M1B 2K9
Canada
204-478-1023
204-452-7721 fax
www.viventia.com

Novovac-M1 246

VivoRx
2825 Santa Monica Blvd.
Suite 104
Santa Monica, CA 90404
310-264-7768
310-453-6948 fax

BetaRx 382

Vivus
545 Middlefield Rd.
Suite 200
Menlo Park, CA 94025
650-934-5200
www.vivus.com

Alibra *451, 576*
Alista *479, 570*
alprostadil/prazosin hydrochloride 451, 576
TA-1790 . . . .*452, 478, 577*

Watson Pharmaceuticals
311 Bonnie Circle
Corona, CA 91720
909-270-1400
909-270-1096 fax
www.watsonpharm.com

estradiol/progestin 389, 494, 566
oxybutynin .481
progestin 563
testosterone . .293, 390, 391, 478, 495, 566,
    570, 579

Wyeth-Ayerst
555 East Lancaster Avenue
St. Davids, PA 19087
610-971-5400
610-995-4668 fax
www.ahp.com/wyeth.htm

17-beta estradiol/trimegestone . .389, 391,
    493, 566, 568
AIP-001 75
Alesse *515*
anti B-7 humanized antibodies . . .51, 156,
    325, 458
CCI-779 176
conjugated estrogen tablets .389, 391, 566,
    568
DAB-452 144
Enbrel *23, 505, 525*

ERA-923 165
etanercept 23, 505, 525
ethinyl estradiol/trimegestrone 561
FluMist *328, 340, 370*
GAR-936 299
HCI-436 . . . . .310, 428
levonorgestrel/ethinyl estradio 515
Meningitec *94, 331, 345*
Premarin/Trimegesterone *389, 391, 566, 568*
rhIL-11 . . . . .204, 414
rPSGL-Ig 38
trimegestone/ethinyl estradiol 563
TSE-424 . . . . .496, 569
vaccine, meningococcal C conjugate . .94,
    331, 345

Wyeth-Lederle Vaccines
One Great Valley Pkwy.
Suite 30
Malvern, PA 19355
610-647-9452
610-995-4668 fax
www.ahp.com

APL400-020 V-B 62, 240, 297
APL400-024Px 306, 520, 564, 578
Genevax-HBV *315, 433*
GeneVax-HIV-Px *294, 324*
Genevax-HSV-Px *306, 520, 564, 578*
Genevax-TCR *62, 240, 297*
vaccine, HIV 294, 324
vaccine, parainfluenza 329, 371
vaccine, viral hepatitis (HBV) . . .315, 433

Xcyte Therapies
2203 Airport Way S.
Suite 300
Seattle, WA 98143
206-262-6200
206-262-0900 fax
www.xcytetherapies.com

T-cells/Xcellerate technology 278, 476

Xenova
260 Littlefield Avenue
South San Francisco, CA 94080
44-0-1753-706600
44-0-1753-706607 fax
www.xenova.co.uk

XR5000 . . . . .87, 161, 201, 236, 58
XR9576 189

XOMA Corporation

2910 7th St.
Berkeley, CA 94710
510-644-1170
510-644-0539 fax
www.xoma.com

anti-CD11a, hu1124 ....459, 524
Neuprex 93, 301, 331, 355, 373, 553
opebecan, rBPI-21, recombinant human bactericidal/permeability-increasing protein 93, 301, 331, 355, 373, 553

XTL Biopharmaceuticals

972-8-940-5134
972-8-940-5017 fax
Becker@xtlbio.com
www.xtlbio.com

XTL-001 ....315, 433

Yamanouchi Pharmaceutical

Shaklee Terraces
444 Market Street
San Francisco, CA 94111
925-924-2000
925-924-2412 fax
www.yamanouchi.com

YM-087, conivaptan 26, 214, 369, 390, 456
YM-177, celecoxib 493, 510
YM-294, oprelvekin 69, 282
YM-337 29
YM-511 ....175, 564, 572
YM-529, minodronate 67, 175, 250
YM-598 ....275, 472, 592
YM-617, tamsulosin 484, 572
YM-872 119
YM-905 482
YM-992 141

YM Biosciences

5045 Orbitor Dr.
Building 11/Suite 400
Mississauga, ON L4W 4Y4
Canada
905-629-9761
905-629-4959 fax
www.ymbiosciences.com

monoclonal antibody 211
Norelin 273, 470, 590
Tesmilifene 273, 470, 590
TheraCIM 211

vaccine, EGF cancer 235
YMB-6H9 ....201, 411

Zambon Group S.p.A.

Via Lillo del Duca, 10
20091 Bresso
Italy
39-0-2-665241
39-0-2-66501492 fax
www.zambon.it

MSI-Albuterol 362

Zarix Inc

1235 Westlakes Drive
Suite 200
Berwyn, PA 19312
610-240-7878
610 240-7999 fax
www.zarix.com

nolatrexed dihydrochloride 222
Thymitaq 222

Zonagen

2408 Timberloch Place
Suite B4
The Woodlands, TX 7380
713-367-5892
218-363-8996 fax
www.zonagen.com

phentolamine mesylate 451, 577
Vasofem 479, 570
Vasomax 451, 577

Therapeutic Indications Index

Use this index to quickly reference drug development activity for a specific illness. Scientific names are set in standard type and potential trade names are set in italics.

Acne

5-aminolevulinic acid 515
Alesse 515
Atrisone 515
clindamycin 515
dadsone topical gel 515
levonorgestrel/ethinyl estradiol ...515
Levulan Photodynamic Therapy ...515
MBI 594AN 515
ResiDerm, Zindaclin 515
tazarotene 515
Tazorac 515

Acquired Immune Deficiency Syndrome (AIDS) and AIDS-Related Infections

Advantage-S 292
AIDS gene therapy 287
Aidsvax 294
ALVAC-HIV 1 287
AMD-3100 287
Anadrol-50 291
Andractim 288
Anticort 291
BMS-232632 287
C319-14/6 287
Cachexon 290
capravirine 288
Coactinon 288
CPI-1189 288
diclofenac 288
dihydrotestosterone 288
DMP-450 288
dOTC 287
emivirine 288
EWBH Treatment 289
GEM-92 289
GeneVax-HIV-Px 294
HMR-4004 289
interleukin-12 (IL-12) 289
L-glutathione 290
memantine 290
nelfinavir, AG1661 290
nitazoxanide (NTZ) 290
nitrone radical trap (NRT) 290
Oralease 288
Oramed 287
oxymetholone 291
perthon/abavca 291
Perthon 291
Priftin 292
PRO 367 291
PRO 542 291
procaine HCl 291
Proleukin Interleukin-2 and
   standard anti-HIV therapy 291
Protectaid 293
Provir 292
Remune 290
ribozyme gene therapy 292
rifapentine, MDL-473 292
Serostim 292
somatropin, r-hGH 292
SP-303 292
SPC3 292
T-1249 292
Tenofovir DF 293
tenofovir disoproxil fumarate 293
testosterone 293
thalidomide 293
Thalomid 293
vaccine, HIV-1 gp-120 prime-boost ..294
vaccine, HIV 294
WF10 294

Acromegaly

pegvisomant 381, 487

674/Therapeutic Indications Index

Somavert *381, 487*

Acute Respiratory Distress Syndrome (ARDS)
LiquiVent *355*
lucinactant 355
Neuprex *355*
opebecan, rBPI-21, recombinant
 human bactericidal/
 permeability-increasing protein 355
perflubron 355
Surfaxin *355*
TP10 355
ZD-8321 356

Addictions
amino-cyclopropane carboxylic acid ..125
DOV 216303 125
NS-2359 125

Adenomatous Polyposis Coli
Aptosyn *153*
exisulind 153

Affective Disorders
CE-1050 125

Alcohol Dependence
acamprosate 125
DOV 216303 125
IP501 125

Allergy
AIC .... .296, 550
brompheniramine/
 pseudoephedrine HCl .... .294, 549
cetirizine HCl 549
Conquer-A *294, 549*
CpG compound .... .295, 549
desloratadine,
 descarboethoxyloratadine 295, 549
Hu-901 .... .295, 549
IDEC-152 .... .295, 549
ketofifen fumarate .... .295, 550
levocetirizine .... .295, 550
MPL vaccine adjuvant .... *.296, 550*
norastemizole 550
vaccines, allergy 550
xyzal, xusal .... *.295, 550*
Zaditen .... *.295, 550*
Zyrtec *549*

Alopecia
GI 198745 .... .381, 516

Alzheimer's Disease
Abilitat *75*
acetyl-L-carnitine 75
AIP-001 75
Alcar *75*
Ampalex *75*
AN-1792 75
Arecoline *79*
Aricept *75*
aripiprazole, OPC-14597, OPC-31 ...75
CEP-1347 75
CX-516, BDP-12 75
donepezil hydrochloride, E2020 75
DPC-543, DMP-543 76
dronabinol 76
FK960 76
galantamine hydrobromide 76
GT-2331 76
leteprinim potassium, AIT-082 76
Marinol *76*
memantine 77
Memantine *79*
Memex *77*
modafinil 77
Neotrofin *76*
NGD 97-1 77
nicotinamide adenine
 dinucleotide (NAD) 77
NS-2330 78
NXY-059 78
Perceptin *76*
phenserine 78
propentofylline, HWA-285 78
Provigil *77*
quetiapine fumarate 78
Reminyl *76*
Seroquel *78*
SIB-1553A 78
SR-57746 79
TAK-147 79
TVP-1012, rasagiline mesylate 79

Amyotrophic Lateral Sclerosis (ALS)
AVP-923 .... .79, 487
brain derived neurotrophic factor,
 BDNF .... .80, 487
SR-57746 .... .80, 487

Anal Fissures
Anogesic *403, 516*
nitroglycerin ointment .... .403, 516

Anemia

Cordox *49*
CPC-111 49
decitabine 49
Dynepo *49*
erythropoietin 49
Flocor *50*
gene-activated erythropoietin ... 49
hemoglobin glutamer-250 (bovine) ...49
Hemopure *49*
MARstem *51*
MDX-33 49
novel erythropoiesis stimulating
 protein (NESP) 50
poloxamer 188 N.F., CRL-5861 50
Procrit *49*
pyridoxalated hemoglobin
 polyoxyethylene (PHP) 50
RF-1010 50
RF-1012 50

Angina
abciximab, c7E3 13
amlodipine besylate 13
Angiomax *13*
AR69931 13
bivalirudin 13
Cardizide SR *13*
Cromafiban *14*
diltiazem HCl/hydrochlorothiazide 13
esprolol 14
fibrinogen-receptor antagonist 14
GP II b/II a 14
human albumin microspheres 14
Norvasc *13*
Optison *14*
PEG-hirudin 14
ranolazine, CVT-303 14
ReoPro *13*
RSR13 15
Tedangin *15*
tedisamil 15
TP-9201 15

Angiogenesis Inhibitor, Cancer
NM-3 153

Anorexia
SR-27897B 125

Anxiety Disorders
amino-cyclopropane carboxylic acid ..126
BuSpar *126*
buspirone HCl 126
buspirone 126

Therapeutic Indications Index/675

CRF receptor antagonist
  (partnered), NBI-37582 126
CRF receptor antagonist
  (proprietary) 126
DU125530 126
flesinoxan 127
fluvoxamine maleate 127
Fluvoxamine-CR 127
GW 150013 127
LY-354740 127
MK-869 127
NAD299 127
NGD 91-1 127
NGD 91-2 127
NGD 91-3 128
NGD 98-1 128
NKP 608 128
NS-2710 128
pagoclone 128
paroxetine 128
Paxil, Seroxat 128
PH94B 128
Siramesine 129
SR-142801, osanetant 128
substance P antagonist candidates ...129
sunepitron, CP-93,393 129
vomeropherin, PH-80 129

Arrhythmia
amindarone-best, SR-33589 15
Amio-Aqueous IV 15
amiodarone HCl 15
azimilide 16
CVT-510 16
DTI-0009 16
GW 473178 16
SB 207266 16
SB 424323 17
SB-237376 16
Stedicor 16
Tedangin 17
tedisamil 17

Aspergillosis
FK463, echinocandin 296, 356, 551
Nyotran 296, 356, 551
nystatin, AR-121 ....296, 356, 551

Asthma
(R,R)-formoterol 356
Aerobid 357
albuterol 356
Albuterol 362
anti-interleukin-5 MAb (Anti-IL-5) ..356
Ariflo 360
Asmanex 359
Budoxis, Oxis 358
CDC 801 357
CpG compound 357
cromolyn sodium 357
DNK 333 357
EPI-2010 357
Flixotide, Flovent 358
flunisolide 357
fluticasone propionate 358
Foradil 358
formoterol 358
GW 328267 358
IDEC-152 358
Intal HFA-227 357
interleukin-4 (IL-4) 359
IPL 576,092 359
LDP-977 359
mepolizumab, SB 240563 359
mometasone furoate 359
MSI-Albuterol 362
Nuvance 359
omalizumab 359
PDE4i, SCH351591 360
pumactant 360
salbutamol 360
salmeterol xinafoate 360
salmeterol/fluticasone propionate ...360
SB 207499 360
SB 683698, TR 14035 361
SCH55700 361
SelCIDs 357
Seretide, Advair 360
Serevent 360
SR-140333 361
Symbicort pMDI 362
Symbicort Turbuhaler 361
T3 361
TBC-1269 361
Theolan 361
theophylline 361
Ultrahaler 360
Ventolin 356
very late antigen-4 inhibitor (VLA-4) .362
Xolair 359

Atopic Dermatitis
ADL 2-1294 ....296, 516
bexarotene 516
Elidel 297, 517
HCT 1026 516
LDP-392 296
pimecrolimus, ASM 981 ...297, 517
Prograf 297, 517
tacrolimus hydrate 297, 517
Targretin-capsule 516

Attention Deficit/ Hyperactivity Disorder (ADHD)
+DDMS 81
Adderall 83, 132
altropane 80, 129
Aricept 81, 130
CNS stimulant 80, 130
d-methylphenidate HCl ...81, 130
donepezil hydrochloride, E2020 ..81, 130
GT-2331 ....81, 130
GW 320659, 1555U88 ...81, 130
Inversine 81, 130
mecamylamine HCl 81, 130
methylphenidate HCl 82, 131
methylphenidate 81, 82, 130, 131
MethyPatch 81, 130
modafinil 82, 131
MR Racemate 82, 131
Perceptin 81, 130
Provigil 82, 131
Ritalin LA 82, 131
SIB-1508Y 82, 131
SLI 381 ....83, 132
SPD 420 ....83, 132
SPD 503 ....83, 132
tomoxetine 83, 132

Autism
secretin 132

Autoimmune Diseases
AGT-1 297
APL400-020 V-B 297
CDC 801 297
Genevax-TCR 297
SelCID 297
VX-148 298

Bacterial Infection
ABT-773 298
amikacin 298
amoxicillin/clavulante potassium ...298
Augmentin SR 298
Avelox 301
AZD2563 298
C. difficile vaccine, CdVax ...298
Campyvax 304
CDC 801 298
Cidecin 299
daptomycin 299

676/Therapeutic Indications Index

DepoAmikacin 298
DiffGAM 300
ETEC vaccine 299
evernimicin 299
Factive 299
galasomite 299
GAR-936 299
gatifloxacin 299
gemifloxacin mesylate 299
H. pylori vaccine 300
HMR-3647, RU-64,004 300
immune globulin (IG-IV) 300
immune globulin (IgG) 300
Ketek 303
lomefloxacin HCl 300
LY333328 300
Maxaquin 300
MBI 226 301
Mikasome 298
MK-826, carbapenem 301
moxifloxacin 301
Neuprex 301
opebecan, rBPI-21, recombinant
  human bactericidal/
  permeability-increasing protein 301
Oritavancin 300
Priftin 302
Protegrin IB-367, rinse, gel 301
Pseudostat 304
psoralen, S-59 302
quinupristin/dalfopristin 302
rifapentine, MDL-473 302
rifaximin 302
roxithromycine, RU-28,965 302
Saccharomyces boulardii 303
SelCID 298
streptogamin 303
Synercid 302
Synsorb Cd 303
Synsorb PK 299
telithromycin 303
Tequin 299
typhoid vaccine 303
V-Glycopeptide, BI-397 304
vaccine, Campylobacter 304
vaccine, DPT/Haemophilus
  influenzae tyype B 304
vaccine, Pseudomonas infection 304
vaccine, S. pneumoniae 305
vaccine, Shigella flexneri and sonneii ..305
vaccine, Streptococcus pneumoniae ..305
Ziracin 299

Benign Prostatic Hyperplasia

alfuzosin 447
alfuzosin 575
GI 198745 ....447, 575
S-doxazosin 447, 575
Xatral 447
Xatral 575

Bipolar Disorders

Carbatrol 134
GW 273293 133
MK-869 133
NPS 1776, alifatic amide 132
olanzapine 133
quetiapine fumarate 133
Risperdal 133
risperidone 133
Seroquel 133
SPD 417, carbamazepine 134
Topamax 134
topiramate tablet 134
Zyprexa 133

Bladder Cancer

arsenic trioxide (ATO) 153, 447
BCI-Immune Activator 155, 449
CI-1042, ONYX-015 ....153, 447
cytostatics 153, 448
eflornithine, DFMO
  (difluoromethylornydil) ...154, 448
EMD 82633 ....154, 448
gallium maltolate 154, 448
gemcitabine HCl 448
Gemzar 448
INGN-201, adenoviral p53 ...154, 448
MCC 155, 449
MDX-447, H-447 ....155, 449
Trisenox 153, 447
valrubicin 155, 449
Valstar 155, 449
ZD-0473/AMD 473 ....155, 450

Blood Cancer

LGD-1550 ....17, 156

Bone Fractures

Chrysalin 487
synthetic peptide 487
TAK-778-SR 488

Bone Marrow Transplant

anti B-7 humanized antibodies ...51, 156
immune globulin intravenous 51, 156
keratinocyte growth factor-2
  (KGF-2) 51, 156
Leucotropin 52, 156
lisofylline, CT-1501R 51
MDX-22 52
ProTec 51
recombinant human GM-CSF ...52, 156
Repifermin 51, 156
tresperimus 52, 157
Venoglobulin-S 51, 156

Bone Metastases

zoledronate 157, 488
Zometa 157, 488

Brain Cancer

Adenoviral p53 ....84, 158
Avonex 84, 158
Cereport 161
CI-1042, ONYX-015 ....83, 157
cidofovir 83
docetaxel hydrate 84, 157
Gliadel 86, 159
hypericin 84
INGN-201 ....84, 158
interferon beta-1a 84, 158
interleukin-4 (IL-4) fusion toxin,
  NBI-3001 ....85, 158
Lucanthone 161
marimastat, BB-2516 ....85, 158
matrix metalloprotease inhibitor
  (MMP) 85
MDX-447, H-447 ....85, 159
motexafing adolinium 86, 159
Prinomastat 85, 159
prolifeprosan 20/carmustine 86, 159
RSR13 ....86, 160
SU101/BCNU 87, 160
SU101 ....86, 160
T67 ....87, 160
Taxotere 84, 157
Temodar 87, 160
temozolomide 87, 160
thalidomide 87, 160
Thalomid 87, 160
VIMRxyn 84
Vistide 83
Xcytrin 86, 159
XR5000 ....87, 161

Breast Cancer

alitretinoin, ALRT-1057 161
anastrozole, ZD-1033 161
Angiozyme 162
Annamycin 162
anti-angiogenic ribozyme 162

Therapeutic Indications Index/677

APC8024 162
Aposyn/Taxotere *165*
Apotsyn/Xeloda *165*
Aptosyn *165*
AR-522 162
arcitumomab 162
Arimidex *161*
B-vax *174*
bexarotene 162
Bonviva *167*
capecitabine/docetaxel 163
CEA-Cide *167*
CEA-Scan *162*
CI-1033 163
cisplatin/epinephrine 163
Combidex *173*
CP-358,774 163
Detox *173*
docetaxel hydrate 163
Doxil, Caelyx *164*
Doxil/Taxotere *164*
doxorubicin HCl 164
doxorubicin/docetaxel 164
eflornithine, DFMO
   (difluoromethylornydil) 164
EMD 82633 164
ERA-923 . . . .*165*
Evista *171*
exisulind/capecitabine 165
exisulind/docetaxel 165
exisulind 165
Faslodex *167*
Femara *169*
FK-317 165
FLT3 ligand 166
G3139/docetaxel 166
gemcitabine HCl 166
Gemzar *166*
Genasense/Taxotere *166*
GeneVax *174*
GnRH Pharmaccine *174*
goserelin acetate 166
GPX-100 166
HER-2/neu dendritic cell vaccine 166
Herceptin *173*
HumaSPECT/BR *174*
ibandronate 167
ICI-182,780 167
IMC-C225, CPT-11 167
IMMU-MN14, anti-CEA 167
INGN 241 (mda-7) 167
INGN-201, adenoviral p53 168
interleukin (IL) 168
IntraDose *163*

Irofulven *170*
ISIS 2503 .168
ISIS 3521 .168
ISIS 5132, CGP 69846A 169
letrozole 169
marimastat, BB-2516 169
MARstem *173*
MDX-210 .169
MDX-447, H-447 170
MGI-114, hydroxymethylacylfulvene,
   HMAF .170
Mobist *166*
MPI-5020 .170
MultiKine *168*
Ovidrel *171*
paclitaxel/carboplatin/trastuzumab . . .170
Panretin *161*
pure anti-estrogen 171
r-hCG 171
raloxifene, LY-139481 171
RFS-2000 .171
Rubitecan *171*
SD/01 171
SERM III 171
SGN-15/Taxotere 172
squalamine 172
T64 172
T67 172
Targretin-capsule *162*
Taxol/Paraplatin/Herceptin *170*
Taxotere *163*
tgDCC-E1A, RGG 0853 173
TheraFab *173*
Theratope *174*
trastuzumab 173
TriAb *174*
vaccine, anti-cancer 174
vaccine, breast cancer 174
vaccine, cancer 174
votumumab 174
Xeloda/Taxotere *163*
YM-511 175
YM-529, minodronate 175
ZD-0473/AMD 473 175
Zoladex IVF *166*

Bronchitis

Avelox *363*
HP-3 362
INS365 363
moxifloxacin 363
Pseudostat *363*
vaccine, Pseudomonas infection 363
vaccine, respiratory syncytial virus . . .363

Burns and Burn Infections

ADL 2-1294 517
Fibrostat *517*
VM-301, OAS 1000 517

Cancer/Tumors (Unspecified)

A4, prodrug 175
ABX-EGF .175
AE-941 175
Angiocol *189*
Angiostatin with radiation therapy *187*
Aposyn/Taxotere *179*
Aranesp *177*
AZD3409 .176
AZD6474 .176
BB-3644 176
BNP 1350 .176
Cachexon *182*
Carn 750 .176
CarraVex *176*
CCI-779 176
CEA-Cide *181*
cisplatin/epinephrine 176
Combretastatin *175*
CP-461 177
D1927 . . . .*177*
D2163, BMS 275291 . . . .*177*
darbepoetin alfa 177
DHA-paclitaxel 184
Doxil, Caelyx *177*
doxorubicin HCl 177
DX-8951 178
E21R 178
E7010 178
ecteinascidin, ET-743 178
EGF-receptor specific monoclonal
   antibody 178
EMD 82633 178
exisulind/docetaxel 179
farnesyl protein transferase inhibitor . .179
FK-317 179
FLT3 ligand 179
fluoropyrimidine, S-1 179
GEM-231 .180
GPX-100 180
GW 572016 180
HP-4 180
human endostatin protein 180
ILX-651 181
Imagent *184*
IMMU-MN14, anti-CEA 181
INGN 241 (mda-7) 181
INGN-201, adenoviral p53 181
interferon alfa-2b 181

IntraDose *176*
Iressa *190*
Irofulven *183*
ISIS 5132, CGP 69846A 182
Karenitecin *176*
L-glutathione 182
LDP-341, PS-341 182
LGD-1550 182
LY231514, antifolate 183
MDAM (γ-methylene-10-
  deazaaminopterin) 183
MGI-114, hydroxymethylacylfulvene,
  HMAF 183
MGV 183
Mobist *179*
monoclonal antibody (Mab),
  anti-VEGF 184
Neovastat *175*
O6-Benzylguanine (BG) 184
OC144-093 184
Onco TCS *189*
Palonosetron *188*
PEG-camptothecin 184
PEG-Intron *181*
perfluorohexane emulsion 184
phenoxodiol 185
PI-88 185
PKC 412 185
Prothecan *184*
R115777 185
raltitrexed, ZD-1694 185
Ras pathway inhibitor 186
Reolysin *187*
rhEndostatin *180*
S-8184 186
SB 596168 186
SGN-10 .... *188*
squalamine 186
T607 186
T64 186
Tapet *189*
Taxoprexin *184*
Temodar *187*
temozolomide 187
thalidomide 187
Thalomid *187*
TNP-470 187
Tomudex *185*
Triapine *188*
troxacitabine, BCH-4556 187
Troxatyl *187*
vincristine 189
Vitaxin *188*
VNP 20009 189
VX-853 189
XR9576 189
ZD-0101, CM-101 190
ZD-0473/AMD 473 190
ZD-1839 190
ZD-9331 190

Candidiasis
FK463, echinocandin 305
Nyotran *305*
nystatin, AR-121 305

Cardiac Ischemia
enoxaparin sodium 17
Lovenox/Clexane *17*
RSR13 17
TP10 17
vascular endothelial growth factor-2
  gene therapy (gtVEGF-2) 18

Cardiac Surgery
ancrod 18
antithrombin III, rhATIII 18
BCX-1470 18
blood substitute 18
Hemolink *18*
heparinase I 19
Imagent *19*
Neutralase *19*
PEG-hirudin 19
perfluorohexane emulsion 19
pexelizumab 19
rNAPc2 20
TP10 20
Vascugel *20*
Viprinex *18*

Cataracts
MDX-RA 539

Cervical Dysplasia/Cancer
arsenic trioxide (ATO) 190, 559
CI-1042, ONYX-015 .... 190, 559
difluoromethylornithine (DFMO) ...191,
  559
HspE7 .... 191, 559
Irofulven *192, 560*
LGD-1550 .... 191, 559
MEDI-517 .... 191, 560
MGI-114, hydroxymethylacylfulvene,
  HMAF 192, 560
MX6 .... 192, 560
TA-CIN 192, 560
TA-HPV 192, 560
Trisenox *190, 559*
vaccine, cervical cancer 192, 561
ZD-0473/AMD 473 .... 192, 561

Chemotherapy
MK-663 193
polymer platinate, AP5280 193

Cholesterol, High Levels
AGI-1067 20
BAY 13-9952 20
cerivastatin sodium 20
Certa *20*
CETP vaccine, CETi-1 21
Cholestagel/Zocor *21*
colsevelam/simvastatin 21
Crestor *22*
estrogen/pravastatin 21
ezetimibe 21
Lovastatin XL *21*
Premarin/Pravachol *21*
Urso *21*
ursodiol 21
ZD-4522, S-4522 22

Chronic Fatigue Syndrome
2CVV 87, 305
Ampligen *88, 306*
galantamine hydrobromide ... 88, 305
poly I:poly C-12-U 88, 306
Reminyl *88, 305*

Chronic Obstructive Pulmonary Disease (COPD)
albuterol 363
AR-C68397AA 364
AR-C89855 364
Ariflo *365*
Budoxis, Oxis *364*
DNK 333 364
Flixotide, Flovent *364*
fluticasone propionate 364
formoterol 364
GW 328267 364
HP-3 365
LTB 019 365
oxandrolone, CO221 365
salmeterol xinafoate 365
salmeterol/fluticasone propionate 365
SB 207499 365
SB 223412 366
Seretide, Advair *365*
Serevent *365*
Symbicort pMDI *366*

Therapeutic Indications Index/679

Symbicort Turbuhaler .... .366
TBC-11251 .... .366
ThGRF 1-44 .... .366
Ventolin .... .363
Viozan .... .364
ZD-8321 .... .366
ZD4407 .... .367

Colon Malignancies
APC8024 .... .193, 403
GL-331 .... .193, 403
Irofulven .... .194, 404
ISIS 2503 .... .193, 403
ISIS 5132, CGP 69846A .... .193, 403
MDX-210 .... .194, 404
MGI-114, hydroxymethylacylfulvene,
    HMAF .... .194, 404
SGN-15/Taxotere .... .194, 404
SR-48692 .... .194, 404
TLK286 .... .405

Colon Polyps
Aptosyn .... .195, 405
exisulind .... .195, 405
Urso .... .195, 405
ursodiol .... .195, 405

Colorectal Cancer
Avicine .... .196, 406
capecitabine .... .195, 405
CEA-Cide .... .198, 408
Cea-Tricom .... .200, 410
CeaVac/TriAb .... .200, 410
CeaVac .... .200, 410
CI-1042, ONYX-015 .... .195, 405
cisplatin/epinephrine .... .195, 406
CTP-37 .... .196, 406
declopramide .... .196, 406
FMdC .... .196, 406
G3139/irinotecan .... .196, 406
G3139/mitoxantrone .... .196, 406
Gastrimmune .... .200, 411
GBC-590 .... .197, 407
Genasense/Irinotecan ...... .196, 406
Genasense/Mitoxantrone .... .196, 406
HSPPC-96 .... .197, 407
HuC242-DM1/SB-408075 .... .197, 407
Hycamtin .... .199, 409
IMC-1C11 .... .197, 407
IMC-C225, CPT-11 .... .197, 407
IMMU-MN14, anti-CEA .... .198, 408
IntraDose .... .195, 406
Iressa .... .201, 411
Irofulven .... .198, 408

MDX-220 .... .198, 408
MGI-114, hydroxymethylacylfulvene,
    HMAF .... .198, 408
NeuTrexin .... .199, 409
Oncophage .... .197, 407
Onyvax 105 .... .201, 411
Onyvax CR .... .200, 410
raltitrexed, ZD-1694 .... .198, 408
RFS-2000 .... .198, 408
Rubitecan .... .198, 408
SB 408075 .... .199, 409
T67 .... .199, 409
TBA-CEA .... .199, 409
Tomudex .... .198, 408
topotecan HCl .... .199, 409
trimetrexate glucuronate/
    leucovorin .... .199, 409
troxacitabine, BCH-4556 ... .199, 409
Troxatyl .... .199, 409
UFT/leucovorin calcium .... .410
Urso .... .200, 410
ursodiol .... .200, 410
vaccine, anti-cancer ...... .200, 410
vaccine, anti-gastrin ..... .200, 411
vaccine,105AD7 .... .201, 411
VNP 40101M .... .201, 411
Xeloda .... .195, 405
XR5000 .... .201
YMB-6H9 .... .201, 411
ZD-0473/AMD 473 .... .201, 411
ZD-1839 .... .201, 411

Conduct Disorder
Risperdal .... .134
risperidone .... .134

Congestive Heart Failure
Adentri .... .23
Atacand .... .22
Avapro .... .22
Blopress .... .23
BMS-186295, SR-47436 (irbesartan) ...22
BMS-186716, omapatrilat .... .22
BMS-193884 .... .22
candesartan cilexetil .... .22, 23
Captelan .... .23
captopril .... .23
carvedilol .... .23
Coreg .... .23
Corlopam .... .24
CVT-124 .... .23
Diovan .... .26
Enbrel .... .23
endothelin A receptor antagonist 23

etanercept .... .23
Etomoxir .... .26
fenoldopam mesylate, SK&F-82526 ...24
HMR-1883/1098 .... .24
Natrecor .... .24
nesiritide .... .24
ranolazine, CVT-303 .... .24
SB 217242 .... .25
Serostim .... .25
SLV 306 .... .25
somatropin, r-hGH .... .25
TBC-11251 .... .25
TBC-3711 .... .25
TCV-116, candesartan cilexetil .. .25
toborinone .... .25
valsartan .... .26
Vanlev .... .22
VAS 991 .... .26
YM-087, conivaptan .... .26

Connective Tissue Diseases
dimethyl sulfoxide, DMSO .... .488

Constipation
neurotrophin-3, NT-3 .... .412
prucalopride .... .412
Resolor .... .412
tegaserod .... .412
Zelmac .... .412

Contraception
Amylin .... .561
BufferGel .... .562
Contraceptive Patch .... .561
ethinyl estradiol/trimegestrone . .561
etonogestrel .... .562
Evra .... .562
glyminox vaginal gel .... .561
immunocontraception .... .561
Implanon .... .562
levonorgestrel/ethinyl estradiol . .562
levonorgestrel .... .562
Nestorone .... .563
norgestimate/ethinyl estradiol tablet ..562
norgestimate/ethinyl estradiol
    transdermal patch .... .562
Ortho EVRA .... .562
Ortho-Eldose .... .562
polyacrylic acid .... .562
PREVEN2 .... .562
PRO 2000 Gel .... .562
progestin, ethynylestradiol ..... .563
progestin .... .563
Protectaid .... .563

680/Therapeutic Indications Index

Savvy .... .561	thalidomide 414	NBI-37582 .... .135
Seasonale .... .564	*Thalomid* *414*	CRF receptor antagonist (proprietary) 135
trimegestone/ethinyl estradiol ..... .563		CX-619, ORG-24448 .... .135
	Cystic Fibrosis	DU125530 .... .135
Coronary Artery Disease	8-cyclopentyl 1,3-dipropylxanthine,	duloxetine HCl, LY-248686 ..... .135
Ad5FGF4 .... .26	CPX .... .367	*Eldepryl* .... *.139*
AI-700 .... .26	alfa inhalation solution .... .367	*Escitalopram* .... *.134*
BioByPass .... .28	alpha-1 antitrypsin (AAT) ...... .367	flesinoxan .... .136
cariporide mesylate, HOE-642 ..... .27	CFTR, GR-213487B .... .367	fluoxetine HCl .... .136
Cromafiban .... .27	gamma interferon .... .367	fluoxetine/olanzapine .... .136
enoxaparin sodium/tirofiban ..... .27	HP-3 .... .367	gepirone .... .136
eptifibatide .... .27	INS365 .... .368	*Geppar (proposed to PTO)* ..... *.136*
Evista .... .28	INS37217 respiratory .... .368	GW 597599 .... .136
Fiblast .... .28	*Merrem* .... .369	GW 650250 .... .136
Generx .... .26	protegrin IB-367, aerosol .... .368	GW-650250A, NS-2389 .... .136
GP IIb/II a .... .27	*Pseudostat* .... .369	INN-00835 .... .136
human albumin microspheres ...... .27	*SuperVent* .... .368	JO-1784, CI-1019 .... .137
Integrilin .... .27	tgAAV-CF .... .368	LU 26-054, SSRI .... .137
Lovenox/Aggrastat .... .27	tyloxapol .... .368	MK-869 .... .137
monoclonal antibody (Mab),	vaccine, Pseudomonas infection ... .369	moclobemide .... .137
anti-VEGF .... .28		NAD299 .... .137
MRE0470 .... .28	**Cytomegalovirus (CMV) Retinitis**	nefazodone metabolite .... .137
Optison .... .27	*Cymeval* .... .306, *539*	neurokinin antagonist .... .137
raloxifene, LY-139481 .... .28	*Cytovene* .... .306, *539*	NGD 98-1 .... .137
trafermin .... .28	ganciclovir 306, 539	NK-1 .... .137
vascular endothelial growth	ISIS-13312 .... 306, 539	NPS 1506 .... .138
factor-121 (VEGF) .... .28	vaccine, cytomegalovirus 306, 539	NS-2389 .... .138
vascular endothelial growth	valganciclovir 306, 539	OPC-14523 .... .138
factor-2 gene therapy (gtVEGF-2) ... .28		ORG-12962 .... .138
VEGF121 .... .29	**Decubitus Ulcers (Bed Sores)**	ORG-34167 .... .138
YM-337 .... .29	VM-301, OAS 1000 .... .517	ORG-34517 .... .138
		Osanetant .... *.134*
Crohn's Disease	**Dementia**	paroxetine .... .138
5D12 .... .412	*Aricept* .... *.88*	*Paxil, Seroxat* .... *.138*
Antegren .... *.413*	donepezil hydrochloride, E2020 ..... .88	*Prozac* .... *.136*
budesonide .... .412	dronabinol .... .88	R 107474 .... .138
CBP-1011 .... .412	galantamine hydrobromide .... .89	R-fluoxetine .... .139
CDC-801 .... .412	*Marinol* .... *.88*	SB 243213 .... .139
CDP-571, BAY 10-356 .... .413	NGD 97-1 .... .89	SB 659746A, EMD 68843 ...... .139
Colirest .... .412	olanzapine .... .89	selgiline .... .139
Entocort .... *.412*	propentofylline, HWA-285 .... .89	*Serzone-ER* .... *.137*
Humicade .... *.413*	*Reminyl* .... *.89*	SLV 308 .... .139
ISIS-2302 .... .413	TAK-147 .... .89	SR-142801, osanetant .... .139
LDP-02 .... .413	*Zyprexa* .... *.89*	SR-46349 .... .139
natalizumab .... .413		SR-48692 .... .140
r-hTBP-1 .... .414	**Depression**	SR-58611 .... .140
Rebif .... *.414*	5-HT1A partial agonist .... .134	substance P antagonist candidates ... .140
recombinant human interferon	amino-cyclopropane carboxylic acid .. .134	TAK-637 .... .140
beta-1a .... .414	antidepressant .... .134	*TritAb* .... *.140*
rhIL-11 .... .414	*Ariza* .... *.134*	YKP-10A .... .140
SelCID .... *.412*	befloxatone .... .134	YKP-10A .... .141
SMART Anti-Gamma Interferon	citalopram HBr .... .134	YM-992 .... .141
Antibody .... .414	CP-122,721 .... .135	*Zyp/Zac* .... *.136*
tazofelone .... .414	CRF receptor antagonist (partnered),	

Therapeutic Indications Index/681

Diabetes Mellitus Types 1 and 2
AC2993 LAR 381
AC2993 381
Actos 385
AERx diabetes management system ..381
AI-401 381
AJ-9677, TAK-677 382
AR-H049020 382
Avandia 386
AZ 242 (AR-H039242) 382
Basen 387
BetaRx 382
Blopress 382
candesartan cilexetil 382
CLX-0901 382
Diamyd 387
DPC-444 382
DPP 728/LAF 237 382
Exendin-4 383
exendin 383
GI 262570 383
GW 427353 383
inhaled insulin 383
insulin 383
KRP-297 383
leptin 383
MBX-102 384
metformin hydrochloride, ADX-155 ..384
Metformin XT 384
metformin/sulfonylureas 384
NBI-6024 384
NN 1215 384
NN 1998, Insulin (r-human) 384
NN 2344, DRF-2593 384
NN 304, insulin detemir 384
NN 414 384
NN 4201, NNC-42-1001 385
NN 622, DRF-2725 385
NNC-90-1170, NN 2211 385
NovoNorm 386
Oralgen 383
orlistat 385
pimagedine HCl 385
pioglitazone HCl 385
pramlintide 385
pulmonary insulin 386
pyrazinoylguanidine (PZG) 386
repaglinide 386
RF-1051 386
rosiglitazone 386
SB 418790 386
Symlin 385
voglibose 387
Xenical 385

Diabetes Prevention
acetyl-L-carnitine 387
Alcar 387

Diabetic Foot Ulcers
becaplermin 387, 518
Regranex 387, 518
therapeutic, wound healing ...387, 518
transforming growth factor beta-2
 (TGF-b2) 387, 518
VM-301, OAS 1000 ....388, 518

Diabetic Kidney Disease
EXO-226 388

Diarrhea
Campyvax 416
DB-075 415
DiffGAM 415
ETEC vaccine 415
immune globulin (IgG) 415
nitazoxanide (NTZ) 415
OPHE001 415
Provir 416
saccharomyces boulardii 415
SP-303 416
vaccine, campylobacter 416
vaccine, Shigella flexneri and sonneii .416

Diet and Nutrition
Cachexon 416
L-glutathione 416

Dupuytren's Disease
collagenase for injection 488
Cordase 488

Ear Infections
NE-1530 551
vaccine, Streptococcus pneumoniae ..551

Effects of Chemotherapy
amifostine 202
amlexanox liquid 202
CP-99142 202
dimethyl sulfoxide, DMSO 202
Ethyol 202
keratinocyte growth factor (KGF) ...202
keratinocyte growth factor-2 (KGF-2) 203
Leucotropin 203
MK-869 203
myeloid progenitor inhibitory
 factor (MPIF) 203
OraRinse 202
Protegrin IB-367, Rinse, Gel ...203
recombinant human GM-CSF ...203
Repifermin 203
RF-1012 204
rhIL-11 204
SB 251353 204
SD/01 204
VML-670 204
Wobe-Mugos-E 204

Emphysema
(R,R)-formoterol 369
alpha-1-proteinase inhibitor ...369

Endometrial Cancer
aminopterin 205
Faslodex 205
GnRH Pharmaccine 205
ICI-182,780 205
MDX-220 205

Endometriosis
abarelix, PPI-149 564
Abarelix-Depot F 564
GnRH Pharmaccine 564
YM-511 564

Epilepsy
fosphenytoin sodium injection ..90
GABA agonist, anxiolytic 90
gabapentin 90
ganaxolone, CCD-1042 90
GW 273293 90
Neurontin 90
NPS 1776, alifatic amide 89
porcine neural cells, focal epilepsy 90
pregabalin 91
remacemide 91
retigabine 91
SB 204269 91
SPD 418 91
SPD 421 91
Topamax 91
topiramate tablet 91
TVP-1901 92

Erectile Dysfunction
(S)-sibutramine 452, 577
Alibra 451, 576
alprostadil/prazosin
 hydrochloride 451, 576
alprostadil 450, 575
alprostadil 450, 575
Alprox-TD, Befar 450, 575

682/Therapeutic Indications Index

apomorphine HCl 451, 576
BMS-193884 . . . . .451, 576
BMS-223131 . . . . .451, 576
Cialis 451, 576
Daproxetine 452, 577
IC351 . . . . .451, 576
Invicorp .452, 578
phentolamine mesylate 451, 577
PT-141 . . . . .452, 577
TA-1790 .452, 577
TAK-251, apomorphine 452, 577
testosterone 452, 577
Topiglan .450, 575
Tostrex 452, 577
Transdermal testosterone gel 452, 577
Uprima 451, 576
vardenafil 453, 578
Vasomax 451, 577

Esophageal Cancer

cisplatin/epinephrine 205, 416
flavopiridol, HMR-1275 . . . . .206, 417
Gastrimmune 206, 417
IntraDose 205, 416
vaccine, anti-gastrin 206, 417

Esophageal Disorders

Aptosyn 417
exisulind 417
V-Echinocandin 417

Eye Disorders/Infections

ADL 2-1294 539
ALT-711 539
batimastat, ISV-120 540
cidofovir 540
Cystavision 540
cysteamine hydrochloride 540
Dehydrex 542
dexamethasone 540
diclofenac, ISV-205 540
INS365 ophthalmic 541
INS37217 respiratory 541
intravitreal hyaluronidase 541
IontoDex 540
Keraform 542
ketotifen fumarate 541
LY-333531 541
octreotide acetate 541
piroxicam 542
PKC 412 542
Posurdex 542
proparacaine .542
Sandostatin LAR 541

Surodex 540
ToPreSite 542
Vitrase 541
Zaditen 541

Female Hormonal Deficiencies/Abnormalities

Estratest 388
estrogens/methyltestosterone 388

Fungal Infections

AmBisome 518, 519
amphotericin B 518
BMS-207147 .518
C319-14/6 519
ciclopirox olamine 519
FK463, echinocandin 519
liposomal amphotericin B 519
Loprox 519
Oramed 519
posaconazole 519
V-Echinocandin 519
Vfend 519

Gallbladder Disorders

GI 181771 417
Urso 418
ursodiol 418

Gastric Cancer

docetaxel hydrate 206, 418
fluoropyrimidine, S-1 . . . . .206, 418
Gastrimmune 207, 419
HSPPC-96 . . . . .206, 418
Iressa 208, 420
Liposomal Encapsulated Paclitaxel . . .419
MDX-210 . . . . .207, 419
MDX-220 . . . . .207, 419
murine monoclonal antibody . . .207, 419
Oncophage 206, 418
RFS-2000 . . . . .207, 419
Rubitecan 207, 419
Taxotere .206, 418
Theragyn 207, 419
vaccine, anti-gastrin 207, 419
ZD-1839 . . . . .208, 420

Gastric Ulcers

AG-1749, lansoprazole 420

Gastroenteritis

Campyvax 420
Elangesic 420
ibuprofen 420

vaccine, campylobacter 420

Gastroesophageal Reflux Disease (GERD)

(+)-norcisapride 420
AR-H047108 .421
KC-11458 421
lansoprazole .421
R 149524 421
reflux inhibitor 421
SLV 305 421
SLV 311 421
Takepron 421
tegaserod 421
vaccine, anti-gastrin II 422
YH-1885, SB 641257 422
Zelmac 421

Gastrointestinal Diseases and Disorders, Miscellaneous

ADL 8-2698 .422
AG-1749, lansoprazole 422
ALX-0600 422
AR-H047108 .422
C. difficile vaccine, CdVax 422
Emitasol, Pramidin 423
H. pylori vaccine 423
intranasal metoclopramide 423
keratinocyte growth factor (KGF) 423
lansoprazole .423
LeuTech 424
MB-U820 423
MK-826, carbapenem 423
Oralex 423
radiolabeled monoclonal antibody . . .424
rifaximin 424
scopolamine 424
Serostim 424
SLV 305 424
SLV 311 424
somatropin, r-hGH 424
Takepron 423
tarazepide 425
tegaserod 425
Zelmac 425

Gastroparesis

Emitasol, Pramidin 425
intranasal metoclopramide 425

Genital Herpes

APL400-024Px 306, 520, 564, 578
Docosanol 307, 520, 565, 578
Genevax - HSV-Px 306, 520, 564, 578

Therapeutic Indications Index/683

GW 419458, DISC-HSV 306, 520, 564, 578
resiquimod 307, 520, 565, 578
Simplirix 307, 520, 565, 579
TA-HSV 307, 520, 565, 578
vaccine, genital herpes 307, 520, 565, 579

Genital Warts
Alferon N Gel 308, 521
HspE7 ....307, 521
interferon (IFN) alfa-n3 ....308, 521
PEN203 ....308, 521
Polyphenon E 308, 521
TA-GW pharmaccine 308, 521

Glaucoma
AGN 192024 542
Alphagan 543
brimidine tartrate 543
CAT-152 543
diclofenac, ISV-205 543
latanoprost 543
Lumigan 542
memantine 543
Xalatan 543

Growth Hormone Deficiencies/Abnormalities
growth hormone releasing factor (GRF) 388
NN 703, NNC 26-0703, r-Somatropin 388
Nutropin Depot 389
pralmorelin 388
somatropin 389

Gynecological Infections
MK-826, carbepenem 565

Head and Neck Cancer
Allovectin-7 213
bexarotene 208
CI-1033 208
CI-1042, ONYX-015 208
cisplatin/epinephrine 208
CP-358,774 209
diclofenac 209
docetaxel hydrate 209
EMD 82633 209
gene therapy, interleukin-2 209
HumaRAD-HN 213
IMC-C225, CPT-11 210
INGN-201, adenoviral p53 210

interleukin (IL) 210
interleukin-12 gene therapy 210
IntraDose 208
LGD-1550 211
MDX-447, H-447 211
MG98 211
monoclonal antibody 211
MultiKine 210
Oralease 209
OSI-774 211
p53 gene therapy 212
porfiromycin 212
Promycin 212
T64 212
Targretin-capsule 208
Taxotere 209
tgDCC-E1A, RGG 0853 212
TheraCIM 211
troxacitabine, BCH-4556 212
Troxatyl 212
ZD0473 213

Heart Disease
abciximab, c7E3 29
BB-10153 29
Cidecin 29
daptomycin 29
human albumin microspheres 30
human muscle cells, cardiac disease ...30
LDP-01 30
Levovist 31
liposomal prostaglandin E1, PGE-1 ...30
Liprostin 30
OPC-18790 30
Optison 30
ReoPro 29
Resten-NG 31
TP-9201 30
Tranilast 31

Helicobacter Pylori
bismuth subcitrate/metronidazole/ tetracycline 425
Helicide 425
Helivax 425
NE-0080 425
vaccine, Helicobacter pylori 425

Hemochromatosis
ICL 670 52

Hemophilia
Alphanate 31, 52
antihemophilic factor 31, 52

Coagulin-B 32, 53
factor VIII gene therapy 31, 32, 53
NovoSeven 32, 53
r-FVIIa 32, 53

Hemorrhage
Corleukin NIF 53
fibrin sealant 54
hemoglobin 54
PolyHeme 54

Hemorrhoids
Anogesic 426
nitroglycerin ointment 426

Hepatic Encephalopathy
ABT-594, epibatidine 426

Hepatitis
ACH-126,443 ....308, 426
adefovir dipivoxil, GS-840 ....308, 426
Albuferon 314, 432
Alferon N Injection 311, 429
anti-hepatitis B 309, 426
anti-hepatitis C 309, 427
BMS-200475 ....309, 427
Ceplene 311, 429
cidofovir 309, 427
clevudine 309, 427
Coviracil 309, 427
EHT899 ....309, 427
emtricitabine 309, 427
Entecavir 309, 427
GENEVAX-HBV 315, 433
HBVIg 310, 428
HCI-436 ....310, 428
HE2000 428
Hepagene 314, 433
hepatitis A 310, 428
hepatitis B immune globulin 310, 428
hepatitis B immunotherapy, HBV/MF59 ....310, 428
hepatitis C protein 310, 428
Heptazyme 312, 430
IDN-6556 ....310, 428
immune globulin intravenous ...311, 429
immune globulin 310, 429
immunostimulatory sequences (ISS) candidate 311, 429
immunotherapeutic, AML 311, 429
Infanrix 313, 431
interferon (IFN) alfa-n3 ....311, 429
interferon alfa-2b/ribavirin 311, 430
interferon alfa-2b 311, 429

684/Therapeutic Indications Index

interleukin-10 . . . . .312, 430
interleukin-12 (IL-12) 312, 430
IP501 . . . . .312, 430
ISIS-14803 . . . . .312, 430
LY466700 . . . . .312, 430
MIV-210 .312, 431
Nabi Civacir 310, 429
Norvir/ABT-378 431
Nothav 310, 428
Omniferon 313, 432
OST 577 .313, 431
Ostavir 313, 431
PEG-Intron/Rebetol 311, 430
PEG-Intron 311, 429
Pegasys .313, 431
peginterferon alfa-2a 313, 431
PeNta-HepB-IPV, vaccine 313, 431
Rebif 313, 431
recombinant human interferon
  beta-1a 313, 431
ritonavir 431
SB M00026 . . . . .313, 431
Tenovil 312, 430
thymalfasin 313, 431
Twinrix-three doses 314, 432
Urso 314, 432
ursodiol .314, 432
vaccine, HCV/MF59,
  hepatitis C 314, 432
vaccine, hepatitis B DNA 314, 433
vaccine, hepatitis B 314, 433
vaccine, hepatitis B 314, 433
vaccine, hepatitis E 314, 432
vaccine, hepatitis 314, 432
vaccine, viral hepatitis (HBV) . . .315, 433
Venoglobulin-S 311, 429
Vistide 309, 427
VML 600, R-848 . . . . .315, 433
VP 50406 . . . . .315, 433
VX-497 . . . . .315, 433
XTL-001 .315, 433
Zadaxin .313, 431

Herpes Labialis Infections
ME-609 .315, 522

Herpes Simplex Infections
AG-701 .316, 522
vaccine, genital herpes 316, 522
valaciclovir 316, 522
Valtrex, Zelitrex 316, 522

Herpes Zoster Infections
ADL2-1294 . . . . .316, 522

Histiocytoma
piritrexim 213

HIV Infection
abacavir 316
ACH-126,443 316
AIDS gene therapy 316
Aidsvax 324
aldesleukin, interleukin-2 (IL-2) 317
Alferon LDO .321
Alferon N Injection 321
ALVAC-HIV 1 317
AMD-3100 317
Ampligen 322
Anticort 323
BCX-34 317
BMS-232632 317
capravirine 318
Coactinon 318
Coviracil 318
DAPD 318
difluoromethylornithine (DFMO) . . .318
DMP-450 318
emivirine 318
emtricitabine 318
Epivir 321
EWBH treatment 319
Gallium maltolate 319
GEM-92 319
GeneVax-HIV-Px 324
GW 433908 .319
HGP-30W 320
HGTV-43 320
HIV-1 immunogen 320
HMR-4004 320
interferon (IFN) alfa-n3 321
interferon (IFN) alfa-n3 321
interleukin (IL) 321
lamivudine 321
MIV-150 321
mozenavir dimesylate 321
Multikine 321
pentafuside, T-20 321
poly I:poly C-12-U 322
PRO 140 322
PRO 2000 Gel 322
PRO 367 322
PRO 542 322
procaine HCl 323
Proleukin Interleukin-2 and
  standard anti-HIV therapy 323
Proleukin 317
Remune 320
ribozyme gene therapy 323
T-1249 323
Tenofovir DF 324
tenofovir disoproxil fumarate 324
vaccine, HIV-1 gp-120 prime-boost . .325
vaccine, HIV .324
vaccine, HIV .324
vaccine, HIV .324
VIR201 324
VX-175 325
WF10 325
Ziagen 316

Hormone Deficiencies
Serostim 389
somatropin, r-hGH 389

Hormone Replacement Therapy/Menopause
17-beta estradiol/trimegestone 389
conjugated estrogen tablets 389
estradiol, 17-beta 389
estradiol/progestin 389
estradiol 389
Estrasorb 389
Estrogel 389
Premarin/Trimegesterone 389
testosterone .390
Tostrelle 390
transdermal testosterone gel 390
17-beta estradiol/trimegestone 566
conjugated estrogen tablets 566
estradiol, 17-beta 566
estradiol/progestin 566
estradiol 566
Estrasorb 566
Estratest 566
Estrogel 566
estrogens/methyltestosterone 566
Premarin/trimegestone 566
testosterone .566
Tostrelle 567
transdermal testosterone gel 567

Huntington's Disease
NeuroCell-HD 92
porcine fetal cells 92
remacemide .92

Hypercalcemia
zoledronate 54, 213
Zometa .54, 213

Hyperlipidemia
BMS-201038 .32

Hypertension
Atacand 33, 453
Beraprost 34, 455
BMS-186716, omapatrilat 32, 453
bosentan 32, 453
candesartan cilexetil 33, 453
Captelan 33, 453
captopril 33, 453
CS-866 . . . . .33, 454
diltiazem HCl 33, 454
Diovan 35, 455
GW 660511 . . . . .33, 454
isradipine 33, 454
lercanidipine 33, 454
Sitaxsentan 34, 454
SLV 306 . . . . .34, 454
SPP 100 . . . . .34, 455
TBC-3711 . . . . .34, 455
TCV-116C .34, 455
telmisartan 34, 455
Tracleer 32, 453
UT-15 . . . . .35, 455
valsartan 35, 455
Vanlev 32, 453
Verzem 33, 454

Hyponatremia
YM-087, conivaptan . . .214, 369, 390, 456

Ichthyosis
glyceryl monolaurin, T-100 522
Glylorin 522

Ileus
prucalopride 434
Resolor 434

Immunosuppressive
AI-502 325
AlloMune 327
anti B-7 humanized antibodies 325
Anti-LFA-1, odulimomab 325
BTI-322, MEDI-507 326
Certican 326
everolimus 326
FTY 720 326
ISAtx247 326
monoclonal antibody, ABX-CBL 326
Nipent 327
Nuvion 327
organ transplantation system 327
pentostatin 327
SDZ RAD 327
SMART anti-CD3 327

SR-31747 327
thalidomide 327
Thalomid 327
VAS981 328

In-stent Restenosis
AGI-1067 35
Antrin/Photoangioplasty 35
liposomal prostaglandin E1, PGE-1 . . .35
Liprostin 35

Infertility
follitropin alpha 567
Gonal-F 567
goserelin acetate 567
LHRH, luteinizing hormone-
    releasing hormone antagonist 567
Ovidrel 567
r-hCG 567
r-hLH 567
Zoladex IVF 567

Inflammatory Bowel Disease
Aliminase 434
Antegren 436
APC 2059 434
Balsalazide 437
budesonide 434
Carn 1000 434
CBP-1011 435
CDP-571, BAY 10-356 435
Colirest 435
Elangesic 435
Entocort CR 434
Humicade 435
ibuprofen 435
ISIS-2302 435
keratinocyte growth factor-2
    (KGF-2) 435
LDP-02 436
LeuTech 436
mesalamine 436
natalizumab 436
NCX 1015 436
Pentasa 436
radiolabeled monoclonal
    antibody 436
Rebif 437
recombinant human interferon
    beta-1a 437
Repifermin 435
rofleponide 437
tazofelone 437

Influenza
adjuvanted influenza 328, 370
Fluad 328, 370
FluMist 328, 370
Pseudostat 329, 371
Relenza 329, 371
RWJ 241947 . . . . .328, 370
RWJ 270201 . . . . .328, 370
vaccine, DPT/Haemophilus
    influenzae type B 328, 370
vaccine, influenza 328, 370
vaccine, influenza 329, 370
vaccine, nasal proteosome
    influenza 329, 371
vaccine, parainfluenza 329, 371
vaccine, Pseudomonas infection .329, 371
zanamavir 329, 371

Insomnia
epalon, CCD-3693 92
NBI-34060 92
NGD 96-1 92
racemic zoplicone 93
Zopiclone 93

Irritable Bowel Syndrome (IBS)
cilansetron 437
Dexloxiglumide 438
NK-2 antagonist 437
Saredutant 437
TAK-637 438
tegaserod 438
Zelmac 438

Kaposi's Sarcoma
Col-3 . . . . .214, 329
IM862 . . . . .214, 330
Metastat .214, 329
thalidomide 214
Thalomid 214

Keratoses
bexarotene 522
Targretin-gel 522

Kidney Disease
5G1.1 456
Adentri 456
Aranesp 456
Corlopam 457
CVT-124 456
darbepoetin alfa 456
doxercalciferol 456
fenoldopam mesylate, SK&F-82526 . .457

686/Therapeutic Indications Index

Hectorol Capsules 456
icodextrin, Extraneal 457
Icodial 457
Lambda 457
lanthanum carbonate 457
LJP-394 457
midodrine HCl 457
novel erythropoiesis stimulating
   protein (NESP) 458
NOX-100 458
pimagedine HCl 458
ProAmatine 457
triacetyl uridine 458

Kidney Transplant Surgery

5c8 (Anti CD-40 ligand antibody) . . .458
AlloMune 460
anti B-7 humanized antibodies 458
anti-CD11a, hu1124 459
Anti-LFA-1, odulimomab 459
Antova 458
BTI-322, MEDI-507 459
ISIS-2302 459
organ transplantion system 460
SMART Anti-CD3 460

Labor and Delivery

SR 49059 569

Laryngeal Tumors/Disorders

cidofovir 214, 551
Vistide 214, 551

Leukemia

Adriamycin 57, 217
aldesleukin, interleukin-2 (IL-2) . .54, 214
aminopterin 54, 215
Annamycin 54, 215
AR-522 . . . . .54, 215
arsenic trioxide (ATO) 55, 215
Atragen 60, 219
BCX-34 . . . . .55, 215
Campath 58, 218
Ceplene 217
Ceplene 57
clofarabine 55
Clofarabine 61, 220
CTLA4-Ig 55, 215
daunorubicin citrate 55, 216
DaunoXome 55, 216
decitabine 56, 216
denileukin diftitox 56, 216
flavopiridol, HMR-1275 . . . . . . .56, 216
G3139 .56, 216

G3139 .57, 216
Genasense/Mylotarg 56, 216
Genasense 57, 216
gene therapy, leukemia 57, 217
GL-331 .57, 217
Glivec .57, 217
GPX-100 . . . . .57, 217
Gvax 61, 220
histamine dihydrochloride 217
imatinib, STI 571 . . . . .57, 217
immunotherapeutic AML 57
interferon alfa-2b 58, 218
L-Vax 61, 220
LDI-200 . . . . .58, 218
LDP-03 .58, 218
liposomal ether lipid 58, 218
lisofylline, CT-1501R 59
MDX-22 . . . . .59, 218
Nipent .59, 218
Ontak .56, 216
PEG-Intron 58, 218
Pegasys 59, 218
peginterferon alfa-2a 59, 218
pentostatin 59, 218
Proleukin 54, 214
ProTec 59
RFS-2000 . . . . .59, 219
Rubitecan 59, 219
SMART M195 . . . . .60, 219
tiazofurin 60, 219
Tiazole .60, 219
TLC ELL-12 . . . . .58, 218
TNP-470 60
tretinoin 60, 219
Trisenox/dexamethasone 60
Trisenox 55, 215
troxacitabine, BCH-4556 . . . . . . .61, 219
Troxatyl 61, 219
vaccine, cancer 61, 220
Vasogen IMT 61, 220

Limb Preservation and Amputation

AS-013 .36, 390
Circulase 36, 390

Liver Cancer

AFP-Scan 221
cisplatin/epinephrine 220
Combidex 222
Doxil, Caelyx 221
doxorubicin HCl 221
Gastrimmune 222
imaging agent 221

IntraDose 220
Irofulven 221
MGI-114, hydroxymethylacylfulvene,
   HMAF 221
MTC-DOX 221
nolatrexed dihydrochloride 222
pivaloyloxymethylbutyrate 222
Pivanex 222
thymalfasin .222
Thymitaq 222
vaccine, anti-gastrin 222
Zadaxin 222

Liver Disease

human liver cells 438
interleukin-10 (IL-10) 438
IP501 438
NovoSeven .438
r-FVIIa 438
Tenovil 438

Liver Transplant Surgery

human liver cells 439

Lung Cancer

AE-941 223
alitretinoin, ALRT-1057 223
Aposyn/Taxotere 227
Aptosyn/Gemzar 227
Aptosyn/Navelbine 227
Aptosyn/Taxotere/carboplatin 234
Aptosyn 227
arcitumomab 223
BAM-002 223
BAY 12-9566 223
BEC2 224
bexarotene .224
biricodar dicitrate, VX-710 224
blood substitute 224
BLP-25 224
BMS-182751, JM-216 225
CEA-Cide 229
CEA-Scan .223
CeaVac/TriAb 235
CI-1033 225
CI-1042, ONYX-015 225
cisplatin/vinblastine/amifostine 225
CP-358,774 225
decitabine .226
DENSPM 226
diarysulfonylurea, ILX-295501 226
diethylnorspermine 226
docetaxel hydrate 226
Doxil, Caelyx 226

Therapeutic Indications Index/687

doxorubicin HCl 226
exisulind/docetaxel 227
exisulind/gemcitabine HCl 227
exisulind/vinorelbine tartrate
    injection 227
exisulind 227
flavopiridol, HMR-1275 228
FMdC 228
gemcitabine HCl 228
Gemzar 228
GL-331 228
Gvax 235
Hemolink 224
HuC242-DM1/SB-408075 228
HuN901-DM1 .228
Hycamtin 234
IMC-C225, CPT-11 228
IMMU-MN14, anti-CEA 229
Incel 224
Incel 236
INGN 241 (mda-7) 229
INGN-201, adenoviral p53 229
INS316 229
Iressa 236
Irofulven 232
ISIS 2503 229
ISIS 3521 230
ISIS 5132, CGP 69846A 230
liposomal ether lipid 230
marimastat, BB-2516 230
MDX-210 231
MDX-220 231
MDX-447, H-447 231
MGI-114, hydroxymethylacylfulvene,
    HMAF 232
Neovastat 223
NX 211 232
Onco TCS 235
OSI-774 232
paclitaxel/carboplatin/amifostine 232
Panretin 223
pivaloyloxymethylbutyrate 232
Pivanex 232
Prinomastat .231
Rebif 233
recombinant human interferon
    beta-1a 233
RSR13 233
SB 249553 233
squalamine 233
SU-101 233
T64 233
T67 234
Targretin-capsule 224

Taxotere 226
tirapazamine/cisplatin 234
Tirazone 234
TLC ELL-12 230
topotecan HCl 234
TriAb/TriGem 235
troxacitabine, BCH-4556 234
Troxatyl 234
vaccine, anti-cancer 235
vaccine, cancer 235
vaccine, EGF cancer 235
vincristine 235
VX-710 236
XR5000 236
ZD-0473/AMD 473 236
ZD-1839 236

Lung Disease
Avelox 371
Flocor 371
moxifloxacin .371
poloxamer 188 N.F., CRL-5861 371
ribavirin 372
TBC-11251 372
vaccine, respiratory syncytial virus . .372
Virazole 372

Lymphoma, non-Hodgkin's
aldesleukin, interleukin-2 (IL-2) 236
arsenic trioxide (ATO) 237
Atragen 240
bectumomab 237
Bexxar 239
CpG 7909 237
daunorubicin citrate 237
DaunoXome .237
epratuzumab 237
FLT3 ligand 237
Fludara 238
fludarabine phosphate 238
G3139/cyclophosphamide 238
Genasense/cyclophosphamide 238
HSPPC-96 238
IDEC-Y2B8, In2B8 238
LymphoCide .237
LymphoScan 237
Mobist 237
Nipent 239
Onco TCS 240
Oncolym 240
Oncophage 238
pentostatin 239
Pretarget 240
Proleukin 236

ribozyme gene therapy 239
Rituxan 239
rituximab/chemotherapy 239
SMART 1D10 antibody 239
subject-specific immunotherapy 238
tositumomab .239
tretinoin 240
Trisenox 237
vincristine 240
Zevalin 238

Lymphomas
AlloMune 63, 241
APL400-020 V-B 62, 240
arsenic trioxide (ATO) 62
BCX-34 . . . . .62, 241
Beta LT 64, 242
bexarotene 241
Clofarabine 64
daunorubicin citrate 62
DaunoXome 62
denileukin diftitox 62, 241
FLT3 ligand 63, 241
Genevax-TCR 62, 240
gullium maltolate 63
hypericin 63
Mobist 63, 241
Ontak 62, 241
organ transplantation system 63, 241
Targretin-capsule 241
TNP-470 63
Trisenox 62
vaccine, cancer 64, 242
vaccine, lymphoma 64, 242
Vaxid 64, 242
VIMRxyn 63

Macular Degeneration
AE-941 543
AMD Fab 544
anecortave acetate 544
EYE-001, NX-1838 544
matrix metalloprotease
    inhibitor (MMP) 544
motexafin lutetium 544
Neovastat 543
Optrin 544
PhotoPoint - SnET2 544
Prinomastat .544
SnET2 544

Malaria
tafenoquine, SB 252263 330
vaccine, malaria 330

vaccine, malaria 330

Male Hormonal Deficiencies/Abnormalities
Andractim *390, 579*
Androsorb *391, 579*
dihydrotestosterone 390, 579
testosterone 391, 579
testosterone 391, 579
Tostrex *391, 580*
Transdermal testosterone gel 391, 580

Malignant Melanoma
Ampligen *244*
CancerVax, C-VAX 242
Ceplene *243*
cisplatin/epinephrine 242
DENSPM *243*
diarysulfonylurea, ILX-295501 242
diethylnorspermine 243
gene therapy, IL-2 and
  superantigen gene (SEB) 243
gene therapy, interleukin-2 243
Gvax *245*
histamine dihydrochloride 243
HSPPC-96 243
IM862 243
interferon alfa-2b 244
IntraDose *242*
M-Vax *245*
Melacine *245*
Oncophage *243*
PEG-Intron *244*
Pegasys *244*
peginterferon alfa-2a 244
poly I:poly C-12-U 244
RFS-2000 ....*244*
Rubitecan *244*
thymalfasin 244
TriGem *245*
troxacitabine, BCH-4556 244
Troxatyl *244*
vaccine, anti-cancer 245
vaccine, cancer 245
vaccine, GMK 245
vaccine, melanoma 245
vaccine, melanoma 245
Zadaxin *244*

Manic Disorders
quetiapine fumarate 141
Seroquel *141*

Melanoma

aldesleukin, interleukin-2 (IL-2) 246
Allovectin-7 ....*247*
CpG 7909 246
DISC GM-CSF 246
G3139/dacarbazine 246
Genasense/dacarbazine *246*
Novovac-M1 246
Proleukin *246*
SB 249553 246
T64 247
vaccine, melanoma 247

Memory Loss
SIB-1508Y 36, 93

Meningitis
cytarabine liposome injection 330
DepoCyt *330*
Meningitec *94, 331*
Neuprex *93, 331*
Nyotran *93, 331*
nystatin, AR-121 ....93, 331
opebecan, rBPI-21, recombinant
  human bactericidal/
  permeability-increasing protein .93, 331
vaccine, meningococcal C conjugate ..94,
  331
vaccine, meningococcus C 94, 331
vaccine, Streptococcus pneumoniae ..331

Menopause
17-beta estradiol/trimegestone ..391, 568
Androsorb *568*
calcitonin 568
conjugated estrogen tablets 391, 568
estrogen 391, 568
estrogen 392, 568
Macritonin *568*
Premarin/Trimegesterone *391, 568*
testosterone 568
Tostrelle *392, 568*
transdermal testosterone gel 392, 568
TSE-424 569
Vivelle-Dot *391, 568*
Vivelle/Menorest *392, 568*

Mesothelioma
Aroplatin *247*
Onconase *247*
ranpirnase 247

Migraine and Cluster Headaches
ALX-0646 94
Botox *94*

botulinum toxin type A,
  AGN-191622 94
CNS-5161 94
dotarizine 95
eletriptan 95
esprolol 95
frovatriptan 95
ganaxolone, CCD-1042 95
GW 468816 96
Imigran, Imitrex *97*
Migrastat *96*
MT 100 96
MT 400 96
MT 500 96
Naramig, Amerge *96*
naratriptan 96
propranolol 96
Relpax *95*
s-fluoxetine 96
selective serotonergic agent 96
sumatriptan 97
zolmitriptan 97
zolmitriptan 97
zolmitriptan 97
zolmitriptan 97
zolmitriptan 97
zolmitriptan 98
Zomig Aura *98*
Zomig Cluster *97*
Zomig FM *97*
Zomig IN *97*
Zomig *97*

Multiple Myeloma
AE-941 ....64, 247
APC8020 ....64, 248
arsenic trioxide (ATO) 65, 248
Beta LT *67, 249*
BrevaRex MAb *66, 249*
CDC 801 ....65, 248
Ceplene *65, 248*
histamine dihydrochloride 65, 248
LDP-341, PS-341 ....65, 249
liposomal ether lipid 66, 249
monoclonal antibody 66, 249
Mylovenge *64, 248*
Neovastat *64, 247*
SelCIDs *65, 248*
skeletal targeted radiotherapy
  (STR) 66, 249
thalidomide 66
Thalomid *66*
TLC ELL-12 ....*66, 249*
Trisenox/dexamethasone *66*
Trisenox *65, 248*

Therapeutic Indications Index/**689**

vaccine, cancer 67, 250
Wobe-Mugos-E 67, 250
YM-529, minodronate 67, 250

Multiple Sclerosis
AnergiX.MS *101*
Antegren *100*
Avonex *99*
Betaseron *98*
CDC 801 98
Copaxone (oral) *98*
Copaxone *98*
Deskar *100*
fampridine 98
glatiramer acetate 98
glatiramer acetate 98
interferon beta-1a 99
interferon beta-1b 98
IR208 99
micellar paclitaxel 99
modafinil 99
natalizumab 100
NBI-5788, MSP-771 100
Neurelan *98*
NeuroVax *99*
pirfenidone 100
Provigil *99*
SelCID *98*
T-cell receptor vaccine 100
thalidomide 101
Thalomid *101*
TM27, ATM027, TCAR 101

Musculoskeletal Diseases
benzestrom 488
Botox *489*
botulinum toxin type A,
  AGN-191622 489
Esterom *488*
recombinant human bone
  morphogenic protein-2 (rhBMP-2) .489

Mycosis Fungoides
HOE-351 ....250, 523
Lamisil *250, 523*
terbinafine 250, 523

Myeloma
gallium maltolate 250

Myocardial Infarction
abciximab, c7E3 36
Amiscan *38*
AMISTAD-II 36

AMP-579 36
cariporide mesylate, HOE-642 36
Diovan *38*
eptifibatide 37
fibrinogen-receptor antagonist ...37
H376/95 37
human muscle cells, cardiac disease ...37
Integrilin *37*
lanoteplase, BMS-200980 37
Lotrafiban *38*
Pallacor *36*
pexelizumab 37
ReoPro *36*
rPSGL-Ig 38
SB 214857 38
TP10 38
valsartan 38

Neuroblastoma
vaccine, allogenic and autologous
  neuroblastoma cells 101, 251

Neurodegenerative Disease
leteprinim potassium, AIT-082 ...101
Neotrofin *101*

Neurologic Disorders
+DDMS 102
dimethyl sulfoxide, DMSO 102
Rebif *102*
recombinant human interferon
  beta-1a 102

Neuropathy, Diabetic
Avapro *103, 392*
BMS-186295, SR-47436
  (irbesartan) 103, 392
LY-333531 ....103, 392
memantine 103, 392
timcodar dimesylate 103, 392
Timcodar *103, 392*
zenarestat 103, 393

Neuropathy
AVP-923 102
leteprinim potassium, AIT-082 ...102
Neotrofin *102*

Obesity
Axokine *394*
bromocriptine, ER-230 393
ecopipam 393
Ergoset *393*
GI 181771 393

GW 427353 393
leptin 393
orlistat 393
RF-1051 393
SB 418790 394
SR-141716 394
Xenical *393*

Obsessive-Compulsive Disorders
fluvoxamine maleate 141
Fluvoxamine-CR *141*

Ocular Hypertension
AGN 192024 545
Lumigan *545*

Oral Cavity Cancer
Allovectin-7 ....*251*

Orthopedic Surgery
hemoglobin glutamer-250 (bovine) ..489
Hemopure *489*
ORG-31540/SR-90107A 489

Orthopedics
recombinant human bone morphogenic
  protein-2 (rhBMP-2) 490

Osteoarthritis
asimadoline 490
BAY 12-9566 490
Benefen *491*
CI-1004 490
COX 189 490
Dirame *492*
etodolac 490
Fortical Injection *492*
ibuprofen 491
insulin-like growth factor-I (IGF-I) ..491
ketoprofen 491
Ketotop *491*
Lodine *490*
matrix metalloprotease inhibitor
  (MMP) 491
MK-663 491
ML3000 492
nabumetone Q 492
Orthovisc *492*
Prinomastat *491*
propiram 492
recombinant salmon calcitonin ..492
topical testosterone gel 492
valdecoxib 493
VX-740, pralnacasan 493

690/Therapeutic Indications Index

YM-177, celecoxib 493

Osteomyelitis
LeuTech 493
radiolabeled monoclonal antibody ...493

Osteoporosis
17-beta estradiol/trimegestone 493
ALX1-11 493
Bonviva 495
calcitonin 494
Estalis 494
estradiol/norethisterone acetate 494
estradiol/progestin 494
estrogen 494
estrogen 494
HCT 1026 494
ibandronate 495
lasofoxifene 495
Macritonin 494
NE-58095, risedronate sodium 495
Neosten 495
parathyroid hormone, PTH 495
SB 273005 495
sodium fluoride 495
testosterone 495
TSE-424 496
Vivelle, Menorest 494
Vivelle-Dot 494
zoledronate 496
Zometa 496

Otitis Media
gatifloxacin 552
Levaquin 552
levofloxacin 552
NE-1530 552
Tequin 552

Ovarian Cancer
Amdray 255
APC8024 251
BAY 12-9566 251
biricodar dicitrate, VX-710 251
BMS-182751, JM-216 252
CEA-Cide 253
CP-358,774 252
diarysulfonylurea, ILX-295501 252
docetaxel hydrate 252
EMD 82633 252
FLT3 ligand 253
FMdC 253
gemcitabine HCl 253
Gemzar 253

HER-2/neu dendritic cell vaccine 253
HMFG1 257
Hycamtin 256
hyperteria/doxorubicin 253
IM862 253
IMMU-MN14, anti-CEA 253
Incel 251
Incel 257
INGN-201, adenoviral p53 254
Irofulven 255
marimastat, BB-2516 254
MDX-210 254
MDX-220 254
MGI-114, hydroxymethylacylfulvene,
  HMAF 255
Mobist 253
murine monoclonal antibody 255
NX 211 255
O-Vax 257
OvaRex 257
p53 tumor suppressor gene 255
PSC 833, valspodar 255
RFS-2000 255
Rubitecan 255
squalamine 256
SU-101 256
Taxotere 252
tgDCC-E1A, RGG 0853 256
Theragyn 255
topotecan HCl 256
troxacitabine, BCH-4556 256
Troxatyl 256
vaccine, tumor cell suspension 257
valrubicin 257
Valstar 257
VX-710 257
XR5000 258
ZD-0473/AMD 473 258

Pain, Acute or Chronic
ABT-594, epibatidine 104, 496
acetaminophen/
  dextromethorphan 104, 496
ADX-153 ....104, 496
asimadoline 104, 497
AVP-923 497
BCH-3963, LEF576 ....104, 497
benzestrom 105, 497
Botox 497
botulinum toxin type A,
  AGN-191622 497
bupivacaine 105, 498
clonadine gel 105, 498
COX 189 ....105, 498

CT-3 ....105, 498
DepoBupivacaine 105, 498
dexamethasone 105, 498
diclofenac 106, 498
Dirame 109, 502
DPI-3290 ....106, 499
Durasgesic 106, 499
Esterom 105, 497
etodolac 106, 499
fentanyl transdermal system 106, 499
fentanyl 106, 499
GW 406381 ....106, 499
HCT 3012 ....107, 499
HydrocoDex 104, 496
hydromorphone 107, 500
IontoDex 105, 498
ketoprofen patch 107, 500
LEF 107, 500
Lidocaine 110, 503
Lodine 106, 499
MH-200, morphine
  hydrochloride 107, 500
MK-663 ....107, 500
Morphelan 108, 501
morphine sulfate 108, 501
morphine 107, 500
nabumetone Q 108, 501
Naropin 109, 502
nasal ketamine 501
NCX 4016 ....108, 501
NCX 701 ....108, 501
neurotrophin-3, NT-3 ....108, 501
NO-naproxen 109, 501
OxycoDex 109, 502
oxycodone 88
oxycodone hydrochloride/
  dextromethorphan hydrobromide ..109, 502
pancrelipase 109, 502
pregabalin 109, 502
propiram 109, 502
ropivacaine HCl 109, 502
RSD 921 ....110, 502
Topamax 110, 503
topical testosterone gel 503
topiramate tablet 110, 503
Viokase 109, 502
ZD-4953 ....110, 503
ziconotide, SNX-111 88

Pancreatic Cancer
Avicine 259, 395, 439
BAY 12-9566 258
CEA-Cide 260, 396, 441

Therapeutic Indications Index/691

CEP-701 . . . . .258, 394, 439
CI-1042, ONYX-015 . . . . . . .258, 394, 439
CTP-37 . . . . .259, 395, 439
DENSPM *259, 395, 439*
diethylnorspermine 259, 395, 439
Gastrimmune *262, 398, 443*
GBC-590 . . . . .259, 395, 440
gemcitabine HCl 259, 395, 440
Gemzar *259, 395, 440*
Gvax *262, 399, 443*
HSPPC-96 . . . . .259, 395, 440
HuC242-DM1/SB-408075 . .259, 395, 440
IMC-C225, CPT-11 . . . . . . .260, 396, 440
IMMU-MN14, anti-CEA . . .260, 396, 441
Irofulven *261, 397, 442*
ISIS 2503 . . . . .260, 396, 441
ISIS 5132, CGP 69846A 260, 396, 441
marimastat, BB-2516 . . . . . .261, 397, 441
MDX-210 . . . . .261, 397, 442
MDX-220 . . . . .261, 397, 442
MGI-114, hydroxymethylacylfulvene,
 HMAF 261, 397, 442
Oncophage *259, 395, 440*
pancrelipase 399
RFS-2000 . . . . .262, 398, 442
Rubitecan *262, 398, 442*
SR-27897B 262, 398, 442
troxacitabine, BCH-4556 . . .262, 398, 443
Troxatyl *262, 398, 443*
vaccine, anti-gastrin 262, 398, 443
vaccine, cancer 262, 399, 443
Viokase *399*
virulizin 263, 443

Pancreatic Disorders
pancrelipase 444
Viokase *444*

Panic Disorders
esprolol 141
fluoxetine HCl 141
pagoclone .142
Prozac *141*

Parasites and Protozoa
nitazoxanide (NTZ) 332
Quilimmune-M *332*
roxithromycine, RU-28,965 332
vaccine, malaria 332

Parathyroid Disease
AMG 073 .399
calcimimetics 399

Parkinson's Disease
altropane .110
apomorphine 110
brasofensine, NS-2214, BMS-204756 .111
CEP-1347 .111
Comtan *111*
CPI-1189 .111
Duodopa *112*
Eldepryl *113*
entacapone 111
etilevodopa, TV-1203 111
FKBP-neuroimmunophilin ligands . . .111
leteprinim potassium, AIT-082 111
levodopa/carbidopa 112
modafinil .112
N-0923 112
Neotrofin *111*
NeuroCell-PD *112*
neurotrophin-3, NT-3 112
nitrone radical trap (NRT) 112
porcine fetal cells 112
Provigil *112*
remacemide 113
ReQuip *113*
Rilutek *113*
riluzole 113
ropinirole .113
selegiline .113
SIB-1508Y 113
SLV 308 113
spheramine 114
TVP-1012, rasagiline mesylate 114
Zelapar *113*

Peripheral Arterial Occlusive Disease
Abbokinase *39*
AngioMARK *39*
Antrin/Photoangioplasty *39*
Genvascor *39*
ifetroban sodium, BMS-180291 39
MS-325 39
prourokinase 39

Peripheral Vascular Disease
AC3056 40
AGI-1067 40
AngioMARK *41*
avasimibe 40
Beraprost *41*
BioByPass *42*
CP-529,414 40
Dromos *41*
Fiblast *41*
ifetroban sodium, BMS-180291 40
iloprost 40
MS-325 41
propionyl-L-carnitine 41
SB 435495 .41
trafermin 41
UT-15 42
vascular endothelial growth
 factor-121 (VEGF) 42
VasoCare *41*
VEGF121 42

Peyronie's Disease
collagenase for injection 460, 580
Cordase *460, 580*

Pneumonia
amikacin 372, 552
Avelox *373*
cefditoren pivoxil 372, 552
DB-289 . . . . .373, 552
HMR-3647, RU-64,004 . . . . . . .373, 552
Merrem *374, 553*
Mikasome *372, 552*
MK-826, carbepenem 373, 552
moxifloxacin 373
Neuprex *373, 553*
opebecan, rBPI-21, recombinant
 human bactericidal/
 permeability-increasing protein 373, 553
protegrin IB-367, rinse, gel 374, 553
Quilimmune-P *374, 554*
quinupristin/dalfopristin 374, 553
Synercid *374, 553*
vaccine, pneumococcal
 infections 374, 554
vaccine, respiratory syncytial
 virus 374, 554
vaccine, Streptococcus pneumoniae . .554

Post-Traumatic Stress Disorders
fluoxetine HCl 142
paroxetine .142
Paxil, Seroxat *142*
Prozac *142*

Premature Ejaculation
paroxetine HCl 580

Premenstrual Syndrome
vomeropherin, PH-80 . . . . .142, 569

Pressure Ulcers
oxandrolone, CO221 523

692/Therapeutic Indications Index

Prostate Cancer

3-month Leuprogel 269, 466, 586
30-day Leuprogel 269, 466, 586
abarelix depot, PPI-149 . . .263, 460, 580
Abetafen. 272, 470, 590
abiraterone acetate 263, 460, 580
ABT-627 . . . . .263, 461, 580
AdjuVax-100a 274, 471, 591
APC8015 . . . . .264, 461, 581
Apomine 274, 471, 591
Aposyn/Taxotere 266, 463, 583
Apra 264, 462, 581
Aptosyn/LHRH agonist 266, 463, 583
Aptosyn 266, 463. 583
arsenic trioxide (ATO) 264, 461, 581
Atragen 272, 469, 589
Avicine 264, 462, 582
bicalutimide 264, 461, 581
Casodex 264, 461, 581
CEP-2563 . . . . .264, 461, 581
CEP-701 . . . . .264, 461, 581
Combidex 273, 470, 590
CT-2584 . . . . .264, 462, 581
CTP-37 . . . . .264, 462, 582
CV706 . . . . .265, 462, 582
CV787 . . . . .265, 462, 582
cVax-Pr 265, 462, 582
CyPat 272, 469, 589
DCVax 274, 471, 591
Doxil, Caelyx 265, 462, 582
doxorubicin HCl 265, 462, 582
DPPE 265, 463, 582
eflornithine, DFMO
   (difluoromethylornydil) . .266, 463, 583
exisulind/docetaxel 266, 463, 583
exisulind 266, 463, 583
FK-317 . . . . .266, 464, 584
G3139/androgen blockade . .267, 464, 584
G3139/docetaxel 267, 464, 584
G3139/mitoxantrone 267, 464, 584
gallium maltolate 267, 465, 584
GBC-590 . . . . .267, 464, 584
*Genasense/androgen
   blockade* 267, 464, 584
Genasense/mitoxantrone 267, 464, 584
Genasense/Taxotere 267, 464, 584
GeneVax 274, 472, 591
GnRH Pharmaccine 273, 471, 590
Gvax 274, 471, 591
IM862 . . . . .267, 465, 585
IMC-C225, CPT-11 . . . . . . .268, 465, 585
INGN-201, adenoviral p53 . .268, 465, 585
interleukin (IL) 268, 465, 585
Iressa 275, 472, 592
Irofulven 270, 467, 587
ISIS 5132, CGP 69846A 268, 466, 585
LDI-200 . . . . .269, 466, 586
Leuplin 3M DPS 273, 471, 591
leuprolide acetate 269, 466, 586
Leuvectin 272, 470, 589
liposomal ether lipid 269, 466, 586
MDX-210 . . . . .270, 467, 587
MDX-220 . . . . .270, 467, 587
Metastron 271, 468, 588
MGI-114, hydroxymethylacylfulvene,
   HMAF 270, 467, 587
MultiKine 268, 465, 585
Norelin 273, 470, 590
Onyvax P 274, 471, 591
p53 gene therapy 270, 467, 588
phenoxodiol 270, 467, 587
Prinomastat 269, 469, 586
Prostvac 274, 472, 592
Provenge 264, 461, 581
PSMA - P1/P2 . . . . .271, 468, 588
Quadramet 271, 468, 588
samarium Sm 153 lexidronam
   pentasodium 271, 468, 588
SGN-15/Taxotere 271, 468, 588
SPD 424 . . . . .271, 468, 588
SR-48692 . . . . .271, 468, 588
strontium-89 chloride
   injection 271, 468, 588
SU-101 . . . . .271, 469, 589
Tesmilifene 273, 470, 590
TLC ELL-12 . . . . .269, 466, 586
tretinoin 272, 469, 589
Trisenox 264, 461, 581
troxacitabine, BCH-4556 . . .272, 469, 589
Troxatyl 272, 469, 589
vaccine, adjuvant 274, 471, 591
vaccine, cancer 274, 471, 472, 591
vaccine, prostate cancer
   (rV-psa) 274, 472, 592
YM-598 . . . . .275, 472, 592
ZD-0473/AMD 473 . . . . . . .275, 472, 592
ZD-1839 . . . . .275, 472, 592

Prostate Disorders

lomefloxacin HCl 472, 592
Maxaquin 472, 592
pygeum africanum 472, 592
Tadenan .472, 592

Psoriasis and Psoriatic Disorders

ABX-IL8 523
ADL 2-1294 .523
AE-941 523
alitretinoin, ALRT-1057 524
Amevive 528
anti-CD11a, hu1124 524
bexarotene .524
Birex 529
BTI-322, MEDI-507 524
efalizumab monoclonal antibody 525
Enbrel 525
etanercept 525
HCT 1026 525
HuMax-CD4 525
hypericin 526
IDEC-114 526
IDEC-131 526
interleukin-10 526
IR502 526
ISAtx247 526
ISIS-2302 527
maxacalcitol 527
MEDI-507 527
micellar paclitaxel 527
NCX 1022 527
Neovastat 523
Nuvion 528
paclitaxel 528
Panretin 524
PEN203 528
Primatized .526
PVAC 528
recombinant human lactoferrin
   (rhLF) 528
recombinant LFA-3/IgG1
   Human Fusion Protein 528
SMART anti-CD3 528
ST630 528
T-cell receptor vaccine 529
Targretin-capsule 524
tazarotene 529
Tazorac 529
Tenovil 526
VAS 972 529
verteporfin .529
VIMRxyn 526
VX-148 529
Xanelim 525
Zorcell 526

Psychosis

DTA 201 142
DU127090 .142
Lu 35-139 143
SR-142801, osanetant 143
SR-48692 143

Therapeutic Indications Index/693

Pulmonary Fibrosis
Avonex 375
Deskar 375
interferon, beta-1a 375
pirfenidone 375

Red Blood Cell Disorders
flumecinol 67
psoralen, S-59 67
Zixoryn 67

Renal Cell Carcinoma
AE-941 ....275, 473
aldesleukin, interleukin-2
   (IL-2) 275, 473
Ampligen 278, 476
Aroplatin 279, 477
arsenic trioxide (ATO) 275, 473
Atragen 278, 476
Avrend 276, 473
CD40 ligand 276, 473
Ceplene 276, 474
DENSPM 276, 474
diarysulfonylurea, ILX-295501 ..276, 473
diethylnorspermine 276, 474
EMD 82633 ....276, 474
GL-331 ....276, 474
histamine dihydrochloride 276, 474
HSPPC-96 ....277, 474
IMC-C225, CPT-11 ......277, 475
interleukin-12 (IL-12) 277, 475
Irofulven 277, 475
Leuvectin 279, 476
MDX-210 ....277, 475
MGI-114, hydroxymethylacylfulvene,
   HMAF 277, 475
Neovastat 275, 473
Oncophage 277, 474
Pegasys 278, 475
peginterferon alfa-2a 278, 475
poly I:poly C-12-U 278, 476
Proleukin 275, 473
T-cells/Xcellerate technology 278, 476
tretinoin 278, 476
Trisenox 275, 473
troxacitabine, BCH-4556 ..278, 476
Troxatyl 278, 476
vaccine, kidney cancer 279, 477

Respiratory Failure
LiquiVent 375
lucinactant 375
perflubron 375
Surfaxin 375

Reversible Obstructive Airways Disease
Foradil 376
formoterol 376

Rheumatoid Arthritis
5G1.1 503
ABX-IL8 503
AGIX-4207 504
AGT-1 504
AnergiX.RA 509
anti-IFNg 504
BB-2827 504
CCR2b 504
CDC 801 504
CDP 870 505
CDP-571, BAY 10-356 505
COX 189 505
Enbrel 505
etanercept 505
etodolac 505
HuMax-CD4 506
Humicade 505
IDEC-151 506
IL-1ra/Anakinra 506
interleukin-1 (IL-1) trap 506
IR501 506
ISAtx247 506
Kineret 506
LF 15-0195 507
Lodine 505
micellar paclitaxel 507
MK-663 507
Nipent 507
pentostatin 507
Prograf 509
r-hTBP-1, recombinant human
   tumor necrosis factor-binding
   protein 1 508
Ravax 506
Rebif 508
recombinant human interferon
   beta-1a 508
SB 273005 508
SB 683698, TR 14035 508
SCIO-469 508
SelCID 504
sTNF-RI, soluble tumor necrosis
   factor-a receptor type I 508
T-cell receptor vaccine 509
tacrolimus hydrate 509
thalidomide 509
Thalomid 509
vaccine, rheumatoid arthritis ..509
valdecoxib 509
VX-740, pralnacasan 509
VX-745 510
YM-177, celecoxib 510
ZD2315 510

Rhinitis
AG7088, anti-rhinoviral agent ...332, 554
Claritin/Singulair 333, 555
desloratadine,
   descarboethoxyloratadine 332, 554
DNK 333 ....333, 555
fluticasone/salmeterol 333, 555
loratadine/montelukast sodium ..333, 555
norastemizole 333, 555
omalizumab 333, 555
rofleponide palmitate 333, 555
Xolair 333, 555

Sarcoma
Apra 279
CT-2584 279
disaccharide tripeptide glycerol
   dipalmitoyl 279
HSPPC-96 280
ImmTher 279
Incel 280
Oncophage 280
T64 280
VX-710 280

Scar Tissue
Fibrostat 530

Schizophrenia and Schizoaffective Disorders
Abilitat 143
amisulpride, SL 91.1076 143
Ampakine 144
Ampalex 144
aripiprazole, OPC-14597, OPC-31 ...143
blonanserin, AD-5423 144
CX-516, BDP-12 144
CX-516, BDP-12 144
DAB-452 144
EMD-57445 144
iloperidone 144
M100907 144
neuroleptic 144
NGD 94-4 145
NK-1 145
olanzapine 145
ORG-23430 145
ORG-5222 145

694/Therapeutic Indications Index

quetiapine fumarate 145
Risperdal *145*
risperidone 145
SC-111 146
Seroquel *145*
Solian *143*
SR-141716 146
SR-142801, osanetant 146
SR-31742 146
SR-46349 147
SR-48692 147
Zomaril *144*
Zyprexa *145*

Seborrhea
ciclopirox olamine 530
Loprox *530*

Sepsis and Septicemia
anti-tumor necrosis factor-alpha 333
antithrombin III 334
atelimomab 334
CytoTAb *333*
drotrecogin alfa 334
E5531 334
GW 270773 335
IC14 335
Pafase *335*
pyridoxalated hemoglobin
   polyoxyethylene (PHP) 335
recombinant human activated
   protein C (rhAPC) 335
SB 249417 335
Segard *334*
tifacogin 335
Zovant *334*

Sexual Dysfunction
Alista *479, 570*
alprostadil 477, 569
apomorphine HCl 477, 569
Cialis *478, 570*
Daproxetine *479*
emprox *569*
Estratest *477, 570*
estrogens/methyltestosterone 477, 570
IC351 . . . . .478, 570
midodrine HCl 478
NMI-870 . . . . .478, 570
ProAmatine *478*
TA-1790 478
testoterone 478, 570
Topiglan *477*
Tostrelle *479, 570*

transdermal testosterone gel 479, 570
Vasofem *479, 570*

Shingles
vaccine, zoster 479

Sinus Infections
AG7088, anti-rhinoviral agent . . .376, 555
Avelox *376*
Bactroban *376, 556*
moxifloxacin .376
mupirocin 376, 556
SB 275833 . . . . .376, 556

Sjogren's Syndrome
IFNalpha *479*
interferon alpha 479

Skin Cancer
CpG 7909 280
eflornithine, DFMO
   (difluoromethylornydil) 280
FK-317 281
interleukin-12 gene therapy 281
Metvix PDT *281*

Skin Infections/Disorders
5G1.1 530
ADL 2-1294 530
AIC *532*
ALT-711 530
Cidecin *530*
daptomycin 530
HCT 1026 531
hypericin 531
Merrem *532*
MK-826, carbepenem 531
quinupristin/dalfopristin 531
Synercid *531*
transforming growth factor
   beta-2 (TGF-b2) 531
VIMRxyn *531*

Skin Wounds
becaplermin 532
dexamethasone 532
IontoDex *532*
keratinocyte growth factor-2
   (KGF-2) 532
Regranex *532*
Repifermin *532*

Sleep Disorders
BMS-214778 .114

doxylamine 114
epalon, CCD-3693 114
GABA agonist, anxiolytic 114
Gaboxadol *115*
GT-2331 114
modafinil 115
NBI-34060 115
Perceptin *114*
Provigil *115*
sodium oxybate (GHB) 115
SR-46349 115
thGRF 1-44 115
Xyrem *115*

Smoking Cessation
CP-526,555 . . . . .147, 376
GW 468816 . . . . .147, 376
LY-354740 . . . . .147, 377
nicotine addiction product 147, 377
SR-141716 . . . . .147, 377

Spinal Cord Injuries
fampridine 116, 510
leteprinim potassium, AIT-082 510
Neotrofin *510*
Neurelan *116, 510*
neurotrophin-3, NT-3 . . . . .116, 510
recombinant human bone morphogenic
   protein-2 (rhBMP-2) 116, 510

Staph Bacterial Infections
hyperimmune globulin 335
MBI 853NL *336*
Nabi StaphVAX *336*
Nabi-Altastaph *335*
Ramoplanin Oral *336*
SA-IGIV 336
vaccine, Staphylococcus aureus 336

Strokes
Abbokinase *119*
ancrod 116
Aptiganel *117*
Argatroban *119*
BB-10153 116
CerAxon *116*
citicoline sodium 116
clomethiazole 117
corleukin NIF 117
Cromafiban *117*
GP IIb/IIa 117
H376/95 117
ion-channel blocker 117
LBS-neurons .117

Therapeutic Indications Index/695

LDP-01 118
leteprinim potassium, AIT-082 118
licostinel, ACEA-1021 118
Neotrofin *118*
nitrone radical trap (NRT) 118
NPS 1506 118
NS-1209, SPD-502 118
NXY-059 119
porcine neural cells, stroke 119
prourokinase 119
SB 249417 119
TP-9201 119
Viprinex *116*
YM-872 119
Zendra *117*

Substance Abuse
lofexidine 148
Medisorb Naltrexone *148*
methadone/dextromethorphan 148
naltrexone 148
TA-CD *148*
therapeutic, substance abuse 148
vaccine, cocaine 148

Systemic Fungal Infections
Nyotran *533*
nystatin, AR-121 533

Systemic Lupus Erythematosus
5c8 (Anti CD-40 ligand
   antibody) 479, 533
Antova *479, 533*
Aslera *480, 533*
GL-701, prasterone 480, 533
IDEC-131 ....480, 533
LJP-394 ....480, 533

Thrombocytopenia
5c8 (anti CD-40 ligand antibody) .68, 281
Antova *68, 281*
argatroban 68
CBP-1011 ....68, 282
Colirest *68, 282*
MDX-33 ....68, 282
PI-88 ....68, 282
psoralen, S-59 ....69, 282
YM-294, oprelvekin 69, 282

Thrombosis
ancrod 42
Angiomax *43*
antithrombin III, rhATIII 42
AR69931 42

Argatroban *45*
AZD 6140 (AR-C126532) 42
bivalirudin 43
CCI-1004 43
desirudin/recombinant hirudin 43
DPC-444 43
enoxaparin sodium 43
Fibrimage *45*
Flocor *44*
GW 473178 43
Lovenox/Clexane *43*
melagatran 43
NCX 4016 44
ORG-31540/SR-90107A 44
poloxamer 188 N.F., CRL-5861 44
Revasc *43*
rNAPc2 44
SR-34006 45
technetium-99m-labeled FBD 45
Viprinex *42*
ZD4927 45

Thyroid Cancer
arcitumomab 283, 399
CEA-Scan 283, 399

Tinea Capitis
Lamisil *534*
terbinafine 534

Tourette's Syndrome
Inversine *120*
mecamylamine HCl 120

Traumatic Brain Injuries
Aptiganel *120*
dexanabinol, HU-211 120
ion-channel blocker 120

Tuberculosis
CDC 801 ....336, 377
SelCID 336, 377

Turner's Syndrome
human growth hormone 400

Ulcers
Ambicin *444*
Elangesic *444*
ibuprofen 444
nisin 444

Urinary Incontinence
(S)-sibutramine 482

ABT-232, NS-49 480
chondrocyte-alginate gel suspension ..480
Chondrogel *480*
darifenacin 481
duloxetine HCl, LY-248686 481
HCT 1026 481
I-OXY/ UROS Infusor 481
midodrine HCl 481
oxybutynin 481
ProAmatine *481*
S-oxybutynin 482
SB 223412 482
TAK-637 482
trospium chloride 482
Trospium *482*
YM-905 482

Urinary Tract Infections
amikacin 482, 571
chondrocyte-alginate gel
   suspension 483, 571
Chondrogel *483, 571*
Cidecin *483, 571*
CIPRO *483, 571*
ciprofloxacin 483, 571
daptomycin 483, 571
Factive *483, 571*
gemifloxacin mesylate 483, 571
Mikasome *482, 571*
MK-826, carbepenem 483, 571
vaccine, urinary tract infection ..483, 572
YM-617, tamsulosin 484, 572

Uterine Fibroids
goserelin acetate 572
YM-511 572
Zoladex FIB *572*

Vaccines
A streptococcus vaccine 337
AdjuVax-100a *341*
Aidsvax *343, 347*
BLP-25 337
C. difficile vaccine, CdVax 337
ChimeriVax JE *340*
Detox *340*
Epstein-Barr virus vaccine 337
ETEC vaccine 337
FluMist *340*
gene therapy, IL-2 and
   superantigen gene (SEB) 337
GeneVax *342*
Gvax *341*
H. pylori vaccine 338

696/Therapeutic Indications Index

hepatitis vaccine 338
HER-2/neu dendritic cell vaccine 338
HGP-30W 338
Infanrix 339
IR208 338
IR501 338
IR502 338
Melacine 345
Meningitec 345
MPL vaccine adjuvant 340
N. meningitidis A/C 339
Nabi StaphVAX .347
NeuroVax 338
Onyvax 105 341
Onyvax CR 340
Onyvax P 340
PeNta-HepB-IPV, vaccine 339
Peru-15 339
Prostvac 346
Pseudostat 346
QS-21 339
Quilimmune-M .345
Quilimmune-P .346
raltitrexed, ZD-1694 339
Ravax 338
Rotarix 339
rotavirus vaccine 339
Simplirix 342
StreptAvax 337
T-cell peptide vaccines 339
Td-IPV 340
tetanus/diphtheria booster 340
Tomudex 339
Twinrix-2 doses .338
Twinrix-three doses 343
typhoid vaccine 340
vaccine, 105AD7 341
vaccine, adjuvant 341
vaccine, allogeneic and autologous
    neuroblastoma cells 341
vaccine, cancer, (pSa) 342
vaccine, cancer .341
vaccine, DPT/Haemophilus
    influenzae type B 342
vaccine, Epstein-Barr virus 342
vaccine, genital herpes 342
vaccine, GMK 343
vaccine, hepatitis 343
vaccine, HIV-1 gp-120 prime-boost . .343
vaccine, HIV 343
vaccine, HIV 343
vaccine, HPV-16 VLP 344
vaccine, HPV 343
vaccine, human papilloma virus 344

vaccine, influenza 344
vaccine, malaria 344, 345
vaccine, melanoma 345
vaccine, meningitis B 345
vaccine, meningococcal C conjugate . .345
vaccine, meningococcus C 345
vaccine, MMR-varicella 346
vaccine, pneumococcal infections 346
vaccine, prostate cancer (rV-psa) 346
vaccine, Pseudomonas infection 346
vaccine, respiratory syncytial virus . .346
vaccine, Shigella flexneri and sonneii . .347
vaccine, Staphylococcus aureus 347
vaccine, Streptococcus pneumoniae . .347
vaccines, allergy 341
yellow fever vaccine 347
Zorcell 338

Vaginal Infection
Alferon N Gel 572
interferon (IFN), alfa-n3 572

Vancomycin Resistant Enterococci (VRE)
Ramoplanin Oral 347

Vascular Diseases
AngioMARK 45
ApoA-I Milano 45
MS-325 45

Venous Leg Ulcers
ifetroban sodium, BMS-180291 534

Vestibular Hypofunction
scopolamine 120, 556

Viral Infection
Alferon N Gel 348
Arilvax 351
BMS-200475 347
ChimeriVax JE .349
cidofovir 348
cidofovir 348
Entecavir 347
Epstein-Barr virus vaccine 348
HumaSPECT/Infectious Diseases 351
interferon (IFN) alfa-n3 348
MEDI-517 348
OST 577 348
Ostavir 348
pleconaril 349
psoralen, S-59 349
ribavirin 349

T611 349
thymalfasin 349
vaccine, DPT/Haemophilus
    influenzae type B 350
vaccine, Epstein-Barr virus 350
vaccine, HPV-16 VLP 350
vaccine, HPV 350
vaccine, human papilloma virus 350
vaccine, respiratory syncytial virus . .350
vaccine, rotavirus 351
Virazole 349
Vistide 348
votumumab 351
VP 14637 351
VX-148 351
yellow fever vaccine 351
Zadaxin 349

White Blood Cell Disorders
alitretinoin, ALRT-1057 69
LDI-200 69
Panretin 69
psoralen, S-59 70
RF-1012 70
SD/01 70
SMART M195 70

Wounds
Apligraf 534
imaging agent, entire body 534
P53 534
therapeutic, wound healing 534
VM-301, OAS 1000 535

Scientific and Trade Name Index

Contained in this index are the names of all of the therapies profiled in the second edition. Scientific names are set in standard type and potential trade names are set in italics.

(+)-norcisapride 420
(R,R)-formoterol 356, 369
(S)-sibutramine 452, 482, 577
+DDMS 81, 102
17-beta estradiol/trimegestone ..389, 391, 493, 566, 568
2CVV 87, 305
3-month Leuprogel 269, 466, 586
30-day Leuprogel 269, 466, 586
5-aminolevulinic acid 515
5-HT1A partial agonist 134
5c8 (Anti CD-40 ligand antibody) 68, 281, 458, 479, 533
5D12 412
5G1.1 ....456, 503, 530
8-cyclopentyl 1,3-dipropylxanthine, CPX 367
A streptococcus vaccine 337
A4, prodrug 175
abacavir 316
abarelix depot, PPI-149 ....263, 460, 580
abarelix, PPI-149 564
Abarelix-Depot F 564
Abbokinase 39, 119
abciximab, c7E3 ....13, 29, 36
Abetafen 272, 470, 590
abiraterone acetate 263, 460, 580
ABT-232, NS-49 480
ABT-594, epibatidine 104, 426, 496
ABT-627 ....263, 461, 580
ABT-773 298
ABX-EGF 175
ABX-IL8 ....503, 523
AC2993 LAR 381
AC2993 381

AC3056 40
acamprosate 125
acetaminophen/dextromethorphan ..104, 496
acetyl-L-carnitine 75, 387
ACH-126,443 ....308, 316, 426
Actos 385
Ad5FGF4 26
Adderall 83, 132
adefovir dipivoxil, GS-840 ......308, 426
Adenoviral p53 ....84, 158
Adentri 23, 456
adjuvanted influenza 328, 370
AdjuVax-100a 274, 341, 471, 591
ADL 2-1294 .296, 316, 516, 517, 522, 523, 530, 539
ADL 8-2698 422
Adriamycin 57, 217
Advantage-S 292
ADX-153 ....104, 496
AE-941 ....64, 175, 223, 247, 275, 473, 523, 543
Aerobid 357
AERx diabetes management system ..381
AFP-Scan 221
AG-1749, lansoprazole 420, 422
AG-701 ....316, 522
AG7088, anti-rhinoviral agent ..332, 376, 554, 555
AGI-1067 ....20, 35, 40
AGIX-4207 504
AGN 192024 ....542, 545
AGT-1 ....297, 504
AI-401 381
AI-502 325
AI-700 26
AIC 296, 532, 550
AIDS gene therapy 287, 316
Aidsvax 294, 324, 343
AIP-001 75
AJ-9677, TAK-677 382

698/Scientific and Trade Name Index

Albuferon *314, 432*
albuterol 356, 363
Albuterol *362*
Alcar *75, 387*
aldesleukin, interleukin-2 (IL-2) . .54, 214, 236, 246, 275, 317, 473
Alesse *515*
alfa inhalation solution 367
Alferon LDO *321*
Alferon N Gel *308, 348, 521, 572*
Alferon N Injection *311, 321, 429*
alfuzosin 447, 575
Alibra *451, 576*
Aliminase *434*
Alista *479, 570*
alitretinoin, ALRT-1057 .69, 161, 223, 524
AlloMune *63, 327, 241, 460*
Allovectin-7 . . . .*213, 247, 251*
alpha-1 antitrypsin (AAT) 367
alpha-1 proteinase inhibitor 369
Alphagan *543*
Alphanate *31, 52*
alprostadil/prazosin hydrochloride451, 576
alprostadil 450, 477, 569, 575
Alprox-TD, Befar *450, 575*
ALT-711 . . . . .530, 539
altropane 80, 110, 129
ALVAC-HIV 1 . . . . .287, 317
ALX-0600 .422
ALX-0646 94
ALX1-11 493
Ambicin *444*
AmBisome *518, 519*
AMD Fab .544
AMD-3100 . . . . .287, 317
Amdray *255*
Amevive *528*
AMG 073 .399
amifostine 202
amikacin 298, 372, 482, 552, 571
amindarone-best, SR-33589 15
amino-cyclopropane carboxylic acid 125, 126, 134
aminopterin 54, 205, 215
Amio-Aqueous IV *15*
amiodarone HCl 15
Amiscan *38*
AMISTAD-II 36
amisulpride, SL 91.1076 143
amlexanox liquid 202
amlodipine besylate 13
amoxicillin/clavulante potassium 298
AMP-579 36
Ampakine *144*

Ampalex *75, 144*
amphotericin B 518
Ampligen *88, 244, 278, 306, 322, 476*
Amylin *561*
AN-1792 75
Anadrol-50 . . . .*291*
anastrozole, ZD-1033 161
ancrod 18, 42, 116
Andractim *288, 390, 579*
Androsorb *391, 568, 579*
anecortave acetate 544
AnergiX.MS *101*
AnergiX.RA *509*
Angiocol *189*
AngioMARK *39, 41, 45*
Angiomax *13, 43*
Angiostatin with radiation therapy 187
Angiozyme *162*
Annamycin *54, 162, 215*
Anogesic *403, 426, 516*
Antegren *100, 413, 436*
anti B-7 humanized antibodies . . .51, 156, 325, 458
anti-angiogenic ribozyme 162
anti-CD11a, hu1124 . . . . .459, 524
anti-hepatitis B 309, 426
anti-hepatitis C 309, 427
anti-IFNg .504
anti-interleukin-5 MAb (Anti-IL-5) . .356
Anti-LFA-1, odulimomab 325, 459
anti-tumor necrosis factor-alpha 333
Anticort *291, 323*
antidepressant 134
antihemophilic factor 31, 52
antithrombin III, rhATIII 18, 42
antithrombin III 334
Antova *68, 281, 458, 479, 533*
Antrin/Photoangioplasty *35, 39*
APC 2059 .434
APC8015 . . . . .264, 461, 581
APC8020 . . . . .64, 248
APC8024 . . . . .162, 193, 251, 403
APL400-020 V-B 62, 240, 297
APL400-024Px 306, 520, 564, 578
Apligraf *534*
ApoA-I Milano 45
Apomine *274, 471, 591*
apomorphine HCl 451, 477, 569, 576
apomorphine 110
Aposyn/Taxotere . .*165, 179, 227, 266, 463, 583*
Apotsyn/Xeloda *165*
Apra *264, 279, 462, 581*
Aptiganel *117, 120*

Aptosyn/Gemzar *227*
Aptosyn/LHRH agonist *266, 463, 583*
Aptosyn/Navelbine *227*
Aptosyn/Taxotere/carboplatin *234*
Aptosyn *153, 165, 195, 227, 266, 405, 417, 463. 583*
AR-522 . . . . .54, 162, 215
AR-C68397AA 364
AR-C89855 364
AR-H047108 . . . . .421, 422
AR-H049020 382
AR69931 . . . . .13, 42
Aranesp *177, 456*
arcitumomab 162, 223, 283, 399
Arecoline *79*
argatroban .68
Argatroban *45, 119*
Aricept *75, 81, 88, 130*
Ariflo *360, 365*
Arilvax *347, 351*
Arimidex *161*
aripiprazole, OPC-14597, OPC-31 75, 143
Ariza *134*
Aroplatin *247, 279, 477*
arsenic trioxide (ATO) 55, 62, 65, 153, 190, 215, 237, 248, 264, 275, 447, 461, 473, 559, 581
AS-013 . . . . .36, 390
asimadoline 104, 490, 497
Aslera *480, 533*
Asmanex *359*
Atacand *22, 33, 453*
atelimomab 334
*Atragen*60, 219, 272, 240, 278, 469, 476, 589
Atrisone *515*
Augmentin SR *298*
Avandia *386*
Avapro *22, 103, 392*
avasimibe 40
Avelox *301, 363, 371, 373, 376*
Avicine *196, 259, 264, 395, 406, 439, 462, 582*
Avonex *84, 99, 158, 375*
AVP-923 . . . . .79, 102, 487, 497
Avrend *276, 473*
Axokine *394*
AZ 242 (AR-H039242) 382
AZD 6140 (AR-C126532) 42
AZD2563 .298
AZD3409 .176
AZD6474 .176
azimilide 16
B-vax 174
Bactroban *376, 556*

Scientific and Trade Name Index/699

Balsalazide 437
BAM-002 223
Basen 387
batimastat, ISV-120 540
BAY 12-9566 ....223, 251, 258, 490
BAY 13-9952 20
BB-10153 ....29, 116
BB-2827 504
BB-3644 176
BCH-3963, LEF576 ....104, 497
BCI-Immune Activator 155, 449
BCX-1470 18
BCX-34 ....55, 62, 215, 241, 317
BEC2 224
becaplermin 387, 518, 532
bectumomab 237
befloxatone 134
Benefen 491
benzestrom 105, 488, 497
Beraprost 34, 41, 455
Beta LT 64, 67, 242, 249
BetaRx 382
Betaseron 98
bexarotene 162, 208, 224, 241,
 516, 522, 524
Bexxar 239
bicalutimide 264, 461, 581
BioByPass 28, 42
Birex 529
biricodar dicitrate, VX-710 ...224, 251
bismuth subcitrate/metronidazole/
 tetracycline 425
bivalirudin 13, 43
blonanserin, AD-5423 144
blood substitute 18, 224
Blopress 23, 382
BLP-25 ....224, 337
BMS-182751, JM-216 ....225, 252
BMS-186295, SR-47436 (irbesartan) ..22,
 103, 392
BMS-186716, omapatrilat 22, 32, 453
BMS-193884 ....22, 451, 576
BMS-200475 ....309, 427, 347
BMS-201038 32
BMS-207147 518
BMS-214778 114
BMS-223131 ....451, 576
BMS-232632 ....287, 317
BNP 1350 176
Bonviva 167, 495
bosentan 32, 453
Botox 94, 489, 497
botulinum toxin type A,
 AGN-191622 ....94, 489, 497

brain derived neurotrophic factor, BDNF .
 80, 487
brasofensine, NS-2214,
 BMS-204756 111
BrevaRex MAb 66, 249
brimonidine tartrate 543
bromocriptine, ER-230 393
brompheniramine/
 pseudoephedrine HCl 294, 549
BTI-322, MEDI-507 .....326, 459, 524
budesonide 412, 434
Budoxis, Oxis 358, 364
BufferGel 562
bupivacaine 105, 498
BuSpar 126
buspirone HCl 126
buspirone 126
C. difficile vaccine, CdVax ..298, 337, 422
C319-14/6 ....287, 519
Cachexon 182, 290, 416
calcimimetics 399
calcitonin 494, 568
Campath 58, 218
Campyvax 304, 416, 420
CancerVax, C-VAX 242
candesartan cilexetil ..22, 23, 33, 382, 453
capecitabine/docetaxel 163
capecitabine 195, 405
capravirine 288, 318
Captelan 23, 33, 453
captopril 23, 33, 453
Carbatrol 134
Cardizide SR 13
cariporide mesylate, HOE-642 ...27, 36
Carn 1000 434
Carn 750 176
CarraVex 176
carvedilol 23
Casodex 264, 461, 581
CAT-152 543
CBP-1011 ....68, 282, 412, 435
CCI-1004 43
CCI-779 176
CCR2b 504
CD40 ligand 276, 473
CDC 801 ....65, 98, 248, 297,
 298, 336, 357, 377, 412, 504
CDP 870 505
CDP-571, BAY 10-356 .....413, 435, 505
CE-1050 125
CEA-Cide 167, 181, 198,
 229, 253, 260, 396, 408, 441
CEA-Scan 162, 223, 283, 399
Cea-Tricom 200, 410

CeaVac/TriAb 200, 235, 410
CeaVac 200, 410
cefditoren pivoxil 372, 552
CEP-1347 ....75, 111
CEP-2563 ....264, 461, 581
CEP-701 .....258, 264, 394, 439, 461, 581
Ceplene 57, 65, 217, 243, 248,
 276, 311, 429, 474
CerAxon 116
Cereport 161
cerivastatin sodium 20
Certa 20
Certican 326
cetirizine HCl 549
CETP vaccine, CETi-1 21
CFTR, GR-213487B 367
ChimeriVax JE 340, 349
Cholestagel/Zocor 21
chondrocyte-alginate gel
 suspension 480, 483, 571
Chondrogel 480, 483, 571
Chrysalin 487
CI-1004 490
CI-1033 ....163, 208, 225
CI-1042, ONYX-015 ....83, 153, 157,
 190, 195, 208, 225, 258, 394, 405, 439,
 447, 559
Cialis 451, 478, 570, 576
ciclopirox olamine 519, 530
Cidecin 29, 299, 483, 530, 571
cidofovir ..83, 214, 309, 348, 427, 540, 551
cilansetron 437
CIPRO 483, 571
ciprofloxacin 483, 571
Circulase 36, 390
cisplatin/epinephrine 163, 176, 195,
 205, 208, 220, 242, 406, 416
cisplatin/vinblastine/amifostine 225
citalopram HBr 134
citicoline sodium 116
Claritin/Singulair 333, 555
clevudine 309, 427
clindamycin 515
Clofarabine 61, 64, 220
clomethiazole 117
clonadine gel 105, 498
CLX-0901 382
CNS stimulant 80, 130
CNS-5161 94
Coactinon 288, 318
Coagulin-B 32, 53
Col-3 ....214, 329
Colirest 68, 282, 412, 435
collagenase for injection 460, 488, 580

colsevelam/simvastatin 21
Combidex 173, 222, 273, 470, 590
Combretastatin 175
Comtan 111
conjugated estrogen tablets 389, 391, 566, 568
Conquer-A 294, 549
Contraceptive Patch 561
Copaxone 98
Cordase 460, 488, 580
Cordox 49
Coreg 23
corleukin NIF 53, 117
Corlopam 24, 457
Coviracil 309, 318, 427
COX 189 ....105, 490, 498, 505
CP-122,721 135
CP-358,774 ....163, 209, 225, 252
CP-461 177
CP-526,555 ....147, 376
CP-529,414 40
CP-99142 202
CPC-111 49
CpG 7909 ....237, 246, 280
CpG compound 295, 357, 549
CPI-1189 ....111, 288
Crestor 22
CRF receptor antagonist (partnered), NBI-37582 ......126, 135
CRF receptor antagonist (proprietary) 126, 135
Cromafiban 14, 27, 117
cromolyn sodium 357
CS-866 ....33, 454
CT-2584 ....264, 279, 462, 581
CT-3 ....105, 498
CTLA4-Ig 55, 215
CTP-37 .196, 259, 264, 395, 406, 439, 462, 582
CV706 ....265, 462, 582
CV787 ....265, 462, 582
cVax-Pr 265, 462, 582
CVT-124 ....23, 456
CVT-510 16
CX-516, BDP-12 ....75, 144
CX-619, ORG-24448 135
Cymeval 306, 539
CyPat 272, 469, 589
Cystavision 540
cysteamine hydrochloride 540
cytarabine liposome injection 330
cytostatics 153, 448
CytoTAb 333
Cytovene 306, 539

d-methylphenidate HCl 81, 130
D1927 177
D2163, BMS 275291 177
DAB-452 144
dadsone topical gel 515
DAPD 318
Daproxetine 452, 479, 577
daptomycin 29, 299, 483, 530, 571
darbepoetin alfa 177, 456
darifenacin 481
daunorubicin citrate 55, 62, 216, 237
DaunoXome 55, 62, 216, 237
DB-075 415
DB-289 ....373, 552
DCVax 274, 471, 591
decitabine 49, 56, 216, 226
declopramide 196, 406
Dehydrex 542
denileukin diftitox 56, 62, 216, 241
DENSPM 226, 243, 259, 276, 395, 439, 474
DepoAmikacin 298
DepoBupivacaine 105, 498
DepoCyt 330
desirudin/recombinant hirudin 43
Deskar 100, 375
desloratadine, descarboethoxyloratadine 295, 332, 549, 554
Detox 173, 340
dexamethasone 105, 498, 532, 540
dexanabinol, HU-211 120
Dexloxiglumide 438
DHA-paclitaxel 184
Diamyd 387
diarysulfonylurea, ILX-295501 ..226, 242, 252, 276, 473
diclofenac, ISV-205 ....540, 543
diclofenac 106, 209, 288, 498
diethylnorspermine 226, 243, 259, 276, 395, 439, 474
DiffGAM 300, 415
difluoromethylornithine (DFMO)191, 318, 559
dihydrotestosterone 288, 390, 579
diltiazem HCl/hydrochlorothiazide 13
diltiazem HCl 33, 454
dimethyl sulfoxide, DMSO ..102, 202, 488
Diovan 26, 35, 38, 455
Dirame 109, 492, 502
disaccharide tripeptide glycerol dipalmitoyl 279
DISC GM-CSF 246
DMP-450 ....288, 318
DNK 333 ....333, 357, 364, 555

docetaxel hydrate ..84, 157, 163, 206, 209, 226, 252, 418
Docosanol 307, 520, 565, 578
donepezil hydrochloride, E2020 ....75, 81, 88, 130
dotarizine 95
dOTC 287
DOV 216303 125
doxercalciferol 456
Doxil, Caelyx 164, 177, 221, 226, 265, 462, 582
Doxil/Taxotere 164
doxorubicin HCl 164, 177, 221, 226, 265, 462, 582
doxorubicin/docetaxel 164
doxylamine 114
DPC-444 ....43, 382
DPC-543, DMP-543 76
DPI-3290 ....106, 499
DPP 728/LAF 237 382
DPPE 265, 463, 582
Dromos 41
dronabinol 76, 88
drotrecogin alfa 334
DTA 201 142
DTI-0009 16
DU125530 ....126, 135
DU127090 142
duloxetine HCl, LY-248686 .....135, 481
Duodopa 112
Duragesic 106, 499
DX-8951 178
Dynepo 49
E21R 178
E5531 334
E7010 178
ecopipam 393
ecteinascidin, ET-743 178
efalizumab monoclonal antibody 525
eflornithine, DFMO (difluoromethylornydil) ..154, 164, 266, 280, 448, 463, 583
EGF-receptor specific monoclonal antibody 178
EHT899 ....309, 427
Elangesic 420, 435, 444
Eldepryl 113, 139
eletriptan 95
Elidel 297, 517
EMD 82633 ....154, 164, 178, 209, 252, 276, 448, 474
EMD-57445 144
Emitasol, Pramidin 423, 425
emivirine 288, 318

Scientific and Trade Name Index/701

emprox 569
emtricitabine 309, 318, 427
Enbrel 23, 505, 525
endothelin A receptor
  antagonist 23
enoxaparin sodium/tirofiban 27
enoxaparin sodium 17, 43
entacapone 111
Entecavir 309, 347, 427
Entocort CR 434
Entocort 412
epalon, CCD-3693 ....92, 114
EPI-2010 357
Epivir 321
epratuzumab 237
Epstein-Barr virus vaccine 337, 348
eptifibatide 27, 37
ERA-923 165
Ergoset 393
erythropoietin 49
Escitalopram 134
esprolol 14, 95, 141
Estalis 494
Esterom 105, 488, 497
estradiol, 17-beta 389, 566
estradiol/norethisterone acetate 494
estradiol/progestin 389, 494, 566
estradiol 389, 566
Estrasorb 389, 566
Estratest 388, 477, 566, 570
Estrogel 389, 566
estrogen/pravastatin 21
estrogen 391, 392, 494, 568
estrogens/methyltestosterone 388,
  477, 566, 570
etanercept 23, 505, 525
ETEC vaccine 299, 337, 415
ethinyl estradiol/trimegestrone 561
Ethyol 202
etilevodopa, TV-1203 111
etodolac 106, 490, 499, 505
Etomoxir 26
etonogestrel 562
evernimicin 299
everolimus 326
Evista 28, 171
Evra 562
EWBH treatment 289, 319
Exendin-4 383
exendin 383
exisulind/capecitabine 165
exisulind/docetaxel 165, 179, 227,
  266, 463, 583
exisulind/gemcitabine HCl 227

exisulind/vinorelbine tartrate
  injection 227
exisulind 153, 165, 195,
  227, 266, 405, 417, 463, 583
EXO-226 388
expected to be Abilitat 75, 143
EYE-001, NX-1838 544
ezetimibe 21
Factive 299, 483, 571
factor VIII gene therapy 31, 32, 53
fampridine 98, 116, 510
farnesyl protein transferase
  inhibitor 179
Faslodex 167, 205
Femara 169
fenoldopam mesylate,
  SK&F-82526 ....24, 457
fentanyl transderm al system 106, 499
fentanyl 106, 499
Fiblast 28, 41
Fibrimage 45
fibrin sealant 54
fibrinogen-receptor antagonist 14, 37
Fibrostat 517, 530
FK-317 ......165, 179, 266, 281, 464, 584
FK463, echinocandin 296, 305,
  356, 519, 551
FK960 76
FKBP-neuroimmunophilin ligands ...111
flavopiridol, HMR-1275 .....56, 206,
  216, 228, 417
flesinoxan 127, 136
Flixotide, Flovent 358, 364
Flocor 44, 50, 371
FLT3 ligand ...63, 166, 179, 237, 241, 253
Fluad 328, 370
Fludara 238
fludarabine phosphate 238
flumecinol 67
FluMist 328, 340, 370
flunisolide 357
fluoropyrimidine, S-1 ....179, 206, 418
fluoxetine HCl 136, 141, 142
fluoxetine/olanzapine 136
fluticasone propionate 358, 364
fluticasone/salmeterol 333, 555
fluvoxamine maleate 127, 141
Fluvoxamine-CR 127, 141
FMdC 196, 228, 253, 406
follitropin alpha 567
Foradil 358, 376
formoterol 358, 364, 376
Fortical Injection 492
fosphenytoin sodium injection 90

frovatriptan 95
FTY 720 326
G3139/androgen blockade ..267, 464, 584
G3139/cyclophosphamide 238
G3139/dacarbazine 246
G3139/docetaxel 166, 267, 464, 584
G3139/irinotecan 196, 406
G3139/mitoxantrone ..196, 267, 406, 464,
  584
G3139 ....56, 57, 216
GABA agonist, anxiolytic 90, 114
gabapentin 90
Gaboxadol 115
galantamine hydrobromide 76, 88,
  89, 305
galasomite 299
gallium maltolate 63, 154, 250,
  267, 319, 448, 465, 584
gamma interferon 367
ganaxolone, CCD-1042 ....90, 95
ganciclovir 306, 539
GAR-936 299
Gastrimmune 200, 206, 207,
  222, 262, 398, 411, 417, 419, 443
gatifloxacin 299, 552
GBC-590 ....197, 259, 267,
  395, 407, 440, 464, 584
GEM-231 180
GEM-92 ....289, 319
gemcitabine HCl 166, 228, 253,
  259, 395, 440, 448
gemifloxacin mesylate 299, 483, 571
Gemzar ..166, 228, 253, 259, 395, 440, 448
Genasense/androgen blockade 267, 464, 584
Genasense/cyclophosphamide 238
Genasense/dacarbazine 246
Genasense/Irinotecan 196, 406
Genasense/Mitoxantrone 196, 267,
  406, 464, 584
Genasense/Mylotarg 56, 216
Genasense/Taxotere 166, 267, 464, 584
Genasense 57, 216
gene therapy, IL-2 and superantigen
  gene (SEB) 243, 337
gene therapy, interleukin-2 .....209, 243
gene therapy, leukemia 57, 217
gene-activated erythropoietin 49
Generx 26
Genevax-HBV 315, 433
GeneVax-HIV-Px 294, 324
Genevax-HSV-Px 306, 520, 564, 578
Genevax-TCR 62, 240, 297
GeneVax 174, 274, 342, 472, 591
Genvascor 39

702/Scientific and Trade Name Index

gepirone ...136	*Hemolink* ...*18, 224*	ICI-182,780 ...167, 205
Geppar (proposed to PTO) ...*136*	*Hemopure* ...*49, 489*	ICL 670 ...52
GI 181771 ...393, 417	*Hepagene* ...*314, 433*	icodextrin, Extraneal ...457
GI 198745 ...381, 447, 516, 575	heparinase I ...19	*Icodial* ...*457*
GI 262570 ...383	hepatitis A ...310, 428	IDEC-114 ...526
GL-331 ...57, 193, 217, 228, 276, 403, 474	hepatitis B immune globulin ...310, 428	IDEC-131 ...480, 526, 506, 533
GL-701, prasterone ...480, 533	hepatitis B immunotherapy, HBV/MF59 ...310, 428	IDEC-152 ...295, 358, 549
glatiramer acetate ...98	hepatitis C protein ...310, 428	IDEC-Y2B8, In2B8 ...238
Gliadel ...*86, 159*	hepatitis vaccine ...338	IDN-6556 ...310, 428
Glivec ...*57, 217*	*Heptazyme* ...*312, 430*	ifetroban sodium, BMS-180291 ...39, 40, 534
glyceryl monolaurin, T-100 ...522	HER-2/neu dendritic cell vaccine ...166, 253, 338	*IFNalpha* ...*479*
Glylorin ...*522*	*Herceptin* ...*173*	IL-1ra/Anakinra ...506
glyminox vaginal gel ...561	HGP-30W ...320, 338	iloperidone ...144
GnRH Pharmaccine ...174, 205, 273, 471, 564, 590	HGTV-43 ...320	iloprost ...40
Gonal-F ...567	histamine dihydrochloride ...65, 217, 243, 248, 276, 474	ILX-651 ...181
goserelin acetate ...166, 567, 572	HIV-1 immunogen ...320	IM862 ...214, 243, 253, 267, 330, 465, 585
GP IIb/IIa ...14, 27, 117	*HMFG1* ...*257*	*Imagent* ...*19, 184*
GPX-100 ...57, 166, 180, 217	HMR-1883/1098 ...24	imaging agent, entire body ...534
growth hormone releasing factor (GRF) ...388	HMR-3647, RU-64,004 ...300, 373, 552	imaging agent ...221
GT-2331 ...76, 81, 114, 130	HMR-4004 ...289, 320	imatinib, STI 571 ...57, 217
Gvax ...*61, 220, 235, 245, 262, 274, 341, 399, 443, 471, 591*	HOE-351 ...250, 523	IMC-1C11 ...197, 407
GW 150013 ...127	HP-3 ...362, 365, 367	IMC-C225, CPT-11 ...167, 197, 210, 228, 260, 268, 277, 396, 407, 440, 465, 475, 585
GW 270773 ...335	HP-4 ...180	*Imigran, Imitrex* ...*97*
GW 273293 ...90, 133	HspE7 ...191, 307, 521, 559	*ImmTher* ...*279*
GW 320659, 1555U88 ...81, 130	HSPPC-96 ...197, 206, 238, 243, 259, 277, 280, 395, 407, 418, 440, 474	IMMU-MN14, anti-CEA ...167, 181, 198, 229, 253, 260, 396, 408, 441
GW 328267 ...358, 364	Hu-901 ...295, 549	immune globulin (IG-IV) ...300
GW 406381 ...106, 499	HuC242-DM1/SB-408075 ...197, 228, 259, 395, 407, 440	immune globulin (IgG) ...300, 415
GW 419458, DISC-HSV ...306, 520, 564, 578	human albumin microspheres ...14, 27, 30	immune globulin intravenous ...51, 156, 311, 429
GW 427353 ...383, 393	human endostatin protein ...180	immune globulin ...310, 429
GW 433908 ...319	human growth hormone ...400	immunocontraception ...561
GW 468816 ...96, 147, 376	human liver cells ...438, 439	immunostimulatory sequences (ISS) candidate ...311, 429
GW 473178 ...16, 43	human muscle cells, cardiac disease 30, 37	immunotherapeutic, AML ...57, 311, 429
GW 572016 ...180	*HumaRAD-HN* ...*213*	*Implanon* ...*562*
GW 597599 ...136	*HumaSPECT/BR* ...*174*	*Incel* ...*224, 236, 251, 257, 280*
GW 650250 ...136	*HumaSPECT/Infectious Diseases* ...*351*	*Infanrix* ...*313, 339, 431*
GW 660511 ...33, 454	HuMax-CD4 ...506, 525	INGN 241 (mda-7) ...167, 181, 229
GW-650250A, NS-2389 ...136	*Humicade* ...*413, 435, 505*	INGN-201, adenoviral p53 ...154, 168, 181, 210, 229, 254, 268, 448, 465, 585
H. pylori vaccine ...300, 338, 423	HuN901-DM1 ...228	INGN-201 ...84, 158
H376/95 ...37, 117	*Hycamtin* ...*199, 234, 256, 409*	inhaled insulin ...383
HBVIg ...*310, 428*	*HydrocoDex* ...*104, 496*	INN-00835 ...136
HCI-436 ...310, 428	hydromorphone ...107, 500	INS316 ...229
HCT 1026 ...481, 494, 516, 525, 531	hypericin ...63, 84, 526, 531	INS365 ophthalmic ...541
HCT 3012 ...107, 499	hyperimmune globulin ...335	INS365 ...363, 368
HE2000 ...428	hyperteria/doxorubicin ...253	INS37217 respiratory ...368, 541
Hectorol Capsules ...*456*	I-OXY/ UROS Infusor ...481	insulin-like growth factor-I (IGF-I) ...491
Helicide ...*425*	ibandronate ...167, 495	
Helivax ...*425*	ibuprofen ...420, 435, 444, 491	
hemoglobin glutamer-250 (bovine) ...49, 489	IC14 ...335	
hemoglobin ...54	IC351 ...451, 478, 570, 576	

Scientific and Trade Name Index/703

insulin .... .383
Intal HFA-227 ....*357*
Integrilin *27, 37*
interferon (IFN) alfa-n3 ...308, 311, 321, 348, 429, 521, 572
interferon alfa-2b/ribavirin 311, 430
interferon alfa-2b .... .58, 181, 218, 244, 311, 429
interferon alpha .... .479
interferon beta-1a .... .84, 99, 158, 375
interferon beta-1b .... .98
interleukin (IL) .... .168, 210, 268, 321, 465, 585
interleukin-1 (IL-1) trap .... .506
interleukin-10 .... .312, 430, 438, 526
interleukin-12 (IL-12) .... .277, 289, 312, 430, 475
interleukin-12 gene therapy ..... .210, 281
interleukin-4 (IL-4) fusion toxin, NBI-3001 .... .85, 158
interleukin-4 (IL-4) .... .359
IntraDose *163, 176, 195, 205, 208, 220, 242, 406, 416*
intranasal metoclopramide 423, 425
intravitreal hyaluronidase .... .541
Inversine *81, 120, 130*
Invicorp *452, 578*
ion-channel blocker .... .117, 120
IontoDex *105, 498, 532, 540*
IP501 ....*125, 312, 430, 438*
IPL 576,092 ....*359*
IR208 ....*99, 338*
IR501 ....*338, 506*
IR502 ....*338, 526*
Iressa *190, 201, 208, 236, 275, 411, 420, 472, 592*
Irofulven *170, 183, 192, 194, 198, 221, 232, 255, 261, 270, 277, 397, 442, 404, 408, 467, 475, 560, 587*
ISAtx247 ....*326, 506, 526*
ISIS 2503 ....*168, 193, 229, 260, 396, 403, 441*
ISIS 3521 ....*168, 230*
ISIS 5132, CGP 69846A *169, 182, 193, 230, 260, 286, 396, 403, 441, 466, 585*
ISIS-13312 ....*306, 539*
ISIS-14803 ....*312, 430*
ISIS-2302 ....*413, 435, 459, 527*
isradipine .... .33, 454
JO-1784, CI-1019 .... .137
Karenitecin *176*
KC-11458 .... .421
Keraform *542*

keratinocyte growth factor (KGF) .... .202, 423
keratinocyte growth factor-2 (KGF-2) .... .51, 156, 203, 435, 532
Ketek *303*
ketoprofen patch .... .107, 500
ketoprofen .... .491
ketotifen fumarate .... .295, 541, 550
Ketotop *491*
Kineret *506*
KRP-297 .... .383
L-glutathione .... .182, 290, 416
L-Vax *61, 220*
Lambda *457*
Lamisil *250, 523, 534*
lamivudine .... .321
lanoteplase, BMS-200980 37
lansoprazole .... .421, 423
lanthanum carbonate .... .457
lasofoxifene .... .495
latanoprost .... .543
LBS-neurons .... .117
LDI-200 ...... .58, 69, 218, 269, 466, 586
LDP-01 .... .30, 118
LDP-02 .... .413, 436
LDP-03 .... .58, 218
LDP-341, PS-341 ..... .65, 182, 249
LDP-392 .... .296
LDP-977 .... .359
LEF .... .107, 500
leptin .... .383, 393
lercanidipine .... .33, 454
leteprinim potassium, AIT-082 ...76, 101, 102, 111, 118, 510
letrozole .... .169
Leucotropin *52, 156, 203*
Leuplin 3M DPS *273, 471, 591*
leuprolide acetate .... .269, 466, 586
LeuTech *424, 436, 493*
Leuvectin *272, 279, 470, 476, 589*
Levaquin *552*
levocetirizine .... .295, 550
levodopa/carbidopa .... .112
levofloxacin .... .552
levonorgestrel/ethinyl estradiol .... .515, 562
levonorgestrel *562*
Levovist *31*
Levulan Photodynamic Therapy *515*
LF 15-0195 .... .507
LGD-1550 ....17, 156, 182, 191, 211, 559
LHRH, luteinizing hormone-releasing hormone antagonist .... .567

licostinel, ACEA-1021 .... .118
Lidocaine *110, 503*
liposomal amphotericin B .... .519
Liposomal Encapsulated Paclitaxel ...419
liposomal ether lipid .... .58, 66, 218, 230, 249, 269, 466, 586
liposomal prostaglandin E1, PGE-1 .... .30, 35
Liprostin *30, 35*
LiquiVent *355, 375*
lisofylline, CT-1501R .... .51, 59
LJP-394 .... .457, 480, 533
Lodine *106, 490, 499, 505*
lofexidine .... .148
lomefloxacin HCl .... .300, 472, 592
Loprox *519, 530*
loratadine/montelukast sodium .... .333, 555
Lotrafiban *38*
Lovastatin XL *21*
Lovenox/Aggrastat *27*
Lovenox/Clexane *17, 43*
LTB 019 ....*365*
LU 26-054, SSRI *137*
Lu 35-139 ....*143*
Lucanthone *161*
lucinactant .... .355, 375
Lumigan *542, 545*
LY-333531 .... .103, 392, 541
LY-354740 .... .127, 147, 377
LY231514, antifolate .... .183
LY333328 .... .300
LY466700 .... .312, 430
LymphoCide *237*
LymphoScan *237*
M-Vax *245*
M100907 .... .144
Macritonin *494, 568*
marimastat, BB-2516 .... .85, 158, 169, 230, 254, 261, 397, 441
Marinol *76, 88*
MARstem *51, 173*
matrix metalloprotease inhibitor (MMP) .... .85, 491, 544
maxacalcitol .... .527
Maxaquin *300, 472, 592*
MB-U820 .... .423
MBI 226 .... .301
MBI 594AN .... .515
MBI 853NL *336*
MBX-102 .... .384
MCC .... .155, 449
MDAM (γ-methylene-10-deazaaminopterin) .... .183

704/Scientific and Trade Name Index

MDX-210 . . . . .169, 194, 207, 231, 254, 261, 270, 277, 397, 404, 419, 442, 467, 475, 587
MDX-220 . . . . . . .198, 205, 207, 231, 254, 261, 270, 397, 408, 419, 442, 467, 587
MDX-22 . . . . .52, 59, 218
MDX-33 . . . . .49, 68, 282
MDX-447, H-447 . .85, 155, 159, 170, 211, 231, 449
MDX-RA 539
ME-609 . . . . .315, 522
mecamylamine HCl 81, 120, 130
MEDI-507 527
MEDI-517 . . . . .191, 348, 560
Medisorb Naltrexone 148
Melacine 245, 345
melagatran 43
memantine 77, 103, 290, 392, 543
Memantine 79
Memex 77
Meningitec 94, 331, 345
mepolizumab, SB 240563 359
Merrem 369, 374, 532, 553
mesalamine 436
Metastat 214, 329
Metastron 271, 468, 588
metformin hydrochloride, ADX-155 . .384
Metformin XT 384
metformin/sulfonylureas 384
methadone/dextromethorphan 148
methylphenidate HCl 82, 131
methylphenidate 81, 82, 25130, 131
MethyPatch 81, 130
Metvix PDT 281
MG98 211
MGI-114, hydroxymethylacylfulvene, HMAF 170, 183, 192, 194, 198, 221, 232, 255, 261, 270, 277, 397, 442, 404, 408, 467, 475, 560, 587
MGV 183
MH-200, morphine hydrochloride 107, 500
micellar paclitaxel 99, 507, 527
midodrine HCl 457, 478, 481
Migrastat 96
Mikasome 298, 372, 482, 552, 571
MIV-150 321
MIV-210 . . . . .312, 431
MK-663 . . . . .107, 193, 491, 500, 507
MK-826, carbapenem 301, 373, 423, 483, 531, 552, 565, 571
MK-869 . . . . .127, 133, 137, 203
ML3000 492
Mobist 63, 166, 179, 237, 241, 253

moclobemide 137
modafinil 77, 82, 99, 112, 115, 131
mometasone furoate 359
monoclonal antibody (Mab), anti-VEGF 28, 184
monoclonal antibody, ABX-CBL 326
monoclonal antibody 66, 211, 249
Morphelan 108, 501
morphine sulfate 108, 501
morphine 107, 500
motexafin lutetium 544
motexafing adolinium 86, 159
moxifloxacin 301, 363, 371, 373, 376
mozenavir dimesylate 321
MPI-5020 170
MPL vaccine adjuvant 296, 340, 550
MR Racemate 82, 131
MRE0470 28
MS-325 . . . . .39, 41, 45
MSI-Albuterol 362
MT 100 96
MT 400 96
MT 500 96
MTC-DOX .221
MultiKine 168, 210, 268, 321, 465, 585
mupirocin 376, 556
murine monoclonal antibody 207, 255, 419
MX6 . . . . .192, 560
myeloid progenitor inhibitory factor (MPIF) 203
Mylovenge 64, 248
N-0923 112
N. meningitidis A/C 339
Nabi Civacir 310, 429
Nabi StaphVAX 336, 347
Nabi-Altastaph 335
nabumetone Q 108, 492, 501
NAD299 . . . . .127, 137
naltrexone .148
Naramig, Amerge 96
naratriptan 96
Naropin 109, 502
nasal ketamine 501
natalizumab 100, 413, 436
Natrecor 24
NBI-34060 . . . . .92, 115
NBI-5788, MSP-771 100
NBI-6024 384
NCX 1015 .436
NCX 1022 .527
NCX 4016 . . . . .44, 108, 501
NCX 701 . . . . .108, 501
NE-0080 425
NE-1530 . . . . .551, 552

NE-58095, risedronate sodium 495
nefazodone metabolite 137
nelfinavir, AG1661 290
Neosten 495
Neotrofin 76, 101, 102, 111, 118, 510
Neovastat 64, 175, 223, 247, 275, 473, 523, 543
nesiritide 24
Nestorone .563
Neuprex 93, 301, 331, 355, 373, 553
Neurelan 98, 116, 510
NeuroCell-HD 92, 112
neurokinin antagonist 137
neuroleptic 144
Neurontin 90
neurotrophin-3, NT-3 . . . . .108, 112, 116, 412, 501, 510
NeuroVax 99, 338
Neutralase .19
NeuTrexin 199, 409
NGD 91-1 127
NGD 91-2 127
NGD 91-3 128
NGD 94-4 145
NGD 96-1 92
NGD 97-1 . . . . .77, 89
NGD 98-1 . . . . .128, 137
nicotinamide adenine dinucleotide (NAD) 77
nicotine addiction product 147, 377
Nipent 59, 218, 239, 327, 507
nisin 444
nitazoxanide (NTZ) 290, 332, 415
nitroglycerin ointment 403, 426, 516
nitrone radical trap (NRT) . .112, 118, 290
NK-1 . . . . .137, 145
NK-2 antagonist 437
NKP 608 128
NM-3 153
NMI-870 . . . . .478, 570
NN 1215 384
NN 1998, Insulin (r-human) 384
NN 2344, DRF-2593 384
NN 304, insulin detemir 384
NN 414 384
NN 4201, NNC-42-1001 385
NN 622, DRF-2725 385
NN 703, NNC 26-0703, r-Somatropin 388
NNC-90-1170, NN 2211 385
NO-naproxen 109, 501
nolatrexed dihydrochloride 222
norastemizole 333, 550, 555
Norelin 273, 470, 590

Scientific and Trade Name Index/705

norgestimate/ethinyl estradiol tablet . .562
norgestimate/ethinyl estradiol
   transdermal patch 562
Norvasc *13*
Norvir/ABT-378 . . . .*431*
Nothav *310, 428*
novel erythropoiesis stimulating
   protein (NESP) 50, 458
NovoNorm *386*
NovoSeven *32, 53, 438*
Novovac-M1 246
NOX-100 . . . .*458*
NPS 1506 .118, 138
NPS 1776, alifatic amide 89, 132
NS-1209, SPD-502 118
NS-2330 78
NS-2359 125
NS-2389 138
NS-2710 128
Nutropin Depot *389*
Nuvance *359*
Nuvion *327. 528*
NX 211 . . . . .232, 255
NXY-059 . . . . .78, 119
Nyotran . . .*93, 296, 305, 331, 356, 533, 551*
nystatin, AR-121 . . . . . .93, 296, 305, 331,
   356, 533, 551
O-Vax 257
O6-Benzylguanine (BG) 184
OC144-093 184
octreotide acetate 541
olanzapine 89, 133, 145
omalizumab 333, 555, 359
Omniferon *313, 432*
Onco TCS *189, 235, 240*
Oncolym *240*
Onconase *247*
Oncophage *197, 206, 238, 243,*
   259, 277, 280, 395, 407, 418, 440, 474
Ontak *56, 62, 216, 241*
Onyvax 105 . . . .*201, 341, 411*
Onyvax CR *200, 340, 410*
Onyvax P *274, 340, 471, 591*
OPC-14523 138
OPC-18790 30
opebecan, rBPI-21, recombinant
   human bactericidal/permeability-
   increasing protein 93, 301, 331,
   355, 373, 553
OPHE001 415
Optison *14, 27, 30*
Optrin *544*
Oralease *209, 288*
Oralex *423*
Oralgen *383*
Oramed *287, 519*
OraRinse *202*
ORG-12962 138
ORG-23430 145
ORG-31540/SR-90107A 44, 489
ORG-34167 138
ORG-34517 138
ORG-5222 145
organ transplantation system 63, 241,
   327, 460
Oritavancin *300*
orlistat 385, 393
Ortho EVRA *562*
Ortho-Eldose *562*
Orthovisc *492*
Osanetant *134*
OSI-774 .211, 232
OST 577 . . . . .313, 348, 431
Ostavir *313, 348, 431*
OvaRex *257*
Ovidrel *171, 567*
oxandrolone, CO221 . . . . .365, 523
oxybutynin 481
OxycoDex *109, 502*
oxycodone hydrochloride/
   dextromethorphan
   hydrobromide 109, 502
oxycodone 88
oxymetholone 291
p53 gene therapy 212, 270, 467, 588
p53 tumor suppressor gene 255
P53 . . . .*534*
paclitaxel/carboplatin/amifostine 232
paclitaxel/carboplatin/trastuzumab . . .170
paclitaxel 528
Pafase *335*
pagoclone 128, 142
Pallacor *36*
Palonosetron *188*
pancrelipase 109, 399, 444, 502
Panretin *69, 161, 223, 524*
parathyroid hormone, PTH 495
paroxetine HCl 580
paroxetine 128, 138, 142
Paxil, Seroxat *128, 138, 142*
PDE4i, SCH351591 360
PEG-camptothecin 184
PEG-hirudin 14, 19
PEG-Intron/Rebetol *311, 430*
PEG-Intron 58, 181, 218, 244, 311, 429
Pegasys . . .*59, 218, 244, 278, 313, 431, 475*
peginterferon alfa-2a 59, 218, 244,
   278, 313, 431, 475
pegvisomant 381, 487
PEN203 . . . . .308, 521, 528
PeNta-HepB-IPV, vaccine . .313, 339, 431
pentafuside, T-20 321
Pentasa *436*
pentostatin 59, 218, 239, 327, 507
Perceptin *76, 81, 114, 130*
perflubron 355, 375
perfluorohexane emulsion 19, 184
perthon/abavca *291*
Perthon *291*
Peru-15 339
pexelizumab 19, 37
PH94B 128
phenoxodiol 185, 270, 467, 587
phenserine 78
phentolamine mesylate 451, 577
PhotoPoint - SnET2 . . . .*544*
PI-88 . . . . .68, 185, 282
pimagedine HCl 385, 458
pimecrolimus, ASM 981 . . . . . . .297, 517
pioglitazone HCl 385
pirfenidone 100, 375
piritrexim 213
piroxicam 542
pivaloyloxymethylbutyrate 222, 232
Pivanex *222, 232*
PKC 412 . . . . .185, 542
pleconaril 349
poloxamer 188 N.F., CRL-5861 44, 50, 371
poly I:poly C-12-U .88, 244, 278, 306, 322,
   476
polyacrylic acid 562
PolyHeme *54*
polymer platinate, AP5280 193
Polyphenon E *308, 521*
porcine fetal cells 92, 112
porcine neural cells, focal epilepsy 90
porcine neural cells, stroke 119
porfiromycin .212
posaconazole .519
Posurdex *542*
pralmorelin 388
pramlintide 385
pregabalin 91, 109, 502
Premarin/Pravachol *21*
Premarin/Trimegesterone *389, 391, 566, 568*
Pretarget *240*
PREVEN2 562
Priftin *292, 302*
Primatized *526*
Prinomastat . . .*85, 159, 231, 269, 469, 491,*
   544, 586
PRO 140 322

Scientific and Trade Name Index

PRO 2000 Gel 322, 562
PRO 367 .291, 322
PRO 542 .291, 322
ProAmatine 457, 478, 481
procaine HCl 291, 323
Procrit 49
progestin, ethynylestradiol 563
progestin 563
Prograf 297, 509, 517
Proleukin Interleukin-2 and
 standard anti-HIV therapy 291, 323
Proleukin 54, 214, 236, 246, 275,
 317, 473
prolifeprosan 20/carmustine 86, 159
Promycin 212
proparacaine 542
propentofylline, HWA-285 . . . . . .78, 89
propionyl-L-carnitine 41
propiram 109, 4952, 502
propranolol 96
Prostvac 274, 346, 472, 592
ProTec 51, 59
Protectaid 293, 563
protegrin IB-367, aerosol 368
protegrin IB-367, rinse, gel 203, 301,
 374, 553
Prothecan 184
prourokinase 39 119
Provenge 264, 461, 581
Provigil 77, 82, 99, 112, 115, 131
Provir 292, 416
Prozac 136, 141, 142
prucalopride 412, 434
PSC 833, valspodar 255
Pseudostat 304, 329, 346, 363, 369, 371
PSMA - P1/P2 . . . . .271, 468, 588
psoralen, S-59 . . .67, 69, 70, 282, 302, 349
PT-141 .452, 577
pulmonary insulin 386
pumactant 360
pure anti-estrogen 171
PVAC 528
pygeum africanum 472, 592
pyrazinoylguanidine (PZG) 386
pyridoxalated hemoglobin
 polyoxyethylene (PHP) 50, 335
QS-21 339
Quadramet 271, 468, 588
quetiapine fumarate 78, 133, 141, 145
Quilimmune-M 332, 345
Quilimmune-P 346, 374, 554
quinupristin/dalfopristin302, 374, 531, 553
R 107474 138
R 115777 185

R 149524 421
R-fluoxetine .139
r-FVIIa 32, 53, 438
r-hCG 171, 567
r-hLH 567
r-hTBP-1 . . . . .414, 508
racemic zoplicone 93
radiolabeled monoclonal
 antibody 424, 436, 493
raloxifene, LY-139481 . . . . .28, 171
raltitrexed, ZD-1694 . . .185, 198, 339, 408
Ramoplanin Oral 336, 347
ranolazine, CVT-303 . . . . .14, 24
ranpirnase 247
Ras pathway inhibitor 186
Ravax 338, 506
Rebif 102, 233, 313, 414,
 431, 437, 508
recombinant human activated
 protein C (rhAPC) 335
recombinant human bone
 morphogenic protein-2
 (rhBMP-2) 116, 489, 490, 510
recombinant human
 GM-CSF 52, 156, 203
recombinant human interferon
 beta-1a 102, 233, 313, 414,
 431, 437, 508
recombinant human lactoferrin
 (rhLF) 528
recombinant LFA-3/IgG1
 Human Fusion Protein 528
recombinant salmon calcitonin 492
reflux inhibitor 421
Regranex 387, 518, 532
Relenza .329, 371
Relpax 95
remacemide 91, 92, 113
Reminyl 76, 88, 89, 305
Remune .290, 320
Reolysin 187
ReoPro 13, 29, 36
repaglinide 386
Repifermin 51, 156, 203, 435, 532
ReQuip 113
ResiDerm, Zindaclin 515
resiquimod 307, 520, 565, 578
Resolor .412, 434
Resten-NG 31
retigabine 91
Revasc 43
RF-1010 50
RF-1012 . . . . .50, 70, 204
RF-1051 . . . . .386, 393

RFS-2000 . . . . .59, 171, 198, 207,
 219, 244, 255, 262, 398, 408, 419, 442
rhEndostatin 180
rhIL-11 .204, 414
ribavirin 349, 372
ribozyme gene therapy 239, 292, 323
rifapentine, MDL-473 . . . . .292, 302
rifaximin 302, 424
Rilutek 113
riluzole 113
Risperdal 133, 134, 145
risperidone 1133, 134, 145
Ritalin LA 82, 131
ritonavir 431
Rituxan 239
rituximab/chemotherapy 239
rNAPc2 . . . . .20, 44
rofleponide palmitate 333, 555
rofleponide .437
ropinirole 113
ropivacaine HCl 109, 502
rosiglitazone 386
Rotarix 339
rotavirus vaccine 339
roxithromycine, RU-28,965 . . . . .302, 332
rPSGL-Ig 38
RSD 921 . . . . .110, 502
RSR13 . . . . .15, 17, 86, 160, 233
Rubitecan 59, 171, 198,
 207, 219, 244, 255, 262, 398, 408, 419, 442
RWJ 241947 . . . . .328, 370
RWJ 270201 . . . . .328, 370
S-8184 186
S-doxazosin 447, 575
s-fluoxetine 96
S-oxybutynin 482
SA-IGIV 336
Saccharomyces boulardii 303, 415
salbutamol 360
salmeterol xinafoate 360, 365
salmeterol/fluticasone
 propionate 360, 365
samarium Sm 153 lexidronam
 pentasodium 271, 468, 588
Sandostatin LAR 541
Saredutant 437
Savvy 561
SB 204269 91
SB 207266 16
SB 207499 . . . . .360, 365
SB 214857 38
SB 217242 25
SB 223412 . . . . .366, 482
SB 243213 139

Scientific and Trade Name Index/707

SB 249417 .119, 335
SB 249553 .233, 246
SB 251353 204
SB 273005 .495, 508
SB 275833 .376, 556
SB 408075 .199, 409
SB 418790 .386, 394
SB 424323 17
SB 435495 41
SB 596168 186
SB 659746A, EMD 68843 139
SB 683698, TR 14035 . . . . .361, 508
SB M00026 . . . . .313, 431
SB-237376 16
SC-111 146
SCH55700 361
SCIO-469 508
scopolamine 120, 424, 556
SD/01 . . . . .70, 171, 204
SDZ RAD 327
Seasonale 564
secretin 132
Segard 334
SelCID 65, 98, 248, 297,
  298, 336, 357, 377, 412, 504
selective serotonergic agent 96
selgiline .113, 139
Seretide, Advair 360, 365
Serevent .360, 365
SERM III 171
Seroquel 78, 133, 141, 145
Serostim 25, 292, 389, 424
Serzone-ER 137
SGN-10 188
SGN-15/Taxotere 172, 194, 271,
  404, 468, 588
SIB-1508Y 36, 82, 93, 113, 131
SIB-1553A 78
Simplirix 307, 342, 520, 565, 579
Siramesine 129
Sitaxsentan 34, 454
skeletal targeted radiotherapy
  (STR) 66, 249
SLI 381 . . . . .83, 132
SLV 305 .421, 424
SLV 306 . . . . .25, 34, 454
SLV 308 .113, 139
SLV 311 .421, 424
SMART 1D10 antibody 239
SMART anti-CD3 . . . . .327, 460, 528
SMART Anti-Gamma
  Interferon Antibody 414
SMART M195 . . . . .60, 70, 219
SnET2 544

sodium fluoride 495
sodium oxybate (GHB) 115
Solian 143
somatropin, r-hGH 25, 292, 389, 424
somatropin 389
Somavert 381, 487
SP-303 . . . . .292, 416
SPC3 292
SPD 417, carbamazepine 134
SPD 418 91
SPD 420 .83, 132
SPD 421 91
SPD 424 . . . . .271, 468, 588
SPD 503 .83, 132
spheramine 114
SPP 100 . . . . .34, 455
squalamine 172, 186, 233, 256
SR 49059 569
SR-140333 361
SR-141716 . . . . .146, 147, 377, 394
SR-142801, osanetant . .128, 139, 143, 146
SR-27897B 125, 262, 398, 442
SR-31742 146
SR-31747 327
SR-34006 45
SR-46349 . . . . .115, 139, 147
SR-48692 . . . . .140, 143, 147, 194,
  271, 404, 468, 588
SR-57746 . . . . .79, 80, 487
SR-58611 140
ST630 528
Stedicor 16
sTNF-RI, soluble tumor necrosis
  factor-a receptor type I 508
StreptAvax 337
streptogamin .303
strontium-89 chloride
  injection 271, 468, 588
SU-101/BCNU 87, 160
SU-101 . . . . .86, 160, 233, 256
  271, 469, 589
subject-specific immunotherapy 238
substance P antagonist
  candidates 129, 140
sumatriptan 97
sunepitron, CP-93,393 129
SuperVent 368
Surfaxin .355, 375
Surodex 540
Symbicort pMDI 362, 366
Symbicort Turbuhaler 361, 366
Symlin 385
Synercid 302, 374, 531, 553
Synsorb Cd 303

Synsorb PK 299
synthetic peptide 487
T-1249 . . . . .292, 323
T-cell peptide vaccines 339
T-cell receptor vaccine 100, 509, 529
T-cells/Xcellerate technology 278, 476
T3 361
T607 186
T611 349
T64 . . . . .87, 160, 172, 186,
  199, 212, 233, 234, 247, 280, 409
TA-1790 . . . . .452, 478, 577
TA-CD 148
TA-CIN .192, 560
TA-GW pharmaccine 308, 521
TA-HPV 192, 307, 520, 560, 565, 578
tacrolimus hydrate 297, 509, 517
Tadenan .472, 592
tafenoquine, SB 252263 330
TAK-147 . . . . .79, 89
TAK-251, apomorphine 452, 577
TAK-637 . . . . .140, 438, 482
TAK-778-SR .488
Takepron 421, 423
Tapet 189
tarazepide 425
Targretin-capsule 162, 208, 224,
  241, 516, 524
Targretin-gel .522
Taxol/Paraplatin/Herceptin 170
Taxoprexin 184
Taxotere 84, 163, 206, 209,
  226, 252, 418, 157
tazarotene 515, 529
tazofelone 414, 437
Tazorac .515, 529
TBA-CEA 199, 409
TBC-11251 . . . . .25, 366, 372
TBC-1269 361
TBC-3711 . . . . .25, 34, 455
TCV-116, candesartan cilexetil 25
TCV-116C 34, 455
Td-IPV 340
technetium-99m-labeled FBD 45
Tedangin .15, 17
tedisamil .15, 17
tegaserod 412, 421, 425, 438
telithromycin 303
telmisartan 34, 455
Temodar 87, 160, 187
temozolomide 87, 160, 187
Tenofovir DF 293, 324
tenofovir disoproxil fumarate . . .293, 324
Tenovil 312, 430, 526

Tenovil *438*
Tequin *299, 552*
terbinafine 250, 523, 534
Tesmilifene *273, 470, 590*
testosterone 293, 390, 391, 452, 478, 495, 566, 568, 570, 577, 579
tetanus/diphtheria booster 340
tgAAV-CF 368
tgDCC-E1A, RGG 0853 . . . .173, 212, 256
thalidomide 66, 87, 101, 160, 187, 214, 293, 327, 414, 509
Thalomid *66, 87, 101, 160, 187, 214, 293, 327, 414, 509*
Theolan *361*
theophylline 361
TheraCIM *211*
TheraFab *173*
Theragyn *207, 255, 419*
therapeutic, substance abuse 148
therapeutic, wound healing 387, 518, 534
Theratope *174*
thGRF 1-44 . . . . .115, 366
thymalfasin 222, 244, 313, 349, 431
Thymitaq *222*
tiazofurin 60, 219
Tiazole *60, 219*
tifacogin 335
timcodar dimesylate 103, 392
Timcodar *103, 392*
tirapazamine/cisplatin 234
Tirazone *234*
TLC ELL-12 . . . . .58, 66, 218, 230, 249, 269, 466, 586
TLK286 405
TM27, ATM027, TCAR 101
TNP-470 . . . . .60, 63, 187
toborinone .25
tomoxetine 83, 132
Tomudex *185, 198, 339, 408*
Topamax *91, 110, 134, 503*
topical testosterone gel 492, 503
Topiglan *450, 477, 575*
topiramate tablet 91, 110, 134, 503
topotecan HCl 199, 234, 256, 409
ToPreSite *542*
tositumomab 239
Tostrelle *390, 392, 479, 567, 568, 570*
Tostrex *391, 452, 577, 580*
TP-9201 . . . . .15, 30, 119
TP10 . . . . .17, 20, 38, 355
Tracleer *32, 453*
trafermin 28, 41
Tranilast *31*

transdermal testosterone gel 390, 391, 392, 452, 479, 568, 570, 567, 577, 580
transforming growth factor beta-2 (TGF-b2) 387, 518, 531
trastuzumab 173
tresperimus 52, 157
tretinoin 60, 219, 240, 272, 278, 469, 476, 589
TriAb/TriGem *235*
TriAb *174*
triacetyl uridine 458
Triapine *188*
TriGem *245*
trimegestone/ethinyl estradiol 563
trimetrexate glucuronate/ leucovorin 199, 409
Trisenox/dexamethasone 60, 66
Trisenox *55, 62, 65, 153, 190, 215, 237, 248, 264, 275, 447, 461, 473, 559, 581*
TritAb *140*
trospium chloride 482
Trospium *482*
troxacitabine, BCH-4556 . . . .61, 187, 199, 212, 219, 234, 244, 256, 262, 272, 278, 398, 409, 443, 469, 476, 589
Troxatyl *187*
Troxatyl *61, 199, 212, 219, 234, 244, 256, 262, 272, 278, 398, 409, 443, 469, 476, 589*
TSE-424 . . . . .496, 569
TVP-1012, rasagiline mesylate 79, 114
TVP-1901 92
Twinrix-2 doses *338*
Twinrix-three doses *314, 343, 432*
tyloxapol 368
typhoid vaccine 303, 340
UFT/leucovorin calcium 410
Ultrahaler *360*
Uprima *451, 576*
Urso *21, 195, 200, 314, 405, 410, 418, 432*
ursodiol 21, 195, 200, 314, 405, 410, 418, 432
UT-15 . . . . .35, 42, 455
V-Echinocandin 417, 519
V-Glycopeptide, BI-397 304
vaccine, 105AD7 . . . . .201, 341, 411
vaccine, adjuvant 274, 341, 471, 591
vaccine, allergy 341, 550
vaccine, allogenic and autologous neuroblastoma cells 101, 251, 341
vaccine, anti-cancer 174, 200, 235, 245, 410

vaccine, anti-gastrin II 422
vaccine, anti-gastrin 200, 206, 207, 222, 262, 398, 411, 417, 419, 443
vaccine, breast cancer 174
vaccine, campylobacter 304, 416, 420
vaccine, cancer 61, 174, 64, 67, 220, 235, 242, 245, 250, 262, 274, 341, 342, 399, 471, 472, 591
vaccine, cervical cancer 192, 561
vaccine, cocaine 148
vaccine, cytomegalovirus 306, 539
vaccine, DPT/Haemophilus influenzae type B 304, 328, 342, 350, 370
vaccine, EGF cancer 235
vaccine, Epstein-Barr virus 342, 350
vaccine, genital herpes 307, 316, 342, 520, 522, 565, 579
vaccine, GMK 245, 343
vaccine, HCV/MF59, hepatitis C .314, 432
vaccine, Helicobacter pylori 425
vaccine, hepatitis B DNA 314, 433
vaccine, hepatitis B 314, 433
vaccine, hepatitis E 314, 432
vaccine, hepatitis 314, 343, 432
vaccine, HIV-1 gp-120 prime-boost 294, 325, 343
vaccine, HIV 294, 324, 343
vaccine, HPV-16 VLP 344, 350
vaccine, HPV 343, 350
vaccine, human papilloma virus 344, 350
vaccine, influenza 328, 344, 370
vaccine, kidney cancer 279, 477
vaccine, lymphoma 64, 242
vaccine, malaria 330, 332, 344, 345
vaccine, melanoma 245, 247, 345
vaccine, meningitis B 345
vaccine, meningococcal C conjugate 94, 331, 345
vaccine, meningococcus C . . .94, 331, 345
vaccine, MMR-varicella 346
vaccine, nasal proteosome influenza 329, 371
vaccine, parainfluenza 329, 371
vaccine, pneumococcal infections 346, 374, 554
vaccine, prostate cancer (rV-psa) 274, 346, 472, 592
vaccine, Pseudomonas infection . .304, 329, 346, 363, 369, 371
vaccine, respiratory syncytial virus . . .346, 350, 363, 372, 374, 554
vaccine, rheumatoid arthritis 509
vaccine, rotavirus 351

Scientific and Trade Name Index/709

vaccine, S. pneumoniae 305
vaccine, Shigella flexneri and sonneii 305, 347, 416
vaccine, Staphylococcus aureus ..336, 347
vaccine, Streptococcus pneumoniae ..305, 331, 347, 551, 554
vaccine, tumor cell suspension 257
vaccine, urinary tract infection ..483, 572
vaccine, viral hepatitis (HBV) ...315, 433
vaccine, zoster 479
vaccine 200, 274, 410, 340, 410, 471, 591
valaciclovir 316, 522
valdecoxib 493, 509
valganciclovir 306, 539
valrubicin 155, 257, 449
valsartan 26, 35, 38, 455
Valstar 155, 257, 449
Valtrex, Zelitrex 316, 522
Vanlev 22, 32, 453
vardenafil 453, 578
VAS 972 529
VAS 981 328
VAS 991 26
Vascugel 20
vascular endothelial growth factor-121 (VEGF) 28, 42
vascular endothelial growth factor-2 gene therapy (gtVEGF-2) 18, 28
VasoCare 41
Vasofem 479, 570
Vasogen IMT 61, 220
Vasomax 451, 577
Vaxid 64, 242
VEGF121 ....29, 42
Venoglobulin-S 51, 156, 311, 429
Ventolin 356, 363
verteporfin 529
very late antigen-4 inhibitor (VLA-4) 362
Verzem 33, 454
Vfend 519
VIMRxyn 63, 84, 526, 531
vincristine 189, 235, 240
Viokase 109, 399, 444, 502
Viozan 364
Viprinex 18, 42, 116
VIR201 324
Virazole 349, 372
virulizin 263, 443
Vistide 83, 214, 309, 348, 427, 551
Vitaxin 188
Vitrase 541

Vivelle, Menorest 392, 494, 568
Vivelle-Dot 391, 494, 568
VM-301, OAS 1000 ....388, 517, 518, 535
VML 600, R-848 ....315, 433
VML-670 204
VNP 20009 189
VNP 40101M 201, 411
voglibose 387
vomeropherin, PH-80 .....129, 142, 569
votumumab 174, 351
VP 14637 351
VP 50406 ....315, 433
VX-148 ....298, 351, 529
VX-175 325
VX-497 ....315, 433
VX-710 ....236, 257, 280
VX-740, pralnacasan 493, 509
VX-745 510
VX-853 189
WF10 ....294, 325
Wobe-Mugos-E 67, 204, 250
Xalatan 543
Xanelim 525
Xatral 447, 575
Xcytrin 86, 159
Xeloda/Taxotere 163
Xeloda 195, 385, 393, 405
Xolair 333, 555, 359
XR5000 ....87, 161, 201, 236, 58
XR9576 189
XTL-001 ....315, 433
Xyrem 115
xyzal, xusal 295, 550
yellow fever vaccine 347, 351
YH-1885, SB 641257 422
YKP-10A 140
YKP-10A 141
YM-087, conivaptan 26, 214, 369, 390, 456
YM-177, celecoxib 493, 510
YM-294, oprelvekin 69, 282
YM-337 29
YM-511 ....175, 564, 572
YM-529, minodronate 67, 175, 250
YM-598 ....275, 472, 592
YM-617, tamsulosin 484, 572
YM-872 119
YM-905 482
YM-992 141
YMB-6H9 ....201, 411
Zadaxin 222, 244, 313, 349, 431
Zaditen 295, 541, 550
zanamavir 329, 371
ZD-0101, CM-101 190

ZD-0473/AMD 473 ....155, 175, 190, 192, 201, 236, 258, 275, 411, 450, 472, 561, 592
ZD-1839 ....190, 201, 208, 236, 275, 411, 420, 472, 592
ZD-4522, S-4522 22
ZD-4953 ....110, 503
ZD-8321 ....356, 366
ZD-9331 190
ZD0473 ....213, 450
ZD2315 510
ZD4407 367
ZD4927 45
Zelapar 113
Zelmac 412, 421, 425, 438
zenarestat 103, 393
Zendra 117
Zevalin 238
Ziagen 316
ziconotide, SNX-111 88
Ziracin 299
Zixoryn 67
Zoladex FIB 572
Zoladex IVF 166, 567
zoledronate 54, 157, 213, 488, 496
zolmitriptan 97, 98
Zomaril 144
Zometa 54, 157, 213, 488, 496
Zomig Aura 98
Zomig Cluster 97
Zomig FM 97
Zomig IN 97
Zomig 97
Zopiclone 93
Zorcell 338, 526
Zovant 334
Zyp/Zac 136
Zyprexa 89, 133, 145
Zyrtec 549

Pediatric Manufacturers Index

Contained in this index are sponsor companies and contact information followed by a listing of the drugs they are manufacturing. Scientific names are set in standard type and potential trade names are set in italics.

3M Pharmaceuticals
3M Center
Building 275-3W-01
St. Paul, MN 55144-1000
651-733-1100
651-736-2133 fax
www.mmm.com

beclomethasone dipropionate 597
Qvar Oral Inhalation 597

Abbott Laboratories
100 Abbott Park Rd.
Abbot Park, IL 60064-3537
847-937-6100
847-937-1511 fax
www.abbott.com

ABT-773 602
cefditoren pivoxil 625

Agouron Pharmaceuticals
10350 No. Torrey Pines Rd.
La Jolla, CA 92037
800-585-6050
858-622-3298 fax
www.agouron.com

delavirdine mesylate 616
Rescriptor 616

Alkermes
64 Sidney St.
Cambridge, MA 02139
617-494-0171
617-621-7856 fax
www.alkermes.com

Cereport 606

Allergan
2525 DuPont Dr.
P.O. Box 19534
Irvine, CA 92623-9534
714-246-4500
714-246-5499 fax
www.allergan.com

Alphagan 614
Botox 607
botulinum toxin type A, AGN-191622 607
brimonidine tartrate 614

Alpha Therapeutic
5555 Valley Blvd.
Los Angeles, CA 90032
800-421-0008
323-227-7027 fax
www.AlphaTher.com

Alphanate 633
antihemophilic factor 633

Alza Corporation(Sequus Pharmaceuticals)
950 Page Mill Road
Palo Alto, CA 94303
650-494-5000
650-494-5151 fax
www.alza.com

Duragesic 624
fentanyl transdermal system 624

Baxter Healthcare
One Baxter Parkway

712/Pediatric Manufacturers Index

Deerfield, IL 60015
847-948-2000
www.baxter.com

vaccine, Group C Meningococcus ... .603
Certiva-IPV .... .633
vaccine, acellular pertussis .... .625
vaccine, DPT and Polio .... .633
vaccine, Group B streptococcus ..... .603

Antex Biologics
300 Professional Dr.
Gaithersburg, MD 20879
301-590-0129
301-590-1251 fax
www.antexbiologics.com

Campyvax .... .604
Campyvax .... .631
Helivax .... .614
vaccine, campylobacter .... .604
vaccine, Campylobacter .... .631
vaccine, Haemophilus influenzae ...624
vaccine, Helicobacter pylori .... .614

Ascent Pediatrics
187 Ballardvale Street
Suite B-125
Wilmington, MA 01887
978-658-2500
978-658-3939 fax
www.ascentpediatrics.com

albuterol .... .597
Pediavent .... .597

ASTA Medica AG
Weismellerstrasse 45
Frankfurt-am-Main
Germany
60314
011-0351-25555-0
011-0351-2555-404 fax
www.astamedica.de

Azelastine .... .613

AstraZeneca
1800 Concord Pike
P.O. Box 15437
Wilmington, DE 19850-5438
800-456-3669
302-886-2972 fax
www.astrazeneca.com

Accolate .... .599
anastrozole, ZD-1033 .... .626
Arimidex .... .626
Atacand .... .618
budesonide .... .628
Budoxis, Oxis .... .598
candesartan cilexetil .... .618
felodipine .... .618
formoterol .... .598
lisinopril .... .618
metoprolol succinate .... .618
Naropin .... .597
Naropin .... .624
Plendil .... .618
Pulmicort Respules .... .599
Rhinocort Aqua .... .628
ropivacaine HCl .... .597
ropivacaine HCl .... .624
Toprol-XL .... .618
zafirlukast .... .599
Zestril .... .618
zolmitriptan .... .622
zolmitriptan .... .623
Zomig Aura .... .623
Zomig .... .622

AVANT Immunotherapeutics
119 4th Ave.
Needham, MA 02494-2725
781-433-0771
781-433-0626 fax
www.avantimmune.com

TP10 .... .606
TP10 .... .625

Aventis Pasteur
Discovery Drive
Swiftwater, PA 18370-0187
800-VACCINE
570-839-4287 fax
www.aventispasteur.com

vaccine, Hepatitis A .... .615
vaccine, HIB/Hep B/IPV/DtaP ..... .615
vaccine, HIB/Hep B/IPV/DtaP ..... .633
vaccine, meningococcal conjugate ...604
vaccine, respiratory syncytial virus ...627

Aventis
P. O. Box 9627
Kansas City, MO 64134
800-362-7466
816-231-5804 fax

www.hoechst.com, www.aventis.com

Arava .... .628
cromolyn sodium .... .597
ebastine .... .628
enoxaprarin sodium .... .630
Intal HFA-227 .... .597
Kestine .... .628
Ketek .... .603
leflunomide .... .628
Lovenox Injection .... .630
Priftin .... .617
quinupristin/dalfopristin .... .625
rifapentine, MDL-473 .... .617
Sabril .... .612
streptogamin .... .602
Synercid .... .625
telithromycin .... .603
vigabatin .... .612

Bayer Corporation
400 Morgan Lane
West Haven, CT 06516-4175
203-812-2000
203-812-5554 fax
www.bayer.com

Baycol .... .607
cerivastatin sodium .... .607
CIPRO .... .631
ciprofloxacin .... .631

Bio-Technology General
70 Wood Ave. South
Second Floor
Iselin, NJ 08830
732-632-8800
732-632-8844 fax
www.btgc.com

Oxandrin .... .623
oxandrolone, CO221 .... .608
oxandrolone, CO221 .... .626
oxandrolone .... .623
Oxsodrol .... .620
recombinant human superoxide dismutase
   (rhSOD) .... .620

BioChem Pharma
275 Armend Frappier
Laval, Quebec H7V 4A7
Canada
450-681-1744
450-978-7755 fax

www.biochempharma.com

vaccine, influenza 619, 632

Biocodex
1910 Fairview Ave. E.
Suite 208
Seattle, WA 98102
206-322-5663
206-323-2968 fax
www.biocodex-usa.com

Saccharomyces boulardii 608

BioNumerik Pharmaceuticals
8122 Datapoint Dr.
Suite 1250
San Antonio, TX 78229
(210) 614-1701
(210) 614-0643
210-614-1701
210-615-8030 fax

BNP 1350 605
Karenitecin 605

Bristol-Myers Squibb
345 Park Avenue
New York, NY 10154
212-546-4000
212-546-4020 fax
www.bms.com

gatifloxacin 602
gatifloxacin 623
Glucovance 611
glyburide/metformin 611
Tequin 602
Tequin 623

Cangene Corporation
104 Chancellor Matheson Road
Winnipeg, MB R3T 5Y3
Canada
877-226-4363
204-487-4086 fax
www.cangene.com

human growth hormone 630
d-methylphenidate HCl 600

Cell Pathways
1300 South Potomac Street
Ste. 110
Aurora, CO 80012
877-231-4567
303-755-2252 fax
www.cellpathways.com

Aptosyn 613
exisulind 613

Celltech Chiroscience plc
216 Bath Road
Slough, Berkshire 5L1 4EN
UK
011-44-753-534655
011-44-753-536632 fax
www.celltech.co.uk

gemtuzumab ozogamicin 620
Mylotarg 620

Centocor
200 Great Valley Pkwy.
Malvern, PA 19355-1307
888-874-3083
610-889-4701 fax
www.centocor.com

infliximab 609
Remicade 609

Cephalon
145 Brandywine Pkwy.
West Chester, PA 19380
610-344-0200
610-344-0065 fax
www.cephalon.com
modafinil 601
Provigil 601

Chiron Corporation
4560 Horton Street
Emeryville, CA 94608
510-655-8730
510-655-9910 fax
corpcomm@cc.chiron.com
www.chiron.com

vaccine, DPT/Haemophilus influenzae
   type B 603
vaccine, DPT/Haemophilus influenzae
   type B 604
vaccine, DPT/Haemophilus influenzae
   type B 619
vaccine, DPT/Haemophilus influenzae
   type B 633
vaccine, DPT/Haemophilus influenzae
   tyype B 632
vaccine, meningococcus C 621
vaccine, meningococcus C 632

CoCensys
201 Technology Dr.
Irvine, CA 92618
949-753-6100
949-790-8710 fax
dslade@cocensys.com
www.cocensys.com

ganaxolone, CCD-1042 612

Curis
45 Moulton St.
Cambridge, MA 02138
617-876-0086
617-876-0866 fax
www.curis.com

chondrocyte-alginate gel suspension ..632
Chondrogel 632

CytRx Corporation
154 Technology Pkwy.
Norcross, GA 30092
770-368-9500
770-368-0622 fax
www.cytrx.com

Flocor 629
poloxamer 188 N.F., CRL-5861 629

Discovery Laboratories
350 South Main Street
Suite 307
Doylestown, PA 18901
215-340-4699
215-340-3940 fax
www.discoverylabs.com

lucinactant 621
SuperVent 610
Surfaxin 621
tyloxapol 610

Du Pont
1007 Market St.
Wilmington, DE 19898
800-441-7515
302-892-8530 fax
www.dupont.com

DMP-777 627

Eisai
6-10 Koishikawa
4 Chome Bunkyo-ku
Tokyo, 112-88
JAPAN
011-81-03-3817-5015
011-81-03-3811-3077 fax
webmaster@eisai.co.jp
www.eisai.co.jp

Aciphex 613
Aricept 600
donepezil hydrochloride, E2020 600
rabeprazole sodium, E3810 613

Elan Pharmaceutical Research
1300 Gould Drive
Gainesville, GA 30504
888-638-7605
770-534-8247 fax

CNS stimulant 600
Theolan 598
theophylline 598

Eli Lilly
Lilly Corporate Center
Indianapolis, IN 46285
800-545-5979
317-277-6579 fax
www.lilly.com

multiple-drug resistance inhibitor ...605
recombinant human activated protein C
 (rhAPC) 628
tomoxetine 601

Endorex Corporation
28101 Ballard Road
Suite F
Lake Forest, IL 60045
847-573-8990
847-573-9285 fax
TheProTeam@aol.com
www.endorex.com

disaccharide tripeptide glycerol dipalmitoyl 628
ImmTher 628

Escalon Medical
351 East Conestoga Road
Wayne, PA 19087
800-433-8197
262-821-9927 fax
www.escalonmed.com/

povidone-iodine 612

Forest Laboratories
909 Third Ave.
New York, NY 10022
800-947-5227
212-750-9152 fax
www.frx.com

Aerobid 598
flunisolide 598

Fujisawa Healthcare
Three Parkway North
Parkway North Center
Deerfield, IL 60015
800-888-7704
847-317-7296 fax
www.fujisawa.com

pralmorelin 614

Genaera Corporation
5110 Campus Drive
Plymouth Meetin, PA 19464
610-941-4020
610-941-5399 fax
www.genaera.com

squalamine 606

Genentech
One DNA Way
South San Francisco, CA 94080
800-225-1000
650-225-6000 fax
webmaster@gene.com
www.gene.com

Nutropin Depot 617
omalizumab 598
omalizumab 628
somatropin 617
Xolair 628

Genzyme Surgical
One Kendall Square
Cambridge, MA 02139
617-652-7500
617-494-6561 fax

CV Seprafilm Adhesive Barrier 607

Genzyme Corporation
One Kendall Square
Building 1400
Cambridge, MA 02139
617-252-7500
617-374-7368 fax
www.genzyme.com

agalsidase beta 613
Aldurazyme 622
alpha-1-iduronidase 622
Fabrazyme 613
recombinant human alpha-glucosidase 625

GlaxoSmithKline
New Horizons Ct.
Great West Road
Brentford, Middlesex
United Kingdom
TW89 EP
919-248-2100, 888-825-5249
011-44-181-975-2764 fax
www.gsk.com

abacavir 615
amoxicillin/clavulanate 602
amoxicillin/clavulanate 623
Augmentin ES 602
Augmentin ES 623
carvedilol 609
Coreg 609
hepatitis vaccine 615
HeXa-HepB-IPV/Hib 615
HeXa-HepB-IPV/Hib 633
Imigran, Imitrex 622
Infanrix 615
Infanrix 631
Infanrix 633
Infanrix 633
lamivudine 615
paroxetine 626
Paxil, Seroxat 626
PeNta-HepB-IPV, vaccine 631
PeNta-HepB-IPV, vaccine 633
Rotarix 628
rotavirus vaccine 628
sumatriptan 622
Twinrix-2 doses 615
vaccine, meningitis B 621

Pediatric Manufacturers Index/**715**

vaccine, meningitis B 632
vaccine, MMR-varicella 632
vaccine, MMR-varicella 633
vaccine, N. meningitidis A/C 621
vaccine, S. pneumoniae 604
Zeffix *615*
Ziagen *615*

Hoffmann-La Roche
340 Kingsland St.
Nutley, NJ 07110
800-526-6367
973-562-2206 fax
www.rocheusa.com

CellCept *619*
Fortovase *617*
mycophenylate mofetil 619
saquinavir 617
orlistat 623
Xenical *623*

Immune Response Corporation
5935 Darwin Court
Carlsbad, CA 92008
800-491-0153
760-431-8636 fax
www.imnr.com

HIV-1 immunogen 616
Remune *616*

Inex Pharmaceuticals
8900 Glanlyon Pkwy.
Suite 100
Burnaby, British Columbia V5J-5J8
Canada
604-419-3200
604-419-3201 fax
www.inexpharm.com

Onco TCS *606*
vincristine 606

Janssen Pharmaceutica
1125 Trenton-Harbourtown Rd.
P.O. Box 200
Titusville, NJ 08560-0200
800-526-7736
609-730-2616 fax
www.jnj.com

farnesyl transferase inhibitor 605
prucalopride 619

R115777 605
Resolor *619*
Risperdal *608*
risperidone 608

Layton Bioscience
105 Reservoir Road
Atherton, CA 94027
650-854-6614
650-854-4776 fax
www.laytonbio.com

Inversine *600*
Inversine *630*
mecamylamine HCl 600
mecamylamine HCl 630

LeukoSite
215 First Street
Cambridge, MA 02142
617-621-9350
617-621-9349 fax
information@leukosite.com
www.leukosite.com

LDP-392 599

Ligand Pharmaceuticals
10275 Science Center Dr.
San Diego, CA 92121
858-550-7500
858-550-7506 fax
www.ligand.com

alitretinoin, ALRT-1057 605
Panretin *605*

Massachusetts Biologic Laboratories
305 South St.
Jamaica Plain, MA 02130
617-983-6300
617-983-6301 fax

immune globulin (IG-IV) 624

Medeva plc
10 St. James Street
London SW1A 1EF
United Kingdom
44-0-1372-364000
44-0-1372-364167 fax
www.medeva.co.uk

methylphenidate HCl 601

MedImmune
35 W. Watkins Mill Road
Gaithersburg, MD 20878
301-417-0770
301-527-4207 fax
www.medimmune.com

MEDI-507 614
palivizumab 604, 608, 609
Synagis *604, 608, 609*

Merck & Co.
1 Merck Dr.
P.O. Box 100
Whitehouse Station, NJ 08889-0100
800-422-9675
908-735-1253 fax
www.merck.com

lovastatin 607
Mevacor *607*

Milkhaus Laboratory
48 Main Street
Boxford, MA 01921
978-887-2086
www.milkhaus.com

HP-3 609

Nabi
5800 Park of Commerce Blvd. NW
Boca Raton, FL 33487
800-635-1766
561-989-5890 fax
www.nabi.com

HBVIg *614*
hepatitis B immune globulin 614
hyperimmune globulin 629
Nabi-Altastaph *629*

Neose Technologies
102 Witmer Road
Horsham, PA 19044
215-441-5890
215-441-5896 fax
info@neose.com
www.neose.com

NE-1530 611
NE-1530 624

Neurocrine Biosciences
10555 Science Center Drive
San Diego, CA 92121
619-658-7600
619-658-7601 fax
www.neurocrine.com

NBI-6024 611

Novartis
556 Morris Avenue
Summit, NJ 07901
973-781-8300
973-781-8265 fax
www.novartis.com

benazepril hydrochloride 617
Elidel 599
Foradil 598
Foradil 627
formoterol 598
formoterol 627
Glivec 620
imatinib, STI 571 620
Lamisil 630
Lotensin 617
methylphenidate 600
methylphenidate 601
pimecrolimus, ASM 981 599
Ritalin LA 600
Ritalin QD 601
rufinamide, RUF 331 612
SDZ RAD 630
terbinafine 630

Noven Pharmaceuticals
11960 SW 144th St.
Miami, FL 33186
800-340-7302
305-251-1887 fax
www.noven.com

methylphenidate 600
MethyPatch 600

Organon
375 Mt. Pleasant Ave.
West Orange, NJ 07052
800-241-8812
973-325-4589 fax
r&d@organon.com
www.organon.com

Mirtazapine 610

rapacuronium bromide 629
Raplon 629
Remeron Tablets 610

Orphan Medical
13911 Ridgedale Dr.
Suite 475
Minnetonka, MN 55305
888-867-7426
612-514-9209 fax
pservices@orphan.com
www.orphan.com

sodium oxybate (GHB) 607
Xyrem 607

Pfizer
235 E. 42nd St.
New York, NY 10017-5755
212-573-2323
860-441-1895 fax
www.pfizer.com

cetirizine HCl 597
fosphenytoin sodium injection 611
gabapentin 612
inhaled insulin 611
Neurontin 612
sertraline HCl 610
sertraline HCl 626
Zoloft 610
Zoloft 626
Zyrtec 597

Pharmacia Corporation
95 Corporate Dr.
P.O. Box 6995
Bridgewater, NJ 08807
908-901-8000
webmaster.int@am.pnu.com
www.pharmacia.com

Detrol 631
Genotropin 614
Linezolid 602
Somatropin 614
thrombopoietin 629
Tolterodine 631
Zyvox 602

Progenics Pharmaceuticals
777 Old Saw Mill River Road
Tarrytown, NY 10591
888-425-2122

914-789-2817 fax
clinicaltrials@progneics.com
www.progenics.com

PRO 542 616

Protherics
1207 17th Ave. South
Suite 103
Nashville, TN 37212
888-327-1027
615-320-1212 fax
www.protherics.com

TritAb 610

Questcor
2714 Loker Ave. W.
Carlsbad, CA 92008
510-732-5551
510-732-7741 fax
www.questcor.com

Cordox 629
CPC-111 629

R.W. Johnson Pharmaceutical Research Institute
920 Route 202 South
P.O. Box 300
Raritan, NJ 06689
908-704-4000

Levaquin 624
levofloxacin 624
tramadol hydrochloride 624
Ultram 624

Repligen Corporation
117 4th Ave.
Needham, MA 02494
800-622-2259
781-453-0048 fax
info@repligen.com
www.repligen.com

secretin 602

Shire Pharmaceuticals
East Anton
Andover, Hants SP105RG
UK
240-453-6400
240-453-6404 fax

Pediatric Manufacturers Index/717

www.shiregroup.com

SPD 420 601
SPD 503 601

Sigma-Tau Pharmaceuticals
800 South Frederick Ave.
Suite 300
Gaithersburg, MD 20877
800-447-0169
301-948-3679 fax
aa@sigmatau.com
www.sigmatau.com

Cystavision 612
cysteamine hydrochloride 612

Skye Pharma
10450 Science Center Drive
Suite 100
San Diego, CA 92121
858-625-2424
858-625-2439 fax
www.depotech.com

cytarabine liposome injection 621
DepoCyt 621

St. Jude Children's Research Hospital
332 N. Lauderdale St.
P.O. Box 318
Memphis, TN 38101-0318
901-495-3300
901-495-3122 fax
lin.ballew@stjude.org
www.stjude.org

vaccine, allogenic and autologous
   neuroblastoma cells 623, 631

Synsorb Biotech
1204 Kensington Road, NW
Calgary, Alberta T2N 3P5
Canada
403-283-5900
403-283-5907 fax
www.synsorb.com

galasomite 602
Synsorb Pk 602

Takeda Chemical Industries
Millbrook Business Center
475 Half Day Road
Suite 500
Lincolnshire, IL 60069
847-383-3000
847-383-3050 fax
www.takeda.com/index-e.html

TNP-470 606
TNP-470 620
TNP-470 621

TAP Pharmaceuticals
2355 Waukegan Road
Deerfield, IL 60015
800-621-1020
847-374-4540 fax

cefditoren pivoxil 597
cefditoren pivoxil 604
cefditoren pivoxil 630
Lansoprazole 612
Prevacid 612
Spectracef 597
Spectracef 604
Spectracef 630

Targeted Genetics
1100 Olive Way
Suite 100
Seattle, WA 98101
206-623-7612
206-223-0288 fax
targen@targen.com
www.targen.com

tgAAV-CF 610

Triangle Pharmaceuticals
4 University Place
4611 University Drive
Durham, NC 27707
919-493-5980
919-493-5925 fax
www.tripharm.com

Coactinon 615
Coviracil 616
emivirine 615
emtricitabine 616

Trimeris
4727 University Drive
Suite 100
Durham, NC 27707
919-419-6050
919-419-1816 fax
info@trimeris.com
www.trimeris.com

pentafuside, T-20 616

Wyeth-Ayerst
555 East Lancaster Avenue
St. Davids, PA 19087
610-971-5400
610-995-4668 fax
www.ahp.com/wyeth.htm

Effexor XR 610
Enbrel 627
etanercept 627
FluMist 619
Meningitec 621
vaccine, meningococcal C conjugate ..621
venlafaxine HCl 610

Wyeth-Lederle Vaccines
One Great Valley Pkwy.
Suite 30
Malvern, PA 19355
610-647-9452
610-995-4668 fax
www.ahp.com

vaccine, parainfluenza 619
vaccine, respiratory syncytial virus ...626

XOMA Corporation
2910 7th St.
Berkeley, CA 94710
510-644-1170
510-644-0539 fax
www.xoma.com

Neuprex 622
opebecan, rBPI-21, recombinant
   human bactericidal/
   permeability-increasing protein 622

Zambon S.p.A.
Via Lillo del Ducay 10
20091 Bresso
Italy
39-02-665241
39-02-66501492 fax
www.zambongroup.com

MSI-Albuterol 599

Pediatric Therapeutic Indications Index

Use this index to quickly reference drug development activity for a specific illness. Scientific names are set in standard type and potential trade names are set in italics.

Acute Pharyngitis
cefditoren pivoxil 597
Spectracef 597

Allergy
cetirizine HCl 597
Zyrtec 597

Anesthesia
Naropin 597
ropivacaine HCl 597

Asthma
Accolate 599
Aerobid 598
albuterol 597
beclomethasone dipropionate 597
Budoxis, Oxis 598
cromolyn sodium 597
flunisolide 598
Foradil 598
formoterol 598
formoterol 598
Intal HFA-227 597
MSI-Albuterol 599
omalizumab 598
Pediavent 597
Pulmicort Respules 599
Qvar Oral Inhalation 597
Theolan 598
theophylline 598
Xolair 598
zafirlukast 599

Atopic Dermatitis
Elidel 599
LDP-392 599
pimecrolimus, ASM 981 599

Attention Deficit/ Hyperactivity Disorder (ADHD)
Aricept 600
CNS stimulant .600
d-methylphenidate HCl 600
donepezil hydrochloride, E2020 600
Inversine 600
mecamylamine HCl 600
methylphenidate 600, 601
methylphenidate HCl 601
MethyPatch 600
modafinil 601
Provigil 601
Ritalin LA 600
Ritalin QD 601
SPD 420 601
SPD 503 601
tomoxetine 601

Autism
secretin 602

Bacterial Infection
ABT-773 602
amoxicillin/clavulanate 602
Augmentin ES .602
galasomite 602
gatifloxacin 602
Ketek 603
Linezolid 602
streptogamin 602
Synsorb Pk 602
telithromycin 603
Tequin 602
vaccine, DPT/Haemophilus
 influenzae type B 604
vaccine, Group B streptococcus 603

720/Pediatric Therapeutics Indications Index

vaccine, Group C Meningococcus 603
vaccine, meningococcal conjugate 604
vaccine, S. pneumoniae 604
Zyvox 602

Bone Marrow Transplant
palivizumab 604
Synagis 604

Bronchitis
cefditoren pivoxil 604
Spectracef 604

Campylobacter Infection
Campyvax 604
vaccine, campylobacter 604

Cancer/Tumors
alitretinoin, ALRT-1057 605
BNP 1350 605
Cereport 606
farnesyl transferase inhibitor 605
Karenitecin 605
multiple-drug resistance inhibitor ..605
Onco TCS 606
Panretin 605
R115777 605
squalamine 606
TNP-470 606
unkown 605

Cardiac Surgery
CV Seprafilm Adhesive Barrier 607
TP10 606

Cataplexy
sodium oxybate (GHB) 607
Xyrem 607

Cerebral Palsy
Botox 607
botulinum toxin type A,
    AGN-191622 607

Cholesterol (High Levels)
Baycol 607
cerivastatin sodium 607
lovastatin 607
Mevacor 607

Chronic Obstructive Pulmonary Disease
oxandrolone, CO221 608

Clostridium difficile
Saccharomyces boulardii 608

Conduct Disorder
Risperdal 608
risperidone 608

Congenital Heart Disease
palivizumab 608
Synagis 608

Congestive Heart Failure
carvedilol 609
Coreg 609

Crohn's Disease
infliximab 609
Remicade 609

Cystic Fibrosis
HP-3 609
palivizumab 609
SuperVent 610
Synagis 609
tgAAV-CF 610
tyloxapol 610

Depression
Effexor XR 610
Mirtazapine 610
Remeron Tablets 610
sertraline HCl 610
TritAb 610
venlafaxine HCl 610
Zoloft 610

Diabetes Mellitus Types 1 and 2
Glucovance 611
glyburide/metformin 611
inhaled insulin 611
NBI-6024 611

Ear Infections
NE-1530 611

Epilepsy
fosphenytoin sodium injection 611
gabapentin 612
ganaxolone, CCD-1042 612
Neurontin 612
rufinamide, RUF 331 612
Sabril 612
vigabatin 612

Esophageal Infections
Lansoprazole 612
Prevacid 612

Eye Disorders/Infections
Azelastine 613
Cystavision 612
cysteamine hydrochloride 612
povidone-iodine 612

Fabry Disease
agalsidase beta 613
Fabrazyme 613

Familial Adenomatous Polyposis Coli
Aptosyn 613
exisulind 613

Gastroesophageal Reflux Disease (GERD)
Aciphex 613
rabeprazole sodium, E3810 613

Glaucoma
Alphagan 614
brimonidine tartrate 614

Graft Versus Host Disease
MEDI-507 614

Growth Hormone Deficiencies/Abnormalities
Genotropin 614
pralmorelin 614
Somatropin 614

Helicobacter Pylori Infection
Helivax 614
vaccine, Helicobacter pylori 614

Hepatitis
HBVIg 614
hepatitis B immune globulin 614
hepatitis vaccine 615
HeXa-HepB-IPV/Hib 615
Infanrix 615
lamivudine 615
Twinrix-2 doses 615
vaccine, Hepatitis A 615
vaccine, HIB/Hep B/IPV/DtaP ...615
Zeffix 615

HIV/AIDS

Pediatric Therapeutics Indications Index/721

abacavir 615
Coactinon 615
Coviracil 616
delavirdine mesylate 616
emivirine 615
emtricitabine .616
Fortovase 617
HIV-1 immunogen 616
pentafuside, T-20 616
Priftin 617
PRO 542 616
Remune 616
Rescriptor 616
rifapentine, MDL-473 617
saquinavir 617
Ziagen 615

Hormone Deficiencies
Nutropin Depot 617
somatropin 617

Hypertension
Atacand 618
benazepril hydrochloride 617
candesartan cilexetil 618
felodipine 618
lisinopril 618
Lotensin 617
metoprolol succinate 618
Plendil 618
Toprol-XL 618
Zestril 618

Ileus
prucalopride .619
Resolor 619

Influenza
FluMist 619
vaccine, DPT/Haemophilus
   influenzae type B 619
vaccine, influenza 619
vaccine, parainfluenza 619

Kidney Transplant Surgery
CellCept 619
mycophenylate mofetil 619

Leukemia
gemtuzumab ozogamicin 620
Glivec 620
imatinib, STI 571 620
Mylotarg 620
TNP-470 620

Lung Disease
Oxsodrol 620
recombinant human superoxide
   dismutase (rhSOD) 620

Lymphomas
TNP-470 621

Meconium Aspiration Syndrome
lucinactant 621
Surfaxin 621

Meningitis
cytarabine liposome injection 621
DepoCyt 621
Meningitec 621
vaccine, meningitis B 621
vaccine, meningococcus C 621
vaccine, N. meningitidis A/C 621

Meningococcemia
Neuprex 622
opebecan, rBPI-21, recombinant
   human bactericidal/
   permeability-increasing protein 622

Metabolic Disease
Aldurazyme 622
alpha-1-iduronidase 622

Migraine and Cluster Headaches
Imigran, Imitrex 622
sumatriptan 622
zolmitriptan 622
Zomig 622
Zomig Aura .623

Muscular Dystrophy
Oxandrin 623
oxandrolone .623

Neuroblastoma
vaccine, allogenic and autologous
   neuroblastoma cells 623

Obesity
orlistat 623
Xenical 623

Otitis Media
amoxicillin/clavulanate 623
Augmentin ES 623
gatifloxacin 623
Levaquin 624

levofloxacin .624
NE-1530 624
Tequin 623
vaccine, Haemophilus influenzae 624

Pain, Acute or Chronic
Duragesic 624
fentanyl transdermal system 624
Naropin 624
ropivacaine HCl 624
tramadol hydrochloride 624
Ultram 624

Pertussis
immune globulin (IG-IV) 624
vaccine, acellular pertussis 625

Pneumonia
cefditoren pivoxil 625
quinupristin/dalfopristin 625
Synercid 625

Pompe's Disease
recombinant human
   alpha-glucosidase 625

Post-Surgical Complications
TP10 625

Post-Traumatic Stress Disorder
sertraline HCl 626
Zoloft 626

Pressure Ulcers
oxandrolone, CO221 626

Psychiatric Disorders
paroxetine 626
Paxil, Seroxat 626

Pubertal Gynecomastia
anastrozole, ZD-1033 626
Arimidex 626

Respiratory Failure
vaccine, respiratory syncytial virus . . .626

Reversible Obstructive Airways Disease
Foradil 627
formoterol 627

Rheumatoid Arthritis
Arava 628

DMP-777 627
Enbrel *627*
etanercept 627
leflunomide 628

Rhinitis
budesonide 628
ebastine 628
Kestine *628*
omalizumab 628
Rhinocort Aqua *628*
Xolair *628*

Rotavirus Prophylaxis
Rotarix *628*
rotavirus vaccine 628

Sarcoma
disaccharide tripeptide glycerol
    dipalmitoyl 628
ImmTher *628*

Sepsis
recombinant human activated
    protein C (rhAPC) 628

Sickle Cell Disease
Cordox *629*
CPC-111 629
Flocor *629*
poloxamer 188 N.F., CRL-5861 629

Staph Bacterial Infections
hyperimmune globulin 629
Nabi-Altastaph *629*

Surgery
rapacuronium bromide 629
Raplon *629*

Thrombocytopenia
thrombopoietin 629

Thrombosis
enoxaprarin sodium 630
Lovenox Injection *630*

Tinea Capitis
Lamisil *630*
terbinafine 630

Tonsillitis
cefditoren pivoxil 630
Spectracef *630*

Tourette's Syndrome
Inversine *630*
mecamylamine HCl 630

Transplantation
SDZ RAD 630

Turner's Syndrome
human growth hormone 630

Urinary Incontinence
Detrol *631*
Tolterodine 631

Urinary Tract Infections
CIPRO 631
ciprofloxacin 631

Vaccines
Campyvax *631*
Infanrix *631*
PeNta-HepB-IPV, vaccine 631
vaccine, allogenic and autologous
    neuroblastoma cells 631
vaccine, Campylobacter 631
vaccine, DPT/Haemophilus
    influenzae tyype B 632
vaccine, influenza 632
vaccine, meningitis B 632
vaccine, meningococcus C 632
vaccine, MMR-varicella 632

Vesicoureteral Reflux Disease
chondrocyte-alginate gel suspension ..632
Chondrogel *632*

Viral Infection
Certiva-IPV *633*
HeXa-HepB-IPV/Hib 633
Infanrix *633*
PeNta-HepB-IPV, vaccine 633
vaccine, DPT and Polio 633
vaccine, DPT/Haemophilus
    influenzae type B 633
vaccine, HIB/Hep B/IPV/DtaP 633
vaccine, MMR-varicella 633

von Willebrand's Disease
Alphanate *633*
antihemophilic factor 633

Pediatric Scientific and Trade Name Index

Contained in this index are the names of all of the therapies profiled in the second edition. Scientific names are set in standard type and potential trade names are set in italics.

abacavir	.615
ABT-773	.602
Accolate	.599
Aciphex	.613
Aerobid	.598
agalsidase beta	.613
albuterol	.597
Aldurazyme	.622
alitretinoin, ALRT-1057	.605
alpha-1-iduronidase	.622
Alphagan	.614
Alphanate	.633
amoxicillin/clavulanate	.602, 623
anastrozole, ZD-1033	.626
antihemophilic factor	.633
Aptosyn	.613
Arava	.628
Aricept	.600
Arimidex	.626
Atacand	.618
Augmentin ES	.602, 623
Azelastine	.613
Baycol	.607
beclomethasone dipropionate	.597
benazepril hydrochloride	.617
BNP 1350	.605
Botox	.607
botulinum toxin type A, AGN-191622	607
brimonidine tartrate	.614
budesonide	.628
Budoxis, Oxis	.598
Campyvax	.604, 631
candesartan cilexetil	.618
carvedilol	.609
cefditoren pivoxil	.597, 604, 625, 630
CellCept	.619
Cereport	.606
cerivastatin sodium	.607
Certiva-IPV	.633
cetirizine HCl	.597
chondrocyte-alginate gel suspension	.632
Chondrogel	.632
CIPRO	.631
ciprofloxacin	.631
CNS stimulant	.600
Coactinon	.615
Cordox	.629
Coreg	.609
Coviracil	.616
CPC-111	.629
cromolyn sodium	.597
CV Seprafilm Adhesive Barrier	.607
Cystavision	.612
cysteamine hydrochloride	.612
cytarabine liposome injection	.621
d-methylphenidate HCl	.600
delavirdine mesylate	.616
DepoCyt	.621
Detrol	.631
disaccharide tripeptide glycerol dipalmitoyl	.628
DMP-777	.627
donezepil hydrochloride, E2020	.600
Duragesic	.624
ebastine	.628
Effexor XR	.610
Elidel	.599
emivirine	.615
emtricitabine	.616
Enbrel	.627
enoxaprarin sodium	.630
etanercept	.627
exisulind	.613
Fabrazyme	.613
farnesyl transferase inhibitor	.605
felodipine	.618

724/Pediatric Scientific and Trade Name Index

fentanyl transdermal system 624
Flocor *629*
FluMist *619*
flunisolide 598
Foradil *598, 627*
formoterol 598, 598, 627
Fortovase *617*
fosphenytoin sodium injection 611
gabapentin 612
galasomite 602
ganaxolone, CCD-1042 612
gatifloxacin 602, 623
gemtuzumab ozogamicin 620
Genotropin *614*
Glivec *620*
Glucovance *611*
glyburide/metformin 611
HBVIg *614*
Helivax *614*
hepatitis B immune globulin 614
hepatitis vaccine 615
HeXa-HepB-IPV/Hib 615, 633
HIV-1 immunogen 616
HP-3 609
human growth hormone 630
hyperimmune globulin 629
imatinib, STI 571 620
Imigran, Imitrex *622*
ImmTher *628*
immune globulin (IG-IV) 624
Infanrix *615, 631, 633*
infliximab 609
inhaled insulin 611
Intal HFA-227 . . . .*597*
Inversine *600, 630*
Karenitecin *605*
Kestine *628*
Ketek *603*
Lamisil *630*
lamivudine 615
Lansoprazole *612*
LDP-392 599
leflunomide 628
Levaquin *624*
levofloxacin 624
Linezolid *602*
Lipitor . . . .*Pfizer*
lisinopril 618
Lotensin *617*
lovastatin 607
Lovenox Injection *630*
lucinactant 621
mecamylamine HCl 600, 630
MEDI-507 614

Meningitec *621*
methylphenidate HCl 601
methylphenidate 600, 601
MethyPatch *600*
metoprolol succinate 618
Mevacor *607*
Mirtazapine 610
modafinil 601
MSI-Albuterol *599*
multiple-drug resistance inhibitor . . .605
mycophenylate mofetil 619
Mylotarg *620*
Nabi-Altastaph *629*
Naropin *597, 624*
NBI-6024 611
NE-1530 .611, 624
Neuprex *622*
Neurontin *612*
Nutropin Depot *617*
omalizumab 598, 628
Onco TCS *606*
opebecan, rBPI-21, recombinant
 human bactericidal/
 permeability-increasing protein 622
orlistat 623
Oxandrin *623*
oxandrolone, CO221 . . . . .608, 626
oxandrolone .623
Oxsodrol *620*
palivizumab 604, 608, 609
Panretin *605*
paroxetine 626
Paxil, Seroxat *626*
Pediavent *597*
PeNta-HepB-IPV, vaccine 631, 633
pentafuside, T-20 616
pimecrolimus, ASM 981 599
Plendil *618*
poloxamer 188 N.F., CRL-5861 629
povidone-iodine 612
pralmorelin 614
Prevacid *612*
Priftin *617*
PRO 542 616
Provigil *601*
prucalopride .619
Pulmicort Respules *599*
quinupristin/dalfopristin 625
Qvar Oral Inhalation *597*
R115777 605
rabeprazole sodium, E3810 613
rapacuronium bromide 629
Raplon *629*
recombinant human activated

protein C (rhAPC) 628
recombinant human
 alpha-glucosidase 625
recombinant human superoxide
 dismutase (rhSOD) 620
Remeron Tablets *610*
Remicade *609*
Remune *616*
Rescriptor *616*
Resolor *619*
Rhinocort Aqua *628*
rifapentine, MDL-473 617
Risperdal *608*
risperidone 608
Ritalin LA *600*
Ritalin QD *601*
ropivacaine HCl 597, 624
Rotarix *628*
rotavirus vaccine 628
rufinamide, RUF 331 612
Sabril *612*
Saccharomyces boulardii 608
saquinavir 617
SDZ RAD 630
secretin 602
sertraline HCl 610, 626
sodium oxybate (GHB) 607
Somatropin 614, 617
SPD 420 601
SPD 503 601
Spectracef *597, 604, 630*
squalamine 606
streptogamin .602
sumatriptan 622
SuperVent *610*
Surfaxin *621*
Synagis *604, 608, 609*
Synercid *625*
Synsorb Pk *602*
telithromycin .603
Tequin *602, 623*
terbinafine 630
tgAAV-CF 610
Theolan *598*
theophylline 598
thrombopoietin 629
TNP-470 . . . . .606, 620, 621
Tolterodine 631
tomoxetine 601
Toprol-XL *618*
TP10 . . . . .606, 625
tramadol hydrochloride 624
TritAb *610*
Twinrix-2 doses *615*

tyloxapol .... .610
Ultram .... *.624*
vaccine, acellular pertussis .... .625
vaccine, allogenic and autologous
   neuroblastoma cells .... .623, 631
vaccine, campylobacter .... .604, 631
vaccine, DPT and Polio .... .633
vaccine, DPT/Haemophilus influenzae
   type B .... .603, 604, 619, 632, 633
vaccine, Group B streptococcus ...... .603
vaccine, Group C Meningococcus .... .603
vaccine, Haemophilus influenzae .... .624
vaccine, Helicobacter pylori .... .614
vaccine, Hepatitis A .... .615
vaccine, HIB/Hep B/IPV/DtaP .. .615, 633
vaccine, influenza .... .619, 632
vaccine, meningitis B .... .621, 632
vaccine, meningococcal C conjugate .. .621
vaccine, meningococcal conjugate .... .604
vaccine, meningococcus C ...... .621, 632
vaccine, MMR-varicella .... .632, 633
vaccine, N. meningitidis A/C .... .621
vaccine, parainfluenza .... .619
vaccine, respiratory syncytial
   virus .... .626, 627
vaccine, S. pneumoniae .... .604
venlafaxine HCl .... .610
vigabatin .... .612
vincristine .... .606
Xenical .... *.623*
Xolair .... *.628*
Xyrem .... *.607*
zafirlukast .... .599
Zeffix .... *.615*
Zestril .... *.618*
Ziagen .... *.615*
zolmitriptan .... .622, 623
Zoloft .... *.610, 626*
Zomig Aura .... *.623*
Zomig .... *.622*
Zyrtec .... *.597*
Zyvox .... *.602*

Appendixes

Useful Websites 728

About CenterWatch 733

   About Center for Clinical Research Practice (CCRP) 733

   Our Commitment and Guarantee 733

   Contact Information 733

   Periodicals 734

   Books and Directories 734

   Patient Education Services 735

   Training and Education Publications 736

   Information Services 736

   TrialWatch Site-Identification Service 737

Useful Websites

Surfing the Web using the many search engines available may help you find more clinical study data or information about research and development. To help facilitate your search, we are providing some Web sites that are more focused on research and clinical trials.

General Clinical Trial Web Sites:
Americas Doctor www.americasdoctor.com
Centers for Disease Control and Prevention www.cdc.gov
Center for Drug Evaluation and Research (FDA) www.fda.gov/cder
CenterWatch www.centerwatch.com
ClinicalTrials.gov www.clinicaltrials.gov
ClinMark.com www.clinmark.com
Drkoop www.drkoop.com
Drug Information Association www.diahome.org
MedExplorer.com www.medexplorer.com
Medscape www.medscape.com
MyDrugRep www.mydrugrep.com
Pharmaceutical Information Network www.pharminfo.com
Pharmaceutical Research and Manufacturers Association www.phrma.org
RxSheets www.rxsheets.com
VitalSpring www.vitalspring.com
WebMD www.webmd.com

Cardiovascular/Hematology
American College of Cardiology, CardioSource http://www.cardiosource.com/
American Heart Association www.americanheart.org
American Society of Hematology http://www.hematology.org/
American Society of Hypertension http://www.ash-us.org/
Children's Health Information Network www.tchin.org
Global Cardiology Network http://www.globalcardiology.org/
Heart Failure Online www.heartfailure.org
National Heart, Lung and Blood Institute http://www.nhlbi.nih.gov/index.htm
Rush Children's Hospital Heart Center www.rchc.rush.edu

Neurology/Psychiatry
Alzheimer's Association www.alzheimers.org
American Academy of Neurology www.aan.com
The American Psychiatric Association www.psych.org
American Psychological Association http://www.apa.org
At Health http://www.athealth.com
Behavior Online http://www.behavior.net
Internet Mental Health http://www.mentalhealth.com

Mental Health InfoSource http://www.mhsource.com
Mental Health Net http://mentalhelp.net
National Institute for Mental Health http://www.nimh.nih.gov
National Institute of Neurological Disorders and Stroke (NINDS) www.ninds.nih.gov
Neurosciences on the Internet www.neuroguide.com

Oncology
American Association for Cancer Research http://www.aacr.org/
American Cancer Society http://www.cancer.org/frames.html
American Lung Association http://www.lungusa.org
American Society of Clinical Oncology http://www.asco.org/
CancerOption.com www.canceroption.com
Cancer Research Institute http://www.cancerresearch.org
Coalition of National Cancer Cooperative Groups http://www.ca-coalition.org/
Eastern Cooperative Oncology Group http://ecog.dfci.harvard.edu/
Leukemia Research Foundation http://www.leukemia-research.org
Lymphoma Foundation of America http://www.lymphoma.org
National Alliance of Breast Cancer Organizations http://www.nabco.org/
National Breast Cancer Organization www.y-me.org
National Cancer Institute http://www.nci.nih.gov/
NCI's CancerNet http://cancernet.nci.nih.gov
National Childhood Cancer Foundation http://www.nccf.org
National Comprehensive Cancer Network http://www.nccn.org/
National Ovarian Cancer Coalition www.ovarian.org
OncoLink http://www.oncolink.upenn.edu
Oncology Nursing Society http://www.ons.org/
Pancreatic Tumor Study Group http://www.mdanderson.org/~pancpgrm/
Pediatric Oncology Group www.pog.ufl.edu
Prostate Cancer Resource Network http://www.pcrn.org

Immunology/Infectious Diseases
AIDS Clinical Trials Information Service http://www.actis.org
AIDS.org http://www.aids.org/immunet/home.nsf/page/homepage
American Academy of Allergy, Asthma and Immunology http://www.aaaai.org/
Infectious Diseases Society of America http://www.idsociety.org/
International Clinical Epidemiology Network http://www.inclen.org
Johns Hopkins University Division of Infectious Diseases http://www.hopkins-id.edu/
National Foundation for Infectious Diseases http://www.nfid.org/
National Institute of Allergy and Infectious Diseases http://www.niaid.nih.gov/
National Jewish Center for Immunology and Respiratory Medicine http://www.njc.org/
The Vaccine Page www.vaccines.com

Pulmonary and Respiratory
American Association for Respiratory Care http://www.aarc.org/
American College of Chest Physicians http://www.chestnet.org/
American Lung Association http://www.lungusa.org
Center for Disease Control, Division of Tuberculosis Elimination http://www.cdc.gov/nchstp/tb/default.htm
The National Association for Medical Direction of Respiratory Care http://www.namdrc.org/home.html
National Heart, Lung and Blood Institute http://www.nhlbi.nih.gov/index.htm

Endocrinology and Metabolism
American Diabetes Association www.diabetes.org; Canadian www.diabetes.ca

American Dietetic Association www.diabetesnet.com/organiz.html
American Medical Association – Diabetes www.ama-assn.org/insight/spec_con/diabetes/diabetes.htm
The Centers for Disease Control – Diabetes www.cdc.gov/health/diabetes.htm
The Cystic Fibrosis Foundation www.cff.org
The Endocrine Society www.endo-society.org
International Diabetes Center onhealth.com/ch1/condctr/diabetes/item,30.asp
National Diabetes Information Clearinghouse (associated with the National Institute of Health) www.niddk.nih.gov/health/diabetes/ndic.htm
The Thyroid Foundation of America www.tsh.org

Gastroenterology/Urology
American College of Gastroenterology http://www.acg.gi.org/
American Gastroenterological Association www.gastro.org
American Journal of Kidney Diseases www.ajkd.org
Childhood Diarrhea, Centers for Disease Control www.cdc.gov/od/oc/parents
Crohn's and Colitis Foundation of America www.ccfa.org
Digestive Disorders Foundation of the UK www.digestivedisorders.org.uk
Irritable Bowel Syndrome Self-Help Group www.ibsgroup.org
The International Society for Peritoneal Dialysis www.ispd.org
National Institute of Diabetes and Digestive and Kidney Diseases www.niddk.nih.gov
National Kidney Foundation www.kidney.org
National Digestive Diseases Information Clearinghouse: Diarrhea www.niddk.nih.gov/health/digest/pubs/diarrhea/diarrhea.htm

Musculoskeletal
Access America for Seniors – Health and Nutrition Pages www.seniors.gov/health.html
American Association of Retired Persons – Health and Wellness Pages www.aarp.org/indexes/health.html
American AutoImmune Related Diseases Organization www.aarda.org
The American College of Rheumatology www.rheumatology.org/index.asp
Arthritis Foundation www.arthritis.org
Duquesne University www.duq.edu/PT/RA/TableOfContents.html
International Osteoporosis Foundation www.osteofound.org
National Osteoporosis Foundation www.nof.org
National Institute of Arthritis and Musculoskeletal and Skin Diseases www.nih.gov/niams
National Institute on Aging www.nih.gov/nia
National Institutes of Health – Osteoporosis and Bone-Related Diseases www.osteo.org
Osteoporosis Imperfecta Foundation www.oif.org
Osteoporosis Society of Canada www.osteoporosis.ca/index.shtml
Rheumatoid Arthritis Information Network www.htinet.com/rain/rainindex.html
U.S. Food and Drug Administration – Older Persons www.fda.gov/oc/olderpersons

Dermatology, Opthalmology and Otolaryngology
American Academy of Ophthalmology http://www.eyenet.org/aao_index.html
American Academy of Otolaryngology-Head and Neck Surgery http://www.entnet.org/
American Optometric Association www.aoanet.org
American Society for Dermatological Surgery www.asds-net.org
Association for Research in Otolaryngology http://www.aro.org/
Association for Research in Vision and Ophthalmology http://www.arvo.org/arvo/
Glaucoma Research Foundation www.glaucoma.org
Harvard Skin Disease Research Center dermatology.bwh.harvard.edu/sdrc_home.html
Loyola University Dermatology Medical Education www.meddean.luc.edu/lumen/MedEd/medicine/dermatology/title.htm

National Eye Institute www.nei.nih.gov
National Psoriasis Foundation www.psoriasis.org
Prevent Blindness America www.preventblindness.org
University of Texas – Skin Diseases Research Center
www.swmed.edu/home_pages/derma/coretitl.htm

Gender-Specific Diseases
American Society of Reproductive Medicine http://www.asrm.org/
CDC, Center for Reproductive Health http://www.cdc.gov/nccdphp/drh/mrh_mens.htm
Society for Women's Health Research http://www.womens-health.org/
The Men's Health Network http://www.menshealthnetwork.org/
National Women's Health Resource Center http://www.healthywomen.org
National Women's Health Information Center http://www.4woman.org/
OB/GYN.net, The Universe of Women's Health http://www.obgyn.net/

Pediatric
Pediatric Information http://www.pedinfo.com/
Baby's Doctor http://www.babysdoc.com/
American Academy of Pediatrics http://www.aap.org/
Kids Health http://www.kidshealth.com/
PediHeart http://www.pediheart.org/
Autism society of America http://www.autism-society.org/
National Institute of Health http://www.nimh.nih.gov/publicat/adhd.cfm
Elizabeth Glaser Pediatric AIDS foundation http://www.pedaids.org/
Pediatric Cancer Research Foundation http://www.pcrf-kids.com/
Pediatric Database http://www.icondata.com/health/pedbase/

About CenterWatch

CenterWatch is a Boston-based publishing company that focuses on the clinical trials industry. We provide a variety of information services used by pharmaceutical and biotechnology companies, CROs, SMOs, and investigative sites involved in the management and conduct of clinical trials. CenterWatch also provides educational materials for clinical research professionals, health professionals and for health consumers. Some of our top publications and services are described below. For a comprehensive listing with detailed information about our publications and services, please visit our web site at www.centerwatch.com.

Center for Clinical Research Practice (CCRP)

The Center for Clinical Research Practice (CCRP) is a division of CenterWatch that provides educational materials and programs focusing on regulatory requirements and on safe and ethical practices in clinical research. Investigators, coordinators, administrators, IRB members and staff, and other health professionals involved in the conduct and management of clinical research use CCRP's publications and services. For more information please visit www.ccrp.com

Our Commitment and Guarantee

Our publications and services offer the highest quality news and information available. Subscribers to the CenterWatch Newsletter receive sharp discounts on most other periodicals, books and directories. We offer sharp discounts on quantity subscriptions and orders. To learn more about our quantity orders, please contact us at (617) 856-5900. If at any time a reader decides to cancel their subscription to a CenterWatch periodical, CenterWatch will refund the entire paid subscription.

Contact Information

Kenneth A. Getz, President & Publisher, kenneth.getz@centerwatch.com
Joan A. Kroll, Director of Marketing & Sales, joan.kroll@centerwatch.com

CenterWatch
22 Thomson Place, 36T1
Boston, MA 02210
617-856-5900
617-856-5901 fax

Periodicals

CenterWatch
A monthly newsletter that provides pharmaceutical and biotechnology companies, CROs, SMOs, research centers and the investment community with in-depth business news, feature articles on trends, original research and analysis, as well as grant lead information for investigative sites.

CenterWatch Europe
A quarterly electronic newsletter dedicated to providing news, information and analyses on the clinical trials industry in the European Union. *CenterWatch Europe* presents in-depth stories, data and analyses for sponsors, CROS and investigator sites involved in managing and conducting clinical research.

CWWeekly
A weekly fax and electronic newsletter that reports on the top stories in the clinical trials industry. Each weekly newsletter includes business headlines, financial information, market intelligence, drug pipeline and clinical trial results from the prior week.

JobWatch
A web-based resource at www.centerwatch.com that provides a comprehensive listing of career and educational opportunities in the clinical trials industry. Companies use *JobWatch* regularly to identify qualified clinical research professionals.

Research Practitioner
An award-winning journal published every other month, filled with informative and pertinent articles about clinical research practice and methods. A continuing education component is included with each issue of *Research Practitioner*, so readers can apply for CEUs or CME credits.

Books and Directories

An Industry in Evolution
A 300 page source book of charts, data tables and statistics on the clinical trials industry. The material is presented in a well organized and easy-to-reference format. This important and valuable resource is used for developing business strategies and plans, for preparing presentations and for conducting business and market intelligence.

The 2001/2002 CenterWatch Directory of the Clinical Trials Industry
A comprehensive directory with over 1,000 pages of contact information and detailed company profiles for a wide range of organizations and individuals involved in the clinical trials industry. Considered the authoritative reference resource to organizations involved in designing, managing, conducting and supporting clinical trials.

The Investigator's Guide to Clinical Research
A 250-page step-by-step resource filled with tips, instructions and insights for health professionals interested in conducting clinical trials. *The Investigator's Guide* is designed to help the novice clinical investigator get involved in conducting clinical trials. The guide is also a valuable resource for experienced investigative sites looking for ways to improve and increase their involvement and success in clinical research.

Protecting Study Volunteers in Research
Recommended by the National Institutes of Health and the Office of Health and Human

Services, *Protecting Study Volunteers in Research* is a 250-page manual designed to assist clinical research professionals in providing the highest standards of safety and ethical treatment for their study volunteers. Written specifically for academic institutions and IRBs actively involved in clinical trials, the manual is also applicable to independent investigative sites. The book has been developed in accordance with the ACCME. Readers can apply for CME credits or Nursing Credit Hours. An exam is provided with each manual.

A Guide to Patient Recruitment: Today's Best Practices and Proven Strategies
A 350-page book designed to help clinical research professionals involved in managing and conducting clinical trials, improve the effectiveness of their patient recruitment efforts. Written by Diana Anderson, Ph.D., with contributions from 15 industry leaders, this guide offers real world, practical recruitment strategies and tactics. It is considered an invaluable resource for educating staff on ways to improve patient recruitment and retention.

The Directory of Drugs in Clinical Trials
A comprehensive directory of new, leading-edge medications currently in research, this directory offers a glimpse at new and upcoming treatment options in Phase I to III clinical trials. The Directory provides easy reference information on more than 2,000 drugs in active clinical trials across a variety of clinical conditions. Detailed information is provided on each drug listed.

Profiles of Service Providers on the CenterWatch Clinical Trials Listing Service™
The CenterWatch web site (www.centerwatch.com) attracts tens of thousands of sponsor and CRO company representatives every month that are looking for experienced CROs and investigative sites to manage and conduct their clinical trials. No registration is required. Sponsors and CROs use this online directory free of charge. The CenterWatch web site offers all contract service providers—both CROs and investigative sites—the opportunity to present more information than any other Internet-based service available. This service is an ideal way to secure new contracts and clinical grants.

Patient Education Services

Volunteering For A Clinical Trial
An easy-to-read, six-page patient education brochure designed for research centers to provide consistent, professional and unbiased educational information for their potential clinical study subjects. The brochure is IRB approved. Sponsors, CROs and investigative sites use this brochure to inform patients about participating in clinical trials. *Volunteering for a Clinical Trial* can be distributed in a variety of ways including direct mailings to patients, displayed in waiting rooms, or as handouts to guide discussions. The brochure can be customized with company logos and custom information.

The New Medical Therapies Report Series
Reports in the *New Medical Therapies* series are concise and easy-to-read. They are filled with thorough and in-depth information on clinical trial activities and drugs in development for specific illnesses and medical conditions. Reports are updated every 6 to 12 months to maintain their timeliness. An invaluable resource for clinical research and healthcare professionals interested in educating their patients about clinical trials, as well as for consumers and patients interested in staying informed about new and promising treatments being developed for their specific illness or medical condition. Reports are available in: Osteoporosis, Prostate Cancer, Depression, Diabetes, Addictions, HIV/AIDS, Breast Cancer, Migraine, Lung Cancer, Alzheimer's; Colorectal Cancer and Hypertension/Heart Disease.
A Word from Study Volunteers: Opinions and Experiences of Clinical Trial Participants
A straightforward and easy-to-read ten-page pamphlet that reviews the results of a survey

conducted among more than 1,000 clinical research volunteers. This brochure presents first hand experiences from clinical trial volunteers. It offers valuable insights for anyone interested in participating in a clinical trial.

The CenterWatch Clinical Trials Listing Service™

Now in its sixth year of operation, The CenterWatch Clinical Trials Listing Service™ provides the largest and most comprehensive listing of industry-sponsored clinical trials on the Internet. In 2001 alone, the CenterWatch web site—along with numerous coordinated online and print affiliations—is expected to reach more than 5 million Americans. The CenterWatch Clinical Trials Listing Service' provides an international listing of nearly 40,000, ongoing and IRB-approved phase I - IV clinical trials.

Training and Education Publications

Foundations for Clinical Research

An independent study course for health professionals involved in the management and conduct of clinical trials. This course provides a solid introduction to research practice today from biomedical experimentation to protocol design, to the implementation and management of clinical research. Continuing education is available with this study course. Includes a textbook, workbook, workbook answer key, sample clinical protocol and sample investigator's brochure. A perfect resource for new or moderately experienced members of the research staff at investigative sites, sponsors or CROs.

Foundations of Human Subject Protection

An independent study course that covers the basic ethical concepts and regulatory requirements of human subject protection. This course will teach you how to conduct clinical research in an ethical and scientific manner and know how to apply sound ethical judgement. Specifically written for IRB members, staff, clinical researchers and healthcare professionals involved in the conduct and management of clinical research.

Regulatory Reference

A handy and comprehensive compilation of the federal regulations, guidance documents, and principles that form the basis of how clinical trials are conducted. The reference book is designed to be not only a source book, but also a tool to help clinical research professionals do their jobs better. The Regulatory Reference, printed as a 297-page manual and is supplied on 2 diskettes in Word for Windows, is fully searchable.

Standard Operating Procedures for Good Clinical Practice at the Investigative Site

Designed to be customized for your research facility, this easy-to-use template is based on the ICH/GCP Consolidated Guidelines and the Code of Federal Regulations and is pertinent to the day-to-day conduct of clinical research. The printed template is provided in a 3-ring binder and on 2 diskettes (in Word 95/97) for installation on your computer.

Information Services

Research Reports and Custom Market Research Services

CenterWatch publishes compilation reports that are based on large primary market research projects. We also conduct custom market research studies for sponsors, CROs and investigative sites. The CenterWatch staff brings unprecedented experience and insight into the clinical trials industry.

CenterWatch Content Solutions Services

CenterWatch offers sponsors, CROs and investigative sites a variety of customized information that can be used for educational, informational and promotional purposes. CenterWatch customized content solutions provide numerous advantages and benefits. Specifically, we can help you:

- Educate and inform your colleagues, staff and contract partners—CROs and investigative sites about critical trends and issues that may impact their performance
- Stimulate new ideas and practices among your colleagues and business partners
- Raise employee and partner performance standards managing and conducting trials, upholding ethical and safety requirements, complying with regulatory mandates and guidelines
- Build awareness and educate health professionals and the patient community about the value of clinical research
- Promote your company's brand name and leadership role in educating the clinical research community

CenterWatch offers custom content in print and electronic "online" formats. Our printed publications offer branding opportunities with custom covers, color inserts, and custom content. And, our electronic content can be used on both Internet and Intranet platforms.

TrialWatch Site-Identification Service

Several hundred sponsor and CRO companies use the TrialWatch service to identify prospective investigative sites to conduct their upcoming clinical trials. Every month, companies post bulletins of their phase I through IV development programs that are actively seeking clinical investigators. These bulletins are included in the *CenterWatch* newsletter—our flagship publication that reaches as many as 25,000 experienced investigators every month. Use of the TrialWatch service is FREE.